Therapeutic Kinesiology

Musculoskeletal Systems, Palpation, and Body Mechanics

MARY ANN FOSTER

PEARSON

Boston   Columbus   Indianapolis   New York   San Francisco   Upper Saddle River

Amsterdam   Cape Town   Dubai   London   Madrid   Milan   Munich   Paris   Montreal   Toronto

Delhi   Mexico City   Sao Paulo   Sydney   Hong Kong   Seoul   Singapore   Taipei   Tokyo

Publisher: Julie Levin Alexander
Editor-in-Chief: Marlene McHugh Pratt
Executive Editor: John Goucher
Assistant Editor: Nicole Ragonese
Development Editor: Mary Anne Maier
Editorial Assistant: Erica Viviani
Director of Marketing: David Gesell
Executive Marketing Manager: Katrin Beacom
Managing Production Editor: Patrick Walsh
Production Project Manager: Christina Zingone-Luethje
Operations Specialist: Lisa McDowell

Design Director: Maria Guglielmo
Media Editor: Amy Peltier
Media Project Manager: Lorena Cerisano
Media Coordinator: Ellen Martino
Full-Service Project Management: Michelle Gardner
Photographer: Rick Giase
Illustrator: Body Scientific International
Composition: Laserwords Maine
Printer/Binder: Courier/Kendallville
Cover Printer: Lehigh-Phoenix Color/Hagerstown

Credits: (Icons) **Key Terms**, YorkBerlin/Shutterstock.com; **Exploring Techniques**, musicman/Shutterstock.com; **Guidelines**, arttizarus/Shutterstock.com; **Self-Care**, discpicture/Shutterstock.com; **Bone Palpation**, DM7/Shutterstock.com; **Muscle Palpation**, DM7/Shutterstock.com
(Chapter Openers) **Chap 4**, michaeljung/Shutterstock.com; **Chap 6**, Elena Elisseeva/Shutterstock.com; **Chap 9**, RCB Shooter/Shutterstock.com; **Chap 12**, ruigsantos/Shutterstock.com; **Chap 14**, John Lumb/Shutterstock.com; **Chap 17**, LouLouPhotos/Shutterstock.com

Notice: The authors and the publisher of this volume have taken care that the information and technical recommendations contained herein are based on research and expert consultation, and are accurate and compatible with the standards generally accepted at the time of publication. Nevertheless, as new information becomes available, changes in clinical and technical practices become necessary. The reader is advised to carefully consult manufacturers' instructions and information material for all supplies and equipment before use, and to consult with a health care professional as necessary. This advice is especially important when using new supplies or equipment for clinical purposes. The authors and publisher disclaim all responsibility for any liability, loss, injury, or damage incurred as a consequence, directly or indirectly, of the use and application of any of the contents of this volume.

This text provides information about therapeutic kinesiology for massage. It does not offer medical advice or treatment. The exercises in this book are meant to be done by and on healthy people.

Cataloging-in-Publication Data on file with the Library of Congress

10 9 8 7 6 5 4 3 2 1

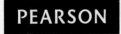

www.pearsonhighered.com

ISBN-13: 978-0-13-507785-6
ISBN-10:   0-13-507785-0

Dedication

This book is dedicated to the power, splendor, and sublime grace of the human body and its movement capacity, and to the dancers, athletes, and natural movers whose performances continually inspire my work.

Brief Contents

Dedication   iii
Acknowledgments   vii
About the Author   ix
Reviewers   x
Preface   xi

PART 1   KINESIOLOGY FOUNDATIONS   1

Chapter 1   Introduction to Therapeutic Kinesiology   2

Chapter 2   The Skeletal System   22

Chapter 3   Joint Motion   48

Chapter 4   The Muscular System   70

Chapter 5   The Neuromuscular System   96

Chapter 6   Biomechanics   128

Chapter 7   Posture   152

Chapter 8   Gait   182

Chapter 9   Basic Palpation Skills   208

PART 2   PALPATION AND PRACTICE   227

Chapter 10   The Thorax and Respiration   228

Chapter 11   The Ankle and Foot   264

Chapter 12   The Knee   330

Chapter 13   The Hip and Pelvis   370

Chapter 14   The Spine   436

Chapter 15   The Head and Neck   484

Chapter 16   The Shoulder Girdle   546

Chapter 17   The Arm and Hand   606

Chapter 18   Body Mechanics and Self-Care   672

Glossary   G-1
Chapter Review Answers   A-1
Index   I-1

Acknowledgments

The marvel that is the human body has always filled me with awe and wonder. As a child, I spent hours observing, sketching, and even trying to move like my siblings and friends, fascinated by the contours of their physiques and the uniqueness of each person's movement patterns. My study of dance and anatomy only deepened this appreciation. It also initiated many years of study and practice in the fields of massage and somatics. During this time, I began writing to share more widely the concepts I continue to use and discover in my teaching and practice.

One area of particular interest to me is the kinesiological foundation of body mechanics. I have explored this interest over the years while teaching numerous types of movement classes for massage therapists and bodyworkers, developing experiential kinesiology course material, writing articles about movement studies in massage, and producing the sourcebook *Somatic Patterning*. In short, it feels as if my entire career to this point has been a preparation for writing this kinesiology text.

This project began one day during a lunch with two colleagues who are also writers: Mary Rose, developer of Comfort Touch®, and Anne Williams, education director at Associated Bodywork and Massage Professionals (ABMP). At the time, we were discussing a book proposal I had developed for a body mechanics text based on kinesiology, which Anne suggested I send to Mark Cohen, then executive editor for Health Professions at Pearson. I did so, and later, when Mark and I were discussing the proposal, he asked if I knew anyone who wanted to write a kinesiology text. A few days after we spoke, a light bulb went on in my head and I thought: why not flip the two? Instead of writing a body mechanics book based on kinesiology, I could write a kinesiology book that covers body mechanics. So I submitted this proposal and *Therapeutic Kinesiology* was born.

I want to express my deep gratitude to Mark for initiating *Therapeutic Kinesiology,* for pushing the proposal through in record time, and, most of all, for hiring my favorite editor and friend, Mary Anne Maier, as development editor for the project. Mary Anne and I have a well-established working relationship that we were able to take to new heights with *Therapeutic Kinesiology.* I am deeply indebted to her for her generous enthusiasm, infinite support, and creative skills, plus her gentle but firm guidance in shaping this manuscript and her hours of work to bring it to fruition.

My appreciation and thanks also go out to the many professionals at Pearson who worked on this text, especially to John Goucher, executive editor, and Nicole (Nikki) Ragonese, assistant editor, who have both been a delight to work with and who assembled a great team of artists. They brought in photographer Rick Giase and his assistant Marie Griffin Dennis, who cheerfully produced hundreds of spectacular photos. Pearson also brought the impeccably organized Marcelo Oliver and his highly talented and productive team of anatomical artists at Bodyscientific to the project, including Carol Hrejsa (project manager), Katie Burgess, Paul Kelly, Kristen Oliver, Esther Pulley, and Liana Bauman. Thank you all for your attention to detail, beauty, and realism, and for bringing to life the phantasmagoria of visions rattling around in my imagination with your spectacular photos, art, and figures.

I especially want to thank my patient and supportive husband, Gary Burns, who knew exactly when *not* to interrupt me and who endured many days, weeks, and months of abandonment and many nights of sleep interrupted by an insomniac writer slipping out to peck away at the keyboard. Thanks also go to Mary Rose, my close friend and generous writing partner (we cowrote the "Talk about Touch" column for *Massage and Bodywork Magazine*). Mary lent a hand in many ways, such as introducing me to Nancy Smith, director of the aerial dance company Frequent Flyers. Thank you to Nancy and her brilliant group of performers, among whom Nicole

Predki, Lynda White, Linn Wilder Muir, Danielle Hendricks (the barefoot runner gracing the cover), Valerie Morris, and Angela Delsanter graciously modeled for this text.

Thanks also go to Stephen West, model and fellow experiential kinesiology teacher while I was at the Boulder College of Massage, and to the yoga instructors Stephen brought in to model: Yuki Tsuji-Hoening, Luke Iwabuchi, and Thomas Crown; to professional model Todd Roe (who posed for the surface anatomy figures); to models Arelis Diaz and Renu Poduval, both talented massage practitioners and kinesiology students who have assisted me in many ways; to Christopher Walken, Marilyn Palmer, and Emma Burns (my daughter-in-law), who all stepped in to model on short notice; to video models Natalie Morgan, Sasha Viers, Jennine Amato, and Roger Patterson; to Fred Schulerud and Mark Nelson for posing for drawings; and to all my movement and massage students and colleagues over the years who have provided me with scores of opportunities to develop this material. This text has been a joy to write because I love this topic so much.

In closing, I want to acknowledge my parents, Kathryn and Lewis, who gave me the focus and persistence I needed to complete a massive undertaking such as this text. I particularly want to acknowledge my father, who, during this writing process, went through a long and painful illness, then passed away in February 2011. I am sad he will not see this book but want to thank him for his generous and faithful support for many of my creative endeavors over the years, especially when the going got tough!

About the Author

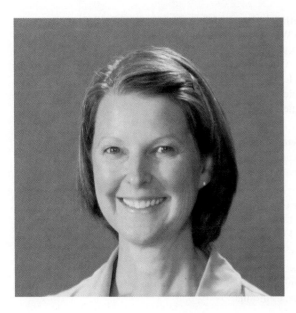

Mary Ann Foster, BA, CMT, is a certified massage therapist who has been in private practice in the Denver/Boulder area since 1981. She has a BA in Body–Mind Therapies and specializes in movement instruction for health care professionals with an emphasis on postural muscle training, body mechanics, self-care, and client education.

An avid researcher and writer, Mary Ann is the author of *Somatic Patterning: How to Improve Posture and Movement and Ease Pain* (2004, EMS Press) and writes regularly for *Massage and Bodywork Magazine.* She developed somatic patterning out of diverse studies in therapeutic massage, Laban movement analysis, Rolfing® movement integration, Body–Mind Centering®, cranial-sacral therapy, Hakomi Body-Centered Therapy, and graduate studies in somatic psychology.

Mary Ann has taught movement and kinesiology classes at a number of colleges and massage schools since 1986, including the Boulder College of Massage Therapy and Naropa, and has worked with diverse populations, including nurses, dancers, and yoga and Pilates teachers, as well as physical and occupational therapists. She has taught seminars on a national level and teaches master classes in neuromuscular patterning for manual therapists and professional movement teachers.

Mary Ann's students describe her as a clear and enthusiastic instructor with an innovative and knowledgeable presentation. In her seminars, she encourages students to cultivate body awareness and efficient movement through therapeutic and experiential exercises. She runs the National Certification Board for Therapeutic Massage and Bodywork-approved professional courses for manual therapists, providing students with cutting-edge tools for neuromuscular patterning.

You can contact Mary Ann at her website at www.somatic-patterning.com.

Reviewers

Jeff Bockoven, LMT
Iowa Massage Institute
Des Moines, Iowa

Kathleen Crawford, LMT
Massage Shoppe
St. Charles, Missouri

Nancy W. Dail, BA, LMT, NCTMB
Downeast School of Massage
Waldoboro, Maine

Brian D. Humphrey, MS
Mount Vernon Nazarene University
Mount Vernon, Ohio

Wolfgang Luckmann, BA
Florida State College
Jacksonville, Florida

Tara G. McManaway, MDivLMT
College of Southern Maryland
La Plata, Maryland

Erika Monge, LMT
Dade Medical College
St. Hialeah, Florida

Kenneth J. Nelan, RM/T, STL, MA, NCBTMB Provider
Sacred Wandering Continuing Education
Tucson, Arizona

Bernadette Della Bitta Nicholson, MS, LMT
Springfield Technical Community College
Springfield, Massachusetts

Lou Peters, BS, LMT, CNMT
American Institute of Alternative Medicine
Columbus, Ohio

Carole Goya Rifflard, LMT, BS, Med
Keiser University
Stuart, Florida

Suzanne Shonbrun, BA
California Institute of Massage and Spa Services
Sonoma, California

Jean M. Wible, RN, BSN, NCTMB, LMT, HTCP
Community College of Baltimore County
Baltimore, Maryland

Preface

Kinesiology is the study of human movement patterns. When you think of human movement, it is easy to picture athletes or dancers performing amazing physical feats. But the truth is that every human body is in nearly constant motion—whether a person is working, playing, or even relaxing. You'll find that our primary focus in *Therapeutic Kinesiology* is on the movement activities that people do every day.

Each of us has memories of powerful body experiences. If you were to ask a group of people to recall the most exciting or relaxing body experience they ever had, you'd hear vivid tales of everything from hang-gliding above a craggy landscape to enduring hours of labor while giving birth to simply lying on a sun-drenched beach soaking up rays. People tend to recall the physical experiences that are emotionally transformative—exhilarating, rejuvenating, or deeply relaxing.

An experiential study of therapeutic kinesiology can be just as transformative. In fact, we can compare the experiential study we're about to undertake to a world tour. We explore the seemingly familiar world of the human body and its movement patterns in ways that can make you feel like you're in all new territory, ripe for fascinating discoveries. As you traverse the amazing movement landscape and explore tissue layers that generate movement, one of your primary tools for transforming your understanding will be your own internal process of *experiential learning*—feeling your muscles, bones, and joints and their movements within your own body. This will be especially important because, as you'll discover, when you couple the learning process with body experiences, it is much easier to truly understand new concepts and remember them.

To ensure an exciting and successful journey, we've packed numerous special features into this text in a handful of clear and easily recognized forms. These include features geared to those of you who like to learn through experiential, body-centered channels and who like practicing what you learn. Use these features to help you navigate through the fascinating world of therapeutic kinesiology.

INTRODUCTORY PICTURES AND STORIES

A good guidebook often begins with pictures and interesting tales that get you psyched about the places you are going to visit. Similarly, each chapter in the first half of *Therapeutic Kinesiology* begins with a body story that was handpicked to introduce you to the kinesiology concepts and biomechanical elements that are discussed in that chapter. We often return to these stories at the end of each chapter as a way to encapsulate very specifically the concepts just presented.

SELF-CARE EXERCISES AND CAUTIONS

A trip can be ruined in an instant by an injury or illness. Injury is a special concern for massage therapists, who need to take care of their own physical well-being by learning to work with good posture and efficient movement. Doing so ensures you will have a productive career free from injury and pain. To help you avoid injuries and body problems in your massage studies and career, we include a *Self-Care* feature that offers 44 different exercises for stretching, posture, and neuromuscular patterning.

We also place *Cautions* in strategic locations, often at the beginning of self-care, technique, or palpation boxes, to help you explore new ideas, movements, and hands-on exercises in a manner that protects you, your practice partners, and your clients. As massage therapists and bodyworkers, we are privileged that people allow us to work with their bodies. With this honor comes the responsibility of all health care professionals to "above all, do no harm." The cautions in the text remind you of this guiding principle when needed.

BRIDGE TO PRACTICE AND EXPLORING TECHNIQUE

Many educational journeys are deepened by interacting with and working alongside the locals. To help you apply the knowledge and experience you'll gain on your journey through the study of therapeutic kinesiology to your subsequent massage practice, we include two features, *Bridge to Practice* and *Exploring Technique*. The *Bridge to Practice* feature presents short tips and ideas on how to apply this material to the actual practice of massage and bodywork. The *Exploring Technique* feature provides 33 different exercises to walk you through step-by-step applications of kinesiology concepts to hands-on procedures. Both of these features provide valuable guidelines for making the study of kinesiology relevant to the practice of massage and bodywork. For this reason, we encourage you to take frequent short breaks along your way to ponder these tips and practice these techniques.

When you are learning new procedures from the Exploring Technique *exercises, make sure to practice them with a partner first and become adept at using them before putting them to use with clients.*

GUIDELINES AND TRIGGER POINT ILLUSTRATIONS

An educational journey can also be enhanced by visits to historical sites. With this intent, we include discussions throughout the text that source the neuromuscular practices most widely used in the massage and bodywork field—for example, muscle energy techniques and trigger point therapy. The *Guidelines* feature provides 16 different boxes throughout Part 1 with steps, tips, and checklists for making assessments, for working with client issues, and for applying techniques. *Trigger Point* figures throughout the second half of the text provide images of trigger point locations and pain referral patterns in more than a hundred of the muscles that we cover.

COMMUNICATION TIPS

The ability to communicate effectively with people you encounter can make or break a successful trip. As a professional massage and bodywork therapist, you will need to become fluent in the language of the body. To help you translate the rich dialect of the body into effective communication skills with your class partners and clients, we've tucked communication tips into the narrative throughout the text. You'll find brief communication tips for translating the language of kinesiology into common vernacular for your clients, cueing your clients on doing specific movements during exercises, getting effective feedback about body sensations, and communicating with other professionals.

PALPATION

When traveling through new locations, it can help to have a consistent daily routine. In our journey through the parts of the body in the second half of the text, we have laid down similar routes to travel in your explorations of each section so that you can relax and enjoy a predictable routine. Each second-half chapter begins with a study of bones, then looks at the joint structures and their movement, and ends with a study of the muscles. In addition, a *Palpation* feature walks you through the diverse terrain of the musculoskeletal system. Over 70 palpation exercises with clear color

photos and beautiful anatomical drawings laid over them will guide you through the varied geography of the bony landmarks and muscles in each part of the body.

SCOPE OF PRACTICE

Each allied health field has its own scope of practice. What differentiates massage and bodywork therapy from physical therapy is our scope of practice.

Massage is a system of structured touch, palpation, or movement of the soft tissue that is done to enhance or restore general health or well-being. **Bodywork** is not as easily defined. The definition that we use here is based on the context of our topic, meaning where kinesiology is used in therapeutic massage. Bodywork is a general term for any system of massage that works with the movement systems in the body to improve and restore the body's overall structure and function. In this sense, bodywork is the holistic application of the therapeutic massage modalities to the movement systems of the body, specifically the neuromusculoskeletal system. **Manual therapy** refers to any type of therapy that involves the application of hands-on techniques to a client or patient. Throughout this text, the terms *massage and bodywork* and *manual therapy* are used interchangeably. In the same vein, the terms *massage and bodywork therapist* and *practitioner* will also be used interchangeably.

The focus of this text is on the practical applications of therapeutic kinesiology in massage and bodywork training and practice. It is geared toward students and practitioners who want to develop the skills to assess and facilitate healthy, whole-body patterns of posture and movement and improve overall skeletal alignment and muscular balance in their clients. Massage therapists need to understand joint and muscle structures and functions to practice effective massage, so we also cover palpation skills as a foundation for manual techniques that use passive joint motions as well as active and resisted movements. In addition, we emphasize **self-study** so that you can apply kinesiology principles in practical exercises for improving your own posture, ease of motion, and body mechanics.

Because the application of specific exercises and hands-on techniques to specific joint or muscle injuries or pathologies constitutes physical therapy, such applications are not included in this text. This does not mean that these applications are not valid, but rather that they fall under orthopedic massage treatment protocols, which need to be practiced under medical supervision and are outside of the holistic scope of this text.

Applications in *Therapeutic Kinesiology* are based on a general, nonmedical assessment and treatment of tissues involved in movement, specifically the skeletal, muscular, and neuromuscular systems. Such applications are foundational to the practice of massage and bodywork. These applications, as well as the palpation skills presented in this text, can also used in orthopedic treatment protocols by physical therapists, physical therapy assistants, and physiotherapists who specialize in the practice of manual therapy.

OVERVIEW OF THE TEXT

Therapeutic Kinesiology is organized into two major parts.

Part 1 lays the foundation for understanding, restoring, and facilitating healthy and normal patterns of posture and movement through massage and bodywork.

- **Chapter 1** introduces *basic kinesiology concepts and terms* relevant to our study and to a massage and bodywork practice.
- **Chapters 2, 3, 4, and 5** on the *skeletal system, joint motion, muscular system, and neuromuscular system* cover the body systems that generate, coordinate, and carry out bodily movements.
- **Chapters 6, 7, and 8** provide concepts and information about *biomechanics, posture, and gait* and relate these topics to body mechanics.
- **Chapter 9** introduces *basic palpation and tissue layering skills* with a focus on the skills that we'll be putting to use in numerous palpation exercises in Part 2.

Part 2 offers a well-organized study of the bones, joints, and muscles, illustrated with beautiful full-color photographs, precise anatomical drawings, and clear mechanical drawings. These chapters are presented in a specific order that reflects the Ida P. Rolf method for developing structural integrity of the myofascial systems in the body. Each chapter in Part 2 includes palpation exercises to help you become comfortable with locating bony landmarks and exploring joint structures and motions, as well as learning the locations, actions, and trigger points of the muscles.

- **Chapter 10** begins with the *thorax and respiration* because full and healthy breathing is critical to optimal alignment and efficient movement.
- **Chapters 11, 12, and 13** on the *foot and ankle, knee, and pelvis* explore joints and muscles of the lower limbs and their roles in the weight support and locomotion of the whole body.
- **Chapters 14 and 15** on the *spine* and the *head and neck* look at core structures in the trunk, cranium, and jaw with an emphasis on vertebral alignment and muscular balance.
- **Chapters 16 and 17** on the *shoulder girdle* and the *arm and hand* examine the muscles and joints of the upper limb that allow a broad range of motion and the unique dexterity of the hands.
- **Chapter 18** on *self-care and body mechanics* summarizes many of the concepts presented throughout the text to prepare you for a transition into practice.

Each chapter throughout the text begins with a list of **objectives** and **key terms** to orient you as we start on a new part of our journey. We've tried to highlight the key terms in bold where they are defined and are most relevant to the material around them, so you may encounter a term earlier in the text that is not highlighted or defined until later in the chapter. Key terms can also be found in the **glossary.**

To help you pause and consider where you have been and what you have learned during the individual stages of this journey, each chapter concludes with a bulleted list of **summary points to remember** and a series of **questions and answers** for study and review.

GUIDELINES FOR SUCCESS

To help you get the most out of your exploration of the body's movement terrain, here are some general guidelines for a successful learning journey.

Relax into this study. Many students shudder with fear at the mere mention of a kinesiology class or test. The anxiety grows particularly intense if students have had difficulty in previous science classes.

Remember that your real goal in undertaking this journey—to learn sound clinical skills and become the best practitioner possible—is far more important than the individual facts you'll memorize along the way. The more thoroughly you actually understand concepts, as opposed to just memorizing facts, the easier it will be to remember what you have learned.

The best way to get a massage client to relax is to be relaxed yourself. Similarly, the more you relax into this study, the deeper this information will sink into your body-based memory logs. Relaxing into this material will give you the most productive trip possible into the world of body movement as it applies to massage therapy.

Slow down and cultivate body awareness. We often think of physical awareness as being centered in the sense organs of the head—eyes, nose, ears, and mouth. Yet the entire body is filled with sensory nerves. In fact, the entire body is a sense organ! Rather than being aware with the sense organs of your head, can you be aware with another part of your body? Can your knee be aware? Can your foot become an organ of perception?

The muscles are especially rich in sensory receptors. The sensory experience becomes even richer when two bodies contact each other through touch. Every person has millions and billions of sensory cells throughout the body that can tune in like antennae to the subtleties of massage and bodywork.

Try this simple exercise that demonstrates how to fine-tune sensory awareness: Touch your hand to your face. Now touch your hand back *with* your face. Which part is touching and which is being touched?

As you read this material, practice differentiating your body experience from your mental experience. Notice when your awareness is centered in your thoughts and when it is centered in body awareness. It only takes a momentary pause to sense where your attention is centered. This simple body–mind practice is meditative, and it will improve your understanding as well as your massage and bodywork skills.

Take frequent breaks to allow for body-based learning. A common complaint from massage students is that they feel overwhelmed and rushed in their classes. It's easy to become so focused on learning how to assess and treat a problem that we forget to take the time to actually feel what we touch or to notice our partner's response. To keep yourself from becoming road-weary, we recommend that you study this material in short, enjoyable excursions. Think of reading as a mental workout and take the time to let your brain recuperate between exertions.

When learning is linked to physical experience, we are more likely to remember what we learn. It's impossible to read vivid descriptions of body-based experiences without having some kind of internal resonance in your own body. The more actively you apply what you read to a physical experience, the easier the material will be to remember, especially if you are a kinesthetic learner. To ground this knowledge in your body, take pause here and there to actually practice the movements you are reading about.

Study one section at a time and use your imagination. Pause after reading and studying a few pages to take in and fully experience the kinesiology terrain. Take a break every few minutes to stand up and move around. Stretch, breathe, do whatever your body needs most in that moment. In addition, take a moment here and there to apply the tools you find in this book to your own self-care. This will improve your ability to slow down and feel the subtleties of movement in your own body and also in your client's body.

Cultivate communication skills and a client-centered focus. Communication skills are vital to success. Effective communication is especially important in the massage and bodywork field because it is client-centered. We want to make sure our clients tell us what they feel, particularly when they are uncomfortable with something we do. Clients might believe in a "no pain, no gain" approach and silently suffer during massage techniques that cause them discomfort. We need to tell clients up front that our hands-on work should not cause them pain or discomfort and ask them to tell us immediately if they feel either. This way, clients know what to expect and can relax under our hands-on pressure.

During this study, communicate openly with your practice partner. Ask your partner for feedback and listen carefully to it. By checking out your experience with your partner, it will become obvious that individuals interpret touch through their own personal filters and biases. These personal interpretations make effective communication both more difficult and a more important skill for a massage therapist to develop.

Let the entire world be your kinesiology lab. Observe and study movement patterns wherever you find them—at the airport, the mall, or the bank. Take a sideways glance at someone walking by and ponder what occurs to you about the person's body pattern. Then look again and you will see more. Or sit in a park and watch people's movements as they go by. Look at general patterns or pick a specific focus. For example, notice how many people look down as they walk, or notice the directions that people swing their arms.

When you find yourself stuck in traffic or in an airplane seat, make a postural study of your own body. Practice contracting and relaxing certain muscles to shift and improve your alignment. Continue the self-study as you work out, hike, bike, or do any other type of activity. Even while washing dishes, notice how you move and how you generate pressure to scrub a pan. With focused attention, simple tasks can become movement-efficiency studies. As you practice daily observation of yourself and other people, your observational skills and understanding of body movement will grow.

Therapeutic Kinesiology has been created as a practical guide for skills-based learning rather than as a technical manual. We developed it specifically for a new generation of students, educators, and practitioners who want and need science textbooks that are relevant to the practice of massage and bodywork. The many experiential exercises in this text are positioned like signposts and rest stops along a highway; they are relevant to specific material in that section and provide numerous opportunities for practical applications and experiential learning activities.

Many hours of work and careful thought have gone into making *Therapeutic Kinesiology* economical and lightweight. Wherever possible, we used images and photos to illustrate concepts and exercises in order to avoid lengthy explanations. In addition, we carefully and deliberately placed a lot of information within this single text to help accommodate a student budget.

Therapeutic Kinesiology combines three books into one—kinesiology, palpation, and body mechanics.

- The **kinesiology section** provides you with a knowledge base about human movement and the skills that make kinesiology concepts relevant to massage and bodywork.
- The **palpation exercises** lead you through an experiential study and working knowledge of functional anatomy to help you develop a tactile foundation for hands-on skills.

- The **body mechanics material** throughout the text, including a dedicated body mechanics chapter at the end of the book, equip you with practical and experiential knowledge of your own body so that you can work effectively, avoid injury, and enjoy a healthy and successful career.

Therapeutic Kinesiology equips you with everything you'll need to have an enjoyable, safe, and productive experiential study trek into the vast territory of the human body and its movement patterns. Bon voyage!

PEARSON
myhealthprofessionskit™

Additional resources are available for students and instructors at www.myhealthprofessionskit.com. Use this address to access the companion website created for this textbook. Simply select "Massage Therapy" from the choice of disciplines. Find this book and log in using your username and password to access the content.

Content available to students includes:

- Videos showing various palpation exercises
- Labeling exercises to test knowledge of various muscles and anatomy

- Key terms flashcards
- Lists of the OIAs for the different muscle groups

Additional content is available for instructors, including:

- Power Point Presentations
- Image Library
- Test Questions
- Instructor's Manual

Contents

Dedication   iii
Acknowledgments   vii
About the Author   ix
Reviewers   x
Preface   xi

PART 1   KINESIOLOGY FOUNDATIONS   1

Chapter 1   Introduction to Therapeutic Kinesiology   2
Chapter Objectives   3
Key Terms   3
1.1   Basic Concepts and Movement Patterns   4
1.2   Orienting Space within the Body   9
1.3   Orienting the Body in Space   11
1.4   Therapeutic Kinesiology   15
Conclusion   18
Summary Points to Remember   18
Review Questions   19

Chapter 2   The Skeletal System   22
Chapter Objectives   23
Key Terms   23
2.1   Elements of Connective Tissue   25
2.2   Tissues Making Up the Skeletal System   28
2.3   Joint Classifications   34
2.4   Skeletal Alignment and Gravity   39
Conclusion   44
Summary Points to Remember   44
Review Questions   45

Chapter 3   Joint Motion   48
Chapter Objectives   49
Key Terms   49
3.1   Osteokinematics: Types of Joint Movement   50
3.2   Arthrokinematics: Movement at Joint Surfaces   56
3.3   Range of Motion   61
3.4   Clinical Applications for Joint Movement   63
Conclusion   67
Summary Points to Remember   67
Review Questions   68

Chapter 4   The Muscular System   70
Chapter Objectives   71

Key Terms   71
4.1   Structural Features of Skeletal Muscles   72
4.2   Contractile Structures and Mechanisms in Muscles   76
4.3   The Continuity of Muscle and Fascia   81
4.4   Muscle Tension and Contractile Forces   86
4.5   Changing Roles of Muscles   88
Conclusion   92
Summary Points to Remember   92
Review Questions   93

Chapter 5   The Neuromuscular System   96
Chapter Objectives   97
Key Terms   97
5.1   Overview of the Nervous System   98
5.2   Sensory Receptors   105
5.3   Reflexes and Basic Movement Pathways   111
5.4   Movement Applications in Neuromuscular Techniques   115
Conclusion   124
Summary Points to Remember   125
Review Questions   126

Chapter 6   Biomechanics   128
Chapter Objectives   129
Key Terms   129
6.1   General Terms and Concepts   130
6.2   The Laws of Motion   134
6.3   Force   135
6.4   Levers   142
Conclusion   148
Summary Points to Remember   149
Review Questions   149

Chapter 7   Posture   152
Chapter Objectives   153
Key Terms   153
7.1   Components of Upright Posture   154
7.2   Muscle Patterns in Upright Posture   162
7.3   Faulty Postures   165
7.4   Postural Assessments   169
7.5   Therapeutic Applications for Postural Education   174
Conclusion   177
Summary Points to Remember   178
Review Questions   179

Chapter 8   Gait   182
Chapter Objectives   183
Key Terms   183
8.1   Components of Gait   184
8.2   Muscle Activity in Gait   194
8.3   Atypical Gait Patterns   196
8.4   Gait Assessment   201
Conclusion   204
Summary Points to Remember   205
Review Questions   206

Chapter 9   Basic Palpation Skills   208
Chapter Objectives   209
Key Terms   209
9.1   The Science of Palpation   210
9.2   The Art of Palpation   211
9.3   Palpation Tips   213
9.4   Tissue Layering   215
Conclusion   224
Summary Points to Remember   224
Review Questions   225

**PART 2   PALPATION AND
            PRACTICE   227**

Chapter 10   The Thorax and Respiration   228
Chapter Objectives   229
Key Terms   229
Muscles in Action   230
10.1   Bones of the Thorax   231
        The Thorax   233
10.2   Joints and Ligaments of the Thorax   235
        Costal Joints   237
10.3   Muscles of Respiration   238
        The Diaphragm   244
        Intercostals   248
        Scalenes   253
10.4   Respiratory Motion and Restrictive Patterns   255
        *Serratus Posterior Superior and Serratus Posterior
        Inferior*   257
Conclusion   260
Summary Points to Remember   261
Review Questions   262

Chapter 11   The Ankle and Foot   264
Chapter Objectives   265
Key Terms   265
Muscles in Action   266
11.1   Bones of the Ankle and Foot   268
        Tibia and Fibula   271
        Tarsals   275
        Metatarsals and Phalanges   277
11.2   Joints and Ligaments of the Ankle and Foot   279
        Subtalar and Transverse Tarsal Joints   289

        Intertarsal and Tarsometatarsal Joints   291
        Metatarsophalangeal and Interphalangeal Joints   293
11.3   Muscles of the Ankle and Foot   294
        *Tibialis Anterior, Extensor Digitorum Longus,
        and Extensor Hallucis Longus*   298
        Gastrocnemius and Soleus   303
        *Tibialis Posterior, Flexor Digitorum Longus,
        and Flexor Hallucis Longus*   307
        Peroneus Longus and Peroneus Brevis   312
        *Extensor Digitorum Brevis and Extensor Hallucis
        Brevis*   316
        *Abductor Hallucis, Flexor Digitorum Brevis,
        and Abductor Digiti Minimi*   319
        Quadratus Plantae and Lumbricals   322
        *Flexor Hallucis Brevis, Adductor Hallucis,
        and Flexor Digiti Minimi Brevis*   325
Conclusion   327
Summary Points to Remember   327
Review Questions   328

Chapter 12   The Knee   330
Chapter Objectives   331
Key Terms   331
Muscles in Action   332
12.1   Bones and Accessory Structures of the Knee   333
        The Knee   336
        Menisci and Bursae in the Knee   339
12.2   Joints and Ligaments of the Knee   340
        Ligaments of the Knee   343
12.3   Muscles of the Knee   355
        Rectus Femoris and Vasti Muscle Group   360
        *Biceps Femoris, Semitendinosus,
        and Semimembranosus*   363
        Popliteus   366
Conclusion   366
Summary Points to Remember   367
Review Questions   367

Chapter 13   The Hip and Pelvis   370
Chapter Objectives   371
Key Terms   371
Muscles in Action   372
13.1   Bones of the Hip and Pelvis   375
        Hips and Pelvis   381
13.2   Joints and Ligaments of the Hip and Pelvis   384
        Sacral Ligaments and Sacral Motion   397
13.3   Muscles of the Hip and Pelvis   399
        Sartorius and Tensor Fascia Latae   403
        *Adductor, Longus, Adductor Brevis, Pectineus, Graci-
        lis, and Adductor Magnus*   408
        *Gluteus Maximus, Gluteus Medius, and Gluteus
        Minimus*   414
        Iliacus and Psoas Major   418
        "Deep Six" Lateral Hip Rotators   424
Conclusion   432
Summary Points to Remember   433
Review Questions   434

Chapter 14 The Spine   436
Chapter Objectives   437
Key Terms   437
Muscles in Action   438
14.1   Bones of the Spine   440
14.2   Joints and Ligaments of the Spine   443
    The Vertebrae   444
14.3   Muscles of the Spine   459
    Splenius Capitis and Splenius Cervicis   461
    Erector Spinae: Spinalis, Longissimus,
        and Iliocostalis   465
    Transversospinalis: Multifidi and Semispinalis Capitis
        and Cervicis   468
    Rectus Abdominis, Obliques, and Transversus
        Abdominis   475
    Quadratus Lumborum   479
Conclusion   481
Summary Points to Remember   482
Review Questions   482

Chapter 15 The Head and Neck   484
Chapter Objectives   485
Key Terms   485
Muscles in Action   486
15.1   Bones of the Head and Neck   488
    Cranial Bones and Bony Landmarks   492
    Facial Bones and Bony Landmarks   496
15.2   Joints of the Head and Neck   499
    Ears, Nose, Hyoid, and Throat Structures   499
    Cranial Sutures   502
    Temporomandibular Joint Structures and Motion   507
15.3   Muscles of the Head and Neck   509
    Frontalis, Occipitalis, and Temporalis   515
    Masseter, Lateral Pterygoid, and Medial Pterygoid   520
    Suprahyoids and Infrahyoid Muscles   532
    Suboccipitals   535
    The Sternocleidomastoid   539
Conclusion   542
Summary Points to Remember   543
Review Questions   544

Chapter 16 The Shoulder Girdle   546
Chapter Objectives   547
Key Terms   547
Muscles in Action   548
16.1   Bones of the Shoulder Girdle   550
    Bony Landmarks of the Shoulder Girdle   552
    Scapula   555
16.2   Joints and Ligaments of the Shoulder Girdle   558
    Acromioclavicular and Sternoclavicular Joints   567
16.3   Muscles of the Shoulder Girdle   573
    Trapezius, Latissimus Dorsi, and Teres Major   577
    Rotator Cuff Muscles: Supraspinatus, Infraspinatus,
        Subscapularis, and Teres Minor   583

    Rhomboids, Serratus Anterior, and Levator
        Scapula   588
    Pectoralis Major, Pectoralis Minor, and
        Subclavius   595
    Deltoid and Coracobrachialis   600
Conclusion   603
Summary Points to Remember   603
Review Questions   604

Chapter 17 The Arm and Hand   606
Chapter Objectives   607
Key Terms   607
Muscles in Action   608
17.1   Bones of the Arm and Hand   610
    Elbow and Forearm   612
    Carpals   616
    Metacarpals and Phalanges   620
17.2   Joints and Ligaments of the Arm and Hand   620
17.3   Muscles of the Arm and Hand   631
    Biceps Brachii, Brachialis, and Brachioradialis   636
    Triceps Brachii and Anconeus   640
    Supinator and Pronator Teres   644
    Flexor Carpi Ulnaris, Flexor Carpi Radialis, Pal-
        maris Longus, and Flexor Digitorum Superficialis
        and Profundus   648
    Extensor Carpi Radialis Longus, Extensor Carpi
        Radialis Brevis, Extensor Carpi Ulnaris, Extensor
        Digitorum, and Extensor Indicis   653
    Flexor Pollicis Longus, Extensor Pollicis Longus,
        Extensor Pollicis Brevis, and Abductor Pollicis
        Longus   658
    Adductor Pollicis, Flexor Pollicis Brevis, Abductor
        Pollicis Brevis, and Opponens Pollicis   661
    Interossei and Lumbricals   665
    Abductor Digiti Minimi, Opponens Digiti Minimi, and
        Flexor Digiti Minimi Brevis   667
Conclusion   669
Summary Points to Remember   669
Review Questions   670

Chapter 18 Body Mechanics and Self-Care   672
Chapter Objectives   673
Key Terms   673
18.1   Skeletal Alignment   674
18.2   Relaxation, Breathing, and Fluidity   679
18.3   Moving Around the Massage Table   681
18.4   Force Applications and Hand Use   685
18.5   Ergonomics and Equipment   692
Conclusion   698

Glossary G-1
Chapter Review Answers A-1
Index I-1

All text in italics refer to muscle and bone palpation exercises.

Special Features

GUIDELINES

Chapter 3
Naming Joint Actions   55
Steps in Passive Range of Motion Stretching   65
Contraindications to Practicing Passive Joint Motion
  with Clients   65

Chapter 5
Elements to Track While Observing Active
  Movement   118
Steps for Using Passive Motion   118
Steps for Using Resisted Motion   119

Chapter 6
Balancing Stability with Mobility   148

Chapter 7
The Use of Imagery in Postural Education   158
Checklist for Assessing Posture   172
Client Communication around Postural Problems   174
Helping Clients Develop Postural Awareness   176

Chapter 8
Working with Clients Who Have Balance Issues   193
Intake of Clients with Antalgic Gait Patterns   198
General Gait Assessments   202
Specific Gait Assessments   203

Chapter 9
Palpation Tips Summary   215

EXPLORING TECHNIQUES

Chapter 2
Tactile Explorations of Viscosity with Corn Starch   27
Joint Approximation   37
Axial Compression Tests to Assess Lines of Force   43

Chapter 3
Exploring Roll, Glide, and Spin in Joint Motion   58
Placing Your Client's Joints in a Loose, Resting
  Position   60

Chapter 4
Viscoelasticity and Plasticity in Myofascia   85

Chapter 5
Muscle Approximation   107

Slow Movement to Relax Head and Neck
  Muscles   110
Trigger Point Therapy   121
Muscle Energy Stretch Techniques   122

Chapter 6
Stress and Strain in Myofascial Release   142

Chapter 9
Static Contact   218
Palpating the Skin   219
Palpating Superficial Fascia   219
Palpating Deep Fascia   220
Palpating Muscle   221
Palpating Tendons and Ligaments   223
Palpating Bone and Periosteum   223

Chapter 10
Following Rib Motion   239

Chapter 11
Restoring Arches in Stiff, Flat Feet   280
Passive Range of Motion for the Ankle   286

Chapter 12
Passive Range of Motion for the Knee   352
Tibiofemoral Rotations   353

Chapter 13
Passive Range of Motion for the Hip   391
Stretching the Iliotibial Band   401
Quadriceps Length Assessment and Stretch   429
Hamstring Length Assessment and Stretch   430

Chapter 15
Passive Range of Motion for the Neck   511
Tracing the Facial Muscles   528

Chapter 16
Passive Range of Motion for the Shoulder   562
Assessing the Neutral Position of the Shoulder
  Girdle   570
Treating the Levator Scapula   591

Chapter 17
Passive Range of Motion for the Wrist   627

Chapter 18
Push-Hands Exercise   689
Pull-Back Exercise   690

SELF-CARE EXERCISES

Chapter 6
Balancing Your Body with Reverse Actions   133
Overcoming On-the-Job Inertia   134
Exercises for Grounding and Countersupport   136
Efficient Use of Force in Pressure Applications   139
Pushing and Pulling with a Partner   146
Lifting a Heavy Object   148

Chapter 7
Postural Sway for Fluid Body Mechanics   155
Lower Back Protection with the Transversus
    Abdominis   165
Training the Postural Stabilizers   175
Centering Your Body over Your Feet   177

Chapter 8
Using a Rocker Base in Massage   186
Exercises for Lower Limb Alignment   190
Improving Sagittal Tracking of the Lower Limb   197

Chapter 10
Breath Support for Shoulder Girdle and Thoracic
    Spine   240
Locating, Tracking, and Stretching the Diaphragm   242
Coordinating Diaphragmatic Breathing with IAP   246
Breathing to Release Tension   258
Exploring Muscle Patterns in Upper Chest Breathing   259

Chapter 11
Stretching the Gastrocnemius and Soleus   303
Strengthening the Intrinsic Muscles of the Feet   321

Chapter 12
Correcting Genu Recurvatum (Hyperextended
    Knees)   350
Tracking and Guiding Menisci Motion   356

Chapter 13
Seated Pelvic Rock   379
Stretching the Lateral Hip Rotators   423
Exercises for the Perineal Muscles   427
Stretching the Hip Muscles   431

Chapter 14
Arcing Exercise for Spinal Movement   451
Waiter's Bow Exercise for Neutral Spine   455
Stretching the Posterior Spinal Ligaments   457
Correcting a Lumbar Sway Back with Lumbar Multifidus
    Training   469
Stretching and Strengthening the Spinal Extensors   470

Chapter 15
Temporomandibular Patterning and Stretching   508
Stretching the Neck   512
Neuromuscular Patterning to Engage the Neck
    Stabilizers   541

Chapter 16
Neuromuscular Patterning for the Scapulohumeral
    Rhythm   572
Stretching the Levator Scapula   588
Stretching the Pectoralis Muscles   597
Finding Scapula Neutral   602

Chapter 17
Grip Strength and Joint Alignment for Massage   631
Stretching the Wrists and Thumbs   668

Chapter 18
Stretching Chest Muscles and the Thoracic Spine   678
Checklist for Body Mechanics in Massage   697

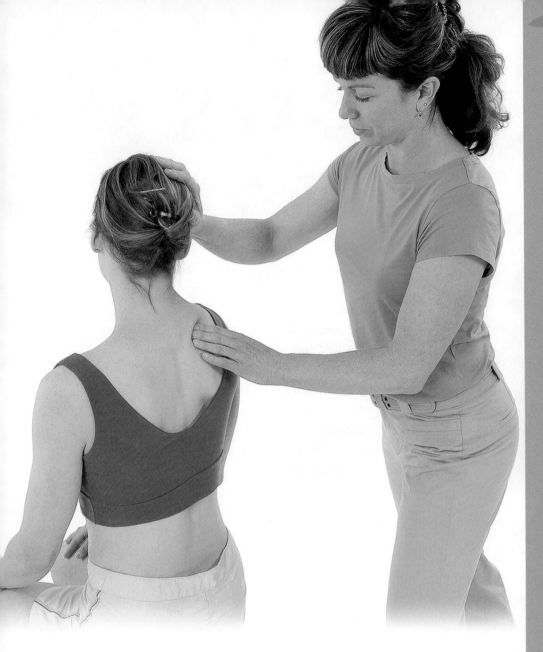

PART

1

Kinesiology Foundations

Chapter 1

Introduction to Therapeutic Kinesiology

Chapter 2

The Skeletal System

Chapter 3

Joint Motion

Chapter 4

The Muscular System

Chapter 5

The Neuromuscular System

Chapter 6

Biomechanics

Chapter 7

Posture

Chapter 8

Gait

Chapter 9

Basic Palpation Skills

1 Introduction to Therapeutic Kinesiology

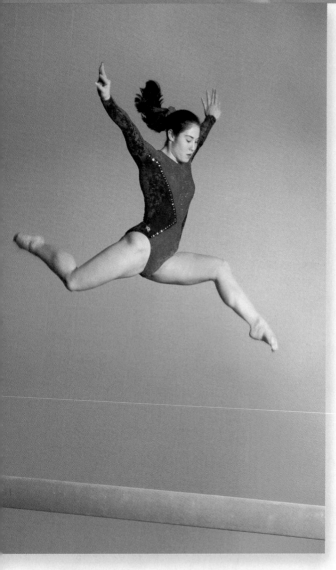

CHAPTER OUTLINE

Chapter Objectives

Key Terms

1.1 Basic Concepts and Movement Patterns

1.2 Orienting Space within the Body

1.3 Orienting the Body in Space

1.4 Therapeutic Kinesiology

Conclusion

Summary Points to Remember

Review Questions

Gymnastics is a sport that harmonizes dynamic movement with rhythm. The amazing range of movement demonstrated by top gymnasts reflects the summit of human movement potential. Olympic gymnasts captivate and dazzle audiences worldwide with their mesmerizing performances.

Gymnastics first developed in ancient Greece as an integral and required part of childhood education. Greek leaders believed it facilitated a unity of body and mind, so they built gymnasiums in every city. These ancient gyms were actually outdoor courtyards where young athletes could combine exercise with leisure and politics and where they trained for public games, which began the Olympic tradition.

Although the original Olympic Games ended in 393 A.D., the tradition was revived in Germany during the early part of the 19th century. Johann Friedrich Gutsmuths (1759–1839) developed a comprehensive system of exercise designed to improve strength, flexibility, and balance. One of Gutsmuths's students named Pehr Henrik Ling (1776–1839) further developed a group of therapeutic exercises into a floor routine that coordinated the rhythmic use of hoops, clubs, and small balls. Ling also created a complementary series of passive stretches and range of motion exercises designed to improve circulation and release muscle tension, which evolved into Swedish massage. By creating an integral link between gymnastic movements and Swedish massage, Ling's work highlights the key role of kinesiology in the study and practice of massage and bodywork therapies.

CHAPTER OBJECTIVES

1. Define kinesiology and biomechanics.

2. Describe the difference between statics and dynamics, and between mobility and motility.

3. Define force. Name two internal and two external forces that generate or affect movement.

4. Define mass.

5. Describe a kinetic chain using several examples.

6. List movement patterns of early motor development, naming the four neurological actions and five neurological pathways.

7. Define the terms *neuromuscular* and *musculoskeletal*.

8. Name the correct terms to identify general areas of and locations in the body.

9. Name the three axes and the three cardinal planes. Describe how they relate to each other.

10. Describe the anatomical position and its relevance to the study of kinesiology.

11. List the body systems directly involved in the production of human movement.

12. Define active technique, passive technique, and neuromuscular patterning.

KEY TERMS

Active technique	Force	Mobility
Anatomical position	Frontal/coronal plane	Motility
Anterior-posterior axis	Gravity	Musculoskeletal
Bilateral axis (medial-lateral axis)	Horizontal/transverse plane	Neuromuscular patterning
Biomechanics	Kinesiology	Passive technique
Diagonal plane	Kinetic chain	Sagittal/median plane
Dimensional balance	Mass	Standing position
Dynamics	Mechanics	Vertical/longitudinal axis

Imagine having a massage and leaving it feeling relaxed and renewed, standing taller and straighter, and walking out pain-free. To create this type of experience for clients, massage and bodywork practitioners need to understand and promote balanced movement in the body. We learn about balanced movement through the study of **kinesiology,** which is the science of human movement. Unlike many other sciences, this broad topic encompasses a number of overlapping fields, all of which help to describe some aspect of body movement. These include anatomy, biomechanics, geometry, physics, and physiology. Practical applications of kinesiology also cover a broad spectrum of movement sciences such as physical education, sports science, and dance. Kinesiology is a core science in massage education and practice.

Because the leading cause of disability in working adults is musculoskeletal pain that limits normal movement, and a primary reason that people seek therapeutic massage and bodywork is for pain relief, it is imperative that we understand kinesiology in order to help our clients restore normal, pain-free movement.[1] It might be surprising to learn that every single massage stroke we use has the potential to move the client's muscles and joints toward or away from optimal alignment and normal motion.

There are many different approaches to the study of this broad topic, ranging from hands-off book learning to hands-on manual therapy. Regardless of the approach, kinesiology courses always require learning the names, locations, and functions of all the muscles and joints. Although the mere thought of learning all these facts can be daunting, it's helpful to realize that the study of kinesiology can also be fun, interesting, and even exciting. It comes to life when we put our hands on the body and actually feel the motion of tissues.

The approach to kinesiology in this book was developed specifically for the massage and bodywork student. It balances cognitive learning with experiential learning by presenting kinesiology concepts with simple explanations, memorable metaphors, and rich images of movement patterns. It also balances a study of the clinical applications of kinesiology with the practice of therapeutic massage by integrating active movement exercises with logical hands-on exercises.

If you are the type of student who finds the volume of information in kinesiology intimidating, it helps to back away from the specifics when you find yourself too deeply buried in the details and take a global perspective once again, thinking about how each part fits into the whole pattern. To help us keep the larger picture in mind, this study is built on an organizing principle of volleying between general to specific, of examining the body from both a global and local perspective. The emphasis is on looking at how the function of each part contributes to or detracts from the structural integrity and movement efficiency of the entire body.

1.1 BASIC CONCEPTS AND MOVEMENT PATTERNS

The human body is our primary vehicle for the journey through life. Like any other vehicle, the body has many moving parts that function according to basic mechanical principles. **Mechanics** is a branch of physics that deals with force and mass in relation to moving bodies. The application of mechanics to human movement is called **biomechanics.**

Understanding basic biomechanics concepts helps us in two ways. First, it allows us to differentiate normal movement patterns from dysfunctional patterns in order to better help our clients. And second, it gives us the foundation for improving our own body-use patterns as we work in order to avoid injury from faulty movement habits.

Biomechanics is divided into two main areas of study: *statics* and *dynamics*.

- **Statics** applies to situations in which the body is balanced, stable, and not moving. A person's whole body can be moving through space yet remain static in form. For example, the gymnast in the opening figure holds a static posture through the height of her jump. A study of statics includes topics such as skeletal alignment, center of gravity, and postural muscle control.
- **Dynamics** applies to situations in which the body is unbalanced and moving. A dynamic body is a body that is changing shape, such as an acrobat performing a floor routine. A study of dynamics examines the forces that act on the body to initiate movement and alter movement while the body changes positions.

Think of statics in terms of the elements of posture in a resting body. A working knowledge of statics is important during manual therapy because we often need to position our bodies in a stable posture in order to apply sustained pressure or stretch.

Think of dynamics in terms of the elements that affect the body while it is actively moving, as it bends and turns through shifting shapes and positions. We need to understand the dynamic effects of movement on the body to make intelligent choices about how we can effectively move and manipulate bodily tissues during manual therapy. In addition, a working knowledge of basic dynamics concepts helps us move our bodies efficiently as we practice massage and bodywork.

1.1.1 Posture Is Intrinsically Dynamic

It is easy to mistake a static posture for the absence of motion. In reality, the living body never stops moving. Even during sleep, there is always intrinsic movement in the body. Internal movement in the body is called **motility.** Movement of the body through space is called **mobility.**

Posture is intrinsically dynamic because even when we are seemingly standing still, the inner workings of the body systems generate and power ongoing internal rhythms.

Living tissue is a quiet symphony of physiological rhythms, a cacophony of internal flows. You need only lay your ear on a friend's belly to hear the nonstop activity of the physiological rhythms. Each organ system moves to its own rhythm, such as the respiratory pump of the lungs, the circulatory pulse of the heart and blood, and the digestive peristalsis of the intestines. In addition to the metabolic whirlwind of activity in the body systems, a group of *equilibrium responses* (ER) located in the inner ear continually adjusts and resets muscle tone as part of a dynamic postural balancing act (discussed in the chapter on the neuromuscular system).

1.1.2 Kinetics and Kinematics

The dynamic aspect of biomechanics is further divided into kinetics and kinematics. **Kinetics** is the study of forces that act on the body to produce or change motion. **Kinematics** is the analysis and measurement of movement in terms of mechanical elements such as velocity, speed, and force. The complex mathematical formulas central to kinematics are beyond the scope of this study.

Force describes any element that generates or alters movement. Internal forces include muscular contractions and reflex actions. External forces include elements such as wind, water, or friction that push, pull, or drag the body. The most constant external force is **gravity,** which is the attraction of anything with weight toward the earth. External forces can increase or decrease the muscular effort needed to generate a movement. For example, it's much easier to ride a bike with the wind behind us than to ride against the wind. Likewise, it's much easier to apply deep pressure in massage when leaning into the hands because we add the force of gravity and body weight to muscular effort.

A basic law of nature is that for every force there is an equal and opposite counterforce. Similarly, for every kinetic force, there is a counterforce to movement. Examples of internal counterforces to movement are ligaments that limit a joint's motion or muscle contractions that oppose a movement. Examples of external counterforces are elements such as wind resistance or a boggy terrain.

How fast and how far a body moves in space depends on the strength of the forces that produce the motion and the counterforces that resist the motion. The rate of any motion can either accelerate or decelerate. For example, motion speeds up while racing down a hill on a bike or skis. Once the bike hits the bottom of the hill and starts heading up another hill, the movement of the bike begins to slow down.

Anything that takes up space and has weight is said to have **mass.** The bigger and denser the mass, the more energy is needed to move it. The mass of a body

defines the person. The muscles serve as the workhorses of "mass transportation," so to speak, moving the body through space. Muscular contractions generate pulls on the bones to lever the body parts or the entire body through space.

1.1.3 Mechanical Forces of Movement in Manual Therapy

One of the most important reasons for massage and bodywork students to study kinesiology is to understand how the forces applied in manual therapy affect the body in the same way that the mechanical forces of posture and movement affect the body. Each hands-on technique we use in massage and bodywork creates a force intended to create a specific change in the tissue being manipulated. Understanding how different hands-on techniques alter various tissues in specific ways helps us to make logical choices about which types of hands-on techniques to use when, where, for how long, and in what direction.

Neuromuscular techniques involve the application of forces with the intention of restoring normal movement to the body. Each tissue has properties that make it stress resistant to the forces of movement. Tissues respond to **load,** a mechanical force of pressure or weight, according to their structural properties. Bones, the densest tissue in the body, hold up well under the compressive loads of heavy weight or strong pressure. Muscles and tendons, which are far more elastic than bone, elongate well under tensional loads that stretch the tissue.

A manual therapist practices deep tissue work to improve skeletal alignment and muscular balance with the goal of restoring normal movement to the body. Given the role of tissue manipulation techniques in our work, it is important to consider the stress properties of specific tissues when choosing what type of forces to apply in manual therapy. We will revisit this important topic in the chapters on the skeletal, joint, muscular, and neuromuscular systems.

1.1.4 Kinetic Chains

Movement is rarely isolated in one muscle or joint. Instead, basic and familiar movement patterns of the human body occur along chains of action, passing from one joint to the next in a predictable sequence. This sequence is defined as a **kinetic chain,** which is a combination of successive joints linked by a series of muscles along a movement pathway. A number of kinetic chains have been identified. Although the joints, muscles, and nervous system always function together in an interconnected fashion, kinesiologists have described kinetic chains from different viewpoints:[2]

- An *articular chain* views the series of connected joints along a movement pathway.

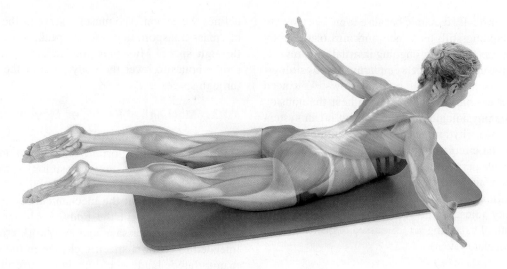

FIGURE 1.1
Extensor chain

- A *muscular chain* views the group of muscles that function together to produce a common action, such as the extensor chain or the flexor chain.

- A *neurological chain* views the neurological links of muscles that contract in an ordered sequence during developmental movement patterns, reflexive movements such as a flexor withdrawal reaction, and postural stabilization functions.

Kinetic chains are often described by the actions they produce. For example, the *extensor chain* of muscles runs along the back of the body from the head to the bottom of the feet (Figure 1.1 ■). It does, however, cross to the front of the body above the knee, at the quadriceps (which are knee extensors). We see the power of the extensor chain in actions such as the graceful arc of the body in a swan dive. In contrast, the *flexor chain* is what curls the trunk and limbs during a cannonball dive. The flexor chain of muscles runs along the front of the body from the jaw and neck down through the abdominals and front of the legs to the toes (Figure 1.2 ■). The flexor chain crosses to the back of the body above the knee, at the hamstrings (which are knee flexors). Having knee flexors and extensors located on the opposite side of the body in relation to other flexors and extensors along these chains allows the knee to bend in the opposite direction of the spine, hip, and ankle.

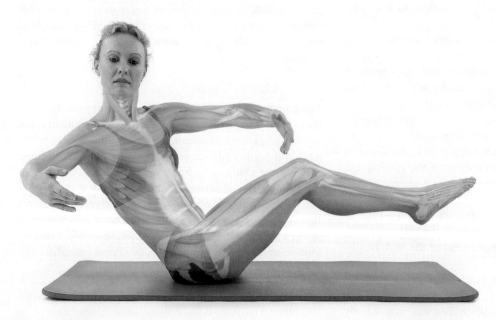

FIGURE 1.2
Flexor chain

A group of postural muscles work as a kinetic chain to maintain the position of one joint in relation to another in an upright body. These differ from chains of muscles that produce movement because they contract simultaneously rather than sequentially. In contrast, muscles in a kinetic chain that produce movement function in synchrony by contracting sequentially, generating coordinated movement patterns by transferring contractile forces along a series of linked joints. It is important to understand the relationship between kinetic chains, muscular balance, and muscular dysfunction. An efficient, coordinated movement reflects **muscular balance**—the relative equality of muscle length and strength between opposing muscles.

Conversely, tightness or weakness in one muscle along the kinetic chain reduces the efficiency of movement in the entire chain. This is important to understand because musculoskeletal pain can occur in an area of the body far from the movement dysfunction that is causing the pain. Vladimir Janda, a Czech neurologist, describes this process of muscular imbalance as a "chain reaction."[3] He explains how muscular pain can occur in a different location than the muscular imbalances causing the overall functional movement pathology. Unless the overall muscular imbalance is addressed in treatment, localized muscular pain can be temporarily relieved with massage or bodywork, yet it persists because of the faulty movement pattern.

The first step to restore healthy function in a kinetic chain is to understand healthy movement patterns, a topic that is expanded on throughout this text. The foundation for healthy motor patterns is formed during early motor development, which we look at in the next section.

1.1.5 Developmental Movement Patterns

In the first year of life, every person goes through the same basic series of developmental movement patterns. Early motor patterns are crucial to normal brain development and neuromuscular organization. Specialists refer to them as *neurological patterns* and classify them into two categories.[4] There are four **neurological actions:** *yield, push, reach,* and *pull.*

The neurological actions organize the quality of a movement pattern.

- *Yielding* sets a baseline of tone for all subsequent actions. All efficient movement begins from a relaxed state. Likewise, in manual therapy, any movement a practitioner asks the client to do will be more efficient if the client can begin the action from a place of yielding. In addition, the quality of touch improves when both the practitioner and client can relax and yield into it.
- *Pushing* compresses the body into itself, shortening the muscles and compressing the joints. A person with strong push patterns tends to have shorter, more condensed muscles, with sumo wrestlers showing us an extreme of this pattern. Pushing establishes lines of force along a series of linked joints, thereby increasing a person's proprioception in the body. To maximize force and minimize effort, practitioners need to pay attention to lines of force during deep tissue applications in order to effectively use full-body push patterns.
- *Reaching* extends the body out into space, taking slack out of the fabric of the soft tissues while lengthening the muscles and the joints. People with strong reach patterns, such as ballerinas, tend to develop elongated muscles.
- *Pulling* occurs as we reach and grasp something to pull it toward us or pull the body toward it. A practitioner pulls the client when stretching a limb or placing traction on the body. You can minimize stretch injuries during pulling activities by maintaining length in both the flexor and extensor muscles of the trunk to keep the spine straight.

The neurological actions occur along a series of five **neurological pathways:** *radial, spinal, homologous, homolateral,* and *contralateral.* The neurological pathways are seen in the shape of a movement pattern. These developmental pathways are most obvious in the skeletal organization of the human body. Like a starfish, the human body has five limbs—the spine, the two lower limbs, and the two upper limbs.

- **Radial** movement occurs when the limbs and spine simultaneously flex and extend in equal relationship to the center of the body. Skydivers extend the body in a radial pattern as soon as they jump from the plane into a flying position.
- **Spinal** movement sequences along the spine. Most human movement patterns involve some kind of spinal motion, but rarely is a body action isolated to the spine alone. Belly dancers may move their arms and legs, but they emphasize spinal undulations.
- **Homologous** means the same on both sides. A frog or rabbit hops in a homologous pattern. Homologous movement is marked by the symmetrical use of both arms and/or both legs, such as when a person works out on a rowing machine or a gymnast swings on parallel bars.
- **Homolateral** means the same on one side. Shot-putters move with a homolateral pattern when flexing the arm and leg on the same side, then extending them together as they throw. **Ipsilateral** is synonymous with homolateral.
- **Contralateral** movement sequences diagonally through the trunk between one arm and the opposite leg. All human gait patterns—walking, running, skipping, even cross-country skiing—are contralateral and involve a cross-crawl opposition of one arm with the opposing leg.

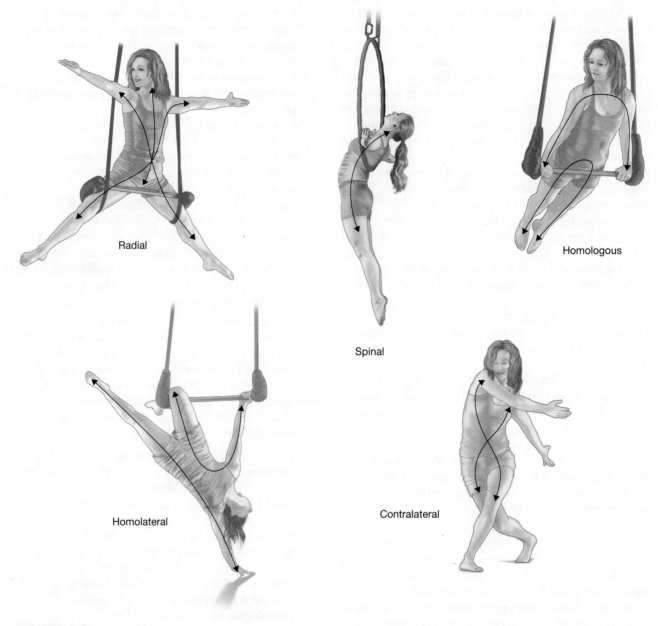

Radial

Spinal

Homologous

Homolateral

Contralateral

FIGURE 1.3
Basic neurological pathways

Most body movement patterns combine a sequence of several of the neurological actions and pathways. Single pathways and actions crystallize during many sports activities and can be observed in still shots of athletes and dancers (Figure 1.3 ■). The crystallization of each pathway gives the body a clear shape, such as the star-shaped radial extension of the gymnast pictured on the opening page of this chapter.

These patterns also manifest in daily activities. A person reaches with the head when carefully listening to a quiet passage during a symphony or focusing through binoculars to see a rare bird from a distance. Most people use a lower homologous push of the feet and a spinal reach with the head to stand from a seated position. Walking requires a contralateral swing of the arm with the opposite leg.

Gaps or weaknesses in any stage of early motor development shape adult posture and movement patterns. For example, when the spinal reach from the head is weak, the neck tends to collapse and the trunk loses height. A person with this pattern might suffer from discomfort or back pain from spinal compression and needs to learn to reach the head up to activate the postural muscles that elongate the neck. Likewise, we can teach clients suffering from discomfort and pain from a collapsed posture simple reach patterns that will elongate their joints. In later chapters, we will revisit the integration of active client movement into manual therapy using these simple actions and pathways, such as reaching from the head or pushing with the feet.

1.1.6 Whole-Body Patterns

Learning kinesiology requires a study of single joint and muscle actions, yet rarely does a single muscle or joint move in isolation. Movement occurs in whole-body patterns. In everything we do, in every daily activity, many muscles and joints contract and stretch and bend and twist in synchrony. All the parts are wired to each other, and the nervous system unifies the whole system to coordinate functional patterns. Even a simple gesture such as raising an arm while standing still recruits muscular activity clear down in the motor units of the legs and feet.

A movement pattern can be either simultaneous or sequential. In a **simultaneous movement,** the whole body moves at the same time. For example, when a person trips while walking, the entire body flinches at once to prevent a fall. In a **sequential movement,** the action travels through the body from one joint to the next. Sequential movements are more common in daily activities. Take, for example, reaching for a pen. The hand initiates the action. The reach elongates the arm and shoulder. If the pen sits a few feet away, the action will sequence into the spine and hips as the person leans forward to reach the edge of his desk. If the pen sits out of reach, the person will need to make a weight shift, moving the trunk to get the pen.

The muscular system is a unified system in which all the parts work in synchrony toward a single goal. In this sense, all muscles act as one muscle. We need to study how the parts work together. The direction of this study can go from the parts to the whole or the whole to the parts—from local to global or global to local. **Local** refers to the structures or movement patterns of a specific joint or muscle. **Global** refers to larger patterns, such as kinetic chains, developmental movement patterns, and whole-body movements. Our emphasis will be on looking at global patterns first, then breaking the study down into local parts. During this study, we oscillate between looking at global and local patterns, to see the bigger picture and to see where and how the parts fit together within the bigger picture.

1.2 ORIENTING SPACE WITHIN THE BODY

In this section, we go over the names and locations of various parts of the body. We also look at terminology that is used to describe one part of the body in relation to another. Keep in mind that kinesiology is a study of organic tissues and evolving concepts. This point is emphasized because it is easy to lose sight of the fact that joint and muscle structures and functions vary from body to body. Although most people have essentially the same parts and patterns, physical structures can vary from person to person. For example,

up to 40 percent of the population lacks certain muscles (the psoas minor and the palmaris longus), and many people have an extra rib or an extra vertebra.

Also keep in mind that there are regional variations in the general terms and concepts used to identify certain body parts. When appropriate, variations in terms are identified.

Here are the definitions of a few general terms needed to begin this study:

- **Neuromuscular** refers to the coordinated functions of the nervous system and the muscular system.
- **Musculoskeletal** refers to the coordinated function of the muscular system and the skeletal system.

1.2.1 Areas of the Body

Body parts and regions are usually named according to their general anatomical locations, although many terms used in popular language differ from medical terms (Figure 1.4 ■). To most people, *leg* means the entire lower limb. Yet talk to an orthopedist about the leg and she will assume that leg references the area below the knee. To make sure we are all referring to the same region of the body, here is a brief review of general terms.

The area from the hip to the knee is the *thigh.* The area from the knee to the foot is the *leg.* The entire structure from the hip joint to the foot is the *lower extremity* (LE) or *lower limb.*

The area from the shoulder to the elbow is called the *arm.* The area from the elbow to the wrist is the *forearm.* The entire structure from the shoulder joint to the hand is the *upper extremity* (UE) or *upper limb.*

The *pelvic girdle* is made up of the pelvic bones, the sacrum, and the thighs. The *shoulder girdle* is made up of the clavicles, the scapulae, and the arms.

The *torso* or *trunk* spans a region that begins at the top of the rib cage and ends at the bottom of the pelvis. The head and neck rest on top of the torso.

Many more terms refer to different areas of the body. They are introduced in subsequent chapters where appropriate.

1.2.2 Anatomical Position

The human body moves relative to space. During dynamic movements, such as running or vaulting, the entire body changes position in space and individual parts change position in relation to each other. Given the changing shape and position of a moving body, all references to movement are made in relation to a stationary, universal position called the *anatomical position.*

The anatomical position was originally named after the position of a cadaver lying on a dissection table. In this position, the palms face up and the weight of the feet turns the legs out. Stand a cadaver up, and this body is now in the **anatomical position** (Figure 1.5 ■). The anatomical position serves as a universal reference point from which we

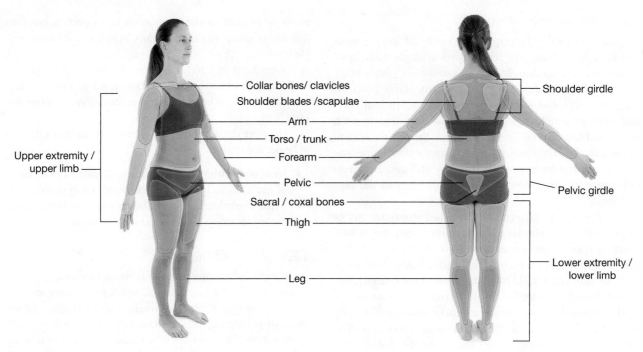

FIGURE 1.4
Areas of the body

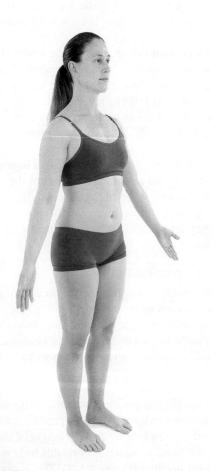

FIGURE 1.5
Anatomical position

describe the position and movement of all parts. For example, when referring to hip flexion, unless otherwise stated, it is assumed that the hip is flexing from the anatomical position. In the more natural **standing position,** the arms typically hang with the palms facing the trunk (Figure 1.6 ■).

1.2.3   Directional Terms

Directional terms are used to describe the location of some body parts in relation to others. Unless otherwise stated, directional terms refer to the body parts when they are in the anatomical or standing position.

- Medial and lateral refer to the location of a body part in relation to the *midline* of the body. **Medial** means closer to midline; **lateral** means farther away from midline. The lower back is medial in relation to the sides of the hips, whereas the crest of the hip is lateral to the spine.
- **Anterior** refers to a part that is closer to the front of the body; **posterior** refers to a part closer to the back of the body. The navel is anterior to the spine, whereas the gluteal muscles are posterior to the spine.
- **Proximal** means closer to the trunk; **distal** means farther away from the trunk. For example, the hand is distal to the elbow; the shoulder is proximal to the hand. The four ball-and-socket joints in the hips and shoulders are referred to as the *proximal joints* because they connect the limbs to the trunk and are therefore the joints closest to the trunk.
- **Superior** means above; **inferior** means below. The head is superior to the trunk, and the navel is inferior to the chest. In a standing position, the head is superior to the pelvis. In a person hanging upside down

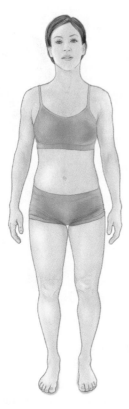

FIGURE 1.6

Standing position

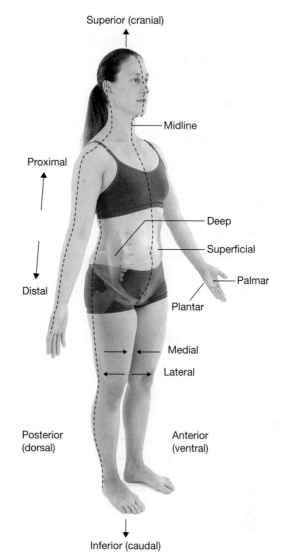

FIGURE 1.7

Directional terms

from gravity boots, the opposite is true—the pelvis is superior to the head.

- The terms **caudal** (which comes from the root "tail") and **cranial,** or **cephalad** (which comes from the root "cephal" or "head"), denote positions that are relative to the spine and the trunk. The head is always located in a cranial position to the trunk, regardless of whether a person is hanging upside down, lying down, or standing up. A caudal massage stroke always moves toward the pelvis. The terms caudal and cranial have traditionally been more commonly used in reference to four-legged animals, but they are being used with more frequency in the massage world today.
- **Dorsal** refers to the top of the foot. **Ventral** is synonymous with anterior. Dorsal and ventral are also used in reference to the back and belly of animals. A shark has a dorsal fin. The belly of a four-legged animal is the ventral surface.
- **Plantar** refers to the bottom of the foot. We plant the plantar surface of the foot on the ground when we step on it. **Palmar** refers to the surface on the palms of the hands (an easy one to remember!).
- **Superficial** refers to areas or structures that are closer to the surface of the body. **Deep** refers to areas or structures located farther away from the surface. The

heart is deep to the chest wall; the skin is superficial to the heart (Figure 1.7 ■).

1.3 ORIENTING THE BODY IN SPACE

The trunk of a tree grows upward and the taproot goes straight down. Similarly, the body of a human being orients to the space around it. A person stands with feet planted on the ground while the spine and head reach toward the sky. Yet unlike a tree, a person can stand on his hands or flip through the air. Given this mobility of a human body, spatial terms are used relative to the position or movement of the body. For example, an upright, extended spine is oriented along a vertical axis. The vertical axis of the body moves with the body. Whether a person is standing up or lying down, if the spine is extended, it is still oriented along a vertical axis.

1.3.1 Axes and Planes

Space is three-dimensional. A **plane** corresponds to each of these dimensions in space, so there are three primary, or cardinal, planes. An **axis** is a straight line that is perpendicular to a plane. Each dimension is oriented along one of three axes (singular: *axis*). The ceiling and floor of a room are oriented in one plane, the walls facing each other in one direction are oriented along another plane, and the other two facing walls are in the third plane.

The three primary axes are straight lines going up and down, front to back, and side to side that intersect at one point (Figure 1.8 ■). Each of the three axes makes up one of the X, Y, and Z coordinates. The three axes correlate with the *height, width,* and *depth* of a mass.

1. The **medial-lateral axis** or **bilateral axis** runs between the right and left sides of the body.
2. The **anterior-posterior axis,** or **AP axis,** runs between the front and back of the body.
3. The **vertical axis** or **longitudinal axis** runs up and down the body along the relative line of gravitational pull.

The three planes are referred to as the sagittal, horizontal, and frontal planes. The planes are most obvious in the cube (Figure 1.9 ■). The two sides of the cube are oriented in the **sagittal (median) plane,** the top and bottom are oriented in the **horizontal (transverse) plane,** and the front and back are oriented in the **frontal (coronal) plane.**

Each plane intersects with the other two planes at a right angle. The frontal (front and back) and sagittal (sides of the cube) planes are oriented along the line of

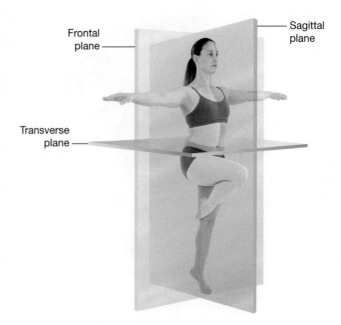

FIGURE 1.9

The three cardinal planes

gravity's pull. An easy way to remember the three planes is that the sagittal plane is like the side of a house, the horizontal plane is like a tabletop, and the frontal plane is like a front door.

Theoretically, there are an infinite number of planes. For example, horizontal planes can stack to infinity like cards in a deck. The three planes that intersect at the center of a cube or body are called the **cardinal planes.** Each plane bisects the body mass into equally weighted halves, so the place where the cardinal planes meet defines the center of weight in the body. The cardinal planes divide the body into halves as follows:

1. The sagittal plane bisects the body between the right and left sides.
2. The horizontal plane bisects the body between the upper and lower halves.
3. The frontal plane bisects the body between the front and the back.

Each plane rotates along an axis; the axis is perpendicular to the plane (Figure 1.10 ■). As an object turns in a plane, it rotates around an axis that is perpendicular to that plane.

1. The sagittal plane rotates along the medial-lateral axis like a wheel turning along its central axle.
2. The horizontal plane rotates along the vertical axis like a merry-go-round spinning around its center.
3. The frontal plane rotates along the anterior-posterior (AP) axis like a windmill turning in the breeze.

The plane in which the body is moving is always relative to the direction in which the body is facing. Flexion and extension of the spine always produce body movement

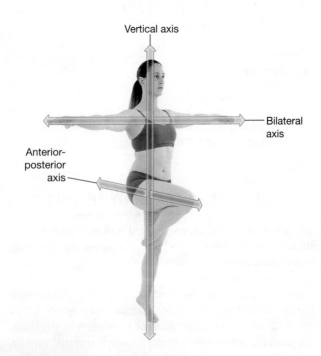

FIGURE 1.8

The three primary axes

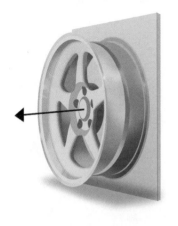

Sagittal plane

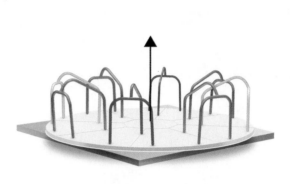

Horizontal (transverse) plane

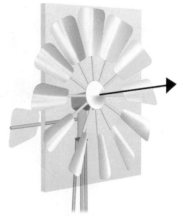

Frontal (coronal) plane

FIGURE 1.10

Mechanical movement in each plane

in the sagittal plane (Figure 1.11a ■). Examples of sagittal movement include a child doing a somersault and a gymnast doing a forward or backward flip. Twisting of the spine always produces movement in the horizontal plane (Figure 1.11b ■). Examples of horizontal plane movement include an ice skater spinning and a golfer swinging a club. Lateral flexion of the spine always produces movement in the frontal plane (Figure 1.11c ■). Examples of frontal plane movement include a person turning a cartwheel and doing jumping jacks.

1.3.2 Diagonal Planes

A **diagonal axis** of a cube is a line that goes from the high-front-right corner of the cube to the lower-back-left corner. A cube has three diagonal axes, and these meet in the exact center of the box. A **diagonal plane** runs perpendicular to each diagonal axis in the cube (Figure 1.12 ■).

Many muscles are oriented along approximately diagonal axes of the body. Take, for instance, the sternocleido-mastoid muscles (SCM) in the neck (Figure 1.13 ■). When

it functions normally, the SCM orients along a diagonal axis, from the back-high to the low-front. Particularly in a tall person with a long neck and well-aligned posture, the SCM brings a graceful poise to the posture. It lifts the back of the head and lifts the upper anterior rib cage. In a person with a forward-head posture, the SCM pulls the back of the head down and forward, shortening and bending the neck.

There are several terms to describe diagonal views of an anatomical image:

- **Anterolateral** refers to a view from an anterior and lateral direction in relation to the body part being viewed (see Figure 1.15).
- **Posterolateral** refers to a view from a posterior and lateral direction.
- **Anteromedial** refers to a view from an anterior and medial direction.
- **Posteromedial** refers to a view from a posterior and lateral direction.

FIGURE 1.11

Spinal movement in each plane:
a) Sagittal plane b) Horizontal plane
c) Frontal plane

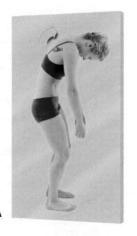

A

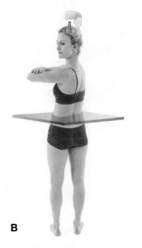

B

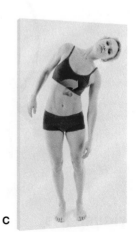

C

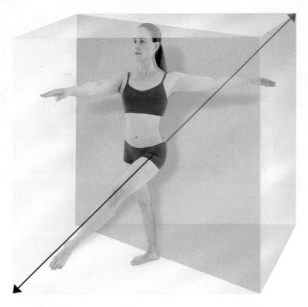

FIGURE 1.12

A diagonal axis and plane

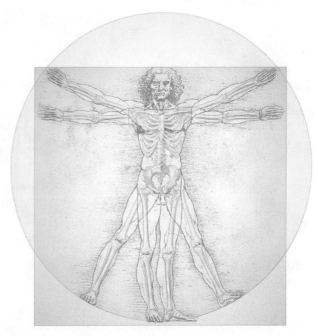

FIGURE 1.14

Leonardo da Vinci's *Vitruvian Man*

1.3.3 Dimensional Balance

The basic spatial configuration of the human body is the **dimensional cross**—the intersection between the width of the arms and length of the spine and lower extremities. Leonardo da Vinci depicted the proportional beauty and symmetry of the dimensional cross in his famous drawing of the human body called the *Vitruvian Man*

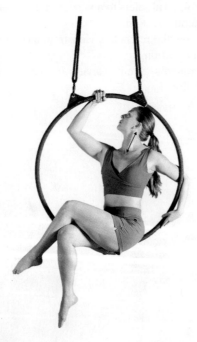

FIGURE 1.13

Some muscles are oriented along the **diagonal axis**

(Figure 1.14 ■). But muscular tensions can shorten and bend the body, distorting these natural proportions. For example, people develop rounded shoulders, hunched rib cages, bowlegs, or head-forward postures because of faulty postural habits.

Every massage stroke we do has direction, so each stroke provides us with an opportunity to move the client's body toward improved alignment and dimensional balance. When the body has **dimensional balance,** it has symmetry and proportion in its height, width, and depth. Each segment of the body aligns above and is supported by the segment below it (Figure 1.15a ■). As simple a move as bringing the legs directly under the body (meaning kneecap under the hip socket) puts the femur into the natural medial rotation that occurs in extension. When we apply massage strokes in a direction that improves alignment, the client receives a passive education about optimal skeletal alignment.

Like snags in a sweater, chronically contracted muscles associated with faulty postures pull and shorten certain areas of the body, tipping body segments off center (Figure 1.15b ■). This results in a distortion of the dimensional balance of the body, reducing its overall structural integrity. In contrast, when the joints are optimally aligned, the muscles have a normal length, and the body has dimensional balance, the body posture is in a state of **structural integrity.** The term "structural integration" was originally coined by Ida Rolf to name the somatic therapy she developed that is now called *Rolfing*®.[5] We will revisit the topics of dimensional balance and structural integrity throughout the text.

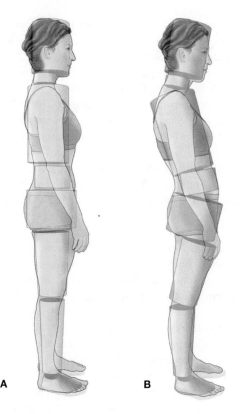

FIGURE 1.15

a) Optimal alignment results in **dimensional balance** in the body.
b) Faulty posture reduces dimensional balance.

1.4 THERAPEUTIC KINESIOLOGY

The approach to kinesiology presented here is *therapeutic* because applications are made to improve the overall posture and movement of the client and practitioner alike. The student's own body often proves to be one of the most effective learning labs in this study. A story illustrates this point: A massage therapist described how, until she experienced the physical sensation of certain postural muscles contracting to support her lower back, she had thought of those muscles as just abstract images in an anatomy book. During a strenuous long-distance run in the mountains while loaded down with a heavy pack, a familiar low back pain started to bother her. She then recalled a stabilizing isometric exercise from massage school that students learned to improve body mechanics and began to practice it as she ran. After a few minutes of contracting the deep muscles along her spine, her stride became easier and the pain completely subsided.

You are encouraged to approach therapeutic kinesiology firsthand during your studies by actually experiencing what integrated joint and muscle functions feel like in your own body. Not only will your body reap the benefits of your newfound knowledge, just as the massage therapist in this story put her knowledge to use, but learning will be easier if your cognitive study is reinforced with body experiences.

1.4.1 A Multi-Systems Approach

All body movement involves a complex coordination among the nervous system, the muscular system, and the skeletal system, plus their associated connective tissues such as ligaments, cartilages, and fascias. The integrated application of therapeutic kinesiology requires a multi-systems approach (Figure 1.16 ■). To help restore normal alignment and movement to the body, we need to understand the relationships among the body systems associated with movement.

When there is a body problem associated with posture or movement dysfunctions, such as chronic muscular pain, we can determine which system or systems are involved by listening to the client's descriptions of physical symptoms. For example:

- Pain from muscles feels achy and diffuse, and decreases with movement.
- Pain from nerves feels sharp and throbbing, and increases with movement.
- Pain from joints is constant, occurs in the problem joint, and occurs independent of movement.

Movement is about relationships between moving parts. When one part becomes more balanced, it naturally follows that the whole body gains more balance. Conversely, when one part of the body is held in chronic muscle contraction, the whole body pattern changes. When addressing movement dysfunctions, consider which tissues or body systems are causing the problem. Movement dysfunction can be caused by muscular imbalances, joint stability dysfunctions, faulty movement patterns, and even nerve compression from restrictions and tensions in surrounding tissues. Throughout the text, we revisit the premise of taking a multi-systems approach to therapeutic kinesiology.

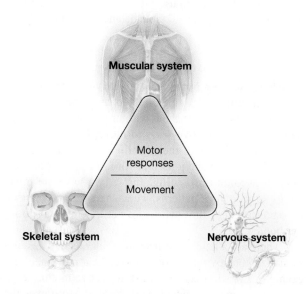

FIGURE 1.16

Body systems that coordinate movement responses

1.4.2 Pattern Recognition as a Therapeutic Skill

Pattern recognition is an innate human ability that can be honed into a therapeutic skill through the study of kinesiology. When we notice someone walking at a distance, the eye takes in the whole pattern or character of the walk. The mind registers the shape and configuration of the entire person. This is why it is easy to recognize friends simply from how they move without seeing their faces.

The unconscious mind picks up more about another person's patterns than we usually recognize consciously. The shape and motion of a friend's stance and gait patterns become familiar to us at a gut level. In addition, the eye is drawn to "held" areas—those parts of the body where skeletal muscles reflexively hold and guard to protect areas of chronic pain. Movement flows around rather than through held areas, which reduces the efficiency of the entire pattern.

Watch world-class athletes performing sports or dance, and the seamless form of their patterns of movement stands out. Their superb form is marked by qualities of efficiency, balance, and spatial clarity. In contrast, watch a person walking past with a noticeable limp, and the asymmetry and imbalance of the gait call for attention. Upon closer observation, muscular imbalances and joint restrictions of the movement dysfunction become obvious. Our minds may even begin to speculate about what injury or trauma this person suffered to cause the problem, and how much pain he or she endures.

Short of illness or sudden injury, many of the body problems that people seek massage and bodywork to alleviate come from the stress and pain caused by faulty posture and movement habits. These problems are easy to observe. By learning to recognize normal movement, we can assess patterns that fall outside the normal range and need attention. In this way, we can use pattern recognition as a rudder to guide our clients toward more balanced posture and more efficient movement.

1.4.3 Neuromuscular Patterning

Whenever we ask our clients to actively participate in a session, either through directed awareness or active movement, we provide them with an opportunity to learn new and more effective ways to move. If we are calling for client motion with the intention of reorganizing and improving muscle and joint functions, the process is called **neuromuscular patterning.** Just as we have the innate ability to recognize patterns, we change our neuromuscular patterns every time we figure out a better way to use our bodies.

There are a number of neuromuscular techniques used in manual therapy that involve active client movement. For example, a practitioner might ask for active motion to get a muscle to contract, which activates muscle reflexes that then cause the muscle to relax, making it easier to stretch.

In one case, a client suffered from hip pain caused by a chronically inhibited gluteal muscle, which failed to fire and contract. As a result, other muscles worked harder and their chronic overuse put pressure on the nerves in her hip, causing chronic pain. Passive bodywork was effective in helping the chronically overused muscles to relax. But the relief was only temporary. The pain pattern returned until the client learned to actively fire and contract the gluteal muscles.

As a clinical skill, patterning integrates therapeutic kinesiology into manual therapy. Patterning can help a client to change the faulty body habits associated with musculoskeletal pain and repetitive injuries. We use patterning in massage every time we help our clients find new and easier ways to posture and move. The chronic muscular tensions clients receive bodywork to alleviate have developed to support them in some way. When we help our clients release chronic tensions that function as their support systems, we need to help them establish new support systems. Neuromuscular patterning replaces old, harmful patterns with new and more efficient patterns. For instance, clients with whiplash injuries frequently develop chronic muscular holding in the neck. If we release this muscular holding, then we need to help them find a new way to support their neck. Establishing a new pattern can be as simple as having the client slowly and in a relaxed manner turn the head several times before getting up. This simple motion can reorganize new and more efficient muscle patterns to support the head and neck.

The kind of touch used in patterning bodywork to guide a client through a new and more efficient movement pattern is called **patterning touch.** Take note that neuromuscular patterning differs from neuromuscular re-education used by physical therapists to treat specific joint and muscle pathologies. Patterning touch is used to improve overall muscle function and movement efficiency.

1.4.4 Passive and Active Techniques

To restore normal motion to the body using neuromuscular patterning, manual therapists often combine passive and active techniques. **Passive techniques** include all hands-on methods that do not require clients' participation. Conversely, **active techniques** include any hands-on methods requiring clients' active participation, such as having them contract or relax certain muscles, or having them move in a certain way (Figure 1.17a ■). All neuromuscular patterning involves the use of active techniques. Obviously, applying active techniques effectively requires a working knowledge of kinesiology and basic biomechanics.

Combining active technique with massage and bodywork has many benefits. It helps clients to improve body awareness, which is the first step in changing a faulty posture or movement habit. It reorganizes the neuromuscular pathways, which improves movement efficiency.

FIGURE 1.17

Samples of active techniques: a) A practitioner guides a client through a more efficient movement range using patterning touch. b) A practitioner provides resistance for the client to push against in order to contract a specific muscle.

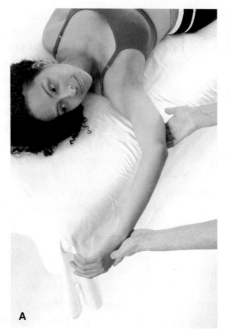

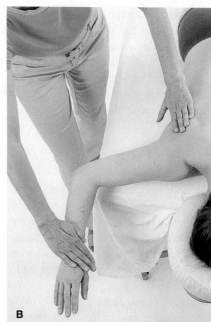

And it helps clients gain active control over how they use their muscles, which they need to improve posture and movement.

Using active technique also makes our work easier because the combination of our efforts and those of the client more than doubles the effect of the work. For example, if we are trying to help a client release muscle tension, the tissues respond more readily when the client actively focuses on relaxing. After all, muscle patterns are under the control of the client. No amount of massage and bodywork will change the muscle patterns if the client is unable to actively take charge of this change. In this sense, the manual therapist is a facilitator and guide to change while the client's awareness and will are the actual agents of change.

Active movements such as subtle pushes and reaches, pelvic tilts, and spinal flexion are easy for clients to do while they are lying down. Active technique applied while the client is on the table is the experiential foundation of client education. Probably the most commonly used active technique is resisted movement, in which a practitioner facilitates the contraction of a target muscle by having the client move against resistance (Figure 1.17b ■). In the chapter on the neuromuscular system, we look at different types of active techniques and discuss why and how to use them.

1.4.5 The Somatic Nature of Physical Patterns

Somatics is a term used in the massage and bodywork field to describe the complementary and alternative therapies that address the body in all its realms—physical, emotional, mental, and energetic.[6] Every pattern of the body has a mental and emotional correlate. The physical patterns of posture and movement outwardly manifest hidden patterns of thoughts and feelings. This is the somatic nature of physical patterns; they reflect a deep body-mind connection. In this context, the term "body-mind" is used synonymously with the term "somatic."

A human being is somatic by nature. For example, an energetic, buoyant stride usually reflects a happy emotional state. In contrast, a heavy, plodding gait often reflects a depressed emotional state. Recognizing the depth of the somatic connection to posture and movement is important when working to change body patterns and practicing neuromuscular patterning. If you are going to take a somatic approach to massage and bodywork, you will need to consider the integral connections among the body, mind, and emotions.

When chronic muscular tensions underlying faulty posture and movement habits are slow to change, they could be serving important psychological functions in a person's life. Skeletal muscles can develop chronic contractions in reaction to trauma or to cope with stressful thoughts and feelings.[7] You can work to release tight muscles and facilitate the contraction of inhibited muscles with active movement, yet neuromuscular patterns rooted in psychological holding and defense mechanisms can be slow to change. Still, many clients want to change their body patterning and will appreciate learning new ways to move through the therapeutic application of active techniques.

Although all of us have relatively similar anatomical structures, each person you work with will have a unique somatic pattern that will respond to your work in its own way. As a massage and bodywork practitioner, you will want to keep the somatic nature of physical patterns in mind when challenged by stubborn, unyielding muscular tensions in your clients. On the other hand, it is extremely gratifying when you are able to help your clients make deep somatic changes in their body patterns using the skills we will be exploring throughout this text.

CONCLUSION

The sport of gymnastics embodies many of the basic concepts of kinesiology that we have covered here. An adept gymnast is able to hold a static posture during incredibly dynamic aerial routines. The gymnastic performer displays superb control over muscular coordination, utilizing the forces of gravity, momentum, and weight to efficiently and powerfully swing, throw, and flip across the floor and over equipment. Each gymnastic move sequences along a clear kinetic chain or movement pathway of adjacent joints linked by a series of contiguous muscles.

A gymnast also demonstrates an advanced and innate ability to move with precise neurological actions and pathways, yielding to relax before pushing, reaching, and

pulling the body through space with strength and agility. The gymnast inhabits every part of the body, from fingertips to toes and head to tail, knowing exactly where and how the body is moving in space. He or she gauges distance and speed during each flip and jump, then executes that move with a dimensional clarity in the plane of action. A dimensional balance can also be observed in the body of the gymnast, who skillfully maintains structural integrity and proportion between the trunk and limbs during a broad range of dynamic movements.

The spatial clarity, dimensional balance, and structural integrity that a gymnast embodies are the same goals a practitioner holds in the practice of massage and bodywork. To use effective body mechanics, you need to know where your body is in space, move with full-body patterns that sequence along complete movement pathways, and balance push and reach patterns. To improve balance and integrity in the client's body, you need to be clear about the direction and kind of force used in each massage stroke.

As you progress through this book, you'll learn to apply kinesiology to palpation manual therapy with a multi-systems approach that integrates skills in pattern recognition, neuromuscular patterning, and active techniques into your hands-on techniques.

SUMMARY POINTS TO REMEMBER

1. Kinesiology is the study of the science of human movement with an emphasis on joint and muscle function. Biomechanics is the application of the physics of force and mass (anything that has weight and takes up space) to the study of human movement.

2. The study of biomechanics is divided into statics and dynamics. Statics applies to the biomechanics of the stable, stationary body; dynamics applies to the biomechanics of the moving body. Motility describes the internal movements of the body and mobility describes the movement of the body through space.

3. Force describes elements that generate or alter movement. Forces are either internal (muscular contractions and reflexes) or external (gravity, wind, or water pressure). Load is a mechanical force (pressure or weight) of relevance to manual therapies because tissues respond to loading from hands-on work according to their mechanical properties.

4. Mass is anything that has weight and takes up space.

5. A kinetic chain is a series of successively linked joints that are connected by a series of muscles and connective tissue along a movement pathway. For example,

the extensor chain includes the muscles and joints generally located along the back of the body.

6. Patterns of movement organized during early motor development fall into two categories: neurological actions (yield, push, reach, and pull) and neurological pathways (radial, spinal, homologous, homolateral, and contralateral).

7. Neuromuscular describes the coordinated function of the nervous system and muscular system. Musculoskeletal describes the coordinated function of the muscular system and skeletal system.

8. When discussing the body, areas of the body (e.g., torso, leg, forearm, thigh, arm) and the relative position of the body (e.g., standing, sitting, prone, supine, side-lying) are identified. Directional terms (e.g., medial, lateral, anterior, posterior, proximal, distal) are used to describe the location of one part of the body in relation to another part.

9. The three primary axes (bilateral, anterior-posterior, and vertical) and three cardinal planes (horizontal, frontal, and sagittal) intersect in a cube. Each axis intersects its respective cardinal plane at a right angle.

10. The anatomical position is a position of the body in which the weight-bearing joints are in extension and the palms face forward. Unless otherwise specified, all descriptions of anatomical parts or joint motion refer to the body in the anatomical position.
11. The body systems directly involved with movement are the nervous system, the muscular system, and the skeletal system.
12. Active techniques require active client participation, usually in the form of movement. Passive techniques are performed by the practitioner on the client's body without the client's active participation. Neuromuscular patterning is an active technique in which the practitioner has the client actively move with the intention of reorganizing and improving the nervous system coordination of muscular functions.

REVIEW QUESTIONS

1. Define kinesiology and biomechanics.
2. True or false (circle one). Statics is associated with the elements of movement; dynamics is associated with the elements of posture.
3. The difference between mobility and motility is that
   a. mobility refers to the movement of the body through space and motility refers to intrinsic physiological movements within the body.
   b. mobility refers to extrinsic movements around the body and motility refers to the movement of the body through space.
   c. mobility refers to intrinsic physiological movements within the body and motility refers to the movement of the body through space.
   d. mobility refers to intrinsic physiological movements within the body and motility refers to the movement of the fluids within the joints.
4. Name three forces that act on the body to generate or affect movement.
5. Acceleration and deceleration refer to the
   a. mass or size and weight of a moving body.
   b. changing velocity of a moving body as it speeds up or slows down.
   c. location in space through which a moving body is traveling.
   d. location in space at which a moving body comes to rest.
6. A kinetic chain is a series of
   a. successively linked fascial membranes that form connective tissues.
   b. unrelated muscles and joints that make a movement pathway.
   c. successively linked extremities that make a movement pathway.
   d. successively linked muscles and joints that make a movement pathway.

7. True or false (circle one). Load is a mechanical force such as pressure or weight.
8. True or false (circle one). A swan diver springs off the diving board using a lower homologous push pattern and an upper homologous reach pattern.
9. What is the difference between a sequential and a simultaneous movement?
10. Using directional terms, one would say the head is _____ to the trunk. The lower limbs are _____ to the shoulders. The abdomen is _____ to the spine. The skin is _____ to the organs
11. When we run our hand along the spine, we touch the
    a. anterior or ventral surface of the body.
    b. posterior or dorsal surface of the body.
    c. posterior or ventral surface of the body.
    d. anterior or dorsal surface of the body.
12. The difference between the anatomical position and the standing position is that
    a. in the anatomical position the palms face forward and in the standing position the palms face toward the body.
    b. in the anatomical position the palms face backward and in the standing position the palms face toward the body.
    c. in the anatomical position the palms face forward and in the standing position the palms face away from the body.
    d. in the anatomical position the palms face forward and in the standing position the palms face backward.
13. True or false (circle one). Running occurs in the sagittal plane.
14. The axis of a plane is a line around which a plane turns that is
    a. diagonal to the plane.
    b. perpendicular to a diagonal.
    c. parallel to the plane.
    d. perpendicular to the plane.

15. Neuromuscular describes the coordinated movement functions between the
    a. nervous system and skeletal system.
    b. nervous system and muscular system.
    c. muscular system and skeletal system.
    d. muscular system and circulatory system.

16. The three body systems involved in the coordination and generation of posture and movement patterns are
    a. the nervous system, the circulatory system, and the muscular system.
    b. the nervous system, the muscular system, and the joint system.
    c. the nervous system, the muscular system, and the skeletal system.
    d. the neuromuscular system, the fascial system, and the skeletal system.

17. True of false (circle one). Passive massage changes neuromuscular pathways.

18. The knowledge of the mechanical effects of movement on bodily tissues is important for a manual therapist to understand because they are
    a. different from the effects of movement forces on the bodily tissues and understanding these effects can inform clinical decisions.
    b. the same effects of static positioning on the bodily tissues and understanding these effects is relevant to the position in which to place a client.
    c. the same as the effects of movement forces on the bodily tissues and understanding these effects can inform clinical decisions.
    d. different from the effects of movement forces on the bodily tissues and understanding these effects has no relevance on clinical decisions.

Notes

1. Mense, S., Simons, D., & Russell, J. (2001). *Muscle Pain: Understanding Its Nature, Diagnosis, and Treatment.* Baltimore: Lippincott, Williams & Wilkins.
2. Page, P., Frank, C., & Lardner, R. (2010). *Assessment and Treatment of Muscle Imbalance: The Janda Approach.* Champaign, IL: Human Kinetics.
3. Ibid.
4. Cohen, B. (1993). *Sensing, Feeling, and Action: The Experiential Anatomy of Body-Mind Centering,* A compilation of articles from *Contact Quarterly* Nothampton, MA: Contant Editions.
5. Rolf, I. (1977). *Rolfing: The Structural Integration of Human Structures.* New York: Harper & Row.
6. Hanna, T. (1979). *The Body of Life.* New York: Knopf; Hanna, T. (1979). *Somatics: Rediscovering the Mind's Control of Movement, Flexibility, and Health.* Reading, MA: Addison-Wesley.
7. Jacobson, E. (1967). *The Biology of Emotions: New Understanding Derived from Biological Multidisciplinary Investigation: First Electrophysiological Measurements.* Springfield, IL: Charles C. Thomas.

PEARSON
myhealthprofessionskit™

Use this address to access the Companion Website created for this textbook. Simply select "Massage Therapy" from the choice of disciplines. Find this book and log in using your username and password to access interactive activities, videos, and much more.

CHAPTER

2 The Skeletal System

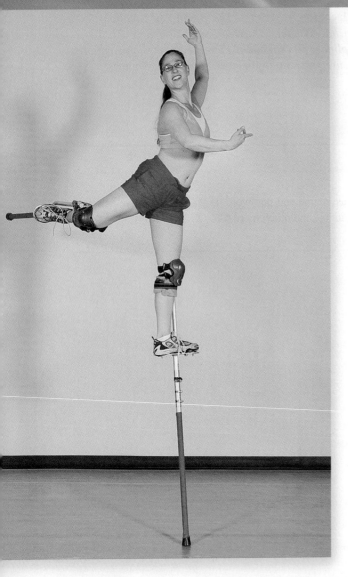

CHAPTER OUTLINE

Chapter Objectives

Key Terms

2.1 Elements of Connective Tissue

2.2 Tissues Making Up the Skeletal System

2.3 Joint Classifications

2.4 Skeletal Alignment and Gravity

Conclusion

Summary Points to Remember

Review Questions

Colorful clowns and performers on stilts are an enduring entertainment at circuses, street shows, and parades. One daring acrobat even crossed a high wire on stilts with someone balanced on his shoulders. Although it may look easy, stilt walking challenges a surety of balance. To learn stilt walking, a novice finds her footing while practicing small steps holding onto a wall or rope. From there, she learns to pivot and turn on one leg.

Stilts also have down-to-earth functions. Fruit pickers, tree pruners, and drywallers sometimes work at heights from stilts. Even some sheepherders use stilts to drive their flocks across swampy terrain. Extreme sports enthusiasts harness the energy of springs

on jumping stilts. These curved-metal springs allow daredevils to bounce along in 9-foot strides, spring over large vehicles in a single bound, and power-jog at 20 miles per hour.

The skeletal system provides a stilt-like internal scaffolding for structural support in the body. Bones have been compared to struts and spacers on a vertical scaffold for soft tissues. Although hard and mineralized, living bone also has a degree of flex and give that allows it to absorb compressive forces and transfer forces along a kinetic chain. By directing these forces along well-aligned pathways, we can harness the kinetic energy in bones to get an energizing spring in every step.

CHAPTER OBJECTIVES

1. List the structures and functions of the skeletal system.

2. List the three elements found in connective tissues and the types of connective tissues.

3. Describe how manual therapy can affect the tissue properties of thixotropy and viscosity.

4. Define and contrast the properties elasticity and plasticity.

5. Describe and contrast the two types of bone tissue.

6. Define and describe the process of bone remodeling.

7. List the five types of bone and provide an example of each type.

8. Name and describe two properties of bone and describe how bone fractures.

9. List and describe 13 types of bony landmarks.

10. Describe two types of cartilage and name three connective tissues in the skeletal system.

11. Describe a bursa and its function.

12. Name and describe the three classifications of joints in the body.

13. Describe a synovial joint and list six types of synovial joints with examples of each.

14. Name and contrast the degrees of movement in axial joints with nonaxial joints.

15. Define the line of gravity and the center of gravity.

16. Define joint neutral and describe its relationship to optimal posture.

17. Name and describe five types of mechanical stress.

 KEY TERMS

Appendicular skeleton	Joint approximation	Remodeling
Axial skeleton	Joint neutral	Shear
Bony landmarks	Line of force	Synovial joint
Center of gravity (COG)	Line of gravity (LOG)	Synovial sheath
Collagen	Mechanical stresses	Tension
Degree of motion	Optimal posture	Thixotropic
Elasticity	Piezoelectric effect	Torque
Fracture	Plasticity	Viscosity

The **skeletal system** provides a bony framework for the body much like the girders and beams provide a steel framework for a skyscraper, although the comparison ends there. The human skeleton is an architectural masterpiece of living bone and working joints against which all man-made structures pale in comparison. Being able to visualize the design features of this bony support system helps us to conceptualize how to align the body through massage and bodywork.

The skeletal system is made up of bones, joints, and other associated tissues. A human body possesses, on average, about 206 bones, although occasionally people have extra bones in the spine, rib cage, hands, or feet. The skeleton has axial and appendicular divisions (Figure 2.1 ■). The **axial skeleton**—which includes 80 bones in the head, vertebral column, thorax and sternum, and sacrum and coccyx—makes up the central axis of the trunk and head. The **appendicular skeleton**—which includes 126 bones in the lower limbs and pelvic bones and the upper limbs and shoulder girdle—make up the "appendages" attached to the trunk.

Bones are durable yet adaptable. The unique composition of bones lends them a resilience and sturdiness comparable to steel, an elasticity that will flex under high compressive loads, and an ability to continually remodel and reshape in response to functional demands.

The five main functions of the skeletal system are support, protection, storage, blood production, and movement. This study focuses on the two functions most related to a study of kinesiology, the support and movement roles served by the bones and joints.

In this chapter, we explore the composition and properties of tissues in the skeletal system, look at how these

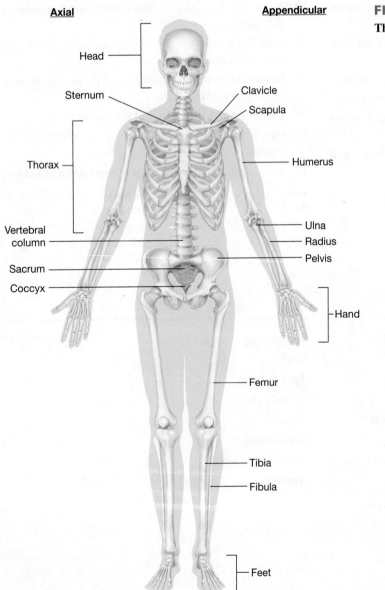

Axial   **Appendicular**

Head
Sternum
Clavicle
Scapula
Thorax
Humerus
Vertebral column
Ulna
Radius
Pelvis
Sacrum
Coccyx
Hand
Femur
Tibia
Fibula
Feet

FIGURE 2.1

The human skeleton

tissues respond to the mechanical stresses of movement and manual therapies, and study the shapes and types of joints in the body. Because connective tissues are the major building block of the skeletal system, this chapter begins with an examination of connective tissues' elements and properties.

2.1 ELEMENTS OF CONNECTIVE TISSUE

Tissue describes a group of similar cells and extracellular substances that form a definite body structure to carry out a specific function. Connective tissue is the most abundant tissue in the body; it permeates every body system. There are four types of **connective tissue:**

1. Blood
2. Bone
3. Cartilage
4. Connective tissue proper

It may seem confusing that blood and bone are classified in the same tissue category. This is the case because, although they may differ in composition, they share the three elements found in all connective tissues—*cells, fluid,* and *fibers.* Blood is primarily made up of fluid and cells, whereas cartilage and bone are made up of mostly fibers and cells.

Connective tissue proper provides a binding and supportive matrix for every bodily structure. There are two types of connective tissue proper:

- **Loose connective tissue** such as superficial fascia and adipose
- **Dense connective tissue** such as deep fascia and ligaments

By understanding the composition of connective tissues in the skeletal system, a practitioner can recognize how each tissue will respond to different massage and bodywork techniques. While reading this section, you are encouraged to visualize the connective tissues on a cellular level in order to imagine how various types of hands-on work can affect each one.

2.1.1 Connective Tissue Building Blocks: Cells, Fibers, and Fluids

Every connective tissue has various types and combinations of the same three elements: cells, fibers, and fluids (see Table 2.1 ■). A cell is the most basic functional unit in a living body. The kinds of cells found in each connective tissue vary according to the type of tissue. *Erythrocytes* (red blood cells) and *leukocytes* (white blood cells) float in the plasma of blood, *osteocytes* (bone cells) reside between the fibers and minerals of bone, and *chondrocytes* (cartilage cells) make up cartilage.

Connective tissue cells and fibers reside within a fluid called **ground substance**—a viscous gel that consists of water, amino sugar molecules, and solutes. The amino sugars in ground substance are highly charged molecules that attract and hold water molecules. The capacity of charged molecules to draw water is called **hydrophilic,** which means "water-loving." The hydrophilic nature of ground substance keeps connective tissue hydrated and turgid. A turgid tissue such as joint cartilage functions like a semiliquid shock absorber to resist compression, which increases joint durability.

There are three basic types of connective tissue fibers: *collagen, elastin,* and *reticular* fibers. **Collagen** is the most abundant protein in mammals and the most prolific fiber in the skeletal system. A single collagen fiber is made up of three collagen molecules, or *fibrils,* spiraled around each other like strands in a rope. Single fibers group in bundles called *fascicles.* Mature collagen fibers exhibit the tensile strength of steel; it takes a force a thousand times its own weight to stretch a

TABLE 2.1 Composition and Features of Connective Tissues

Type of CT	Cells	Ground Substance	Fibers	Types/Features
Blood	White blood cells, red blood cells	Extensive fluid transport system	Minimal	The only liquid tissue
Bone	Osteocytes, osteoblasts, osteophytes	Minimal	Extensive network of collagen	Spongy and compact, calcium and minerals harden bone
Cartilage	Chondrocytes, chondroblasts	Minimal but more than bone	Collagen, elastin	Hyaline, fibrocartilage
Loose connective tissue	Fibroblasts (which produce fibers), macrophages, adipocytes	Extensive fluid bed serves as reservoir for nutrients	Collagen, reticular and elastin	Aerolar (superficial fascia), adipose, reticular (in lymph nodes, spleen, bone marrow)
Dense connective tissue	Fibroblasts	Minimal	Mostly collagen	Regular (ligaments and tendons), irregular (fascia, aponeurosis)

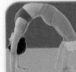

BRIDGE TO PRACTICE
Working with Stiff, Unyielding Tissues

Resistance tends to meet resistance and flow meets flow. If you find yourself pushing against the stiffness of the client's body, you may become stiff yourself. When your client's tissues feels stiff and unyielding, look for those places in your client's body and your own body where the tissues feel pliable and fluid. Focus your attention on these fluid aspects of your client's body to counterbalance a focus on releasing its rigidity.

collagen fiber. Connective tissues continually undergo regenerative processes; old fibers break down and new fibers are produced.

Both single fibers and collagen fascicles are connected by a series of horizontal cross-links (Figure 2.2 ■). The closer together the fascicles are, the tighter the latching of the cross-links and the less sliding capacity between fascicles. In contrast, the more hydrated the connective tissue, the farther apart the fascicles and the more pliable the cross-links.

Elastin fibers are found in vast quantities in tissues that need to stretch, such as the skin, the urinary bladder, and the blood vessels. They can stretch up to one and a half times their resting length. Depending on genetic makeup, a minimal amount of elastin fibers can be found in the ligaments and joint capsules of some people, making their joints more flexible.

Reticular fibers are thin, delicate fibers that provide a loose supportive framework in organs such as the liver and the spleen, although they are not found in the skeletal system. A loose, fluffy webbing of collagen and reticular fibers that resembles cotton candy attaches the skin to superficial fascia.

2.1.2 Connective Tissue Properties

Because of their composition, connective tissues possess certain properties that respond to the mechanical forces of movement and bodywork. Properties vary according to the cell–fluid–fiber ratios in each connective tissue. We briefly discuss the properties affecting the skeletal system. Because dense connective tissue, particularly fascia, weaves through every body system, we revisit these properties in subsequent chapters when discussing joint motion, stretching, and deep tissue bodywork applications.

2.1.2.1 THIXOTROPY AND VISCOSITY

Ground substance is a thick viscous fluid that, like gelatin, is **thixotropic.** This means that it responds to variances in temperature by changing from a gel to a sol (liquid) and back again. When warmed, ground substance becomes thin and watery; when chilled, it becomes viscous and thick. This is why exercise loosens the muscles and joints. The heat generated by muscular contractions during vigorous workouts warms the body. Massage practitioners take advantage of the thixotropic property of connective tissue fluids by warming a client's body with hot packs or general massage at the beginning of a session.

Ground substance also exhibits the property of **viscosity**—the time-dependent property of a thick fluid substance to resist and dampen pressure. An object sinks through a viscous fluid more or less slowly, depending on the thickness of the fluid. Viscous fluids in the body resist compression and reduce joint friction in a manner similar to how fluids function in hydraulic brakes. Imagine filling a syringe with a viscous fluid. The faster the plunger is pushed, the higher the fluid pressure. The thicker the fluid, the greater the resistance and the longer it takes to plunge through the fluid. This will be important for you to remember when practicing deep tissue techniques; pressure needs to be applied slowly and gradually to overcome fluid resistance in dense connective tissues.

2.1.2.2 ELASTICITY AND PLASTICITY

Elasticity is the property of tissue to recoil or rebound after being deformed by a mechanical force. Like a rubber band, elastic tissue rebounds to its original shape after undergoing deformation. Although collagen itself is not elastic, it is crimped in wave-like folds that straighten when compressed or stretched. The crimping arrangement of collagen fibers contributes to the elasticity of dense connective

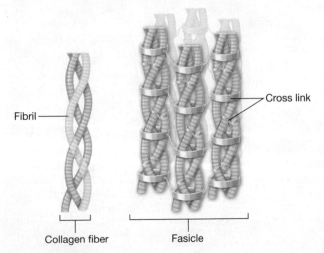

Fibril

Cross link

Collagen fiber   Fasicle

FIGURE 2.2
Collagen fibers

EXPLORING TECHNIQUE
Tactile Explorations of Viscosity with Corn Starch

This corn-starch exploration is used widely in massage and bodywork schools to provide students with a tactile experience of the viscous properties of connective tissues. To practice it on your own, you will need a box of corn starch, a pan, some water, a large, thick balloon, and a funnel.

1. Fill a bowl or pan with a box of corn starch. Then slowly add water and mix to a thick, gooey consistency.
2. Sink your hands into the mix and massage this substance, exploring its properties of viscosity (Figure 2.3a ■). Contrast pushing versus sinking, noticing how long it takes for this

substance to yield to pressure (Figure 2.3b ■). *When you sink slowly, does the substance yield? When you sink your hands into it too fast, do you notice how it breaks up?*
3. Use the funnel to pour some of the corn-starch mixture into a balloon, filling the balloon as full as you can get it. Squeeze the air out of the balloon and tie the end in a knot to seal it. Explore squeezing and kneading the balloon, which mimics the elastic skin of the body.
4. To clean up afterward, add water to the cornstarch until it becomes watery. Then wash it down a sink or flush it down a toilet.

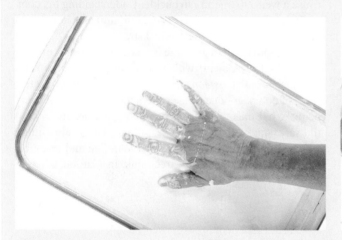

FIGURE 2.3a

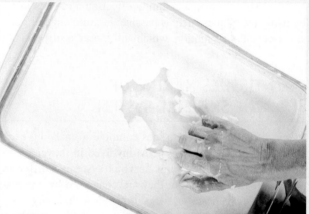

FIGURE 2.3b

tissues (Figure 2.4 ■). Every type of dense connective tissue demonstrates some measure of elasticity.

Tissues can only stretch so far before they reach their **elastic limit.** At this limit, the tissues can no longer return to their original shapes and undergo plastic changes. This describes the property of **plasticity**—an irreversible deformation of a tissue that occurs in response to forces that exceed its elastic limit. An elastic waist band illustrates these two properties. When it is new, its elasticity gives your pants a snug fit. But as it wears out, its elastic fibers undergo plastic changes, causing your pants to sag and eventually slide right off.

2.1.2.3 THE PIEZOELECTRIC EFFECT

Dense connective tissues generate electrical potentials in response to mechanical stresses. This phenomenon is called the **piezoelectric effect.** Like a living crystal, molecules in bones and dense connective tissues move according to changes in electrical gradients. Compression or tension from movement, stretching, and even bodywork

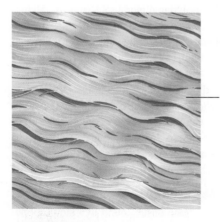

Dense regular connective tissue (found in ligaments)

FIGURE 2.4
Crimping in collagen fibers contributes to their elasticity.

BRIDGE TO PRACTICE
Effects of Friction and Deep Pressure on Dense Connective Tissue

Cross-fiber friction and deep tissue massage break immature collagen bonds and create space between connective tissue fibers in muscles. This allows ground substance to flush back into the interfiber and intercellular spaces, hydrating the tissues. It also creates a piezoelectric effect that triggers absorption of more fluid into the ground substance. After you apply these techniques to your client's tissue, take a short pause to allow time for the fluids to hydrate the tissues.

stimulates the piezoelectric effect, changing the electrical charge of hydrophilic (water-loving) molecules, which causes connective tissues to absorb moisture. The dynamic loading of joint surfaces from cyclic motion also causes joint cartilage to absorb water, keeping movable joints healthy. You can create a similar effect on a client's joints by using techniques such as passive, intermittent compression or oscillating motion, which will loosen a stiff joint.

2.2 TISSUES MAKING UP THE SKELETAL SYSTEM

Many different types of tissues combine to make up each body system. The body systems involved in movement—the skeletal, muscular, and nervous systems—differ in structure and function, but they are connected by a pervasive connective tissue network that binds them together. We now look at the tissues of the skeletal system, which include bone, cartilage, and dense connective tissues such deep fascias, ligaments, and joint capsules.

2.2.1 Bone

Bone is the densest, strongest tissue in the body. Like all connective tissues, it is made of living cells (in the case of bone, osteocytes), ground substance, and fibers. All bone is a combination of about one-third organic matter—the living cells that regenerate it and make it somewhat flexible—and two-thirds inorganic matter—the nonliving mineral salts (mostly calcium and phosphate crystals) embedded in a matrix of collagen fiber. Bone has a minimal amount of ground substance, yet its high fiber and mineral content makes it extremely rigid and durable.

Bones function as stiff lever arms for motion. The **stiffness** of a tissue is measured by how much load it takes to elongate that tissue within an elastic range. With a tensile strength comparable to steel, bone can withstand high compression loads with minimal elastic response. In fact, compression strengthens bones. Weight-bearing exercise is essential to maintaining skeletal system health because it stimulates bone growth.

2.2.1.1 COMPACT AND SPONGY BONE

There are two kinds of bone tissue found in a single bone: *compact* and *spongy* bone. The elements making up each type of bone differ in arrangement, which gives each one

distinct architectural features that equip bones to bear maximal weight with minimal structures. For example, the densest bone tissue, compact bone, is the thickest in the middle of the shaft of a long bone where bending forces would cause a weaker structure to buckle. Understanding the composition of each type of bone tissue illuminates how bones hold up so well under mechanical stress.

Compact (cortical) bone is made up of groups of bone cells called *osteocytes,* which are arranged in dense ring-like shapes called *osteons* (Figure 2.5 ■). A thin, protective layer of compact bone tissue covers the outer layer of every bone. What makes compact bone compact are its osteons that are stacked in tall dense pillars. These are tightly grouped in concentric rings called *lamellae* and resemble the growth rings of a mature tree trunk. In addition, adjacent

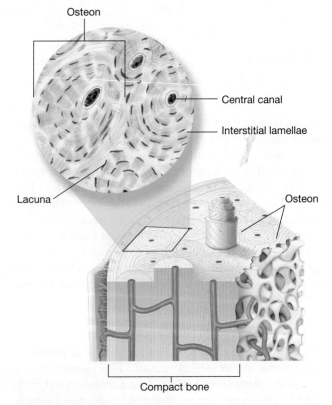

FIGURE 2.5
Osteons in compact bone

lamellae possess oblique fibers that run along opposite diagonals, which strengthen compact bone.

Spongy (cancellous) bone lies under compact bone. It is composed of a loosely arranged lattice of osteocytes that resemble a sponge—hence, the name. At first glance, the osteocytes appear to be randomly arranged in a disorganized fashion, yet the cells actually align along the lines of tension called *trabeculae* ("small beams"). The trabeculae are organized in rows of thin plates and beams that resemble flying buttresses in a Gothic cathedral. The trabeculae function as a system of bony struts that allow for optimal load distribution in multiple directions (Figure 2.6 ■).

Examine an old deer or elk bone and the difference between compact and spongy bone becomes obvious (Figure 2.7 ■). On the outside, the compact bone appears as a white, dense layer with steely shine similar to glass; on the inside, the spongy bone resembles a honeycomb of sharp glass-like projections that make the bone look like a petrified sea sponge. The unique composition of each type of bone tissue outfits it to best absorb and transfer mechanical stresses in a manner specific to that layer. The osteon pillars in compact bone function like springs in a mattress to resist compressive stress: the alternating diagonal fibers of the lamellae resist torsion (twisting) in both directions. The trabeculae in spongy bone distribute mechanical stress throughout the inside of the bone along multiple tracts.

2.2.1.2 TYPES OF BONE

Bones come in many different shapes and sizes, with contours that resemble the organic forms found in rock formations. Although individual bones might appear formless, each shape reflects a type of bone that evolved to perform a specific function. For example, the somewhat flat yet slightly

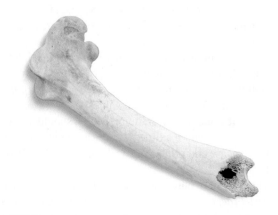

FIGURE 2.7

Notice the difference between the **compact bone** on the outside and the **spongy bone** on the inside of this old deer bone.

dished form of cranium bones and ribs cradle and protect vulnerable organs such as the brain and lungs. In contrast, the slightly bowed shafts of the long strong bones in the lower limbs bear weight while allowing for minimal flex.

Although the shapes and sizes of individual bones vary, each bone is identified as one of five types (Figure 2.8 ■):

1. The **long bones** have a tubular *shaft* and round convex or concave *condyles* on each end. Long bones are

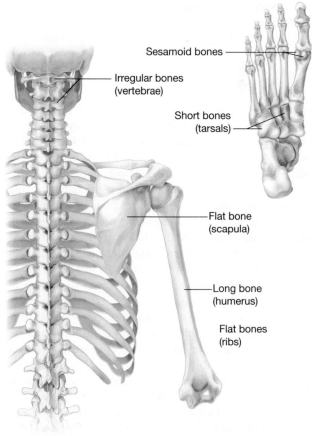

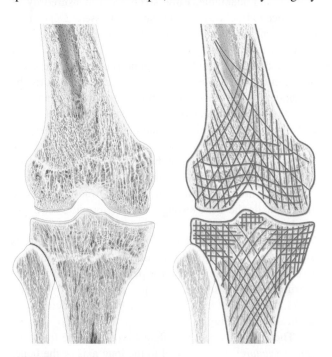

FIGURE 2.6

The **trabeculae** in spongy bone organizes along lines of tension.

FIGURE 2.8

Types of bones

found in the legs and arms, the hands and feet, and the fingers and toes. *Clavicles* (collar bones) are also considered long bones.

2. The **short bones** tend to be more block-shaped. Short bones fit tightly together in areas that need maximal stability with minimal mobility, such as the *carpals* and *tarsals* of the wrists and ankles.

3. The **flat bones** of the cranium, pelvis, shoulder blades, and sternum curve a little to shape around the organs they encase and protect. The *ribs* are also classified as flat bones.

4. The **irregular bones** of the axial skeleton include the *vertebrae, coccyx,* and *sacrum.* Their irregular shapes allow for diverse functions. For example, the processes in each vertebra serve as attachments for tendons and ligaments: the vertebral foramen houses the spinal cord, and smaller foramens allow the passage of peripheral nerves from the spinal cord into the trunk. Some cranial bones at the base of the skull and several facial bones, such as the jaw, are also classified as irregular bones.

5. The **sesamoid bones** resemble the shape of sesame seeds. These small, round bones lie under tendons near joints. They are strategically placed in vulnerable, high-use areas to protect adjacent tissues from friction during motion. For example, the *patella* on the front of the knee deflects the pull of the quadriceps muscle away from the joint. Without it, the large and powerful quadriceps tendon would wear a groove in the bone. Also, two small sesamoid bones under the ball of the foot protect the tendons acting on the big toe from undue compression.

2.2.1.3 BONE REMODELING

Although it is easy to view bones as solid tissue, bone is extremely dynamic because it continually undergoes **remodeling**—a regenerative process that involves the reabsorption of old tissue and the production of new tissue. Mechanical stress stimulates the remodeling, causing *osteoclasts* (specialized bone cells) to break down and absorb old and damaged bone, while *osteoblasts* produce and lay down new bone (Figure 2.9 ■). Remodeling occurs in response to functional demands. According to Wolff's law, bone thickens in areas that function under high stress and breaks down and reabsorbs in areas that function under low stress.

A newborn's bones remodel at 10 times the rate of an adult's bones. Remodeling accelerates in response to injury or when increased loads are regularly placed upon the skeletal structure, as in weightlifting. Bony projections increase in size where muscles and tendons consistently pull on them. Bones also thicken in areas that function under greater stress and are more vulnerable to fractures, such as the center of long bones in the lower limb. Conversely, bones tend to demineralize and weaken in bedridden or sedentary people due to the lack of stress.

Bones need to work under load (weight or force) to be healthy. Gravity is a constant force on the bones. Consider

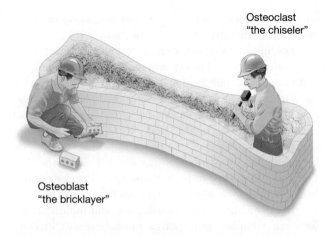

FIGURE 2.9

Bone remodeling: Osteoclasts break down old bone while oesteoblasts build new bone.

what would happen if gravity decreased by half; the body would probably evolve to a taller and thinner skeleton. On the other hand, if gravity doubled, the body would probably evolve a shorter and thicker skeleton. In the absence of gravity, the bones demineralize and weaken. Astronauts suffer this condition after extended stays in outer space. These points underscore the circular relationship between gravity and bone strength. The human body needed gravity's pull to evolve and strengthen its skeletal system; conversely, the human body needs a skeletal system to stand upright and move in the Earth's gravitational field.

2.2.1.4 BONE STRENGTH AND ELASTICITY

Bones exhibit several properties that make them highly durable and adaptable. **Bone strength** is measured by its resistance to fracture from mechanical stresses.[1] Deposits of calcium and other minerals harden and strengthen the bony matrix. **Bone elasticity** defines its ability to deform under stress and then reform to its original shape after the stress has been removed. The elasticity of a bone is measured by the amount of deformation it can withstand under load.

Of all the connective tissues, bone has the strength and elasticity to make it rigid and highly resistant to deformation. Bone can withstand far more compressive force than soft tissue, and it heals better than soft tissue. Even though bone is incredibly strong, it is still susceptible to **fractures** (breaks) from trauma. But a fracture in bone always heals the bone stronger than its previous strength level, whereas a ligamentous tear always heals weaker. When a person suffers a complete fracture, the break is usually cast to straighten the bone so that it remodels in a functional position. When a person breaks a weight-bearing bone, the sooner the injured party stands up and walks, the quicker the stimulus for bone remodeling and the faster the healing.

There are a number of different types of bone fractures. *Linear fractures* occur parallel to the long axis of the bone, while *transverse fractures* occur perpendicular to the long axis. *Spiral fractures* twist the bone and *oblique fractures* occur diagonally to the long axis of a bone. Other common classifications of bone fractures are listed below.

- *Partial fracture:* The break is incomplete.
- *Complete fracture:* The break is completely through the bone.
- *Nondisplaced fracture:* The bones retain a normal alignment.
- *Displaced fracture*: The bones shift out of a normal alignment.
- *Stress fracture:* A microscopic fracture, often from compression stresses.
- *Comminuted fracture*: The bone splits into multiple pieces.
- *Compacted fracture*: The bone fragments are driven into each other.
- *Greenstick fracture*: A partial fracture, usually in a child's bone, that breaks one side of the bone while bending the other side.
- *Compound (open) fracture*: A break that protrudes through the skin.
- *Pott's fracture*: A fracture in the distal end of the fibula.
- *Colles' fracture*: A fracture in the distal end of the radius.

Bone absorption can exceed bone formation, decreasing bone density and strength. This leads to a condition called **osteoporosis,** which causes bones to become brittle and susceptible to fracture. Osteoporosis is common in post-menopausal women due to decreased estrogen levels. Since bone remodeling slows down with aging, seniors, especially women, are advised to practice weight-bearing exercise and to take calcium and vitamin D supplements. Manual therapists need to be careful working on clients with osteoporosis because deep pressure to areas like the rib cage could crack their ribs.

2.2.1.5 BONY LANDMARKS

All bones exhibit a set of markings that reflect their basic functions. For example, *tubercles* and *ridges* form under the attachments of muscles and tendons and *foramens* and *grooves* develop as passageways for blood vessels and nerves.

The **bony landmarks,** also called bone markings, serve as signposts to guide a massage and bodywork student through the vast tissue landscapes during tactile exercises. There are different categories and types of bony landmarks (Figure 2.10 ■). The names of bony landmarks reflect their shapes and functions. Although it is usually unnecessary to learn the names of all the bone markings, recognizing them and being able to locate them during palpation will make the names easier to remember because many of the names are descriptive of their shapes.

There are a number of bony landmarks that provide attachments for muscles, tendons, and ligaments. There are also a number of bony landmarks found in and around joints. To understand specific joint structures and functions, you will want to become familiar with the following bony landmarks:

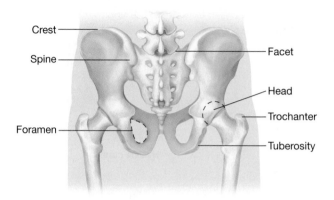

FIGURE 2.10

How many **bony landmarks** in this figure can you identify from the list below?

- *Condyle:* Round knuckle-like knob found on the end of long bone
- *Facet:* Shallow, almost flat articular surface
- *Head:* Round projection attached to a neck of long bone
- *Crest:* Narrow, sharp ridge
- *Epicondyle:* Prominent raised knob above condyle
- *Fossa:* Shallow bowl-like depression
- *Foramen:* Hole or opening
- *Groove:* Linear depression
- *Line:* Less prominent ridge
- *Process:* Prominent knob
- *Ridge:* Raised edge or lip
- *Spine:* Sharp projection
- *Tubercle:* Rough, rounded projection
- *Tuberosity:* Small process
- *Trochanter:* Large, rough process

We revisit these bony landmarks in later chapters by locating them during specific palpation exercises.

2.2.2 Cartilage

Cartilage in the skeletal system can be compared to rubber gaskets and shocks in cars. This highly resilient connective tissue lines the articular surfaces of movable joints to protect them from excessive wear. Cartilage disks are also found inside joints.

There are three types of cartilage in the body: hyaline cartilage, fibrocartilage, and elastic cartilage (Figure 2.11 ■). The most flexible of the three, elastic cartilage, is found in the few areas of the body that need to bend, such as the outer ear. Only hyaline cartilage and fibrocartilage are found in the skeletal system.

Hyaline cartilage is also called *articular cartilage* because it covers the two articulating surfaces of bones in freely movable joints. You can observe hyaline in the glassy blue-white tissue covering the end of a chicken leg. The moderate water content in hyaline cartilage renders it a perfect load-bearing surface for resisting joint compression and reducing friction. Both the *larynx* in the neck and the *costal arch* along the front of the rib cage are examples of hyaline cartilage.

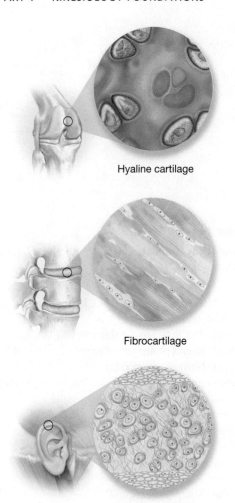

FIGURE 2.11
Three types of cartilage

Fibrocartilage makes up shock-absorbing disks found in joints that work under high compressive loads, such as the *menisci* of the knees and the *intervertebral disks* in the spine. Fibrocartilage resembles hyaline cartilage in structure only with far less water and many more fibers. The matrix of a fibrocartilage disk is composed of thick interwoven layers of collagen fibers arranged in concentric rings.

Most tissues receive cellular nourishment from their blood supply. All types of cartilage lack a blood and nerve supply; as a result, cartilage is unable to repair itself when damaged. Joint cartilage receives its nutrients from a viscous lubricant called **synovial fluid,** which fills the space within freely movable joints.

The duration and magnitude of forces applied to cartilage during joint motion affect the rate that fluid flows both into and out of this resilient tissue. Intermittent joint loading during movement creates a milking action that circulates synovial fluid around cartilage, underscoring the vital importance of motion and exercise to joint health.

Compressive loading also squeezes fluid out of cartilage during motion: it gradually seeps back once the load is removed.[2,3] This is why a person is taller in the morning than at night, the disks in the spine imbibe (absorb water) and hydrate during sleep. Bodywork techniques that stimulate synovial fluid circulation include general joint mobilization and articulation techniques, such as passive range of motion, rhythmic rocking, and joint approximation.

2.2.3 Dense Connective Tissues

Dense connective tissues make up the connecting and stabilizing fabric of the skeletal system, such as fascias, ligaments, tendons, and joint capsules (Figure 2.12 ■). There are three types of dense connective tissue: regular, irregular, and elastic. Only regular and irregular dense connective tissues are found in the skeletal system.

Regular dense connective tissue has collagen fibers oriented in parallel bundles that can withstand high tension and transfer muscular pulls along the direction of their fibers. It is found in tendons and ligaments.

Irregular dense connective tissue has collagen fibers arranged in a crosshatched, multilayered sheet that is strong yet elastic in multiple directions. It is the primary component of fascias and joint capsules.

2.2.3.1 FASCIA AND PERIOSTEUM

Fascia is a strong pervasive type of dense irregular connective tissue that wraps and binds all tissues. Many interconnected layers of fascia envelop and connect every single muscle, bone, nerve, and organ in the body. To observe fascia, look for that milky, filmy tissue that covers the muscles on chicken or beef. Fascia can be compared to plastic wrap. It is durable yet supple and can be thin or thick depending on its location and function. The different fascias are named by their locations: *deep fascia* lies right below superficial fascia

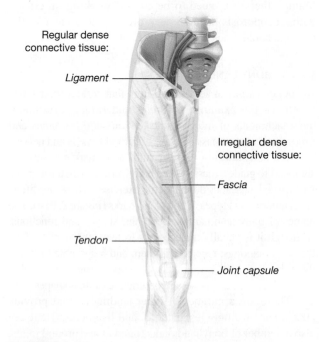

FIGURE 2.12
Fascia

Compact bone

Yellow marrow

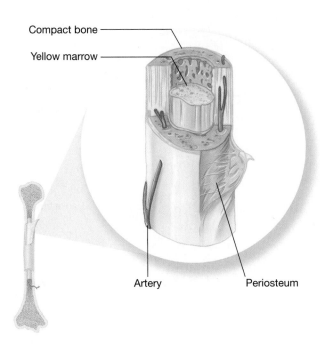

Artery

Periosteum

FIGURE 2.13
Periosteum

and covers muscles, *visceral fascia* wraps visceral organs, and a thick *plantar fascia* protects the soles of the feet.

Fascia covering bones, called **periosteum,** provides attachments for muscles and tendons (Figure 2.13 ■). Periosteum is rich in sensory nerves and can be sensitive to manual manipulation. Previous bone fractures may be tender to touch, although tissue mobilization over old breaks can reduce pain and tenderness in the periosteum. Like all fascias, periosteum exhibits elasticity. It can be stretched by massaging it directly against the bone.

2.2.3.2 LIGAMENTS, TENDONS, AND JOINT CAPSULES

A **ligament** connects and binds bone to bone. These short bands of dense connective tissue provide passive restraints that limit joint motion beyond a normal range.

The arrangement of collagen fibers varies slightly in tendons and ligaments. In a **tendon,** the fibers organize in parallel bundles along the pull of its muscle. In ligaments and joint capsules, the fibers orient in several oblique

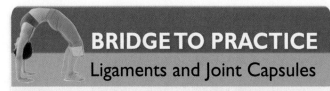

BRIDGE TO PRACTICE
Ligaments and Joint Capsules

Avoid deep work on overstretched ligaments and joint capsules because this could stretch the loose tissue even more, which will exacerbate joint instability.

directions. This allows ligaments to resist stress along different lines of tension created when a joint bends or twists. There are some elastin fibers in ligaments, and these make them more pliable and elastic than tendons.

A **joint capsule** surrounds synovial joints like a collar. It is made up of two layers of dense irregular connective tissue that have a degree of elasticity that permits movement in the joint. The capsule also protects the joint by limiting motion beyond a certain range. The strong outer layer of the capsule provides a passive restraint to motion, contributing to the joint's stability. The inner layer of the capsule is lined with a serous membrane (a membrane that secretes fluid) called a *synovium,* which secretes synovial fluid.

Both ligaments and joint capsules need to demonstrate a certain degree of elasticity in order for a movable joint to bend and twist. If these tissues become stiff due to dehydration or fibrous buildup, cross-fiber friction and deep linear stripping techniques can loosen them and restore joint elasticity. In contrast, too much tension on the ligaments and joint capsules or poor posture can stretch these tissues beyond their elastic limits, creating irreversible plastic changes that lead to joint instability.

2.2.3.3 MISCELLANEOUS JOINT STRUCTURES

Bursae are small fibrous sacs filled with synovial fluid. They are located around freely movable joints (Figure 2.14 ■). Bursae are sandwiched between two structures that slide across each other during joint movement, usually under tendons. A single bursa works like a ball-bearing to reduce

BRIDGE TO PRACTICE
Releasing Fascial Restrictions around Bone

In areas where the bone is close to the skin, the skin and superficial fascia can become glued (stuck) to the periosteum, compressing structures in the intermediary layers and restricting motion in them. This can be problematic in areas like the ankle, where

gluing can restrict the sliding movement of tendons between the skin and bone. You can loosen such restrictions by applying slow, deep massage directly on top of the bone, moving the skin and superficial fascia against it.

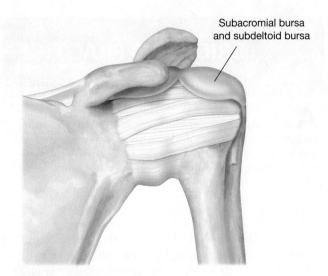

FIGURE 2.14
Bursae

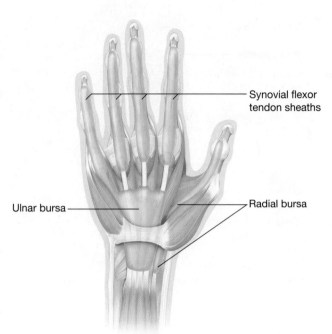

FIGURE 2.15
Synovial sheaths over tendons

friction; it provides a fluid pad for the tendon to slide across as the muscle contracts and pulls on the bone. Bursae can be injured by a blow or from excessive friction, which can lead to inflammation and a painful condition called *bursitis*.

Synovial sheaths are like elongated double-layered tubes of bursa that wrap around tendons (Figure 2.15 ■). They resemble buns around hot dogs, providing a protective liquid casing that reduces wear and friction on the sliding tendons. Inflammation to synovial sheaths of the tendons, which usually occurs due to excessive friction or a direct blow to the sheath, is called *tenosynovitis*. This condition often occurs with inflammation of a tendon, which is called *tendonitis*.

Injured or inflamed bursae tend to be sore even to a light touch. The palpation of an inflamed bursa or synovial sheath could increase a client's pain. If these structures generate pain, avoid palpating them or putting any pressure on them during massage and bodywork. To locate an injured bursa or sheath, have the client show you where it is.

2.3 JOINT CLASSIFICATIONS

One bone articulates with an adjacent bone at a **joint,** also called an *articulation*. There are three general classifications of joints; each classification reflects both the structure and function of that type of joint (see Table 2.2 ■). Just like the joints in a piece of furniture, some lack motion, others allow a small degree of motion, and others are freely movable.

Most of the joints that lack motion or permit some motion are found in the axial skeleton, where the joints serve weight-bearing and stabilization functions. In contrast, most of the *freely movable* joints are found in the four limbs, which evolved for diverse movement functions, the lower limbs for support and locomotion and the upper limbs for mobility and complex hand articulations.

As a massage practitioner, you can learn to visualize the different types of joints and their range of motion in order to recognize normal motion patterns and move clients within a normal range. Although rarely used in practice, the names of joint classifications—*synarthrosis, amphiarthrosis,* and *diarthrosis*—could show up on state and national exams.

2.3.1 Fibrous Joints

A **synarthrosis** is a **fibrous joint** in which two bones are firmly bound together by a strong yet thin layer of dense connective tissue (Figure 2.16 ■). The fibrous joints are located in areas where bones protect underlying organs, for example, the sutures in the cranium. Fibrous joints allow the transference of force from one bone to the next, although they permit very little movement, if any at all. Fibrous joints are generally described as nonmovable joints.

Two other classifications of fibrous joints include the *gomphosis* peg-in-socket joints of the teeth, and the *syndesmosis* joints of the forearm and the leg. A syndesmosis is made up of a dense interosseous membrane that binds the two long bones, such as the tibiofibular joint, which allows for a slight amount of gliding and rotation (Figure 2.16).

2.3.2 Fibrocartilage Joints

An **amphiarthrosis** is a **fibrocartilage joint** with a fibrocartilage disk sandwiched between two bones connected by dense connective tissues. Also called **cartilaginous joints,** they are found in areas where the bones need to provide support and shock absorption, yet also allow some flexibility, so they are described as semimovable joints. Examples include the intervertebral joints along the front of the spine and the pubic symphysis along the anterior pelvic rim (Figure 2.17 ■).

TABLE 2.2 Joint Classifications

Classification	Joint Structure	Range of Motion	Example
Synarthrosis	Fibrous Suture	None or slight	Sutures in cranium
Gomphosis	Peg and socket	None	Socket of teeth
Syndesmosis	Ligamentous	Slightly movable	Distal tibiofibular joint
Amphiarthrosis	Cartilaginous or fibrocartilage	Semimovable	Pubic symphysis Intervertebral joints
Diarthrosis	Synovial	Freely movable	Hips, shoulders, elbows, knees, fingers, and toes

2.3.3   Synovial Joints

A **diarthrosis** is a **synovial joint.** All synovial joints have a joint cavity, which is space between the articulating bones that is filled with synovial fluid. This space allows a range of free motion; hence, synovial joints are classified as freely movable joints.

Synovial joints are the most abundant type of joints in the body. They are located primarily in areas that need to be able to move freely in the course of daily activities, such as the back of the spine, the limbs, and the jaw.

2.3.3.1   SYNOVIAL JOINT STRUCTURES AND FLUID

Of the three classifications of joints, the synovial joints have the most complex structure and functions. Although there are six types of synovial joints that come in a variety of shapes and sizes, they all share five distinctive features (Figure 2.18 ■):

- A *joint capsule* that forms a sleeve-like cuff connecting two articulating bones
- A *joint cavity* enclosed by the capsule
- *Hyaline cartilage* covering the articulating surfaces of the bones

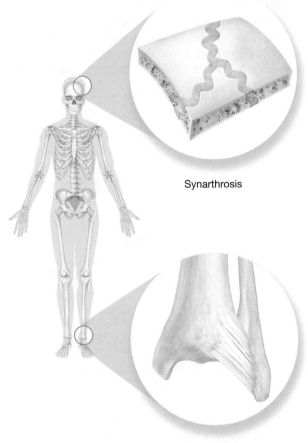

Synarthrosis

Syndesmosis

FIGURE 2.16
Fibrous joints

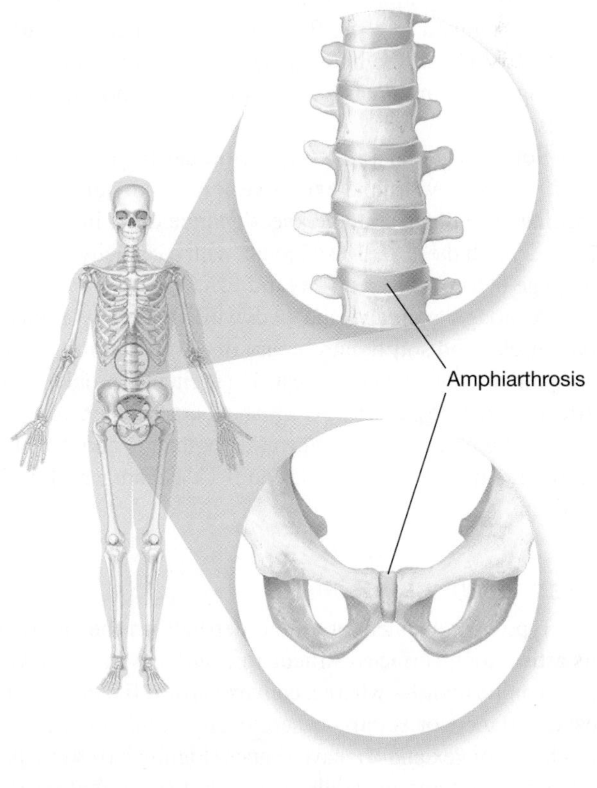

Amphiarthrosis

FIGURE 2.17
Fibrocartilage joints

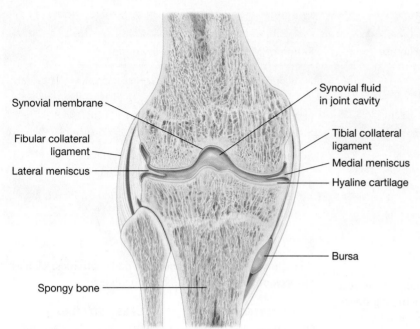

FIGURE 2.18
Synovial joint: diarthrosis

Synovial membrane

Fibular collateral
ligament

Lateral meniscus

Spongy bone

Synovial fluid
in joint cavity

Tibial collateral
ligament

Medial meniscus

Hyaline cartilage

Bursa

- A *synovial membrane* inside the joint capsule that secretes synovial fluid
- *Synovial fluid* filling the cavity within the capsule

Synovial fluid serves several functions. It lubricates the joint, reduces friction between articulating surfaces, and nourishes cartilage within the joint. Synovial fluid also works as a liquid shock absorber, resisting compressive loads much like the fluids in a water bed that cushion the weight of the body. This is particularly important in weight-bearing areas such as the knees and the spinal joints.

Some synovial joints have fibrocartilage disks that equip them to withstand excessive wear from compressive loading. The menisci in the knees and the disks in the jaws provide both these well-used joints with a capacity for high mileage before their treads wear down.

Although massage and bodywork generally focuses on muscles and soft tissues, injury or dysfunction in any of the joint structures could be causing a client's problem and affecting muscle patterns. As a manual practitioner, you will want to be able to make general assessments about which structure, muscles or joints, could be causing a client's problem.

2.3.3.2 JOINT SURFACE SHAPES

The type of movement at a joint depends on the shape of its articulating surfaces. Articulating surfaces in a synovial joint can be **ovoid**—where a convex surface fits into a concave surface—or **sellar**—where each articulating surface has both convex and concave shapes (Figure 2.19 ■). Sellar articulations come in saddle shapes or a shape that resembles two mounds with a valley in between.

The curved articular surfaces in the ovoid joints allow for a rolling and gliding motion of one bone against another. The deeper articular surfaces of the ball-and-socket joints resemble the shape of a globe. They connect in a stable fit and allow for motion in the multiple directions a globe can turn. The saddle-shaped surfaces of many hinge joints allow for a bending motion in two directions, similar to how a horseback rider can rock forward, back, and sideways in a saddle.

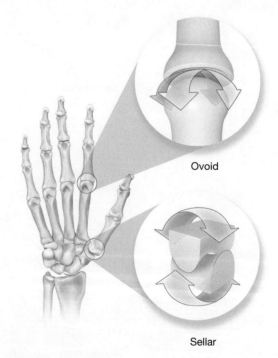

Ovoid

Sellar

FIGURE 2.19
Shapes of joint surfaces

EXPLORING TECHNIQUE
Joint Approximation

Joint approximation is a manual technique in which a joint is first compressed, then decompressed. Loading and unloading the synovial joints with approximation can stimulate fluid circulation in hyaline cartilage, which may explain why clients who suffer from arthritic joint pain get relief with gentle joint approximation. We use it in this exercise to explore the shape of the articulating surfaces and to stimulate fluid circulation in the articular cartilage.

Caution: If practicing this technique on someone with arthritic joints, it is important to be very gentle. Avoid squeezing the joint itself or pulling on the joint, which could exacerbate inflammation and pain.

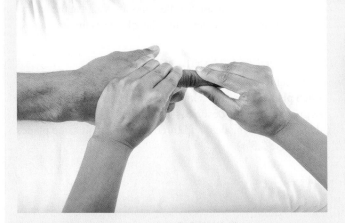

FIGURE 2.20a

1. Begin with the joints in the fingers or toes. Gently but firmly hold the bones on either side of the joint (Figure 2.20a ■). Slowly compress the distal bone into the proximal bone. Once compressed, move the distal bone slightly to rock its articular surface against the proximal articular surface. The movement will be minimal.

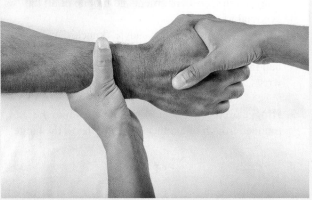

FIGURE 2.20c

3. Approximate the wrist by slowly compressing the hand into the forearm (Figure 2.20c ■). As you compress the wrist, keep in mind that you are compressing many joints: the metacarpals into the carpals, the distal carpals into the proximal carpals, and the proximal carpals into the ulna. Once compressed, gently move the wrist in a small range of motion, sensing how many different ways the many bones in the wrist can be approximated.

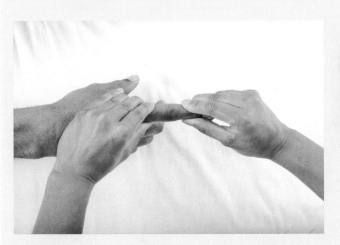

FIGURE 2.20b

2. Next, slowly release the compression (Figure 2.20b ■). You will feel the joint spring back out into your distal hold. Give it very light traction to encourage more space in the joint.

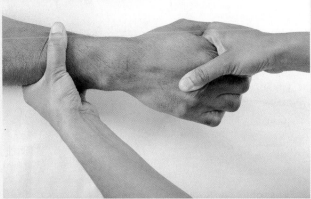

FIGURE 2.20d

4. Slowly release the compression of the wrist and then apply light traction (Figure 2.20d ■). As you apply traction, make sure to keep the palm of the hand in the same plane as the palmar surface of the forearm to avoid twisting and straining the wrist. Practice approximation on other joints. As you practice on several different joints, you will begin to feel differences in the shape and amount of movement in each joint.

It is helpful for practitioners who practice joint motion or compression techniques to be able to visualize the shape of the articulating surfaces to understand how the bones fit together in order to move them within a safe range.

2.3.3.3   SIX TYPES OF SYNOVIAL JOINTS

The synovial joints are classified according to the shape of their articulating surfaces, which determines their range of motion. The six types of synovial joints are (Figure 2.21 ■):

1. **Ball-and-socket:** A ball-like spherical head of one bone sits in the cup-like socket of another bone. Ball-and-socket joints are found in the hips and shoulder. They are the most congruent and mobile of all the synovial joints.
2. **Ellipsoid** or **condyloid** (condyle "knuckle"): Two oval articular surfaces fit together like a rounded half ball in a shallow dish. Ellipsoid joints are found in the wrists, lower ankle, and the knuckles of fingers and toes.
3. **Hinge:** A bony cylinder of one bone fits into the rounded trough of another bone, similar to the hinge on a door. Hinge joints are found in the knees, elbows, fingers, and toes.
4. **Plane** or **gliding:** Made up of the connection between two slightly curved but nearly flat articular surfaces. Because plane joints allow minimal motion, they are located in areas of the body that need stability, such as the spine, wrist, and foot.
5. **Pivot:** The rounded end of one bone projects into a ring-like shape of another bone. Pivot joints are found in the forearm and at the base of the skull.
6. **Saddle:** Two articulating surfaces, each shaped like the riding saddle for a horse, fit together in a reciprocal, interlocking relationship. Saddle joints are found at the base of the thumb and where the clavicle meets the sternum.

2.3.3.4   DEGREES OF MOTION

Synovial joints can move in zero, one, two, or three planes. Each plane of motion is known as a **degree of motion.** One degree of motion describes movement in one plane, two degrees in two planes, and three degrees in all three planes (see Table 2.3 ■).

FIGURE 2.21

Six types of synovial joints

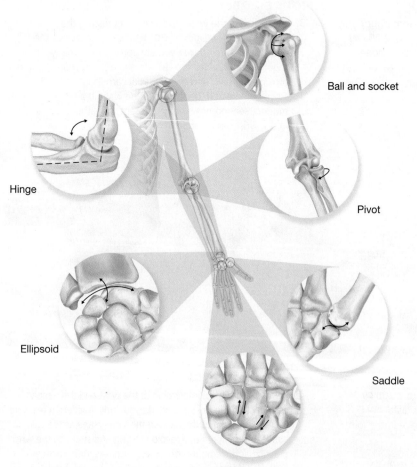

Ball and socket

Pivot

Hinge

Saddle

Ellipsoid

Plane (gliding)

TABLE 2.3 Degrees of Motion in Synovial Joints

Degrees of Motion	Numbers of Axes	Type of Joint	Type of Motion	Example
0	Nonaxial	Plane (Gliding)	Glide	In between the carpals and tarsals
1	Uniaxial	Hinge Pivot	Flex/extend Rotate right or left	Elbow, ankle, fingers, toes
2	Biaxial	Ellipsoid (Condyloid) Saddle	Flex/extend, abduct/adduct Flex/extend, abduct/ adduct Rotate and oppose	Wrist, knuckles of the ankles and toes Base of the thumb
3 or more	Triaxial or multiaxial	Ball-and-socket	Flex/extend, abduct/adduct, rotate	Hips and shoulder

Nonaxial joints do not bend around an axis. They have zero degrees of motion. For example, the bones in the plane joints between the small bones in the wrists and ankles slide across each other in the same plane. Because nonaxial joints are found in areas where the body needs more stability than mobility, their sliding motion is minimal.

Uniaxial joints move in one plane, like a door hinge. Because we can only actively move the hinge joints, such as the elbows and fingers, in one plane around one axis, they are classified as uniaxial joints. They have one degree of motion. Note that it is possible to passively rotate hinge joints, although rotation is considered an accessory motion that lies outside the normal range of motion.

Biaxial joints move in two planes along two axes. Ellipsoid joints, such as the wrists, can move along two axes, either up and down or sideways, making them biaxial joints. Biaxial joints have two degrees of motion.

Triaxial (multiaxial) joints have the greatest range of motion of all the synovial joints; they can move freely in all three planes. For example, the ball-and-socket joints of the hips and shoulder can move in multiple directions through all three planes, so they have three degrees of movement.

To visualize the axis of movement in a joint, imagine a pin along its axis of rotation. For example, most doors open and close around a pin inside the hinge that runs along the vertical axis. In the ankle hinge, which can only flex and extend, the pin runs from side to side along a bilateral axis of motion.

2.4 SKELETAL ALIGNMENT AND GRAVITY

The human body is literally anchored to the Earth by gravity. The gravitational pull is so constant that we barely notice it until a change of dynamics catches our attention. For example, when we lose our grip and drop something heavy or inadvertently step off a short ledge, gravity's downward force can be startling. Weight is relative to gravity; that is, gravity gives mass weight. Without gravity all bodies would become weightless and float. In addition, without gravity the human body would not need an axial bony framework to counter gravity's pull.

The narrower and more vertical a structure, the less energy it takes to hold it up. Hence, the human skeleton is the most efficient design on the planet for standing because it is the most vertically stacked of all animal skeletons. In an upright position, our three bony masses—head, rib cage, and pelvis—stack one on top of another. The head sits on top of the thorax, the thorax over the pelvis, and all three align over the feet.

2.4.1 Center of Gravity, Line of Gravity, and Optimal Posture

The **center of gravity** (COG) of a mass is that point around which all parts are exactly balanced: it is the same as the center of weight. The **line of gravity** (LOG) is the direction of gravity's force; it is, basically, a plumb line. Our uniquely upright skeleton aligns the body along a single vertical axis.

- The *COG in the skull* lies several inches behind the "third eye" on the forehead, slightly above and between the eyebrows.
- The *COG in the chest* lies several inches above the diaphragm, anterior to the 10th thoracic vertebra, midway between front and back below the heart.
- The COG in the *pelvis* lies behind and below the navel, directly in front of the sacrum. It is usually lower on women because of greater width and weight in the pelvic girdle.

In **optimal posture,** the COG of each weight-bearing body part aligns as close to the LOG as possible

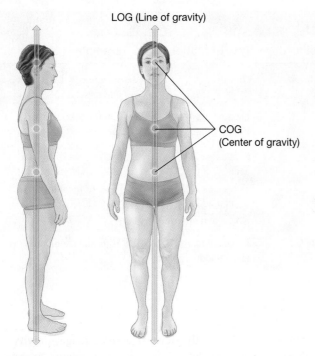

FIGURE 2.22
COGs align along LOG

(Figure 2.22 ■). This allows gravity to flow through the center of a standing body. Optimal posture aligns the skeletal system in a position of *mechanical advantage,* which equalizes gravity's downward pull on the bones with the upward countersupport of the axial skeleton.

When a person demonstrates optimal posture, all the weight-bearing joints of the spine and lower limbs extend. Joints in the extended position are in what is referred to as **joint neutral** because they are straight, being neither bent nor twisted. Joint neutral serves as a reference point for optimal skeletal alignment.

Short of injury or developmental disability, joint alignment is determined by muscle patterns. Clients receive massage and bodywork for help with muscle problems. You can assess skeletal alignment by looking at how the joints align in relationship to neutral. The resting alignment of people's bones and joints reflects their muscle-use patterns. Places where the bones deviate from a joint-neutral alignment in a standing posture indicate areas of muscular imbalance. This type of visual assessment provides information on which direction a massage stroke needs to go to help move the bones back to neutral. For example, if the lower back hyperextends in an excessive lordotic curve, the tissues in the lower back will be chronically shortened and need to be lengthened to bring lumbar vertebrae back to joint neutral.

The farther a joint bends or twists away from neutral, the more mechanical stress there is on that joint in a stationary posture. Specifics about the neutral position of each

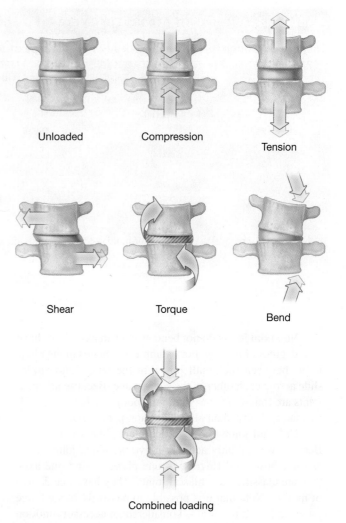

FIGURE 2.23
Mechanical stresses

joint, along with a discussion about how muscle patterns affect joint neutral and how a practitioner can work with these patterns, are presented in later chapters.

2.4.2 Mechanical Stresses

Five **mechanical stresses**—compression, tension, shear, torque, and bend—act on the skeletal system in both posture and movement. Although they affect all tissues, the effect of mechanical stresses on the vertebral bodies and disks of the spine can be especially damaging, which is how they are depicted in these images (Figure 2.23 ■). Mechanical stresses place a load on the tissue. **Unloaded** refers to the hypothetical state of a structure that exists in absence of mechanical stress. However, because the pull of gravity is constant, forces are always acting on body structures, so the tissues are always loaded to some degree.

1. **Compression** occurs when two forces press into the center of a structure from opposite directions.

Weight-bearing joints of the body compress under the body's own weight in an upright posture. They also compress while carrying a load or during push patterns. When standing, the load of our own body weight and gravity compresses the joints in the spine and the lower limbs, and the counterforce comes from structural and postural mechanisms that maintain upright posture.

2. **Tension** occurs when two forces pull on a structure from opposite directions. In an optimal posture, a person keeps the head lifted, which creates an upright tensional pull that counters gravity. Tension occurs in the joints during reaching and stretching motions, both of which take the slack out of the joint capsules and surrounding connective tissues. Traction (distraction) also increases tensile stresses in joint structures.

3. **Shear** occurs when two parallel forces press into different ends of a structure from opposite directions, resulting in a shearing motion. Shear occurs in a very small range during the sliding movement in nonaxial plane joints. Shear also occurs in the spinal joints during activities that displace a body mass horizontally, such as when a person cranes the head forward to look at a computer screen.

4. **Torque** occurs when two forces perpendicular to the axis of the structure turn in opposite directions, resulting in rotation. Torque occurs in the joints during rotational movements, such as turning the head to look back.

5. **Bend** combines tensile and compressive stresses. When a joint bends, the concave side of the bend is under compression while the convex side is under tension. All joints bend during axial movements that close the angle of the joint.

Combined loading occurs when two or more forces act on a structure at the same time. The joints are engineered to withstand mechanical stresses of combined loading within a normal range of motion. For example, the body is always under compressive stress due to the combined forces of gravity and body weight. In a person with optimal posture, compression has a minimal affect on the weight-bearing joints. But in a bent or twisted posture, the combination of compression with bending increases wear on the joints.

A practitioner can minimize the effects of stress on the joints by using manual techniques to improve the alignment of the client's skeletal system. Every massage stroke can potentially move the client toward joint neutral, lengthening shortened muscles to help move the bones to a position of optimal posture.

2.4.3   Lines of Force

The skeletal structure evolved to work under compression. To minimize joint compression while maximizing support in an upright posture, the weight of each body mass—head, thorax, and pelvis—must be borne as close to the LOG as possible. A stilt walker has to stack her joints and align each body mass over her leg to balance on a single stilt (Figure 2.24 ■). To explore this concept, balance a heavy book on top of your head. To keep it from falling, you will need to carry the load right in the center of your head. You will also need to keep your spine, hips, and legs aligned directly under your head to allow the weight of the book to transfer through the center of your body along a line of force defined by the axial compression.

A **line of force** is the pathway along which a force passes from one joint to the next along a kinetic chain (Figure 2.25 ■). For every force there is an equal and opposite counterforce. Take, for example, walking. While stepping, the heel strikes the ground and a counterforce pushes back up into your body. The striking force and counterforce travels through the joints along a pathway that defines a line of force. The pathway depends on skeletal alignment, which in turn depends on muscle-use patterns.

BRIDGE TO PRACTICE
Moving Joints toward Neutral with Massage and Bodywork

Before massaging your client, look at how his or her body rests when supine on the table, visualizing the skeleton at rest. How close are the joints to a neutral alignment? If you up-ended your client in this exact position, would he or she end up in an optimal posture?

This type of visual assessment can give you information on which direction to take a massage stroke. As you massage your clients, ask yourself: *Which direction does a massage stroke need to go to help move the bones toward their optimal alignment?*

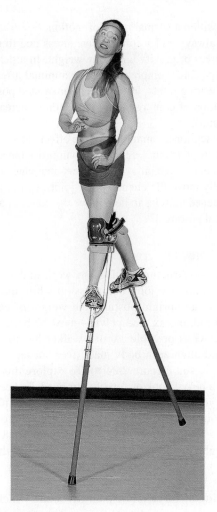

FIGURE 2.24
A stilt walker has to balance the COGs in her three body masses.

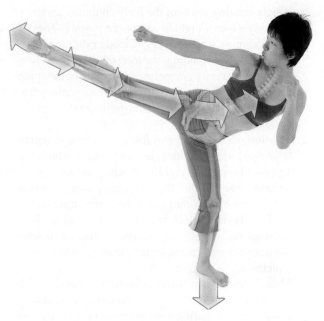

FIGURE 2.25
Lines of force and counterforce

Ideally, compressive forces transfer through the center of the weight-bearing joints while walking. If any joint along the extensor chain is chronically bent, compressive stress from the load will crash into the corner of the bent joint. Chronic muscular contractions bend joints away from a neutral alignment. As practitioners, we can stretch the muscles to straighten the joints. We can also teach clients how to use muscles in ways that better align the joints. The first step in this educational process is to help our clients become aware of their skeletal alignment. One simple way

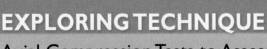

EXPLORING TECHNIQUE
Axial Compression Tests to Assess Lines of Force

Use this simple compression test to assess the alignment of the thorax over the pelvis and legs, to help your partner feel how compression translates through the joints from the shoulders to the feet, and to feel when the upper body balances over the lower body and the base of support.

Caution: Do not perform this test on anyone who has pain from a spinal disk problem.

1. Have your partner stand comfortably with her feet under her hips. Have her sense where on her feet she feels her weight is balanced. Stand behind your partner and lightly press down on both of her shoulders.

   Press lightly and release several times. The joints should feel springy. Ask your partner where in the body she feels the compression. If the body masses stack vertically, it will go all the way to her feet. Wherever the spine chronically bends (usually in the lower back) compression pools. Most people feel the lower back bend, which indicates that the thorax is behind rather than over the base of support (Figure 2.26a ■).

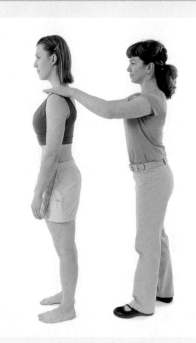

FIGURE 2.26b

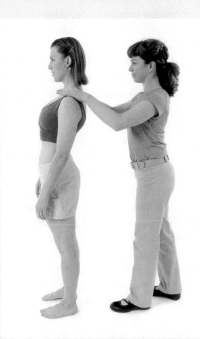

FIGURE 2.26a

2. Next, have your partner close her eyes, then subtly sway back and forth, keeping both her feet flat and shifting her weight from heels and toes (Figure 2.26b ■). Tell your partner to sense the place where it feels like her thorax comes over the pelvis, and stop there. Then repeat the compression test. She will feel the compression in her feet if her thorax is actually aligned over her base of support.

3. You can also practice this compression test with your partner lying face up on a massage table. Lightly push up on her feet several times, using a rocking motion (Figure 2.26c ■). Make sure to leave her heels resting on the table to keep the axial joints in the same plane. Ask your partner to notice where she feels the compression and rocking in her skeletal system. Also observe which parts of your partner's body move and which parts look stiff. Lastly, ask your partner what she feels. This will give you both a reading on how the forces of compression travel through her body.

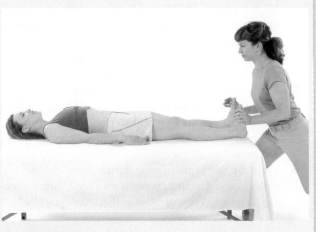

FIGURE 2.26c

to do this is with compression. Simply push down on the shoulders while your client is standing or up through the feet while your client is lying down, and ask the client to feel how the force travels through the body.

CONCLUSION

Stilt walking can help us to remember a few main points about the skeletal system. Stilts highlight the uniquely axial upright nature of the human skeleton. To balance at this height, a person needs to align the COG of each part of her skeleton over the base of support and keep her hips and knees in a joint-neutral relationship. The place where the stilts attaching to her lower legs are comparable to fibrous nonmovable joints with the straps functioning as dense connective tissue binding the stilts to her legs. The soles of her shoes provide

cushioning between her feet and the stilts, similar to how fibrocartilage disks absorb shock in a synovial joint.

To step, the stilt walker lifts and flexes her leg. The length of her leg exaggerates the bend in the freely movable hinge joint of the knee and the ball-and-socket joint of the hip. It is important that she keep her hips lined up with her knees so that the stilts don't cross and trip her up. To turn, she spins her body on the peg at the end of the stilt, rotating it like a pivot joint.

The alignment lessons of stilt walking apply to general body movement and to bodywork as well. It is important to keep the axial skeleton vertically aligned when we are upright to minimize mechanical stress on the spine. Similarly, every stroke and technique we use in a massage and bodywork session can be done in a direction that helps move the joints toward optimal skeletal alignment.

SUMMARY POINTS TO REMEMBER

1. The skeleton is made up of 206 bones and all the associated structures including the joints and associated tissues. The skeleton is divided into the axial skeleton (head, vertebral column, thorax, sternum, sacrum, and coccyx) and appendicular skeleton (lower limbs, pelvic bones, upper limbs, and shoulder girdle). The five main functions of the skeleton are support, movement, protection, storage, and blood production.

2. Connective tissue (CT) is the most abundant tissue in the body. All CTs are composed of cells, fibers (collagen, elastin, and reticular fibers), and ground substance. There are four types of CT: blood, bone, cartilage, and connective tissue proper (dense or loose).

3. Connective tissue responds to the mechanical forces of movement and bodywork because of certain of its properties, such as thixotropy (the ability to change from a gel to a liquid when heated or put under pressure) and viscosity (the ability of a thick fluid to resist and dampen pressure).

4. Elasticity refers to the ability of tissues to recoil or rebound after being deformed by a mechanical force. Tissues can only stretch to their elastic limit. Once they reach this limit, further stretch will induce plastic changes, which are irreversible. Plasticity refers to the irreversible deformation of tissue in response to forces that exceed its elastic limit.

5. There are two types of bone tissue: compact bone and spongy bone. Compact bone forms a hard, thin, protective layer made up of bone cells (osteocytes), which

are tightly packed into units called osteons. Deep to this layer resides spongy bone, which has cells that are loosely packed in geometric rows (trabeculae) along lines of tension.

6. Bone is a dynamic tissue that responds to mechanical stress in an ongoing process called remodeling. In this process, specialized cells called osteoclasts break down and absorb old, damaged bone cells while osteoblasts produce new bone.

7. Bones come in different shapes and sizes. There are five types of bone: long (femur), short (carpal), flat (sternum), irregular (vertebra), and sesamoid (patella).

8. The shape and markings of a bone reflects its function. There are different types of bony landmarks, such as condyles, facets, processes, fossae, or tubercles.

9. The property of bone strength is measured by a bone's resistance to mechanical stress. Bone elasticity is its ability to deform under stress. Although bones can withstand high levels of compressive stress, they are susceptible to fractures (breaks) from severe stress or cumulative traumas.

10. The skeletal system has two types of cartilage: hyaline cartilage covers the articulating surfaces of synovial joints and fibrocartilage is found in the shock-absorbing disks. Dense connective tissues in the skeletal system include ligaments, joint capsules, and periosteum (fascia covering bone).

11. A bursa (plural: *bursae*) is a small, fluid-filled sac embedded in tissues around a joint, usually under

tendons, in order to reduce friction around freely movable joints.

12. There are three main types of joints in the skeletal system. A fibrous, synarthrotic joint is nonmovable; a fibrocartilage, amphiarthrotic joint is semimovable; and a synovial, diarthrotic joint is freely movable and the most abundant type of joint in the body.

13. A synovial joint has a cuff-like joint capsule, a cavity filled with synovial fluid, a synovial membrane that produces fluid, and articulating surfaces lined with hyaline cartilage. There are six types of synovial joints: ball-and-socket, ellipsoid (condyloid), hinge, plane (gliding), pivot, and saddle.

14. Synovial joints move in either one plane (uniaxial), two planes (biaxial), or three or more planes (triaxial or multiaxial). Plane joints are nonaxial (they do not bend), hinge joints are uniaxial, ellipsoid joints are biaxial, and ball-and-socket joints are multiaxial.

15. When assessing skeletal alignment and joint motion, the effects of gravity need to be considered. In optimal skeletal alignment, the center of gravity (center of mass) in the head, thorax, and pelvis align on a plumb along the line of gravity (the direction of gravity's force) over the base of support.

16. Five mechanical stresses generated by internal forces and external forces affect the skeletal system: compression, tension, shear, torque, and bend.

17. A line of force is the pathway along which a force travels through the body.

REVIEW QUESTIONS

1. The two divisions of the skeletal system are the
   a. axial skeleton (which includes the head, spine, ribs, sternum, upper limbs, and shoulder girdle) and the appendicular skeleton (which includes the lower limbs and pelvic bones, sacrum, and coccyx).
   b. axial skeleton (which includes the head, spine, lower limbs, and pelvic bones) and the appendicular skeleton (which includes the ribs, sternum, sacrum, coccyx, and the upper limbs and shoulder girdle).
   c. axial skeleton (which includes the lower limbs and pelvic bones and the upper limbs and shoulder girdle) and the appendicular skeleton (which includes the head, spine, ribs, sternum, sacrum, and coccyx).
   d. axial skeleton (which includes the head, spine, ribs, sternum, sacrum, and coccyx) and the appendicular skeleton (which includes the lower limbs and pelvic bones and the upper limbs and shoulder girdle).

2. The three elements found in every connective tissue are
   a. cells, ground substance, and collagen.
   b. cells, ground substance, and fibers.
   c. cells, ground substance, and elastin.
   d. cells, ground substance, and osteons.

3. What type of connective tissue fiber is the most abundant in the skeletal system and what is one of its properties?

4. Define and contrast two connective tissue properties: elasticity and plasticity.
   a. Elasticity is the ability of tissues to return to their original shape after being deformed. Plasticity is deformation of tissues beyond their elastic limit, which results in irreversible changes.
   b. Elasticity is the inability of tissues to return to their original shape after being deformed. Plasticity is deformation of tissues beyond their elastic limit, which results in irreversible changes.
   c. Elasticity is the ability of tissues to return to their original shape after being deformed. Plasticity is deformation of tissues beyond their elastic limit, which results in reversible changes.
   d. Elasticity is the ability of tissues to return to their original shape after being deformed. Plasticity is regeneration of tissues beyond their plastic limit, which results in irreversible changes.

5. What are the two types of bone tissue and where are they located?

6. What are trabeculae, which type of bone tissue are they found in, and what function do they serve?

7. Name the five types of bones and give one example of each.

8. The two substances that make bones rigid and strong are
   a. mineral deposits and elastin fibers.
   b. mineral deposits and reticular fibers.
   c. mineral deposits and collagen fibers.
   d. mineral deposits and calcium.

9. Bone remodeling is a regenerative process in bone tissues in which cells called
   a. osteoclasts break down and reabsorb old bone tissue while cells called osteoblasts produce and lay down new bone tissue.
   b. osteoblasts break down and reabsorb old bone tissue while cells called osteophytes produce and lay down new bone tissue.
   c. osteoblasts regenerate and rebuild old bone marrow while cells called osteoclasts produce and lay down new bone marrow.
   d. osteoclasts break down and reabsorb periosteum tissues while cells called osteoblasts produce and lay down new periosteum layers.

10. Name three bone markings and describe them.

11. Name the two types of cartilage found in the skeletal system and give one example of where each type is found.

12. Structures in the skeletal system made up of dense connective tissues include
    a. ligaments, tendons, fascias, joint capsules, and ground substance.
    b. ligaments, tendons, fascias, joint capsules, and synovial fluid.
    c. ligaments, tendons, fascias, joint capsules, and periosteum.
    d. ligaments, tendons, fascias, joint capsules, and collagen.

13. Match three types of joints—fibrous, fibrocartilage, and synovial—with their range of movement:
    a. freely movable
    b. nonmovable
    c. semimovable

14. True or false (circle one). The synovial joints are the most abundant types of joints in the body.

15. Five structures found in all synovial joints include a joint
    a. capsule, joint cavity, fibrocartilage disk, synovial membrane, and synovial fluid.
    b. capsule, joint cavity, elastic cartilage, synovial membrane, and synovial fluid.
    c. capsule, joint cavity, hyaline cartilage, synovial membrane, and synovial fluid.
    d. capsule, joint cavity, connective tissue, synovial membrane, and synovial fluid.

16. The six types of synovial joints are the
    a. ball-and-socket, ellipsoid, hinge, plane, saddle, and nonaxial joints.
    b. ball-and-socket, ellipsoid, hinge, plane, pivot, and biaxial joints.
    c. ball-and-socket, ellipsoid, hinge, plane, pivot, and triaxial joints.
    d. ball-and-socket, ellipsoid, hinge, plane, saddle, and pivot joints.

17. True or false (circle one). A triaxial ball-and-socket joint can only move in three planes.

18. The center of gravity of an object or body mass is
    a. a vertical line through a mass.
    b. the center of weight in a mass.
    c. the velocity of a moving mass.
    d. the base of support of a mass.

Notes

1. Steindler, A. (1972). *Kinesiology of the Human Body: Under Normal and Pathological Conditions.* Springfield, IL: Charles C. Thomas.
2. Norkin, C., & Levangie, P. (2005). *Joint Structure and Function: A Comprehensive Analysis* (3rd ed.). Philadelphia: F. A. Davis.
3. Alter, M. (2004). *Science of Flexibility* (3rd ed.). Champaign, IL: Human Kinetics.

PEARSON
myhealthprofessionskit™

Use this address to access the Companion Website created for this textbook. Simply select "Massage Therapy" from the choice of disciplines. Find this book and log in using your username and password to access interactive activities, videos, and much more.

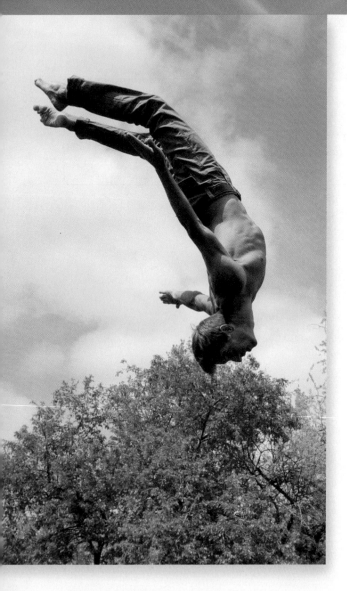

CHAPTER

3 Joint Motion

CHAPTER OUTLINE

Chapter Objectives

Key Terms

3.1 Osteokinematics: Types of Joint Movement

3.2 Arthrokinematics: Movement at Joint Surfaces

3.3 Range of Motion

3.4 Clinical Applications for Joint Movement

Conclusion

Summary Points to Remember

Review Questions

Jumping on a trampoline has become a popular backyard sport. It provides lots of exercise and requires minimal skill to master. To bounce safely with control, a jumper aims for the center of the trampoline, with his spine straight and the legs underneath. Upon impact, his legs naturally bend to absorb shock and push down to thrust the body back up.

A trampoline novice should bounce slowly until the up-and-down motion feels natural. To spring higher and higher, he pushes down with greater force while increasing lift by moving the arms in a swimming breaststroke. Control develops from practicing crisp body poses during the peak of suspension such as jumping jacks, pike bends, and toe-touch splits. Gifted jumpers who can easily perform flips and twists might head for a career in the circus.

CHAPTER OBJECTIVES

1. Define a joint and describe its function.

2. Describe the difference between osteokinematic and arthrokinematic joint motion.

3. Define and contrast linear, rotary, and curvilinear motion.

4. Define axial motion and list the axial motions that occur in each plane.

5. Describe nonaxial motion and list two nonaxial motions and two combined motions.

6. Define and contrast an open kinetic chain and a closed kinetic chain.

7. Name and describe three types of movement between the articulating surfaces in a joint.

8. Explain the convex–concave rule of joint motion.

9. Explain the difference between a close-packed and loose-packed joint position.

10. Define range of motion and list four elements that affect it.

11. Define joint stability and list the passive and active restraints that maintain stability.

12. Define joint mobility, hypermobility, hypomobility, and instability.

13. Define active, passive, and resisted joint motion.

14. Define and contrast sprains and strains.

15. Name and define three types of normal end-feel to joint motion.

KEY TERMS

Accessory movement	End-feel	Passive motion
Active restraints	Hypermobility	Passive restraints
Articulation	Hypomobility	Physiological movement
Backward rotation	Joint play	Range of motion (ROM)
Closed kinetic chain	Joint stability	Resisted range of motion
Close-packed position	Linear motion	Rotary motion
Concave–convex rule	Loose-packed position	Sprain
Curvilinear motion	Open kinetic chain	Strain

In the last chapter we covered the skeletal system. The amazing thing about this collection of bones is its ability to move. Movement occurs at the place where two bones meet, called a **joint** or **articulation.** During movement, the bones serve as levers, the joints as fulcrums, and the muscles as the power source. Imagine what it would be like to move around without bones. We would be reduced to inching along like a worm or slug. Fortunately, the human body evolved this uniquely upright system of linked joints and bony levers that allows us to move with a level of control and efficiency that stands without rival in the animal world.

Many of the pain-causing muscular problems for which people receive bodywork invariably affect joint motion in some way. This is why the study of human kinesiology is an important part of massage training. It is necessary to understand variances in joint structures and ranges of motion to be able to move a client's joints within a normal range. It is also essential to be able to accurately visualize the shape of the articulating surfaces in the joints and how these surfaces move across each other to effectively use passive motion with your clients.

Skeletal joints demonstrate features comparable to the mechanical joints used in furniture, architecture, and machines. For example, sutures in the skull resemble the dovetail joints found in wooden tables, the elbows and knees resemble the hinges found on doors, and the hips and shoulders resemble the ball joints found in the axle of a car. Although there are only six types of freely movable synovial joints in the human body, they total over 250. The collective motion of the synovial joints allows for a repertoire of human movement that far exceeds any movement system found in manmade designs.

This chapter begins with a study of two categories of joint motion. *Osteokinematics* covers the observable movements of the joints through space. *Arthrokinematics* covers the unseen movements between the articulating surfaces of the bones inside the joints. Then we explore different aspects of range of motion, such as stability and mobility, active and passive movements, and what constitutes a normal and abnormal range of motion. The chapter ends with an overview of clinical applications for using joint motion in both active and passive ranges, with general guidelines for moving synovial joints within safe and effective parameters.

3.1   OSTEOKINEMATICS: TYPES OF JOINT MOVEMENT

Osteokinematics refers to different types of joint movements. Axial and nonaxial joint motions were introduced in the chapter of the skeleton. Recall that axial motion always pivots around an axis, bending or twisting a joint. During axial motion, the moving bone inscribes a circular arc through space. The axis of motion is always perpendicular to the arc or plane of motion. For example, when kicking a ball, the leg swings at the hip in a sagittal plane, flexing along a bilateral axis (Figure 3.1 ■).

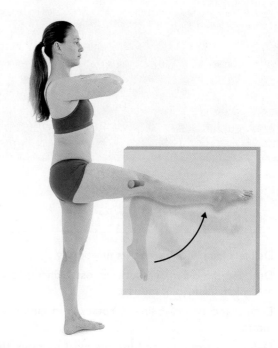

FIGURE 3.1

Axial motion in the sagittal plane occurs around a bilateral axis.

In contrast, during nonaxial motion, the articulating surfaces of the moving bones glide or slide across each other. Nonaxial joint motion usually occurs in conjunction with an axial motion. Take, for example, the coordinated movement of the shoulder and scapula. Raise one arm overhead and notice how the shoulder moves around the axis at the joint while the scapula slides in a nonaxial motion across the ribs (Figure 3.2 ■).

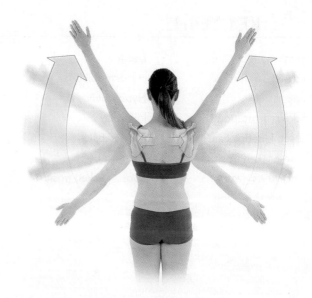

FIGURE 3.2

Axial and nonaxial joint motions usually occur together.

3.1.1   Linear, Rotary, and Curvilinear Motion

There are several different types of motion that are defined by the pathways the moving bone or moving body takes through space (Figure 3.3 ■). Keep in mind when looking at these different types of motions that they can be an action at a single joint or the movement of the entire body through space. **Linear motion** or **translatory motion** describes movement along a straight path, such as sledding down a hill or pushing a book across a table. The gliding motion in a plane joint is also linear. A bodyworker uses linear motion during long, straight effleurage or stripping strokes.

    Rotary motion describes the circular movement around a fixed point, such as a turning windmill or the rotating spokes on a wheel. In rotary joint motion, such as elbow, knee, or hip flexion, a bone or body part moves around a fixed point or axis. It is also called **angular motion** because rotary motion bends the moving joint into an angle. During angular motion, each point along the moving part moves in the same direction at the same time, except over an uneven distance. Because a rotary motion pivots in an arc around an axis, a rotary motion is always an axial motion.

    Curvilinear motion describes movement along a curved pathway, such as the long arc of a music conductor's gesture or the sweeping curve of a skier banking a bend. Many curvilinear actions involve some combination of linear and rotary motions. Take, for example, the action of waxing a car. The hand moves along both curvilinear and linear pathways while the shoulder and elbow joints flex and extend in rotary, angular motions.

3.1.2   Axial Movements in Each Plane

All the movements below describe axial motion in a single plane. Since axial motion occurs around a fixed point, the axial motions described below are all rotary motions.

Sagittal plane movements

- **Flexion:** A movement that bends and closes the angle of a joint (Figure 3.4 ■).
- **Extension:** The opposite of flexion, a movement that bends and opens the angle of a joint (Figure 3.4). A return from flexion. The neutral position of the joint.
- **Hyperextension:** Movement that extends a joint behind the frontal plane (Figure 3.4).
  Note: Since the knee or the elbow have a limited range of motion past extension, excessive hyperextension in either of these joints is considered pathological and should be avoided because it can stress and even injure joint structures. In contrast, because the hips and shoulders can extend behind the body, hyperextension is a normal part of their range.
- **Dorsiflexion:** A movement of the foot toward the dorsal surface of the leg, closing the angle of the ankle past 90 degrees (Figure 3.5a ■).
- **Plantarflexion:** A movement of the ankle toward the planter surface of the foot, opening the angle of the ankle past 90 degrees (Figure 3.5b ■). When the ankle is at 90 degrees, it is in neutral.

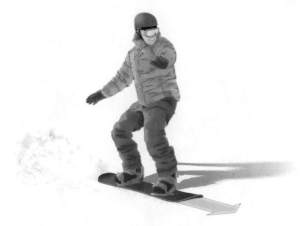

Linear

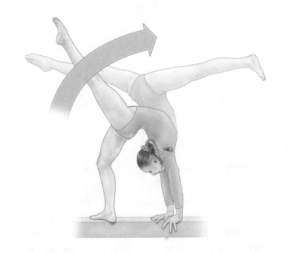

Rotary

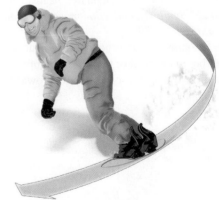

Curvilinear

FIGURE 3.3
Three different types of motion

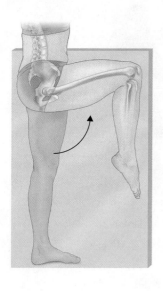
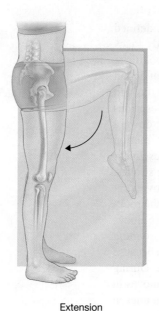
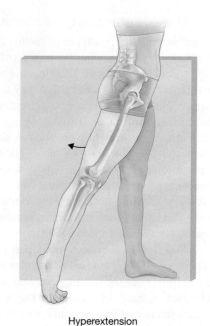

Flexion   Extension   Hyperextension

FIGURE 3.4

Range of movement in the sagittal plane.

Frontal plane movements

- **Abduction:** A movement of the limb away from the midline of the body (Figure 3.6a ■).
  Note: Since the terms abduct and adduct sound similar, most teachers call them "A-B-duction or A-D-duction," putting an emphasis on the difference.
- **Adduction:** A movement of the limb toward the midline of the body (Figure 3.6b ■).
  Note: Here's an easy way to remember which is which. To "abduct" is to take away: aliens abduct humans. Similarly, abduction moves the limbs away from midline. In contrast, adduction begins with the root "add." Similarly, adduction moves or "adds" a limb toward the midline.
- **Lateral flexion:** A side-bending movement of the spine either to the right or to the left (Figure 3.7 ■).
- **Inversion:** Turning the sole of the foot toward midline (Figure 3.8a ■).

- **Eversion:** Turning the sole of the foot away from midline (Figure 3.8b ■).

Horizontal plane movements

- **Lateral (external) rotation:** A movement of an appendicular joint such as the hip or shoulder as it turns away from midline of the body, in an outward direction (Figure 3.9a ■).
- **Medial (internal) rotation:** A movement of an appendicular joint such as the hip or shoulder as it turns toward the midline of the body, in an inward direction (Figure 3.9b ■).
- **Right** and **left rotation:** A movement of the spine or head turning either right or left (Figure 3.10 ■).

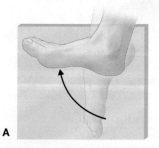
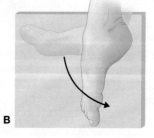

A   B

FIGURE 3.5

Dorsflexion and plantarflexion

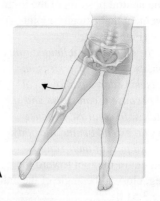
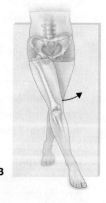

A   B

FIGURE 3.6

a) **Abduction** of the hip
b) **Adduction** of the hip

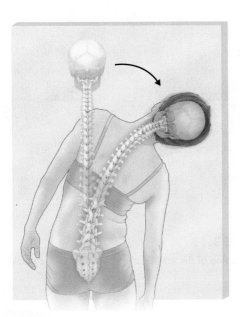

FIGURE 3.7
Lateral flexion of the spine

- **Backward** and **forward rotation:** A rotation of the pelvis in the horizontal (transverse) plane (Figure 3.11 ■).
- **Horizontal flexion** (horizontal adduction) and **horizontal extension** (horizontal abduction): Movements of the shoulder joint from 90 degrees flexion to a horizontal position in front of the body (Figure 3.12 ■).

3.1.3 Nonaxial Movements

Nonaxial movement involves one articulating surface gliding across another, similar to two blocks sliding across each other. Because plane joints cannot bend or rotate along an axis, they move with a nonaxial, gliding motion.

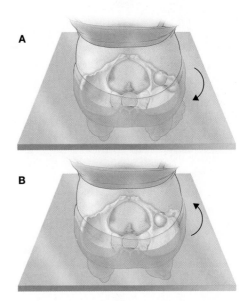

FIGURE 3.9
a) **Lateral rotation** of the right hip b) **Medial rotation** of the right hip

The shoulder blades and jaw also demonstrate nonaxial movements. When a person shrugs the shoulders, the shoulder blades or *scapulae* slide up along the rib cage. This gliding motion is called **elevation** of the scapulae. The jaw, or *temporomandibular joint* (TMJ), elevates when the mouth is closed from an open position. **Depression** describes the return action of either the scapulae or the jaw, lowering the shoulders or opening the mouth.

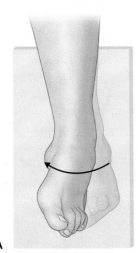
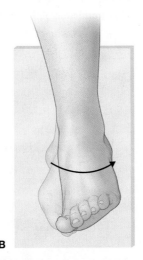

FIGURE 3.8
a) **Inversion.** b) **Eversion**

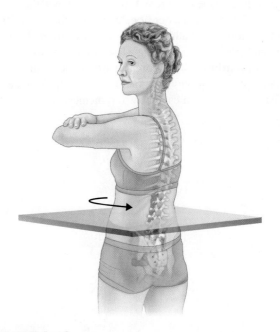

FIGURE 3.10
Left rotation of the spine

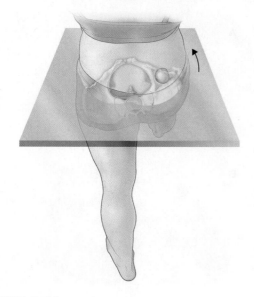

FIGURE 3.11
Forward rotation of the pelvis

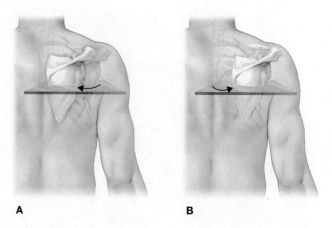

A   **B**

FIGURE 3.13
a) **Retraction** of the scapula b) **Protraction** of the scapula

Retraction (adduction) draws the scapulae together in back; **protraction** (abduction) pulls them around to the front (Figure 3.13a-b ■). A person rowing a boat retracts the shoulders when pulling back on the oars and protracts when pushing forward. A shy teen often protracts the scapulae to fold the chest and withdraw, whereas a soldier retracts the scapulae and arches the spine to push the chest out in the military posture.

3.1.4 Combined and Miscellaneous Movements

Circumduction is a combined movement that inscribes a cone-like shape (Figure 3.14 ■). It combines the movements of flexion and extension, lateral and medial rotation, and abduction and adduction. A cowboy circumducts the arm and elbow while twirling a lasso to rope a cow.

Supination of the forearm turns the palm of the hand from a downward facing position to face up (Figure 3.15a ■). An easy way to remember the *sup*ination

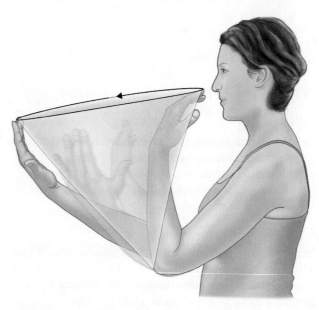

FIGURE 3.14
Circumduction of the elbow

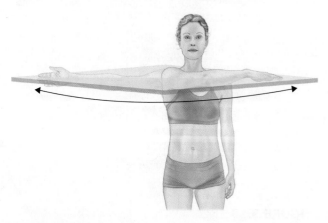

FIGURE 3.12
Horizontal flexion and extension of the shoulder

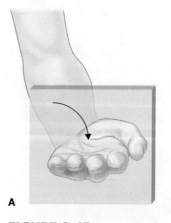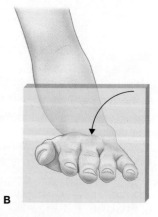

A   **B**

FIGURE 3.15
a) **Supination**. b) **Pronation**.

GUIDELINES
Naming Joint Actions

1. When referring to a joint motion, make sure that the reference includes two facts:
   - The name of the moving joint
   - The name of the direction that it is moving, such as "hip flexion," "knee extension," or "lateral rotation of the shoulder."
2. Build rapport with your clients by referring to joints using common names rather than confusing them by using technical terms, but use anatomical terms for joints in written reports or case studies, or when conferring with other health professionals (although they, too, may use the common names).
   - Common names: *Hip, shoulder, elbow,* and *knee*
   - Anatomical names: *Coxofemoral, glenohumeral, humeroulnar,* and *tibiofemoral joints*

3. Begin movement descriptions of joint actions with the joint relative to the standing or anatomical position, unless otherwise specified. This means that movement terms such as "flexion," "extension," and "rotation" always describe actions that begin with the joint in extension.
4. Make sure to use the correct terms to describe joint and muscle actions. It is a common mistake to say a "muscle flexed." Remember the following rules:

   - *Joints flex and extend.*
   - *Muscles contract and relax.*

action is to imagine a person turning the palm up to carry a bowl of *soup*. **Pronation** is the reverse action; the palm turns down (Figure 3.15b ■).

The **supine position** refers to the position of the body when a person is lying on the spine. To remember this position, think "supine on the spine." The **prone position** is just the opposite. It refers to the face-down position of a person lying on the belly. Just like the pronation turns the belly of the forearm down, to lie prone is to lie on the belly. Supination and pronation of the foot and ankle involve the coupled movement of two joints in the foot and ankle, which is covered in the foot chapter.

When the arm is lifted to the side (abducted), the scapula follows with the motion of **upward rotation,** which is a combination of elevation, rotation, and protraction (Figure 3.16 ■). As the arm is lowered, the scapula moves in **downward rotation,** a combination of depression, retraction, and rotation.

The natural movements that people use during the course of a day, such as standing from a seated position or bending over to pick something up, are referred to as **activities of daily living** (ADL). Most ADL are combined movements through a series of joints and rotations. For example, tossing a ball involves the combined shoulder movements of flexion, adduction, and lateral rotation.

Many kinesiology books focus on the movements of athletes and performers. These trained and skilled movers provide wonderful examples of outstanding human performance; however, it is also important to understand the basic movement patterns that people commonly do

in their ADL. People need functional movement patterns to be able to move efficiently through daily activities—such as bending, lifting, and turning—to avoid pain and injury. Manual therapists need to understand functional movement patterns because we may be moving our clients through these patterns during table work. Because performing daily activities with faulty form leads to the common body problems that people tend to seek massage and bodywork to alleviate, these patterns are addressed throughout this text.

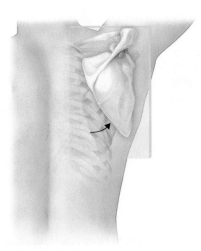

FIGURE 3.16
Upward rotation of the scapula

3.1.5 Closed and Open Kinetic Chains

Recall from the introductory chapter that a *kinetic chain* is a succession of movement through bony segments linked together by movable joints. When one end of the chain is fixed, it is called movement in a **closed kinetic chain** (Figure 3.17a ▪). For example, when standing up from a seated position, both feet are fixed or closed on the ground. In contrast, when one end of the chain is free or open, it is called an **open kinetic chain** (Figure 3.17b ▪). When extending the knee from a seated position, the leg moves as the free end of an open chain.

Another way to describe open and closed chains is to name which end of the limb—*distal* or *proximal*—is stationary or moving—is *fixed* or *free*. When reaching across a table, the distal end of the moving arm is free. When standing from a seated position, the distal ends of the lower limbs are fixed.

Movement in a closed chain creates a predictable sequence along a series of linked joints. During a deep knee bend, it is natural to expect that the ankles, knees, and hips will all bend together. The lower limb is unique in that its flexor and extensor muscles crisscross between the anterior and posterior sides of the body. As a person extends the legs from a deep knee bend, extensor muscles contract on the posterior hip, anterior thigh, posterior calf, and anterior ankle and foot. This crisscrossing chain of muscles allows the knee to bend and straighten in the opposite direction of the hip and ankle, like an accordion opening and closing. It also allows the joints of the lower limb to simultaneously fold and unfold under the trunk, a pattern crucial for efficient walking, running, jumping, and making level changes such as climbing steps.

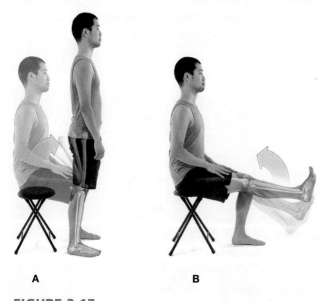

A   **B**

FIGURE 3.17

a) **Closed kinematic chain.** b) **Open kinematic chain.**

The way that movement sequences along a kinetic chain depends on muscular balance as well as individual body patterning. A person with healthy and strong muscles will crouch then jump with simultaneous and even flexion, then extension, of the trunk and lower limbs. In contrast, a person with imbalanced muscles or faulty patterning will probably demonstrate a weak or uncoordinated pattern of movement. In another example, one person turning the head to look behind the body might rotate the vertebral segments of the entire spine. In contrast, another person with a rigid or injured spine might only rotate the spine to the base of the neck.

In manual therapy, passive movement or stretching at one end of a limb or the spine usually creates a predictable sequence along its kinetic chain. For example, when applying strong traction to the foot, we can expect the joints and soft tissues along the entire lower limb to be lengthened. When passively stretching a client's arm overhead, we can expect the stretch to extend through the arm into the shoulder and trunk.

3.2 ARTHROKINEMATICS: MOVEMENT AT JOINT SURFACES

The last section covered osteokinematics, which are movements of a joint such as flexion and extension. This section covers **arthrokinematics,** which refers to the different types of movement that occur *inside* the joint as the articulating surfaces move across each other.

Recall from the chapter on the skeleton that the curved surfaces of the joints fit together in convex–concave pairs that come in ovoid or stellar shapes (see Figure 2.19). Most synovial joints are ovoid joints. The knee and elbow are both stellar joints.

- In an *ovoid joint,* an egg-shaped mound fits into a hollow depression.
- In a *stellar joint,* each joint surface has both convex and concave contours.

When passively moving a joint, it is helpful to understand how the articulating surfaces fit together. The size and shape of the articulating surfaces determine the pathway of motion in each joint. To demonstrate this point, consider how the symmetrical runners on a rocking chair allow for an even rolling motion in one plane. Imagine how unevenly the rocking chair would move if one runner was slightly shorter or had a deeper arc to its curve than the other. It would rock along a curvilinear pathway, tipping to one side as it rolled across an uneven base. Similar dynamics occur during knee and elbow movement because the right and left condyles in both these joints vary in size and shape.

3.2.1 Roll, Glide, and Spin

The articulating surfaces of synovial joints move in one of three ways: rolling, gliding, or spinning (Figure 3.18 ■).

- **Roll:** Occurs when one articulating surface rolls across another, for example, a ball rolling across a table.
- **Glide:** Occurs when one articulating surface slides across another. One bone can turn in place against another bone, similar to a braked tire skidding on ice; or one bone can slide across another, similar to a block sliding down a ramp.
- **Spin:** Occurs when one articulating surface turns on another, for example, a top spinning. Spinning is a pure rotary motion that occurs in very few joints. The ball-and-socket joints of the hips and shoulders spin during rotation, and the head of the radius spins against the humerus during forearm pronation and supination.

The kind of movement that occurs in each joint depends on the shape of the articulating surfaces. Most synovial joints move in some combination of rolling and gliding actions. To feel this, roll the back of your right hand on the palm of your left hand. Then glide the back of your right hand against the palm of your left. Now combine the two by making a fist with your right hand and cupping it with the palm of your left hand. Turn your fist in the center of your right palm by raising and lowering your right elbow. Notice how you need to move your fist with a combined rolling and gliding motion to keep the fist centered in the palm.

If the joints did not glide with rolling, one joint surface would roll off the other and bump into nearby structures. For example, take the movement of the ball-and-socket

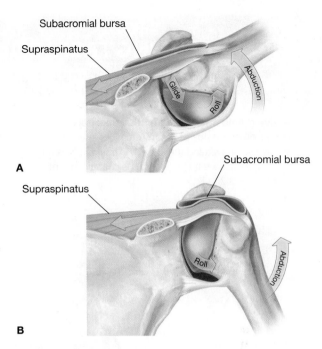

FIGURE 3.19

a) During shoulder abduction, the humeral head both rolls and glides in the glenoid fossa. b) When the humeral fails to glide down, abduction will compress the subacromial space, causing **shoulder impingement.**

joint in the shoulder. When raising the arm, the head of the humerus rolls up while gliding down (Figure 3.19a ■). Without the downward gliding motion, the *humeral head* would roll up and jam against the bony ledge of the *acromion process,* causing shoulder impingement, which is a common ailment (Figure 3.19b ■). Plane joints move with a pure gliding motion because they are nonaxial and cannot bend (Figure 3.20 ■).

Movement occurs between articular surfaces in a joint at the point of contact. In an axial joint, the point of contact is perpendicular to the axis of rotation. During the gliding and rolling actions the axis of rotation continually changes,

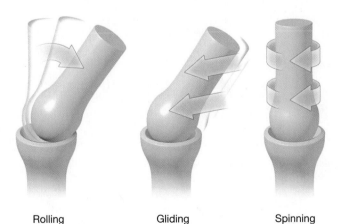

Rolling   Gliding   Spinning

FIGURE 3.18

Arthrokinematics: Three types of movement between joint surfaces.

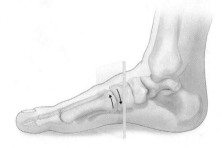

FIGURE 3.20

As weight shifts from the heel to the toes, the tarsal bones glide and sink, flattening the arches.

EXPLORING TECHNIQUE
Exploring Roll, Glide, and Spin in Joint Motion

1. **Active rolling and gliding in the knee:** Place your fingertips on either side of the front of your knee joint. Then slowly flex and extend the knee by lifting and lowering your foot. As your knee moves, sense the changing point of contact (Figure 3.21a ■).

3. **Passive rolling and gliding with the first toe:** Hold your first toe with one hand while stabilizing the first metatarsal bone with your other hand. Slowing flex and extend the joint, noticing how the distal bone rolls and glides against the proximal bone (Figure 3.21c ■).

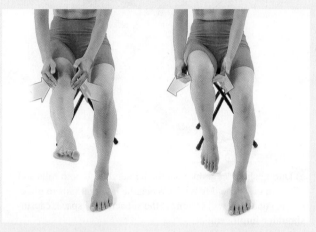

FIGURE 3.21a

FIGURE 3.21c

2. **Active spinning in the hip joint:** Straighten one leg and place your hand over your hip joint. Then roll your foot on your heel. This will laterally and medially rotate your hip, causing it to spin in the socket (Figure 3.21b ■).

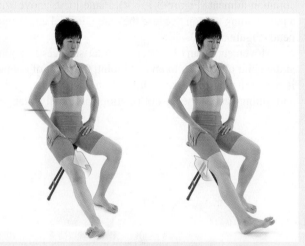

FIGURE 3.21b

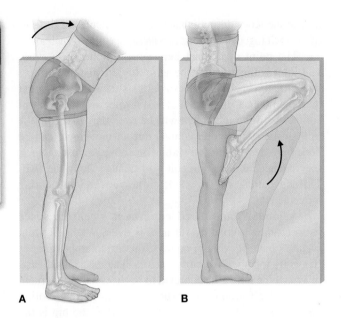

FIGURE 3.22

a) The pelvis is mobile and the femur is stable. b) The femur is mobile and the pelvis is stable.

BRIDGE TO PRACTICE
Passively Moving Joints

When passively moving your client's joints, visualize the irregularly shaped articulating surfaces in each joint. This will help you move each joint in accordance with the mechanics unique to that joint.

---

so it is called the **instantaneous axis of rotation (IAR)**—the changing point of contact between the articular surfaces during joint motion.

- *While rolling,* the point of contact on both articulating surfaces keeps changing. Imagine a paint roller rolling across a wall or two pieces of Velcro tearing apart.
- *While gliding,* the point of contact on one surface remains the same while the contact on the other surface progressively moves along a series of points.
- *While spinning,* the point of contact on both surfaces remains the same.

3.2.2 Concave–Convex Rule

During typical joint motion, a moving bone turns around a stable bone. The nonmoving bone provides a stabilizing joint surface for the moving bone. For example, in a forward bow, the *pelvis moves against the stability of the lower limbs* (Figure 3.22a ■). The action can be reversed. For example, in a standing leg lift, the *lower limb moves against the stability of the pelvis* (Figure 3.22b ■). The inverse action reverses which bone moves and which bone remains stable.

To determine which bone moves in which direction, the concave–convex rule applies. This rule states that:

- *When a bone with the* convex *joint surface moves, the joint surface always moves in the* opposite direction *as the bone.* For example, when a person raises one arm to the side, the convex head of the humerus moves down in the opposite direction of the arm, which moves up (Figure 3.23a ■).
- *When a bone with the* concave *joint surface moves, the joint surface moves in the* same direction *as the bone.* For example, when extending a finger, the concave proximal surface of each phalange moves in the same direction as the finger (Figure 3.23b ■).

3.2.3 Joint Congruency and Incongruency

The organic shapes of bones reflect their functions. The cranial bones fit around the brain to protect it, and the ribs fit around the lungs and heart to protect them and to expand the space

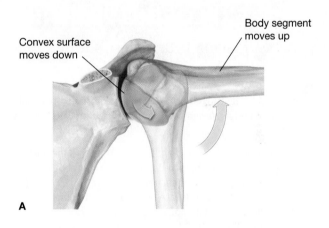

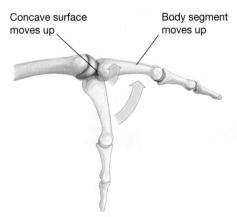

FIGURE 3.23

Concave–convex rule: a) The convex surface of the joint moves in the opposite direction of the moving bone. b) The concave surface of the joint moves in the same direction of the moving bone.

around the lungs during inhalation. The articulating surfaces of joints fit together to move in patterns specific to each joint.

The point of contact between the bones in a synovial joint is **incongruent** because the articulating surfaces rarely match each other in size; one side is usually larger than the other. Compress a synovial joint and the point of contact between the bones will be irregular. Bringing the joint surfaces into total contact during movement can be done only by rocking and sliding one bone against another; they connect at changing points of contact along the IAR. This is what takes place inside most synovial joints during movement.

A joint is considered **congruent** when the space between the articulating surfaces is even. When the joint surfaces have maximum contact, the articulating surfaces fit snugly together like puzzle pieces. The mechanical parts in a machine joint are calibrated to be maximally congruent to minimize friction and ensure a smooth gliding motion between parts. The ball-and-socket joint of the hip is the most congruent joint in the body.

3.2.4 Close-Packed and Loose-Packed Positions

When a joint is in a congruent position, its articulating surfaces have maximal contact. This is called the **close-packed position** of a joint. In the close-packed position, the articulating surfaces reach maximum compression, the joint capsule and supporting ligaments become taut, and the joint becomes maximally stable and difficult to *distract* (to traction or separate). The weight-bearing joints of the knee and hip come into a close-packed position in extension. Given this fact, it seems logical to stand with the legs straight and extended because in the standing position, these weight-bearing joints will be more supportive if they are maximally stable.

In contrast, when a joint is minimally congruent, its articulating surfaces have minimal contact. This is called the **loose-packed position** (or **open-packed position**) of a joint, which is also a resting position. When a joint is in a loose-packed position, its supporting ligaments become slack and its articulating surfaces have minimal contact. The synovial joints of the ankle, knee, and hip come to an

---

EXPLORING TECHNIQUE
Placing Your Client's Joints in a Loose, Resting Position

Placing your clients' limbs in a loose-packed position may help them relax. Here are several ways to do this before you begin a massage.

1. Put a pillow under your client's knees. This takes the ankles, knees, and hips to an open-packed position at about 30 degrees of flexion for each of these joints.
2. Place your client's hands face-down on the abdomen and bend the elbows at an open angle (about 70 degrees), which puts the joints of the upper limbs in a loose-packed position (Figure 3.24a ■).

3. To put your client's spine in a loose-packed position, place your client in a side-lying position and have him or her curl into flexion. Place pillows under your client's head, top arm, and between the knees (Figure 3.24b ■).
4. After you have put your client in a loose-packed position, ask the client if the position feels comfortable. If it does not, have your client move into a comfortable position and notice the position of the upper and lower limbs. *What does the client's preferred resting position tell you about the resting tone of the person's joint capsules and ligaments?*

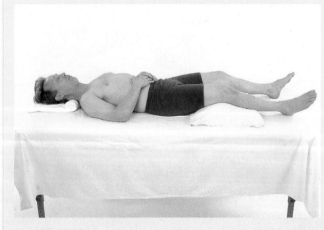

FIGURE 3.24a

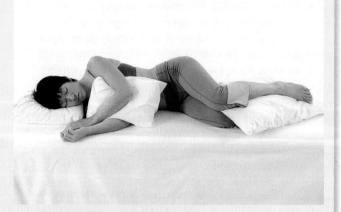

FIGURE 3.24b

open-packed position in a bent-knee posture of about 30 degrees. Passive joint movement should be practiced from a loose-packed position, which is at about 30 degrees of flexion or midway between extreme ranges of motion.[1]

3.3 RANGE OF MOTION

Every freely movable joint has a specific **range of motion (ROM),** which describes the number of degrees in which a joint can move.[2] Range of motion is measured in the degree of the joint angle. In a standing position, the hips extend to 180 degrees. When lifting the knee to the level of the hip, the angle of the hip flexion measures 90 degrees (Figure 3.25 ■).

Range of motion varies among individuals of different genders and ages. In addition, some people are naturally more flexible than others because of genetic predisposition. Women tend to have a greater ROM in the hips and shoulders than men. Age also affects ROM, which usually decreases in seniors due to a loss of elasticity in the connective tissues.

Several structural and functional elements affect the range of motion of a synovial joint:

- The shape of articulating surfaces of the bones
- The elasticity of joint capsules, supporting ligaments, and associated fascias
- The tone, strength, and tightness of any muscles acting on a joint
- Structural injuries, neurological damage, and subsequent guarding against pain

A person's daily activities and habitual body-use habits also affect muscle patterning, which, in turn, affects joint ROM. Muscular holding from physical or emotional pain will restrict joint motion. Inactivity can lead to weak muscles and a fibrous buildup in connective tissues that restrict joint range of motion. That old adage "use it or lose it" holds true for joint and muscle function. When people fail to use a specific range of motion, over time they will lose muscular control and joint flexibility within that range.

Many clients seek massage and bodywork to restore motion to inflexible areas. To achieve this goal, a practitioner will need to know the normal range of motion for each joint and be able to recognize normal and abnormal joint motion. The average ROM for each major joint action is covered in subsequent chapters on specific parts of the body.

3.3.1 Joint Stability and Mobility

There is a functional relationship between joint stability and mobility. Joints need to be mobile enough to move within a normal range, yet stable enough to avoid injury from joint motion outside a normal range.

The **stability** of a joint is defined by its ability to resist displacement. A stable joint can withstand mechanical forces such as compression, torsion, shear, and pull without injury while moving within a normal range. Both passive and active restraints stabilize a synovial joint.

- **Passive restraints** include the joint capsule, supporting ligaments, and associated fascias.
- **Active restraints** include the tendons and muscles acting on that joint and the neurological control a person has over the muscles acting on that joint.

Ligaments and joint capsules contribute about half the total resistance to displacement from movement, whereas tendons only contribute about one-tenth, and muscles contribute the rest.[3]

The **mobility** of a joint describes the range of motion it can be moved without restriction from surrounding structures. The shape of the joint structure affects mobility. The shoulder socket is shallow compared to the hip socket, allowing for a far greater range of mobility. The deeper hip socket is far more stable than the shoulder, which it needs to be able to carry the weight-bearing load of the trunk. Joint mobility is also a measure of flexibility. Muscle tightness can restrict joint mobility. For example, tight hamstring muscles limit the range of hip flexion in many people.

3.3.2 Active and Passive Range of Motion

The range in which people can actively move their joints using their own muscular power defines an **active range of motion (AROM).** The degree to which a person's joints can be passively moved by another person defines a **passive range of motion (PROM).**

A joint can be moved in a greater range with passive motion than with active motion. When a practitioner performs passive joint motion on a client, the client often relaxes the muscles around that joint. This muscular relaxation releases the active restraints, allowing the practitioner to move the joint slightly farther than the client could actively move it.

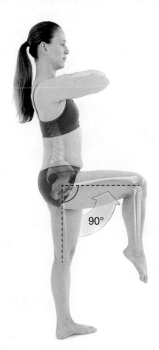

FIGURE 3.25
The range of joint motion is measured by the angle of the joint.

The difference between active and passive range of motion in a normal, healthy joint should be minimal. Any greater difference between the AROM and PROM of a joint can be clinically significant. Here's a case to illustrate the point. Normal hip abduction is 45 degrees. Suppose a client in a side-lying position is only able to lift the leg toward the ceiling (in hip abduction) to 15 degrees, yet you can passively abduct the client's hip to 30 degrees (Figure 3.26a-b ■). There is a 15-degree difference between active and passive range, which is more than minimal. There is also a 15-degree difference between the passive range and the normal range. This indicates a 15-degree restriction to the normal range as well as a 15-degree range in which the client is unable to control the muscles in performing normal hip abduction.

The 15-degree restriction could be coming from passive restraints to hip motion, which you can release with bodywork. The 15-degree range the joint is capable of moving, although the client is unable to make it move, is neurological. This means that the client lacks control over the muscles in this range of abduction, which is a function of the nervous system. To restore this range, the client will need to learn how to move in it, which requires neuromuscular patterning. After releasing the passive restraints, you can guide the client through an increased range of motion using patterning techniques, which are covered in the neuromuscular chapter.

The active range in which a person can move a joint defines its **physiological movement.** For example, the normal range of motion in the fingers is flexion and extension. You could, however, passively rotate the joints in the fingers to a small degree. This range of rotation demonstrates the **accessory movement** of the joint—the range that a person cannot actively move a joint, but in which another person can move it. Accessory motion is also referred to as **joint play.**

Joints can only move so far. At the end of range they hit a *physiological barrier* that prevents further motion. There are three normal physiological barriers to motion:

- Bone hits bone (occurs only in elbow extension and jaw occlusion).
- Joint capsules stretch to their elastic limit (the most common barrier to movement in synovial joints).
- Tissue bumps up against tissue (occurs only in elbow, hip, and knee flexion).

3.3.3 Hypomobility and Hypermobility

Restrictions to joint mobility cause **hypomobility,** which is a limited range of joint motion. Hypomobility can be caused by chronically contracted muscles, fibrous scarring of ligaments or the joint capsule, damage to joint structures, and neurological damage to or lack of control over the muscles acting on a joint. It can also be caused by prolonged infirmity or long-term inactivity.

When a joint becomes hypomobile, it loses its joint play. As a rule, increasing joint motion in one plane always increases motion in all planes. Taking a hypomobile joint through its range of accessory movements can help to restore normal physiological movement in a hypomobile joint.

The opposite of restricted range of motion is too much motion. Some people possess an innate inclination toward **hypermobility,** which is excessive joint motion. Hypermobility is usually due to a laxity of ligaments and joint capsules. Laxity in one joint does not necessarily mean laxity in all the joints. Some activities require hypermobility in specific joint motions, such as in the spines, hips, and feet of dancers and gymnasts. Performers or athletes may even train for hypermobility in certain joints by deliberately overstretching them.

Hypermobility differs from instability. A person with hypermobile joints can usually control the movement of lax joints, such as a gymnast performing a back walkover. In contrast, people with joint instability cannot control joint motion outside of a normal range. Since joint instability

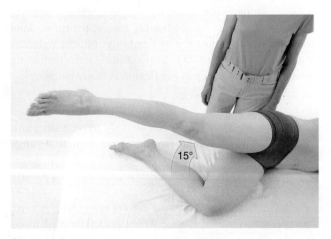
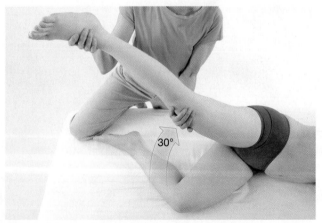

A **B**

FIGURE 3.26

a) Range of abduction during active movement is 15 degrees. b) Range of abduction during passive movement is 30 degrees.

results from the lack of control over muscles stabilizing the joints, this topic is expanded upon in the chapter on muscles.

Hypermobile joints are susceptible to repetitive injuries, which can lead to tissue damage, instability, and joint dislocation. For example, a person with hypermobility in the ankles may develop a habit of rolling out on the feet, spraining ligaments, and straining muscles and tendons. Note the difference between sprains and strains:

- **Sprains** refer to injuries to noncontractile tissues such as ligaments, joint capsules, cartilage, fascias, blood vessels, and bursa.
- **Strains** refer to injuries to contractile tissues such as muscles, tendons, and their attachments to bone. *(One easy way to remember the difference between the two is that strain has a* t, *which stands for tendons.)*

3.4   CLINICAL APPLICATIONS FOR JOINT MOVEMENT

Manual therapy techniques often use active or passive movement of the joints, particularly techniques that work with the muscles. There is a complex interplay between joint proprioceptors, muscle tone, and neuromuscular patterning. Because of this interconnection, moving the joints within their physiological range provides many therapeutic benefits in the practice of massage and bodywork.

Active movement techniques have neurological effects that include:

- Reorganizing firing patterns in muscles and along kinetic chains
- Improving the overall balance and efficiency of neuromuscular patterns
- Releasing chronic muscular holding in overworked muscles

- Accessing reflexes during *muscle energy techniques* (covered in the neuromuscular chapter)

Passive joint movement techniques have mechanical effects that include:

- Increasing range of motion
- Stretching soft tissues around the joint
- Triggering the relaxation response in associated muscles
- Alleviating pain by reducing hypersensitivity to motion
- Improving the lubrication of joint surfaces
- Improving the client's awareness of joint patterns

In this last section, we look at the clinical skills used in massage and bodywork practices that involve joint motion. Although we touch lightly on the use of active and passive range of motion to assess the client's condition, this last section focuses more on *when* and *how* to use active and passive joint motion during a session. We examine the integrated use AROM, PROM, and resisted client motion in a three-tiered client assessment in the neuromuscular chapter.

3.4.1   Active Motion

Active motion includes any movements that clients perform of their own volition. Observing a client's active movements can provide you with a snapshot of information about the client's muscle and joint patterns. You can also observe whether or not clients can move on their own, their willingness to move, and their quality of movement. With active movement, clients demonstrate how far their muscles will actually move the joints, which is a measure of tone, strength, and coordination.

Observing the client's movement at the beginning of the session helps a practitioner to begin to understand the client's problem. During a session, you may want to ask the client to perform an active movement to check the effectiveness of the work. If the restrictions to motion have been successfully released, the range of motion will increase.

BRIDGE TO PRACTICE
Stretching Targeted Tissues Only

Caution: If a person has hypermobile joints, stretching ligaments and joint capsules is contraindicated.

Stretch ligaments and joint capsules only when you are sure that these joint structures restrict joint mobility. A client with joint stiffness due to scarring following a surgery would benefit

from having the ligaments stretched around the restricted joint. However, a hypermobile client who has restricted joint motion due to muscular spasms from an injury needs work that lengthens the muscles while avoiding stretching the joint capsule or the ligaments around the restricted joint. Doing so would increase the hypermobility of the joint, possibly making the condition worse and even leading to joint instability.

If chronic muscular contractions that cause pain during motion have been successfully released, the movement will be pain-free.

Cue an active movement during the client intake by saying, "Show me what movement causes you pain or feels restricted." Then observe the range, quality, and overall pattern of the client's movement pattern. Also, note the client's willingness to move and any symptoms or reactions the client has or reports during the movement.

Clients are often apprehensive about moving when it causes pain. If the client experiences pain during active movement and not during passive movement, this usually indicates some kind of muscular problem. If the client is injured and has tissue damage, the AROM will indicate the range of motion to be avoided or be careful with during the session.

3.4.2 Passive Motion

Passive motion is joint movement that one person performs on another. Passive range of motion techniques involve passively moving a client's joint through a normal range of motion to the end of range. Passive joint stretching is widely used in massage and bodywork to stretch muscles and joint structures in order to increase range of motion.

The direction a joint can be passively moved depends on the degrees of motion in the joint. For example, the knee can flex and extend; therefore, passive motion on the knee can only be performed in flexion and extension. In contrast, the hip can flex, extend, abduct, adduct, and rotate in either direction, so you can passively move the hip joint in six directions through multiple degrees of motion.

Passive range of motion tests can be used to determine which tissues restrict movement and cause pain. We examine AROM and PROM assessment tests in the neuromuscular chapter. For now, know that it is essential to have clients with any type of joint issues to demonstrate their AROMs before taking them through PROMs in the same actions. If the client has any symptoms or pain during active motion, the use of passive motion should be avoided in that range during a session.

3.4.2.1 NORMAL END-FEELS

When a joint reaches the end of its physiological range of motion, something restricts further motion. The quality of the restriction is called the **end-feel** of that joint. Recall that there are three normal restrictions to synovial joint motion: bone, joint capsule, and soft tissues. Each of these three restrictions has a distinct end-feel. End-feel is an important assessment indicator. We look at end-feels in two categories: normal and abnormal/pathological.

A healthy joint exhibits one of the three normal end-feels, which are bony, firm, and soft (Figure 3.27 ■):[4]

- In a **bony end-feel,** movement is restricted because bone meets bones. Only two joints have a normal end-feel that is hard: elbow extension and jaw elevation. When the jaw elevates to close the mouth, teeth meet teeth at end range, which prevents further motion.
- In a **firm** or **capsular end-feel,** the position of the joint stretches the capsule and supporting ligaments to their elastic limits, preventing further motion. Most synovial joints have a capsular end-feel that feels like reaching the elastic limit of thick leather.
- In a **soft end-feel,** tissue meeting tissue, or tissue approximation, prevents further motion. The joints with a soft end-feel—the hip, knee, and elbow—move into deep flexion when a person curls into full-body flexed position.

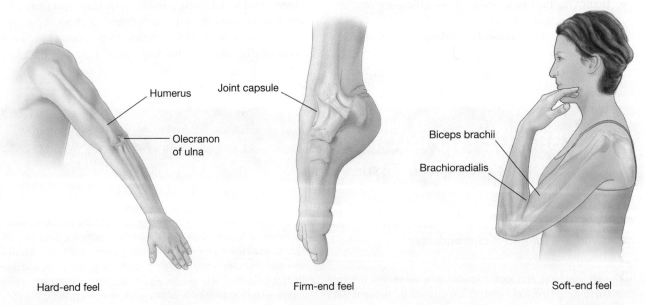

Hard-end feel   Firm-end feel   Soft-end feel

FIGURE 3.27

Three types of **normal end feels** in joint motion

GUIDELINES
Steps in Passive Range of Motion Stretching

1. The client should be relaxed and comfortable.
2. Move only one joint at a time. Move the unaffected side first.
3. Begin with the joint in a neutral position.
4. Hold both sides of the joint. Fully support the joint in a firm but comfortable grasp.
5. Tell the client to inform you of any pain or discomfort the PROM causes.
6. Put traction on the joint before moving it to avoid pain in joint structures that could be compressed and pinched during joint motion.
7. Use one hand to stabilize the nonmoving bone, the other hand to support and move the moving bone in the joint. Move the joint in a linear motion to end range. Never force the motion.
8. Observe the client during the test. *Stop immediately if you notice or the client tells you the motion is causing pain or discomfort.*
9. At end range, stretch the joint a little bit farther. To confirm you have reached end range, ask the client if he or she feels a stretch.
10. Perform a PROM on the same joint on the other side to make a bilateral comparison.

Before stretching any joint to end range, you will want to know the normal end-feels of any joint. Most synovial joints have a firm end-feel. Only the knee, hip, elbows, fingers, and toes have a soft end-feel in flexion. This should be easy to remember because these are all the joints that go into deep flexion when the body is curled in a fetal position. The main joint to avoid stretching in hyperextension is the elbow because it presses bone into bone.

3.4.2.2 ABNORMAL END-FEELS

Many things can restrict joint motion and lead to an abnormal end-feel: pain, injury, muscle tension, neurological damage, and loose bodies (such as chipped cartilage) floating inside the joint. Evaluating the cause of abnormal end-feels is outside the scope of practice of massage and bodywork. However, it is important to be familiar with them to know when a PROM is contraindicated.[5] Here is a list of five abnormal end-feels that you could encounter when moving a joint to end range:

- A **boggy end-feel** is characterized by a mushy, spongy quality, usually from excess fluid or swelling in and around the joint.
- A **hard end-feel** is characterized by an abrupt stop that occurs short of the normal end range, caused by an abnormal growth, a loose body, or bony restriction in the joint.
- A **lax end-feel** lacks an increase in tension; the range of motion goes beyond normal.
- In an **empty end-feel,** or **spasm end-feel,** the joint movement causes pain; therefore, muscular guarding prevents motion beyond a limited range.
- A **fibrotic end-feel** is characterized by a rapid buildup of tension, usually because of fibrotic thickening around the joint, perhaps due to scarring from injuries or surgeries. Joints with fibrotic end-feels that have restricted range of motion need to be stretched, which can be done with passive range of motion stretching and/or *cross-fiber friction* around the joint structures.

GUIDELINES
Contraindications to Practicing Passive Joint Motion with Clients

1. Do not stretch hypermobile joints because the joint structures are already lax. Stretching them will exacerbate the hypermobility.
2. Do not move injured joint structures or surrounding tissues.
3. Do not move any joints that the client does not want to have passively moved.
4. Stop passive joint motion if the client experiences any strong or stabbing joint pain that causes muscular guarding.
5. Stop passive joint motion when encountering an abnormal end-feel, except for a fibrotic end-feel.

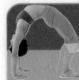

BRIDGE TO PRACTICE
Working with Clients with Movement Restrictions

Clients may report restrictions to movement during an intake interview or on their health histories. When your client has an injury, chronic pain, or some kind of movement restriction, ask the client to demonstrate the limited range of motion to show you which joints are restricted and/or which movements cause pain. If a movement causes pain, avoid taking your client through this range of movement during the session.

3.4.3   Resisted Range of Motion

When you have a client move against applied resistance, this is called **resisted range of motion** (RROM). There are many clinical uses for this technique (Figure 3.28 ■). You might have the client move against resistance to get a certain muscle to bulge so that it can be more easily located during palpation. Resistance can be applied through range of motion to improve the quality of joint motion.

Resisted range of motion tests are also practiced to differentiate contractile from noncontractile tissues as the cause of joint restriction or pain. To use RROM to improve joint function, you need to understand the range of motion in each joint and how the muscles act on that joint. Instructions for RROM are integrated into the muscle palpation exercises in the chapters covering the different areas of the body in Part 2.

3.4.4   Joint Mobilization

Joint mobilization is a therapeutic technique in which a manual therapist uses passive joint motion to restore normal joint position, to stretch a stiff joint, to relieve joint pain limiting active movement, and to help a client recover from an injury or trauma.[6]

Mobilization techniques practiced in physical therapy involve the specific gliding movement of the articular surfaces of a single joint in the direction of restriction or through an accessory range of motion. Restrictions are determined by the specific evaluation tests of the physiological and accessory movements of a joint, the degree of restriction in the joint, and the cause of restriction.

Mobilization techniques practiced in massage and bodywork are more generalized. They focus on overall loosening of joints along a kinetic chain, using rhythmic shaking and jiggling techniques that come out of Swedish massage traditions and/or the Trager method. Rather than being systemized, Trager focuses more on the quality of touch and movement, using gentle movements that emphasize rhythmic rotation, traction, and rocking movements. Gentle and rhythmic joint motion coaxes the client's body to release both mental and muscular control, inducing a state of muscular relaxation. The mobilization of a restricted joint can restore the sequence of movement along a kinetic chain.

3.4.5   Joint Articulation

In the same way that articulate people speak with clarity, power, and persuasion, people with articulate bodies move with patterns of refined, precise control. A simple hand gesture can reflect a subtlety of muscular control that gives the motion a deep, expressive quality. Joints are referred to as articulations, but the term *articulation* also refers to a quality of joint motion. In an articulate action, the joints roll and glide along graded pathways. For example, when lifting the arm, the shoulder muscles contract in an ordered sequence, creating a smooth and even, rather than a choppy and erratic, quality of motion.

Although specific joint mobilization and manipulation techniques lie outside the scope of massage and bodywork, you can still move the client's joint with specificity whenever using passive joint movement. Joint stretching, as taught in most massage programs, usually focuses on the stretch at the end of range. **Joint articulation** as a therapeutic technique is the slow, specific movement of a client's

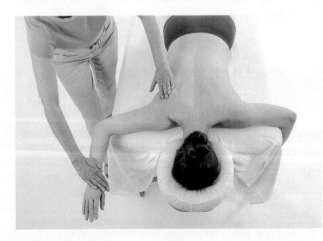

FIGURE 3.28
Resisted range of motion

joint that focuses on the quality of joint motion with the goal of improving joint arthrokinematics.

When practicing joint articulation, move the joints slowly, visualizing the articulating surfaces while also tracking how these surfaces actually move in relation to each other inside the joint. Depending on the shape of the surfaces, some articulations will need to be rotated during passive motion, whereas other joint surfaces will need to be glided or rolled.

Keep in mind that moving a joint too fast is like driving too fast. Speedy drivers miss the signs and turns along the journey and have more accidents. Moving a joint slowly while paying attention to its internal articulation pattern decreases the risk of injuring the client. It also gives the client time to pay attention and to relax into the motion, which improves client awareness and enhances the relaxation response. As mentioned earlier, the joint structures are rich in sensory nerves. If the movement is slow enough, the client's brain will have time to register subtle changes in position and motion and as a result, reset the muscle tone.

CONCLUSION

Jumping on a trampoline provides many examples of the joint movements and concepts discussed in this chapter. As the jumper bounces up and down, he moves in a linear motion that slightly flexes and extends the joints of his lower limbs.

A jackknife folds his hips and body in a sagittal plane via a rotary motion, a twisting flip moves his body along a curvilinear pathway, and a curled flip spins his body in an axial turn.

While bouncing, the feet push down in a closed-chain action against a spring-like surface. The rebound shoots his body into the air in an open-chain action. During the pushoff moment, his joints compress into a close-packed position; during the height of a bounce, his joints reach their most loose-packed position. Jumping jacks pump the jumper's limbs between alternating abduction and adduction movements in the frontal plane, gliding and rolling both his shoulder and hip joints in their sockets. A back drop lands his body in a supine position, while a belly drop lands his in a prone position, both in the horizontal plane.

The force of the trampoline's elasticity rebounds through the elastic tissues around the joints and the shock-absorbing cartilages and fluids within the joints. The elastic suppleness of the joints allows him to bend and rotate the body within a normal physiological range. If he has hypermobile joints, he will be able to throw his legs into the splits at the peak of suspension. A person with hypomobile joints will barely be able to touch his toes.

The therapeutic effects of trampoline jumping can also be approximated during a bodywork session with a rhythmic quality of oscillating motion that passively rolls, glides, and rocks the client's joints with the intention of improving articulation as well as synovial fluid circulation.

SUMMARY POINTS TO REMEMBER

1. A joint, also called an articulation, is a place where two bones meet. A bone provides a lever for movement; a joint provides a fulcrum for movement.

2. Osteokinematics refers to the different types of joint motion. Arthrokinematics refers to the types of movement inside a joint.

3. Linear (translatory) motion follows a straight path. Rotary (angular or axial) motion bends a joint into an angle. Curvilinear motion follows a curved pathway.

4. Axial (rotary) motion occurs around a fixed point. Examples of axial motion include flexion and extension in the sagittal plane, abduction and adduction in the frontal plane, and rotation in the horizontal plane.

5. In a nonaxial motion, one joint surface slides against another joint surface. Examples of nonaxial motions include elevation, depression, protraction, and retraction of the scapula. Most daily activities involve a combination of axial and nonaxial joint motion, such as supination of the forearm and circumduction of the wrist.

6. In an open kinetic chain, the end of a moving part of the body is free. In a closed kinetic chain, the end of a moving part is fixed. The hand and arm move in an open

kinematic chain when waving and in a closed kinetic chain when pushing a cart.

7. The articulating surfaces of a joint can roll, glide, or spin. The arthrokinematics of each joint depend on the shape of its articulating surfaces. For example, ellipsoid joints roll and glide, plane joints glide, and pivot joints spin.

8. The concave–convex rule of joint motion states that when a bone with a convex joint surface moves, the joint surface always moves in the opposite direction of the moving bone. In contrast, when a bone with a concave joint surface moves, the joint surface always moves in the same direction of the moving bone.

9. In a close-packed position, the articulating surfaces of a joint have maximum contact. In a loose-packed (open-packed) position, which is also the resting or neutral position of a joint, the articulating surfaces have the least amount of contact.

10. Range of motion (ROM) describes the degrees in which a joint can move. The ROM is affected by the shape of the joint's surfaces, elasticity of connective tissues around the joint, tone of muscles acting on the joint, and injuries that have occurred to that joint.

11. The stability of a joint is defined by its ability to resist displacement. Stability is maintained by the passive restraints of noncontractile tissues (joint capsules and ligaments) and the active restraints of contractile tissues (muscles and tendons).

12. The mobility of a joint refers to its movement within a normal range. Hypermobility refers to excessive joint motion. Hypomobility is limited joint motion. Instability is the lack of muscular control over joint motion.

13. Active joint motion is generated by a person's muscular activity; passive joint motion is generated by an outside force, such as another person moving the joint; resisted joint motion occurs when a person moves a joint against an external force.

14. A sprain is damage to noncontractile tissue such as a ligament or a joint capsule. A strain is damage to contractile tissues such as a muscle or a tendon.

15. When a joint reaches the end of its range of motion, there is a quality of restriction called the end-feel. A normal joint exhibits three types of end-feel: hard (bone meets bone), firm (joint capsule reaches its elastic limit), and soft (tissue meets tissue).

REVIEW QUESTIONS

1. Match the three types of motions—linear, rotary, and curvilinear—to the following definitions:
   a. a circular movement of a bone around a fixed axis
   b. a movement along a curved pathway
   c. a movement along a straight path

2. Name three joint movements that occur in each plane.

3. Four nonaxial movements of the scapulae and the planes of each motion are
   a. elevation and depression in the horizontal plane plus protraction and retraction in the frontal plane.
   b. elevation and depression in the sagittal plane plus protraction and retraction in the horizontal plane.
   c. elevation and depression in the frontal plane plus protraction and retraction in the sagittal plane.
   d. elevation and depression in the frontal plane plus protraction and retraction in the horizontal plane.

4. Circumduction is
   a. a motion that inscribes a cone-like shape in space.
   b. a circular motion that combines flexion, extension, and supination.
   c. a movement that can only be done at ball-and-socket joints.
   d. a nonaxial gliding motion.

5. True or false (circle one). In a motion that involves an open kinetic chain, the distal end of the moving limb is fixed.

6. The three types of movement that occur between articulating surfaces within a joint are
   a. rolling, spinning, and turning.
   b. sliding, gliding, and rolling.
   c. rolling, gliding, and spinning.
   d. rolling, sliding, and turning.

7. Of the three types of joint movements identified in the last question, identify which one is nonaxial and briefly describe this type of joint motion.

8. True or false (circle one). The concave–convex rule states that when a bone with a concave surface moves, the joint's surface moves in the opposite direction of the bone.

9. Why would massage and bodywork practitioners need to understand the concave–convex rule?

10. The difference between a close-packed and loose-packed position of a joint is that
   a. in a close-packed position, the joint is maximally compressed and the joint capsule and ligaments are taut. In a loose-packed position, the joint capsule and ligaments are slack and there is space between the articular surfaces.
   b. in a close-packed position, the joint is slack and the joint capsule and ligaments are overstretched. In a loose-packed position, the joint capsule and ligaments are slack and the joint is in a resting position.
   c. in a close-packed position, the joint surfaces are fused and the joint capsule and ligaments are taut. In a loose-packed position, the joint capsule and ligaments are slack and there is space between the articular surfaces.
   d. in a close-packed position, the joint is maximally rotated, which makes the joint capsule and ligaments taut. In a loose-packed position, the joint capsule and ligaments are slack and there is space between the articular surfaces.

11. What four factors affect the range of motion?
   a. Range of motion is affected by the type of the joint cartilage, the elasticity of joint tissues, the condition of the muscles around the joint, and injuries and pain.
   b. Range of motion is affected by the shape of the joint surfaces, the innervations of joint tissues, the condition of the muscles around the joint, and injuries and pain.
   c. Range of motion is affected by the shape of the joint surfaces, the elasticity of joint tissues, the condition of the muscles around the joint, and injuries and pain.
   d. Range of motion is affected by the shape of the joint surfaces, the elasticity of joint tissues, the condition of the muscles around the joint, and synovial fluid.

12. Joint stability is
    a. the degree to which a joint can stretch.
    b. the ability of the joint structures to displace from a neutral position.
    c. the capacity of joint restraints to prevent motion beyond a normal range.
    d. the effect of hyaline cartilage to lubricate a joint during joint motion.

13. A person's ankle can be passively flexed to a 100-degree angle but actively flexed to a 90-degree angle because
    a. when the ankle is actively stretched in flexion, the muscles are relaxed so the ankle can move a little bit farther than when the ankle is passively stretched.
    b. when the ankle is passively stretched in flexion, the muscles are contracted so the ankle can move less than when a person actively flexes the ankle.
    c. when the ankle is passively stretched in flexion, the muscles are relaxed so the ankle can move less than when a person actively flexes the ankle.
    d. when the ankle is passively stretched in flexion, the muscles are relaxed so the ankle can move a little bit farther than when a person actively flexes the ankle.

14. True or false (circle one). A hypermobile joint has a restricted range of motion due to some kind of restriction.

15. The difference between a sprain and a strain is that
    a. a sprain is damage to contractile tissues such as ligaments and joint capsules; a strain is damage to noncontractile tissues such as muscles and tendons.
    b. a sprain is damage to noncontractile tissues such as ligaments and joint capsules; a strain is damage to contractile tissues such as muscles and tendons.
    c. a strain is damage to noncontractile tissues such as cartilage and bursae; a sprain is damage to contractile tissues such as muscles and tendons.
    d. a sprain is damage to noncontractile tissues such as spongy and compact bone; a strain is damage to contractile tissues such as smooth muscles.

16. Why would a practitioner ask a client to demonstrate an active movement?

17. Match the three types of normal end-feels—bony, firm, and soft—with the following definitions:
    a. A pliable feel and the end range of motion because soft tissue of another part of the body prevents further motion.
    b. A hard and nongiving feel at the end range of motion because bone meets bone.
    c. A capsular, leathery feel at the end range of motion restricted by the elastic limits of ligaments and the joint capsule, but when held under pressure, moves a little further.

18. It is *not* contraindicated to stretch a joint to end range when a client
    a. reports pain during any range of joint motion.
    b. has restricted joint motion due to tight muscles.
    c. is uncomfortable and does not want to be stretched.
    d. has hypermobile joints due to lax ligaments.

Notes

1. Magee, D. (2007). *Orthopedic Physical Assessment* (5th ed.), Philadelphia: Saunders.
2. Kendall, F., McCreary, E., Provance, P., & Romani, A. (2005). *Muscles: Testing and Function, with Posture and Pain* (5th ed.). Baltimore: Lippincott, Williams & Wilkins.
3. Alter, M. (2004). *Science of Flexibility* (3rd ed.). Champaign, IL: Human Kinetics.
4. Cyriax, J., & Cyriax, P. (1996). *Cyriax's Illustrated Manual of Orthopedic Medicine* (2nd ed.). Edinburgh, UK: Butterworth-Heinemann.
5. Isaacs, E., & Bookhout, M. (2002). *Bourdillon's Spinal Manipulation* (5th ed.). Boston: Butterworth-Heinemann.
6. Maitland, G. (1991). *Peripheral Manipulation* (3rd ed.). Oxford, UK: Butterworth-Heinemann.

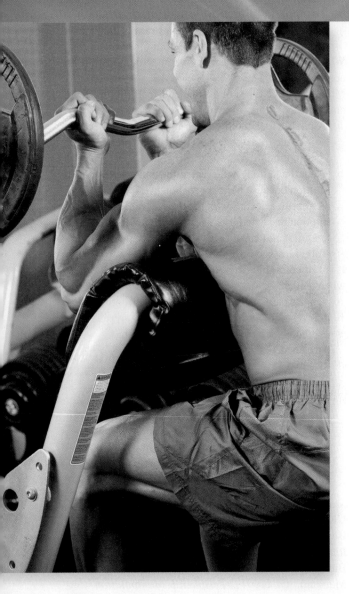

CHAPTER OUTLINE

Chapter Objectives

Key Terms

4.1 Structural Features of Skeletal Muscles

4.2 Contractile Structures and Mechanisms in Muscles

4.3 The Continuity of Muscle and Fascia

4.4 Muscle Tension and Contractile Forces

4.5 Changing Roles of Muscles

Conclusion

Summary Points to Remember

Review Questions

People weight-train for many reasons: to look and feel better, to build strength or muscle mass, or to develop endurance. The muscular system adapts to the specific demands placed on it, therefore it is important to establish goals for training based on the results you desire. Building strength is about increasing the force generation of a muscle, which requires one type of training. Building muscle mass is about increasing the number and size of muscle cells, which requires another type of training. Building endurance is about improving the metabolic efficiency of the muscles, which requires yet another type of training.

Weight trainers determine the best program for each outcome based on the percentage of a maximum load (weight) that a person can lift, or on the number of repetitions a person can do to failure. Lifting high load with few repetitions builds strength; lifting low loads with many repetitions builds endurance and burns fat. Even without a specific program, weight training never has just one outcome; the results always overlap, building some level of endurance, mass, and strength.

Different types of weight training can develop different body types, although the genetic predisposition of a person factors into the equation. Power lifters tend to retain more body fat, whereas body builders with restricted diets develop sculpted musculature.

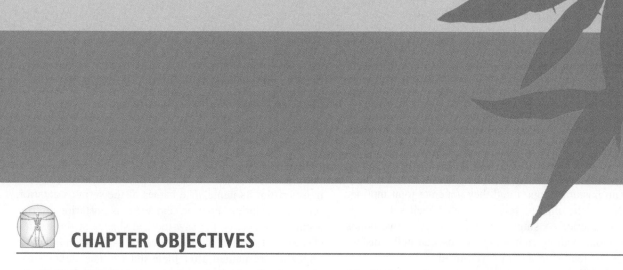

 CHAPTER OBJECTIVES

1. Define the muscular system and describe its main kinesiological functions.

2. List and describe five types of muscle shapes.

3. Define how a muscle is named and the origin and insertion of a muscle.

4. List and define four properties of muscle tissue.

5. Describe the smallest contractile unit and the overall structure of a muscle.

6. Name and describe the theory that explains muscular contraction.

7. Define a motor unit and the all-or-none law.

8. Define the recruitment process with a single muscle.

9. Define muscle tone.

10. Name the energy source for contraction and two ways that muscles metabolize it.

11. Define and contrast muscle spasms, muscle contractures, and muscle fatigue.

12. List and briefly describe three types of contractile fibers in muscle.

13. Define and describe the myofascial system and the manual techniques that address it.

14. Describe passive tension and active tension.

15. List and define three types of contraction and define the length–tension relationship.

16. Describe the different functions that a muscle can perform in movement.

17. Define coordination and describe the process of a coordinated movement.

18. Describe the difference between passive and active insufficiency in biarticular muscles.

KEY TERMS

Adaptive shortening	Excursion	Myofascial system
Agonist	Isometric contraction	Origin and insertion
Antagonist	Long axis of a bone	Prime mover
Biarticular muscles	Mobilizer	Recruitment
Concentric contraction	Motor unit	Stabilizer
Contracture	Muscle fatigue	Stretch weakening
Creep	Muscle tone	Synergist
Eccentric contraction	Myofascial release (MFR)	Tensegrity system

There are three different types of muscle tissue in the body: cardiac muscle (found in the heart), smooth muscle (found in the organs), and skeletal muscle. Of the three, only **skeletal muscle** pulls on the bones of the skeletal system. Around 650 skeletal muscles, plus all their associated connective tissues, fascias, and tendons, make up the **muscular system.** All references to muscle made from here on will refer to skeletal muscles unless otherwise indicated.

Muscles carry out two main movement functions: they maintain postural support and they generate joint motion. Muscles are the ultimate force generator: their sole capacity is contraction. A single muscle attaches to two bones across a joint. During contraction, a muscular pull transfers through the tendon to a bony lever, resulting in joint compression and joint motion.

Understanding *how* the muscular system produces movement is essential for being able to adapt the many massage and bodywork techniques for working with the muscular system to a variety of clinical applications. As we move through this chapter, keep in mind that learning about the muscular system is essential to a study of kinesiology and to all forms of massage and bodywork.

We begin this chapter with an overview of the structural features of the muscular system. After that, we drop down to a microscopic level to examine how muscle cells contract. Then we look at the integral relationship between the muscles and fascia in a myofascial network, at the contractile forces generated by muscles, and at length–tension relationships. This chapter ends with a study of the different types of contractions and the changing roles that a single muscle can play in different actions.

4.1 STRUCTURAL FEATURES OF SKELETAL MUSCLES

The muscular system consists of a continuous network of muscles and connective tissues that lie directly under the skin and cover the entire body like a well-tailored elastic suit. Also, like a patchwork quilt, the skeletal muscles in the body are knitted together as one unified fabric of interconnected elastic panels. The fabric moves in response to the electrical stimulation of the nerves, changing shape as individual muscles contract and pull along the many movement pathways and avenues that make up our human movement repertoire.

All muscles in this complex network function in synchrony to produce coordinated actions. No one muscle acts alone. For muscles to move joints, contractions that shorten working muscles in one area must be matched with the elongation of muscles in other areas.

To picture a topical map of the muscular system, Renaissance artists depicted muscles by painting a three-dimensional global map of muscles called an "ecroche" on a plaster model of the human body. If one stretched the imagination even further and could visualize the model moving, it would be easy to see how the changing muscular tensions in one area of the body translate through the fabric of the entire system (Figure 4.1 ■). The muscular system is the ultimate shape-shifter of the body.

4.1.1 Muscle Names

Rather than simply memorizing the names and locations of the many muscles, a student of kinesiology can pick up clues about the shape, location, size, and function of each muscle from its name. The names of the serratus anterior, serratus posterior superior, and serratus posterior inferior accurately describe the saw-toothed shapes of these muscles as well as their physical locations. The rhomboid and trapezius are named after their shapes. The flexor carpi ulnaris is named after its attachment sites and function—it attaches to the carpal bones of the wrist on the side of the ulnar bone and is a wrist flexor.

Variations in the names and descriptions of muscular structures and functions invariably show up in textbooks. The reason for this is that the taxonomy of names of skeletal muscles was developed by scientists who did not always share the same view of the body. In addition, slight variations in muscular anatomy exist from one person to the next.

Another aspect of naming muscles that can be confusing is that some muscles are named according to their primary movement functions. This can mislead a student to view that movement as the muscle's only action. For example, in the anatomical position, the adductor muscles of the hip attach along a line of pull that favors adduction, although individual adductor muscles also assist the actions of hip flexion and extension.

4.1.2 Muscle Shapes

A muscle's shape reflects its arrangement of fibers and the direction of their pull during contraction. Muscles come in strap, fusiform, rhomboidal, triangular, and pennate shapes (Figure 4.2 ■):

- A **strap muscle** has long, flat, parallel fibers that run the length of the muscle and culminate in a wide, flat tendon. The tendons of strap muscles can be segmented, as in the rectus abdominis.
- A **fusiform muscle** is shaped like a spindle, wide in the belly and tapered on the ends, with parallel fibers that narrow into long and strong cord-like tendons. Fusiform muscles can have more than one part, such as the two-headed biceps brachii.
- A **rhomboidal muscle** is flat with four sides in a quadrate or parallelogram shape. Its parallel fibers culminate in flat tendons that attach along a bony ridge or line.
- A **triangular** (convergent) **muscle** has fibers arranged in a fan-like shape that converge into a point. Its convergent fibers often twist into a spiral shape, as in the pectoralis major and trapezius.
- The **pennate muscles** have fibers that run at oblique angles to their central tendons, like fibers in a feather.

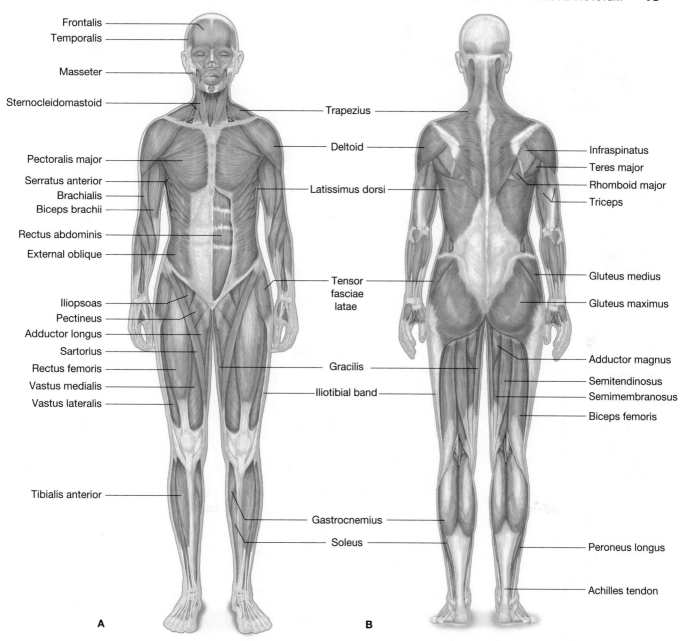

Frontalis
Temporalis
Masseter
Sternocleidomastoid
Pectoralis major
Serratus anterior
Brachialis
Biceps brachii
Rectus abdominis
External oblique
Iliopsoas
Pectineus
Adductor longus
Sartorius
Rectus femoris
Vastus medialis
Vastus lateralis
Tibialis anterior

Trapezius
Deltoid
Latissimus dorsi
Tensor fasciae latae
Gracilis
Iliotibial band
Gastrocnemius
Soleus

Infraspinatus
Teres major
Rhomboid major
Triceps
Gluteus medius
Gluteus maximus
Adductor magnus
Semitendinosus
Semimembranosus
Biceps femoris
Peroneus longus
Achilles tendon

A

B

FIGURE 4.1

Muscular system: a) Anterior view b) Posterior view

BRIDGE TO PRACTICE
Utilizing Muscle Fiber Arrangement

You will want to understand the fiber arrangement of each muscle for several reasons. This information will help you accurately palpate the muscle, figure out its line of pull and joint action when it contracts, and accurately apply manual techniques that run parallel or perpendicular to its fibers.

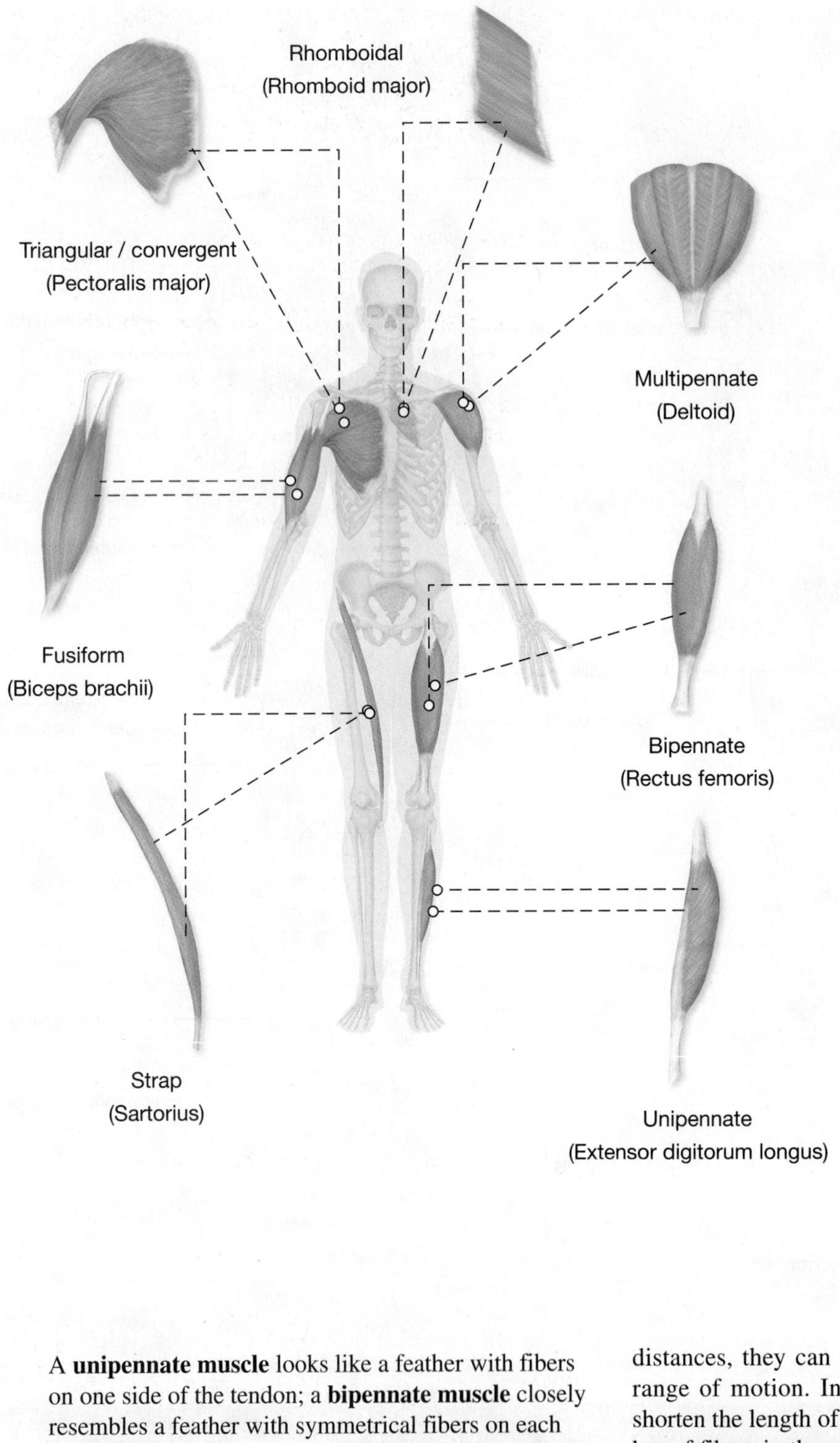

FIGURE 4.2
Types of muscles

Rhomboidal
(Rhomboid major)

Triangular / convergent
(Pectoralis major)

Multipennate
(Deltoid)

Fusiform
(Biceps brachii)

Bipennate
(Rectus femoris)

Strap
(Sartorius)

Unipennate
(Extensor digitorum longus)

A **unipennate muscle** looks like a feather with fibers on one side of the tendon; a **bipennate muscle** closely resembles a feather with symmetrical fibers on each side of the central tendon; and a **multipennate muscle** looks like a fan of overlapping feathers.

The length of the fibers in a muscle determines how far that muscle can move a bone. Muscles with long parallel fibers have the length advantage; muscles with shorter diagonal fibers have the strength advantage. **Excursion** is the distance a muscle can lengthen or shorten (Figure 4.3 ■). The longer the fibers of a muscle, the more capacity it has to pull a bone over a greater distance (Figure 4.4 ■). Because strap and fusiform muscles can contract over longer

distances, they can usually move joints through a larger range of motion. In contrast, pennate muscles can only shorten the length of their fibers, although the greater number of fibers in the cross section of a pennate muscle gives it a capacity for generating a stronger force (Figure 4.5 ■).

Examples of muscle function as it relates to fiber arrangement can be found in the hamstrings and quadriceps. The hamstring muscles cross the hip and knee. The vastus muscles of the quadriceps group cross only the knee. The long parallel fibers of the hamstrings are better suited for shortening along a longer excursion across two joints, whereas the pennate fibers of the vastus muscles are better suited for generating greater force to extend the knees against gravity.

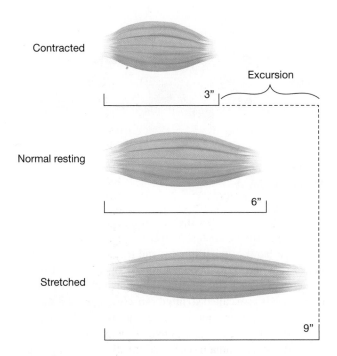

FIGURE 4.3
Excursion of a muscle

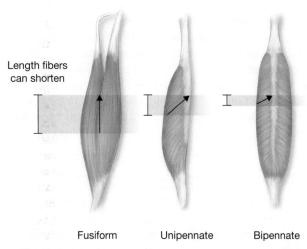

FIGURE 4.5
The **line of pull** in fusiform, unipennate, and bipennate muscles

4.1.3 Muscle Attachments

Muscles can also be named after the bones to which they attach. The sternocleidomastoid attaches to three bony attachment sites: the sternum, clavicle, and mastoid process (Figure 4.6 ■). The frontalis on the forehead attaches to the frontal bone of the cranium.

Each muscle usually attaches to the bones making up a joint in two places, which describe that muscle's origin and insertion.

- The **origin** is traditionally the most proximal attachment site of a muscle. It can also be named as the attachment that remains fixed during a specific motion.
- The **insertion** is traditionally the most distal attachment site of a muscle. It can also be named as the attachment that moves during a specific motion.

Identifying the distal and proximal of some muscles, such as muscles along the spine, is difficult. Other muscles are too short or weak to generate motion, so naming the origin and insertion after a fixed or moving end becomes confusing. To clear up any issues in deciding which end of a muscle is which, muscular attachments are also described as *proximal* and *distal attachments* for muscles in the limbs, or as *inferior* and *superior attachments* for muscles attaching above or below each other along the spine. We use both in this text, identifying muscles by traditional origins and insertions as well as their proximal and distal attachments.

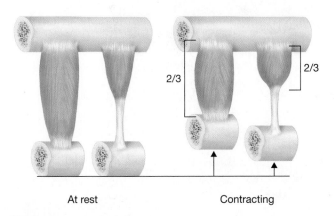

FIGURE 4.4
The length of a muscle's fibers determines how far it can move a bone.

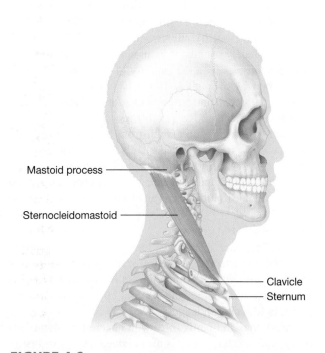

FIGURE 4.6
The sternocleidomastoid is named after its three attachment sites.

In a textbook study of individual muscles, the attachment sites appear to be clear and delineated. In a living body, where one muscle ends and another begins is not always that clear. Variations do exist. Some muscles are absent in certain percentages of the population, and attachment sites vary somewhat according to genetics. Keep the possibility of anomalies in mind when you find muscles during palpation with shapes and attachment sites that depart from general knowledge or textbook illustrations.

4.2 CONTRACTILE STRUCTURES AND MECHANISMS IN MUSCLES

A single muscle contains many bundles of muscle fibers call **fascicles,** which means "little bundle." Each fascicle, in turn, contains 100–150 single muscle cells, or **fibers.** A muscle fiber is the smallest contractile structure in a muscle that can respond to nerve stimulation.

A muscle fiber is capable of only two functions: it can either contract or it can relax. When a muscle fiber contracts, it shortens, although during certain types of contractions, a muscle lengthens. This brings up an important phenomenon that occurs in skeletal muscles: muscles can be elongated when their fibers are pulling toward each other during a contractile response. This is a key point to understand in order to work safely and effectively with muscles during bodywork. We revisit this important point after looking at how muscles actually contract.

4.2.1 Properties of Muscle Tissue

Muscle is an incredibly flexible and adaptable tissue due to four properties: contractility, extensibility, elasticity, and responsiveness. Although other body systems demonstrate some of these properties, no other body systems possess all four. **Contractility** allows muscles to forcibly shorten when adequately stimulated by motor nerves. **Extensibility** provides muscles with the capacity to be lengthened when acted upon by an outside force. **Elasticity** ensures that muscles will recoil and return to their normal resting length after being extended. **Responsiveness** gives muscle tissue the ability to respond to stimuli from both inside and outside the body. Responsiveness is also referred to as *excitability* or *irritability* because a muscle contracts when excited by nerve impulses generated by the nervous system or by artificial stimuli such as an electrical charge.

4.2.2 Muscle Fibers

Muscle fibers are shaped like long cylinders that taper at each end. On average, a fiber is from 1 to 40 millimeters in length and 10 to 100 micrometers in diameter. The longest muscle fiber in the body can run up to 30 centimeters, which is 12 inches in length.

Each muscle fiber is filled with hundreds of thousands of *microfibers.* Each fiber is also divided into segments by a series of transverse lines called *Z-lines.* Each segment

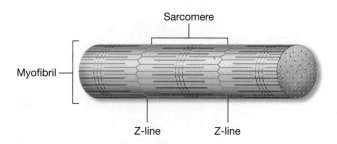

FIGURE 4.7
Muscle sarcomere

between the Z-lines is called a **sarcomere** (Figure 4.7 ■). The Z-lines divide each sarcomere into compartments that look like bands, which line up end to end like a string of boxcars. When viewed under a microscope, the banded sarcomeres give each fiber a striated look, which is why skeletal muscle is also called **striated muscle** (Figure 4.8 ■). The number of bands in a muscle fiber determines its length.

A cell membrane called a *sarcolemma* covers each muscle fiber. The sarcolemma reaches into the fiber with finger-like projections called *T-tubules.* The sarcolemma and T-tubules serve as conduits for electrical currents (Figure 4.9 ■).

4.2.2.1 MICROFILAMENTS IN MUSCLE FIBERS

A single sarcomere contains hundreds of thousands of thin filaments called *microfibers* or *myofilaments.* **Myosin** and **actin** are the two primary contractile proteins found in a sarcomere. Myosin filaments, the thicker of the two, are shaped like golf clubs with heads that can swivel in two directions. The myosin heads are situated at intervals along the length of

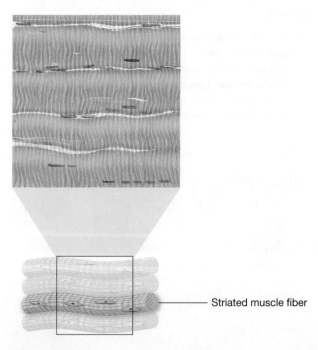

FIGURE 4.8
Striated fibers of a skeletal muscle

FIGURE 4.9

T-tubules permeate a muscle fiber.

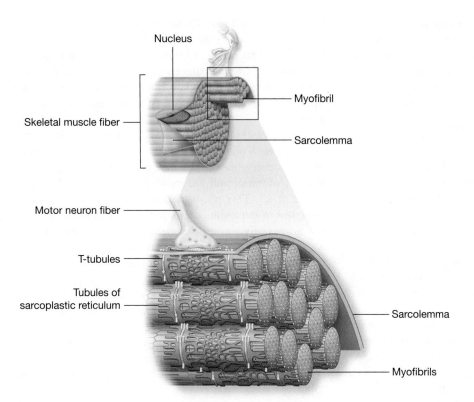

Nucleus

Myofibril

Skeletal muscle fiber

Sarcolemma

Motor neuron fiber

T-tubules

Tubules of sarcoplastic reticulum

Sarcolemma

Myofibrils

the myosin filament, sticking out on all sides. Actin filaments, the thinner of the two, resemble two twisted strings of beads made up of *actin molecules* and a *troponin complex* situated at intervals (Figure 4.10 ■). Six actin filaments overlap and interdigitate with one myosin filament, surrounding it on all sides (Figure 4.11 ■). The myosin heads and troponin complex on the actin serve as crossbridges that chemically bond during muscular contraction, a process that is described shortly.

A coiled elastic filament called **titin** is found between the dense bundles of actin and myosin filaments. The discovery of titin is relatively recent, and its functions are still being investigated.[1] Titin is thought to be a structural component that keeps the cell from being crushed or damaged. When a fiber is stretched to its elastic limit, titin prevents the

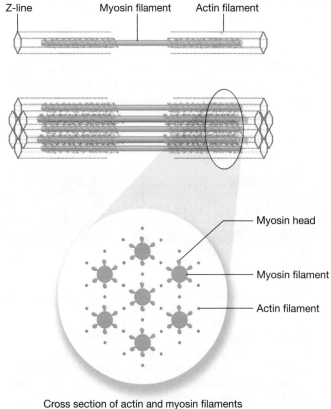

Z-line   Myosin filament   Actin filament

Myosin head

Myosin filament

Actin filament

Cross section of actin and myosin filaments

FIGURE 4.11

Arrangment of actin and myosin filaments

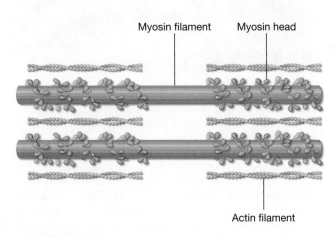

Myosin filament   Myosin head

Actin filament

FIGURE 4.10

Actin and myosin filaments

fiber from being overstretched and torn by providing internal resistance. As a muscle fiber is elongated and stretched, the titin filaments uncoil and straighten. Titin also serves as a connective tissue component that attaches a muscle fiber to surrounding tissues; titin fibers extend out of muscle fibers and anchor them to tendons, ligaments, and even bones.

4.2.2.2 THE SLIDING FILAMENT THEORY OF MUSCLE CONTRACTION

When a motor nerve stimulates a muscle fiber, the nerve sends an electrical impulse into the sarcolemma, which travels down the T-tubules into the cell. The nerve impulse, also called an **action potential,** depolarizes the fiber, creating an electrical charge that triggers a cascade of chemical processes that end in a contractile response. First, the action potential initiates a release of calcium ions (electrically charged molecules) that flood into the cell and open binding sites on the myosin heads and troponin complex in the actin filaments. Once open, the myosin and actin crossbridges on the binding sites chemically bond to each other. Then the myosin heads swivel like an oar on a boat dipping and pulling back, causing the filaments to slide across each other like sliding doors (Figure 4.12 ■). As the filaments slide across each other, the fiber shortens into a contractile response called a **muscle twitch.**

During a single muscle twitch, the crossbridges bind and release once. As long as the motor nerve fires and sends action potentials into the muscle fiber, the crossbridges continue to bind and release. Contraction occurs as the result of successive muscle twitches and grows stronger with each consecutive twitch.

4.2.3 Motor Units

A **motor unit** consists of a motor neuron plus all the muscle fibers it innervates (Figure 4.13 ■). The number and size of the motor units within muscles vary from one to the next. Small muscles that we use for fine motor control, such as those found in the hands and eyes, have as few as 10 fibers per motor unit. Large muscles that generate strong but less articulate contractions, such as the gastrocnemius, have as many as 2,000 fibers in a motor unit. Most muscles contain a mix of small and large motor units.

Fibers within a motor unit cannot contract independently of each other. When a motor neuron fires, its stimuli reach every fiber in the motor unit. Depending on the strength of the stimuli, the motor fibers respond all at once or not at all. This phenomenon is known as the **all-or-none law** of muscular contraction. Nerve stimulation does not necessarily ensure that the motor unit fires because a nerve impulse can be too weak to trigger a contractile response. A motor unit is the smallest functional unit in a muscle.

The fibers within a single motor unit can be dispersed throughout a muscle. A widespread distribution of fibers allows the tension a motor unit generates to spread all the way through a muscle, producing a weak contraction in the entire muscle. The amount of tension a muscle generates during a contraction depends on the number of motor units firing.

During muscular contractions, motor units fire in a round-robin fashion. Some turn on while others turn off, blinking like lights on a marquee. The repetitive and asynchronous firing of many motor units ensures a smooth and gradual muscular contraction. If they all turned on and off at once, the contraction would be jerky and spastic, similar to how alternately pumping a gas and brake pedal would cause a car to lurch and stop. The round-robin firing pattern of motor units also spreads the work throughout the muscle, preventing fatigue in any one place.

BRIDGE TO PRACTICE
Gauging Pressure during Deep Tissue Work

When practicing deep tissue massage, it is important to remember that when a muscle is contracted, the crossbridges are chemically bonded. Because of these chemical bonds, applying deep pressure and stretch to a contracted muscle can create micro-tears in the sliding filaments. This can give your client stiff and achy muscles the day after the session. To prevent tissue damage and client discomfort, make sure your client's muscles relax before applying deep pressure or stretch.

Many clients easily relax under deep pressure, unless the pressure causes pain. If your client winces or contracts, you are probably working too deep and need to lighten your pressure and/or stretch. Gauge your level of pressure so that it hovers in a range where your client can relax.

It also helps to coach your client to actively relax the muscles you're working on. If your client has trouble relaxing the muscles you are working with, there are effective muscle energy techniques you can use to trigger muscular relaxation responses. For example, have your client contract and relax the tight muscle, then stretch it using deep gliding pressure. The post-isometric relaxation response will enhance the stretch.

FIGURE 4.12

Contractile mechanism: actin and myosin fibers bind and pull together during a muscle contraction.

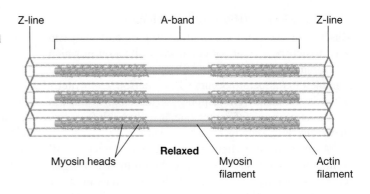

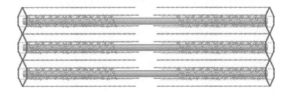

Relaxed

Z-line | A-band | Z-line
Myosin heads | Myosin filament | Actin filament

Fully contracted

4.2.3.1 FREQUENCY OF STIMULATION

The rate of successive nerve impulses stimulating a motor unit determines the strength of the contraction. If a motor unit is stimulated before it relaxes entirely, the subsequent contraction is stronger than the first. As one nerve stimuli follows another, the strength of the contraction grows with each twitch. This phenomenon, called *wave summation,* builds up tension in the muscle. Wave summation ensures a smooth and continuous contraction.

The faster the nerve impulses reach the muscle fibers, the stronger their contractile response. Wave summation continues until a muscle reaches maximum tension and all the motor units are firing. Once at maximum tension, all contractions fuse into one sustained contraction marked by the absence of relaxation, and the muscle becomes rigid. Since a muscle cannot remain contracted and rigid indefinitely, eventually it fatigues, at which time relaxation occurs.

4.2.3.2 RECRUITMENT OF MOTOR UNITS

The process of increasing the number of motor units that are firing in a muscle is called **recruitment,** which is synonymous with *multiple motor unit summation.* Whereas the primary function of wave summation is to ensure a smooth, continuous contraction, the primary function of multiple motor unit summation is to control the force of contraction.

Just as a car accelerates slowly at first, recruitment begins with smaller motor units. If a larger force is needed for the action, larger motor units are then recruited. Larger motor units can contract with up to 50 times the strength of the smaller motor units. This gradual summation allows us to modulate the strength of contraction performed by the same muscle groups during different activities. We use the same muscles to lift a pencil as we do to raise a 20-pound barbell. The difference between the two actions lies in the number of motor units recruited for each action.

Muscles are always contracting on some level. Even when the body is at rest, a number of motor units fire and generate tension in the muscle. The involuntary contractions that occur in resting muscle create **muscle tone.** Muscle tone serves several important functions: it provides postural support, it maintains a state of readiness, and it keeps muscles firm and healthy.

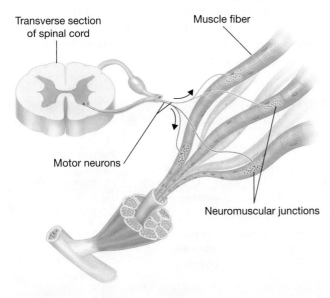

Transverse section of spinal cord

Muscle fiber

Motor neurons

Neuromuscular junctions

FIGURE 4.13

Motor unit

4.2.3.3 MUSCLE CONTRACTURE AND FATIGUE

Muscle can overwork and contract to the point of spasm or **contracture**—a state of continual contraction in which the crossbridges on the sliding filaments fail to unlink. An example of contracture occurs when a person gets writer's cramp in the hand from gripping for too long. Cramps in the leg, another type of contracture, usually result from low blood salts, low calcium, or dehydration.

As mentioned earlier, an overstimulated muscle will eventually reach a state of fatigue. When **muscle fatigue** sets in, the strength of the contraction becomes progressively weaker until the muscle stops contracting due to the physiological inability to produce the energy needed to continue contracting. Its energy supply—oxygen and glucose—has been depleted and metabolic wastes begin to accumulate, causing the muscle to simply stop working. If a person happens to be running around when the lower limb muscles reach fatigue, the legs will simply buckle and go limp as the muscles quit working.

Muscle fatigue can be local or central. Local fatigue is often preceded by a muscle contracture. Central fatigue is more complex. It occurs because of chemical changes in the brain and the motor nerves. Although the specific causes of central fatigue remain unknown, many factors are associated with it, such as chronic pain syndromes that involve sleep disorders, general fatigue and discomfort, and a pattern of tender nodules in the muscles called trigger points.

4.2.4 Energy Sources for Muscle Contraction

The primary source of energy for muscular contraction is *adenosine triphosphate* (ATP), which is the end product of glucose (a simple sugar) metabolism. Muscles store little ATP and need an ongoing supply in order to refuel depleted sources that get used up during contractions.

Muscle fibers produce ATP through two primary metabolic processes: *oxidation* and *glycolysis*. Oxidative fibers use oxygen to metabolize ATP in a process called **aerobic respiration.** Aerobic mechanisms are slow but highly efficient, converting one glucose molecule into 36 ATP molecules.[2] During aerobic respiration, glucose combines with oxygen, producing ATP and the by-products of carbon dioxide and water.

$$\text{Glucose} + \text{oxygen} \longrightarrow \text{ATP} + CO_2 + H_2O$$

In contrast, glycolytic fibers use sugar to metabolize ATP in a process called **anaerobic glycolysis.** During rigorous muscle activity, glycolysis converts glucose to ATP in the absence of oxygen through a chain of chemical reactions. Anaerobic glycolysis produces ATP quickly and burns it just as quickly. It is far less efficient than oxidation through aerobic respiration. Although glycolysis produces only 5 percent as much ATP as oxidation, it burns ATP two to three times as fast.

About 90 percent of the lactic acid that glycolysis produces as a by-product diffuses into the bloodstream within 30 minutes after a workout. The other 10 percent of lactic acid is metabolized by liver, heart, and kidney cells. This information dispels a long-held myth that massage removes lactic acid from the muscles. Although massage can increase local circulation in the capillaries, there is little evidence that massage removes lactic acid from the muscles after exercise.[3]

4.2.5 Types of Contractile Fibers

Three primary types of muscle fibers carry out contractile responses: type I slow fibers, type IIA fast fibers, and type IIB fast fibers. Each fiber is classified according to its speed of contraction and how it metabolizes energy.

Slow fibers convert glucose to ATP through the slow process of oxidation, and are therefore called **slow type I fibers** or *SO fibers,* referring to slow oxidation. Slow fibers are small and red because they have a rich capillary supply and contain more *myoglobin* (cells that bind with oxygen) than fast fibers. Their contractions are slow yet extremely efficient, making them resistant to fatigue. Because of their attributes, slow fibers are suited for activities that require sustained contractions, such as postural support and endurance activities.

In comparison with slow fibers, **fast type IIA** and **type IIB fibers** are larger and faster, yet not as efficient (see Table 4.1■). Because fast fibers lack the rich blood supply of the SO fibers, they appear to be white.

TABLE 4.1 Types of Contractile Fibers

Type of Fiber	Size and Color	Speed and Strength of Contraction	Rate of Fatigue	Metabolic Path	Recruitment Order
Type I fibers slow oxidative (SO fibers)	Small and red	Slow and weak	Fatigue resistant	Aerobic	First
Type IIA fibers fast oxidative-glycolytic (FOG fibers)	Larger and white	Fast and strong	Moderately fatigue resistant	Aerobic and anaerobic glycolysis	Second
Type IIB fibers fast glycolytic (FG fibers)	Largest	Fastest and strongest	Fatigue rapidly	Anaerobic glycolysis	Third

Type IIA fibers convert glucose to ATP through both oxidation and glycolysis and are also called *FOG fibers,* referring to fast oxidative and glycolytic. FOG fibers work during activities that require both endurance and strength, such as long-distance running.

Type IIB fibers only work through glycolysis, so they are also called *FG fibers,* referring to fast glycolytic. FG fibers are the largest and strongest of the three primary types of muscle fibers, yet fatigue the quickest, making them well adapted for quick, rigorous movement. They work during activities that require on–off pumping contractions of the muscles, such as weightlifting.

Every muscle has all three types of fibers, in ratios determined by genetics, use patterns, and location. Limb muscles tend to have an even distribution of slow and fast fibers, except in postural muscles like the soleus muscle in the calf and the vastus muscles above the knee, which have more slow fibers. Trunk muscles involved in postural support also have more slow fibers.

All fibers within a single motor unit are the same type. The speed and strength of a contraction depends on the type of fibers contracting in a motor unit. Fibers develop in accordance with how we use and train our muscles. Muscle fibers can change over time, adapting to body-use patterns. Sustained isometric exercises such as yoga develops slow type I fibers. Endurance exercises develop fast type IIA fibers. Activities requiring strength and speed develop more fast type IIB fibers. As the body ages, fast fibers tend to gradually change into slow fibers.

4.3 THE CONTINUITY OF MUSCLE AND FASCIA

A pervasive network of connective tissue, made up primarily of fascia, weaves the hundreds of muscles and millions of fibers in the muscular system into one interconnected network. Intricate layers and sheaths of deep fascia bind muscle groups to each other, to bones, and across joints (Figure 4.14 ■). Broad, flat, and dense sheets of fascia called **aponeurosis** provide attachment sites and support for intersecting layers of trunk muscles in areas such as the lower back and abdomen. Flat strips of fascia called **retinaculum** wrap the ankles and wrists, holding the tendons close to the bone.

Deep fascias bind all the muscles and bones snugly together, as thick plastic wrap might, into envelopes and compartments that then blend into ligaments and joint capsules (Figure 4.15 ■). Also, fascias connected to muscles and bones are continuous with fascias covering organs. This explains how chronic muscular tensions and scarring can sequence into organ cavities and affect the position of the organs.

The fascial network permeates muscular tissue down to the cellular level. Fascial sheathing called **epimysium** covers a single muscle, **perimysium** wraps each muscle

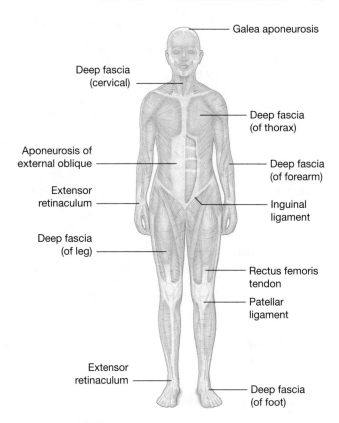

FIGURE 4.14
Continuity of fascia and muscle

fascicle, and a thin layer of **endomysium** surrounds an individual muscle fiber (Figure 4.16 ■). Nerves and blood vessels, also covered with fascias, run within a muscle between fascicular compartments.

Like all cells, a muscle fiber cell is a fluid-filled sac that contains organelles and microfilaments. Inside each cell, a structural scaffolding of connective tissue microfilaments provides a *cytoskeleton* that maintains the dimensional integrity of the cell. This intercellular scaffolding also responds to mechanical stresses around it by shoring up structure, which prevents the cells from being flattened.[4] Fascias wrapping and permeating muscles blend around and through the tendons and into the periosteum around the bone. Connective tissue fibers originating in muscle tissue even extends into bone tissue. This is why we have *avulsion fractures,* where an extreme injury to a tendon breaks away a piece of the bone rather than tearing the tendon off the bone or at the musculotendinous junction.

4.3.1 The Myofascial System

Given the intricately interconnected relationship of muscles with fascia, it is impossible to work with one tissue without affecting the other. We may call this body system the muscular system, but it is more accurately described as a **myofascial system.** Any system that provides support via tensional forces is called a **tensegrity system;** hence the myofascial system is a tensegrity system or network (Figure 4.17 ■). When looking at skeletal alignment, we

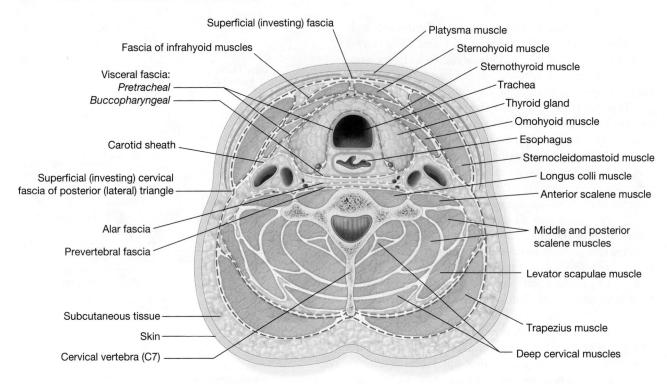

FIGURE 4.15

Fascial compartments in the neck: cross section at C-7

visualize the bones stacking up one on top of another, forming compression members for weight-bearing. In a tensegrity system, bones serve as struts and spacers embedded and floating in a three-dimensional webbing of myofascia.

In a study of kinesiology, it is important to understand the continuity of tissues in the myofascial network to grasp how the forces of movement translate through

the body. The word *tissue* comes from the Latin word *texere*, which means "texture or fabric." The strength and density of a tissue depends on the weave of its fibers. Some tissues, like some fabrics, are thick and tough, such as ligaments and tendons. Other fabrics are loosely woven and airy, such as superficial fascia. Other fabrics are dense and tightly woven, such as deep fascia. The different weaves and warps of the fascias permeate the many layers and bundles of parallel fibers in muscle tissue.

The advantage of this arrangement is that the mechanical stresses of posture and movement transfer throughout the elastic fibers of the myofascial webbing, reducing stress on any one part. The disadvantage of this arrangement, one particularly important for practitioners to note, is that chronic pulls and tension in one area of the myofascia transfer to other parts of the web. Like a snag in a finely woven fabric, scar tissue and myofascial adhesion, as well as chronic muscular holding or laxity, reduce the structural integrity of the entire body. Misalignment in one area of the tissue network affects the alignment and flow of movement through other areas. This dynamic could be compared to how slack ropes and stitched repairs in the tent fabric distort the shape of the whole tent. A pull in one area always translates to another part. Chronic pulls in the tensegrity of the myofascial system always require compensations elsewhere in the webbing. As a result of these compensations, a foot injury can progress

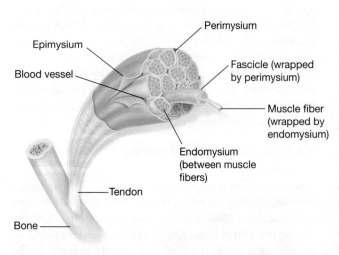

FIGURE 4.16

Cross section of a muscle

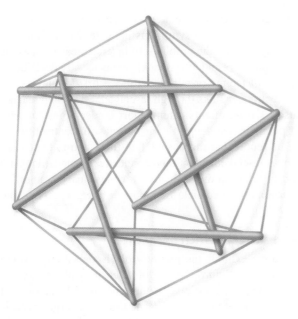

FIGURE 4.17
Tensegrity system

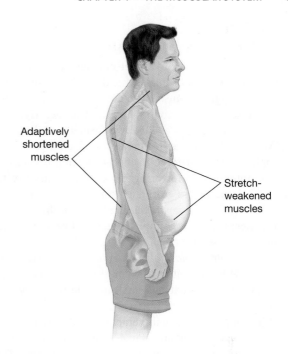

Adaptively
shortened
muscles

Stretch-
weakened
muscles

FIGURE 4.18
The anatomy of **muscular imbalance**

into a lower back or neck problem, which underscores the importance of addressing whole-body patterns during bodywork rather than limiting treatment to areas of pain and injury.

4.3.2 Adaptively Shortened and Stretch-Weakened Muscles

Myofascia is a highly adaptive tissue that undergoes structural changes in response to the demands placed on it. Movement stimulates the remodeling of connective tissues that permeate muscle tissue, resulting in a turnover of collagen fibers. In areas of little or no motion, collagen fibers build up, resulting in muscle stiffness and tightness. Researchers have found that substantial buildup of connective tissues occurs in and around muscle fibers that have been immobilized for as little as 2 days.[5] This explains the stiffness a person feels after several days lying in a sick bed. Muscle tightness limits range of motion, resulting in both muscular and movement imbalances. Severe and long-standing muscle tightness can lead to a condition called *tightness weakness,* which occurs from a combination of fibrous buildup in the muscle, ischemia, and inelasticity.

Muscles held in a shortened position for a prolonged period of time will undergo **adaptive shortening** (Figure 4.18 ■). When a limb is immobilized in a cast for 6 weeks or more in a shortened position, the body begins to reabsorb sarcomeres and the muscle will truly shorten in length. This adaptation occurs because in the shortened position, a muscle can generate little or no active tension upon contraction. To correct the imbalance, the body remodels the length of the muscle. The adaptively shortened muscle

can now spread out to a new resting length and has room to contract in the immobilized position. These structural changes in the muscle are what cause the severe reduction in range of motion that a person experiences when a cast is removed from a limb.

The opposite is also true. Muscles held in an elongated position over a period of time will develop **stretch weakness.**[6] Stretch-weakened muscles form elongated patterns of fibrous buildup and fascial tensions. If a muscle is immobilized in a lengthened position for an extended period of time, the body will generate new sarcomeres that cause the muscle to actually increase in length. Rather than becoming tight and short like adaptively shortened muscles, overstretched muscles become taut, ropy, and stringy due to a buildup of collagen fibers in them.

Postural strain often leads to the development of adaptively shortened and stretch-weakened muscles. When a muscle is chronically short on one side of a joint or trunk, the opposing muscles become overstretched. For example, a hunched, rounded-shoulder posture causes the anterior chest muscles to become adaptively shortened and tight and the posterior midscapular muscles to become stretch weakened and taut. Fascias connected to adaptively shortened and stretch-weakened muscle groups tend to become thick, fibrous, and inelastic. As a result, **fascial adhesions** develop that glue one muscle group to another, restricting range of movement by preventing the sliding motion of muscles, tendons, and even nerves.

4.3.3 Manual Therapy for the Myofascial System

Manual therapies used to effect change in myofascial tissues work with both muscles and fascia, as the term *myofascial* suggests. Muscle is a contractile, living tissue whereas fascia is a noncontractile, inert tissue. **Myofascial release (MFR)**, also called **myofascial mobilization (MFM)**, is a deep tissue technique in which a practitioner applies sustained-force loading to stretch myofascia with the intention of restoring mobility and motility to restricted tissue layers. Although this technique is generally referred to as *myofascial release,* nothing actually releases; the tissues simply stretch and become more mobile. Of course, it can feel like a great release of tension for the client, but *myofascial mobilization* better describes the technique because it restores motion to restricted layers of myofascia so that muscles can slide freely during motion.

When applying manual therapies to myofascia, both the mechanical and neurological aspects of this tissue may need to be addressed. To prepare the tissues for MFM, a kneading stroke such as petrissage (a Swedish massage stroke), which warms the tissues creating a thixotropic effect, will soften myofascia. Swedish massage can also help a client deeply relax the muscles so that they can be effectively massaged and stretched. If clients are unable to relax their muscles, no amount of bodywork can do it for them. In such cases, you can draw on neuromuscular techniques that access the neurological circuitry controlling muscular responses. Neuromuscular therapies require that clients participate in the process, following your cues to contract and relax specific muscles.

Normal length can be restored to adaptively shortened muscles with slow stretching done over a period of several weeks. Stretching slowly and gradually is important to avoid tissue damage from stretch injuries, especially with clients who have recently had casts removed. Their rehabilitation needs to be gradual to allow time for the muscle to adapt to lengthened a position and rebuild lost sarcomeres. It is also important to avoid loosening and elongating stretch-weakened muscles. Massage practitioners frequently make this mistake by stretching tissues around the lower, medial border of already-hypermobile scapulae. Stretching already-overstretched muscles not only exacerbates the strain on them, it disorganizes the entire myofascial network. When a stretch weakness stems from postural strain, a person needs postural muscle education to improve the condition.

To figure out whether to use manual therapies that address muscle or fascia (contractile or noncontractile tissues), pay attention to the quality of the tissues during palpation and to the client's feedback. Muscles are rich in sensory nerves whereas fascia lacks sensory nerves.

When clients report sore areas, tender points, or pain during movement, these symptoms indicate that muscles are probably causing the problem. In layered areas such as the upper shoulders and lower back, clients usually describe an absence of feeling or numbness in the first few layers. As the practitioner sinks through fascial adhesions and reaches muscle tissue, clients often report tender points or trigger points buried deep in their muscles. In contrast, when clients report that the tissues feel thick and tight but not painful, fascial adhesions and connective tissue buildup are probably causing the problem. Thick fascia and connective tissues can feel like inelastic rubber or fiberglass, tough and unyielding.

4.3.3.1 VISCOELASTICITY AND CREEP

Myofascia exhibits the property of **viscoelasticity,** which combines the fluid resistance of viscosity with the spring-like rebound of elasticity. Under sustained force or load over a period of time, viscoelastic tissues undergo **creep**—a progressive stretching that could be thought of as a slow-motion plastic change (Figure 4.19 ■). A lighter load over a longer period of time produces a larger creep. Heat also increases the rate of creep.

Creep beyond the elastic limit creates irreversible plastic changes. This has both its benefits and liabilities in the practice of deep tissue bodywork. Silly putty provides an analogy to contrast how we can stretch viscoelastic tissues in ways that can be either therapeutic or damaging. Yank on silly putty quickly and it will tear in half; pull on it slowly and it yields and stretches. Similarly, applying deep pressure too quickly can trigger protective contractions in the client. As mentioned earlier, the application of deep pressure to contracted muscles can also result in micro-tears to the sliding filaments and cause delayed soreness.

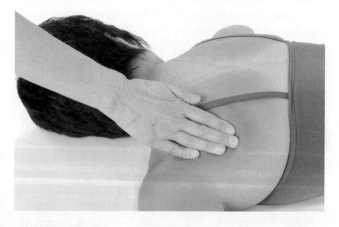

FIGURE 4.19

When myofascial tissues are placed under sustained pressure over a period of time, they undergo a progressive stretch called **creep.**

To create plastic changes in myofascial tissues that are therapeutic rather than damaging, deep pressure should always be applied slowly. The pressure should be gradual enough to induce creep and to give the client time to actively relax and allow the tissues to stretch. The initial part of a stretch under sustained pressure occurs in the elastic range. In order to create lasting changes in the client's tissues, you will need to hold pressure on the tissues until the tissues move beyond their elastic limit into the plastic range.

Sensing when a myofascial stretch shifts from the elastic range to the plastic range is a therapeutic skill that can be developed by paying attention to the quality of give in the tissues. The shift can be sudden and palpable, or slow and gradual. During this transition, the tissues yield, soften, and elongate. Clients can usually feel when their tissues yield and may comment on these changes, so it is helpful to ask for their feedback to verify the shift.

4.3.3.2 PIEZOELECTRIC PROPERTIES OF MYOFASCIA

Deep tissue work has several physiological effects on myofascia that involve changes in the polarity of ions—electrically charged particles. Applying sustained pressure and/or stretch to myofascia triggers a **piezoelectric effect,** which alters the electrical charge in the hydrophilic (water-loving) molecules in fascia, causing them to absorb water. As the tissues hydrate, myofascia becomes more pliable.

The collagen fibers in fascia also act like a semiconductor. When the myofascial network is placed under mechanical stress, electrical currents spread throughout, creating a softening in the system.[7] Another effect that deep pressure stimulates is the turnover of collagen fibers in myofascia. Friction techniques, in which a practitioner rubs against the surface of the tissues with a repetitive motion, also have this effect. Friction evokes a piezoelectric effect that loosens and broadens tissues and assists in the alignment of immature collagen fibers of new scar tissue into linear bundles.

- **Linear friction** or **stripping** along the direction of muscle fibers can help realign randomly crosshatched fibers in scars and injured tissues during the chronic stage of inflammation (Figure 4.20a ■).
- **Cross-fiber** or **transverse friction** applied across muscle, tendon, or ligament fibers will broaden and effectively loosen tight or fibrous tissues (Figure 4.20b ■).[8]

EXPLORING TECHNIQUE
Viscoelasticity and Plasticity in Myofascia

Although terms like *viscoelasticity* and *plasticity* seem remote, you can actually feel these properties during hands-on work. This exploration will help you develop the tactile skills you need to recognize viscoelastic and plastic changes in your client's tissues. Make sure to get your partner's feedback as you explore this exercise in different areas of the body. Explore areas where your partner's muscles are healthy and strong, and also areas that your partner wants to stretch.

1. **To explore the viscous quality of tissue:** Slowly apply pressure to your partner's tissues in a location where there are several layers of myofascia, such as along the lower back or shoulders. Press straight in, perpendicular to the skin, slowly sinking the pads of your fingers into the tissues while sensing the viscosity of fluids in the myofascia. Explore sinking into different areas of the myofascia; notice the different *rates* at which you can sink. In the tissues with a greater fluid content, you will feel more viscous resistance, which necessitates sinking in at a slower rate.

2. **To explore the elastic quality of tissue:** Press your partner's skin to pin it against underlying structures. Then slide the skin in a horizontal direction to stretch it. Notice how far it stretches and when you reach the first sign of resistance, which is the elastic limit. Then release it and watch how it springs back in elastic recoil. Explore stretching the skin in different areas and directions, taking it only to the elastic limit.

3. **To feel the viscoelastic properties of tissue:** Slowly press into the center of the myofascia in muscular areas such as the thigh, forearm, hips, or shoulders, pressing at a 45-degree angle. Again, notice the rate at which you sink (the viscous property) and the amount of pressure you need to slide the tissues to their elastic limits (the elastic property).

4. **To assess when the tissues reach a plastic range:** Choose an area where your partner wants more length, then repeat the last exercise, pressing and stretching the myofascia at a 45-degree angle until it reaches its elastic limit. At this point, maintain the pressure and stretch and wait for creep. When the tissues reach creep, they will become more pliable and stretch even farther, shifting and sliding like stiff fabric softening and stretching. Repeat several times until you can discern what the shift from the elastic into the plastic range feels like.

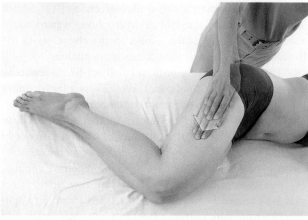

A

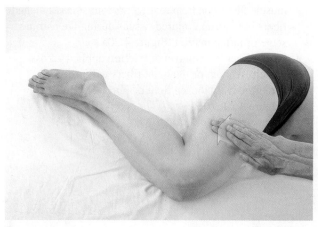

B

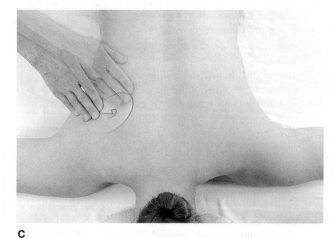

C

FIGURE 4.20

Friction techniques: a) Linear friction (stripping) b) Transverse friction (cross-fiber) c) Circular friction

- **Circular friction** is effective for loosening areas of myofascia crossing joints (Figure 4.20c ■).
- **Pin and stretch** is a combined friction and myofascial release technique in which a practitioner pins one end of a restricted tissue layer or muscle to stabilize it, then uses linear friction to stretch the tissue away from the pinned end.

4.4 MUSCLE TENSION AND CONTRACTILE FORCES

Skeletal muscles move bones by exerting forces that pull on bony levers. As a muscle's tension increases, so too does the force of a muscular pull. Muscle tension is a combination of both passive and active forces. The viscoelastic properties of fascias and connective tissues in associated structures create passive tension in a muscle. The muscle fibers produce contractile forces that result in active tension.

The force a muscle produces when it contracts depends on the resting length of the muscle. Resting tone in a muscle also comes from a combination of active and passive tension, which we look at in this section.

4.4.1 Passive and Active Tension

Passive tension depends on the elasticity of the inert (noncontractile) tissues running parallel to muscle fibers (epimysium, perimysium, endomysium) and the connective tissues in and around nerves and blood vessels. These noncontractile tissues constitute the *parallel elastic components* of a muscle.

In a resting muscle, the parallel components are slack. As the muscle fibers lengthen, the parallel components become taut, stretching like rubber bands. This increases the passive tension of a muscle, storing potential elastic energy. When a muscle contracts from a position of stretch, the elastic recoil of connective tissues contributes to the strength of the contraction. This dynamic also increases an economy of effort in movement activities that involve alternating stretch–shorten cycles of working muscles. It increases force production in rigorous sports activities. For example, a tennis player maximizes muscular tension and force by swinging the racket back before hitting the ball.

When a muscle fiber is stimulated by a motor neuron, it generates **active tension** in a contraction. The contractile pull transfers from the muscle through the tendon to the bone. As contractile tension builds and the muscle shortens, it pulls slack out of the tendon, which then transmits the force of the pull into the bony lever. Because a tendon

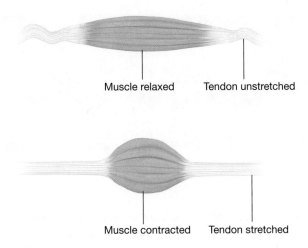

Muscle relaxed   Tendon unstretched

Muscle contracted   Tendon stretched

FIGURE 4.21

The tendon stretches as the muscle contracts.

functions in tandem with its muscle, the connective tissues embedded in a muscle fiber and its tendon constitute the *series elastic component* of a muscle (Figure 4.21 ■). Tendons possess less extensibility than fascias; they can stretch an average of 3–10 percent.[9]

4.4.2 Types of Contraction

There are two main types of contractions: **isotonic** and **isometric** (Figure 4.22 ■). During isotonic contractions, a muscle changes length, either shortening or elongating: During an isometric contraction, the muscle length remains the same (see Table 4.2 ■).

Concentric means "moving toward the center." A **concentric contraction** is isotonic, condensing a muscle into a shortened position. During a concentric contraction, the amount of internal force the muscle produces overpowers the external load or resistance on the muscle. Because the muscle is moving a load during a concentric contraction, the muscle is doing *positive work.*

An opposite dynamic occurs during an **eccentric contraction,** also isotonic, which is traditionally defined as a lengthening contraction. Muscles can actively shorten, but they cannot actively lengthen of their own accord. They can only be lengthened by an external force. During an eccentric contraction, the external load or resistance acting upon the contracting muscle overpowers the strength of the contraction. As a result, the muscle is internally shortening while externally being pulled apart. The sliding filaments still bind, but when they release, they are pulled farther apart. Because an external load is moving the muscle during an eccentric contraction, the muscle is doing *negative work.*

When a muscular force fails to move a joint, the contraction is defined as isometric, which means "same

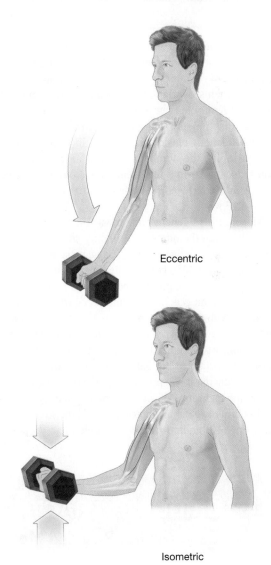

Concentric

Eccentric

Isometric

FIGURE 4.22

Three types of contractions

TABLE 4.2 Types of Contraction		
Type of Muscular Contraction	Length Changes in Muscle during Contraction	Force/Load (Resistance) Relationship
Concentric contraction	Muscle shortens	F is greater than L
Eccentric contraction	Muscle is lengthened	F is less than L
Isometric contraction	Muscle remains the same length	F is equal to L

length." During an **isometric contraction,** a muscle contracts in place. It remains the same length because the force it exerts matches the load or resistance it is pulling on.

4.4.3 Length–Tension Relationship

There is an optimal length from which a muscle can generate maximum tension, which defines the **length–tension relationship.** In a muscle fiber at rest, a certain number of sliding filaments overlap. The amount of overlap depends on whether a muscle fiber rests in a lengthened or shortened position. Adaptive shortening and stretch weakening reduces the optimal length–tension relationship in a muscle. In both these positions, the number of crossbridges available for binding decreases. In a lengthened position, too few fibers overlap; in a shortened position, too many fibers overlap (Figure 4.23 ■).

Muscle fibers generate the most force when there is a balance between the number of binding sites that are occupied and the number that are open. Say a muscle fiber has 100 binding sites total. If 50 binding sites are occupied and 50 are open, half the sites are pulling and the other half are posed to pull. A muscle can generate maximal force when the contraction begins with the muscle in this middle range of its resting length. At the end range of a concentric contraction, a muscle loses its ability to generate tension. As it shortens, 90 binding sites may be occupied but only 10 are open, minimizing the amount of tension it can produce. On the opposite end of the scale, at the end range of an eccentric contraction, a muscle loses its ability to generate more tension. In the stretched position, if only 10 binding sites are occupied and 90 potential

sites are open, only 10 sites are working, which produces a weak force. It is as though the muscle loses its grip.

When stretching a muscle or using a resisted movement technique that requires a muscular contraction against resistance, it is important to pay attention to the position of the joint. There are three general positions to consider (Figure 4.24 ■):

- **Outer range:** When the angle of the joint is open as far as it can go.
- **Midrange:** When the angle of the joint reaches the middle of its range of motion.
- **Inner range:** When the angle of the joint is closed.

To effectively stretch a muscle, position the joint(s) it acts on in outer range. The joint's outer range places the muscle in a maximally lengthened position, which is its weakest position to generate a contraction. On the other hand, to effectively use resisted movement techniques on a muscle, you'll want to position the joint(s) the muscle acts on in midrange, which is the optimal position to generate a contraction because it allows the muscle to generate the most tension. (Resisted movement techniques are discussed in detail in the neuromuscular chapter.)

4.5 CHANGING ROLES OF MUSCLES

A single muscle never works alone. Each muscle contributes its share to the overall coordination of a movement, performing a specific role during movement (see Table 4.3 ■). Like team members, muscles each play in a

BRIDGE TO PRACTICE
Caution with Resisted Movement in Outer Range

Because a muscle is in its weakest position when the joint it acts on is positioned in the outer range of motion and will not be able to generate much force, be careful when asking a client to contract a muscle against resistance with the joint in outer range. For example, when the elbow is completely extended, the biceps brachii is in its weakest position. If you do call for resisted movement with the joint in its outer range, be sure to apply only minimal resistance to avoid muscle strain.

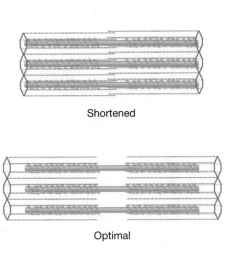

Shortened

Optimal

Lengthened

FIGURE 4.23

Length–tension relationship: The resting length of a muscle fiber affects the amount of tension (contractile force) it can generate.

TABLE 4.3	**Muscle Functions**
Muscle Functions	Definition of Function
Agonist	Initiates the action, the prime mover
Antagonist	Opposes the antagonist
Synergist	Assists the agonist
Neutralizers	Prevent secondary movement of agonist
Stabilizers	Maintain joint neutral, prevent excessive joint play

different position. Some begin the game and move in the center of action and others provide support and backup (Figure 4.25 ■).

4.5.1 Agonist, Antagonist, Synergists, and Neutralizers

The muscle that initiates a joint action is the **agonist,** or **prime mover.** All other muscle roles are defined in relation to the agonist during a specified action. For example, in a straight leg raise that flexes the hip, the quadriceps initiates the movement. It is the agonist or prime mover for hip flexion. During hip extension, the hamstrings take on the role of agonist.

The agonist can work both concentrically and eccentrically, depending on the direction of the movement. During a push-up, as the body moves away from the ground, the triceps work concentrically and shortens to extend the elbows. As the body is lowered to the ground, the triceps

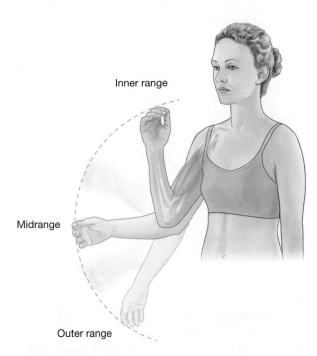

Inner range

Midrange

Outer range

FIGURE 4.24

Range of joint motion

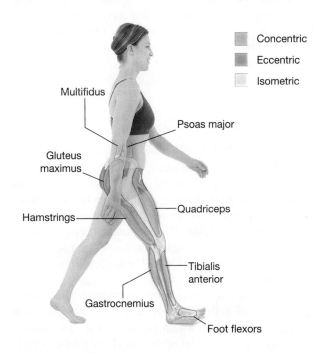

Concentric
Eccentric
Isometric

Multifidus

Psoas major

Gluteus maximus

Hamstrings

Quadriceps

Tibialis anterior

Gastrocnemius

Foot flexors

FIGURE 4.25

Muscular functions during hip flexion

work eccentrically to control the speed of downward motion while resisting gravity.

A muscle assisting the action of the agonist takes on the role of the **synergist,** pulling near the same angle or plane as the agonist. During hip flexion, the psoas major works as a synergist by assisting flexion. During hip extension, the gluteus maximus acts as the synergist by assisting extension.

Muscles that prevent undesired movements of an agonist work as **neutralizers.** Say, for instance, that flexion is the desired action and the agonist both flexes and laterally rotates a joint. A medial rotator will contract to neutralize lateral rotation by the agonist.

The muscle that produces the opposite movement of the agonist is the **antagonist.** An antagonist serves two main roles: it gradually relaxes during the contraction of the agonist in order to permit and control joint movement, and it also acts as a brake on the agonist during sudden, ballistic movements. Its contraction at the end range of a ballistic joint motion will prevent injuries to the joint structures.

When the agonist and the antagonist co-contract, they generate even pulls on a joint in opposite directions, canceling each other out so that no motion occurs. Their combined actions pull the joint into compression, which fixates the joint. In this role, the agonist and antagonist are acting as **fixators** to prevent motion.

Muscles also work in a non-moving body to maintain joint neutral in an optimal postural alignment. In terms of joint stability, muscle functions come under two general classifications of the stabilizers and the mobilizers. The **stabilizers** work independently of joint motion to maintain joint neutral in an upright postural support. They also work during movement to prevent excessive joint play. **Mobilizers** is a general term to describe muscles working as agonists and synergists to generate and carry out joint motion. Stabilizers generally have more slow fibers, mobilizers more fast fibers. Of course, the role of stabilizers and fixators overlap, although the primary stabilizers are always stabilizers while the fixators can move between fixating or movement functions.

4.5.2 Stabilizers, Coordination, and Recruitment Timing

The stabilizers tend to be small, monoarticular (one-joint) muscles that lie close to the joint. Their contractions approximate a joint, drawing its articular surfaces closer together. The stabilizers function like ties that batten down cargo before a ship takes off. They contract prior to motion tightening up a joint to prevent excessive joint play when the body begins moving. Stabilization underlies smooth and coordinated muscle patterns.

Coordination results from the efficient and orderly recruitment of muscles during an action. **Recruitment timing** is the order in which the motor units and muscle groups contract during an action. Smaller motor units and smaller muscles generate less tension and use less energy than larger motor units and larger muscles. An efficient

recruitment strategy based on the conservation of energy has the following attributes:

- The slow fibers fire before the fast fibers.
- The smaller motor units fire before the larger motor units.
- The stabilizers fire before the mobilizers.

4.5.3 Biarticular Muscles

Biarticular muscles cross two joints. The biarticular muscles of the ankles, knees, and hips work together to maximize muscular efficiency during activities such as walking, running, and jumping. The simultaneous flexion and extension of joints in the lower limb and the alternating orientation of the joints makes this economical arrangement possible. The knees flex in the opposite direction as the hips and the ankles. When the hamstrings contract and shorten to flex the knees, they are lengthened at the hip by the contraction of the hip flexors. On the other side of the thigh, the rectus femoris undergoes a similar dynamic. It contracts and shortens to flex the hip while being lengthened at the knee by the action of the knee flexors.

This dual tension shortens the muscle at one end while lengthening it at the other, causing a **parallel shift,** also called a *concurrent movement,* in the muscle (Figure 4.26a ■). Since neither of these muscles changes length, some kinesiologists argue that this is actually isometric contraction, an argument well beyond the scope of this text.

The opposite of the parallel shift is a **countercurrent movement.** During this type of movement, the biarticular muscle acts on both joints at once. If you raise your leg with the knee extended, the rectus femoris pulls on both the hip and knee (Figure 4.26b ■). It flexes the hip while extending the knee, shortening at both ends.

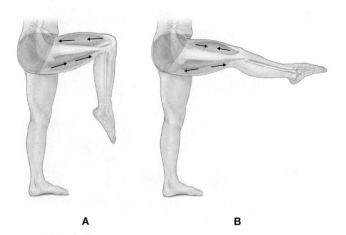

A   **B**

FIGURE 4.26

a) In a **parallel shift,** the agonist and antagonist function like two cords on a pulley, with the hamstrings sliding down and the rectus femoris sliding up, both maintaining their same length.
b) In a **countercurrent shift,** the agonist shortens at both ends while the antagonist is lengthened at both ends.

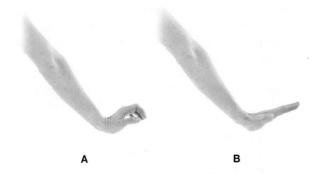

FIGURE 4.27

Demonstration of **passive insufficiency** of the wrist and finger flexors

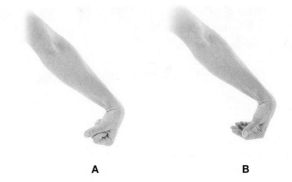

FIGURE 4.29

Demonstration of **active insufficiency** of the wrist and finger flexors

4.5.4   Passive and Active Insufficiency

Muscles crossing more than one joint can only contract or stretch so far. At the extreme range of motion, biarticular and multiarticular muscles reach a point of limited ability to produce or maintain tension. When muscles cannot lengthen far enough to allow maximum ROM in all the joints they cross, they have reached **passive insufficiency.** To feel how this affects range of movement, extend your wrist as far as possible, and you'll notice that the fingers curl. To straighten the fingers, you'll need to decrease the degree of extension in your wrist (Figure 4.27 ■). The fingers flexors can only stretch so far, preventing the wrist and finger joints from reaching full extension at the same time.

Remember this dynamic when performing passive stretches on muscles that cross two or more joints. The location and degree of stretch can be modulated by the number of joints

taken to the end range. To get a thorough stretch in the hamstring muscles, take both the hip and the knee to end range of motion (Figure 4.28 ■). To only stretch muscles crossing the back of the knee, take only the knee to end range of joint motion.

Muscles crossing two or more joints cannot exert enough tension to move all the joints they act on at the same time. When muscles reach a point of maximal shortening and can no longer pull, they have reached **active insufficiency.** To feel how this affects range of movement, keep your wrist straight and make a fist. Now slowly flex the wrist toward end range of motion and notice how your fist begins to open (Figure 4.29 ■).

When a biarticular muscle is maximally shortened and continues to contract, it reaches active insufficiency and can easily cramp. The tendency to cramp is strong in the biarticular muscles of the lower limbs (Figure 4.30 ■).

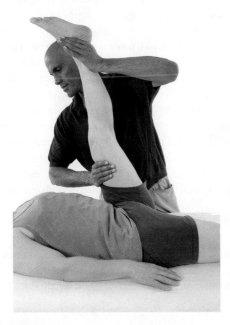

FIGURE 4.28

Passive hamstring stretch on a client

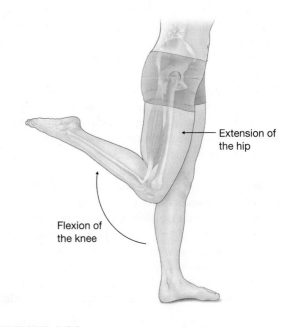

Extension of the hip

Flexion of the knee

FIGURE 4.30

Extending the hip while flexing the knee maximally shortens the hamstrings, which can reach active insufficiency and spasm.

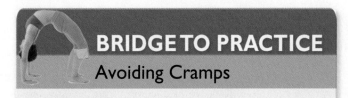

BRIDGE TO PRACTICE
Avoiding Cramps

To avoid triggering a cramp in a client during a session, be careful when asking your clients to move in a range that maximally shortens a biarticular muscle, such as asking a prone client to lift the thigh and extend the hip with the knee bent.

CONCLUSION

It is possible to exercise in many different ways because muscles function under our voluntary control. We can contract or relax them at will, as well as train the order and rate in which they contract. Because of the viscoelastic properties of muscle and connective tissue, we can also place the muscles under pressure or stretch to create irreversible plastic changes in them, which explains how deep tissue massage works.

The muscles and their many associated fascia make up the myofascial system, which wraps the entire body like a three-dimensional suit of elastic fabric. Imagining how this suit fits over the body and how each muscle changes shape during movement can aid the visual learner. Tracing the striated fibers in each muscular panel of this suit can aid the kinesthetic learner.

No single muscle ever acts alone. All muscles work together. In this sense, the myofascial system is actually one muscle and one connective tissue with many parts. It is holistic in nature; tensional pulls generated by muscular contractions in one area always translate to another area of the body. This holistic attribute is of particular relevance for massage and bodywork practitioners to recognize because changing the resting length of one part of the myofascia will affect how movement passes through the entire system.

SUMMARY POINTS TO REMEMBER

1. The muscular system is made up of the skeletal muscles and all their associated connective tissues, fascias, and tendons. The main functions of the muscular system are to provide postural support and protection and to generate joint motion.

2. There are about 650 skeletal muscles in the body, which come in many different shapes, including strap, fusiform, rhomboidal, triangular, and pennate shapes. The length of a muscle determines how far it can move a bone. Excursion describes the distance a muscle can shorten or lengthen.

3. Muscles are named by the actions they produce, their shapes, or the bones or locations to which they are attached. The term *origin* identifies the proximal attachment site of a muscle; the term *insertion* identifies the distal attachment site of a muscle.

4. Muscle tissue has four properties: contractility (the ability to forcibly shorten when stimulated by motor nerves), extensibility (the capacity to be lengthened by an outside force), elasticity (the capacity to return to a normal resting length after being extended), and responsiveness (the ability to respond to stimuli).

5. The smallest contractile unit in a muscle is a single muscle cell, or fiber. Each muscle fiber is a long, microscopic-sized cylinder with many striated segments called sarcomeres, which contains contractile proteins called myosin and actin. Bundles of muscle fibers are called fascicles. Bundles of muscle fascicles make up a single muscle.

6. The sliding filament theory explains how a muscle contracts. It postulates that when a motor nerve stimulates a muscle fiber, it sends an electrical impulse into the muscle cell. This triggers a series of events that culminates in the chemical bonding of myosin and actin filaments, which pull toward each other in a contraction.

7. A motor unit, the smallest functional unit of a muscle, consists of a motor neuron and all the muscle fibers it innervates. When a motor unit receives nerve stimulation, none of its fibers contract if the stimulus is too weak; if the stimulus is strong enough to trigger a contraction, all the fibers in the motor unit contract.

8. Motor units fire in a round-robin fashion, gradually increasing in number in a process called recruitment, which is synonymous with multiple motor unit summation.

9. Muscles always contract on some level to maintain a state of readiness. The degree of involuntary contraction occurring in a resting muscle is called muscle tone.

10. The energy source for muscular contraction is called adenosine triphosphate (ATP). It is produced through

oxidation, an aerobic process in which oxidative fibers metabolize ATP with oxygen. ATP is also produced through glycolysis, an anaerobic process in which glycolytic fibers use glucose, a simple sugar, to metabolize ATP.

11. Muscles that overwork can contract in a continual state, called a spasm or contracture. Muscle fatigue occurs when the energy supply to generate contractions has been depleted. An overstimulated muscle will fatigue, often after a spasm or contracture.

12. The three primary types of muscle fibers are slow type I, fast type IIA, and fast type IIB. Slow fibers contract slowly and weakly, are fatigue resistant, and are found in higher concentrations in postural muscles. Fast fibers contract more quickly and strongly, fatigue rapidly, and are found in higher concentrations in muscles that produce joint motion.

13. The myofascial system is made up of the skeletal muscles and all their associated fascias. It is considered a tensegrity system because it provides a network of support through tensional forces. Myofascial release (MFR) is a manual therapy used to release myofascial restrictions to restore flexibility and improve posture and movement.

14. Passive tension in a muscle comes from the elasticity of noncontractile tissue. Active tension comes from the pull of contractile muscle fibers.

15. In an isotonic contraction, a muscle changes length. There are two types of isotonic contraction: In a concentric contraction, the muscle shortens; in an eccentric contraction, the muscle is lengthened. In an isometric contraction, the muscle remains the same length. The length–tension relationship refers to the optimal length at which a muscle can generate maximum tension.

16. Muscles work in several different roles. The agonist is the prime mover that generates joint motion, the antagonist counters the pull of the agonist, the synergists assist the agonist, and the neutralizers prevent undesired movements.

17. Coordination is the efficient recruitment and firing pattern of the muscles working along a kinetic chain during an action. In a coordinated action, stabilizer muscles contract before mobilizer muscles to prevent excessive joint play during movement.

18. Biarticular muscles cross two joints. A biarticular muscle can reach a state of active insufficiency when it is acting on both joints but is maximally shortened and unable to pull any farther. A biarticular muscle reaches a state of passive insufficiency when it is maximally lengthened across both joints and unable to lengthen any farther. In both states, the muscle is susceptible to a protective spasm or contracture.

REVIEW QUESTIONS

1. Skeletal muscle tissue differs from smooth muscle and cardiac muscle because
   a. it is under involuntary somatic control.
   b. it is under voluntary control and generates joint motion.
   c. it functions in the processes of digestion and elimination.
   d. it is controlled by the autonomic nervous system.

2. Name the three attributes that a muscle called the "flexor digitorum longus" is likely to have given its anatomical name.

3. Name and briefly describe five different shapes that skeletal muscle comes in.

4. True or false (circle one). A fusiform muscle can usually produce a stronger force than a pennate muscle.

5. The origin and insertion of a muscle describe its
   a. distal and proximal attachment sites.
   b. attachment site of tendon to muscle fibers.
   c. attachment site of a pennate fiber to a central tendon.
   d. proximal and distal attachment sites.

6. The four properties of muscle tissue are
   a. extensibility, elasticity, responsiveness, and contractility.
   b. elasticity, excitability, contractility, and extensibility.
   c. elasticity, contractility, extensibility, and irritability.
   d. extensibility, elasticity, conductibility, and irritability.

7. Extensibility, one of the four properties of a muscle tissue, it defined as
   a. the capacity of a muscle to be lengthened by an outside force.
   b. the ability of a muscle to forcibly shorten when stimulated by motor nerves.
   c. the capacity of a muscle to return to a normal resting length after being extended.
   d. the ability of a muscle to respond to stimuli.

8. The smallest contractile unit in a muscle is a
   a. motor unit.
   b. muscle fiber.
   c. sliding filament.
   d. muscle fascicle.

9. True or false (circle one): When a muscle fiber is relaxed, the chemical bonds between the binding sites on the sliding filaments are open.

10. A motor unit is
   a. the smallest structural unit of a muscle fascicle.
   b. a sensory nerve plus all the muscle fibers it innervates.
   c. a motor nerve plus all the muscle fibers it innervates.
   d. a structure that is exactly the same size in all muscles.

11. The differences between slow and fast muscle fibers are that
   a. slow fibers contract slowly with strong contractions and fatigue more quickly. Fast fibers contract quickly with weak contractions and are fatigue resistant.
   b. slow fibers contract slowly with weak contractions and are fatigue resistance. Fast fibers contract quickly with strong contractions and fatigue more quickly.
   c. slow fibers contract slowly with weak contractions and are fatigue resistant. Fast fibers contract slowly with sustained contractions and are fatigue resistant.
   d. slow fibers contract quickly with weak contractions and are fatigue resistant. Fast fibers contract slowly with sustained contractions and fatigue more quickly.

12. What is the myofascial system?

13. Define adaptively shortened and stretch-weakened muscles and briefly describe how faulty postures can lead to these conditions.

14. Because of the property of viscoelasticity, when myofascial tissues are placed under a sustained load, they undergo creep. To induce creep in myofascia during bodywork, a practitioner needs to
   a. apply deep pressure quickly and hold for a short time.
   b. apply light pressure quickly and release immediately.
   c. apply deep pressure slowly and release before stretch occurs.
   d. apply deep pressure slowly and hold past the elastic limit.

15. Match the following types of contraction—eccentric, concentric, isometric, isotonic—to their definitions:
   a. A muscle changes length during contraction due to greater or lesser resistance on it.
   b. A muscle shortens because the force of its contraction is greater than the resistance on the muscle.
   c. A muscle lengthens because the force of its contraction is less than the resistance on the muscle.
   d. A muscle stays the same length because the force of its contraction is equal to the resistance on the muscle.

16. Match the following muscle functions—agonist, antagonist, synergist, neutralizer, stabilizer—to their definitions:
   a. the muscle that assists the prime mover
   b. the muscle that prevents secondary actions of the prime mover
   c. the muscle initiating an action, the prime mover
   d. the muscle that works independent of an action to prevent joint play
   e. the muscle that opposes the prime mover

17. Muscle fatigue is a state in which a muscle
   a. uses sugar to metabolize ATP in order to continue contracting.
   b. uses oxygen in oxidative energy production to continue contracting.
   c. can no longer produce the energy it needs to continue contracting.
   d. becomes saturated with lactic acid and needs to continue contracting.

18. A muscle contracture is a state of
   a. intermittent contraction in which crossbridges on sliding filaments fail to unlink.
   b. constant contraction in which crossbridges on sliding filaments fail to unlink.
   c. constant relaxation in which crossbridges on sliding filaments remain unlinked.
   d. intermittent relaxation in which crossbridges on the sliding filaments unlink.

Notes

1. Alter, M. (2004). *Science of Flexibility* (3rd ed.). Champaign, IL: Human Kinetics.
2. Tortora, G., & Grabowski, S. (2001). *Principles of Anatomy and Physiology* (9th ed.). Menlo Park, CA: Benjamin Cummings.
3. University of California, Berkeley. (2006, April 21). "Lactic Acid Not Athlete's Poison, But An Energy Source If You Know How To Use It." *Science Daily.* Retrieved November 20, 2009, at www.sciencedaily .com /releases/2006/04/060420235214.htm.
4. Ingbar, D. (2003). "Mechanosensation through Integrins: Cells Act Locally But Think Globally." *Proceedings of the National Academy of Sciences USA, 100*(4), 1472–1474.
5. Williams, P., & Goldspink, G. (1984). "Connective Tissue Changes in Immobilized Muscle." *Journal of Anatomy, 138*(2), 343–350.
6. Kendall, F., McCreary, E., & Provance, P. (2005). *Muscles: Testing and Function with Posture and Pain* (4th ed.). Baltimore: Lippincott, Williams & Wilkins.
7. Oschman, J. (2000). *Energy Medicine: The Scientific Basis.* London: Churchill Livingstone.
8. Cyriax, J., & Cyriax, P. (1993). *Cyriax's Illustrated Manual of Orthopedic Medicine* (2nd ed.). Edinburgh, UK: Butterworth-Heinemann.
9. Levangie, P., & Norkin, C. (2005). *Joint Structure and Function: A Comprehensive Analysis* (4th ed.). Philadelphia: F. A. Davis.

PEARSON
myhealthprofessionskit™

Use this address to access the Companion Website created for this textbook. Simply select "Massage Therapy" from the choice of disciplines. Find this book and log in using your username and password to access interactive activities, videos, and much more.

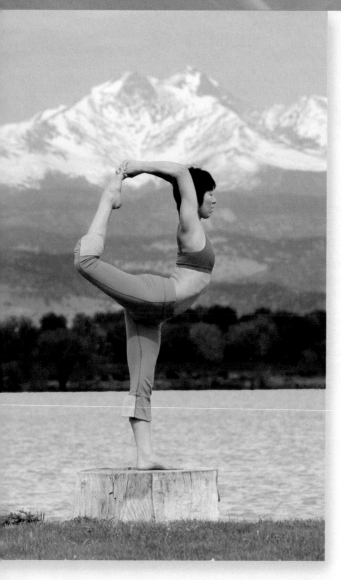

CHAPTER OUTLINE

Chapter Objectives

Key Terms

5.1 Overview of the Nervous System

5.2 Sensory Receptors

5.3 Reflexes and Basic Movement Pathways

5.4 Movement Applications in Neuromuscular Techniques

Conclusion

Summary Points to Remember

Review Questions

Most people associate yoga with a form of stretching, but *yoga* is a Sanskrit word that has many meanings, all of which imply the unity of the body and mind. Yoga is a very old spiritual discipline developed in India where the ancient language of Sanskrit originates. In a yoga practice, a person learns to control and relax the often busy mind through a practice of breathing, conscious stretching postures, and meditation in specific body poses.

Yoga underwent a revival when the counterculture movement and the famous Beatles popularized it in the West in the 1960s and early 1970s. There are more than 30 styles of yoga, each with a different philosophy. Hatha yoga uses slow movements that stretch, align, and detoxify the body during a series of specific postures. Hot yoga is practiced in rooms heated like a sauna. Other schools of yoga focus on power, strength, and endurance, moving quickly through postures and stretches using flowing transitions. Restorative and therapeutic approaches to yoga use a slower pace and a gentler tone with a focus on neuromuscular control of posture and movement, quieting mental chatter, and connecting the body and the mind. Most people who practice yoga on a regular basis enjoy the centering yet energizing benefits of this ancient body–mind practice.

CHAPTER OBJECTIVES

1. Describe and compare the major divisions of the nervous system.

2. Define a neuron and list and describe three types of neurons in the neuromuscular system.

3. List and describe the peripheral nerves and associated connective tissues.

4. Define neural tension and explain its implications in movement and bodywork.

5. Define a sensorimotor loop and describe how it works in faulty movement patterns.

6. Define and compare proprioception and perception.

7. Describe the stretch reflex and a reflex arc.

8. Describe the proprioceptor in tendons and two proprioceptors in joint capsules.

9. Describe specialized proprioceptive organs in the labyrinth of the inner ear.

10. Define the law of reciprocal inhibition and describe how it works in reflex movements.

11. List three types of movement assessment and three conditions they are used to assess.

12. Describe how to make a general assessment about whether a client's pain pattern is generated by contractile or noncontractile tissues.

13. List the reasons for using resisted motion during a session, then describe the steps for performing resisted motion with a client.

14. Define a trigger point and its effects and describe the process of trigger point therapy.

15. List two muscle energy techniques and describe the steps for each.

16. Describe the dynamics of a stretch injury.

KEY TERMS

Crossed extensor reflex

Direct technique

Extensor thrust reflex

Flexor withdrawal reflex

Indirect technique

Muscle energy techniques (METs)

Muscle spindle

Myotatic reflex

Neural tension

Neuromuscular system

Nociceptors

Post-isometric relaxation (PIR) technique

Proprioception

Reciprocal inhibition

Reciprocal inhibition (RI) technique

Reflex arc

Sensorimotor loop

Sensory receptors

Somatic nervous system (SNS)

Stretch injury

Stretch reflex

Synapse

Tendon reflex

Trigger point (TrP)

In the last three chapters, we covered the skeletal, joint, and muscular systems. Now we turn our attention to the complex circuitry connecting the nervous system to the muscular system, which together constitute the **neuromuscular (NM) system.** The neuromuscular system is not actually a body system, per se, but a combination of all the muscles, nerve tissues, and awareness mechanisms that work together to produce human movement.

This chapter is central to the study of kinesiology because it looks at how three body systems work together in the coordination and production of movement. The different roles played by the muscles, bones, and nervous system can be described with a horse and carriage analogy. The muscles, like the horse, generate the power; the skeleton, like the carriage, provides a framework for the moving structures; and the nervous system, like the driver, steers the coach and controls the equine labor.

The horse moves under the direct control of the driver. Similarly, the muscular system functions as the workhorse of the nervous system. Muscles do not operate of their own accord; they cannot make decisions about where or how the body moves. Without the brain and nerves directing motor pathways to determine what moves where and when, skeletal muscles would be rendered inert. The muscular system is intricately wired to the nervous system via billions and trillions of neurons and synapses in the brain and spinal cord, where rapid processing coordinates every single movement we make.

As manual therapists, we need to back up a step and recognize that clients' consciousness is intricately wired to their movement system. To improve a client's range, balance, and economy of effort in motion, we tap into the neuromuscular circuitry through active techniques. For example, a practitioner can increase range of motion using client-assisted stretching. This chapter emphasizes the many active techniques that a practitioner can use to tap into the client's neuromuscular circuitry to effect therapeutic changes in muscle and joint patterns. These techniques capitalize on reflex mechanisms in the neuromuscular system and include active, passive, and resisted movement as well as client-assisted stretching, trigger point therapy, and muscle energy techniques.

This chapter has a lot of guidelines and techniques for applications of therapeutic kinesiology in neuromuscular therapy. The guidelines serve as a general list of directions for applying the techniques effectively. The last section of this chapter covers the use of passive, active, and resisted movement in neuromuscular techniques. You will want to pay special attention to all of the skills in this chapter because you will be using them in the many palpation exercises throughout the second half of the book.

5.1 OVERVIEW OF THE NERVOUS SYSTEM

The nervous system (NS) serves as the central command station for the coordinated and smooth function of each part of the entire body. Every body system takes its working orders from the nervous system. The NS has complex functions and intricate parts, including several major divisions (Figure 5.1 ■). The **central nervous system** (CNS) is made up of the brain and spinal cord. The **peripheral nervous system** (PNS) is every part of the nervous system outside of the CNS, which includes the peripheral nerves and groups of nerve cells in the body called *ganglia;* it is further subdivided into the autonomic nervous system and the somatic nervous system.

The **autonomic nervous system** (ANS) regulates all *involuntary* or "automatic" organ functions. It controls the organs through two divisions: parasympathetic and sympathetic. Each division has an opposite effect on the body. The *parasympathetic division* slows the metabolic engine down for resting and digesting; the *sympathetic division* speeds the metabolic engine up for action, including the freeze, fight, or flight responses.[1] The parasympathetic system regulates slow organ functions such as digestion, elimination, and recuperation. The sympathetic system draws metabolic energy away from the viscera and sends it to muscles, getting the body ready for action by speeding the heart rate and respiration. Many massage modalities, such as Swedish and cranialsacral therapy, tap into ANS circuitry to release autonomic tension, promote the relaxation response, and improve autonomic flexibility—the ability to move from sympathetic tone to parasympathetic tone.

The **somatic nervous system** (SNS) controls the skeletal muscles and *voluntary* movement, so it is also called the *skeletal nervous system. Soma* means "body," and this part of the nervous system coordinates body postures and movements carried out by the workhorses of the muscular system. Neuromuscular techniques, which tap into the SNS circuitry that controls muscle patterns, are often used for the relief of pain and muscle soreness.

Two main reasons that people receive massage are for the restorative effects of relaxation and pain relief from muscle soreness.[2] These reasons are important to remember when practicing neuromuscular (NM) techniques. Therapies such as trigger point pressure and deep tissue stretching can be painful and interfere with relaxation, or they can be incredibly relaxing, but only under certain conditions.

Many of these techniques require the client to actively participate in the process, providing feedback about pain levels, moving in certain ways, or contracting specific muscles against resistance. Active neuromuscular techniques are usually more effective if the client can relax during them by moving slowly, by observing the chain of action, and by using minimal effort.

5.1.1 Neurons

A **neuron** is a *nerve cell* made up of three parts: a *cell body* and long, thin nerve fibers extending out of the side of the cell body called *axons* and *dendrites* (Figure 5.2 ■). The structure of a single neuron reflects the three general

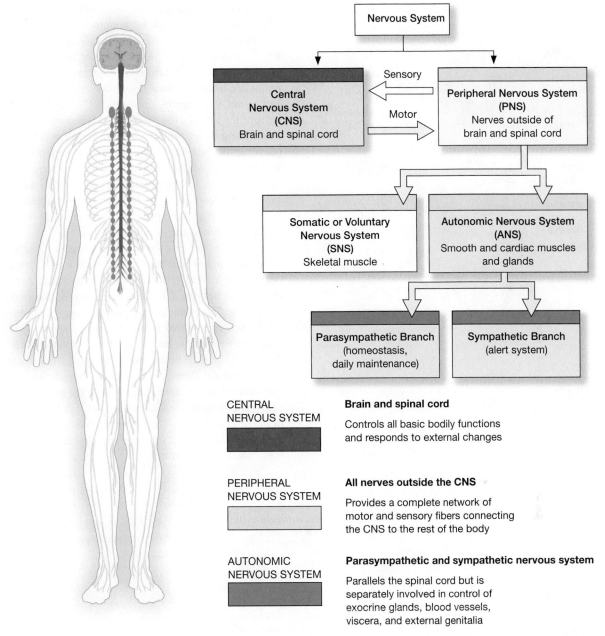

FIGURE 5.1

Divisions of the nervous system

functions of the nervous system: to receive sensory input, to process sensory information, and to send out motor signals.

- *Axons* receive sensory information from the body and the environment.
- *Cell bodies* process and integrate information.
- *Dendrites* deliver motor impulses to the organs and muscles.

There are three functional classifications of neurons—sensory neurons, interneurons, and motor neurons—each defined by the direction in which they transmit nerve impulses.

- **Sensory (afferent) neurons** carry sensory impulses *to* the brain and spinal cord.
- **Interneurons (association neurons)** transfer signals *between* neurons in the brain and spinal cord.
- **Motor (efferent) neurons** carry motor impulses *from* the brain and spinal cord to the muscles.

Neurons connect to other neurons or end organs at a **synapse**—a junction where the impulses pass between neurons in the brain and spinal cord, or pass between an axon and a receptor organ in the body. A synapse between a motor nerve and a muscle fiber is called a *neuromuscular junction* (Figure 5.3 ■). The synapse area of the muscle

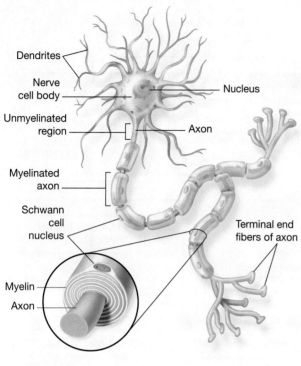

FIGURE 5.2

Neuron

fiber plasma membrane that is adjacent to the axon terminal of the motor nerve is called a *motor end plate*. This junction between nerve tissue and muscle tissue is a key area for the manual therapist to be aware of because it is an area of greater electrical activity in the muscle, where motor points are located. *Motor points* correspond with both trigger points and acupressure points. Usually located in the belly of the muscle, the motor points are important to locate when using direct pressure to treat tender points or trigger points in the muscles. These points can be tender to touch and are places where a palpable twitch can be elicited.[3]

A synapse is like a path we can walk in nature. The more we walk on one path, the stronger the connection at the synapse grows and the faster the velocity of nerve-impulse conduction across the synapse.

A single **nerve** consists of a group of nerve fibers bundled together into cords. In the brain and spinal cord, nerves are called **tracts;** in the body, they are called **peripheral nerves.** The difference between the two is that connective tissues encase peripheral nerves, whereas naked tracts lack connective tissue and operate in a fluid environment. Peripheral nerves are long, creamy-white cords that extend out the brain and spinal cord from nerve roots (Figure 5.4 ■). There are two kinds of peripheral nerves. The **cranial nerves** that branch out of the brain stem innervate cranial and cervical muscles as well as the sense organs in the head and neck. The **spinal nerves** that branch out of the spinal cord at each vertebral segment innervate the body organs and skeletal muscles.

FIGURE 5.3

Neuromuscular junction

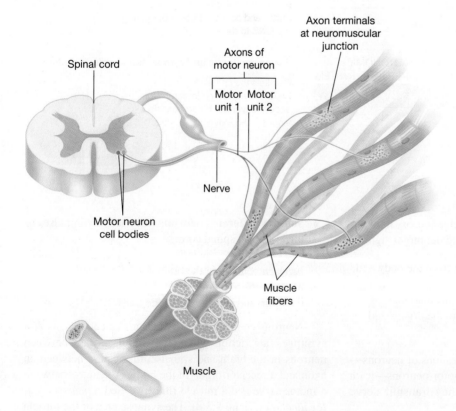

BRIDGE TO PRACTICE
Relaxation and Neuromuscular Therapy

It takes skill to use NM techniques deeply enough to be effective in relieving pain and muscle soreness but still allow your client to relax. You need to work deeply enough to release chronic muscular holding and stretch tissues, but not so deep that you trigger protective guarding in your client.

If you use active techniques during NM treatments, limit the number of these you use during a session so that you can engage your clients' participation now and then without continually interrupting their relaxation process. Also, support and encourage your clients to sink into deep relaxation in between the times when you need to ask for their feedback or ask them to actively participate in the session.

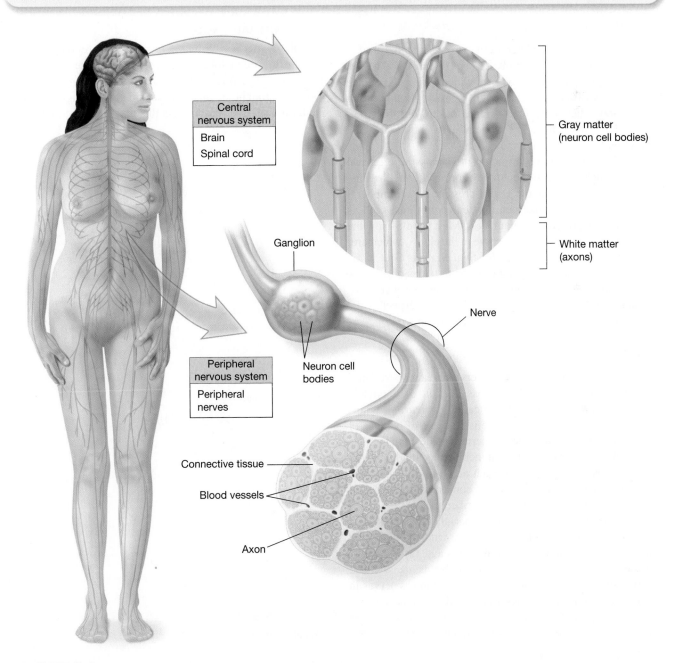

FIGURE 5.4

Nervous system

BRIDGE TO PRACTICE
Getting Feedback about Neurological Symptoms

Whenever you apply deep pressure or stretch to areas that peripheral nerves pass through, especially around joints, make sure to ask your client to report any neurological symptoms that arise, such as tingling, numbness, shooting pains, or sensations of pins and needles.

A general understanding of the anatomical location of peripheral nerves will assist you in working safely around nerves. We revisit this topic as it comes up in the second half of the text.

5.1.2 Peripheral Nerves

A network of peripheral nerves runs from the spinal cord to muscles in the trunk and limbs. Groups of peripheral nerves in different areas of the body are called *nerve plexi*. Each **nerve plexus** (singular) consists of a group of intersecting nerve roots that strategically branch out toward the structures they innervate. The peripheral nerves are embedded between layers of tissues and muscles.

During palpation, you might roll across a peripheral nerve, which will feel like a ropey cord and could be mistaken for a round tendon. Direct pressure on a peripheral nerve is likely to evoke neurological symptoms, such as shooting pain, tingling, or numbness. Most people know the feeling of bumping the ulnar nerve in the elbow, which creates a sharp, zinging pain. The *brachial plexus* is close to the surface and vulnerable during work on the sides of the neck and the upper shoulder (Figure 5.5 ■). It passes between the scalene muscles, then dives under the lateral aspect of the clavicle and over the first rib on its way to the arms.

5.1.2.1 CONNECTIVE TISSUES OF PERIPHERAL NERVES

A cross section of a peripheral nerve reveals a structural organization similar to the cross section of a muscle (Figure 5.6 ■). A fascial sheath called *epineurium* wraps a single nerve. Each single nerve is made up of bundles of nerve fascicles. Each fascicle, in turn, is made up of bundles of single nerve fibers. A fascial membrane called *perineurium* wraps a nerve fascicle. Each nerve fiber is either an axon or a dendrite. A thin layer of connective tissue called *endoneurium* covers a single nerve fiber.

Connective tissues encasing peripheral nerves give them a flexibility and elasticity so they can bend with joint movement and slide between muscles and fascial membranes during movement. When a joint bends, the skin and soft tissues around the joint stretch and compress nerves in that area. Connective tissues around and within nerves create a spongy padding so that a nerve can withstand a certain degree of compression from surrounding tissues.[4]

5.1.2.2 NEURAL TENSION

Peripheral nerves elongate in areas where they bend, primarily around joints. Nerves can elongate from 8 to 20 percent of their resting length before sustaining damage. During a straight leg raise, the sciatic nerve elongates up to 12 millimeters.[5] If nerves lose this extensibility along one

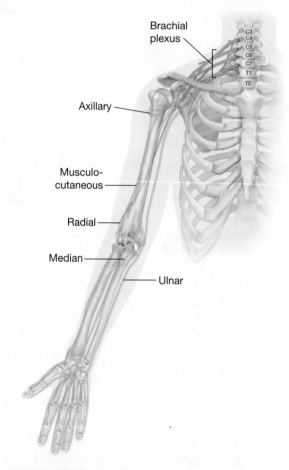

FIGURE 5.5
Brachial plexus

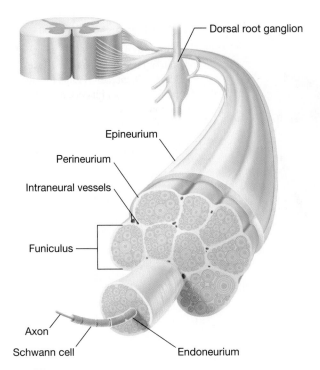

FIGURE 5.6

Peripheral nerve: cross section

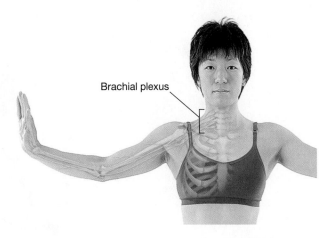

FIGURE 5.7

Arm stretch that puts neural tension on the brachial plexus

area, **neural tension** that equalizes tension along the nerve increases in another area.[6]

Stretching causes neural tension. To experience the continuity of neural tension in the peripheral nerves from your hands to your spine, raise your arms to your sides, then slightly bend your elbows while pulling your fingers back as you slowly push your palms away (Figure 5.7 ■). You should feel a stretch and may even feel tingling in the peripheral nerves to your hand since this stretch places them under tension.

Myofascial restrictions and skeletal misalignments can restrict the sliding motion of peripheral nerves and even compress them, causing nerve entrapment.

It is important to recognize the effects that myofascial restrictions and entrapments place on nerves, particularly when stretching a client with passive motion. Myofascial restrictions create mild symptoms at the end range of motion, such as neural tension and tingling. Nerve entrapments usually create stronger symptoms such as numbness, tingling, pins and needles, and shooting pains during a normal range of motion. Stretching a client with nerve entrapment can put excessive tension on the areas of the nerve that are *not* entrapped, which will exacerbate symptoms. To avoid this, loosen soft tissues around entrapped nerves with massage before performing general stretching.

There are many clinical tests to check for pathologies that develop from neural tension beyond a normal range, such as the *slump test*.[7] In a simplistic version of this test, the practitioner has a patient sit on a table or counter where both feet can hang off. Next, the patient is directed to slump forward and drop the head (Figure 5.8a ■). Then the practitioner slowly lifts the patient's foot, stopping at the first sign of any symptoms

BRIDGE TO PRACTICE
Client Feedback during Passive Joint Movement

Prepare your clients for passive joint movement by stressing how important it is that they report any symptoms of discomfort or pain as soon as the symptoms occur. Then make sure to perform passive joint motions slowly, watching your clients' faces to monitor them for symptoms of pain. Stoic clients are often reluctant to report discomfort. They may hold a "no pain, no gain" belief and suffer silently. On the flip side, hypersensitive clients might interpret normal sensations of tissue stretching as pain and discomfort. In this case, make sure to describe to your client what is and isn't normal sensation.

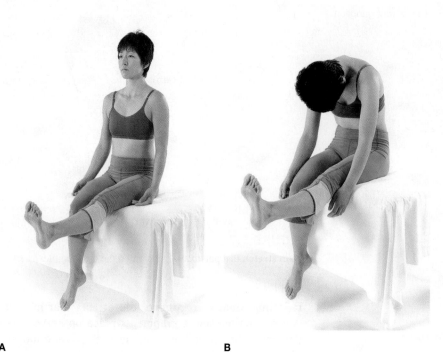

A   **B**

FIGURE 5.8

Slump test: a) Client sits in an upright position, raises leg, then dorsiflexes ankle. b) Client then slumps forward. A positive test will induce neurological symptoms.

of nerve restriction or pathology (Figure 5.8b ■). Pathologies show up as sensitivities or pain along the peripheral nerves, indicating areas where the nerves are under mechanical stress.

Clinical testing for neural tension pathologies may not be within the scope of a massage and bodywork practice. Still, it is important to understand the dynamics of peripheral nerve tension because any passive joint movements performed on clients places their peripheral nerves under tension. If their nerves are already compressed, restricted, or impinged, moving their joints within a small range of normal motion will create symptoms.

5.1.3 Neuromuscular Patterns

During the process of motor development from birth to walking, every person moves through the same series of basic movement patterns. The patterns are push, reach, and pull actions that occur along radial, spinal, homologous, homolateral, and contralateral pathways, which were discussed in the introductory chapter. Every human movement can be described according to these basic patterns. For example, a swimmer doing a butterfly stroke reaches and pulls in an upper body homologous motion; a shot putter throws the shot using a homolateral push with the leg and arm, and a runner swings the arms and legs in opposition in a contralateral gait.

Every movement pattern the body performs involves a sequence of muscular contractions. The neurological program for each pattern is recorded on the "hard drive"

of the *motor cortex*—the part of the brain that stores the programming for neuromuscular patterns. Every time we repeat a certain movement, the motor cortex pulls up the neuromuscular template for that movement and runs it. Just like a nerve synapse, the more a motor pathway is used, the stronger it becomes due to the myelination of motor nerves.

All peripheral nerve axons are covered with *myelin sheaths*—a layer of lipids (fat) that insulate and protect nerves. Myelin also speeds the conduction of nerve impulses away from the central nervous system. The more well traveled a neuromuscular pathway, the thicker the myelin becomes on the motor nerve along this pathway. This explains how certain movement patterns become habitual. The nervous system likes to route movement down well-used pathways. As a result, the motor nerves along dominant tracks, like the surface of major highways, are continually paved and repaved with thicker and thicker myelin sheaths, which speeds the transmission of motor impulses along these routes.

5.1.4 Sensorimotor Loop and Neuromuscular Patterning

Body movement requires continuous coordination between sensory feedback from the neuromuscular system and motor responses through muscular contractions. Movement occurs as the result of a constantly cycling **sensorimotor loop,** which is a continual and almost instantaneous interchange between sensory input and motor output (Figure 5.9 ■). This amazing process occurs through a sophisticated neurological circuitry connecting myriad sensory organs embedded in muscles and joints to motor units.

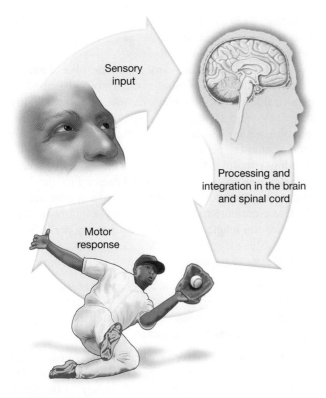

FIGURE 5.9
Sensorimotor loop

It would be impossible for a person to consciously process and control the complex sensorimotor processes that underlie an ongoing production of movement responses. Attempt to write with your nondominant hand and you will appreciate the habitual yet refined circuitry of the neuromuscular system. Fortunately for us, the nervous system coordinates 95 percent of our movement programs at a subcortical level, below the level of our conscious awareness.

Unfortunately, faulty neuromuscular patterns all too easily become habit. Faulty movement patterns cause muscle and joint imbalances, which manifest as posture and movement problems and lead to the chronic pains and repetitive-use injuries that people often seek massage and bodywork to relieve. You can change faulty patterns to improve overall muscle and joint function with neuromuscular patterning exercises.[8]

Patterning involves slowing a faulty movement pattern down enough to become aware of where in the chain of action the faulty muscular response occurs. Sometimes this awareness alone is enough to reorganize a more efficient neuromuscular pathway, but more often a person needs to redirect the movement to improve the pattern. Redirecting the movement can involve both inhibiting a faulty muscular response and facilitating a more efficient response. Say, for example, that every time a man looks down, he feels neck

pain. To change the pattern, he needs to practice moving his neck slowly enough to relax the overworking muscles and also to engage a more effective use of his muscles during movement. You can use patterning touch to guide the new movement, helping him to slowly turn his neck, calling attention to habitual contractions so he can relax them while he moves.

5.2 SENSORY RECEPTORS

Sensory nerves in the musculoskeletal tissues pick up information from a number of **sensory receptors,** which are specialized cells and microscopic organs. They work, in essence, as the eyes and ears of the body. The sensory receptors relay information to the central nervous system for processing. They let the neurons know what's going in the body so that the brain and spinal cord can coordinate appropriate responses.

There are two major classifications of sensory receptors: *interoceptors* and *exteroceptors*. Exteroceptors receive stimuli through the organs of the five senses—the eyes, ears, nose, mouth, and skin. Interoceptors called *visceroceptors* pick up sensory impulses from the organs. Interoceptors called **proprioceptors**—sensory receptors for proprioception—pick up sensory impulses from the musculoskeletal system. Interoceptors throughout the neuromuscular system relay a continuous stream of information through neurons to the motor units for the coordination of instantaneous motor responses.

5.2.1 Proprioception and Perception

Proprioception is an awareness of posture, movement, balance, and the location of the body in space. Proprioceptive organs in the muscles, tendons, and joints receive information from the musculoskeletal system about changes in movement and position. The brain interprets proprioceptive input as **perception** and then coordinates an outgoing stream of motor responses according to how it perceives sensation.

Perceptions are not always accurate. A client may perceive her neck as being straight, when in reality her head tilts to one side but has been off center for so long that her brain registers the tilt as normal. When a neuromuscular pattern shifts, a client might experience perceptual confusion and need to reorient. For example, if you were to straighten this client's neck, she might feel the aligned position as crooked, in which case she could look in the mirror to get accurate visual feedback that overrides her skewed perceptions.

The central nervous system processes proprioceptive information with a degree of efficiency and precision that goes largely unnoticed until errors in perception result in errors in movement. Here is an explanation of the process. We use the same arm muscles to lift a heavy rock as we do to lift a glass of water. We perceive the rock as heavy and the glass as light. The brain sends information about the perceived weight to proprioceptors in the joints, tendons, and muscles to adjust the degree of muscular effort needed for each task. If the perceptions are inaccurate, the movement response will be off. For example, if a person heaves a heavy box up to lift it and the box is actually empty, his effort will send the box flying through the air.

Fortunately for us, our neuromuscular mechanisms run with a perceptual acuity that rarely fails. Proprioceptors in the inner ear continually inform the brain about where the body is located in space, how fast it is moving, and what the orientation of the head and body is relative to the ground. Proprioceptors in the joints determine exactly how far and at what rate the joints need to move to walk down a staircase, and then they reset the muscular tone for walking on flat ground. This smooth interface between proprioceptors and perceptions runs at the edge of our awareness, requiring minimal attention yet allowing us to move through daily activities with ease and accuracy in muscular control.

5.2.2 Muscle Spindles

There are two basic kinds of skeletal muscular cells: extrafusal and intrafusal fibers. **Extrafusal fibers** are the contractile fibers presented in the muscle chapter, the slow and fast fibers making up motor units. Extrafusal fibers are four times the size of the intrafusal fibers and far more

abundant. They are innervated by large-diameter *alpha motor neurons,* which deliver the motor impulses we need to produce muscular contractions.

Intrafusal fibers are sensory muscle fibers found in a **muscle spindle.** Each spindle consists of 2–10 intrafusal fibers inside a connective tissue capsule with a spindle-like shape (Figure 5.10 ■). Muscle spindles are interspersed throughout a muscle, anchored to the extrafusal fibers by endomysium and perimysium, to monitor stretch in the surrounding extrafusal fibers. They are innervated by small-diameter *gamma motor neurons* and respond to stretch by contracting. Although the contractions of a spindle are too weak to contribute to the overall work output of muscle, the change in length is picked up by sensory nerve fibers located inside the spindle cell. Muscle spindles contain two types of sensory nerves:

- One picks up information about length changes in the muscle.
- The other picks up information about the rate of length changes in the muscle.

This fine-tuned sensory apparatus in the spindle fibers function as the overseers of muscular effort. They relay information about extrafusal fiber activity to the CNS, which uses the information to coordinate the degree and speed of muscular contractions needed to carry out any task at hand.

Muscle approximation is a great technique for using reflex mechanisms to lengthen muscles. To **approximate** means to shorten. Muscle approximation involves slowly pushing the two ends of a muscle together to shorten it. The movement mechanically simulates the shortening that occurs during contraction, which produces a relaxation response. Although the mechanism controlling this response is unclear, it is probable that the spindle fibers register the shortened position, which triggers a resetting of the muscle length by inducing a relaxation response.

5.2.2.1 A REFLEX ARC

An extensive part of the sensorimotor circuitry controls reflex activity. *Reflexes* are responses to stimuli that occur automatically, without conscious thought. Muscles can be stimulated by motor impulses coming from the brain and spinal cord or by impulses coming directly from the spindle cell through a **reflex arc.** The reflex arc bypasses more complex neuromuscular pathways for movement. It provides a simple, rudimentary pathway that allows muscles to make immediate adjustments to incoming stimuli, particularly to noxious or threatening stimuli. The knee-jerk test is a great example of a reflex arc in action. Reflex tests are used to diagnose the condition of a neuromuscular pathway. To check the knee-jerk reflex, a doctor taps on the patellar

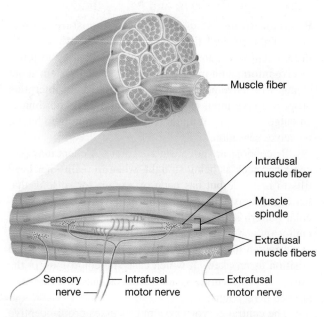

Muscle fiber

Intrafusal muscle fiber

Muscle spindle

Extrafusal muscle fibers

Sensory nerve — Intrafusal motor nerve — Extrafusal motor nerve

FIGURE 5.10

Muscle spindle

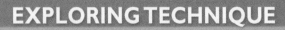

EXPLORING TECHNIQUE
Muscle Approximation

Approximation is a useful hands-on tool to relax and lengthen your client's muscles. You can use it on any muscle anywhere in the body. The way you use this technique will depend on the individual muscle size and shape because you'll need to sculpt your hand around each end of the muscle. For flat muscles, use a broad touch; for thin, spindle-shaped muscles, use a pincher touch.

1. Hold the muscle near its origin and insertion, at the musculotendinous junction.

2. Slowly push the ends of the muscle together to shorten it (Figure 5.11a ■).
3. Keep holding the muscle and wait until you feel the relaxation response. As the muscle relaxes, you'll feel it slowly spring out into your hands. It will take a few seconds because it is a tonic (slow) muscle response.
4. Once you feel the muscle finish relaxing, slowly draw the origin and insertion apart until you feel like you've lengthened the muscle as far as it will allow you to (Figure 5.11b ■).

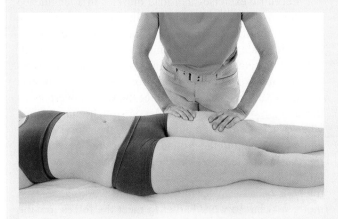

FIGURE 5.11a

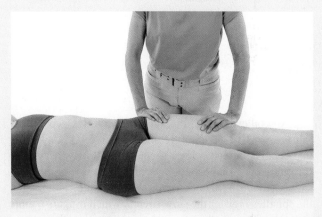

FIGURE 5.11b

tendon right below the knee cap with a mallet, putting the extensor muscles on a quick stretch. When the reflex arc works, the patient's knee extends with a quick kick.

A reflex arc is made up of receptor, sensory nerve, integration center through a single synapse or multiple synapses, a motor nerve, and muscle fibers (Figure 5.12 ■). In a reflex arc, the movement response to the stimuli is always exactly the same.

Reflex arcs ensure instant protective responses to stimuli that could result in tissue damage or death. They operate on auto pilot, moving us away from dangers faster and with more efficiency than conscious thought could possibly coordinate. They free our minds from the ongoing and detailed tasks of keeping the body upright, in control, and on guard to jump out of harms way.

5.2.2.2 THE STRETCH REFLEX

Muscle spindles play a key role in monitoring and responding to stretch through one of the most basic reflex arcs, called a **stretch reflex.** This neural pathway exists between muscle spindles and motor units to control two types of reflex responses: a **tonic** (slow) and **phasic** (fast) stretch reflex. Each types of stretch reflex, also called a **myotatic reflex**, responds to a different speed of muscle stretching.

● A gradual elongation in muscle length elicits a tonic stretch reflex, which results in a slow muscular contraction.
● A quick stretch of a muscle results in a phasic stretch reflex, which triggers protective contractions that prevent the muscle from overstretching and tearing.

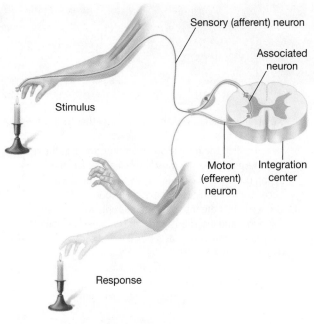

Sensory (afferent) neuron

Associated neuron

Stimulus

Motor (efferent) neuron

Integration center

Response

FIGURE 5.12
Reflex arc

A good example of the tonic stretch reflex occurs during *postural sway,* a subtle and reflexive body swaying that occurs while standing. As the body slowly sways one direction, intrinsic postural muscles on one side of the body slowly stretch. When these muscles reach a certain length, the spindles register the slow stretch, which triggers a tonic stretch reflex resulting in a slow contraction that sways the body in the other direction. This reflex also prevents weight-bearing joints from yielding to the constant pull of gravity and flexing. It keeps the postural muscles active in order to keep the body upright, so it is sometimes referred to as an *antigravity reflex.*

The phasic stretch reflex mediates the knee-jerk response discussed in the last section. It also occurs during a preparatory backswing. As a batter swings, the backswing puts the working muscles on a quick stretch, which results in a reflexive muscular contraction used to hit the ball. The velocity of the preparatory motion determines the rate at which the spindles discharge; and it should match the force and speed of the desired outcome. This explains why a golfer putts with a slow, controlled backswing that matches the swing of the putt. In contrast, a batter uses a quick, strong backswing to match the velocity and force he needs to hit a home run.

5.2.2.3 STRETCH INJURIES

Two scenarios make a muscle susceptible to a stretch injury: when a muscle is put on a stretch while it is contracting concentrically, or when a muscle contracts while it is being stretched or working eccentrically. **Stretch injuries** often occur when a person is lifting or moving a heavy load

and the weight of the load or some other force overpowers the contraction and tears the muscle. For example, a person pulling a stubborn horse on a rope will probably sustain a stretch injury if the horse suddenly rears.

Stretch injuries also occur during ballistic movements that are common to many sports. Punters often suffer stretch injuries in hamstring pulls. As the punter swings his leg back to punt the ball, the hamstrings contract powerfully and quickly. Then, when he swings his leg forward to kick the ball, the powerful contraction of the quadriceps overpower the hamstrings before they are able to lengthen, pulling and perhaps even tearing the hamstrings.

The punter would be advised to train his hamstring muscles to lengthen them past the point at which the stretch reflex reflexively shortens them. To overcome a stretch reflex, the stretch needs to be held for 30 seconds or longer.

Eccentric exercises that load muscles in a lengthened position also put working muscles in a position vulnerable to stretch injuries. For example, some people like to exercise with ankle weights. When starting a straight leg lift with ankle weights from a supine position, the hip flexors are maximally lengthened and prone to a stretch injury. The injury occurs when the load of the weight overpowers the strength of the muscle. A classic stretch injury occurs when a person lifts something heavy, then loses control while lowering it to the ground and drops the weight, tearing the biceps tendon. Muscles are more susceptible to injury during eccentric contractions than concentric contractions because fewer motor units are working, so each motor unit has to work harder to meet the forces moving against it.

5.2.3 Golgi Tendon Organs

A muscle can only contract so far. When a muscle reaches maximum contraction and has shortened as much as it can, the tendons of the muscle begin to stretch. At this point, proprioceptors embedded along the *musculotendinous junction,* called **Golgi tendon organs** (GTOs), register an increased tension on the tendon (Figure 5.13 ■). The GTOs relay this information to the CNS, which triggers an inhibitory response that causes that muscle to relax. Relaxation occurs gradually in order to relieve tension on a tendon.

Although sensory signals from the GTOs are too weak to completely inhibit a motor nerve signal, they play an important role in modulating muscle tension between agonist and antagonist muscles. GTOs serve as a precise gauge of the force that muscles need to actually pull on the bones. Muscles are always contracting on some level, so there is always recruitment of motor units. The GTOs become activated only when the muscles begin pulling on the bones, stretching tendons, and generating joint motion.

There are several important differences between muscle spindles and GTOs (see Table 5.1 ■). Muscle spindles

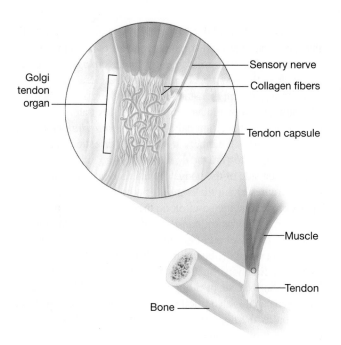

FIGURE 5.13
Golgi tendon organ

respond to changes in the length of muscle fibers and the speed of length changes. GTOs respond to tension in the tendon. Muscle spindles trigger *excitatory nerve impulses,* causing a muscle to contract. In contrast, GTOs trigger *inhibitory nerve impulses* to reduce the number of motor units firing.

The muscle spindles and GTOs together control the rate and degree of joint motion, gradually shortening the muscles on one side of a joint while lengthening the muscles on the other side. Together they create a controlled action between opposing muscles so that they gradually turn a joint, like two ropes in a pulley. As tension in the agonist muscle increases, the GTOs decrease tension in the antagonist by gradually inhibiting motor-unit activity, allowing it to lengthen smoothly in order for even and smooth joint motion to occur.

Forces other than muscular contractions also pull on tendons, affecting GTOs. For example, we can only hang from a hand grip for so long until our body weight causes the tendons to stretch. When they reach a certain length, the GTOs trigger a **tendon reflex** that inhibits muscular contraction, causing us to suddenly lose our grip and drop to the ground.

5.2.4 Joint Proprioceptors

There are several kinds of proprioceptors embedded in connective tissues around the joints that pick up information about mechanical compression. Proprioceptors around joints assist in the coordination of joint motion. Do a simple task such as sitting down from a standing position with your eyes closed, and the joint proprioceptors will give you information about how your joints move during this action. The **Pacinian corpuscles** in the joint capsules detect rapid changes in pressure and vibration. The **Ruffini endings** embedded in the skin around joints detect slow changes in the position or angle of the joint.

The joint proprioceptors also protect the joints from damaging movements. If pain signals coming from joint proprioceptors indicate that moving that joint risks damaging the joint, pain signals can trigger an inhibition of muscular contractions. Here is a case that illustrates this process. A client reported that while walking, every time his knee bent past 10 degrees he felt a shooting pain in his knee and it buckled under him. Medical evaluations determined that the meniscus was torn. Every time he flexed his knee past 10 degrees, a flap of cartilage called a *plica* folded and pinched, which resulted in intense shooting pain. To prevent further damage to the cartilage, his nervous system immediately acted on the message coming from the joint proprioceptors, sending inhibitory signals to turn off the muscles acting on his knee.

Joint proprioceptors can also function as **nociceptors**, which are sensory nerve endings that register extreme changes in temperature or pressure as painful stimuli. (The process of *nociception* is the perception of pain.) The joint proprioceptors only function as nociceptors when extreme changes in temperature, such as blistering heat or frigid cold, or crushing pressure reach a certain threshold. This triggers the coordination of protective reflexes, such as the knee buckling in the case just described.

TABLE 5.1	Comparing Muscle Spindles and Golgi Tendon Organs	
Properties	Muscle Spindles	Golgi Tendon Organs
Triggered by	Changes in muscle length and speed of contraction (muscle stretch)	Increased tension in tendons (tendon stretch)
Neurological effect	Triggers excitatory motor impulse, results in contraction	Triggers inhibitory motor impulse, results in relaxation
Location	Embedded throughout muscle	Embedded in musculotendinous junction
Elasticity	Far more elastic than tendons	Far less elastic than muscle

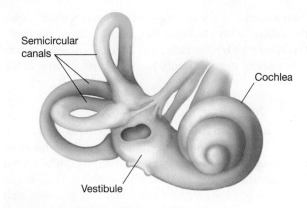

FIGURE 5.14

Labyrinth of the inner ear

5.2.5 Labyrinth and Neck Proprioceptors

The temporal bone in the cranium houses a convoluted maze of chambers and tunnels in the bone called the **labyrinth,** located in the inner ear. The labyrinth contains specialized sensory nerves that register positional changes in the head and neck, resulting in ongoing adjustments in muscular tone related to balance and equilibrium responses.

Three structures inside the labyrinth—an egg-shaped structure called the *vestibule,* three intersecting *semicircular canals,* and a snail-shaped *cochlea*—contain proprioceptors that control balance or equilibrium, spatial orientation, and hearing (Figure 5.14 ■). A periosteum membrane lines the entire bony labyrinth. A thin *endolymph* fluid fills the membrane, and microscopic nerves called *hair cells* that resemble cilia line the membrane. The hair cells are sensitive to the movement of the fluid as the head moves through changes in position and velocity (speed in a specific direction).

Inside the vestibule, two sac-like structures called the *saccule* and *utricle* contain tiny bony crystals called *otoliths* or

"ear stones." The otoliths float within the gelatinous fluid filling these chambers and stimulate the hair cells as they brush pass them. The hair cells register linear changes in velocity, such as the linear acceleration and deceleration you feel when riding in a car that starts and stops along a straight road. The otoliths also stimulate a primitive reflex that responds to changes in head position called the *tonic labyrinthine reflex.* As the otoliths in the inner ear sink in the direction of gravity, the body yields toward the direction the head turns, increasing tone on that side of the body.[9] As the face turns down, flexor tone increases along the front of the body; as the face turns up, extensor tone increases along the back of the body.

The *semicircular canals* register the angular movements of the head and help us maintain a sense of spatial orientation when the head tips at different angles or changes rotational directions, such as when we are riding in a car as it banks a sharp curve, or riding on a tilt-a-whirl ride at a carnival. Each canal is also filled with a thin, clear fluid that shifts direction as the head tilts, stimulating hair cells lining the canal. Each of the three semicircular canals is also oriented in a different plane to register changes in each plane.

In addition to these labyrinth mechanisms for maintaining balance, joint proprioceptors and muscle spindles in the top half of the neck contribute to head-righting reflexes, which rebalance the head to the upright position and align the head with the body during movement. Ideally, a person can retain flexibility and range of motion in the cervical spine so that the head can easily rebalance over the body during a range of movements. Yet as people age, there is a tendency to develop stiff muscles in the neck and lose range of motion in the cervical spine, which can dull equilibrium responses. Also, as the tissues in the inner ear age and stiffen, people can develop balance problems, dizziness, and even nausea. Massage and bodywork can help a client maintain a freedom of movement in the cervical spine, which supports equilibrium responses.

EXPLORING TECHNIQUE
Slow Movement to Relax Head and Neck Muscles

When clients relax enough to allow you to passively move their heads, it shows they really trust you. As clients yield to passive movement of the head and neck, and relax their cervical muscles, their heads will become heavier and move more freely. Passive movement of the head also stimulates the *tonic labyrinthine reflex,* causing a deep relaxation response to spread through the entire body. Here is a simple exercise to do just that.

With your partner in a supine position:

1. Cradle the head under both hands to completely support it (Figure 5.15a ■). Let your hands conform to the shape of the

posterior cranium with an encompassing touch that does not compress the head. Rest the back of your hands on the table.

2. Have your partner close his or her eyes, relax the forehead, and allow or imagine the weight of the head to sink into your hands.

3. Slowly roll the head to one side as though you were pouring liquid sand inside a bowl by slowly tipping the bowl (Figure 5.15b ■). Move gently and at a slow rate that allows your partner to relax. If your partner has trouble relaxing, you may need to move the head with micromovement, barely moving it at all.

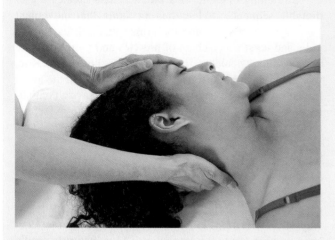

FIGURE 5.15a

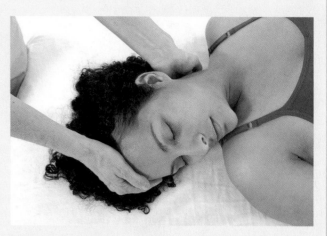

FIGURE 5.15b

4. If your partner has a stiff neck and cannot let you move his or her head, barely lift your hands to lift the head, then relax your hands in a way that encourages your partner to let the weight of the head sink into your hands.
5. As you roll the head to one side, allow any natural movement responses to occur. If a partner's neck and head start

moving automatically in a direction, give them room to move. Avoid holding or moving the head in a manner that prevents natural movements.
6. Next, slowly roll the head to the other side.
7. Repeat several times until your partner can relax the weight of his or her head in your hands and let you move it.

5.3 REFLEXES AND BASIC MOVEMENT PATHWAYS

Neuromuscular pathways are laid down through a gradual process of sensorimotor learning that begins with basic reflexes. Newborns come into the world equipped with a handful of rudimentary reflexes to ensure their survival, such as the rooting reflex that coordinates nursing movements.

From birth to walking, motor pathways develop slowly, beginning with the emergence of basic reflex patterns that are processed in the spinal cord and lower brain center, such as hand-to-eye and hand-to-mouth movements. Over time, these simple reflexes slowly combine to form more complex pathways and the infant begins rolling over and pushing up onto the hands and feet. By the time a toddler can stand up and walk, the basic movement pathways common to all human movement patterns have been organized in the neuromuscular circuitry. Although simple reflex actions disappear as more complex movement patterns emerge, the neuromuscular circuitry controlling reflexes is active during all of our movements.

5.3.1 Reciprocal Inhibition and Reflexes

In a study of animal reflexes, a physiologist named Lord Sherrington first identified a law that explains the firing pattern of opposing muscles during reflex movements. The law of **reciprocal inhibition** describes how a muscle relaxes when the muscle opposing it contracts.[10] Relaxation occurs to a degree that allows for smooth movement at the joint. Sherrington further postulated that agonist/antagonist

muscle pairs share a *reciprocal innervation* by motor neurons located in the spinal cord. The reciprocal innervation of opposing muscle groups allows for the simultaneous excitation of one muscle and inhibition of the other. It also ensures the smooth coordination of movement during rhythmic actions such as chewing or walking.

There are a number of basic reflexes in the human movement range that demonstrate the law of reciprocal inhibition. The **extensor thrust reflex** automatically extends the limbs to catch us when we fall. The **flexor withdrawal reflex** pulls the limbs into quick flexion to move us away from danger such as fire, the edge of a cliff, or a perceived threat. The **crossed extensor reflex** lifts one foot while extending the other leg to prevent us from stepping down onto a sharp nail (Figure 5.16 ■).

Reflexes underlie coordinated movement sequences. For example, the extensor thrust and flexor withdrawal reflexes underlie the muscle and joint patterns active during a push-up or while jumping rope, and the crossed extensor reflexes underlie all gait patterns such as walking, running, or skipping. Hiking on uneven terrain or participating in sports activities that require spontaneous movement patterns, such as team sports or skiing, can keep the reflexes active and sharp. The inhibition of reflexes can stiffen the body and can lead to awkward, uncoordinated movement patterns. Inactive people who have inhibited reflexive movements for many years can and often do develop balance problems as they age, which can lead to fear of falling and muscular guarding that develops around this fear.

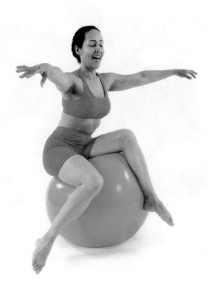

FIGURE 5.16
Reflexive movement

5.3.2 Kinetic Chains

Recall from the introductory chapter that a kinetic chain is a series of successively arranged joints and muscles making up a movement pathway (Figure 5.17 ■). A kinetic chain can be described by the movement pathway it sequences along. Most activities of daily living occur along predicable movement pathways. We get into a car with a homolateral movement that initiates in the foot and extends one side of the body. We reverse directions when walking by turning the head, which sequences into rotation down the spine into the hip and leg. And we watch a plane fly overhead by tipping the head back and extending the spine to look up. In each example, movement initiates at one end of a kinetic chain and sequences along a predictable pathway.

Stretching one end of a kinetic chain creates a predictable sequence of lengthening along that movement pathway. When stretching the arms overhead, the stretch pulls and lengthens a chain of muscles and joints from the arms into the shoulders, trunk, and lower limbs. Likewise, when applying traction on a supine client's feet, if the lower limbs and spine are free of restrictions and have a continuity of tone, the client will feel the lengthening from the feet all the way to the head.

5.3.3 Meridians

In Chinese medicine, **meridians** are channels or pathways in the body along which Ch'i (qi), or energy, flows. A meridian connects every finger and every toe along a linear pathway into the trunk (Figure 5.18 ■). Along each meridian are a number of acupressure points. Acupuncturists needle these points to open the flow of blocked energy along a meridian. It is also interesting to note that the acupressure points follow the pathways of the muscles and nerves. Some of the acupressure points, also called *tonic points,* are known to relieve muscular tension and pain. Many of the tonic points correspond to motor points in muscles, where trigger points build up and where there is the most electrical activity.[11]

Meridians roughly follow muscular and movement pathways along the kinetic chains. The movement of each digit follows a distinct pathway into the trunk. The fingers and toes are like parallel rays. Movement of the thumb and index finger sequences along the biceps line into the chest; whereas movement of the little finger sequences along a triceps line into the scapula and back.

Anatomist and Rolfer Tom Myers has created an "anatomy trains" map depicting the structural aspects of the movement pathways along 12 myofascial meridians.[12] A number of these meridians follow the bodywork recipe formulated by Ida Rolf, a sequence for unlayering myofascial pathways along a series of "Rolf lines." Myers expanded the Rolf lines into 12 anatomy trains, identifying the

BRIDGE TO PRACTICE
Reflexive Movements in Massage Clients

During a massage and bodywork session, clients often make reflexive movements. They show jumpy responses to touch on certain parts of their bodies or automatically withdraw from touch that elicits pain. These innate movements are natural responses that are to be expected, yet many clients feel out of control and embarrassed by the sudden reflexes. As a result, they might hold chronic tension in their bodies to prevent unexpected movements during the session, which works against the goals of the session.

In these situations, it can help to tell your clients that reflexive movement responses are normal and it's okay to allow them to occur. Explain how important reflexes are to protect us by helping us balance when we fall or allowing us to jump out of harm's way. Support reflexive movements when they arise. For example, if you are working on your client's foot and you trigger a flexor withdrawal reflex, follow it by pushing the foot toward the hip to support innate flexion.

FIGURE 5.17

Extensor chain of muscles

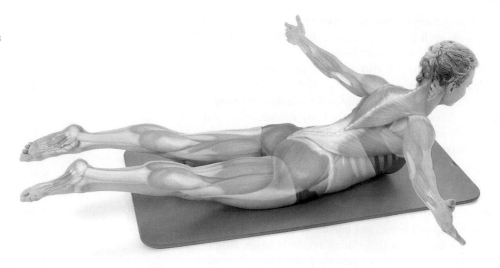

contiguous chain of muscles and connective tissues along each myofascial meridian.[13]

By viewing the movement pathways of the body through a context of kinetic chains and myofascial meridians, we can assess the overall patterns more easily. This is a particularly important skill for practitioners working in the complementary health sciences who make general assessments about the overall health and balance of the neuromusculoskeletal system.

5.3.4 Assessing Kinetic Chains

An assessment of a kinetic chain can provide information about the type of movement a person is performing and the efficiency of muscular coordination in the action. The most obvious assessment is to determine whether a kinetic chain is open or closed. Most body movements are combinations of open- and closed-chain actions. For example, as a person walks, the stance leg works in a closed chain while the swing leg swings in an open chain. The head and upper

FIGURE 5.18

Chinese energy meridians

Major Energy Channels and Important Acupoint Locations

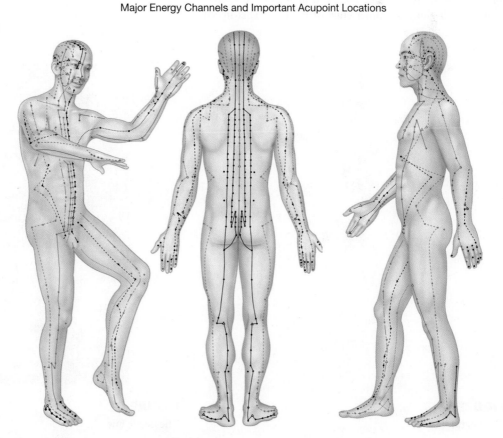

spine nearly always move in an open chain with only a few exceptions, such as when someone does a headstand or a soccer player hits a ball with his head.

Kinetic chains are also assessed according to movement pathways. If we were to paint a body with the primary kinetic chains, the major pathways of movement would appear as lines running along the body's front, back, and sides, with an additional pair of lines crossing the trunk. In the introductory chapter, we looked at the flexor chain and extensor chain of muscles, which create a *front line* (see Figure 1.2) and a *back line* (see Figure 1.1).

A *lateral line* runs along the side of the body through a series of muscles that are connected across joints from the leg, up the hip and trunk, and into the arm (Figure 5.19 ■). We stretch the lateral line during a side bend. A *diagonal line* creates two oblique pathways that cross the trunk and stretch during twisting and contralateral movements (Figure 5.20 ■). The diagonal line follows a kinetic chain activated by the crossed extensor reflex.

Not all movement pathways run along direct pathways of muscles. For example, the *inside line* of the legs is more a line of force and weight support that runs from the medial arches up the inside of the leg, the inner thigh, and through the hips and sacrum into the spine (Figure 5.21 ■). It engages a line of muscles including the flexor digitorum longus and flexor hallucis longus, tibialis posterior, popliteus, medial adductors and vastus medialis oblique; the perineum and lateral hip rotators; and core muscles in the trunk, including the perineum, psoas major, and the deep spinal erectors. The inside line can be observed in skiers and skaters as they push along the inner edge of the foot. This inside

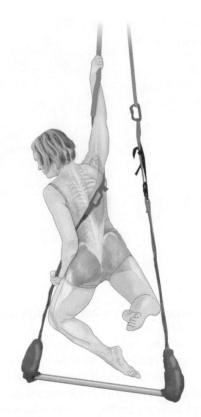

FIGURE 5.20

The diagonal line

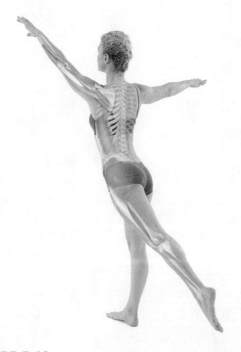

FIGURE 5.19

The lateral line

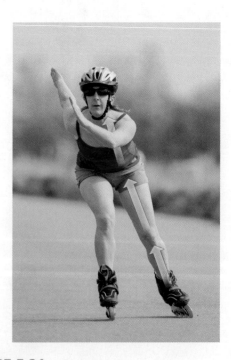

FIGURE 5.21

The inside line

line is most obvious when it is missing or collapsed, as in knock-kneed or bow-legged patterns (see Figure 7.29a-b).

To assess the three-dimensional integrity of the myofascial system, look at the dimensional balance in a group of kinetic chains and ask:

- Is the height, width, and depth of the body proportional and symmetrical? If it is not, along which lines are the soft tissues overstretched or shortened?
- Do the muscles center the weight-bearing joints in extension? If not, where are the muscles stretch weakened and where are they adaptively shortened? How does this affect the meridians?
- How does tone along one pathway relate to its opposing pathway? Are the lateral lines even in length and spatial orientation? Are the inside lines symmetrical? Is the core centered over the feet? Are the flexor and extensor chains balanced in length and tone?
- Is the distal end of the active part of the body moving in an open or closed chain? What part of the body is moving as an open chain? What part of the body is moving as a closed chain?

To determine whether a pathway is balanced and functional, look at the continuity of tone in the muscles along that chain. For example, the continuity of tone along the extensor path can be assessed through three channels:

- *In a palpatory assessment,* run your hands along the pathway and note the continuity of muscular tone or breaks in tone. In a palpation assessment along the spine, which is easy to do with a client during the intake process, run your palms and fingertips down your client's back several times to check the muscles for a continuity of tone.
- *In a postural observation,* look at the client's body from the side. Observe the resting length of the muscles and the position of the joints in relation to neutral. Note where the muscles are stretch weakened or where they are adaptively shortened.
- *In a movement observation,* watch a client do a particular movement, and track the order in which the muscles fire and the joints move along a kinetic chain during a specific action.

To examine how palpatory assessments and posture and movement observations can affect the course of treatment, consider the following case study.

A client complained of chronic pain in the lower neck and between the shoulder blades (Figure 5.22 ■). A general palpation revealed that the spinal muscles in her midthoracic spine, where she had chronic postural flexion, were ropey, taut, and overstretched. Muscles in her cervical spine, where she had chronic hyperextension, were short and tight.

- An *observation of her postural pattern* revealed hyperextension in the lower cervical spine and flexion in the upper and midthoracic spine, which was consistent with the palpatory findings.

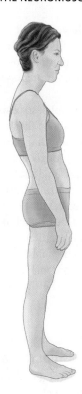

FIGURE 5.22

Assessment question: How does a client's chronic pain relate to her postural pattern?

- The *movement assessment* involved active movement. When the client was asked to look up, she bent her neck in the lower cervical spine, yet the rest of her spine remained immobile. Spinal extension was limited in the mid- and upper thoracic spine. Spinal flexion was severely limited in the neck and lower back.
- The *treatment* involved deep tissue work along her spine to improve a continuity of muscular tone, as well as specific stretching that took her lower cervical spine into flexion and her midthoracic spine into hyperextension.

5.4 MOVEMENT APPLICATIONS IN NEUROMUSCULAR TECHNIQUES

This last section covers the clinical applications of kinesiology and movement studies to neuromuscular techniques in massage and bodywork. Everything else you study in this book is for the purpose of being able to effectively apply these therapeutic techniques covered in this section.

Massage affects the neuromuscular system because it accesses the sensorimotor loop in an elegantly simple yet effective process: Muscle massage helps clients become aware of their muscle tension (sensory input). Once clients can feel their tensions (central nervous system processing), they respond by relaxing their muscles (motor response). When general massage is enough to relax a client's muscular tension, that client possesses a very responsive neuromuscular system and is skilled at relaxation.

When clients cannot relax so easily, there are a number of neuromuscular techniques that will trigger relaxation responses. Rather than learning how to do every one of these techniques on every single muscle in the body, it is far more beneficial to understand the mechanisms underlying each technique. Once you truly grasp these mechanisms, it will be easier to adapt each technique to muscles anywhere in the body. Neuromuscular techniques can be applied locally to relax or even facilitate contractions in specific muscles. They can also be applied globally to improve the overall structural and functional integrity of the body—that is, to improve the ease and efficiency of both posture and movement.

5.4.1 Active, Passive, and Resisted Motion Assessments

The first step in using neuromuscular techniques is to determine whether muscular imbalances, movement restrictions, or pain signals are coming from contractile or noncontractile tissues. The general symptoms a client presents can provide clues about the source of the problem. Three motion tests—active, passive, and resisted—can be used to narrow down the source of a client's problem. The general idea of active, passive, and resisted joint motion was introduced in the joint chapter. These tests work by placing the tissues under specific stresses to recreate the client's symptoms. The tests are performed in succession as a process of elimination. Keep in mind that these tests are for making general assessments about minor joint and muscle problems. They can also identify conditions or areas where manual therapy is contraindicated.

Assessment is progressive. It begins with the client's active movement, followed by passive joint motion, followed by resisted motion. Where and when pain occurs can provide these clues:

- Pain that occurs during active motion points to muscular contraction as the pain generator, but the pain could also be coming from noncontractile tissues in the joint that are compressed during movement.
- Pain that occurs during active motion but not during passive movement usually comes from contractile tissues—from the muscles or tendons.
- Pain that occurs during passive movement but not during resisted movement usually comes from noncontractile structures, such as ligaments, joint capsules, or other joint structures (such as menisci, bursa, synovial lining, blood vessels, or nerves).
- Pain coming from muscular injuries usually radiates along the length of the muscles. In contrast, pain

coming from injuries to joint structures is usually localized within the joint structures. Joint pain can even inhibit the motion.

Motion tests can be applied in many different contexts to achieve a variety of treatment goals, from general loosening to pain relief to improved range of motion. Keep in mind that the same skills for doing motion tests are also used in some neuromuscular techniques.

Motion assessments and techniques can be done a number of ways that fall on a continuum ranging from active to passive (Figure 5.23a-c ■). Table 5.2 ■ describes movement techniques used in manual therapy along this active to passive range of joint motion. Directions for active nonassisted movement and active resisted movement techniques can be found in muscle palpation exercises in Part 2. Directions for passive nonassisted range of motion skills can be found for the major appendicular joints in the bone palpation exercises in Part 2, as well as in some of the Exploring Technique features such as the joint and muscle approximation exercises.

During passive and active assisted movement, it is important to recognize that the movement can go into the direction of ease or discomfort, a direction that either shortens or stretches the tissues. **Direct technique** moves the client in a direction that stretches the tissues and pulls them out of their shortened position. **Indirect technique** moves the client in a direction that takes the tissues into a shortened position. These concepts arise out of osteopathic traditions, although they are broadly used in many therapeutic applications.

Movement therapists call indirect movement techniques "going into the pattern" or "taking over the pattern." By taking the body into its shortened pattern and holding it there, you take over the work of the holding pattern and put the dysfunctional muscles on slack. Indirect technique frees up the energy held in the muscular contraction so that the stretch receptors can reset. Osteopath Lawrence Jones, the founder of a gentle indirect technique called *strain–counterstrain,* emphasizes the importance of holding the shortened position for at least 90 seconds, then *slowly* returning to a neutral position to give the muscles time to reorganize resting tone.[14]

5.4.1.1 ACTIVE MOTION SKILLS

People instinctively guard areas of chronic pain. As a result, movement occurs *around* rather than *through* injured, guarded areas. If a client complains of pain during motion, you can ask the client to demonstrate the movement that causes pain in order to observe where the client chronically holds and restricts joint motion. To avoid further injury, it is important to warn the client to move slowly and use minimal effort while demonstrating problematic movements. Also, compare the range of movement on the symptomatic side with the nonsymptomatic side to assess the normal range and quality of motion for that client.

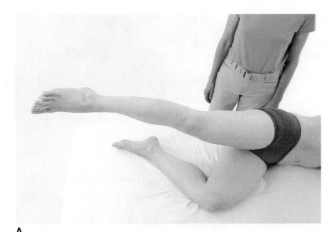

A

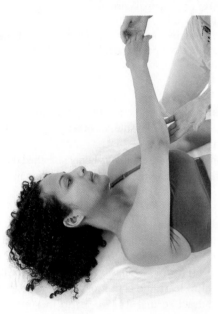

B

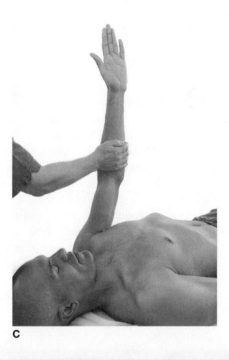

C

FIGURE 5.23

a) **Active nonassisted movement** b) **Active-assisted movement** c) **Active-resisted movement. Each of the following three movement techniques requires a different level of client and/or practitioner involvement.**

TABLE 5.2 **Movement Techniques**		
Technique	Client Participation	Practitioner Participation
Active nonassist	Client actively moves.	Practitioner asks or directs the client to move a certain way.
Active assist	Client moves with practitioner's guidance.	Practitioner assists client movement by providing physical support or guiding the pathway of movement.
Active assisted stretch	Client moves into position of stretch.	Practitioner helps client stretch farther by applying direct pressure, traction, or myofascial stretching.
Active resisted	Client moves against the practitioner's pressure.	Practitioner provides pressure for client to move against.
Passive assist	Client contributes minimal energy toward the desired movement.	Practitioner actively moves the client and coaches the client to contribute minimal effort to moving.
Passive nonassist	Client is totally passive.	Practitioner moves a passive client.

GUIDELINES
Elements to Track While Observing Active Movement

1. **The starting position of the moving joints in relation to joint neutral:** Does the client begin moving from a neutral or from a held, flexed, or rotated joint position?
2. **The place where the movement initiates:** Does the client begin the motion at the hands, feet, head, or pelvis, with the smaller, more articulate muscles?
3. **The overall pattern of movement in joints:** In which joints does movement occur?
4. **The range of motion:** Is the movement within a normal range?
5. **The pathway of motion:** In which order do the joints move?

6. **The quality of motion:** Is the movement smooth or segmental?
7. **The client's willingness to move:** Is the client reluctant to move?
8. **The point at which the symptoms occur:** Where in the range of motion does the client report restriction and/or pain?
9. **The client's reaction to symptoms:** Does the client guard against pain, jump, wince, or push through the restriction and/or pain?
10. **The same movement on the other side of the body:** Does the client move the other side in a normal range?

5.4.1.2 PASSIVE MOTION SKILLS

Passive joint movements are used in massage and bodywork to stretch the soft tissues (especially myofascia), to restore normalcy and balance to the tissues, and to improve range of motion. You can determine whether or not passive joint motion would be appropriate during a session by paying close attention to the client's natural movements during the intake process, noticing patterns of gait and posture, and noticing guarded, nonmoving areas of the client's body. Passive motion is contraindicated on any joint where the client experiences symptoms during active motion (pain, swelling, bruising, numbness, etc.).

Pain during passive joint motion could indicate two types of tissue damage:

- Pain localized in the joint may indicate damage to a ligament, joint capsule, or other joint structures (bursa, cartilage, etc.).
- Pain along a muscle that is being stretched during passive joint movement may indicate dysfunction in that muscle.

5.4.1.3 RESISTED MOTION SKILLS

Resisted motion tests are traditionally used to evaluate the length and strength of a dysfunctional or injured muscle.[15] There are many reasons to use resisted motion in massage and bodywork. Massage students practice resisted movement to learn the action of a muscle or to get a muscle to contract so that it is easier to locate during palpation. Resisted motion tests follow active and passive tests

GUIDELINES
Steps for Using Passive Motion

1. **Get the client's permission to passively move the joint.** Also, tell the client *what* you are going to do and *why* you are going to do it.
2. **Firmly support the area, placing one hand on each side of the joint.** Use one hand to stabilize the supporting bone, the other hand to move the joint. Hold your client in a manner that is firm but gentle and comfortable for the client.
3. **Before moving the joint, place it under light traction.** This prevents you from pinching anything in the joint that could cause pain. Be careful putting too much traction on the fingers, toes, or shoulders because these joints are already highly mobile and susceptible to pain from overstretching.

4. **Instruct your client to inform you immediately during passive joint motion if he or she experiences any pain or discomfort.** Watch your client's face as you perform passive joint movement for any expressions of discomfort or pain, and stop immediately if these occur.
5. **Using linear motion, move the joint slowly and firmly to its end range of motion and hold there.** Then ask your client if he or she feels a stretch (which indicates you've reached end range.)
6. **At the end range, take the stretch a little farther.**
7. **Perform steps 1–6 on the other side to check for symmetry.**

GUIDELINES
Steps for Using Resisted Motion

1. **Give the client simple instructions before using resisted motion:** "Lightly push against the pressure I am applying on your ankle." You can also reverse roles. Rather than having the client push against your resistance, you can have the client resist your movement. In this case you would say, "Hold your elbow here and don't let me move it."

2. **Place the client in a safe position, fully supporting the moving joint.** For example, to perform a resisted motion test on the biceps brachii, you would make sure the client's elbow is supported by the table or your hand.

3. **Instruct the client to use minimal effort while moving:** "Push back lightly with about 10 percent of your effort."

4. **Apply linear pressure that moves the joint in one direction.** Do not twist the joint.

5. **Hold the pressure for several seconds.** Hold the pressure longer if your intention is to facilitate a weak or inhibited muscle, which will allow ample time for the client to increase the strength of contraction.

6. **Ask the client to report any pain or discomfort.** Stop immediately if there is any pain.

7. **Make a bilateral comparison.** Doing so will help you determine what is normal for that client, and also to balance the two sides of the client's body.

Interpreting Findings[16]

- *Strong yet painful contraction:* Indicates a minor injury to muscle or tendon.
- *Weak yet painless contraction:* Depending on the degree, could indicate muscle weakness or indicate a motor nerve dysfunction and require a medical referral.
- *Weak and painful contraction:* Could indicate a serious injury such as a fracture.
- *Reluctance to move:* Clients are often reluctant to move an area when there is serious injury. You can usually identify serious injuries and contraindications to resisted motion during the client-intake process.

to determine whether contractile or noncontractile tissues are causing pain. When a client feels pain during resisted motion but not during a passive motion, the pain generator is most likely a dysfunctional muscle.

Other reasons for using resisted movements include:

- To facilitate an inhibited muscle
- To organize and improve neuromuscular patterns
- To perform muscle energy techniques
- To test a muscle to determine the effectiveness of treatment (the muscle is tested before and after treatment)

During resisted motion, a practitioner applies pressure to a certain area of the client's body and asks the client to push against the pressure. To use resisted movement, a practitioner needs to know the general location of a muscle and what type of joint motion it produces upon contraction. For example, since the biceps brachii produces elbow flexion, to get the biceps to contract, you would have your client flex the elbow against your resistance on the wrist.

A muscle produces the weakest contraction from an outer range, where it is maximally lengthened, and the strongest contraction from an inner range, where it is maximally shortened. Midrange is probably the best position from which to ask for resisted motion. The elbow is in midrange at about 80 degrees of flexion.

Resisted motion can be done against isometric or isotonic contractions, in either a static position or through a range of motion. Isometric contractions occur in a static position, so resisted motion is easy to perform on a bodywork client lying on a table. Isotonic contractions require that a client moves through a range of motion, which works well in sports-massage applications.

- Use concentric contractions during resisted motion to strengthen a weak muscle.
- Use eccentric contractions during resisted motion to lengthen a short, fibrotic muscle.

5.4.2 Trigger Point Therapy

A muscle under chronic tension often develops a **trigger point** (TrP)—a localized irritable nodule in the muscle that, when placed under direct pressure, refers pain to other areas of the body.[17] Pain from trigger points can prevent the muscles from reaching a full range of stretch during motion, restricting motion and reducing both strength and endurance.

Trigger points can be both active and latent:

- *Active trigger points* cause pain and discomfort even in the absence of movement. They also cause stiffness and decreased range of motion, which clients rarely notice.
- *Latent trigger points* increase chronic muscle tension, but clients do not feel them until they are put under direct pressure.

Muscles can also develop **tender points,** which are localized tender points that do not refer pain. Trigger points and tender points both respond to direct sustained pressure, which softens the point and is very effective in relieving muscular pain.

There are four cardinal features of active trigger points:

1. A palpable nodular or band-like hardening in the muscle
2. A highly localized spot of extreme tenderness in a taut band of tissue in the muscle

3. Digital pressure on the spot reproduces the client's distance-pain complaint and triggers a protective reflexive movement called a **jump sign**
4. Direct pressure held on the trigger point relieves pain

Trigger point therapy was initially developed by Dr. Janet Travell, who wrote the classic trigger point texts about myofascial pain and dysfunctions.[18] Direct pressure on the trigger point nodule, applied perpendicularly to the surface of the muscle, is very effective in alleviating pain and inactivating the trigger point (Figure 5.24 ■). You hold pressure

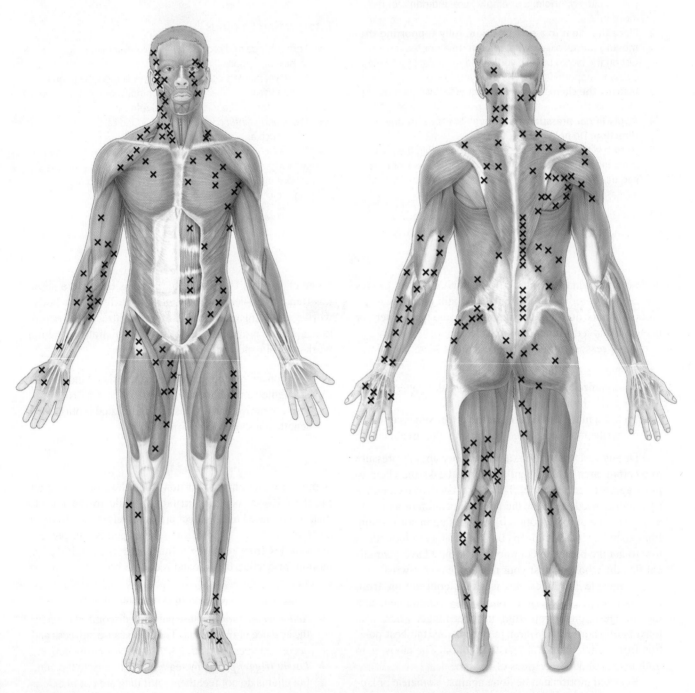

FIGURE 5.24

Trigger points in the body

on the point until the client reports that the pain coming from the area has subsided. This can take anywhere from five to 30 seconds, depending on the depth of the trigger point.

Trigger point therapy affects the neuromuscular system in several ways. It changes muscle patterns, which ultimately changes movement patterns. Also, direct pressure on the point helps clients to locate the source of muscular pain so that they can actively relax those muscles, which in turn makes trigger point therapy more effective as an active technique.

Trigger points are usually found in the belly of muscles, but they can also be found in scar tissues, tendons, ligaments, joint capsules, and other connective tissues. Trigger points located in scar tissues tend to refer burning, prickling, lightning-jab sensations. Trigger points located in the belly of the muscle refer specific muscular pain patterns, usually a generalized, diffuse aching sensation. Multiple trigger points are often peppered throughout one small area in multiple layers of adjacent or overlapping muscles. Trigger point locations and their pain referral patterns will be marked on illustrations of individual muscles in the second half of this text.

5.4.3   Muscle Energy Techniques

Muscle energy techniques (METs) were originally developed by osteopath Fred Mitchell Sr. as a method of joint mobilization that restores a normal range of motion to joints restricted by hypertonic, shortened muscles. METs use active muscular contraction to elicit a relaxation response in a muscle before stretching it, which enhances the stretch. You can use METs on your own muscles while stretching, or with a client to improve stretching.

The traditional manual therapy MET combines body positioning with the client's own muscle contraction. During this process, the practitioner places the client in a position that takes a joint to the end range of its restricted range of motion. Then the practitioner applies resistance for the client to push against to contract and shorten the muscle, restricting range. After the client relaxes the target muscle, the practitioner then stretches this muscle by moving the joint even farther, to its next layer of resistance. Resistance, also called a barrier, is the point at which the joint has reached its end range of motion.

The stretch returns the muscle to its normal resting length, which restores a normal range of motion. METs are based on the principles of post-contraction relaxation response and reciprocal inhibition. The two primary MET methods that Mitchell developed are:

- **Post-isometric relaxation** (PIR), which involves the contract-relax-stretch process of the target muscle that was just described.
- **Reciprocal inhibition** (RI), which involves contracting the antagonist to increase the stretch of the agonist.

EXPLORING TECHNIQUE
Trigger Point Therapy

Because of the specificity of their location in muscles, learning to feel trigger points requires consistent palpation practice. Refer to the trigger point figures in Part 2 chapters for trigger point locations and referral patterns in specific muscles.

1. To locate a trigger point in a muscle, spiral down into the belly of the muscle with direct pressure using your thumbs, fingertips, or elbow. Make sure your pressure is perpendicular to the plane of the muscle (Figure 5.25 ■). To verify whether or not you're on a tender point, look for a jump sign and ask your client for feedback.
2. Hold pressure on the center of the point for up to 10 seconds, or until your client has reported that the pain is subsiding.
3. As the pain subsides and the muscle relaxes and softens, slowly sink deeper into the point to check for latent trigger points buried under active trigger points.
4. Release your pressure when the client reports that the muscle pain has subsided.
5. To address muscle symmetry and leave your client on midline, check the same point on the other side of the body. If it is painful, hold that trigger point until it releases.
6. After trigger points in an area have released, stretch the target muscles with passive myofascial release techniques and/or active muscle energy techniques.

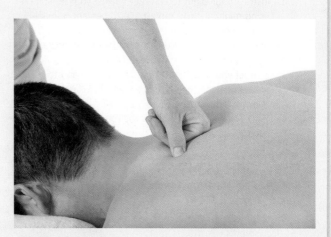

FIGURE 5.25

5.4.3.1 POST-ISOMETRIC RELAXATION AND RECIPROCAL INHIBITION

Post-isometric relaxation is based on the theory that contracting a muscle induces a post-contraction relaxation response, making that muscle easier to stretch. The PIR technique is sometimes referred to as *contract–relax;* it would more accurately be called *contract–relax–stretch,* which describes all three steps in the technique.

The theory behind reciprocal inhibition is that actively contracting the antagonist of a muscle that is being stretched induces a tendon reflex in the agonist, which inhibits its contraction, making the agonist easier to stretch. The RI technique is sometimes referred to as the "contract–relax" technique. Practitioners often use the RI technique right after the PIR technique to further enhance the PIR stretch. Using PIR and RI together is often referred to as "contract–relax–antagonist–contract," or *CRAC* for short, which is an easy way to remember the steps.

PIR stretches can be repeated two or three times, depending on the client's condition and the results of each application. Each situation will be different. Contract–relax can also be practiced with the client in any position—prone, supine, side-lying, or even sitting up. Keep in mind when using any MET to stretch muscles that associated connective tissues are also being stretched.

5.4.3.2 GENERAL APPLICATIONS FOR MUSCLE ENERGY

Muscle energy techniques are widely used in athletic training for stretching effectively, which is a preventive measure to avoid muscle strain and joint sprain caused by tight muscles. They are also widely used in manual therapy to alleviate chronic stiffness and muscular tension, and to treat pain and movement dysfunctions associated with restricted joint motion.

People use METs in their stretch routines by contracting muscles before stretching them. As discussed

---

EXPLORING TECHNIQUE
Muscle Energy Stretch Techniques

The PIR and RI techniques are usually done in the same stretching progression, one right after the other. When you do them in progression, you are performing a CRAC stretch.

PIR stretch: Instruct your client about what you're going to do, *"To stretch your hamstrings, I'm going to lift your leg and ask you to lightly push against my resistance. Then I'll tell you to relax, after which I will stretch your muscles."* Instruct your clients to report abnormal symptoms such as pain or discomfort as soon as they occur. If your client does report abnormal symptoms, stop immediately.

1. Place your client's restricted joint in a position that moves it to the limit of its motion and apply light resistance (Figure 5.26a ■).
2. Instruct your client to contract against your resistance using minimal effort (about 10–20 percent of maximum effort), and hold the contraction for about 5 seconds: *"Lightly and slowly push against my resistance. Good, now hold…hold…keep holding."*
3. Instruct your client to take a deep breath and to completely relax on the exhalation, which will enhance the relaxation response (Figure 5.26b ■).
4. Wait for several seconds for the muscle to relax, then carefully stretch your client's joint a little farther.

RI stretch: While pressing your partner into a stretch, instruct her or him to contract the antagonist. *"Contract your thigh (quads) to pull your leg toward your chest and increase the stretch"* (Figure 5.26c ■).

5. Have your partner completely relax and rest for a few moments.

6. Repeat steps 1–4 up to three times. Then repeat the whole routine on the other side.

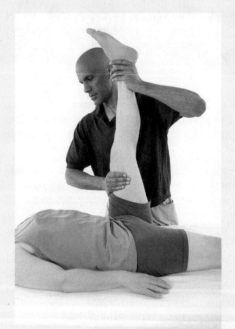

FIGURE 5.26a

a) Client contract agonist (hamstring) against practitioner's resistance.

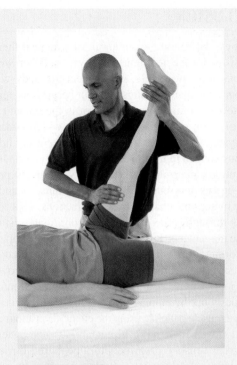

FIGURE 5.26b

b) Client relaxes agonist.

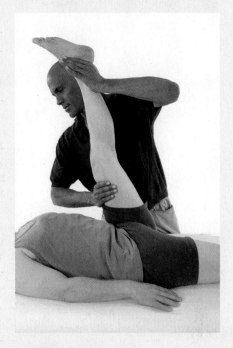

FIGURE 5.26c

c) Client contracts antagonist (quadriceps) as practitioner stretches agonist.

earlier, PIR is based on the fact that a strong contraction will activate the stretch reflex, which elicits a relaxation response. Here is a simple demonstration of using both RI and PIR to effectively stretch the hamstrings.

1. Bend over and touch your toes and notice how far your hamstrings let you stretch.
2. Now stand in a squat position with the spine straight for as long as you can hold it.
3. Then bend over and stretch again. You should be able to bend farther because the squat worked the hamstrings, which should trigger a post-contraction relaxation response.
4. Finally, engage the antagonist by actively contracting your quadriceps while you stretch your hamstrings, which should increase your stretch even more. To do this, pull the muscles up above your knees.

Muscle energy can be utilized in massage and bodywork independently of applied resistance and joint motion. For example, to enhance the effectiveness of myofascial release, have your client contract and relax a muscle before you apply deep tissue pressure to stretch that muscle. When applied directly after resisted movement, an **active pin and stretch** technique is highly effective in releasing stubborn muscle spasms that generate pain. First, the client contracts against your resistance to trigger a post-isometric relaxation response.

Then, you pin one end of a restricted tissue layer, usually a chronically shortened muscle, and have your client actively move to stretch away from your pressure (Figure 5.27 ■).

Muscle energy techniques work well in the seated massage position, especially with neck and shoulder muscles like the levator scapula and scalenes, which are common pain generators in people who work at computers or in seated positions (Figure 5.28a-b ■). When using this combination of techniques in a seated massage, it is important to make sure your client sits up straight in a position of optimal posture. Also, direct your client to contract her or his abdominal muscles and press the feet into the floor to stabilize the trunk during the stretch.

Because muscle energy techniques require active client movement, this combination can be used as part of a neuromuscular patterning session to reorganize neuromuscular pathways and improve the client's movement patterns. The combination of hands-on techniques, active client movement, and postural cues creates synergistic effects. The MET stretches restore length and flexibility to the myofascial system, the active pin and stretch enhances the effect of myofascial release, and the active movement and postural cues improve the overall skeletal alignment and physical coordination. This blend of powerful techniques can help your clients achieve deep and lasting structural changes as well as functional changes in both posture and movement.

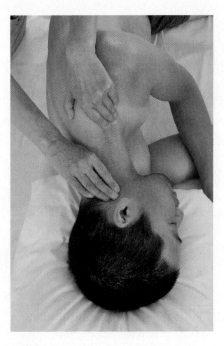

FIGURE 5.27

Pin and stretch technique: Practitioner pins the trapezius myofascia on the client's shoulder, then applies linear friction to stretch the trapezius towards its origin on the cranium.

CONCLUSION

Conscious, deliberate movement during manual therapy is akin to yoga for the neuromuscular system. When we move with conscious awareness, we connect the body with the mind, our muscular functions with our nervous-system control. The autonomic nervous system is the ancient involuntary division of the nervous system, which control the organ systems. The somatic nervous system is under our conscious control in the coordination of all motor activity.

Complex neuromuscular circuitry connects proprioceptive organs and sensory nerves in the muscles and joints with the motor units that generate contractions. This circuitry operates through reflex arcs, which coordinate instinctive, reflexive movements. It is possible to access the complex sensorimotor network, which operates mostly below conscious awareness, using neuromuscular techniques to improve muscle and joint activity in motor functions. The neuromuscular techniques work by tapping into the client's nervous system to change muscle patterns, using the client's conscious awareness and movement to reorganize neuromuscular patterning.

Myriad sensory proprioceptors peppered throughout the musculoskeletal tissues provide a person with constant information about where the body is located in space and how it is moving. They also register pain sensations, particularly those that develop from chronic muscular holding. In this sense, the neuromuscular system is far more than a motor system that moves the body through space. It is a sensory organ that tunes up the body and mind every time a client undergoes the yoga-like practice of yielding into massage and neuromuscular therapy.

FIGURE 5.28

Active pin and stretch technique: a) Practitioner applies resistance for client to contract the levator scapula against. b) Practitioner pins scapular end of levator scapula while client does active stretch away from practitioner's pressure.

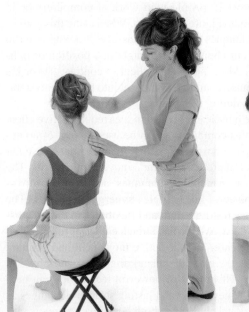

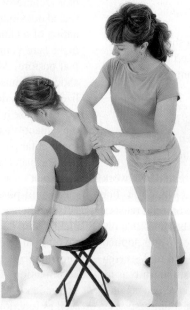

A   B

SUMMARY POINTS TO REMEMBER

1. The central nervous system (CNS) is made up of the brain and spinal cord. The peripheral nervous system (PNS) includes all nerves and ganglia outside the CNS. The PNS has two branches: the somatic or skeletal nervous system (SNS), which controls skeletal muscles and voluntary movement; and the autonomic nervous system (ANS), which controls involuntary functions such as digestion and breathing.

2. A neuron is a nerve cell. There are three types of neurons: a sensory neuron carries information toward the brain and spinal cord; an interneuron passes signals between neurons; and a motor neuron carries signals from the brain and spinal cord to the muscles.

3. The peripheral nerves are made up of tracts (bundles of single nerves). Spinal nerve tracts leave the spinal cord at each vertebral segment, then interconnect in groups called nerve plexi. Each nerve plexus (i.e., brachial, lumbar, sacral) is embedded within myofascial tissues en route to the muscles it innervates.

4. Peripheral nerves are flexible and elastic so that they can slide, bend, and elongate around joints. Myofascial adhesions and chronic muscle contractures can restrict the sliding motion of nerves, leading to entrapment and neural tension (an increase in tension in one area of a nerve to compensate for the loss of extensibility in another area of the nerve).

5. A sensorimotor loop is a continual and almost instantaneous interchange between sensory input and motor output. Sensory fibers called muscle spindles, or intrafusal fibers, pick up information about muscle length changes and the rate of length changes, regulating the muscular effort needed to carry out specific movement. Motor fibers called extrafusal fibers are the slow and fast contractile fibers found in motor units.

6. Proprioception is the reception of input from neuromuscular proprioceptors that provides an awareness of the body's posture, movement, and location in space. Perception is the brain's interpretation of proprioceptive input.

7. The stretch reflex is a protective reflex modulated by spindle fibers that cause a muscle to contract after it stretches a certain length, which prevents overstretching.

8. A reflex arc is the rudimentary sensorimotor circuitry that controls reflexive movements and is made up of a receptor, a sensory nerve, an integration center through single or multiple synapses, a motor nerve, and muscle fibers.

9. When a muscle is contracting eccentrically and the load on the muscle overcomes the force of the contraction, that muscle is susceptible to a stretch injury. A common stretch injury occurs when an agonist contracts before its antagonist can relax, stretching and tearing the muscle while it is contracting.

10. Golgi tendon organs are tendon proprioceptors that register increased tension on tendons and trigger protective inhibitory responses that in turn trigger muscle relaxation and modulate tension between agonist/antagonist muscles. Pacinian corpuscles in joint capsules detect rapid changes in pressure and vibration, and Ruffini endings in joint capsules detect slow changes in the position or angle of a joint.

11. Specialized proprioceptive organs in the labyrinth of the inner ear—the vestibule, the semicircular canals, and the cochlea—control balance and equilibrium, spatial orientation, and hearing.

12. The law of reciprocal inhibition describes how agonist and antagonist muscles work in opposing pairs, one relaxing while the other contracts, during protective, reflexive movements such as the extensor thrust reflex or the flexor withdrawal reflex.

13. Active, passive, and resisted movement assessments are used in manual therapy to assess movement imbalances, movement restrictions, or the source of musculoskeletal pain.

14. Pain caused by joints and ligaments tend to be localized to these structures but can occur during both active and passive movement. Pain from muscles and tendons occurs during active but not passive movement and radiates along the length of the muscle.

15. Resisted movement is used in manual therapy to facilitate relaxation responses for muscular energy techniques. It is also used to facilitate inhibited muscles, organize and improve neuromuscular patterns, and assess muscle function and treatment effectiveness.

16. A trigger point is a localized irritable nodule or band-like hardening that develops in a muscle under chronic tension, which, when placed under direct pressure, creates a jump sign and refers pain. In trigger point therapy, direct pressure is applied to the nodule until the pain subsides, and then the affected muscle is stretched.

17. Post-isometric relaxation (PIR) is a muscle energy technique (MET) in which a target muscle is contracted to induce a relaxation response, then stretched. Reciprocal inhibition (RI) is an MET in which the antagonist is contracted to enhance the stretch of the agonist.

REVIEW QUESTIONS

1. The part of the peripheral nervous system that controls movement is the
   a. somatic nervous system.
   b. brain and spinal cord.
   c. autonomic nervous system.
   d. involuntary nervous system.

2. Match each type of neuron—sensory (afferent) neuron, interneuron, and motor (efferent) neuron—with its function:
   a. The neurons that carry motor impulses from the CNS to the skeletal muscles.
   b. The neurons that carry signals between neurons in the CNS.
   c. The neurons that carry impulses from the body to the CNS.

3. Describe the structure of a peripheral nerve and its associated fascias.

4. True or false (circle one). Peripheral nerves are flexible and elastic; they can elongate and bend around moving joints and slide within fascial pockets between tissue layers.

5. If a nerve looses extensibility in one area, neural tension will
   a. decrease in another area to equalize tension along the nerve.
   b. increase in another area to equalize tension along the nerve.
   c. result in lesions that discolor specific areas of the skin.
   d. have no effect on the extensibility of the peripheral nerves.

6. A definition of proprioception is
   a. the specialized cells and organs classified as sensory receptors.
   b. the brain's perceptual interpretation of proprioceptive input.
   c. an awareness of balance, movement, and the location of the body in space.
   d. the information coming in from the five senses.

7. True or false (circle one). The extrafusal fibers are the sensory muscle fibers found within a muscle's spindle; the intrafusal fibers are the motor muscle fibers found in a motor unit.

8. The two functions of a muscle spindle are
   a. to pick up information about tonic changes in muscles and the rate of tonic changes in muscles.
   b. to pick up information about fiber changes in muscles and the rate of fiber changes in muscles.
   c. to pick up information about phasic changes in muscles and the rate of phasic changes in muscles.
   d. to pick up information about length changes in muscles and the rate of length changes in muscles.

9. Name the components in a reflex arc and describe how they work.

10. True or false (circle one). A tonic stretch reflex, also called an antigravity reflex, causes a muscle put on a slow stretch to undergo a slow contractile response.

11. Describe the dynamics of a stretch injury and give one example.

12. A Golgi tendon organ is a
   a. sensory organ found in tendons that registers changes in muscle tension.
   b. proprioceptor in the musculotendinous junction of the antagonist.
   c. receptor that triggers the muscle to contract.
   d. proprioceptor in the joint ligaments under the tendon.

13. Match each proprioceptor—Pacinian corpuscles, Ruffini endings, nociceptors, and semicircular canals—with their functions.
   a. Picks up extreme changes in temperature and pressure interpreted as pain.
   b. Registers angular movements of the head.
   c. Detects rapid changes in pressure and vibration on a joint capsule.
   d. Detects slow changes in the position or angle of a joint.

14. The theory of reciprocal inhibition describes
   a. how an agonist muscle relaxes when the synergist contracts.
   b. the simultaneous excitation and inhibition of opposing muscles.
   c. how agonist/antagonist contract simultaneously during reflex movements.
   d. the cortical control of muscular contractions during deliberate actions.

15. A client feels aching pain and soreness along a broad area covering the length of the thigh during active hip flexion but not during hip extension or passive hip flexion. The most likely source of pain is
   a. an entrapped nerve.
   b. a sprained ligament.
   c. a hip flexor muscle.
   d. a hip extensor muscle.

16. Name four important safety guidelines for using passive and resisted motion with a client.

17. Identify the statement that describes the muscle energy technique post-isometric relaxation (PIR), also called contract–relax.
    a. A practitioner has a client contract a tight muscle against resistance to induce a relaxation response before the practitioner stretches it.
    b. A practitioner has a client contract the antagonist of the target muscle to induce relaxation of the agonist before the practitioner stretches the target muscle.
    c. A practitioner has a client relax a muscle before stretching it to induce proprioceptive awareness of resting tone.
    d. A practitioner has a client contract the same muscle on the other side of the body before stretching it to induce contralateral muscle response.

18. What is a trigger point and how can it be treated in massage and bodywork?

Notes

1. Marieb, E., & Hoehn, K. (2007). *Human Anatomy and Physiology* (7th ed.). San Francisco: Pearson Benjamin Cummings.
2. Brunner, N. (2009). "Massage Profession Metrics: Consumer Research Overview." Associated Massage and Bodywork Professionals public educator site. Retrieved October 23, 2009, from www.massagetherapy.com/media/metricsoverview.php.
3. Simons, D., Travell, J., & Simons, L. (1999). *Myofascial Pain and Dysfunction: The Trigger Point Manual: Vol. 1. Upper Half of Body* (2nd ed.). Philadelphia: Lippincott, Williams & Wilkins.
4. Shacklock, M. (2005). *Clinical Neurodynamics: A New System of Musculoskeletal Treatment.* Edinburgh, UK: Elsevier.
5. Kapandji, I. A. (1988). *The Physiology of Joints: Vol. 3. The Trunk and Vertebral Column* (5th ed.). Edinburgh, UK: Churchill Livingstone.
6. Magee, D. (2007). *Orthopedic Physical Assessment* (5th ed.). Philadelphia: Saunders.
7. Ibid.
8. Foster, M. (2004). *Somatic Patterning: How to Improve Posture and Movement and Ease Pain.* Longmont, CO: EMS Press.
9. Cohen, B. (1990). *The Evolutionary Origins of Movement.* Amherst, MA: Author.
10. Sherrington, C. (1952). *The Integrative Action of the Nervous System.* London: Cambridge University Press.
11. Rose, M. (2009). *Comfort Touch: Massage for the Elderly and the Ill.* Baltimore: Lippincott, Williams & Wilkins.
12. Myers, T. (2008). *Anatomy Trains: Myofascial Meridians for Manual and Movement Therapists* (2nd ed.). New York: Churchill Livingstone.
13. Myers, T. (2010, Jan/Feb). "Discovery Through Dissection: The Anatomy Trains Perspective." *Massage and Bodywork Magazine,* pp. 34–43.
14. Ibid.
15. Kendall, F., McCreary, E., & Provance, P. (2005). *Muscles: Testing and Function with Posture and Pain* (5th ed.). Baltimore: Lippincott, Williams & Wilkins.
16. Cyriax, J., & Cyriax, P. (1993). *Cyriax's Illustrated Manual of Orthopedic Medicine* (2nd ed.). Edinburgh, UK: Butterworth-Heinemann.
17. Simons, D., Travell, J., & Simons, L. (1999). *Myofascial Pain and Dysfunction: The Trigger Point Manual: Vol. 1. Upper Half of Body* (2nd ed.). Philadelphia: Lippincott, Williams & Wilkins.
18. Ibid.

PEARSON myhealthprofessionskit™

Use this address to access the Companion Website created for this textbook. Simply select "Massage Therapy" from the choice of disciplines. Find this book and log in using your username and password to access interactive activities, videos, and much more.

CHAPTER

6 Biomechanics

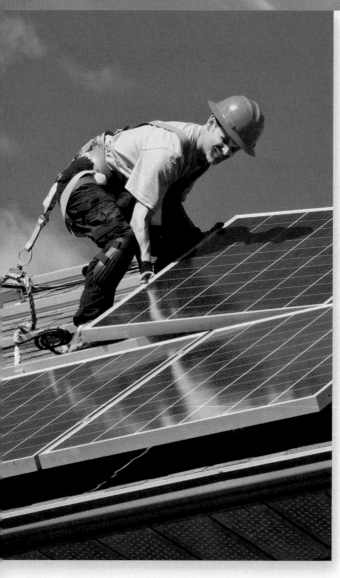

CHAPTER OUTLINE

Chapter Objectives

Key Terms

6.1 General Terms and Concepts

6.2 The Laws of Motion

6.3 Force

6.4 Levers

Conclusion

Summary Points to Remember

Review Questions

Skilled construction workers usually have an instinctive ability to use biomechanical principles in work-related tasks. Their job is physically demanding. Only those with natural abilities and coordination can work day after day in ways that prevent injuries. During the course of a project, a worker often performs a number of different jobs, such as loading and unloading building materials, operating heavy machinery, and using specialized tools. He or she may also dig trenches, erect scaffolding, and build or dismantle construction forms. This type of job demands a high degree of body

awareness and efficiency in body movement, and an ability to work at a steady pace in order to conserve energy and maximize output. The construction worker's movements are usually deliberate and well timed, particularly when moving heavy objects or hazardous materials, balancing on ladders or narrow platforms, or working at dangerous heights or in precarious positions. Each undertaking may require physical strength and fitness, good balance and hand–eye coordination, and an ability to solve mechanical problems.

CHAPTER OBJECTIVES

1. Define velocity, acceleration, and deceleration. Explain how gravity affects velocity during muscular contractions.

2. Define friction. Describe what increases and decreases friction.

3. Define line of pull. Define the mechanical axis of a bone.

4. Define a reverse muscle action and describe how a joint movement can reverse.

5. List and define each of Newton's three laws of motion.

6. Describe a force vector in relation to a muscular contraction.

7. List and describe three types of forces that produce movement.

8. Define torque and describe how muscles work as force couples to produce torque.

9. Describe the force–velocity relationship.

10. Describe the stress–strain curve and its relationship to tissue response under load.

11. Define a lever and its three parts. Identify the output favored by each lever.

12. Describe each type of the three levers and provide an example of each one.

13. Define equilibrium and contrast the three different types of equilibrium.

14. Describe several applications of biomechanics to effective and sound body mechanics.

KEY TERMS

Acceleration

Axis

Concurrent forces

Deceleration

Effort

Equilibrium

Force couple

Force vector

Force–velocity relationship

Friction

Ground reaction force (GRF)

Law of acceleration

Law of action and reaction

Law of inertia

Lever

Line of pull

Linear forces

Mechanical advantage (M Ad)

Momentum

Parallel forces

Resistance

Reverse muscle action

Torque

Velocity

Biomechanics is an interdisciplinary study of the mechanical aspects of human movement. While the human body is far more complex than a system of moving parts, the study of biomechanics clarifies how the laws of motion, levers, and the effects of moving forces apply to the human body.

The emphasis of this chapter is the overall convergence of the static and dynamic forces acting on the body at rest or in motion. We cover some basic biomechanical concepts that apply to the mechanical efficiency of joint and muscle function, specifically to leverage, lines of pull, force transmission, and torque. These concepts are easy to observe and to apply during daily activities, particularly while pushing, pulling, and lifting. Understanding biomechanics is not only vital for helping our clients, but essential for taking care of our own bodies. In fact, research on massage and bodywork practitioners shows that more than 70 percent incur work-related injuries, so efficient body mechanics are essential for career longevity and injury prevention.[1] This chapter provides many practical self-care exercises and tips for applying biomechanical concepts to your own body mechanics. These exercises can improve the effectiveness of your hands-on applications in massage and bodywork as well. They also provide helpful tips that you can share with clients to improve their body-use patterns in their daily and work-related activities.

We begin with a review of the general biomechanics terms and concepts that were introduced in previous chapters.

6.1 GENERAL TERMS AND CONCEPTS

Biomechanics apply to both *statics*—the mechanics of nonmoving systems—and to *dynamics*—the mechanics of moving systems. In the human body, statics relates to posture and dynamics relates to the movement of the body in space. To measure the mechanical aspects of posture and movement, we can look at the three-dimensional intersection of the elements of mass, space, and time.

A *mass* is a quantity of matter in the body. Mass takes up space. The three major masses of the human body—the head, thorax, and pelvis—align along the *line of gravity* (LOG). The LOG can be determined by tying a weight to a string, then hanging it as a plumb line. The force of gravity acts on physical objects or bodies at all times, drawing all masses toward the earth. The point of application of gravity is always in the center of a symmetrical object or mass, which is the *center of gravity* (COG). If an object or mass is asymmetrical, the COG will be located in the center of weight.

When lifting any part of the client's body, it is important to fully support the center of weight in that part of the body. For example, lifting a client's arm by the wrist causes the arm to hang from and distract the wrist. Unless distraction is the intended outcome, it puts tensional stress on the wrist that can be uncomfortable for a client.

To differentiate types of motion, look to the pathway a moving mass makes in space. A *linear motion* travels along a straight line in one direction, whereas a *rotary motion* travels along a curvilinear pathway. Linear and rotary movements usually occur together in a body-movement pattern. Massage and bodywork strokes can involve either linear or rotary force applications, depending on the intention of the stroke. General kneading strokes usually involve curvilinear pathways of motion that sculpt and shape around the tissues, whereas deep tissue work often uses linear pressure.

6.1.1 Velocity, Gravity, and Friction

Velocity combines speed and direction. This includes the speed of a movement or the speed of a contraction. Velocity increases during **acceleration** and decreases during **deceleration.** Although skilled movers such as a Tai Chi master can move with sustained speed, rarely does the speed of a body movement remain constant. It usually slows down or speeds up.

Many forces act on a body to alter the speed and direction of its motion. Wind or a fluid current accelerates the velocity of an object moving in the same direction as it is, whereas friction and gravity decelerate the velocity of a moving object. The type of contraction a muscle produces and the velocity of the contraction depends on the direction of the joint movement in relation to gravity. During movement in an upward direction, the muscles work harder, shortening into concentric contractions to overcome the resistance of gravity. The force of gravity decelerates and slows a movement. This is why it takes more muscular effort to walk up a hill than down a hill. Just the opposite occurs when lowering a weight in a downward direction. The force of gravity accelerates the downward motion. To counter gravity, the muscles contract eccentrically, acting as a brake to control the accelerating velocity of movement in the direction of gravity. Without eccentric contractions in the legs to control the rate of descent, a person walking down a steep hill would lose control and could easily tumble head over heels.

Muscles are more susceptible to injury when working eccentrically because fewer motor units are firing, so each motor unit has to work harder to meet the forces pulling against it. This is why your legs become so sore after a downhill hike; the muscles work harder to prevent acceleration toward the gravitational pull. Similarly, when practicing passive movement on a client, we need to be slow and careful in lowering whatever body part we are moving with control to avoid dropping it.

Friction is the force that occurs between two surfaces that are moving against each other. The rougher the moving surfaces, the more friction that will be created between them and the slower the motion between them. Friction puts a drag on sliding forces. Too much friction prevents motion; too little friction prevents control and stability. For example, it is nearly impossible to slide across most carpets in socks because of friction, yet it is easy to slide across a carpet in slick, nylon booties.

BRIDGE TO PRACTICE
Using Lotion to Reduce Friction

Massage therapists usually use lotion or oil to reduce friction on the skin for gliding strokes. However, you will need some friction to be able to apply adequate pressure into the muscles. Friction aids deep tissue work and myofascial release work where you need traction to pin the tissues in order to stretch them. Many massage clients receive massage to relieve muscle tension. To work more effectively in the muscular system, use lubricants sparingly.

6.1.2 Lines of Muscular Pull

A **line of pull**, or *angle of pull,* is the direction a muscular force exerts upon a joint. The degree of force a muscle exerts depends on the relationship between its line of pull and the mechanical axis of the bone. The **mechanical axis of a bone** is an imaginary line that runs between the centers of the articulating joints on either end of a bone. The mechanical axis may or may not run through the shaft of a bone, depending on the overall shape of the bone (Figure 6.1 ■).

The line of pull in muscles is dynamic; it changes throughout a movement as the angle of the joint opens or closes. The line of pull is assessed at any given point during a motion by the angle of attachment between a muscle's tendon and the mechanical axis of the bone on which it inserts. The closer the line of a muscle's pull is to the mechanical axis of the bone, the weaker the force that muscle can exert on the joint. The contraction of a muscle with a line of pull closer to the mechanical axis of a bone exerts a stabilizing effect on a joint, pulling its articulating surfaces closer together. For example, the predominantly vertical line of pull in the posterior fibers of the psoas major positions it to function as a primary stabilizer of the anterior lumbar vertebra (Figure 6.2 ■).

In contrast, the contraction of a muscle with a line of pull at an angle to the mechanical axis of a bone exerts a mobilizing effect on a joint, producing torque and rotary motion. The psoas major generates joint motion as the hip moves past 30 degrees of flexion. As the angle of attachment reaches a right angle, the rotary force the muscle can exert on the joint increases. When the biceps brachii tendon reaches a 90-degree angle with the forearm during elbow flexion, 100 percent of the biceps contractile forces go into the movement of the joint (Figure 6.3 ■).[2]

Most muscles exert diagonal lines of pull across joints. Muscles oriented along a diagonal axis insert lateral to the midline of the bone. When they contract, they exert forces that simultaneously close the angle of

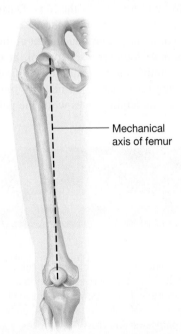

FIGURE 6.1
Mechanical axis of a bone

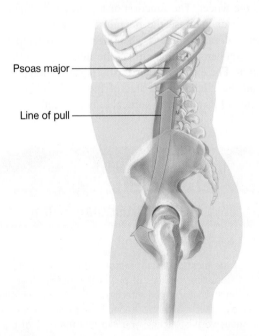

FIGURE 6.2
Line of pull of a muscle

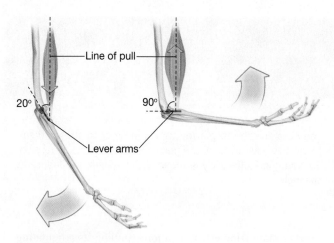

FIGURE 6.3

When the **line of pull** is at a 90-degree angle to the mechanical axis of the bone, 100 percent of a muscle's contractile force goes into the movement of the joint.

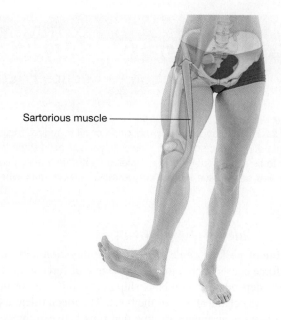

FIGURE 6.4

The orientation of the sartorius muscle gives it a **diagonal line of pull** that produces both hip flexion and lateral rotation.

the joint while rotating the joint. The sartorius runs from the lateral side of the hip to the medial side of the knee, so it simultaneously flexes and laterally rotates the hip (Figure 6.4 ■).

Muscles with broad attachments can have multiple lines of pull. The upper, middle, and lower parts of the trapezius respectively elevate, retract, and depress the scapula (Figure 6.5 ■). During rock climbing, the parts of the trapezius muscle working along a line of pull progressively change during the upward and downward movements of the arms.

Many muscles act as anatomical pulleys, exerting a line of pull that bends around a corner. A pulley consists of a rope wrapped around a groove in a wheel that, when pulled, turns the wheel. The function of a pulley is to change the direction or increase the magnitude of a force. Muscles act as anatomical pulleys when their tendons wrap around bony protuberances that deflect the line of pull away from the joint. For example, the tibialis posterior tendon wraps around the medial malleolus of the ankle, changing the direction of its pull from vertical to horizontal.

6.1.3   Reverse Muscle Action

A muscle action can be reversed. In most joint movements, one bone in the joint moves while the other bone remains fixed. In a **reverse muscle action**, the moving and fixed ends switch roles. To feel a reverse action in the *rectus femoris,* stand up and lift your knee to flex your hip. During standing hip flexion, the distal attachment of the rectus femoris at the knee moves while the proximal attachment at the hip remains fixed. Reverse the action by bowing to bend forward at the hips. During the bow, the distal muscular attachment at the knee remains fixed while the proximal muscular attachment at the hip moves (Figure 6.6a-b ■). Another way to look at this reverse action is to examine the inversion of the fixed (supporting) and moving (articulating) bones in a joint. In standing hip flexion, the femur moves while the pelvis remains

BRIDGE TO PRACTICE
Lines of Muscular Pull in Massage

One of the most important reasons to learn kinesiology is to be able to visualize the lines of pull in the muscles that you are working on so that you can effectively stretch muscles. Lines of pull create pathways of tension along kinetic chains. For example, during many yoga stretches, you can feel the lines of pull and pathways of tension along a series of overlapping muscles and linked joints in your own body.

The long gliding strokes of effleurage follow lines of pull, going with the grain of the muscles, so to speak. When stretching adaptively shortened muscles, you'll want to elongate the tissues along these lines of pull. Even when you are working across muscles using petrissage and cross-fiber strokes, you will need to know the lines of pull in the muscles to know which direction to move.

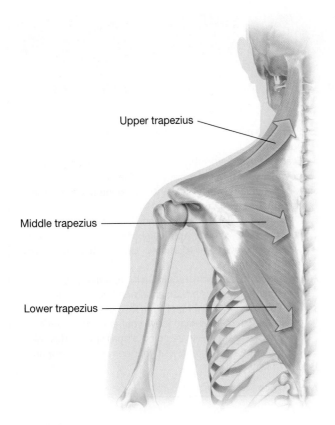

Upper trapezius

Middle trapezius

Lower trapezius

FIGURE 6.5

A muscle can have **multiple lines of pull.**

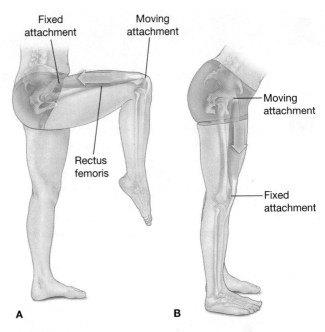

Fixed attachment

Moving attachment

Rectus femoris

Moving attachment

Fixed attachment

A   B

FIGURE 6.6

Reverse muscle action: a) Hip flexion on trunk b) Trunk flexion on hip

---

SELF-CARE

Balancing Your Body with Reverse Actions

To practice massage and bodywork in a way that balances your muscles and joints, consider reversing movements that you use a lot during the session.

1. If you do a lot of pressing and pushing strokes, balance these strokes with lifting and pulling strokes. Push compresses the joints in your hands and arms, while pull stretches them. Alternating push with pull reverses the mechanical stress that push placed on your body as your work.

2. You can apply the same reversal principle to a stretching and workout routine. The practice of massage involves a lot of flexion from bending over the table. In a stretching routine, make sure to stretch your hip, shoulder, and hand flexors to counter this effect. Choose stretches that move the joints in the opposite direction of your working positions to reverse the muscle actions. If you tend to look down as you work, you'll want to stretch the front of your neck and look up (Figure 6.7 ■).

3. Also, consider strengthening the antagonists of the muscles you use a lot in your work. For example, massage uses the flexors and medial rotators of the shoulders, which you can balance by strengthening the lateral rotators and extensors of the shoulders.

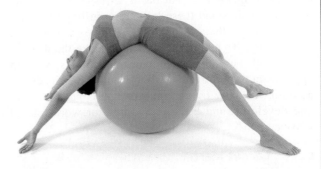

FIGURE 6.7

SELF-CARE
Overcoming On-the-Job Inertia

Many people have jobs that require sitting or standing in one place for a long time. The lack of movement from working in a stationary position can create a feeling of heaviness from inertia. This is particularly problematic for people who sit at desk jobs with poor posture and weak abdominal tone, which compresses the abdominal viscera.

Here are some simple tips you can use and share with your clients to help overcome the inertia that occurs from working in stationary positions:

1. Breathe deeply so that your respiration creates an intrinsic motion in your trunk. Let the inhalation lift the chest and slightly extend the spine and let the exhalation slightly flex the spine. This will help to keep the upper back from sinking into chronic flexion.
2. If you have to sit for long periods, subtly rock back and forth over the ischial tuberosities at the bottom of your pelvis.

3. Every few minutes roll your shoulders; yawn and stretch your arms.
4. Every time you remember to, look up at the ceiling then down at your navel to move your spine in both directions.
5. Move your legs by alternately straightening one knee, then the other, at least 20 times.
6. If you have to stand for long periods, let your body sway a little bit, slowly shifting your weight from your heels to toes or between your feet. Occasionally practice standing on one leg and balancing.
7. Massage and bodywork requires a lot of arm and hand movement, as well as movement around the table. If you find yourself getting stiff and your arms getting tired as you give massage, make sure to move your entire body with every stroke, even if you are doing a small stroke. This will distribute the work throughout your body so that your arms don't overwork.

---

fixed. In a forward bend, the pelvis moves while the femur remains fixed.

Any joint action can be reversed. The same action occurs when we bend the elbows to cover our mouth to cough, and when we pull ourselves up on a chinning bar. The difference between the two actions is that the bones and muscle reverse roles. Another difference is that in the first action, the hand moves toward the body in an open chain; in the second action the body moves toward the hands, which grip the bar in a closed chain.

6.2   THE LAWS OF MOTION

Sir Isaac Newton formulated three laws that explain the patterns of movement that occur all around us all the time. We understand these laws at an instinctive level, having learned them through the many experiences of daily living. By taking the time to analyze the dynamics of each law during common movements, we can apply them to improve overall movement efficiency for activities of daily living, enhance sports performance, and develop sound body mechanics for work-related movement tasks.

6.2.1   Law of Inertia

The first law of motion is the **law of inertia,** which states that *a body at rest or in linear motion tends to stay at rest or in motion unless acted upon by an external force.* **Inertia** is

a property of matter to both resist the initiation of motion and to resist changes in motion. Inertia is measured by the size and weight of a mass. The heavier the mass, the greater its inertia and the more force it takes to set it in motion and to stop it when it is in motion. For example, it takes more force to roll a bowling ball than a soccer ball; it takes more force to lift a heavy table than a book.

Overcoming inertia to stop a rapidly moving body or object requires a lot of force applied quickly or less force applied gradually. A baseball player uses friction to make a quick stop while skidding into home plate whereas a bicyclist gradually brakes into a slower stop. A simple way to apply this law to body mechanics is for manual therapy practitioners to make every movement of the hands a full body motion to prevent inertia from setting into any one area. If a manual technique involves a short stroke, practitioners can rock their whole bodies the same short distance, matching the length of the stroke with the movement of their body.

Unfortunately, many modern injuries result from the impact that inertia creates when a moving vehicle collides with a nonmoving object or body. For example, when a person sitting in a stopped car gets rear-ended, the car lurches forward, causing the seat to slam forward into the stationary passenger, usually snapping the head backward into a whiplash. The opposite dynamic occurs when a bicyclist hits a curb while cruising down a street. The bike crashes to a halt while the cyclist remains in motion and flies off the bike and over the curb.

6.2.2 Law of Acceleration

The second law of motion is the **law of acceleration,** which states that *the distance an object travels when set in motion is proportional to the force causing the movement.* The greater the force, the stronger the acceleration and the farther the object travels. Lightly toss a tennis ball and it moves a short distance. Fast-pitch a tennis ball and it travels a lot farther due to the increased muscular force that sets it in motion.

The forces required to accelerate a mass relate to the weight, density, and size of the mass. This explains why it is difficult to throw a feather; its light mass and weight is easily overcome by external resistance from air. Similarly, a shot putter uses a lot of **power** (strength plus velocity) to throw a lead ball in order to overcome internal resistance from the weight of the ball. Increasing the time in which the force is applied either increases the velocity or decreases the force needed to accelerate the object. A tennis player swings the racket backward to hit the ball on the carry-through strike. This increases the amount of time the racket contacts the ball and moves it forward, which, in turn, increases the force and velocity that moves the ball.

Momentum increases acceleration. **Momentum** is force applied to a moving object that increases its velocity. A javelin thrower runs to gain momentum and increase power in the throw. A farmer throwing hay bales on the bed of a truck capitalizes on momentum by swinging each bale to lift it more easily. Likewise, a manual therapist can load a massage table into a car using less effort by swinging it up rather than lifting it from a dead weight.

The human body is made up of tissues that vary in mass and density and move at different velocities. You may experience these differences by feeling the sensation of the abdominal viscera shifting inside your body while banking a corner in a car or riding an elevator. The denser and more weighted muscles and bones arrive a bit sooner than the less dense viscera. This explains why people often feel the organs drop shortly after going down on an elevator; the viscera take longer to descend.

6.2.3 Law of Action and Reaction

The third law of motion is the **law of action and reaction**, which states that *for every action there is an opposite and equal reaction.* Forces always come in pairs. The reactive force, or counterforce, always occurs in the opposite direction and of an equal magnitude to the active force.

The greater a force, the greater its counterforce will be. Forces and counterforces can be in a static or dynamic balance. When a person carries a heavy suitcase, static forces balance each other. The muscular effort it takes to carry a suitcase matches the weight of the suitcase. In contrast, dynamic forces and counterforces result in motion. A person jumps down on a trampoline and the trampoline pushes back up with an elastic counterforce. The height that the person bounces up matches the force that the person sends down on each jump. A light jump creates a tiny bounce; a forceful jump sends the person bouncing higher.

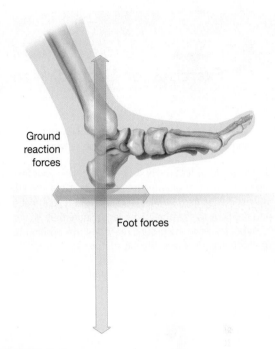

FIGURE 6.8
Ground reaction force

While walking, the foot presses down against the ground, which in turn generates a **ground reaction force** (GRF) that provides resistance in the opposite direction with an equal magnitude (Figure 6.8 ■). The denser the ground, the greater the counterforce, which explains why walking on concrete is easier than walking on sand.

In solving any biomechanical movement problem, the force of gravity, which constantly pulls bodies down, must always be considered. The greater the weight and mass of a body and the closer it is to the earth, the greater the gravitational pull. As objects move away from the earth, the pull of gravity lessens. Although the mass of a body is the same on Earth as on the moon, the astronaut floats because the difference in the gravitational pull changes the weight of the body.

6.3 FORCE

Many forces affect how we move, such as weight, size, strength, and timing. Although these many forces are familiar to most people, defining a force is not that simple. In the first chapter, force was described as an element that generates or alters motion. Forces can be generated internally from muscular contraction, or they can arise from external elements, such as wind, rain, or another body moving against a moving body.

Movement is described in measurable quantities, such as distance, speed, and direction. A **vector** quantity is a combination of two elements, the magnitude and direction of a force. Magnitude is the amount or size of the applied force, which can be measured in pounds of pressure. The direction of a force occurs along a line of action. For

SELF-CARE
Exercises for Grounding and Countersupport

Here is a simple grounding exercise to put Newton's third law of action and reaction into practice while you're working.

1. Stand with your feet under your hips. Imagine your feet like tap roots on a tree growing into the floor. Do a small deep-knee bend (Figure 6.9a ■). Then slowly push your feet down into the floor to straighten your legs (Figure 6.9b ■). As you push down, sense the ground reaction force pushing back up through your core to lift and support your body.

2. While you practice massage and bodywork, occasionally check into your awareness of your feet, then press them into the floor to ground yourself. Let the connection between your feet and the ground be as strong as your connection between your hands and your client.

3. If you are leaning your body's weight into your client to apply pressure, sense the counterforce from the client's body and the table coming up into your hands and arms to support you.

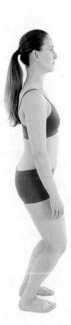

FIGURE 6.9a

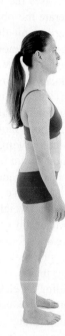

FIGURE 6.9b

example, the direction of gravity is always vertical. Vectors are depicted by arrows that show the direction and length of the force a muscular contraction exerts on a joint. A simple way to figure out in which direction a muscle acts on a joint is by drawing a vector arrow over an image of the muscle. The vector arrow depicts the length of a muscular pull and the direction in which it is pulling, although it does not illustrate the magnitude of an applied force.

6.3.1 Characteristics of Force Vectors

A force always has an exact point of application on an object or body, which is where the force is applied. Gravity always applies force through the center of weight in a mass. Muscular contractions apply force at attachment sites.

To accurately describe a force, the magnitude, direction, and point of application need to be identified. For example, the **force vector** a muscular pull exerts on a bone is measured through three criteria.

- Identify the *point of application* (the muscular attachment site on the moving bone).
- Assess the *direction of force* (the line of muscular pull).
- Measure the *magnitude of force* (the strength of the muscular contraction).

Force vectors from muscular pulls are usually represented by drawing a line from the moving attachment site (point of application) along the length of the muscle (the

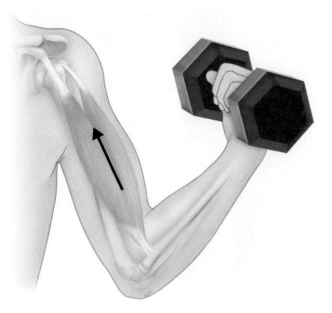

FIGURE 6.10
Force vector

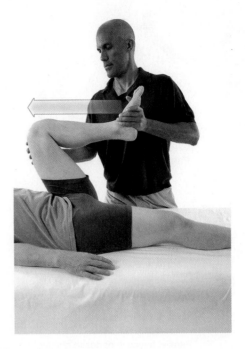

FIGURE 6.11
Linear force application in bodywork

direction and magnitude of the pull) (Figure 6.10 ■). The force vector of a muscle contraction can be determined by running a rubber strap on a skeleton along the length of that muscle.

Most people figure out force vectors intuitively, usually to solve the mechanical problems that show up in daily tasks. For example, imagine pushing a shopping cart when its front right wheel becomes stuck in a large crack in the floor. With a quick glance to assess the depth and width of the crack, you push down on the left back wheel to pop the right front wheel up, then shove the cart forward and to the right to clear the crack. This example demonstrates the kind of intuitive assessments of force vectors (e.g., the direction and magnitude of force needed to liberate the cart from the crack) that we make all the time.

6.3.2 Types of Force

Defining the forces in a movement assessment is not always simple. Many forces act on the body at one time along different vectors from various sources. We've already talked about the contractile forces that produce joint motion and the natural forces that alter movement, such as wind, water, gravity, and friction. Now we look at applied forces that result in movements in specific directions.

Forces always come in pairs. As the law of action and reaction dictates, a force is always met by a counterforce of equal magnitude. A force can be applied toward or away from a body or an object, from a push or a pull generated either inside or outside of the body. Applied forces can be linear, parallel, or concurrent.

Linear forces result from forces applied along the same axis, either toward or away from each other. A linear force can result in translatory motion, such as pushing a box across a floor, or a rotary motion, such as the linear pull of a contracting muscle that bends and rotates a joint. A practitioner uses linear force when applying a massage stroke in a single direction (Figure 6.11 ■).

Parallel forces are separate, linear forces of equal magnitude applied in the same plane, either in the same direction or in opposite directions (Figure 6.12a ■). Two or more parallel forces can work against a single force if it is located in between the parallel forces. Take the example of a person rowing a boat. The parallel forces produced by the oars pull back against the boat and the opposite force the moves the boat forward. Parallel forces applied in opposite directions will produce a rotary motion, a torque. If the rower pulled with the right oar while pushing with the left oar, the boat would turn. In another example, a gymnast pushes down on the parallel bars with both arms, which results in a parallel lift of the spine and trunk in the opposite direction. A massage practitioner using parallel forces torque during wringing strokes, moving the hands in opposite directions with equal pressure (Figure 6.12b ■).

Concurrent forces act on a body or object at the same point of application from different directions (Figure 6.13a ■). We use concurrent forces when we pump a bellows, pressing the two handles of the bellows to create a third resultant force, which is the air current. Laborers often use concurrent forces to move heavy equipment. For example, two workers might lift a pump out of a shallow hole by strapping a rope under it, then standing on opposite sides and pulling along opposite diagonals. They will each

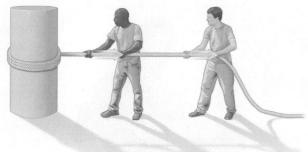

Parallel forces in the same direction

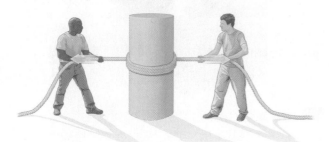

A   Parallel forces in opposite directions

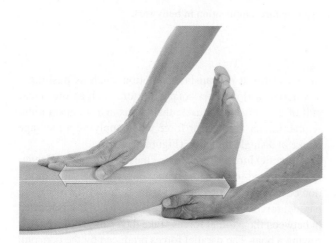

B

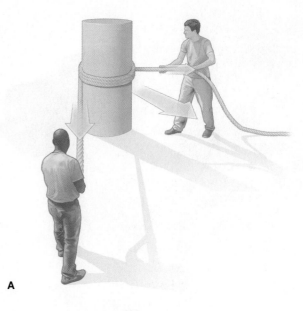

A

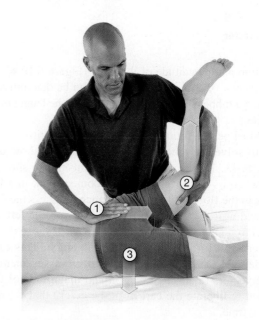

B

FIGURE 6.12

Parallel force applications: a) Equal forces are going the same direction. b) **Parallel force application in bodywork:** The practitioner applies equal forces in opposite directions to stretch the myofascia on the shin.

FIGURE 6.13

a) **Concurrent force application** b) **Concurrent force application in bodywork:** The practitioner (1) presses down on the sacrum while (2) lifting up on the thigh to (3) extend the hip joint.

need to exert an equal amount of force to straighten the strap and lift the pump straight up. It will be difficult to lift the pump if one worker pulls with greater force than the other.

Muscles with divergent fibers that pull on the same joint in different directions generate concurrent forces, and the resultant force generates joint motion. For example, the anterior and posterior fibers of the gluteus medius muscle pull in different directions to produce a resultant force that abducts the hip. The same dynamic occurs when two or more muscles pull on a joint from different

directions to produce a single motion in one direction. A practitioner uses concurrent forces when applying pressure on the client's body in two different directions to create a line of force in a third direction (Figure 6.13b ■).

6.3.3 Torque and Force Couples

Two or more forces applied in opposite directions can create **torque**, a rotational motion around an axis. Torque is the rotary counterpart of linear force. We all use torque in the course of our daily activities to move things more

SELF-CARE
Efficient Use of Force in Pressure Applications

Applying biomechanical principles to body mechanics can help you maximize the efficiency of force applications while minimizing the stress they create on your body. Pushing establishes lines of force through the bones via compression. Pulling establishes lines of pull through the soft tissues via tensional stress. Here are some tips to help you apply the forces of push and pull more efficiently as you work.

1. Face the direction you are pushing or pulling. This will help you absorb the counterforces of compression and stretch more directly into the core of your body. It can also prevent hand, wrist, and back injuries from the strain that occurs on joints as you twist them while you push and pull.

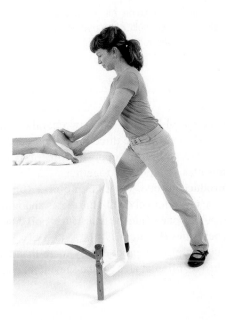

FIGURE 6.14a

2. Push with your whole body from your feet. Make sure to keep your spine straight and at least one leg in extension (Figure 6.14a ■). Push from a lunge position or with both straight legs, aligning your body in a plank position like a person does during a push-up. Pushing with your spine extended allows compression to be absorbed along all the vertebral

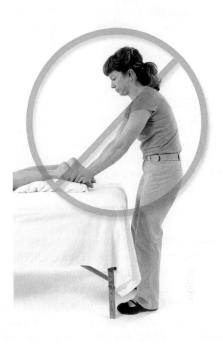

FIGURE 6.14b

segments, which dissipates mechanical stress in any one segment.

3. Avoid pushing with the spine bent into flexion because the compression from the push will stress the spine (Figure 6.14b ■).

(continued)

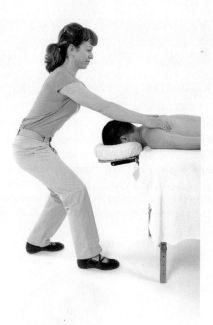

FIGURE 6.14c

4. Pull with your entire body, sitting back like a water skier. Keep your spine straight, your elbows straight but unlocked, and your shoulder girdle anchored to the spine and sacrum by contracting the lower trapezius and latissimus dorsi muscles (Figure 6.14c ■).

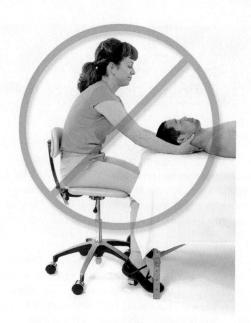

FIGURE 6.14d

5. Avoid bending your spine, hiking your shoulders, or locking your elbows as you pull or the pull will get stuck there and overstretch tissues in that area (Figure 6.14d ■).

easily, twisting a lid off a jar, pulling open a swinging door, or flipping a burger with a spatula (Figure 6.15 ■).

A linear force will push or pull a body in a linear direction, while a muscular torque pivots a joint around an axis of rotation. Torque makes things in the world turn round. The amount of torque produced by a muscular contraction depends on the moment arm of the working muscle. A **moment arm** is the perpendicular distance between the muscular line of pull and the axis of motion in the joint (Figure 6.16 ■). As a muscle contracts and produces joint motion, the angle of attachment changes. Torque is the greatest when the moment arm is 90 degrees, which occurs when the line of pull is perpendicular to the mechanical axis of the bone.

A **force couple** occurs when two parallel forces act simultaneously in opposite directions to produce motion. Like two hands pulling in opposite directions to turn a wheel, muscles contracting together as a force couple always produce torque. An example of a force couple occurs in the posterior pelvic tilt; the rectus abdominis pulls up on the pubic bone while the hamstrings pull down on the ischial tuberosities (Figure 6.17 ■).

Torque can also be produced by more than two muscles attached to different areas of the same joint contracting

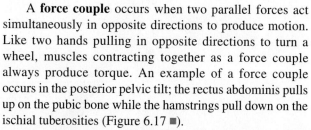

Line of pull

Center of joint

Moment arm

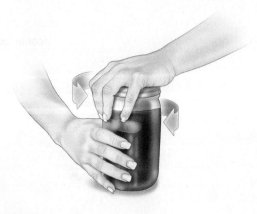

FIGURE 6.15

A **force couple** creates torque.

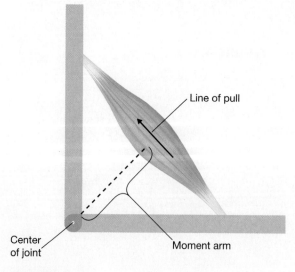

FIGURE 6.16

Moment arm

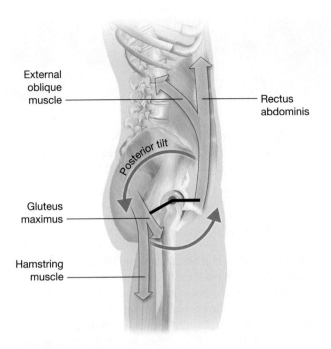

FIGURE 6.17

The hamstrings and rectus abdominis contract together as a **force couple** to tilt the pelvis posteriorly.

simultaneously to generate lines of force in different directions. To picture this, imagine several children spinning a merry-go-round by simultaneously pulling it from different sides. Groups of muscles around the hips, shoulders, and scapulae simultaneously pull in different directions to produce rotation (Figure 6.18 ■).

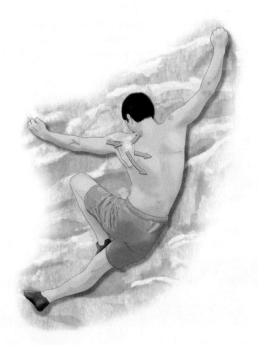

FIGURE 6.18

Torque forces produced by scapular muscles pull in different directions to turn the scapula.

A practitioner uses a force couple when simultaneously working opposing muscles, moving the hands in opposite directions along the agonist and antagonist muscles (see Figure 6.12b). This type of massage stroke is often used in integrative methods of massage for several reasons. It helps clients to feel dimension in their bodies, to feel how muscle groups connect across joints, and to feel how muscles work in coupled pairs.

6.3.4 Force–Velocity Relationship

The speed of a muscular contraction affects the force it generates, creating a **force–velocity relationship.** There is an inverse relationship between the amount of force the muscles can generate and the speed of the contraction:

- As muscular force increases, the speed of contraction decreases.
- As muscular force decreases, the speed of contraction increases.

Moving a lighter load requires less muscular force so the muscles can contract faster. Conversely, moving a heavier load requires more force so the muscles need more time to contract in order to generate the extra force. An example of the force–velocity relationship occurs while switching gears on a bike. The lower the gear, the faster a person can pedal. To generate more force, a person needs to gradually shift to higher gears, which creates more resistance so the pedaling is slower.

6.3.5 Stress–Strain Curve

Stress has many definitions. In a general definition, stress refers to elements that place wear and tear on the body. How a person responds to stress is called a *stress response.* In biomechanics, **stress** is defined as the internal resistance of a tissue to deformation. **Strain** is the change in tissue length due to deformation. The **stress–strain curve** of a tissue is determined by comparing the length of a tissue after being under stress to its original length (Figure 6.19 ■).

Stress and strain are dependent on the type of the tissue, type of load applied, point of load application, direction of force, magnitude of load, and the rate and duration of load. The shape of the stress–strain curve for each tissue will look slightly different depending on the elastic and plastic

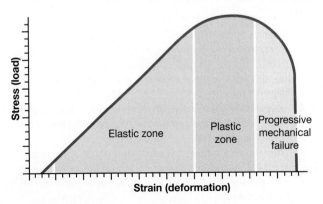

FIGURE 6.19
Stress–strain curve

BRIDGE TO PRACTICE
Force–Velocity Relationship in Manual Therapy

The force–velocity relationship can be put to use in manual therapy in this way. If you want to increase your pressure, slow your movement. By applying pressure slowly, you allow your muscles time to generate greater force. You also give your body ample time to adjust the magnitude of force you are applying and to adjust to the rate at which your client's tissues respond to your touch.

---

properties of the tissue. Tissues respond to mechanical forces according to their structural composition. For example, bones hold up well under compressive stresses, whereas muscles and tendons elongate well under tensional stresses.

The human body evolved to move while under the effects of many forces, but tissues do have their plastic limits. Too much compression, tension, or shearing can deform the tissue to a degree that it cannot recover, causing plastic and permanent changes. To restore chronically shortened myofascias to their normal length, manual therapists apply sustained pressure or tension to tissue to create plastic changes.

6.4   LEVERS

A **lever** is a simple machine that magnifies force and converts force to torque. We use levers during many daily tasks with simple tools such as scissors, can openers, and brooms. A lever consists of a rigid bar (lever arm) that pivots around an axis or fulcrum. Levers operate according to the principles of torque. Force is applied in one direction to move a load in another direction. Every lever has three parts: an axis (fulcrum), effort (force), and resistance (load or weight).

EXPLORING TECHNIQUE
Stress and Strain in Myofascial Release

A challenge in doing deep tissue work effectively is stretching a targeted layer of myofascia without damaging underlying tissues, especially nerves and blood vessels. Whenever you add more pressure, you add more stress, which creates more strain. If you apply too much pressure too fast and injure vulnerable tissues, your client will flinch and guard against pain.

To protect your clients, work slowly, watch your clients' responses to your work, and ask them for feedback about pressure. As myofascia stretches, clients often report feeling a light burning sensation. If your client reports such discomfort from myofascial stretching, explain that this sensation is normal and to be expected, which will help your client relax into myofascial release work.

1. Begin by applying perpendicular pressure to the area of myofascia that you are going to stretch. Sink into this area, pinning against the underlying tissues, pressing in until you feel the first level of resistance. If you are unsure about depth of pressure, ask your client for feedback.
2. Now change the direction of your pressure to a 45-degree angle, shifting in the direction you will be stretching the tissue (Figure 6.20 ■).
3. Then stretch the tissue to its first layer of resistance and hold. Ask your client to consciously relax the muscles under your pressure. Eventually the tissue will soften and stretch even farther.

4. As the tissues yield and stretch, sink straight into the next layer of resistance, then stretch it on a 45-degree angle, hold, and wait until the tissue yields again and stretches.
5. Remove your pressure slowly because elastic tissues have a certain level of rebound and you do not want to shock your client with a quick recoil.
6. Myofascial mobilization is like peeling an onion. Stretch the top layers, then gradually work down through subsequent layers.

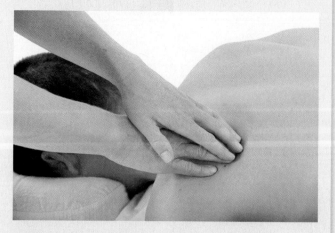

FIGURE 6.20

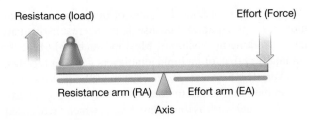

FIGURE 6.21

Effort arm and **resistance arm relationships**

- The **axis** (A) is the *fulcrum* around which a lever pivots.
- The **effort** (E) is the *force* that moves the lever.
- The **resistance** (R) is the *load* or *weight* that the lever moves.

The type of lever depends on the arrangement of these three parts. There are three different types of levers, each having its advantages and disadvantages in the realms of power, speed, or distance.

The distance between the effort and the axis is called the **effort arm** (EA) or lever arm; the distance between the resistance and the axis is called the **resistance arm** (RA) (Figure 6.21 ■).

A first-class lever magnifies force, allowing a relatively small force to be used to move a relatively large load a short distance. The power of a first-class lever is gained at the expense of the range of motion. We use first-class levers in a lot of daily chores, such as prying a cap off a jar with a spoon, weighing portions of food on a balance scale, or cutting paper with scissors (Figure 6.22 ■).

A second-class lever is also very powerful, using minimal effort to move a great amount of resistance, but also sacrifices range of motion to the magnification of effort. Second-class levers are uncommon because they work by carrying the load in between the axis and the effort. Examples can be found in earth-moving machinery that places the load in the middle, such as a backhoe or a wheelbarrow (Figure 6.22).

A third-class lever does just the opposite of the other two. Although they cannot produce a lot of power, a third-class lever such as a broom or shovel can move a smaller load a greater distance (Figure 6.22). A striking implement such as a golf club, tennis racket, and baseball bat also works as a third-class lever. The length of the lever arm allows it to go through a large arc of motion to overcome the relatively smaller resistance of a tennis ball, baseball, or golf ball. The force combination of racket speed and distance multiplies the projectile power of the lever arm, increasing a range of motion at the expense of force.

6.4.1 Levers in the Human Body

Each bone in the body works as a lever, particularly the long bones of the limbs (Figure 6.23a-c ■). Each body segment functions as a lever arm. The joints are the fulcrums of the bony levers in the body, providing pivot points around which movement occurs. Freely movable joints work

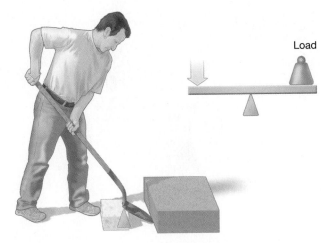

First-class lever

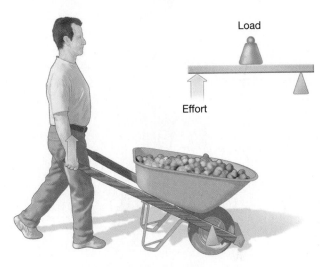

Second-class lever

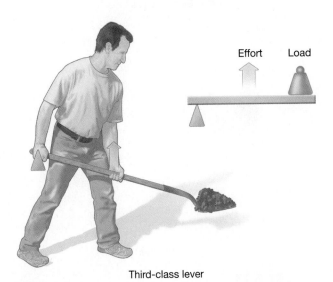

Third-class lever

FIGURE 6.22

The three types of levers

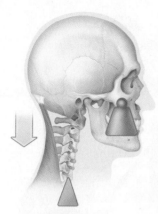

First class

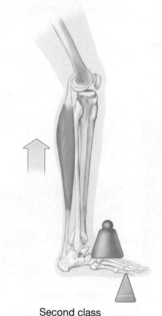

Second class

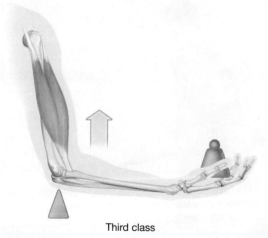

Third class

FIGURE 6.23

Levers in the body

together as a coordinated system of bony levers. Human movement is complex because it is the result of many levers working in synchrony. Most movements involve the cumulative effect of multiple joint levers working together.

Very few first-class levers exist in the body. Most muscles in the limbs attach to bones relatively close to the axis of motion and work as third-class levers, which favor speed, range of motion, and agility. A joint works as a third-class lever when the angle of the joint closes and as a second-class lever when the angle of the joint opens. For example, the biceps brachii functions as a third-class lever during flexion, when the flexors work concentrically, and as a second-class lever during extension, when the flexors work eccentrically (Figure 6.24a-b ■).

As a general rule, the closer the muscular force is to the fulcrum of movement, the greater the range of motion on the distal end of the lever arm. During elbow flexion, the arc of motion at the hand is much greater than the arc of motion closer to the elbow.

The point of resistance in a single lever in a body movement is not easy to identify because of the number of forces acting on the body from different directions. For example, when turning the head, resistance may be regarded as the center of gravity in the head. When turning the head against someone's hand, resistance comes from the center of contact of the hand. The resistance point could also be identified as the contraction of antagonist muscles or restrictions created by ligaments and taut bands.

6.4.2 The Mechanical Advantage of a Lever

These concepts may sound complex, but anyone who is familiar with using simple levers such as shovels or crowbars already knows this information intuitively. For example, when you sweep the floor with a broom, you probably hold the broom with one hand in the middle and the other hand at the end, which increases the efficiency of your lever. Understanding the components of levers can help you solve your own body mechanics issues as they arise. Being able to describe the components of levers can also help you assess client movement problems and explain to your clients more efficient ways to move.

The mechanical advantage of a lever describes its efficiency as a work tool (Figure 6.25 ■). **Work** is defined by how much force it takes to move an object a certain distance.

$$\text{Work} = \text{Force} \times \text{Distance}$$

The **mechanical advantage** (M Ad) of a lever is defined by the ratio between the effort arm (EA) and the resistance arm (RA). In other words, mechanical advantage equals the effort arm divided by the resistance arm.

$$\text{M Ad} = \text{EA} \div \text{RA}$$

- First-class levers can have an M Ad equal to 1 (RA = EA) or greater or lesser than 1.
- Second-class levers always have an M Ad greater than 1 (EA > RA).

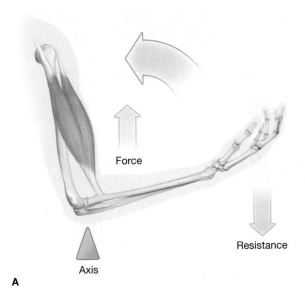

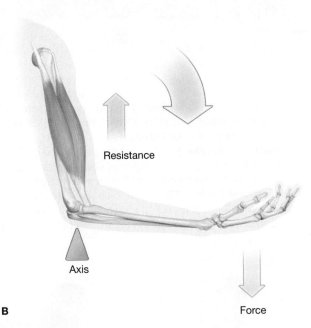

A

B

FIGURE 6.24

a) The biceps work as third-class lever in a concentric contraction. b) The biceps work as second-class lever in an eccentric contraction.

- Third-class levers always have an M Ad less than 1 (RA > EA).

As mentioned earlier, levers are simple machines that magnify force. Levers work to produce strong forces over short distances or weak forces over long distances. Only a first class lever can balance force with distance, which occurs when the axis of the lever is right in the middle. Move the fulcrum toward one end or the other and the EA becomes greater or lesser than the RA.

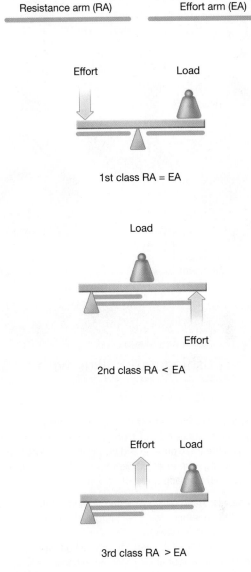

FIGURE 6.25

Mechanical Advantage (M Ad) of levers

Most of the muscles in the human body function as third-class levers, which, like brooms and sports rackets, favor speed and distance rather than work. If the M Ad of levers were measured by speed and distance rather than work output, then the bony levers in the human body, particularly in the limbs, would rate quite high. After all, the human body has evolved a system of levers well adapted for locomotion. In other words, human beings were born to run!

To apply this information to manual therapy, keep in mind that the longer the lever arm (either the EA or RA) that you use, the greater your leverage will be. For example, to bend a prone client's knee, it is easier to lift the client's leg at the ankle rather than in the middle of the calf. Similarly, when performing a resisted movement on the quadriceps, it is more efficient to apply resistance on the ankle than below the knee (Figure 6.26a-b ■).

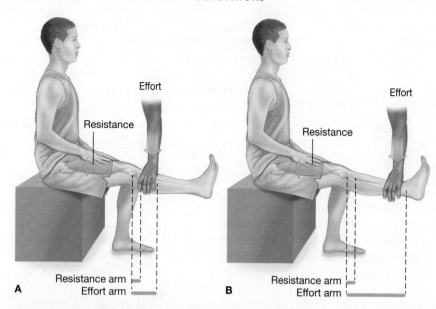

FIGURE 6.26
a) A short effort arm reduces the M Ad of the lever. b) A longer effort arm increases the M Ad of the lever.

SELF-CARE
Pushing and Pulling with a Partner

Pushing establishes lines of force through the bones via compression. Reaching establishes lines of tension through the soft tissues via tension. Practice these pushing and pulling with a massage partner to help you organize more efficient lines of force and lines of pull, which you can then apply to your body mechanics.

1. **Push hands:** Stand facing your partner and lightly touch palms. Now together, slowly lean into each other, supporting each other's weight and finding a balance point in between (Figure 6.27a). Keep your entire body vertical and stable. Lean from your ankle joints. Bend one knee to step back. Then push yourself back up to self-supported standing and repeat several times. *Is your spine straight? Is your chest lifted? Are your elbows lower than your shoulders. Are your lower abdominal muscles contracted? Are your knees and elbows straight but not locked?*

2. **Partner pull backs:** Stand facing your partner and grasp each other's forearms. Now together, slowly lean back, supporting each other's weight and finding a balance point in between (Figure 6.27b). Again, keep your entire body vertically aligned and stable. If you are both balanced and aligned, you should be able to sit down together, then stand back up.

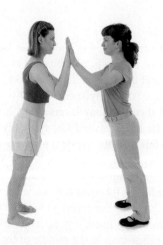

FIGURE 6.27a

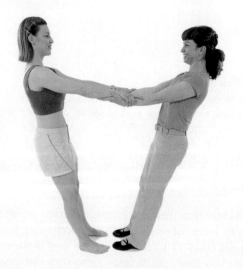

FIGURE 6.27b

6.4.3 Equilibrium, Stability, and Mobility

A body at rest is in a **stable equilibrium** because all forces and torques acting on it balance each other out and add up to zero (Figure 6.28a ■). To move a body from a stable equilibrium, the COG must be lifted. Here are some examples.

A seated person moves out of stable equilibrium by standing; a book is moved out of a stable flat resting position by standing it on one side. An **unstable equilibrium** occurs when a minimal force can shift a body and cause its COG to fall, such as a person balancing on a physioball or standing on one leg (Figure 6.28b ■). A **neutral equilibrium** occurs when the COG of an object or body remains level as it shifts position, such as a rolling ball or a child doing somersaults (Figure 6.28c ■).

To maintain equilibrium, the COG needs to be balanced over the **base of support** (BOS), whatever part of the body is supporting the body weight. The smaller the base of support, the more crucial it is that the COG be balanced along the line of gravity (LOG) over the BOS. If the COG in one part of the body shifts off the LOG, the COGs in other parts will need to shift in the opposite direction to maintain equilibrium (Figure 6.29 ■). This is particularly

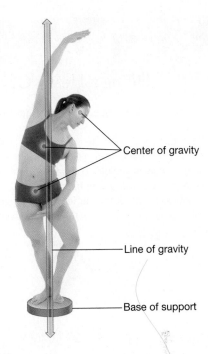

FIGURE 6.29

The COG aligns along the LOG over the **base of support** (BOS).

relevant to the human body because of its narrow BOS. The lower the COG, the more stable a body becomes, especially when the supporting surface where a person is sitting or standing is unstable. A person sitting in a row boat is going to be far more stable than a person standing in a boat. People instinctively widen their BOS to remain more stable, such as staggering the feet in the direction the train is moving. When the train turns a corner the dynamics change, and people have to adjust their position to remain stable.

The higher the COG, the less stable the body. Standing on your tip toes is much less stable than standing with both feet flat on the ground. Two people carrying a canoe might lift it overhead, which is less stable then carrying it lower but allows the weight of the boat to be borne as a top load.

Mobility and stability have an inverse relationship. The greater the stability of a body, the greater effort it takes to overcome inertia and get a body moving. It takes more energy to step forward from a wide stance than a narrow stance where the leg can easily swing under the hip. The greater mobility of a body, the less stability it has. In an activity where we need to move quickly with agility, such as tennis, standing with the feet close together allows us to step freely from the center in any direction. Sprinters and swimmers pose at the starting line in an unstable position so that they can easily and quickly fall off center into a forward motion. Similarly, massage therapists need to be mobile enough to move around the table but stable enough to support themselves as they work.

Understanding basic principles of biomechanics is important for recognizing and solving movement problems. It is also the key to using effective body mechanics

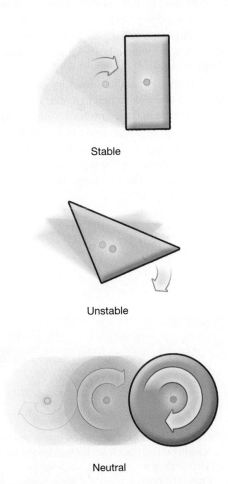

Stable

Unstable

Neutral

FIGURE 6.28
Types of equilibrium

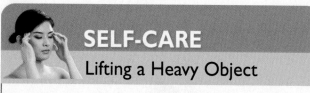

SELF-CARE
Lifting a Heavy Object

1. Contract your lower abdominals to avoid strain on your lower back.
2. Bend your knees and hold the weight as close to your trunk as possible to increase your stability (Figure 6.30 ■).
3. Keep your spine straight to engage the strong erector spinae muscles along your back.
4. To power the lift, push your feet down to come up. This will engage the large, powerful muscles in your hips and pelvis.

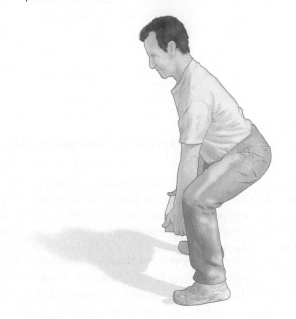

FIGURE 6.30
Proper lifting

in massage and bodywork. By taking a moment to determine the most efficient body-use pattern, you can figure out how to apply biomechanical principles to most work-related tasks, particularly those that require the use of physical force.

CONCLUSION

In a careful observation of skillful construction workers on the job, the biomechanical principles that underlie work-related tasks become obvious. For example, when lowering heavy materials, workers move slowly to control the accelerating speed that the weight of the object creates. To prevent friction that would slow down transport and could damage supplies, large and heavy loads are moved from one location to another on rolling carts. The cart moves along a linear path. By carrying and lifting heavy objects close to the body, a worker maximizes efficiency by moving along the vertical axis of the bony structure and in the line of pull of the primary working muscles.

Reverse muscle actions show up in repetitive, back-and-forth motions such as sawing or pounding nails. The laws of motion show up in many tasks, such as driving heavy moving equipment slowly to control the power of inertia and be able to stop quickly. Counterforces become obvious when watching workers push down while lifting up or push forward while pulling back. The power of momentum assists them to swing a heavy object in order to hike it up to a higher level.

Two workers use parallel forces by keeping both ends of a beam lifted at the same height to carry it. They demonstrate a force couple and the power of torque when pushing with equal force in opposite directions to turn and rotate a large crate. They magnify force by using simple levers such as crowbars or screwdrivers to pry open lids or boxes. And they increase mechanical advantage by using wrenches to turn screws or bolts.

GUIDELINES
Balancing Stability with Mobility

Here are some tips for maintaining a balance between stability and mobility while practicing manual therapy:

1. Maintain a neutral spinal alignment to keep the center of gravity in each body mass aligned and stable.

2. Keep your base of support under you unless you are leaning into a stroke. Putting your front foot under the table will throw your base of support back, so avoid this.
3. Wear shoes that provide traction if you are working on a slippery floor.

SUMMARY POINTS TO REMEMBER

1. Velocity describes the speed and direction of movement. An increase in velocity is acceleration; a decrease in velocity is deceleration. Gravity affects velocity. Eccentric contractions control an increase in velocity during downward movement; concentric contractions overcome a decrease in velocity during upward motion.

2. Friction is a force between two surfaces moving against each other. Friction is greater in motion between rough surfaces and less in motion between smooth surfaces.

3. A line of pull is the direction of force a muscular contraction exerts on a bone. The mechanical axis of a bone is an imaginary line that runs between the centers of the articulating joints on either end of that bone.

4. A reverse muscle action occurs when the moving and fixed ends of a muscle switch roles. A joint movement reverses when the moving bone in one action becomes the fixed bone in another action. For example, the femur moves during standing hip flexion and is fixed during forward bending of the trunk in a standing position.

5. The laws of motion explain the dynamics of a moving body in the field of gravity. The law of inertia states that a body at rest or in linear motion tends to stay at rest or in linear motion until acted upon by an outside force. The law of acceleration states that the distance an object travels when set in motion is proportional to the force causing the motion. The law of action and reaction states that for every action there is an opposite and equal reaction.

6. The force vector of a muscular pull is measured by the point of force application of the force on a joint, the direction of the force, and the magnitude of the force.

7. Forces can be linear (along the same axis), parallel (in the same direction), and concurrent (in different directions).

8. Torque is a rotational movement around an axis created by two forces working in opposite directions. Muscles work as force couples to produce rotational movement when they simultaneously pull on opposite sides of a joint in opposing directions.

9. In a force–velocity relationship, the speed of contraction decreases as a muscular force increases, and the speed of contraction increases as a muscular force decreases.

10. The stress–strain curve explains how the amount and duration of load applied to tissue results in a corresponding level of strain and resulting tissue deformation.

11. A lever is a simple machine that magnifies force and converts force to torque. The arrangement of the three parts of a lever—axis or fulcrum, effort or force, and resistance or load—determines the mechanical advantage of the lever. The bones, joints, and muscles in the human body work together as levers to generate movement.

12. A first-class lever such as a crowbar, where the fulcrum is between the effort and resistance, produces power but limits range of motion. A second-class lever such as a wheelbarrow, where the load is between the effort and fulcrum, magnifies force. A third-class lever such as a broom or a bat, where the effort is between the fulcrum and the load, favors speed and distance but limits force.

13. Equilibrium describes the balance of a resting body or body in motion. Equilibrium is stable when the forces acting on a body are balanced. Equilibrium becomes unstable when minimal force can tip a body or move it. Equilibrium is neutral when the center of gravity of an object remains level as the body moves, as in a rolling ball.

REVIEW QUESTIONS

1. Velocity is a combination of _____ and _____.

2. Define acceleration and deceleration.

3. True or false (circle one). We have to work harder when walking up a hill than down because our muscles are working against gravity.

4. What is the line of pull in a muscular contraction and how does it change during joint motion?

5. A reverse muscle action is
   a. when the moving and fixed ends of a muscle and joint switch roles.
   b. when a muscle elongates rather than shortens during a contraction.
   c. when the fast fibers of a contracting muscle alternate with the slow fibers.
   d. when the moving and fixed ends of a muscle and joint remain the same.

6. Which description describes a reverse muscle action in the gluteal muscle?
   a. The gluteal muscle reverses action when, from a standing position, a person does hip extension, then bends forward at the waist.
   b. The gluteal muscle reverses action when, from a standing position, a person does knee flexion with hip extension, then bends forward at the hips.
   c. The gluteal muscle reverses action when, from a standing position, a person does hip flexion, then bends laterally at the waist.
   d. The gluteal muscle reverses action when, from a standing position, a person does hip flexion, then bends forward at the hips.

7. The law of inertia states that
   a. the distance an object travels when set in motion is proportional to the force causing the movement.
   b. a body at rest or in linear motion tends to stay at rest or in motion unless acted upon by an outside force.
   c. a body at rest or in linear motion tends to stay at rest or in motion unless acted upon by internal compressive force.
   d. for every action there is an opposite and equal reaction.

8. The three factors that describe the force vector of a muscle are the
   a. attachment site of the muscle, the line of muscular pull, and the fibers active during the contraction.
   b. attachment site of the muscle, the line of muscular pull, and the strength of the moving bone.
   c. attachment site of the muscle, the line of muscular pull, and the strength of contraction.
   d. attachment site of the muscle, the line of counter pull, and the velocity of contraction.

9. Concurrent forces are
   a. parallel forces applied in the same direction, either toward or away from each other.
   b. forces that act on a body or object at the same point of application from different directions and create a third resultant force.
   c. separate forces of equal magnitude applied in the same plane, either in the same direction or in opposite directions.
   d. forces that act on a body or object at different points of application from the same direction.

10. Torque occurs when
    a. two or more forces applied in opposite directions create a rotational movement around an axis of motion, such as two hands turning a wheel.
    b. two or more forces applied in the same direction creates a rotational movement around an axis of motion, such as two hands turning a wheel.
    c. two or more forces applied in opposite directions creates a linear movement along an axis of motion, such as two hands sliding a wheel.
    d. two or more forces applied in opposite directions creates a gliding movement along an axis of motion, such as two hands pulling a wheel.

11. True or false (circle one). A force couple occurs when two parallel forces act simultaneously in opposite directions to produce torque.

12. The force–velocity relationship states that
    a. as a muscular force increases, the speed of the contraction decreases.
    b. as a muscular force decreases, the speed of the contraction is constant.
    c. as a muscular force increases, the speed of the contraction increases.
    d. as a muscular force decreases, the speed of the contraction decreases.

13. The stress–strain curve is formulated by comparing the
    a. density of a tissue after being under stress to its original density.
    b. elasticity of a tissue after being under stress to its original elasticity.
    c. length of a tissue after being under stress to its original length.
    d. viscosity of a tissue after being under stress to its original viscosity.

14. Define a lever and describe its three parts.

15. Which type of lever favors speed and distance over power and is commonly found in the human body?

16. True or false (circle one). The shorter the effort arm of a lever, the more powerful the lever.

17. The human body is in the most stable equilibrium when
    a. sitting because the center of gravity in the largest body mass is midway to the ground and the base of support is balanced between the two sides.
    b. standing because the center of gravity in each body part is closest midline and the base of support is under the major body masses.
    c. side-lying because the center of gravity in each body mass is closer to the ground and the base of support is broader.
    d. lying supine because the center of gravity in each body part is closest to the ground and the base of support is broadest.

18. When lifting a heavy object, which of the following statements describes poor body mechanics?
    a. Hold the weight of the object as close to your COG as possible.
    b. Bend the knees and keep the spine straight as you lift.
    c. To engage powerful trunk muscles, pull up with the shoulders as you lift.
    d. To engage powerful hip muscles, push your feet down as you come up.

Notes

1. Greene, L., & Goggins, R. (2006, Feb/Mar). "Musculoskeletal Symptoms and Injuries among Experienced Massage and Bodywork Professionals." *Massage and Bodywork Magazine,* pp. 48–58.

2. Kreighbaum, E., & Barthels, K. (1996). *Biomechanics: A Qualitative Approach for Studying Human Movement.* Needham Heights, MA: Pearson Education.

PEARSON
myhealthprofessionskit™

Use this address to access the Companion Website created for this textbook. Simply select "Massage Therapy" from the choice of disciplines. Find this book and log in using your username and password to access interactive activities, videos, and much more.

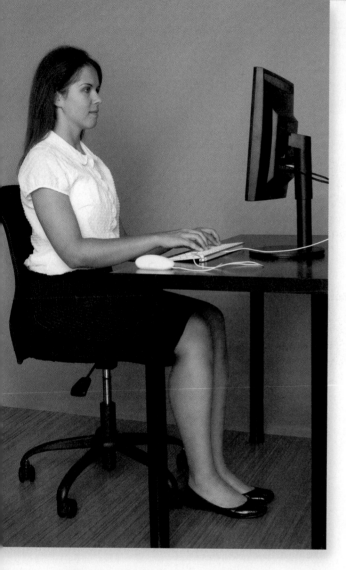

CHAPTER

7 Posture

CHAPTER OUTLINE

Chapter Objectives

Key Terms

7.1 Components of Upright Posture

7.2 Muscle Patterns in Upright Posture

7.3 Faulty Postures

7.4 Postural Assessments

7.5 Therapeutic Applications for Postural Education

Conclusion

Summary Points to Remember

Review Questions

Every day, all over the world, millions of people work from a seated position—at a desk, in front of a computer, and even behind a steering wheel. Workers performing tasks that require hours of focused attention often endure numbing sitting marathons in sacrifice to their livelihoods. Ideally, seated workers have job tasks that require standing up and walking around intermittently so that they move throughout the day.

In the 1800s, 80 percent of laborers worked the land for their bread and butter. Today over 90 percent of the populace earns their livelihood from a seated position, which can add up to 80,000 hours over a lifetime. In addition, we travel to work seated in cars

or buses, then spend our leisure time watching movies or reading in a chair. The human body evolved to move, yet our lifestyles cultivate sedentary activities, causing many people to suffer back pain and musculoskeletal disorders at some point in their lives.

"Active sitting" provides a remedy to this sedentary conundrum. It involves practicing exercises from a chair, such as intermittently rocking the pelvis or stretching the arms and the spine. Most important is standing up every 20 minutes to engage the large muscles of the hips, which improves circulation in the entire body. Whatever exercises you choose to accomplish active sitting, movement is your best therapist.

CHAPTER OBJECTIVES

1. Define posture and describe the components of optimal upright posture.

2. Name two postural reflexes and describe how they work.

3. List and briefly describe architectural features of the spine, pelvis, shoulders, and head.

4. Describe how each of the three movement systems contributes to postural support.

5. Describe how postural muscles work as joint stabilizers.

6. Describe a stability dysfunction and a substitution pattern, and how they affect a pain cycle.

7. Define and contrast primary and secondary postural stabilizers.

8. Discuss why mobilizer muscles function poorly as postural stabilizers.

9. List and define three directions that spinal curvatures deviate from optimal alignment.

10. Name and describe five patterns of faulty posture.

11. List and describe two common alignment problems in the knees.

12. Describe how a postural assessment is made.

13. List five steps for changing faulty posture.

14. Describe how posture affects body mechanics.

KEY TERMS

Anterior pelvic tilt

Axial compression

Core muscles

Eccentric loading

Flat-back posture

Ideokinesis

Joint instability

Kyphotic curve

Kyphotic-lordotic posture

Lordotic curve

Posterior pelvic tilt

Postural stabilizers

Postural sway

Posture

Round-back posture

Scoliosis

Stability dysfunction

Substitution pattern

Sway-back posture

Torticollis

All the chapter topics we've covered so far—bones, joints, muscles, and the neuromuscular system—come together in a study of posture and gait. These two topics relate to everybody and are central to the study of human movement in kinesiology. Everyone has a personal style of sitting, standing, and walking. Whether or not a client brings a specific problem to massage and bodywork, we can begin to understand the general configuration of muscle and joint function by assessing the client's carriage and stride.

Posture is the relative alignment of the body in any position. Posture is also an attitude. "To posture" is to take a stance, to assume a position, which invariably reflects the psychological state of the person living in that body. In this context, posture expresses mood; it outwardly manifests the inner workings of the mind and the emotional interior of an individual. Depression affects both the body and mind, showing up as a sunken, collapsed deportment. In contrast, joy and excitement tend to elevate and lift the posture. This depth of relationship between posture and psychology is important to remember when helping clients to change ineffective postural habits. Manual therapy alone cannot change postural problems rooted in psychological issues. In this case, improving posture will demand a person's commitment to self-awareness and self-improvement.

In the upright human posture, the legs and thighs serve as vertical columns to support the spine. The legs of an elephant also function as columns, yet their limb muscles are puny relative to the muscles in the lower limbs of a human. The larger thigh and leg muscles in the human body accentuate the wider range of postural demands on human beings as compared to other animals. Although posture is generally thought of as a static position, human beings move through a wide variety of postures during the day, from lying down to kneeling to sitting to standing. In this regard, posture is dynamic; it is the dynamic alignment of the joints as a person moves from one position to another.

Many people believe that they inherit faulty postures, or that muscle and joint injuries cause posture and movement dysfunctions. Just the opposite is more often true. The repetitive stress that movement places on a poorly aligned structure is cumulative. Poor posture, over time, damages the tissues and creates mayhem in the body. The chronically flexed postures that develop from habits such as craning the neck in front of a computer or slouching on a couch to watch television have become commonplace in our modern way of life.

An understanding of optimal posture can provide a practitioner with a rudder to steer the direction of a massage and bodywork session. Where and how the posture deviates from vertical reveals areas of muscular imbalances, highlighting where in the body the muscles need to be stretched or toned. Each massage stroke and technique can be applied in a direction or manner that moves the client's body toward improved skeletal alignment and ease of movement.

This chapter begins with a review of the elements of optimal posture, followed by a look at postural muscle functions and joint stabilization, faulty postural patterns, and postural assessments and corrections. Effective body mechanics depend on the underlying efficiency of posture and gait patterns. With this in mind, we'll also look at applying postural principles to self-care applications for both practitioner body mechanics and client education.

7.1 COMPONENTS OF UPRIGHT POSTURE

The first and most important aspect to improve posture is assessing how well the joints are aligned. Recall from Chapter 2 that a person demonstrates an optimal upright posture when the center of gravity (COG) in each body mass is as close to the line of gravity (LOG) as possible. Optimal posture places the weight-bearing joints in an extended, neutral position where they are neither bent nor rotated. The COGs should also align over the base of support (BOS) so that when a person stands, the feet land directly under the pelvis. Other bony landmarks align vertically in ideal posture that can be assessed from the side view (Figure 7.1 ■):

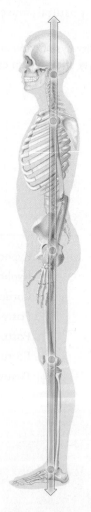

FIGURE 7.1

Bony landmarks that align in **optimal posture**

- The ear and mastoid process
- A point just anterior to the shoulder joint
- A point posterior to the hip joint and greater trochanter a point just anterior to the center of the knee
- A point just anterior to the front of the ankle

7.1.1 Dynamic Postural Reflexes

Upright posture is generally thought of as a position that the body assumes, although it is by no means static. Posture is always dynamic because it is impossible to stand perfectly still. Anyone who played statue as a child might remember how difficult it was to hold the body completely still. This difficulty arises from a reflex called **postural sway,** which creates a subtle swaying motion of the entire body from front to back. As the body sways, subtle contractions of postural muscles occur on one side of the body, which subtly stretch the postural muscles on the other side. The stretch triggers a tonic stretch reflex, creating subtle contractile responses that perpetuate the oscillating motion of postural sway. The talocrural joints of the ankles serve as fulcrums for the swaying motion, causing the whole body to lean like tall grass in a gentle wind. The role of ankle movement in postural sway underlies efficient walking patterns, which will be expanded on in the gait chapter.

In a normal range of postural sway, the arc of motion in the upper body averages a distance of 12 inches in diameter (Figure 7.2 ■). Too much postural sway can indicate a

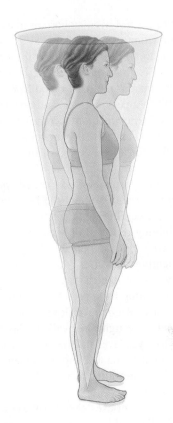

FIGURE 7.2

Range of **postural sway**

SELF-CARE
Postural Sway for Fluid Body Mechanics

Your quality of movement as you give massage usually translates through your hands into your quality of touch. Practicing postural sway is a great way to keep your body fluid and supple yet well aligned. This will not only improve your body mechanics but enhance your quality of touch. Here are the steps for practicing postural sway:

1. **Getting ready:** Begin standing in an upright posture with your pelvis centered over your feet and your spine elongated. This centered posture, or "human stance," is home base, a place to return to whenever you need to take a momentary rest to center and realign your body while giving massage.[1] Stand comfortably with your knees straight but not locked.

2. **Swaying:** With both feet flat on the floor, allow your body to subtly sway.

3. **Use contrast to feel the effects of sway:** If it is difficult to sway, hold your body really still and feel the effort this takes. Then release this effort and you should feel a subtle swaying motion.

4. **Tips for the feet:** As you sway, sense your body's weight slowly shifting between your heels and toes. Make sure your feet are flat on the floor. Avoid curling your toes or lifting your heels. Imagine a ball-bearing in each ankle and sense your body shifting over these ball-bearings so that your ankles become the fulcrum of motion.

5. **Breathing:** Notice how breathing affects swaying. Breathing in tends to slightly extend the spine, which rocks the body forward. Breathing out tends to slightly flex the spine, which rocks the body back.

6. **Practicing during daily activities:** Whenever you find yourself standing for lengthy periods of time, while at work or waiting in line, tune into postural sway to wake up this dynamic reflex.

7. **Integrating with massage:** To begin a massage, center your body in an upright stance. Then sense your postural sway to engage a feeling of inner fluidity. Once you feel the sway, place your hands on your client and sense the sway. Then sway into your hands and begin the massage.

person's lack of control over supporting muscles or a neurological dysfunction; too little sway leads to rigidity and restricted circulation. Postural sway is important because it generates light contractions in the muscles of the calves, which assist the venous return of blood from the legs back to the heart. When a person has a rigid posture that blocks this dynamic reflex, circulation becomes restricted, which can lead to fainting. This often occurs in a crowd of people who are standing for a long period of time, with someone eventually passing out.

Other dynamic postural reflexes called *optical righting* and *head righting reflexes* orient the head to the horizon to sustain upright equilibrium. Structures in the inner ear mediate all righting reflexes; they are constantly at work to keep the head upright and the eyes level. Without these important orienting responses, the nervous system cannot accurately register which way is up, which would be incredibly disorienting for a person, creating severe problems with balance. Righting reflexes can be seen in the head movements of a tightrope walker who makes subtle shifts to keep the eyes level and the neck vertical. Righting reflexes can be felt in the leveling movements of the head and neck when you are sitting in a boat being tossed around by turbulent waves.

Optical righting reflexes also orient the head over the body and level the field of vision. The optical righting reflex can be observed in a baby who is just learning to hold her head up (Figure 7.3 ■). Her head will bob until her eyes meet the gaze of the mother, which stabilizes the head motion. An adult engages the optical righting reflex when holding reading material far enough away from the face that it comes into focus (Figure 7.4 ■).

To feel optical righting, hold your hand so close to your face that your field of vision blurs. Then slowly move your hand and face away from each other until your hand is in a position where you can see it, which should trigger optical righting to lift your head and lengthen your neck. Another great way to engage the optical righting reflexes is

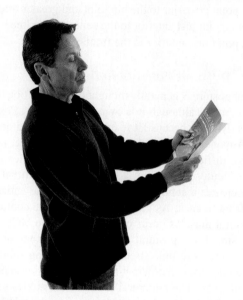

FIGURE 7.4

Optical righting reflex to focus on reading material

to lie over a physioball and keep the neck aligned with the spine while reading in this position for about 20 minutes (Figure 7.5 ■). Because it engages the postural muscles in the neck and restores the cervical curve, this exercise can help a person recover from a stiff neck incurred by looking down for long periods at a workstation.

To sense the head righting reflex, close your eyes and slowly move your head, noticing the position where your head feels aligned over your body, which may take a while to feel. Or do the same while sitting on a physioball with your feet firmly planted on the floor—but only close your eyes if you already have good balance (Figure 7.6 ■). People with balance problems usually become dizzy or nauseous when they close their eyes because they lose the visual support provided by optical righting.

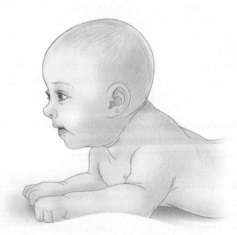

FIGURE 7.3

Optical righting reflex in an infant

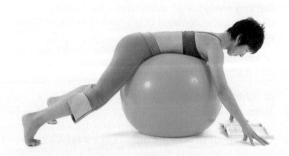

FIGURE 7.5

This exercise engages the optical righting reflex, restores the cervical curve, and tones postural muscles in the neck.

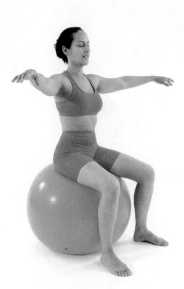

FIGURE 7.6

Balance exercise *Warning: If you have problems with dizziness or balance, do not try this exercise.*

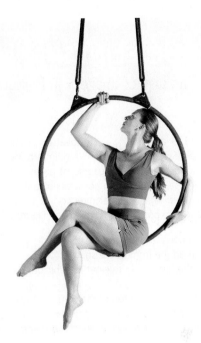

FIGURE 7.7

Notice the refined postural awareness of this dancer.

7.1.2 Skeletal Architecture in a Standing Posture

The human skeleton not only provides a stable inner scaffold upon which the soft tissues attach and around which the body can sway, it is also a well-calibrated structure with specific architectural features. Every single joint and bone in the body possesses a unique structural design. Understanding the architectural analogies for each major body part provides insight into the mechanics of joint structure and function. This also gives a practitioner vivid imagery with which to visualize the ideal movement range of each different part of the body. For example, the three arches of the foot form a flexible architectural vault, the shoulder joint resembles a flywheel, and the ankle joint fits together like a mortise.

Visualization can be a powerful tool for changing patterns of posture and movement because each image creates a gestalt of a total body experience. Dancers develop poise and refined postural awareness from years of practicing fundamental ballet exercises in which they move within an imagery grid of clear lines of spatial tension (Figure 7.7 ■). Dynamic images of movement can be used to shift bony relationships in order to effectively improve skeletal alignment. For example, to help a client lengthen the neck, you could suggest that the client visualize the head floating away from the body.

While there are many different types of images to visualize, research has shown that anatomically sound imagery is more effective in changing body patterns than images based on abstract ideas.[2] The reason for this is that the human brain is so adept at organizing neuromuscular

pathways around ideas of how the body *should* be, that if an abstract image goes against the architectural design of the skeleton, it could create more problems than it was meant to fix. For example, some ballerinas learn that the spine should be straight, so they strive to straighten the back and later suffer body problems due to an unnatural flattening of the spinal curves.

You can give your clients anatomically based images as tools for changing postural patterns. The process of changing posture and movement efficiency with imagery—such as imagining the rib cage breathing like a toy accordion, the hips flexing like a jackknife closing, or the neck lengthening like a balloon floating—is called **ideokinesis.** To equip you with sound imagery for working with posture, we look at some general architectural aspects of the spine and trunk in the next section.

7.1.2.1 THE SPINE AS A CURVED COLUMN

The human spine is a flexible column with three curves. Curved columns are able to absorb shock better than straight ones. To illustrate this point, imagine jumping on a straight wooden board balanced between two concrete blocks. The board will most likely break because it is straight. Had the board been bowed, it would flex and bend under compressive loading. The spine is extremely resilient to vertical loading and compression stresses; the flexible curves in the cervical, thoracic, and lumbar regions allow the spine to bend and flex under pressure. When placed under **axial compression,** which occurs when a person carries a heavy load on top of the head, the curved spine can withstand a greater axial load than a straight bony column.[3]

GUIDELINES
The Use of Imagery in Postural Education

Between 1929 and 1931, an innovative physical educator named Dr. Lulu Sweigard developed a unique body of anatomically based images during the course of an extensive research project on the use of imagery in postural education.[4] Sweigard's research identified nines lines of direction to visualize to evoke effective changes in posture and movement (Figure 7.8 ■):

1. Lengthen down the back of the spine.
2. Lengthen up the front of the spine.
3. Shorten the distance between the pubic bone and the 12th vertebra.
4. Either lift or lower the top of the sternum toward or away from the top of the spine (*the direction of the action depends on the relative position of the sternum to the head*).
5. Narrow the rib cage.
6. Widen across the back of the pelvis.
7. Narrow across the front of the pelvis.
8. Reposition the center of the knee under the center of the hip socket.
9. Shorten the distance between the big toe and heel, especially during walking.

Sweigard had her students use imagery of the lines to guide slow, controlled movements. She also created these guidelines for practicing movement exercises with the goal of improving neuromuscular efficiency:

- Begin each exercise from a position of complete relaxation in order to avoid carrying dysfunctional muscular habits into new actions.
- Inhibit any voluntary effort toward the movement until the image initiates the action. Otherwise, the habitual posture or movement will dominate and perpetuate a faulty pattern.

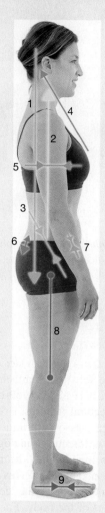

FIGURE 7.8
Sweigard's nine lines of movement

There are two types of normal spinal curves (Figure 7.9 ■):

- A **lordotic curve** is *convex* toward the front in the cervical and lumbar areas.
- A **kyphotic curve** is *concave* toward the front in the thoracic and sacral areas.

The degree of curve in an individual spine will vary according to the shape of the individual vertebrae, which is determined by genetics. Some people have spinal structures with a greater degree of curve than others. Imbalanced muscle tone and postural holding patterns also affect the shape of the spine. Like the coils in a spring under compression, an increase in the degree of curve in one area of

a spine can increase the degree of curve along the entire spine. Conversely, the lengthening and flattening of one curve usually elongates the entire spine. Ideally, the postural muscles stabilize the spinal curves in their maximal length without flattening the structure. Maximal length only occurs when the body masses align along the line of gravity and the postural muscles are engaged.

7.1.2.2 THE PELVIS AS A BRACED ARCH

The bony pelvis structure resembles the braced arch that originated in Roman architecture. In a braced arch, two vertical columns buttress against two diagonal blocks, which in turn hold up a keystone that is wedged in the center. The femurs serve as the vertical columns of the arch; they

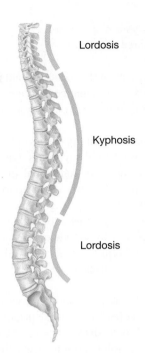

FIGURE 7.9

The spinal curves

Lordosis

Kyphosis

Lordosis

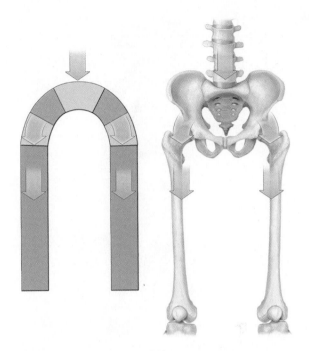

FIGURE 7.10

Pelvis as a braced arch

diagonally buttress into the hip sockets of the pelvic bones, which in turn hold up the sacrum. The sacrum serves as the keystone of the arch (Figure 7.10 ■).

The sacrum resembles an upside-down triangle that transmits force in three directions: up into the spine and down into the two lower limbs. Ground reaction forces from the feet travel up the legs and thighs into the sacrum, where they combine into a single thrust into the spine. Compressive force travels down the spine into the sacrum, which splits the force for transmission down each leg.

Any degree of slant in the columns of an architectural braced arch would compromise the integrity of the structure. The organic tissues in the human body are more adaptable. A wide stance reduces the vertical thrust of the legs into the pelvic bones, so muscles have to work harder to support the trunk. Our most energy-efficient stance is one in which the legs are parallel and the feet are directly under the hip joints.

7.1.2.3   THE SHOULDER GIRDLE AS A YOKE

In an optimal posture, the shoulder girdle balances across the rib cage like a yoke (Figure 7.11 ■). The clavicles and scapulae serve as horizontal struts for the yoke; the arms hang like buckets off each side.

Muscles arising in the neck and shoulders suspend and tether the bones of the shoulder girdle over the rib cage and seat the arms into the shoulder sockets. The balance of the yoke depends on the position of the bony rib cage and spine and the balance of the head over the neck and thorax. Two small joints between each clavicle and the sternum attach the entire yoke to the axial skeleton. The shoulder girdle rides on the waves of respiratory motion expanding

and lifting the shoulders from underneath. If the sternum is lifted and respiratory motion is normal and full, the yoke can balance horizontally across the rib cage. If the sternum and rib cage are sunken and depressed, the shoulders tend to round and sink, dragging the yoke down like a rider on a sagging horse.

7.1.2.4   THE HEAD AS A TOP LOAD

The head rests on the spine as a top load, but only when it centers over the thorax (Figure 7.12 ■). Because the human spine is so adaptable to carrying weight along a vertical column, people from many cultures transport large baskets or other heavy items on top of their heads. There is a lot of wisdom in balancing a book on your head to learn

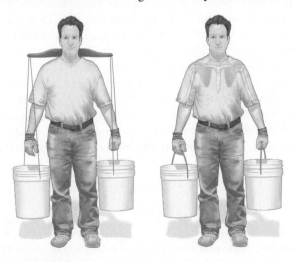

FIGURE 7.11

Shoulder girdle as yoke

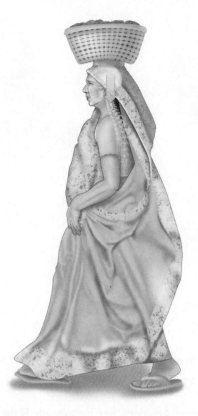

FIGURE 7.12
Head as top load

about posture because doing so requires that you hold the head directly over the trunk so that the weight of the book transfers straight down into the spine.

Ideally, the vertical axis of the head and neck counterbalances the horizontal axis of the shoulder yoke. Because of their integral muscular connections, a postural deviation in the head and neck usually throws the shoulder girdle off its horizontal balance, and any postural deviation in the shoulders throws the neck off. To feel this, pinch your shoulder blades together and notice how this affects the alignment of your head and neck (it usually results in a "chin-poke" or forward head posture where a person thrusts the chin forward), or tip your head back and notice how this shifts your shoulders (it usually causes the shoulders to drop and round). For this reason, it is crucial that the head be aligned directly on top of the thorax for the shoulder girdle to be optimally aligned. It is also crucial that the shoulder girdle be aligned so that the chest can open, the sternum can lift, and the space between the scapulae can widen.

7.1.3 The Role of Movement Systems in Posture

Optimal posture requires a balanced function between the three body systems involved in the production of movement: the skeletal system, muscular system, and nervous

system. Each system contributes to postural support through one of three channels:

- Passive restraints of the ligaments and joint capsules
- Active forces of muscular contractions
- Motor control from the nervous system

The relationship among the joints, muscles, and nervous system in postural support is dynamic. If one leg of this tripod becomes dysfunctional in maintaining an optimal posture, the other two legs need to work harder to take up the slack. When working with a faulty pattern of movement or posture, you need to figure out which one of the three systems fails to provide postural support in order to know which system to treat. The failure could arise from a joint injury, a muscle dysfunction, or a neurological problem.

The ligaments and joint capsules contribute minimally to postural support because in the upright neutral stance, these tissues tend to be slack. They offer the most support at an end range of joint motion, when they work under tension as passive restraints to limit excessive joint play. Collapsed or bent postures place the weight-bearing joints under bending stresses, which puts tension on the passive joint supports. In such flexed postures, the weight of the body literally hangs off the passive restraints, gradually overstretching and weakening the ligaments and joint capsules, causing them to become lax. The cumulative effect is overstretched and weakened ligaments. Bending stresses are the most damaging to the spine because the upper part of the bent area loses it base of support. When the spinal ligaments become too weak to hold the vertebrae together, the muscles have to work harder to provide support. The thoracic spine is especially vulnerable to sustained bending stresses from poor posture since its natural kyphosis already bends toward flexion (Figure 7.13 ■). People with

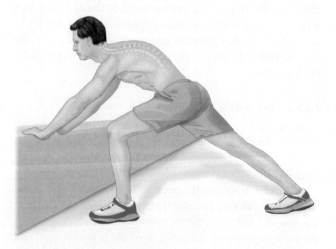

FIGURE 7.13

An **excessive thoracic kyphosis** overstretches the thoracic ligaments and muscles.

BRIDGE TO PRACTICE
Working with Chronic Thoracic Flexion

A client with a chronically flexed thorax can develop back pain from stretch-weakened ligaments or muscles in the midscapular area. When working with clients with this pattern, avoid massage and bodywork techniques that stretch already overstretched soft tissues in this area.

Trigger point therapy can provide pain relief in stretch-weakened muscles, followed by kneading techniques such as petrissage that restore circulation and sensation to numb tissues.

Tissue approximation can also be effective in restoring a normal resting tone to the muscles while increasing a client's awareness of the area, which is a preliminary step in learning exercises that develop motor control.

To maintain bodywork effects, suggest that your client focus on keeping the sternum lifted during the course of daily activities. Extension stretches (see Figure 14.44a) and arcing exercises (see Figure 14.19) are also recommended.

overstretched ligaments from excessive thoracic flexion generally experience chronic pain in the midscapular area.

The muscles, particularly postural muscles, work as active postural supports by generating contractile forces that hold the bones together. Under normal conditions, the postural muscles actively and reflexively contract to keep the body upright. When the passive restraints of ligaments and joint capsules become damaged, additional muscles work overtime to provide a backup system to stabilize injured joints, reducing the overall economy of the postural support system. Flexed postures place the posterior muscles along the thoracic spine under **eccentric loading,** which means that the muscles are contracting eccentrically to support weight. Muscles can become damaged or suffer stretch injuries from being overloaded. This frequently occurs in postural muscles working under sustained eccentric loading.

To feel the difference between concentric and eccentric loading, compare holding a heavy weight like a bowling ball with the elbow bent at 120 degrees (eccentric loading) for several seconds to holding it with the elbow bent at 45 degrees. At 120 degrees, the elbow flexors work under eccentric loading, which requires increased effort and creates more stress than concentric loading. The same dynamic occurs in the forward head posture. The spinal muscles along the thorax become stretch weakened from the weight of the head. At the same time, the muscles overwork and become taut to prevent the upper spine from buckling under the load of the head.

When a person has poor posture, the postural muscles tend to be inactive and fail to provide support. The control of postural muscles is a key strategy in the long-term correction of faulty posture. Control means being able to contract and relax a specific muscle at will. Control prevents poor posture from being carried into daily activities such as bending and lifting, which reduces the overall economy of the muscular system. For example, when the thoracic spine is chronically flexed, other muscles overwork in the

compensatory patterns of cervical and lumbar hyperextension to straighten the spine (see Figure 7.13). To activate postural muscles, a client needs to learn how to reposition the bones into a better alignment, then actively contract specific postural muscles to hold the bones in place. For example, a person with a pattern of chronic thoracic flexion needs to learn how to lift the sternum and engage the spinal muscles in the midscapular region that extend the thoracic spine (Figure 7.14a-b ∎).

Self-care exercises for learning postural muscle control and for improving movement efficiency are presented throughout the text.

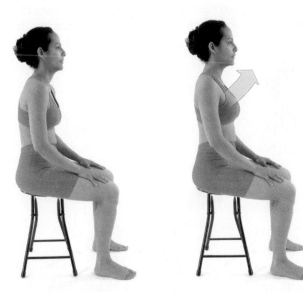

FIGURE 7.14

a) Many people have a postural pattern of **chronic thoracic flexion.** b) To correct a posture of thoracic flexion, lift the sternum.

7.2 MUSCLE PATTERNS IN UPRIGHT POSTURE

The uniquely vertical human posture provides a mechanical advantage over other animals because in the human body the postural muscles work toward a unified goal: that of supporting a single weight-bearing column. A small group of postural muscles co-contract along the core of the body to stabilize the joints they act on when the body is in an upright position. In contrast, the postural muscles of quadrupeds must work harder to support their horizontal spines, which span the distance between their forelegs and hindlegs like a suspension bridge hung between four posts (Figure 7.15 ■). In addition, most quadrupeds stand with their limbs in a partially flexed posture, which is maintained by continuous muscular contractions.

A standing posture is remarkably economical, requiring little muscular effort. Electromyographic studies of muscular activity in a standing posture show that simply standing requires minimal muscular activity, but only if the body masses stack as close to the vertical axis as possible.[5] This economy drops significantly when any one body segment displaces away from the LOG. For example, if the head aligns right over the neck and trunk, its weight transfers directly into the spine. An anterior displacement of the head, as in the head-forward posture, requires increased muscular effort to hold the head up and prevent further anterior displacement. Unless posture is optimally vertical, walking is easier than standing because the body realigns on each step. This explains why clients with chronic pain can tend to be fidgety and shift around in an effort to find a more comfortable position.

In an optimal standing alignment, constant muscular activity has been recorded in the deep spinal muscles, the iliopsoas group, and the soleus and tibialis posterior muscles.[6] Low-grade muscular activity also occurs in lower trapezius and rotator cuff muscles around the shoulder. The supraspinatus continually fires to prevent the downward displacement of the humerus in the glenoid fossa, as do the muscles elevating the mandible, which keep the mouth closed.

Although relatively few muscles work to maintain upright posture, truly vertical posture is a fluctuating event. Add postural sway to the equation and more muscles come into play to provide support, firing in oscillating bursts. During postural sway, intermittent contractions have been found in the gluteus medius, tensor fascia latae, hamstrings, transversus abdominis, and obliques.

7.2.1 Postural Muscles as Joint Stabilizers

The same muscles that provide postural support also stabilize the weight-bearing joints. The isometric contractions of the deep spinal muscles draw the vertebrae closer together to increase axial compression (see Figure 7.17a). Because of their dual function—postural support and joint stabilization—we will refer to postural muscles as **postural stabilizers.**

Recall from Chapter 4 that most muscles have both slow and fast fibers, although the ratio varies from one muscle to the next. Postural muscles tend to have more slow fibers and prime movers tend to have more fast fibers. The slow fibers generate weak but fatigue-resistant contractions, while the fast fibers generate quick and strong contractions that fatigue rapidly. This means that if the right muscles are working, a person will be able to sit or stand for long periods of time without muscle fatigue. If a person feels muscle fatigue and aching from sitting or standing, it is likely that that person is using the wrong muscles for postural support.

The postural muscles work with tonic (slow), sustained contractions, so they should be trained using slow, sustained isometric contractions done in place. In contrast, the prime movers produce phasic (fast), pumping contractions and are trained with ballistic joint motion actions common in weightlifting and many sports activities.

When assessing or working to improve muscle function, consider the recruitment order in which the muscles fire. In an ideal recruitment pattern, the slow muscle fibers contract before the fast fibers; the postural stabilizers contract before the prime movers. If the postural stabilizers are contracted in a stationary posture, when the body does move, the postural stabilizers will be able to restrict joint play outside of a normal range. They function like the cargo ties on a ship, battening down the cargo so it doesn't slip around the deck once the ship takes off.

7.2.1.1 STABILITY DYSFUNCTIONS AND PAIN PATTERNS

In an optimal recruitment pattern, the postural stabilizers contract prior to movement. If the postural stabilizers fail to contract before the body moves, the powerful phasic contractions of the mobilizer muscles can bend the joints outside

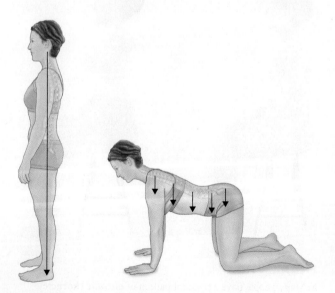

FIGURE 7.15

Lines of gravity in human spine compared to quadruped spine

of their normal range of motion, causing excessive joint play and instability. **Joint instability** is marked by the lack of control of joint motion at the end of range. Hypermobility differs from joint instability because people with hypermobile joints, such as gymnasts, ballet dancers, or yogis, can usually control joint motion outside of a normal range.

Every subsequent movement of an unstable joint increases mechanical stress on the joint capsule as well as its ligaments and tendons. Initially, a person may not notice the problems, but the damaging effects build over time. Eventually the joint structures become so weakened and damaged that the person develops a **stability dysfunction,** which occurs when a person is unable to control joint motion at normal range and causes tissue trauma.

Faulty postures are a major contributing factor to joint instability and the escalation of this problem into a stability dysfunction. When a person has a collapsed or bent spinal alignment, simple movements can further injure the spine by overstretching the ligaments and soft tissues around an unstable joint, causing pain and leading to muscle spasms. At this point, the unstable joint becomes a weak link in the chain of motion, and even a small movement can do serious damage, causing joint injury when a person moves the wrong way. Clients usually report such injuries as puzzling, saying that they were just bending over or turning when something snapped or gave out.

Pain is a major contributing factor to this dynamic because when a person develops chronic or acute pain, muscles acting as postural stabilizers become inhibited and stop firing. Why the stabilizers become inhibited and turn off is largely unknown, but the fact that this occurs is clinically relevant. In one study on subjects with chronic low back pain, only 10 percent of the participants could control the transversus abdominis—a major stabilizer of the lumbar spine—compared to 82 percent of those without chronic pain who could control it.

A benchmark of poor control over the transversus abdominis is abdominal distension, which places a front load on the lumbar spine (Figure 7.16 ■).[7] A distended abdomen also places a downward drag on the thorax, depressing the chest and interfering with normal breathing. This pattern is common among seniors, who tend to lose abdominal tone.

7.2.1.2 SUBSTITUTION PATTERNS

When the postural stabilizers fail, the mobilizer muscles take over their job of postural stabilization and become chronically contracted in a **substitution pattern,** also called a *compensatory* or *adaptive pattern.* The job of postural support requires muscles to work with isometric contractions. When the mobilizers become locked in isometric contractions, they become unavailable for movement, requiring other muscles to work harder and reducing the efficiency of the entire neuromuscular system.

Joint instability creates a twofold muscular dysfunction—one in the postural system and the other with the

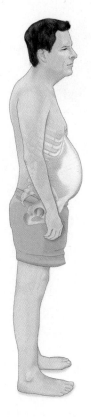

FIGURE 7.16

Poor control over the transversus abdominis is associated with low back pain.

efficiency of movement. Pain from joint instability causes postural stabilizers to turn off and become inhibited. This in turn causes the prime movers to overwork in substitution patterns and to also spasm in reaction to pain. Because muscles acting as prime movers are usually larger muscles that span longer distances and have stronger lever arms, they make poor postural stabilizers (Figure 7.17a-b ■). They fatigue rapidly and become ischemic and fibrous, which causes more pain, further inhibiting the stabilizer

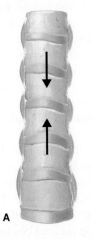
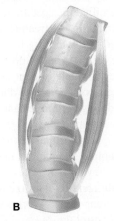

A   **B**

FIGURE 7.17

a) Effect of postural muscle contraction: **axial compression**
b) Effect of prime mover contraction: **joint motion**

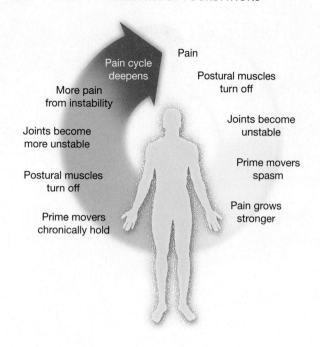

FIGURE 7.18
Dynamics of the **pain cycle**

muscles, leading to more pain and spasm, and escalating the pain cycle (Figure 7.18 ■).

The injurious consequences of stability dysfunctions are complicated by the detrimental effects that substitution patterns have on skeletal alignment and movement efficiency. The fast fibers of prime movers fatigue rapidly when they become chronically contracted while shoring up an unstable posture. A person experiences such imbalances through a gradually increasing set of symptoms, such as trigger points, muscular ache and fatigue, chronic muscle and joint pain, faulty posture, and dysfunctional movement patterns.

7.2.2 Postural Stabilizers and Core Control

Using electromyography (EMG) studies, researchers have identified the specific muscles to train as primary joint stabilizers in the treatment of chronic muscular pain associated with stability dysfunctions.[8] This group of muscles serves as *primary* postural stabilizers, which means that they fire independent of motion. *Secondary* postural stabilizers come into play during movement to *control* the speed and range of movement. *Mobilizers* generate more ballistic joint motion.

A lot of muscles function in more than one role. For example, the gluteus maximus functions in all three roles: the slow-twitch gluteal fibers work isometrically as primary stabilizers to stabilize the hip in a standing posture. The midrange fibers work eccentrically as secondary stabilizers to control the descent of the trunk during forward bending. The fast twitch gluteal fibers work concentrically to mobilize and extend the hip in vigorous locomotive activities such as running.

Many of the primary stabilizers lie close to the joints, particularly along the spine (Figure 7.19 ■). For this reason, they are often referred to as "core" muscles. A kinetic chain of core postural muscles in the pelvis—the transversus abdominis, multifidus, diaphragm, and perineum—form a closed loop that provides a foundation for stability in the entire body. There are also stabilizing muscles in the lower limb. The tibialis posterior lifts the medial arch of the foot and stabilizes the ankle. The vastus medialis oblique, a deep quadriceps muscle above the inside of the knee, keeps the knee stable and the patella tracking correctly.

A person doesn't have to be injured to begin training the **core muscles** as postural stabilizers. Core exercise programs that focus on developing the core muscles to improve form have become popular. One such approach, Pilates, focuses on teaching people to contract the postural muscles in order to maintain a neutral spine while strengthening the larger, more extrinsic muscle groups.

Although extrinsic muscular strength contributes greatly to postural stability, the postural muscles themselves need a different type of training. Muscles are strengthened with weight training, loading the muscles to increase force generation during phasic, pumping actions that move joints. Developing postural stabilizers involves establishing control over them rather than strengthening them. Learning to control a muscle means being able to contract it at will and then keep it contracted in stationary postures and during movement.

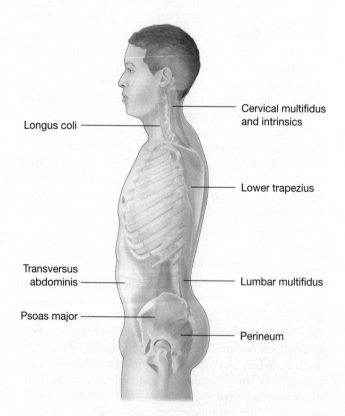

Longus coli

Cervical multifidus and intrinsics

Lower trapezius

Transversus abdominis

Psoas major

Lumbar multifidus

Perineum

FIGURE 7.19

Muscles working as **primary postural stabilizers** in the trunk

SELF-CARE
Lower Back Protection with the Transversus Abdominis

Akey postural muscle that stabilizes the lumbar spine and sacroiliac joints and supports the abdominal viscera is the transversus abdominis. To protect your lower back, make sure to keep this muscle contracted while you work, especially when pushing or pulling. Here is an exercise to train this muscle.

1. Sit or stand in an upright posture. Then place your hands on your lower abdomen between your navel and pubic bone in order to monitor whether or not the transversus abdominis contracts.
2. Let your abdominal wall completely relax so that your belly distends (Figure 7.20a ■).
3. Next, *slowly* draw your lower abdominal wall straight back toward your sacrum with a light isometric contraction (Figure 7.20b ■). Use only one-third maximum effort.
4. Hold it for 10 seconds, then completely relax it.
5. Repeat 10 times.

While you're practicing massage or bodywork, make sure to keep this muscle contracted by pulling in your lower abdomen. It will strengthen your core and stabilize your lower back and sacroiliac joints as you work, protecting them from injury.

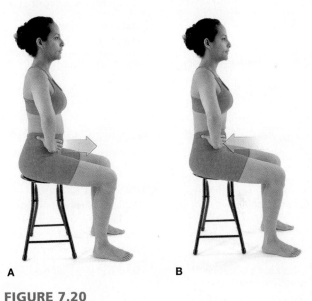

A   B

FIGURE 7.20

Each postural stabilizer provides a specific type of postural support. For example, the transversus abdominis supports the lower abdominal wall, and when it is not contracting, the abdomen distends. You can learn to tell which muscle needs training by the different types of postural patterns that occur when that postural stabilizer fails to fire (Table 7.1 ■). Specific postural functions of the various postural muscles are revisited throughout the chapters in Part 2.

7.3 FAULTY POSTURES

Faulty postural patterns usually fall along a continuum between two extremes: a collapsed, sagging posture or a lifted, military posture. In a collapsed posture, the body lacks support. The spine is sunken and compressed in exaggerated spinal curvatures (see Figure 7.22). In military posture, the upper body is lifted up and back, arching the spine into hyperextension (Figure 7.21 ■). This posture unnaturally raises the thorax, causing the spinal muscles to work overtime to keep the upper body lifted and prevent it from tipping over backward.

Faulty postures increase mechanical stress on the joints, which in turn reduces the overall efficiency of posture and movement. Whenever part of the body displaces out of the line of gravity in one direction, some other part of the body

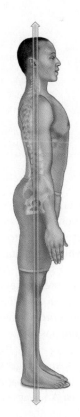

FIGURE 7.21
Military posture

TABLE 7.1 Stabilizer Muscles and Their Actions

Muscle	Postural Stabilizing Function	Action	Hallmarks: How to Tell This Muscle Is Contracting
1. Tibialis posterior	Lifts medial arch and stabilizes ankle	Ankle plantarflexion and inversion	Medial arch remains lifted and stable; when standing on toes, ankle remains centered, does not wobble
2. Soleus	Stabilizes body during forward lean of postural sway	Ankle plantarflexion	Calf muscles contract and bulge above Achilles tendon
3. Vastus medialis oblique	Stabilizes patella	Knee extension with adduction	Bulges on medial side of knee
4. Perineum	Supports pelvic viscera	Elimination and reproduction	Draws the base of pelvis into center, narrows ischial tuberosities
5. Transversus abdominis	Compresses abdominal viscera, stabilizes lumbar spine and sacroiliac joints	Increases intra-abdominal pressure (IAP)	Draws the lower abdominal wall straight back, draws ASIS together and slightly narrows the lower waist
6. Psoas major	Posterior fibers stabilize anterior lumbar spine, seats head of the femur into hip socket (*acetabulum*)	Anterior fibers extend the lumbar spine and assist hip flexion	Bulge of distal tendon in inguinal region, anterior lumbar spine stiffens from increased axial compression
7. Lumbar multifidus	Stabilizes posterior lumbar spine	Assists lumbar extension and rotation	Fills the lamina groove, posterior lumbar spine stiffens from increased axial compression
8. Lower and middle trapezius	Maintains neutral position of scapulae against ribs	Retracts and depresses scapulae	Upper trapezius and neck elongate; scapulae lie flat against ribs along vertical axis
9. Serratus anterior	Works with trapezius to maintain neutral position of scapula	Protracts and upwardly rotates scapula	Lower third tethers inferior angle of scapula to side of middle rib cage
10. Longus coli	Stabilizes anterior cervical spine	Flexes cervical spine	Lengthens and flattens cervical lordosis
11. Cervical multifidus and suboccipitals	Limits excessive cervical flexion and excessive rotation	Assists cervical extension	Stiffens cervical lordosis in maximal length

tips in the opposite direction to restore balance. As a result, nonpostural muscles contract to shore up the off-center alignment, causing these muscles to overwork and become adaptively shortened while their antagonists become stretch weakened.

When assessing postures, a key area to look at is the alignment of the spine. An abnormal degree of curve in the spine is called a *curvature*. Three main types of spinal curvatures occur in faulty postures:

- **Excessive lordosis:** An exaggerated anterior spinal curvature, usually in the lumbar and cervical spine.
- **Excessive kyphosis:** An exaggerated posterior spinal curvature, usually in the thoracic spine.
- **Scoliosis:** A lateral spinal curvature, which can occur anywhere in the spine.

The use of the terms "lordosis" and "kyphosis" can lead to confusion because some kinesiologists use them to refer to normal spinal curves whereas others use these terms to refer to abnormal curvatures. To clarify the meaning, we have qualified these terms with the adjective *excessive*.

Ideally, the pelvis is level. One key marker of faulty posture is the direction in which the pelvis is chronically tilted. Imagine the pelvis as a bony basin or bowl filled with water. When it tilts off of a level position, water will spill out the back or the front. In an **anterior pelvic tilt** (APT), the top of the pelvis tips forward. This pattern often occurs when a person has an excessive lordosis of the lumbar spine. In a **posterior pelvic tilt** (PPT), the top of the pelvis tips backward. This pattern often occurs when a person tucks the pelvis. Both patterns involve muscular imbalances in the hip and pelvic muscles.

Excessive spinal curvatures and postural faults in one part of the body inevitably create secondary compensations in other parts of the body. A challenge in working to restore balance to myofascial tissues under stress from faulty postures is to work with whole-body patterns, addressing both primary and secondary areas of stress. For example, compensations to counterbalance the anterior pelvic tilt can occur in the limbs and the spine. A person might lock the knees and grip the toes, or develop an excessive kyphosis in the thorax and a forward head posture. You can stretch the chronically shortened muscles in the lower back to correct the pelvic tilt, but compensatory patterns in the legs and upper spine will also need to be addressed to balance the entire structure.

7.3.1   Lordotic and Kyphotic Postures

The **kyphotic-lordotic posture** is marked by an anterior pelvic tilt and spinal curvatures, with an excessive lordosis in the lower back and neck and an excessive kyphosis in the upper back (Figure 7.22 ■). People with this posture usually show muscular weakness in deep lumbar extensors (especially the multifidus), hamstrings, and the abdominal muscles. The anterior tilt places the hip joints into chronic flexion, causing muscles acting as hip flexors to become short and tight. Excessive spinal curvatures place a downward drag on the entire structure, causing stretch weaknesses in muscles that labor under excessive eccentric loading. A person could develop *spondylolisthesis* as the fifth lumbar vertebrae displaces anteriorly and slides away from the sacrum. The kyphotic-lordotic posture bends the spine at the apex of each curve so it is also called the "zig-zag posture."

The **sway-back posture** is a postural deviation in which a person tends to lean back, which posteriorly displaces the thorax and sways the spine (Figure 7.23 ■). The backward lean tends to tuck the pelvis into a posterior pelvic tilt, which flattens the lumbar curve and causes the hamstrings to become short and tight. In compensation for the posterior displacement of the thorax, the head displaces anteriorly and the upper thoracic spine flexes, often resulting in a dowager's hump. In addition, the gluteus maximus is weak, creating a flattening of the buttocks.

The **flat-back posture** is marked by a posterior pelvic tilt, which tucks the pelvis, flattening the lumbar spine (Figure 7.24a ■). The hip extensors, particularly the hamstrings, pull the pelvis into a posterior tilt, causing them to become chronically tight and short and the hip flexors to become stretch weakened. The cervical spine develops an excessive lordosis to compensate for flattening in the thoracic and lumbar areas, also leading to a dowager's hump. A variation is a flat-back posture where the lumbar and cervical segments of the spine become flattened and the thoracic curve reverses and becomes lordotic, causing the scapulae to wing (Figure 7.24b ■). This unusual posture is marked by excessive muscular effort to maintain the upright position of the spine, which can cause rigidity.

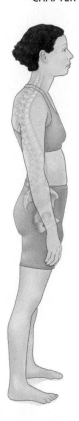

FIGURE 7.22
Kyphotic-lordotic posture

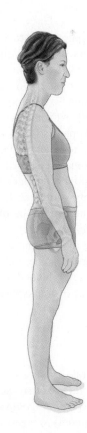

FIGURE 7.23
Sway-back posture

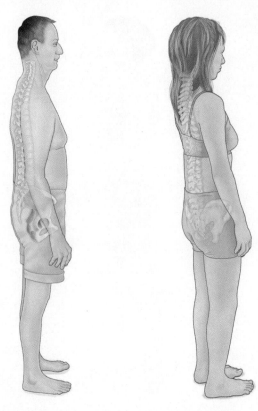

FIGURE 7.24

a) **Flat-back posture** b) **Variation of flat-back posture**

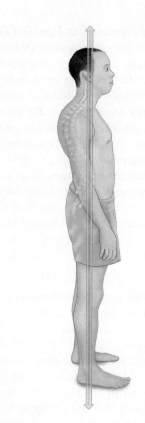

FIGURE 7.25

Round-back kyphotic posture

A **round-back** (kyphotic) **posture** is marked by excessive flexion in the thoracic spine, which creates a hunchback (Figure 7.25 ■). There are two types of round-back postures. In a functional pattern, a person with a normal structure develops a round-back from a collapsed, chronically flexed posture. When the thoracic spine is chronically flexed, the excessive kyphosis forces a person to hyperextend the neck in order to level the head. As a result, the thoracic extensors become stretch weakened while the neck extensors become adaptively shortened. The chest muscles also become adaptively shortened from the rounding of the shoulders. In a congenital type of round-back called *Scheuermann's disease*, the thoracic vertebrae grow into a wedge shape, creating a sharp curve and pointed bend in the middle of the thoracic spine. Scheuermann's disease usually develops during childhood and teen years and is more difficult to correct than a kyphosis caused by faulty postural habits.

7.3.2 Scoliosis

In a scoliosis, the lateral deviation of the spine creates an S-shape curvature (Figure 7.26 ■). Scoliosis can be congenital or acquired. *Congenital scoliosis* involves structural deformities, most commonly wedge-shaped vertebral bodies and a malformed rib cage. When the rib cage becomes malformed, one side is usually much larger than the other

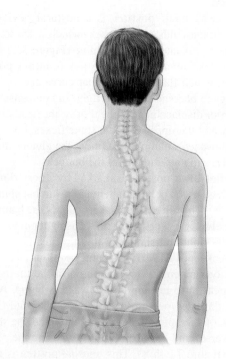

FIGURE 7.26

Scoliosis

side. Depending on the degree of deformity, surgical interventions to straighten the spine may be necessary to remove the compressive stress that severe congenital scoliosis places on the heart and lungs. *Acquired scoliosis* is generally nonstructural and develops from asymmetrical muscle-use patterns, such as work-related habits. For example, a delivery worker who repeatedly moves in and out of a truck from the same side will develop muscle asymmetries in the arms, shoulders, and spine. Also, people with hearing or vision problems on one side tend to habitually turn their heads to point the strong ear or eye toward what they hear or see.

Torticollis is a scoliosis in the cervical spine from damage to the sternocleidomastoid (SCM) muscle in the neck (Figure 7.27 ■). In this postural deviation, also called "wry-neck," the head tilts to the side of the affected SCM.

7.3.3 Alignment Problems in the Lower Limb

A number of postural problems can develop in the spine as compensations to misalignments in the joints of the lower limbs. Some lower limb misalignments are caused by faulty habits, such as locked knees. Others are caused by structural deviations, such as a club foot or a short leg.

Skeletal misalignments in the lower limb affect the alignment of the hips and spine, and postural problems in the trunk can affect lower limb alignment. To feel this, stand up and lock your knees and notice how your pelvis moves into an anterior tilt, or collapse your spine and notice how your weight shifts on your feet.

Common postural problems in the feet include *pes cavus* or *hypersupination,* which lifts the medial arches too high and restricts motion in the ankles, and *pes planus* or *hyperpronation,* which flattens the medial arches of the feet (Figure 7.28a-b ■). Common problems in the knees include

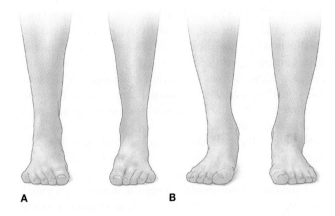

FIGURE 7.28

a) **Supinate feet** b) **Pronated feet**

genu varum, a bow-legged alignment, and *genu valgum,* a knock-kneed alignment (Figure 7.29a-b ■). Unless a person actually has structural deviations, misalignments in the lower limbs can be corrected by learning to move the joints and work the muscles with better alignment. This discussion is expanded in the chapters on the feet and knees.

7.4 POSTURAL ASSESSMENTS

Many massage and bodywork clients want help with their posture, and they expect practitioners to be knowledgeable about skeletal alignment. They often seek our help in alleviating pain and discomfort from chronic muscular contractures that compress their joints and lead to postural

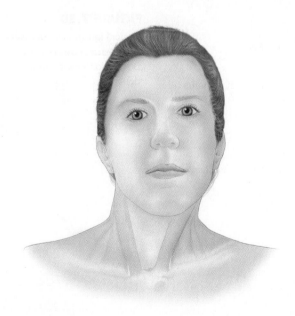

FIGURE 7.27

Torticollis

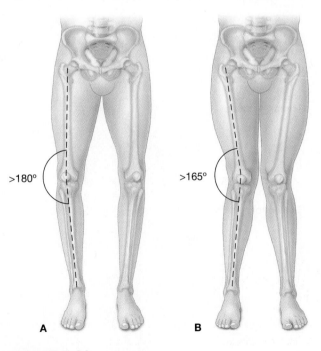

FIGURE 7.29

a) **Genu varum** b) **Genu valgum**

problems. To provide such clients with general guidance in improving posture requires skills in postural assessment.

In massage and bodywork classes, postural assessments are often practiced by having a student in shorts and tank top stand in front in a grid, then comparing bilateral bony markings against horizontal and vertical lines for asymmetries. It could be stressful for a client to be overly scrutinized in this way, so postural assessments with clients are usually more discreet and general. Avoid putting clients on the spot because it could add to any discomfort they already feel. In addition, visual assessments are general and not always accurate. They do, however, provide a great vehicle for studying posture. Palpatory assessments of bilateral bone markings can also be made on a person in a recumbent posture.

A casual assessment of a client's posture can begin the minute the client walks in the door. In a single glance, it is easy to see the overall postural pattern. This is what happens when people recognize friends from a distance by the shape of their posture and movement. First impressions can provide useful information about postural patterns because the eye is drawn to distortions in the overall shape of the body, such as an abnormal curve or asymmetry.

While making postural assessments, take into account individual variations because every person has his or her own pattern of optimal skeletal alignment. Some people will have more prominent spinal curves than others; some people will have larger bone structures; others will have more elastic soft tissues. Also, our clients' perceptions of their own postural patterns are important to consider, particularly when they ask for tools to improve their alignment. With this last point in mind, guidelines for practicing a client-centered postural assessment is covered in this section.

7.4.1 Structural Assessments of Skeletal Alignment

A helpful study of posture can be made by observing the body in a standing position from all four sides. However, as mentioned earlier, taking the time to assess a client's posture in a standing position can make the client feel discomfort from being overly scrutinized. It can also focus clients' attentions on all the things that are wrong with them. Some quick photos of a fully clothed client in a standing position will provide objective feedback that you and the client can observe together. In addition, a transparent grid can be laid over the photos to help see the symmetry or imbalances in the client's body.

It is important to assess alignment from several different views because each position of the body provides a different level of information about skeletal alignment.

- *Observe posture from the front and the back of the body:* Observing your client's body in a standing posture from the front or back provides information about the structural symmetries or asymmetries between the two sides of the body. Bony markings on each side can be compared to see if they are level, such as the crest of the hips, the top of the shoulders, and the elbows or kneecaps (Figure 7.30a-b ■). When one side is higher than another, it is important to look at what is going on in the proximal joints—the hips or shoulders—and in the spine. A shoulder or hip might be hiked or rotated, or the spine might be side-bent in lateral flexion or rotated. When body weight is centered over one leg, this can indicate leg dominance on that side.
- *Observe posture from the sides of the body:* Observing your client's body in a standing posture from the

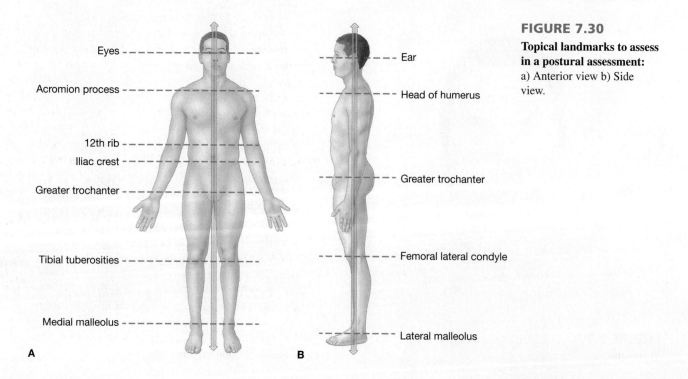

Eyes

Acromion process

12th rib

Iliac crest

Greater trochanter

Tibial tuberosities

Medial malleolus

Ear

Head of humerus

Greater trochanter

Femoral lateral condyle

Lateral malleolus

A

B

FIGURE 7.30

Topical landmarks to assess in a postural assessment: a) Anterior view b) Side view.

sides provides information about functional patterns, showing artifacts of where people hold the body behind midline or ahead of midline as they move (Figure 7.31a-b ■). Midline from the side is the plumb line. Visualize three dots, one in the center of each body mass depicting the center of gravity in each mass, as three floating balloons with a string connecting the dots.

In addition, a person might look aligned from a side view, but if there are spinal rotations, one side could look completely different from the other side. Comparing photos of the two sides of the body placed next to each other will make postural asymmetries and rotations between sides more apparent. Breaks in the verticality of the body from the side view reveals areas where postural muscles fail to provide core support.

- *Observe posture with the body in a supine position:* Observing your client's posture in a recumbent, supine position provides information about joint alignment, muscle resting length, and the client's ability to relax. The components of skeletal alignment in an upright posture apply to the recumbent posture. When assessing a recumbent posture, each vertebra as well as the head, pelvis, and limbs should sink into the table along its own vertical axis (Figure 7.32 ■). The

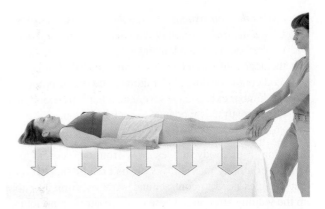

FIGURE 7.32

Horizontal grounding of the body in a recumbent position

feet and legs should line up under the hips, although in a supine position, the weight of the feet will externally rotate the hips supine. The chest should be wide and the shoulders should lie relatively flat. Clients with tight chest muscles will still have rounded shoulders. The spinal curves should be maximally lengthened so that the head, thorax, and pelvis lie relatively level rather than tilted.

- *Compare posture with the body in standing and seated positions:* Observing your client's spine with your client standing, then observing it again with your client seated and comparing the two, provides another level of information. The contrast shows whether spinal misalignments and muscle tensions are caused by lower limb imbalances or by spinal imbalances. For example, if there is torque in the spine while a client is standing but it disappears while the client is sitting, it is highly likely that the torque is coming from joint or muscle imbalance in the lower limbs that transfers into the spine in a standing position.

7.4.1.1 ASSESSING SKELETAL ALIGNMENT AND MUSCULAR FUNCTION

To assess skeletal alignment, look at the joints in relation to joint neutral. Recall from the chapter on joints that joint neutral is an extended position of the joint, one in which a joint is not flexed, hyperextended, or rotated. When looking at the joint alignment, consider where each joint is positioned in relation to a neutral-joint alignment. If the joint deviates from a neutral alignment, there are several components to assess about the joint position.

- *Assess the direction that the joints deviate from a neutral position.* Observe the client's posture and determine which direction the joints deviate from neutral. You might observe, for example: "The client stands with her thoracic spine rounded in flexion, her lumbar spine hyperextended, and her hips flexed and laterally rotated."

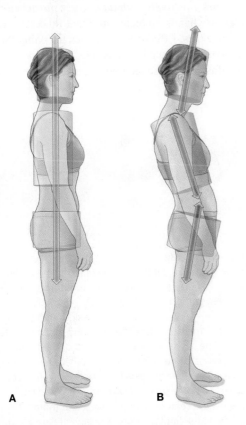

FIGURE 7.31

Alignment of three body masses: a) In an optimal posture, the body masses align along the line of gravity. b) In a faulty posture, the body masses tip into a zig-zag pattern.

- *Assess the approximate degree that the joint deviates from a neutral position on a scale of minimal, moderate, or severe.* When looking at the same client, assess the degree of variance from a joint-neutral position. You could conclude: "Her thoracic flexion is moderate, her lumbar extension is severe, and her hip flexion and lateral rotation is moderate in each direction."

As mentioned earlier, faulty postures involve the deviation of the body masses away from the vertical axis. Whenever a body mass moves off its base of support, certain muscles need to contract and work overtime to shore up the leaning structure. These compensatory contractures work as instinctive righting responses; they prevent the bent body from straying even farther from vertical or buckling. As a result, certain muscles develop dysfunctional patterns that cause them to become adaptively shortened on one side of the body and stretch weakened on the other side. Dysfunctional tight or taut muscles associated with faulty postures usually develop myofascial pain syndromes (trigger points, achiness, and referred pain) and lead to faulty movement patterns. In addition, chronic pain tends to inhibit postural muscles, which makes the overall pattern even worse.

There are three types of muscular dysfunctions to assess a faulty postural pattern when posture deviates from an optimal alignment:

- *Assess which muscles are adaptively shortened:* The areas where the joints are in chronic flexion usually point to places where the muscles are adaptively shortened. When referring to the same hypothetical client used in the joint assessment, you might conclude: "The client's lumbar extensors, hip flexors, and lateral hip rotators look adaptively shortened."
- *Assess which muscles are stretch weakened:* On the opposite side of the body where the muscles are adaptively shortened, muscles are usually stretch weakened. You might notice: "The client's thoracic erector spinae muscles and midscapular muscles look stretch weakened."
- *Assess which postural muscles are inhibited:* Postural muscles that are inhibited will fail to contract and provide adequate support for the skeletal system. A practitioner needs to know which muscles work as postural muscles and how to tell they are not working correctly. Hallmarks for assessing postural muscle function are outlined in Table 7.1. You might see that there is poor tone in muscles located in the lamina groove and that the medial borders of the scapulae wing (stick up) and conclude: "The client's lumbar multifidus and lower trapezius appear to be inhibited."

After making these assessments, you can develop a treatment plan that restores muscles to their normal resting length, which restore the neutral position of the joints. Here are examples of how to work with each type of muscle dysfunction:

To work effectively with adaptively shortened muscles, use hands-on techniques that relax and stretch the muscles. Effective techniques for doing this include basic Swedish massage, trigger point therapy, myofascial release techniques, and muscle energy techniques.

GUIDELINES
Checklist for Assessing Posture

Here are some guidelines for assessing a healthy standing posture. They are based on the ideal neutral position of the joints of the body in extension.

1. The feet are directly under the pelvis and hips.
2. The knees and hips (except the ankles) are extended.
3. The legs are parallel.
4. The kneecaps face forward.
5. Weight is centered on each foot in the tripod between the heel, first toe, and fifth toe.
6. The toes are extended and facing forward.
7. The shoulders are level.
8. The chest is wide both in the front and back.
9. The sternum is lifted. The clavicles are horizontal.
10. The entire rib cage moves with respiration.
11. The scapulae lie flat against the ribs. The medial borders of the scapulae are parallel to the spine. The scapulae are relatively vertical rather than tilted.
12. The arms hang vertically along the sides of the body. The palms of the hands face the body and the thumbs face forward. The hands rest slightly in front of the trunk.
13. The cervical spine and lumbar spine have normal lordotic curves. The thoracic spine has a normal kyphotic curve. The curves do not seem overly kyphotic or flattened.
14. The head is centered over the neck and thorax. The upper palate and occiput are level. The jaw is relaxed.

BRIDGE TO PRACTICE
Observing Postural Patterns

Hone your observation skills of postural patterns in public areas where there are lots of people. Go to a mall or park and sit in a discrete spot where you can observe and study people and their postures. Pick one or two aspects of posture to watch each time you go out. One day you can look at head and shoulder patterns, the next day you can look at abdominal and lower back patterns.

Keep in mind that most people who feel like they are being watched become uncomfortable and disagreeable, so be discreet and polite. Observe certain rules, such as no pointing, staring, or making loud and inappropriate comments. Also, wear sunglasses to avoid making people uncomfortable.

To work effectively with stretch-weakened muscles, be careful not to lengthen already overstretched tissues. Stretch-weakened muscles often develop trigger points and taut bands, so a practitioner could use trigger point pressure followed by cross-fiber techniques to break up taut bands. Then you could use muscle approximation to reset the resting length of a muscle and resisted movement to facilitate contractions that increase muscle tone. All of these techniques will also improve the client's awareness of optimal resting length.

To work effectively with inhibited postural muscles, facilitate postural muscle contraction by directing the client to do light isometrics and subtle intrinsic movements. For example, cue a prone client to lift the face slightly above the face cradle in order to contract the lumbar multifidus, or lift the corner of the shoulder in order to contract the lower trapezius muscles. Because this neuromuscular patterning approach is not widely used, integrating postural muscle activation into hands-on work may require training that is beyond the scope of this text.

7.4.1.2 DETERMINING THE SOURCE OF FAULTY POSTURES

When assessing a body problem related to faulty posture, it is important to take a client history to determine whether a postural pattern developed from an injury or illness or developed as a result of habitual patterns. Postural problems often develop from muscular guarding around an injury such as a sprained joint or a broken bone. A person can also develop postural problems from work-related habits. People with desk jobs where they have to sit all day can develop chronic back pain. People typically develop lower back pain from slouching, and neck and shoulder pain from using a forward head posture while working at a computer or holding a phone against the ear by hiking a shoulder.

Postural deviations can also arise from bony deformities, such as a *hemi-pelvis* (a condition in which one pelvic bone is considerably smaller than the other) or a leg-length discrepancy (a condition in which a long bone of the leg is shorter on one side). If you suspect such a condition, you could suggest that the client be evaluated by an orthopedic specialist. Postural deviations can also be caused by genetic anomalies, such as a Scheumann's kyphosis or *Poland's anomaly* (the absence of the pectoralis major on one side).

BRIDGE TO PRACTICE
Providing Feedback about General Postural Patterns

Glance at a person's posture as if you are taking a snapshot image to gauge the overall pattern that jumps into view. You might see the emotional tone of the pattern first. For example, a person might look anxious or tentative, as if she is afraid of falling.

After you see the general tone, switch your focus back to the anatomy and describe what you see in anatomical terms: "The lumbar spine is in flexion, the shoulders are externally rotated, and the elbows are held up and back." You can also describe the muscular tone of the pattern: "She seems to have high tone along her abdominal flexors, although they look undeveloped and weak."

You can provide clients with such conditions with a massage and bodywork maintenance program to help alleviate pain from muscular imbalances that develop around malformed bones.

7.4.2 Client-Centered Postural Assessments

Massage and bodywork practitioners can tell clients what patterns they observe, but cultivating the clients' ability to see and feel their own patterns is even more important. While the practitioner will have one assessment of a client's posture, the client may perceive his or her posture in a completely different way. Client-centered postural assessments are great for clients who want help in helping themselves.

When making a client-centered postural assessment, you will want to help clients gain a kinesthetic awareness and mechanical understanding of their postural patterns. Help clients do this by pointing out the connection between their physical complaint and their faulty postural pattern. For example, when the client complains of neck pain, noticing a hiked shoulder or a chronically hyperextended neck is clinically relevant because these postural patterns could be causing or exacerbating the pain.

7.5 THERAPEUTIC APPLICATIONS FOR POSTURAL EDUCATION

Ergonomic approaches to postural education focus on adjusting chair and table height to better support ideal skeletal alignment and verticality. Ultimately, though, changing posture is an inside job because it requires that people actually change how they use their bodies. This can only be

achieved through commitment, body awareness, and daily practice. Changing posture involves a series of steps:

- Developing a kinesthetic awareness of the body
- Shifting skeletal alignment into joint neutral
- Training the postural muscles to support joint neutral
- Relaxing and stretching overworked muscles
- Integrating postural awareness into activities of daily living

7.5.1 Body Mechanics

Effective body mechanics are built on good posture. Sitting or standing for long periods will be easier with a well-aligned spine. Lifting, pushing, or pulling with the spine aligned in joint neutral and the postural muscles contracted will help stabilize the spine and establish a direct line of force from the hands to the feet.

To develop more efficient body mechanics, joint positioning in an optimal posture is crucial for mechanical stresses to pass through the center of the joints. At the same time, the postural muscles need to be actively contracted and working to maintain the optimal joint position. Keep in mind that every activity we do trains the muscular system, either for better or worse. If you are slouching as you read this text, you are training your postural muscles for slouching.

Because the postural muscles work independently of motion, they can be trained anywhere, anytime, with subtle isometric contractions done in place. Developing optimal postural support requires commitment and discipline. It can be a struggle to simply remember to pay attention to engaging your postural support system. Some people put red dots on their mirrors, walls, and tables so that every time they see the dot, they are reminded to realign the spine and

GUIDELINES
Client Communication around Postural Problems

It is out of the scope of massage and bodywork practice to diagnose where a client's pain is coming from, although if clients don't recognize that the chronic pains they complain of could be related to a postural problem, you could suggest this possibility. This is especially helpful for clients who want to learn about their body patterns to improve their conditions.

For example, if you notice that a client's right hip looks stiff as he walks in, you can continue a discreet observation of his postural pattern during the intake process. As the client sits, you might notice that he leans back and to the right, hikes his right hip, and laterally flexes his spine to the left. If this client reports that he has pain in his lower back and right hip and neck, and hopes your session can give him relief, you may want to look at

the relationship between his pain pattern, treatment goals, and postural pattern in your treatment plan.

At this point, there are a series of questions you can ask this client that will connect the posture to the pain pattern and help you both decide how to proceed in the session:

1. "Did you have an injury or do you know why your hip hurts?"
2. "Do you think your posture has anything to do with your hip pain?"
3. "Do you feel pain in your hip as you sit leaning back like that?"
4. "Is there any position or activity that relieves your hip pain?"

contract the postural muscles. We suggest working on posture whenever you find yourself sitting or standing, while driving, watching television, or even while standing in line at the bank or grocery store. These stationary activities provide great opportunities to straighten the spine and draw the lower abdomen in, widen the shoulders, and lengthen the neck.

It is also helpful to place full-length mirrors in strategic locations in your treatment room to occasionally look over to check your own alignment. This will be particularly helpful during static force applications, such as when practicing deep tissue work, when optimal posture is crucial to avoid joint and back injuries.

7.5.2 Integrating Postural Education into Bodywork Sessions

The more adept you become at maintaining good posture and engaging your own postural muscles, the more client education tools you can develop.[9] Training postural muscles begins with isometric exercises, which are easy exercises to teach clients as they receive hands-on work. Some forms of bodywork actually integrate postural education with bodywork, such as structural integration and neuromuscular patterning.[10] Ironically, the chronically shortened muscles that learn how to release and stretch with massage and bodywork are often the very muscles that provide the client with support. As a result, deep tissue work can

---

SELF-CARE
Training the Postural Stabilizers

Contract each postural muscle slowly with minimal effort, using only one-third your maximum effort. If you tend to overwork, begin by visualizing each step, which will be enough to begin waking up postural muscle support.

1. **Transversus abdominis:** Slowly draw your lower abdominal muscles right above your pubic bone straight back toward your sacrum.
2. **Lumbar multifidus:** If you tend to have a lumbar sway back, pull your lumbar spine straight back (Figure 7.33a-b ■).
3. **Lower trapezius:** Lift your sternum and widen your chest, then imagine sandbags on the bottoms of your scapulae,

lightly drawing them down with your lower trapezius muscles. Make sure to stay wide between your shoulder blades, so that your shoulder girdle does not migrate behind your body.
4. **Cervical intrinsics:** Lift the back of your head without lowering your chin, which should lengthen your neck and activate the postural muscles in your neck.

Since clients seek massage for relief from back pain associated with poor posture, you can teach your clients these simple isometrics to engage postural muscles while they are on your table.

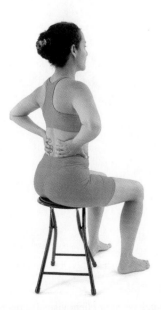

FIGURE 7.33a

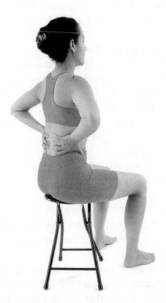

FIGURE 7.33b

actually release a client's postural support system, making the need for postural muscle education in a massage and bodywork session even more crucial. The combination of bodywork with postural education can provide you with powerful tools for helping clients improve their posture.[11]

Integrating neuromuscular patterning into a bodywork session involves coaching the client to contract specific postural muscles while releasing and stretching tight muscles. For example, when a client's lower back muscles become chronically shortened due to an anterior pelvic tilt and weak abdominal muscles, while stretching this area, suggest that the client lightly contract the lower abdomen muscles. The stretch will be more effective because the client is contracting the antagonist muscles. In addition, the client engages a new and more effective neuromuscular pathway, learning to engage the abdominal muscles while lengthening the lower back.

7.5.3 Challenges with Postural Corrections

Sometimes what we do to improve our posture actually makes it worse. This happens when people respond to commands such as "sit up straight" with quick, strong

---

GUIDELINES
Helping Clients Develop Postural Awareness

If your clients want help improving their postures, the first step is to help them develop a greater postural awareness. Here are several guidelines for helping your clients begin to build an awareness of posture through cognitive, visual, and kinesthetic channels:

1. **Explain the basic premises of healthy posture.** Show your client how the head needs to align over the thorax, which needs to align over the pelvis and over the feet (Figure 7.34 ■).
2. **Ask clients to describe their own posture.** This provides information on their level of self-awareness and focus. It also reveals a client's self-image, which, if overly negative, can perpetuate and increase a chronic pain pattern. Guide your client to see the overall pattern, including healthy aspects of his or her posture.
3. **Use photographs to educate your clients.** Take some pictures of your client standing from the front, back, and side, then sit and study them together.
4. **Help clients to assess the tone of their spine.** With your client seated, run your hand down the spinal muscles so that the client can feel the muscular tone. Then ask if the client feels a continuity of muscular tone or differences of tone in different areas.
5. **Use a mirror to help clients assess their own posture.** Have your client stand beside a full-length mirror, look at his or her alignment from the side, and tell you what he or she sees. Then give your client a standing compression test by gently and quickly pushing down on both shoulders, then releasing (see Figure 2.23b of the standing compression test). Explain how the client will feel the compression travel through the body into the feet if he or she is vertically aligned, or will feel the body bend in places where it is not vertically aligned.
6. **At the end of your session, have your clients compare their before and after posture.** Have them move back into the posture they had at the start of the session, then shift into the new posture so that they learn to make a

transition between the old pattern and the new pattern. If there have been postural changes from the session, helping your clients feel these changes will motivate them to continue to improve their posture.

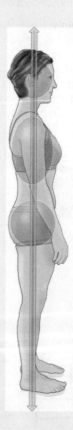

FIGURE 7.34

For healthy posture, have your client visualize the head, thorax, and pelvis stacking over each other along the vertical axis.

SELF-CARE
Centering Your Body over Your Feet

Here are some simple exercises to help you center your body over your feet while engaging the postural muscles you learned about in this chapter.

1. **Getting ready:** Begin in a standing position. Make the adjustments you need to shift your body into an optimal posture, contracting your lower abdomen, tipping your pelvis to a level position, and lengthening your spine.
2. **Exploring foot position:** Once you feel centered in your best posture, close your eyes. Take a few steps in place, landing your feet right under your body. Then open your eyes and look down to see if your feet landed under you.

3. **Improving balance:** Stand on one leg, then bend and straighten the supporting knee (see Figure 12.32a). As you straighten your knees, be careful not to lock it (see Figure 12.32b). Sense when your leg feels straight and your body feels centered over that leg. Repeat on the other side.
4. **Rolling the spine:** From a standing position, slowly flex your neck and roll down your spine, head first, one vertebra at a time into forward bending (see Figures 14.29a-14.29d). Then reverse the motion and roll up, tail (coccyx) first, stacking each vertebra one by one.

contractions in the mobilizer muscles. When a slouching person is admonished to sit up straight, that person usually jerks the spine into a hyperextended position using the mobilizer muscles, which are not suited for sustained contraction. When these muscles tire and begin to ache, the person usually sinks into a slump again.

Many people try to correct postural deviations by overcorrecting in the opposite direction. Many postural corrections create compensatory holding patterns that cause another layer of musculoskeletal imbalances. In other words, what many people do to improve the posture actually makes it worse. For example, a person with rounded shoulders will pull the shoulders back and pinch the scapulae together, thrusting the spine forward. This creates even more muscular tension in the spine without actually improving the position of the shoulder joints. Another common postural problem occurs when people correct a sway in the lower back by tucking the pelvis, which creates muscular holding that restricts the free swinging of the hip joints while walking.

How individuals perceive their posture is probably one of the most important aspects of working with alignment patterns. All parts of the body are connected, and changes to the alignment of one part will invariably shift a person's perception of the entire structure. In addition, posture often reflects emotions and psychological aspects of a person. If you want to integrate postural education into your massage and bodywork practice, you can develop a strong foundation for working effectively with postural patterns by beginning with a study of your own posture. Approaching posture through self-study can also provide you with many tools for self-care. It can enhance your body mechanics,

improve your quality of touch, and support the efficiency of motion in your entire body.

CONCLUSION

An adept practitioner can peek into any office and make a general assessment of individual postures by comparing the joint alignment of each person to joint neutral. The most common seated patterns will probably be the flexed postures and the hyperextended postures. Common standing patterns will probably include locked knees, swayed lower backs or lordosis, and hunched upper backs or kyphosis. There may even be people shifting around in an attempt to find a more comfortable posture.

All of these individuals can shift their sitting or standing positions and contract the right muscles to move the body toward more optimal posture. For example, the flexed person could straighten the spine, lengthen the neck, and contract the lower abdominal muscles. The hyperextended person could lower the bottom ribs, rock the pelvis to a level position, and draw the lumbar spine back to move into a more balanced alignment. The person with locked knees could unlock the knees and practice standing on one leg, which will strengthen the balance over an extended knee. And the person with the hunched upper back could lift the sternum to straighten the thorax, which would also lift the compression off the heart, lungs, and abdominal organs.

All of us can improve our overall physical state of being by paying attention to our posture, which will not only improve the balance of our joints and muscles but will help us to look and feel better as well.

SUMMARY POINTS TO REMEMBER

1. Posture is the relative alignment of the body as well as the taking on of an attitude or stance. In optimal posture, the body masses align along the line of gravity, and specific bony landmarks (i.e., ear, shoulder, hip, knee, and ankle) align vertically.

2. Dynamic postural reflexes such as postural sway and righting reflexes continually rebalance the body and the head around the vertical axis to maintain upright posture.

3. Each major area of the skeleton has specific architectural features that reflect the mechanical functions of joints in that area. The spine is a curved column, the pelvis is a braced arch, the shoulder girdle is a bony yoke, and the head is a top load.

4. Optimal posture requires the balanced functions of the skeletal, muscular, and nervous systems. When assessing postural dysfunction, first determine which body systems are affected by the problem and then determine how the other systems compensate.

5. Postural muscles also work as joint stabilizers by contracting isometrically, pulling the joint surfaces closer to prevent excessive joint play during motion.

6. Stability dysfunctions occur when the postural muscles fail, resulting in joint movement beyond a normal range. Excessive motion can damage joint structures and trigger compensatory muscular contractions called substitution patterns, reducing the overall efficiency of movement and causing more dysfunction, pain, and injury.

7. Primary postural stabilizers fire independently of motion; secondary stabilizers fire during movement to control the speed and range of motion. Primary stabilizers are often called core muscles because they are usually deep or intrinsic muscles.

8. Mobilizer muscles function poorly as postural muscles because they have a predominance of fast fibers that fatigue quickly and ache when isometrically contracted. They also tend to span long distances and are multiarticular, causing them to bend weight-supporting joints when working isometrically. Chronic bending displaces parts of the body away from the vertical axis, which in turn triggers compensatory muscular holding to shore up off-center parts.

9. The spinal curves can deviate from optimal alignment in three directions: an exaggerated lordosis or anterior lumbar curve, an exaggerated kyphosis or posterior spinal curve, and a scoliosis or lateral s-shaped curve.

10. Five faulty postural patterns include a military posture that hyperextends the spine, a kyphotic-lordotic posture that collapses and exaggerates the spinal curves, a sway-back posture in which the thorax leans posteriorly, a flat-back posture that flattens the spine and posteriorly tilts the pelvis, and a round-back posture that increases the thoracic kyphosis.

11. Two common alignment problems in the knees are genu valgum, a knock-kneed alignment, and genu varum, a bow-legged alignment. Both misalignments lead to compensatory postural problems in the feet, pelvis, and spine.

12. A postural assessment involves the evaluation of the symmetry and balance of bilateral bony landmarks relative to horizontal and vertical lines in a standing or sitting body. Joint balance is assessed by identifying the position of a resting joint relative to a neutral alignment. Muscular balance is assessed by identifying which postural muscles are failing to provide core support, which muscles are adaptively shortened, and which muscles are stretch weakened.

13. To change a faulty posture, a person needs to develop body awareness of the faulty pattern, shift skeletal alignment to a joint-neutral position, train postural muscles, relax and stretch overworking muscles, and integrate postural awareness into daily activities.

14. Optimal posture underlies effective body mechanics. Postural education can prevent chronic back pain and can also prevent injury from faulty positioning while lifting, pushing, and pulling.

REVIEW QUESTIONS

1. True or false (circle one). Posture is the relative alignment of the body in only the standing position.
2. Postural sway is a dynamic postural reflex that causes the body to subtly sway
   a. in a standing posture, is caused by phasic stretch reflexes in postural muscles, and assists the venous return of blood from the legs to the heart.
   b. in a seated posture, is caused by active volition in prime movers, and it assists the venous return of blood from the legs to the heart.
   c. in all positions, is caused by tonic stretch reflex in joint proprioceptors, and assists the venous return of blood from the legs to the heart.
   d. in an upright posture, is caused by tonic stretch reflexes in postural muscles, and assists the venous return of blood from the legs to the heart.
3. Head righting is a dynamic postural reflex that
   a. is mediated by the Golgi tendon organs.
   b. orients the body in off-centered position.
   c. triggers contralateral movement responses.
   d. helps keep the head aligned vertically over the body.
4. What architectural structures do the spine, pelvis, shoulder girdle, and head resemble?
5. True or false (circle one). A collapsed posture puts the passive restraints around the joints under tension, which can gradually overstretch them and damage them.
6. Fill in the blank. Upright posture requires minimal muscular activity, but only if the body masses align as close to the _____ as possible.
7. Muscles that provide postural support during movement are classified as
   a. prime movers.
   b. joint stabilizers.
   c. secondary stabilizers.
   d. synergist movers.
8. Muscles that work as primary postural stabilizers
   a. tend to have slow twitch fibers and function with light, isometric contractions, but only during movement.
   b. tend to have slow twitch fibers and function with light, isometric contractions in stationary postures and during movement.
   c. tend to have fast twitch fibers and function with strong, concentric contractions in stationary postures.
   d. tend to have slow twitch fibers and function with eccentric contractions in flexed positions of the spine.
9. Fill in the blank. When the postural stabilizers fail to contract, other muscles contract to compensate in what is called a _____ (*two words*).
10. What is a stability dysfunction?
11. The primary postural stabilizer that compresses the abdominal viscera and protects the lumbar spine and sacroiliac joints is the
    a. transversus abdominis.
    b. external oblique.
    c. iliopsoas muscle group.
    d. internal oblique.
12. Match the terms describing spinal curvatures—lordosis, kyphosis, and scoliosis—with their definitions.
    a. A posterior spinal curve that occurs in the thoracic spine.
    b. An abnormal lateral spinal curve that can occur anywhere in the spine.
    c. An anterior spinal curve that occurs in the lumbar and cervical spine.
13. What is a scoliosis in the neck called?
14. When making a postural assessment of a person in a standing position, which of the following statements is true for a person with optimal posture?
    a. The bilateral bone markings are asymmetrical, the body masses align along a plumb line, and the weight-bearing joints are extended.
    b. The bilateral bone markings are symmetrical, the body mass aligns along a zig-zag line, and the weight-bearing joints are slightly flexed.
    c. The bilateral bone markings are symmetrical, one body mass aligns over another along a plumb line, and the weight-bearing joints are extended.
    d. The bilateral bone markings are symmetrical, the body masses stack along a plumb line, and the weight-bearing joints are hyperextended.
15. Which of the following guidelines is *not* an indicator of a healthy standing posture?
    a. The shoulders and the clavicles are level and horizontal.
    b. The knees and hips are hyperextended and face sideways.
    c. The cervical spine and lumbar spine have normal lordotic curves.
    d. The head is centered over the neck and thorax.

16. True or false (circle one). A faulty posture can be caused by habitual muscular patterns but never by structural deformities such as deviations in the shape or length of the bones.
17. A client-centered postural assessment is one in which the practitioner
    a. helps a client deepen a self-awareness of the personal postural patterns to help the client develop tools for change.
    b. tells a client what his or her postural pattern is and then does bodywork on the client to change the pattern.

c. assesses the client's joint range of motion and then normalizes that range with muscle energy and deep tissue techniques.
d. takes photos of the client's posture at the end of each session to study to determine a treatment plan for the next session.

18. Name two therapeutic applications for postural education.

Notes

1. Foster, M. (2005, April/May). "A Case for the Human Stance." *Massage and Bodywork Magazine,* pp. 72–81.
2. Sweigard, L. E. (1974). *Human Movement Potential: Its Ideokinetic Facilitation.* New York: Harper & Row.
3. Kapandji, I. (1974). *The Physiology of the Joints: Vol. 3. The Trunk and Vertebral Column.* Edinburgh, UK: Churchill Livingstone.
4. Sweigard, L. E. (1974). *Human Movement Potential: Its Ideokinetic Facilitation.* New York: Harper & Row.
5. Basmajian, J., & DeLuca, C. (1984). *Muscles Alive: Their Functions Revealed by Electromyography* (5th ed.). Baltimore: Williams & Wilkins.
6. Ibid.
7. Richardson, C., Jull, G., & Richardson, B. (1995). "A Dysfunction of the Deep Abdominal Muscles Exists in Low Back Pain Patients," *Proceedings of the World Confederation of Physical Therapists,* p. 932.
8. Richardson, C., Jull, G., Hides, J., & Hodges, P. (1999). *Therapeutic Exercises for Spinal Segmental Stabilization: Scientific Basis and Clinical Approach.* London: Churchill Livingstone.
9. For more extensive information about training postural muscles, see Chapter 9 in *Somatic Patterning: How to Improve Posture and Movement and Ease Pain* by M. Foster (2004, Longmont, CO: EMS Press).
10. Rolf, I. (1977). *Rolfing: The Integration of Human Structures.* New York: Harper & Row.
11. Foster, M. (2006, November/December). Muscles and the Postural Flute. *Massage and Bodywork Magazine,* pp. 76–82.

CHAPTER

8 Gait

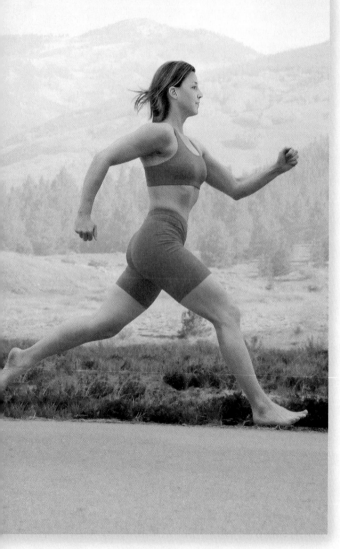

CHAPTER OUTLINE

Chapter Objectives

Key Terms

8.1 Components of Gait

8.2 Muscle Activity in Gait

8.3 Atypical Gait Patterns

8.4 Gait Assessment

Conclusion

Summary Points to Remember

Review Questions

Jogging grew as a popular sport in the 1970s. Soon after, high-tech running shoes flooded the market to provide joggers with foot protection from impact injuries that develop from running on unyielding surfaces such as concrete or asphalt. Human beings have run for centuries either in their bare feet or with minimal footwear, so why the sudden need for fancy footwear? Some runners say there is no need. They claim that shunning their shoes and tackling the turf barefoot has not only reduced and prevented injuries, but has also improved their form.

In an effort to understand these results, researchers have started to make kinematic comparisons between endurance runners with and without shoes.[1] What they've discovered is fascinating.

Runners wearing shoes tend to dorsiflex the ankle and hit the ground heel first, while seasoned barefoot runners plantarflex the ankle and land on the forefoot (the ball of the foot), which greatly reduces compression on impact.

These findings have led to several hypotheses. First, barefoot running increases the sensory feel of the feet moving against the ground and strengthens the foot muscles. Second, it encourages forefoot landing, which improves form. Surprisingly, some researchers think that the comfort and cushioning offered by running shoes may actually be dangerous because it reduces the sensitivity of the feet and encourages a heavy heel strike, increasing injury from excessive impact.

CHAPTER OBJECTIVES

1. Define gait and name another term for gait.

2. Name and define the two phases of gait patterns and the subphases of each.

3. Describe the difference between walking and running.

4. Define step, stride, and step width and identify the average length of each one.

5. Define cadence and describe three different levels of cadence in gait.

6. Describe how the pelvis moves in each plane during a normal walking gait.

7. Discuss the dynamics of contralateral motion in the limbs and trunk.

8. Discuss the role of fall and recovery in gait.

9. Describe the three functions of muscles in the lower limbs motion during gait.

10. Define an antalgic gait and describe how it can be treated with massage and bodywork.

11. List and describe five antalgic gait patterns.

12. List four atypical gait patterns caused by joint dysfunctions and describe each one.

13. Define an ataxic gait and describe two types of ataxic gait patterns.

14. Describe different approaches to gait assessment.

KEY TERMS

Ambulation	Float moment	Psoatic gait
Antalgic gait	Foot angle	Pushoff
Ataxic gait	Foot flat	Stance phase
Cadence	Gait	Step
Cross-extensor reflex	Gluteus maximus lurch	Step width
Double-limb support	Heeloff	Stride
Drop-foot gait	Heel strike	Swing phase
Extensor support moment	Midstance	Trendelenburg gait

Walking is the easiest way to transport the body over short distances. Everybody who uses this convenient and energy-efficient manner of transport has a personal style of walking. Walking is, in essence, posture in motion. People tend to carry the shape of the posture they sit with into movement, which gives their walk a distinct character and cadence. A gait pattern is only as efficient as its underlying posture. A person who sits with hiked shoulders usually stands up and walks with hiked shoulders. A healthy stride begins with a centered, upright stance, which makes understanding the basic components of posture a crucial foundation in the study of gait.

Gait is any locomotive pattern in which the legs transport the body forward in space, such as walking, running, and skipping. Another term for gait is **ambulation.** Whereas most mammals ambulate over four legs, human beings walk in a bipedal gait. "Bi" means "two." Our uniquely bipedal gait is made possible by the biomechanics of an upright spine balanced over two lower limbs.

There are a number of reasons to learn about gait. Gait mechanics underlie all movement patterns, so a study of gait can help a practitioner understand how the human body moves. Gait reveals general patterns of muscle and joint function. The way a client walks can provide clues about past injuries, such as a limp from a sprained joint or a spastic stride from neurological damage. This information, in turn, can help the practitioner figure out a strategy for treatment. The way clients walk also reflects their mental and emotional states because gait, like posture, is influenced by psychology and disposition. A client who arrives with a bouncy, energetic stride probably feels pretty good, whereas a client walking with a cautious weighted shuffle could be struggling with pain, anxiety, or pressing conflicts. Such a manner emphasizes the reality that heavy emotions not only drag down the psyche, but also the body.

In this chapter we look at the basic components of walking and running, including the stance and swing phases; speed and cadence; the synchrony of joint motion in the lower limbs; pelvic movement in each plane; trunk rotation and contralateral limb swing; and the underlying dynamics of fall and recovery in gait. We also look at joint and muscle patterns in each phase of gait, atypical gait patterns, and how to make general assessments for the purpose of learning about this primary human movement. The biomechanics of walking apply to all activities, including body mechanics in massage and bodywork, so we explore ways to employ gait principles for self-care and body mechanics. Our emphasis is on maximizing the efficiency of movement while minimizing stress on the body.

In traditional kinesiology texts, posture and gait are usually covered at the end of the text after all the muscle and joint functions have been presented. We are covering posture and gait in the first half of the book so that we can refer back to these concepts in subsequent chapters on body parts to help explain how each part works in relation to the movement of the entire body. Also, self-care features throughout this chapter provide students with tools for using their bodies efficiently while practicing the palpation exercises in the second half of the text.

8.1   COMPONENTS OF GAIT

Gait is the most well-studied and documented pattern of human movement. The many components of human locomotion come together in a dynamic and complex interplay of movement in all three planes. The pelvis moves in a figure-eight motion that combines a lateral pelvic shift, a forward pelvic tilt, and horizontal rotation. The arms and legs swing in the sagittal plane, causing the upper and lower body to counterrotate at the waist. The feet work against the ground, adapting to uneven terrain, absorbing shock, and driving the body forward with each step.

There are a number of components in walking that, although simplistic, provide unifying principles for a study of whole-body movement patterns:[2]

- Stance and swing phases
- Step and stride length and width
- Cadence
- Joint motion in the lower limbs
- Pelvic movement in each plane
- Trunk rotation and contralateral limb motion
- Reflexive movement cycles of fall and recovery

The loss or exaggeration of any one component is compensated for by changes in the other components. This, in turn, decreases the economy of motion and increases the overall energy required to walk or run. Restrictions or injuries to the knees prove the most costly. A person with knee problems compensates with adjustments in the alignment of all the other joints along the lower limbs. Knee problems can even affect spinal alignment and movement.

8.1.1   Stance and Swing Phases

During each gait cycle, the lower limbs cycle between two alternating phases: a **stance phase** and a **swing phase** (Figure 8.1a-h ■). The stance phase begins when the foot contacts the ground and ends when that same foot leaves the ground. The swing phase occurs when the foot leaves the ground and the lower limb swings forward. On average, 60 percent of walking occurs in the stance phase and 40 percent in the swing phase.

In the stance phase, the lower limb moves in a closed chain with the foot on the ground. The body shifts up, over, and across the foot; the ankle and ball of the foot serve as the primary levers for the stance motion. In a normal walking gait, a person rolls from the heel on heel strike to the toes on pushoff (Figure 8.2a ■). Weight follows a curved path of pressure from the heel, along the lateral arch, and into the ball of the foot (Figure 8.2b ■). Weight loading stretches the arches, creating a rebound that produces elastic energy which propulses the body forward into the next step. Movement at the first metatarsophalangeal joint is critical to completing the pushoff phase of stance.

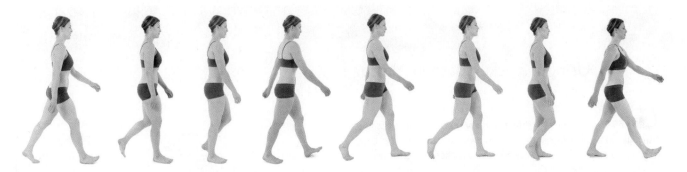

Heel strike	Foot flat	Midstance	Heeloff	Pushoff	Early swing	Midswing	Late swing
		Right leg stance phase				**Right leg swing phase**	
Double support 10%		Single support 40%		Double support 10%		Single support 40%	

FIGURE 8.1

Stance and swing phases of gait

During the swing phase, the opposite dynamic occurs. The foot and lower limb move in an open chain against the stability of the pelvis and trunk. The femur and leg swing at the pelvis, inscribing an arc of motion with the foot.

Each stance phase breaks down into five subphases:

- **Heel strike:** When the heel contacts the ground, the ankle flexes, and the toes hyperextend.
- **Foot flat:** When the whole foot comes into contact with the ground.
- **Midstance:** When the body weight shifts up and over the stance leg.
- **Heeloff:** When the heel lifts off the ground.
- **Pushoff** (or *toe-off*): When the toes push off the ground.

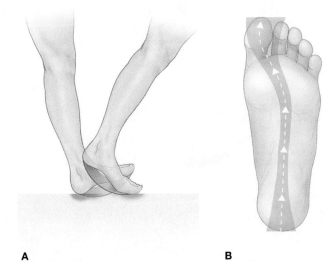

FIGURE 8.2

a) Rolling through the foot b) **Normal path of pressure** on foot during stance phase

Each swing phase breaks down into three subphases:

- **Early swing** (or *acceleration*): When the lower limb swings in a downward arc.
- **Midswing:** When the lower limb swings directly under the hip.
- **Late swing** (or *deceleration*): When the lower limb swings in an upward arc and the knee extends in preparation for heel strike.

Immediately after pushoff, the foot breaks contact with the ground and the leg drops out from under the hip. Just like swinging on a swing set, during this downward arc, the lower limb falls in the direction of gravity and gains momentum, which accelerates the motion. For this reason, the first part of the swing phase is also called *acceleration*.

The lower limb passes under the body at the bottom of the arc, at midswing, and begins the upward arc of the late swing. During this upward motion, the leg swings against gravity and loses momentum. For this reason, the late-swing phase is also called *deceleration*. Early swing and late swing are also referred to as *initial swing* and *terminal swing*.

In the average walking gait, both feet make simultaneous contact with the ground for about 20 percent of the motion cycle. This phase of walking is called a **double-limb support.** During this phase, a person rocks from heel strike on the back foot to push off on the front foot. The feet provide a rocker base to shift weight forward.

You can apply gait principles to your own body mechanics by using a rocker base to move the body forward and back over the feet while giving massage. When using a rocker base in massage, just as a person does when stepping to walk, the body moves through stance-phase mechanics. Applying stance-phase mechanics in massage provides several advantages:

- Shifting weight over a rocker base allows you maximum mobility from which you can easily move in any direction.

SELF-CARE
Using a Rocker Base in Massage

Gait mechanics underlie effective body mechanics in massage. Use this warm-up exercise to explore moving over a rocker base to give massage, the same way you use a rocker motion to walk.

1. **Establishing a rocker base:** Begin in an upright stance. Take a step forward the same way you do when walking (Figure 8.3a ■). Then explore rocking between your front and back foot until the movement feels smooth, using your feet as a rocker base. Make sure to rock all the way from your back heel to your front toes, feeling your back toes bend to lift your body up and over your stance leg. Notice how your pelvis rises up and over your front foot as you rock forward.

2. **Practicing moving on a rocker base:** Begin massaging your client using the rocking motion between your feet to move your entire body and your hands (Figure 8.3b ■). Feel how standing over an extended knee gets you up and over your client (Figure 8.3c ■). Face the direction of your hand movement; this will help you keep your body behind your hands. To reverse your hand movement, rock onto your back foot. To change directions, turn your stance hip and foot to turn your entire body. Move as though your legs and pelvis were driving your arms and hands from behind. Explore rocking from a straight-leg stance into a lunge, then back. Also explore rocking from one lunge position to another.

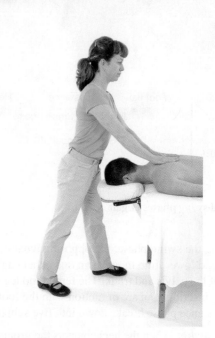

FIGURE 8.3b

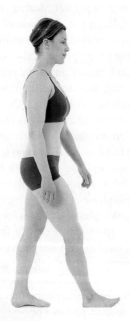

FIGURE 8.3a

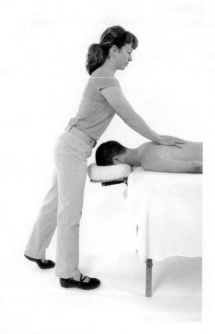

FIGURE 8.3c

3. **Coordinating rocker length with stroke length:** Explore moving your hands with different types of Swedish massage strokes. As you move your hands, rock from one foot to the other, always take a step length that is the same length as your massage stroke (Figure 8.3d ■). Shift your rocker base to follow the pathway along which you move your hands.

   a. During small strokes, rock over your feet using short steps; during long strokes, rock over your feet using long steps.
   b. During linear strokes, move your body in a linear motion.
   c. During curvilinear strokes, move your body in a curvilinear motion.
   d. During petrissage strokes that move in a figure eight, move your pelvis and shift your weight over your feet in a figure-eight motion.

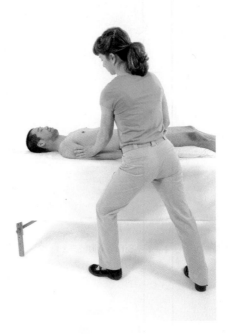

FIGURE 8.3d

- The stance phase has an upright extensor moment. You can return to this neutral posture at any time during a massage when you need to recenter yourself.
- On each forward step, your body rises over the stance leg, which lifts you up and over the client, positioning your upper body to apply pressure down and into the client.

8.1.2   Step and Stride Length and Width

A single **step** begins when the foot makes contact with the ground and ends when the other foot makes contact with the ground. *Step length* is measured between the same location on one foot and on the other foot (Figure 8.4 ■). A measurement of step length can be taken anywhere on the feet as long as it is the same place on both feet. A step length averages between 15 and 18 inches; it is usually longer on a taller person and shorter on a smaller person.

A **stride** equals two steps. *Stride length* is measured at the same point on the same foot over two steps. To measure stride length from footprints on the ground, calculate the distance between the right heels on two consecutive prints. Stride length averages between 30 and 36 inches and will vary according to height and leg length. A stride is also called a *gait cycle*.

Each foot moves along a sagittal pathway or track. The space between the right and left heel equals the **step width** (Figure 8.5 ■). Step width is measured at the heels because most people toe out. An average step width is 2–4 inches, depending on the size of the person. Ideally, each

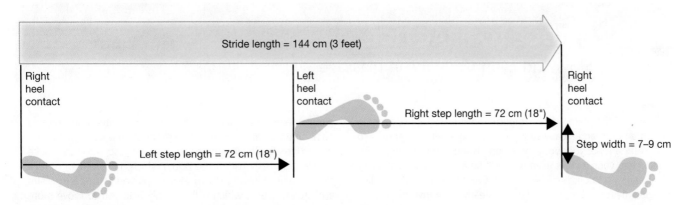

Stride length = 144 cm (3 feet)

Right heel contact

Left heel contact

Right heel contact

Left step length = 72 cm (18")

Right step length = 72 cm (18")

Step width = 7–9 cm

FIGURE 8.4

Step length and stride length

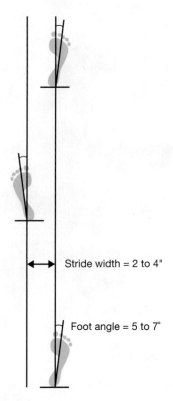

FIGURE 8.5

Step width and foot angle

Stride width = 2 to 4"

Foot angle = 5 to 7°

heel contact occurs right under the hip socket; therefore, step width in a normal gait reflects the width between the coxofemoral joints. The degree of toe-out is called the **foot angle,** which averages 5–7 degrees. The faster a person walks, the smaller the foot angle tends to become.

8.1.3 Cadence

Cadence measures the speed of the gait by the number of steps per minute.

- A slow walking gait cadence is about 70–90 steps per minute.

- An average walking cadence is 100–120 steps per minute.
- An average running cadence is 180 steps per minute, or three steps per second.

Watch a person walk and the rhythm of the gait becomes obvious. The more equal the right and left step lengths, the more symmetrical the bilateral motion and the more even the cadence of the gait. An emphasis in rhythm on one side, which occurs in a limping walk, indicates asymmetrical movements between the two sides of the body and an uneven step length.

As the speed of gait decreases, a person spends less time in the swing phase and more time in the stance phase. The slower people walk, the longer they have double support. Because the body is more stable when both feet are on the ground, people with poor balance tend to walk slowly to extend the double support phase. Women tend to walk slightly faster than men.

As the speed of walking increases, the swing phase also increases until eventually both feet lift off the ground into a **float moment.** A running gait has three phases: a stance, swing, and float phase. The float phase is what distinguishes running from walking. A runner spends about 40 percent of the gait in the stance phase, 60 percent in the swing phase, and 20 percent in the float phase.

8.1.4 Joint Motion in the Lower Limb

Ambulation moves the three main joints of the lower limb—the hip, knee, and ankle—through a revolving chain of flexion and extension. The range and timing of motion in each joint varies from one individual to the next.[3] Here is a summary of the typical joint activity that occurs during each phase of a walking gait (Figure 8.6 ■). Degrees are not exact; they are only given to help with the visualization process.

- *During heel strike,* the hip flexes about 30 degrees and the ankle moves to a neutral position (a 90-degree angle).
- *From heel strike to foot flat,* the ankle plantarflexes about 5 degrees to lower the foot to the ground.

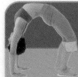

BRIDGE TO PRACTICE
Slow and Even Cadence in Massage

One of the prerequisites of efficient gait is walking or running with an even and steady cadence. This same principle applies to the efficiency of your body movement as you give massage. If you can keep your rhythm even, you will be able to move smoothly through transitions between strokes. Even stimulating strokes like tapotement can be practiced with a steady, even rhythm.

Moving with a slow and steady rhythm as you give massage will not only benefit your client. The two primary reasons

people receive massage are for the relief of stress and muscle pain. One crucial element in stress reduction is learning to slow down, literally slowing the heart rate and respiration to induce a relaxation response in the body, which, in turn, can reduce muscle pain. Slowing down also helps you to impart a calm and steady touch, which will not only help you to move more efficiently, but give you ample time to check in with your body as you work.

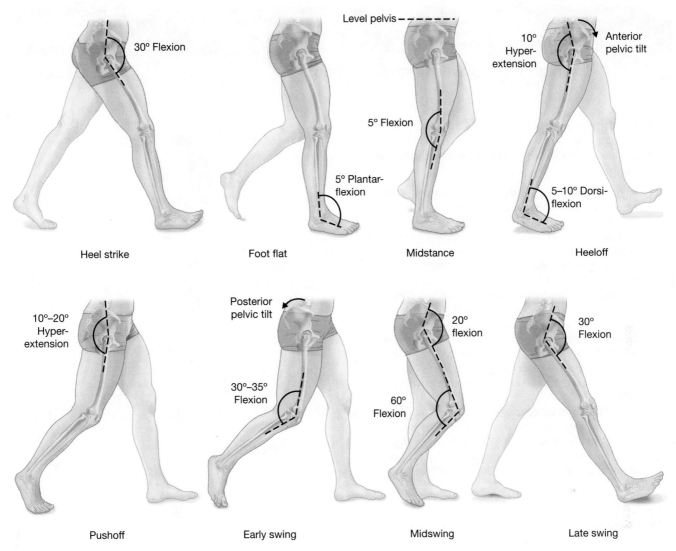

FIGURE 8.6

Joint actions in gait

- *From foot flat to midstance,* as the body shifts up and over the standing leg, the ankle dorsiflexes about 5 degrees. During midstance, the pelvis is level. After midstance, the body begins to lean forward over the ankle and the hip and knee both extend in an **extensor support moment,** which prevents the lower limb from buckling as the body moves over the stance leg.
- *During heeloff,* the ankle dorsiflexes from 5 to 10 degrees as the body leans into pushoff, causing the pelvis to tilt anteriorly.
- *During pushoff,* the toes hyperextend, the knee extends, and the hip hyperextends from 10 to 20 degrees. After pushoff, the swing phase begins.
- *During early swing,* the hip and knee fall into flexion and the knee flexes about 30 degrees, causing the pelvis to tilt posteriorly as the leg swings forward.
- *During the swing phase,* the hip moves from hyperextension to flexion; the knee flexes to about 60 degrees and the ankle flexes so that the foot clears the ground.

- *During late swing,* the hip flexes about 30 degrees, the knee extends, and the ankle dorsiflexes as the foot reaches into heel strike.

In an optimal alignment, the center of the hip, knee, and ankle face the same direction during the entire gait cycle. Although the hips, knees, ankles, and metacarpophalangeal joints flex and extend as hinge joints during gait, each joint has some degree of rotation. For example, the tibia and femur counterrotate at the knee during both flexion and extension. The combined rotations of joints in the lower limb are finely calibrated to produce synchronous motion in the sagittal plane.

If any one joint rotates outside of its normal range and deviates from its ideal track in the sagittal plane, the alignment of all the other joints will be affected. Genu varum (a bow-legged alignment) puts a torque in the knees that laterally twists the tibias, supinates the ankles, twists the forefoot, and abducts the hip joints. Poor alignment during gait increases mechanical stress and causes undue wear and tear on the articular cartilage

SELF-CARE
Exercises for Lower Limb Alignment

When you're giving a massage, it's important to keep the joints of your lower limbs aligned so that you do not twist your knees or ankles. Explore these simple exercises and guidelines for optimal alignment.

1. **Aligning your legs:** Stand in front of a mirror in shorts and bare feet so you can see your ankles and knees. Imagine four dots, one on each joint of one of your lower limbs— the hip, knee, ankle, and second metatarsal (Figure 8.7a ■). In an optimal alignment, the dots should line up under your hips. Look in the mirror and assess your alignment. Adjust your legs so that your dots line up.

2. **Aligned knee bends:** Do a small knee bend and watch your joints flex as you move (Figure 8.7b ■). Slowly push down with both feet to come back up and extend your legs. Spread your toes on the ground as you push. Avoid popping up or locking your knees. *Do your four dots stay aligned in the same plane? Are your feet under your hips? Can you keep your spine straight, as though it were moving down an elevator shaft?*

3. **Aligned lunges:** Lunge forward on one leg. As you lunge, watch your alignment to make sure your joints are in the same plane (Figure 8.7c ■). Your knee should be aligned with your foot. If you had headlights shining out of each dot, they would all shine in the same direction.

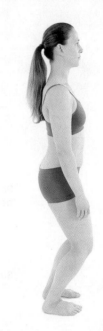

FIGURE 8.7b

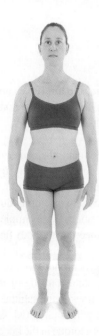

FIGURE 8.7a

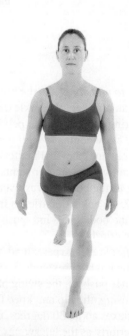

FIGURE 8.7c

a. Lunge on the other leg and check your alignment on that side. Make sure your knee doesn't fall to either side, out of alignment with your hip and foot (Figure 8.7d ■).

b. Explore lunging in different directions, making sure to turn your trunk and entire leg in the direction of your lunge by rotating from the hip.

As you are giving massage, use the same mechanics for leg movement as you did in each of these exercises.

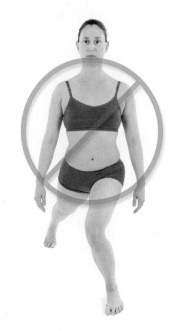

FIGURE 8.7d

of the joints in a manner similar to how tire treads on poorly balanced car wheels wear down unevenly and prematurely.

8.1.5   Pelvic Movement in Each Plane

In a normal walking gait, the pelvis simultaneously rotates in all three planes.[4]

- *Sagittal plane movement of the pelvis:* The pelvis tilts in the sagittal plane during gait activities, rocking 5 degrees forward and backward in anterior and posterior pelvic tilts. This motion is best observed by watching a person walk from a side view. From heel strike to foot flat, the pelvis rises about 5 centimeters (about 2 inches), lifting the trunk up and over the stance leg like a wave cresting. If a fluorescent glow dot was placed on the side of the hip, from a side view the pelvic motion would create a light tracer that looked like a wavy line (Figure 8.8 ■).

- *Frontal (coronal) plane movement of the pelvis:* The pelvis makes a lateral pelvic shift and lateral pelvic tilt in the frontal plane. These sideways movements are best observed by observing a person walk from the front or back view. As weight shifts between the feet, the pelvis makes a lateral shift that averages 4 centimeters (slightly over 1½ inches). The hip over the swing leg abducts while the stance leg adducts, causing the swing hip to dip down about 5 degrees in a lateral pelvic tilt (Figure 8.9 ■). Women usually make a slightly wider lateral shift than men because their pelvic bones are wider.

- *Horizontal (transverse) plane movement of the pelvis:* The pelvis also rotates forward with the swing leg when weight shifts from the back foot to the front foot (Figure 8.10 ■). Pelvic rotation in the horizontal plane is difficult to view; an ideal vantage point would be watching a person walk from above. Early gait researchers were known to put mirrors on the ceiling

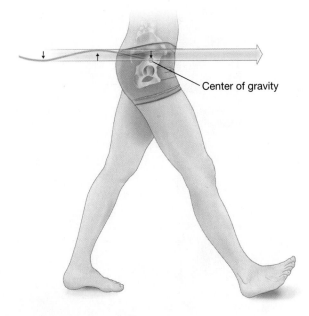

Center of gravity

FIGURE 8.8
Vertical oscillation of pelvis in sagittal plane

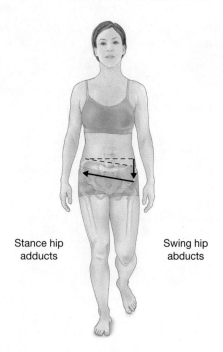

Stance hip
adducts

Swing hip
abducts

FIGURE 8.9
Lateral pelvic shift and pelvic tilt

to measure forward and backward rotation during gait, which averages about 8 degrees (4 degrees on each side). If rotation is restricted, both the arc of the swing leg and the length of the step will be shorter. Conversely, shorter steps reduce both horizontal pelvic rotation and the arc of the swing leg.

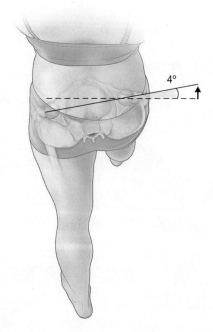

4°

FIGURE 8.10
Horizontal rotation of pelvis

8.1.6 Trunk Rotation and Contralateral Limb Motion

In a normal gait pattern, the arms and legs swing in the sagittal plane in a contralateral pattern. As one leg swings forward, the opposite arm swings back, causing the upper body and lower body to rotate in opposite directions. The pelvis rotates anteriorly, moving with the swing leg; the shoulder girdle counterrotates in the posterior direction, moving with the backward swinging arm.

If we had to consciously direct every step we take, as an injured person often does during rehabilitation, walking would be a slow and measured process requiring focused attention and lots of effort. Fortunately for us, the nervous system coordinates the bulk of our movement patterns below our conscious awareness through reflexes. This frees the brain for the cognitive functions, allowing the body to move somewhat on autopilot. The faster we move, the more our reflexes kick in to coordinate neuromuscular pathways. The **cross-extensor reflex** coordinates the contralateral pattern—the simultaneous flexion of one leg with the extension of the other. When a person steps on a nail, this reflex ensures a lightning-quick response, causing the person to jerk that limb away from the nail and extend the other leg for support.

When the pace of walking reaches a certain cadence, a complex combination of reflexes coordinates the contralateral swing of the arms and the legs. It would be difficult to walk at a fast pace or run without swinging the limbs in opposition. During a slower pace, this level of coordination does not occur, so arms may simply hang motionless, or nearly so, at the sides of the body.

The forward propulsion of the body increases during a quicker pace due to a combination of several forces:

- The pendular swinging of the legs adds momentum to the gait.
- Ground reaction forces from pushoff in the stance foot shift the body up and forward, setting the swing leg into motion.
- Arm swing and trunk rotation also contribute thrust to the forward drive of the body. (This last point explains why strength training in the core and the upper body improves the efficiency of walking and running.)

8.1.7 Fall and Recovery

Walking is a process of losing balance and catching oneself with a reflexive step. As the body leans forward into each step, the loss of balance causes one leg to reflexively flex to catch the body and recover balance (Figure 8.11 ■). Each step is actually a dynamic sequence of fall and recovery, which leads to the next step, and so on into a progression of forward strides.

Walking for an adult seems simple and controlled, although it takes years for a child to learn this control and balance. The loss of balance and subsequent fall-and-recovery sequence is most obvious when a baby first discovers the

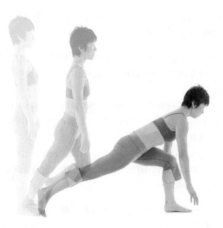

FIGURE 8.11

Falling forward into a reflexive step

standing posture. A baby learns to walk from the precarious balance of standing, then teetering and falling, and finally creating the pitter-patter of first steps. Each time the baby topples over, one leg after the other shoots out in a protective stepping reflex through a revolving series of steps. The loss of balance and thrill of discovery create a momentum that drives the immature little body across the room until the baby catches

him- or herself on a chair or wall. This learning process continues to evolve until about age 7, when the coordination, balance, and control of the adult gait pattern emerges.

While walking, a person continually surrenders a state of vertical balance to the uncertainty of the next step. Walking is not as extreme an action as stepping off a cliff, but it has a touch of this free fall into space. To allow the body to fall off balance into one step after another requires a degree of trust in the ground support. Imagine walking across a bed of slippery rocks or across an old and seemingly rotted wooden bridge. Caution would lead to muscular holding, which is rooted in the precarious ground support and the subsequent fear of falling.

Walking also requires a degree of trust in the body and its motor skills. The joints in the human body are well calibrated for vertical balance. The grace and efficiency of the gait pattern depends on the perfect stacking of the joints in the momentary upright stance phase. When ideally stacked, our joints fall into precise fit like vertical tumblers falling into place. Any postural misalignment or part of the body that a person chronically holds reduces the subsequent efficiency of the gait patterns and can fuel the fear of falling. This happens during the aging process as motor skills decline and balance becomes an issue, underscoring the importance of movement and exercise throughout a lifetime.

 GUIDELINES
Working with Clients Who Have Balance Issues

It is important for you to be aware if your clients have balance issues in order to adjust the environment and session accordingly. Many people develop balance issues from inactivity, a decline in motor skills, and the subsequent fear of falling. Older clients with tipsy balance and osteoporosis could easily break a hip in a fall.

Balance issues will usually be obvious. As clients walk in, you will notice that they walk slowly and cautiously; they may even have a cane or walker. Here are some guidelines to help clients with poor balance issues feel more comfortable so that they can relax muscular holding associated with a fear of falling.

1. Always greet new clients at the door. If a client has an obvious problem with balance, offer an arm to assist that client as needed.
2. Make sure your environment is safe and well lit. Shovel snow from walkways and throw salt over icy areas. Put up signs that clearly mark steps. Make sure all steps are sturdy and stable. Place traction strips across slippery steps, such as wood or vinyl steps. Secure loose carpets or rugs to the floor so that a client cannot stumble over them.
3. Put questions on your health history that identify balance issues, such as questions about loss of balance, tendency to fall, low blood pressure, dizziness, ringing in the ears, osteoporosis, and a history of strokes.

4. Equilibrium structures are located in the inner ear, therefore clients with balance problems often have limited range of motion in the neck. They could become disoriented or dizzy during passive joint motion. Check with your client before passively moving any parts of the client's body, especially the head and neck.
5. Avoid doing quick, passive movements on any client with equilibrium issues because it may be difficult for such a client to adjust to rapid changes in position.
6. Keep a small stool under your massage table to help infirm clients or clients with balance issues get on and off the table. If your clients needs assistance getting up and off the table but prefer getting up in privacy, ask them if they want you to pull out the stool for them to step down on before you leave the room. Also, remove any pillows, bolsters, or equipment that could get in their way as they are making the transition to standing and walking out the door.
7. Escort clients with poor balance to the door, and even to their car, if needed. If this is not possible, inquire about having such clients bring someone to the session who can assist them when needed.

8.2 MUSCLE ACTIVITY IN GAIT

Early gait studies published in the 19th century were made by attaching reflective tape or light tubes along the sides of the body, then taking a series of closely timed photographs to track segmented joint motion.[5] This technique was improved upon by a modern researcher who left the shutter open in the camera, then flashed a light at a speed of 20 times per second so that the segmented joint motion could be seen in a single photograph.[6]

Modern gait laboratories employ higher-tech methods to study ambulation, with electromyography (EMG) studies to measure firing patterns in muscles, pressure plates in the floor to measure ground force generated by foot–floor contact, and high-speed synchronized cameras that collect data from three directions. This information is then collated into biomechanical statistics about gait for use in athletic training and the ergonomic design of furniture, shoes, and equipment. It also helps a student of kinesiology to visualize joint and muscle patterns in a gait sequence.

Although data obtained about muscles from electromyographic studies is quite extensive, it is still difficult to tell how much force a muscle is generating or why it is contracting at a certain time. In addition, EMG studies rarely measure activity in the deeper muscles, such as the iliopsoas group or perineum muscles at the base of the pelvis.

During gait pattern, the lower limb muscles work in three main capacities:

- *Isometric contractions* stabilize and support the lower limb in a static position, especially during the stance phase.
- *Concentric contractions* generate a propulsive force to accelerate lower limb motion, especially during the swing phase.
- *Eccentric contractions* provide a restraining force to decelerate lower limb motion, especially during the swing phase.

The muscular activity in each phase of the gait cycle is logical, so it is easier to learn about the muscle patterns in gait by thinking about them logically than through memorization (Table 8.1 ■). Generally speaking, muscle patterns can be determined by the angle joint and the relationship of limb alignment to the body.

- If the angle of the joint is *closing,* muscles acting on that joint are working in concentric contractions.
- If the angle of the joint is *opening,* muscles acting on that joint are working in eccentric contractions.
- If the angle of the joint is *static,* muscles acting on that joint are working in concentric contractions.

The firing patterns of muscles presented in this section reflect their activity during a normal walking gait.

TABLE 8.1 Gait Muscle Patterns

Gait Phase Interval	Joint and Action Key: ext, extension; flex, flexion; HE, hyperextension	Concentric Muscle Activity	Eccentric Muscle Activity
Midswing to heel strike	Hip–ext to flex Knee–flex to ext Ankle–dorsiflexion	Quadriceps Iliopsoas Tensor fascia latae Anterior adductors Dorsiflexors	Gluteus maximus Hamstrings Plantarflexors (gastrocnemius, soleus, tibialis posterior)
Heel strike to midstance	Hip–flex to ext Knee–ext to slight flex Ankle–neutral (at 90°)	Hamstrings as hip extensors Vastus muscles Dorsiflexors	Rectus femoris Plantarflexors
Midstance to heeloff and pushoff	Hip–ext to HE Knee–flex to ext Ankle–plantarflexion	Hamstrings Gluteus maximus Posterior adductors Plantarflexors Peroneals (fibularis group)	Quadriceps Dorsiflexors
Pushoff to early swing	Hip–ext to HE Knee–ext to flex Ankle–neutral (90°)	Hamstrings as knee flexors Gluteus maximus Dorsiflexors	Gluteus medius and minimus
Early swing to midswing	Hip–HE to ext Knee–flex Ankle–neutral (90°)	Gluteus medius and minimus Dorsiflexors Knee flexors	Gluteus maximus Hamstrings

8.2.1 Muscle Activity in the Stance Phase

To simplify assessment of muscle firing patterns in the hip and knee during the stance phase, it helps to break the arc of movement into three categories: when the lower limb is behind the body, when the lower limb is over the body, and when the lower limb is in front of the body (Figure 8.12 ■). When the hip and knee extend behind the body, concentric contractions occur along the back of these joints and eccentric contractions along the front. Just the opposite pattern occurs when the hip flexes and knee extends in front of the body. Here is a more detailed breakdown:

- *During heel strike:* Isometric contractions occur in the hip extensors to stabilize the stance hip and prevent flexion. Concentric contractions occur in both the hip flexors and knee extensors. Concentric contractions also occur in the dorsiflexors to hyperextend the toes at the metacarpophalangeal joints. Eccentric contractions occur in the hip extensors, knee flexors, and plantarflexors to decelerate the forward swinging motion of the lower limb.
- *During foot flat:* Eccentric contractions occur in the dorsiflexors to lower the forefoot toward the floor. Concentric contractions occur in the knee flexors to prepare the joint for loading.
- *During midstance:* Isometric contractions occur in the hip abductors to stabilize the hip and prevent excessive adduction. Isometric contractions also occur in the knee extensors and plantarflexors to stabilize the ankle.

- *During heeloff:* Concentric contractions occur in the plantarflexors to raise the heel. Concentric contractions occur in hip and knee extensors to hyperextend lower limb.
- *During pushoff:* Concentric contractions occur in the hip extensors, plantarflexors, and the dorsiflexors of toes to hyperextend the metacarpophalangeal joints. Eccentric contractions occur in both the hip flexors and dorsiflexors after the toes leave the ground and the swing phase begins.

8.2.2 Muscle Activity in the Swing Phase

To simplify assessment of muscle firing patterns in the hip and knee during the swing phase, it helps to break the arc of movement into three categories: when the lower limb is behind the body, when the lower limb is directly under the body, and when the lower limb is in front of the body (Figure 8.13 ■). Again, when the hip and knee extend behind the body, concentric contractions occur along the back of these joints and eccentric contractions along the front. Just the opposite pattern occurs when the hip flexes and knee extends in front of the body. Here is a more detailed breakdown:

- *During early swing:* Concentric contractions occur in the hip extensors, knee flexors, and dorsiflexors, keeping the knee and ankle flexed. Eccentric contractions occur in the hip flexors.

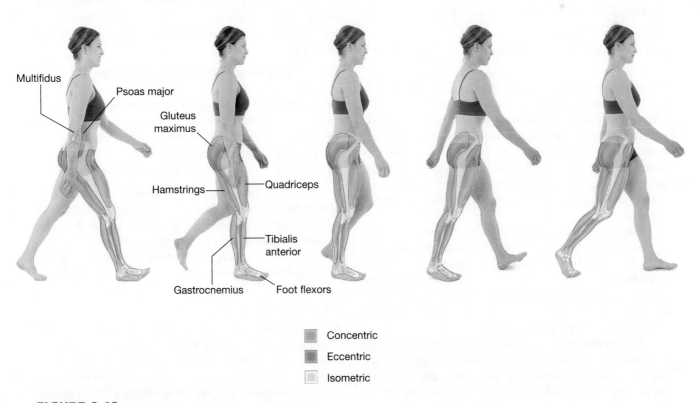

Concentric

Eccentric

Isometric

FIGURE 8.12

Muscle actions in gait: stance phase

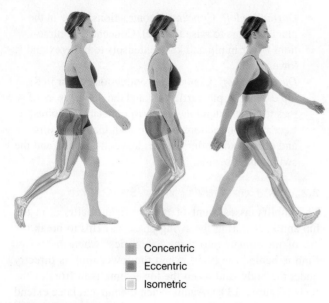

□ Concentric
■ Eccentric
□ Isometric

FIGURE 8.13
Muscle actions in gait: swing phase

- *During midswing:* Concentric contractions continue in the knee flexors and dorsiflexors to make sure the foot clears the ground. Eccentric contractions occur in the hip extensors to decelerate the motion.
- *During late swing:* Concentric contractions occur in the hip flexors and knee extensors to prepare for heel strike. Eccentric contractions occur in the hip extensors and plantarflexors to decelerate hip flexion and dorsiflexion in preparation for heel strike.

8.2.3   Muscle Activity in the Trunk and Shoulders

There is minimal activity in the trunk muscles during gait. Ideally, the spinal stabilizers—transversus abdominis, multifidus, psoas major, longus coli, and suboccipitals—work with light isometric contractions to keep the spine relatively stable during the entire gait cycle. (For a review of the stabilizer muscles, see Table 7.1). In addition, muscle activity has been found in the erector spinae during two periods of the gait cycle: at the end range of both hip flexion and hip hyperextension.

The external obliques and internal obliques also work as secondary stabilizers to control trunk rotation. The obliques play a key role in transmitting rotational forces from the limbs through the waist, transferring motion between the upper and lower body. When the oblique muscles are weak or inhibited, rotation in the waist during the gait cycle will be restricted or absent.

The lower trapezius and the serratus anterior should be active to stabilize the shoulder girdle and scapula during the entire arc of arm swing. The glenohumeral flexors are remarkably quiet during shoulder flexion: If the shoulders are rounded, the latissimus dorsi and infraspinatus are active during shoulder extension.

When observing gait from the front or the back, the space between the lower limbs should remain relatively parallel, about the same width as the feet. This indicates muscle integrity along the inside line of the lower limb. This inside line supports the core of the body, which will be evident in alignment of the trunk directly over the stance foot. When observing gait from the side, during midstance the pelvis and spine should align directly over the stance foot, and the stance knee and hip should completely extend. This indicates balance between the flexor and extensor chains of muscles along the front and back of the body.

8.3   ATYPICAL GAIT PATTERNS

Atypical gait patterns occur for a number of reasons: pain from movements in a specific range; muscle weakness, tightness, or paralysis; joint damage or fusion; bone deformation; and neurological effects.

All of us have something unique about our gait. Short of injury, muscle or joint dysfunction, or neurological damage, the unique traits that occur in atypical gait patterns are usually caused by faulty postural patterns. Any deviations from an ideal posture require muscular effort that a person carries into walking. If a person has a sway back while standing, he or she will usually walk with a sway back. If a person pinches the scapulae together while standing, he or she will usually walk with a retraction in the scapulae that pulls the elbows behind the body. Any degree of postural holding will reduce the efficiency of walking. Here are some common holding patterns that affect gait:

- Swinging the arms sideways or holding the shoulders still
- Taking extra-wide steps or extra-narrow steps
- Walking with a pigeon-toed stride
- Walking with the legs turned out like a ballerina
- Popping up on the toes on each step
- Walking with an exaggerated lateral hip swing

Excessive motion in any one plane reduces the range of motion in another plane. A sideways arm swing will result in excessive trunk rotation, which reduces the range of sagittal motion. An exaggerated up and down motion from popping up on the toes on each step reduces the step length and forward momentum.

8.3.1   Antalgic Gaits

Any kind of gait dysfunction that occurs as a self-protective measure to avoid a painful range of motion constitutes an **antalgic gait,** which is characterized by a shortened stance phase.[7] For example, a person with hip arthritis often hold the hips in chronic flexion while walking to avoid pain on extension; a person with chronic headaches or whiplash tends to walk gingerly with a stiff spine to reduce the

SELF-CARE
Improving Sagittal Tracking of the Lower Limb

This exercise will improve sagittal tracking in the joints of your hips, knees, ankles, and toes while you walk. It will also improve muscular coordination in your legs so your joints flex and extend in unison. It is one of the original Rolfing movement exercises called "toes up, toes down."

1. **Getting ready:** Begin sitting in a chair in an upright position with your shoes off: put both feet flat on the floor. Make sure your thighs and feet are aligned with your hip joints.
2. **Toe movement:** Starting with one foot, raise all five toes while keeping the ball of your foot on the ground (Figure 8.14a ■). Your arches should stretch. Then lower your toes. Raise your toes again, this time watching them to make sure all five toes lift at once. It's common for either the big toe or little toe to lead. If this happens, repeat until you lift all five toes in unison.

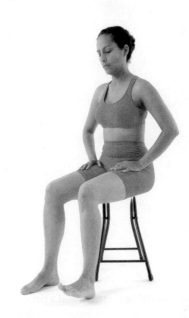

FIGURE 8.14b

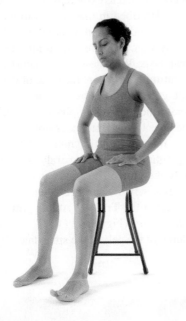

FIGURE 8.14a

3. **Toe and ankle movement:** Add another step. First lift your toes, then lift your ankle, then reverse the sequence (Figure 8.14b ■). Practice this sequence—toes up, ankle up, ankle down, toes down—several times with one foot. Watch your knee as you move, making sure your knee stays aligned with your ankle and hip as though the entire limb were sandwiched between two narrow walls. If your knee moves out of line, place your palms on either side of it to stabilize it (Figure 8.14c ■).
4. **Comparing sides:** After doing the exercise on one foot, compare your feet by standing up and walking around. Notice whether this foot and knee feel any different from the other side and how. Most people feel this side is more aligned.

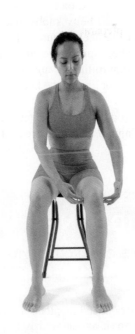

FIGURE 8.14c

5. Repeat steps 1–3 with the other foot. Then get up and walk around again to integrate the movement of both sides into your gait.

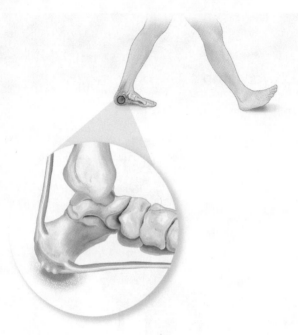

FIGURE 8.15
Heel spur

painful reverberation of heel strike; and a person with lower back pain tends to restrict trunk rotation to avoid irritating movement in the problem area.

Antalgic gaits occur with *plantar fasciitis*—the inflammation of the fascia on the sole of the foot—and with *heel spurs*—small bony knobs that develop on the calcaneus bone of the heel (Figure 8.15 ■). People with plantar fasciitis or heel spurs develop a flat-footed gait to avoid sharp pain from rolling through the foot and stretching the plantar fascia or having the heel spur press into the soft tissue.

People develop antalgic gait patterns from instinctive guarding around injured or pained areas of the body. This can even occur with minor injuries that a person might brush off as inconsequential without realizing that he or she is subconsciously walking around the injured area. If a relatively healthy client who is free from injury demonstrates an atypical gait, you can inquire about pain patterns to determine if the gait is antalgic in nature. Antalgic gaits can and often do develop below a level of conscious awareness due to the pain from the accumulative effects of poor posture.

Antalgic gait patterns always involve compensatory muscular holding. If a client has an injury in one leg or hip, it is probable that muscles on the other side of the body are overworking and symptomatic. For example, one client had an accident that seriously deformed his tibia on the right leg, making that leg shorter. As a result, he received massage and bodywork for chronic muscle pain and trigger points that developed in his lower back, both hips, and the other limb.

8.3.2   Muscle Dysfunctions in Gait

A study of atypical gait patterns will prepare you to identify the muscular imbalances that occur in compensatory patterns. You are encouraged to explore walking in each of the atypical patterns described in this section to feel how that gait affects muscles and joints in other parts of the body.

Some gait dysfunctions are due to muscle weakness, tightness, or paralysis. Weakness in the hamstrings results in **genu recurvatum gait,** where the knee of the stance leg locks into hyperextension (Figure 8.16 ■). Because hamstrings decelerate the late-swing phase, hamstring weakness causes the knee to snap into extension.

Weakness, **paresis** (partial muscle dysfunction or paralysis), or **plegia** (total muscle paralysis) in the abductors, particularly the gluteus medius, can cause the stance hip to lurch sideways into excessive adduction. Weakness on one side results in the **Trendelenburg gait,** also called the *gluteus medius lurch* (Figure 8.17 ■). To counterbalance the sideways lurch of the pelvis, the spine laterally bends to

GUIDELINES
Intake of Clients with Antalgic Gait Patterns

If your client has concerns and symptoms you suspect are associated with an antalgic gait, you can work with the muscular compensations in the gait pattern.

1. Find out the cause of the antalgic gait.
   - Is it coming from an injury or a postural pattern?
   - When did it start?
   - What range of motion causes pain and why?
   - What muscles contract during that range?

2. Obtain information about injuries affecting gait from your client's health history. If an injury is serious enough to have warranted medical attention, ask your client to provide you with information from a medical evaluation that explains the condition.
3. Develop a treatment plan that will offer clients with antalgic gait pattern relief from chronic pain due to compensatory muscular holding.

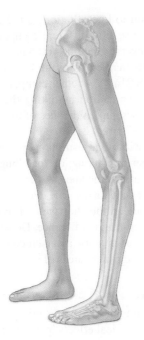

FIGURE 8.16

Genu recurvatum (hyperextended knee)

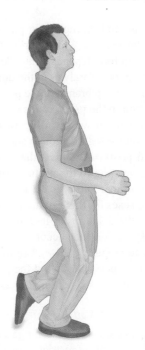

FIGURE 8.18

Gluteus maximus lurch

the affected side. Bilateral weakness or dysfunction in the gluteus medius causes excessive lateral hip motion, resulting in a **waddling gait.** The Trendelenburg gait occurs to varying degrees, depending on the severity of abductor dysfunction.

The gluteus maximus stabilizes the hip in extension in midstance. Weakness in the gluteus maximus muscle results in a loss of control over hip extension, causing

the stance hip to jackknife into flexion on heel strike, then lurch into hyperextension on midstance. This creates an extreme backward-then-forward rocking motion of the trunk on the hips called the **gluteus maximus lurch** (Figure 8.18 ■).

Weakness in the dorsiflexors causes a **steppage gait** or **drop-foot gait,** causing the toes to drop and slap down on the ground on each step (Figure 8.19 ■). To avoid dragging

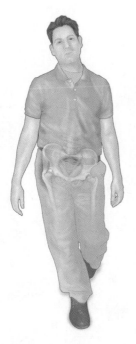

FIGURE 8.17

Trendelenburg gait (gluteus medius lurch)

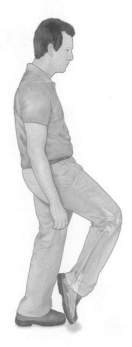

FIGURE 8.19

Drop-foot gait

the foot on the ground during swing phase, a person with drop foot lifts the knee very high during the swing phase. The degree of drop foot depends on the degree of dysfunction in the dorsiflexors. Paralysis to the dorsiflexors occurs with damage to the deep branch of the peroneal nerves.

A dysfunction in the psoas can lead to a **psoatic gait,** during which a person walks in hip flexion and lateral rotation of the stance leg, as though she or he were bowing. The flexed position tightens the extensors muscles along the spine, leading to the postural compensations of an exaggerated lumbar and cervical lordosis and an anterior pelvic tilt. Causes for this gait include inflammation to the bursa under the distal psoas tendon, psoas tendonitis, or visceral dysfunction that occurs in relationship with the psoas muscle (Figure 8.20 ■).[8] In all cases, chronic hip flexion helps a person to avoid the painful stretch of the hip flexors and iliopsoas during hip extension.

8.3.3 Limitations to Joint Range of Motion

Atypical gaits develop when the range of motion in the joints of the lower limb is restricted or absent. This can be caused by joint injuries, fusion, or bony deformities, conditions that are usually painful and require orthopedic treatment.

Hip joint restrictions from severe arthritis or fusion lead to a "bell-clapper" gait in which a person swings the leg forward with an extreme posterior pelvic tilt, then steps onto the stance leg with an extreme anterior tilt, jerking the pelvis back and forth to compensate for the lack of hip motion. This gait strains the lumbar spine and often leads to secondary joint problems.

Restriction to knee flexion as the result of injury or fusion leads to several different compensatory gaits. One compensation is the **circumducted gait,** in which a person swings the affected leg from the hip in an arc around the body (Figure 8.21a ■). Another compensation is to hold the affected leg in abduction by hiking the hip. A third compensation is to rise up on the toes of the unaffected leg in a **vaulting gait** (Figure 8.21b ■).

A person with ankle restriction or fusion takes on a "peg-legged" manner of walking, or "paddling" by swinging the foot in an arc around the knee. A person with a hemi-pelvis, a smaller coxal bone on one side, has a limping gait in which the pelvis drops on the short side. The same type of gait occurs with a leg-length difference. Depending on the severity of the bony asymmetry, a person could develop scoliosis as well as chronic pain in areas of compensatory holding.

8.3.4 Neurological Effects in Gait

Neurological impairment from injury, stroke, or disease can cause neurological effects in gait such as spasticity and rigidity. Such impairments lead to a lack of control over some aspect of the gait cycle, depending on which muscle groups are affected.

An **ataxic gait** occurs when there has been damage to the cerebellum. This can lead to *hypotonia* (low muscle tone) and decreased muscle strength or hypertonic muscles and spasticity. Neurological damage and poor muscular coordination result in unsteady balance with either a limp and flaccid quality of movement or a tight, spastic quality. An ataxic walk is characterized by difficulty with motor control and a widened base to compensate for balance problems.

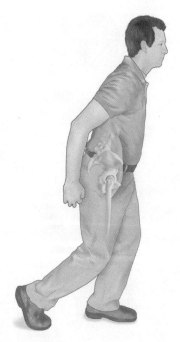

FIGURE 8.20

Psoatic gait

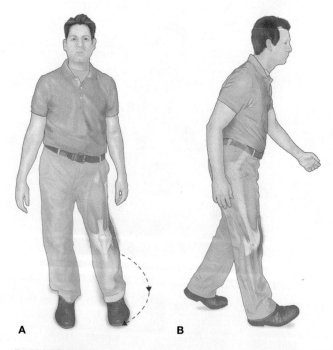

A   **B**

FIGURE 8.21

a) **Circumducted gait** b) **Vaulting gait**

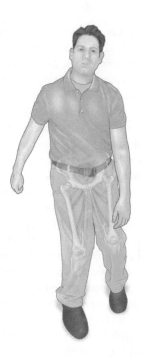

FIGURE 8.22
Scissors gait

There are many conditions that lead to ataxia, such as Down's syndrome, developmental disabilities, and Marfan's syndrome (a genetic disorder affecting connective tissues), to name a few. Cerebral palsy (CP) results in hypertonic muscles and spasticity of several different types. It can affect one side of the body, the lower body, or the entire body. People with spastic CP in the lower limbs often have a **crouched gait**, walking with the legs and hips in chronic flexion and with an exaggerated lateral arm swing and trunk rotation. Adductor dysfunction or paralysis can lead to a **scissors gait** that causes the knees to cross in a scissor-like motion (Figure 8.22 ■).

The **Parkinsonian gait** is marked by chronic flexion in the trunk, lower limbs, and elbows, all of which restrict range of motion, impair reflexes, and cause balance issues. People with this gait take short, jerky steps and step primarily on the toes and forefoot. They have difficulty starting and stopping due to muscular rigidity.

Massage clients with gait impairment due to neurological dysfunctions tend to respond well to relaxation techniques that calm the nerves and allow spastic or rigid muscles to rest. Muscle energy techniques tend to be inappropriate for such clients because of the damage to the neuromuscular circuits.

8.4 GAIT ASSESSMENT

Although each person walks and runs with the same basic components, gait patterns can be as unique as individual personalities. The way a person walks reflects that individual's character and psychological state. This explains how it is possible to recognize friends from a distance by the shape or rhythm of their gait; people intuitively recognize the overall shape and style of a person's body patterns.

Innate pattern recognition abilities equips you with a basic tool to begin a gait assessment, which is also an effective learning exercise in the study of human kinesiology. Gait assessment can help you see how all the parts move together. Additionally, an assessment of gait can provide you with general information about a client's muscle and joint patterns, which will be invaluable when planning the course of a session.

8.4.1 General and Specific Gait Assessments

The first impression we get when we see a person walking provides a snapshot image of the overall pattern. The eye sees the whole body when the gait is symmetrical, efficient, and flowing. Conversely, the eye is easily drawn to distortions in shape and restrictions in flow, which is why it is helpful to take note of your first impression when practicing gait observation. As we continue to observe the person walking, the various components of gait start to become obvious, such as the cadence, specific joint actions, alternating phases of limb motion, and trunk rotation.

Before looking at assessment, let's discuss where and how to observe gait as a learning exercise. Airports, malls, and public parks where a lot of people are walking by make great laboratories for observing and assessing gait patterns. Keep in mind, though, that most people are sensitive to being watched.

When you practice gait observation in public places, it is prudent to be discreet, respectful, and professional. When we take classes outside for gait observation, students often wear sunglasses and sit in a circle so it is not obvious we are viewing people. Inappropriate behaviors such as pointing, staring, mimicking gait patterns, or loud talking about patterns are unprofessional and strictly prohibited.

When studying gait patterns, make sure to focus on recognizing normal and healthy body mechanics in gait, taking care to notice balance, symmetry, a full range of joint motion, normal firing patterns in the muscles, and a completion of each cycle of gait. This will train you to identify and appreciate healthy patterns. It will also allow you to give positive feedback to a self-berating type of client who becomes overly focused on negative patterns and body problems.

Self-study of gait is an important way to build compassion. Most people have quirky or awkward movement habits that cause an affected gait. These are easy to point out in other people, but not always so easy to see in your own body, so watch yourself walking toward a full-length mirror or window. Better yet, video yourself walking from the front, back, and side, then watch the video and answer the questions in the general and specific gait assessments found below.

Because it is natural to identify the overall pattern of gait before targeting specific elements, two sets of guidelines for gait assessment—general and specific—are presented in this section. Use these questions as a guide for studying gait patterns in a public place, for self-study, or for conducting a gait laboratory in a class or with a partner.

8.4.2 Therapeutic Applications for Gait Assessments

Gait assessment can provide information about joint and muscle function that can help you develop a treatment plan for individual sessions. Because people tend to take on an affected, unnatural gait when being observed or put on the spot, begin a discreet gait assessment as your client walks into your office.

As your client walks, observe the overall pattern and assess these levels of the pattern—movement pathways, joints, muscles, and underlying posture:

1. Which joints have restricted motion and need stretching? Which joints have too much motion and need stabilization?
2. Which muscles are adaptively shortened? Which muscles are stretch weakened? Which muscles need stretching or strengthening? Which muscles need to be brought under conscious control to improve the overall movement pattern?
3. Which pathway of movement (kinetic chain) is affected by the gait? (See "Kinetic Chains" in the introductory chapter and "Assessing Kinetic Chains" in the neuromuscular chapter.)
4. What is the underlying posture that is carried into gait?

Here are several examples of what you might find during gait observations:

- When a client has a bow-legged gait, muscles along the inside line and core pathway will be adaptively shortened. The feet will be chronically pronated. If a client complaining of chronic foot pain has a flat-footed walk, it is logical to assume that the arches lack motion and the intrinsic muscles of the foot need work. In a flat-footed gait pattern, a person usually fails to roll through the foot, so the end ranges of the stance phase—heel strike and pushoff—tend to be missing in the gait. In this case, make sure to work to restore flexibility to the arches and a more centered alignment to the knees and hips.
- When a client walks more heavily on one foot, he or she may have a lateral bend in the spine that shortens muscles and compresses joints along the lateral pathway. In this case, consider working with the client in a side-lying position to first lengthen muscles and decompress joints on the shortened side.
- When a client walks with a pattern of chronic flexion, a heavy heel strike, and a posterior pelvic tilt, flexor muscles along the front of the body will be adaptively shortened while muscles along the back pathway will be stretch weakened. In this case, you may want to start the session with your client supine so that you can stretch tight flexor muscles.

8.4.3 Gait Education in Bodywork

As mentioned in the introductory chapter, human beings have a natural and innate ability for pattern recognition. This means that recognizing inefficiencies in gait is perhaps one of the easiest steps in addressing faulty body patterns. As a massage and bodywork practitioner, you can integrate client education about gait into bodywork with these practical tools:

GUIDELINES
General Gait Assessments

Get together with a friend or class partner and watch each other walk. Answer these assessment questions. Be aware of when your answers are objective or subjective. An objective finding is some aspect of gait that two or more people could observe and agree on. A subjective answer is an intuitive impression or opinion.

1. What is the overall quality of the gait (e.g., is it bouncy, fast, measured, confident, awkward, or tipsy)?
2. What part of the body is your attention drawn to and why?
3. What is the underlying posture of the gait?
4. What is the energetic pattern of the gait (e.g., the energy could be heavy, light, bent, cautious, jumpy, guarded,

internally focused, externally focused, sympathetic dominance, or parasympathetic dominance)?
5. What moves and what holds as your partner walks? Does he or she tend to walk around a certain part of the body?
6. What is the rhythm and cadence of the gait?
7. Is the gait symmetrical?
8. Does your partner lean back or does any part of the body move sideways?
9. Does one part of the body arrive before another (e.g., in the head-forward posture, the face arrives first; in the posterior pelvic tilt, the hips tend to arrive first)?

GUIDELINES
Specific Gait Assessments

When making gait assessments of yourself or a partner, first make a general assessment of the gait pattern and then make a specific assessment. With a partner, take turns watching each other walk and answer the specific questions below. Then share your findings with each other.

Feet:

1. Are your partner's feet pigeon-toed or toed out?
2. Do your partner's feet chronically supinate (which leads to high arches) or pronate (which leads to flat feet)?
3. What is the foot angle? What degree do the toes point to the side?
4. If your partner's feet are misaligned, to what degree? Also, which muscles are adaptively shortened and stretch weakened by the pattern?
5. Does your partner roll through the entire foot into pushoff? Do your partner's toes bend to 90 degrees on pushoff?
6. What is your partner's step width?
7. Does the foot on the swing leg extend into heel strike?
8. Is the heel strike on the front leg simultaneous with the pushoff on the back leg?

Knee and Limb Alignment:

9. Are your partner's feet, ankles, knees, and hips facing forward and moving along a sagittal track? If not, what direction does each joint move?
10. Does your partner have a pattern of genu valgum (knock-kneed) or genu varum (bow-legged)? To what degree?
11. Do your partner's thighs swing under the pelvis in the sagittal plane? If not, in what direction do they move? Do your partner's hip joints swing freely?
12. What are the step and stride lengths? Are the steps symmetrical? If not, how are they asymmetrical and to what degree?
13. Right after midstance, is there an extensor support moment where the knee, hip, and spine extend together?

Pelvis:

14. Does your partner's pelvis rock forward and backward in an anterior and posterior tilt? Is the tilt limited or exaggerated? If so, by how much?

15. Does your partner's pelvis rotate horizontally, moving forward with the swing leg? Is the rotation limited or exaggerated? If so, by how much?
16. Does your partner's pelvis make a lateral shift, swinging side to side? Is the shift limited or exaggerated? If so, by how much?

Arms and Trunk:

17. Do your partner's arms move in sagittal plane? If not, in what direction do they move?
18. Do your partner's arms swing freely at the shoulders? If not, where are they restricted?
19. Do your partner's arms swing in opposition to the legs?
20. Do your partner's pelvis and thorax counterrotate?
21. Is there an ease of rotation in your partner's thorax? Are your partner's spine and ribs supple and responsive to the movement of the lower limbs? If not, are they held and rigid?

Head and Neck:

22. Does your partner's head ride over the thorax?
23. Does your partner's head move freely, subtly bobbing on top of the neck?
24. Are your partner's eyes looking out on the horizon? If not, where does he or she look while walking?

Once you and your partner have answered these questions as objectively as possible about each other's gait, you might explore taking on each other's gait patterns to get a feeling for the pattern. Needless to say, you'll want to employ a high level of professionalism for this to be a helpful learning experience for both of you rather than a hurtful mimicry.

Begin by taking turns walking behind each other and exploring how to recreate the gait mannerisms of your partner. Get a general sense of how movement in one part of the body affects movement in another part. Next, explore exaggerating or restricting certain components of the gait. Then take note of how this affects other parts of the body and how muscles and joints have to work differently to exaggerate or restrict the pattern.

- *Begin gait education during the client intake process.* During your client intake process, ask your clients if they think the way they walk has a relationship to the body issues they want your help with. If they want help with gait patterns, ask them to explain how their body issues relate to their walking patterns and describe the pattern or demonstrate it by walking around to show you.

- *Relate the client's condition to the gait pattern.* Relate the information the client shared with you during the intake process and what you observed in the client's gait to the body issues or symptoms for which the client is seeking help. The more insights clients can glean about their own body patterns, the more self-help tools they will develop. For example, if a flat-footed client can feel how he fails to roll through the foot, then he knows what he needs to do to change the pattern. As he walks, you can help him focus on rolling through the foot, bending his toes behind him during the pushoff phase. With practice, this intake process will eventually take less than 10 minutes, leaving plenty of time for hands-on work.

- *Integrate problems with gait into the treatment plan.* By explaining the relationship between the client's gait pattern and muscle problems, you can then share the treatment plan by relating the movement pattern to goals for the bodywork sessions. For example, you might say. "I'm going to focus on restoring motion in your arches by loosening the muscles along the legs and spine that have become chronically shortened. I also want to help stretch your hip flexors and extensors so your legs can swing more freely as you walk."

- *Use feedback about gait to cultivate the client's body awareness.* To build self-awareness, ask your client about his or her gait pattern before sharing your feedback. You might ask, "How would you describe your gait?" When giving a client feedback about what you observe in the gait, keep your feedback simple, short, and direct so that the client focuses more on body awareness than on trying to understand your feedback.

- *Provide positive feedback first to build your client's resources.* Provide positive feedback about the gait first, especially with self-critical clients who tend to focus on what's wrong with them. You could say, "You have good pushoff, which shows your extensors are strong." This will help a self-critical client shift from a focus on problems toward solutions. When giving constructive feedback about faulty patterns, be objective by describing what you actually see rather than interpreting what you see. For example, you might say, "It looks like you walk with your weight back on your heels," rather than, "You're holding back because you're afraid of taking charge and moving forward."

- *Help your client integrate changes from hands-on work into the gait pattern.* At the end of the session, help the client integrate the table work you've done into gait with a brief walk around the room. Doing this utilizes neuromuscular patterning; in other words, the client reorganizes the way her muscles and joints function by actively moving with a focused self-awareness. As the client walks, suggest that she tune into this new feeling several times a day, such as bending the toes or rolling completely through the foot as she walks. This will help clients build self-awareness skills and integrate the effects of massage and bodywork into a new, more effective movement pattern.

With practice, you can implement gait education into your hands-on sessions in a minimal amount of time. Remember to keep your suggestions brief and simple, focusing on only one or two aspects of gait so that you help your clients without confusing them with a lot of technical information. By limiting what you share to one or two simple suggestions for improving gait, you'll help your clients to more easily implement your suggestions in their daily activities.

CONCLUSION

The research findings comparing the biomechanics of runners who wear shoes with those of barefoot runners have provided a new outlook on gait mechanics. It's been long accepted that heel strike initiates the stance phase, although the forefoot landing in barefoot runners significantly reduces compression on impact. There are still a lot of questions to be answered about the implications of barefoot running, but the research process is a great learning tool.

Students of kinesiology are encouraged to undertake their own research of gait patterns through observational analysis. This is easy to do because the world provides us with a rich laboratory of people walking all around us. There are so many components of gait to observe. Simply pick one a week to observe. For example, spend a week watching the subphases of stance and swing, and notice which subphase is the most obvious and which most people tend to skip over. Another interesting study is to watch for the float phase in all the runners you notice out in public. As you observe runners with poor form, ponder this question: Would that person be better off walking fast than jogging with faulty mechanics?

Another aspect to consider is how the underlying postural pattern affects the efficiency of the gait. During the gait cycle, the body should return to an upright posture in the extensor support moment, which is the moment right after foot flat when the body leans into the next step. If a person is unable to stand up straight, how does this affect the whole-body pattern? Or, if a person is unable to bend the big toe for pushoff, what compensations occur elsewhere in the body? Try walking without bending your big toes and see what happens in the rest of your body.

A study of compensatory patterns in gait will definitely improve your skills in assessing joint and muscle patterns. Restrictions in joint motion often lead to adaptively shortened muscles, which cause the aches and pain that clients seek massage and bodywork to relieve. Guaranteed, if you want to continually unfold new levels of understanding of posture and gait you need only make the world your learning laboratory to begin honing your observational skills. These skills can enhance your practice as well as your own body awareness and efficiency.

SUMMARY POINTS TO REMEMBER

1. Gait, or ambulation, is any locomotive pattern in which lower limb movement transports the body, including walking and running.

2. There are two main phases in bipedal gait: the stance and swing phases. During all five subphases of the stance phase—heel strike, foot flat, midstance, heeloff, and pushoff—the foot contacts the ground. During all three subphases of the swing phase—early swing, midswing, and late swing—the foot is off the ground.

3. Double-limb support, where both feet contact the ground, occurs in a walking gait about 20 percent of the time. A float moment, where both feet are off the ground, occurs in a running gait about 20 percent of the time and differentiates running from walking.

4. A stride is made up of two steps; the average step length is between 15 and 18 inches and the average stride length is 30–36 inches. Stride width is the space between the right and left heels; the average step width is between 2 and 4 inches.

5. Cadence is a measure of the number of steps per minute. A slow walking cadence is 90 steps per minute; an average walking cadence is 120 steps per minute; an average running cadence is 180 steps per minute.

6. In a normal gait pattern, the pelvis rocks anteriorly and posteriorly in the sagittal plane and moves up and down about 2 inches. It rotates in the frontal plane about 1½ inches as weight shifts laterally, and it rotates forward in the horizontal plane with the swing leg.

7. As weight shifts from the right side to the left side of the body, the upper body and lower body counterrotate with each other in a contralateral pattern. During a normal-to-fast gait, the arms and legs swing in opposition, contributing to the rotation of the trunk.

8. Gait is a process of continual fall and recovery. During gait patterns, a person leans forward and loses balance, then recovers balance in a revolving chain of oppositional lower limb movement. Ninety percent of the neuromuscular coordination in a gait pattern occurs on a reflexive level, below the level of conscious awareness.

9. Lower limb muscles function in three capacities during ambulation. Concentric contractions accelerate joint motion and close the angle of the joints. Eccentric contractions decelerate joint motion and open the angle of the joints. Isometric contractions stabilize the joints to prevent excessive joint play during gait.

10. An antalgic gait pattern occurs as a self-protective measure to avoid a painful range of motion. Massage and bodywork can help relieve compensatory muscular holding in antalgic gait patterns.

11. Gluteus medius dysfunction causes excessive lateral hip motion called the Trendelenburg gait. Gluteus maximus dysfunction leads to extreme backward/forward hip motion called the gluteus maximus lurch. Dorsiflexor dysfunction causes a steppage gait or drop-foot gait. Psoas muscle dysfunction causes chronic hip flexion in a psoatic gait.

12. Joint damage, movement restrictions, or fusion in the knee can lead to a stiff-legged, circumducted, or vaulting gait; ankle injury or fusion can lead to a peg-legged or paddling gait; a hemi-pelvis (smaller coxal bone on one side) or leg-length differences can lead to spinal scoliosis and a limping gait.

13. An ataxic gait is a dysfunction caused by neurological effects and marked by restricted range of motion, poor balance, a lack of muscular control, and short, jerky steps. Ataxic gait can be caused by hypotonia from muscle flaccidity, and by muscular spasticity common in conditions such as cerebral palsy and Parkinson's disease.

14. Gait assessment can be general, looking at the quality of the overall pattern, or specific, identifying normal and dysfunctional range of joint motion during each phase of gait, as well as normal and dysfunctional muscle firing patterns.

REVIEW QUESTIONS

1. True or false (circle one). Gait is also called ambulation.
2. The subphases in the stance phase are
   a. foot flat, midstance, toe-off, heel strike, and midswing.
   b. foot flat, midswing, late swing, heel strike, and midstance.
   c. heel strike, foot flat, midstance, heeloff, and pushoff.
   d. heel strike, foot flat, midswing, heeloff, pushoff.
3. What is double-limb support in gait?
4. What differentiates running from walking is that during running there is a float moment in which
   a. both feet are off the ground at the same time.
   b. the feet are on the ground at the same time.
   c. both legs swing forward at the same time.
   d. both feet lightly touch the ground at the same time.
5. Name the three phases of the swing phase and briefly describe each one.
6. An average step length
   a. can be measured by the distance in a footprint between the right heel and the left heel.
   b. can be measured by the distance in a footprint between the right heel and the right heel.
   c. can be measured by the distance in a footprint between the right heel and the left toes.
   d. can be measured by the distance in a footprint between the right heel and the left toes.
7. True or false (circle one). Men tend to walk with a slower cadence than women.
8. An extensor support moment is the part of the stance phase
   a. during toe-off when the back knee bends and the weight of the lower limb initiates the swing phase.
   b. during the heel strike when the spine extends as a protective measure to dissipate the shock of heel compression.
   c. when the body loses its vertical balance and the knees and hips of both lower limbs lock simultaneously to prevent falling.
   d. when hip and knee extend to prevent the lower limb from buckling as the body leans forward during limb loading.
9. Match the plane that the pelvis moves through—horizontal, sagittal, or frontal— during ambulation with the following three actions:
   a. right or left pelvic rotation
   b. lateral pelvic shift and lateral pelvic tilt
   c. anterior and posterior pelvic tilt
10. If the swing phase is restricted, the step length will be _____ and anterior pelvic rotation will be restricted.
11. During a normal-to-fast gait, the arms and legs swing in a contralateral pattern, which means that they
    a. swing perpendicular to each other.
    b. swing in synchrony with each other.
    c. swing in opposition to each other.
    d. swing together on the same side.
12. True or false (circle one). During the heel strike of the stance phase, the hip flexors contract eccentrically while the hamstrings on the same side contract concentrically.
13. Name and describe the gait dysfunction that occurs when the gluteus maximus is dysfunctional.
14. Which joint actions occur during midstance in the stance limb?
    a. The hip flexes, the knee flexes, and the ankle dorsiflexes.
    b. The hip extends, the knee extends, and the ankle dorsiflexes.
    c. The hip flexes, the knee extends, and the ankle dorsiflexes.
    d. The hip extends, the knee extends, and the ankle plantarflexes.
15. During midstance, what joint actions occur in the hips?
    a. The stance hip adducts and the swing hip abducts.
    b. The stance hip abducts and the swing hip adducts.
    c. The stance hip adducts and the swing hip adducts.
    d. The stance hip abducts and the swing hip abducts.

16. What muscle stabilizes the lateral side of stance hip and what atypical gait occurs when this muscle becomes dysfunctional?
    a. The gluteus medius stabilizes the stance hip and the Trendelenburg gait with excessive flexion in the stance hip called the "gluteus maximus lurch."
    b. The gluteus maximus stabilizes the stance hip and the Trendelenburg gait with excessive hyperextension in the stance hip called the "gluteus maximus lurch."
    c. The gluteus minimus stabilizes the stance hip and the Trendelenburg gait with excessive abduction in the stance hip called the "gluteus minimus lurch."
    d. The gluteus medius stabilizes the stance hip and the Trendelenburg gait with excessive adduction in the stance hip called the "gluteus medius lurch."

17. An antalgic gait is any gait dysfunction that occurs as a
    a. learned holding pattern to avoid a hypermobile range of motion.
    b. self-protective measure to avoid a painful range of motion.
    c. self-protective measure to avoid an awkward range of motion.
    d. self-protective measure to avoid a unstable range of motion.

18. Briefly describe four approaches to gait assessment.

Notes

1. Lieberman, D., et al. (2010). Foot Strike Patterns and Collision Forces in Habitually Barefoot versus Shod Runners. *Nature, 463,* 531–535.
2. Saunders, J., Inman, V., & Eberhart, H. (1953). The Major Determinants in Normal and Pathological Gait. *Journal of Bone and Joint Surgery, 35A,* 543–558.
3. Levangie, P., & Norkin, C. (2005). *Joint Structure and Function: A Comprehensive Analysis* (4th ed.). Philadelphia: F. A. Davis.
4. Magee, D. (2007). *Orthopedic Physical Assessment* (5th ed.). Philadelphia: Saunders.
5. E. Muybridge conducted gait research using light tubes and sequence photography, which was published in 1887 in Philadelphia at the University of Pennsylvania. His work, titled *Human and Animal Locomotion* was republished in 1979 in New York by Dover Press.
6. Murray, M., & Gore, D. (1981). Gait of Patients with Hip Pain or Loss of Hip Joint Movement. In J. Black & J. Dumbleton (Eds.), *Clinical Biomechanics: A Case History Approach.* New York: Churchill Livingstone.
7. Magee, D. *Orthopedic Physical Assessment.*
8. DiGiovanna, E., Schiowitz, S., & Dowling, D. (2005). *An Osteopathic Approach to Diagnosis and Treatment* (3rd ed.). Baltimore: Lippincott, Williams & Wilkins.

9 Basic Palpation Skills

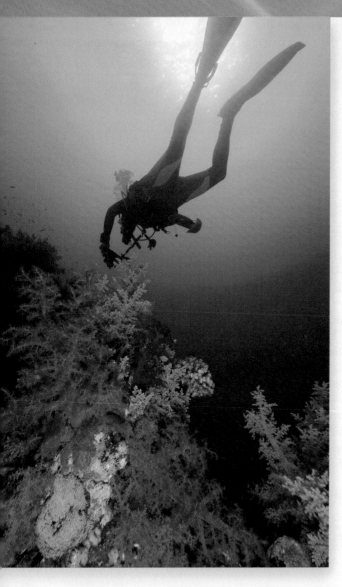

CHAPTER OUTLINE

Chapter Objectives

Key Terms

9.1 The Science of Palpation

9.2 The Art of Palpation

9.3 Palpation Tips

9.4 Tissue Layering

Conclusion

Summary Points to Remember

Review Questions

Six million people descend into the incredible undersea world of diving each year. Whether for work or play, deep-sea diving offers an exciting and sometimes dangerous plunge into a vast aquatic sphere of exotic marine life and unknown riches. Beneath the surface lurks a wealth of sunken treasures, inland caves, and coral reefs. Seasoned divers experience many adventures, from thrilling encounters with sharks to wondrous sightings of exotic fish and coral to mysterious floats through blue holes. All divers must use certain safety precautions: They descend slowly to adapt to water pressure, holding their noses and gently blowing to equalize pressure in the ears and sinuses. They also ascend slowly to prevent the blood gases from forming bubbles that could be fatal.

Just as a diver slowly sinks down into a watery milieu, so a massage and bodywork practitioner slowly presses through the skin with her hands while mentally submerging into the anatomy that resides below. Beneath the skin lies a diverse terrain of many different tissue layers, textures, and sensitivities. The practitioner also takes safety precautions, moving slowly while paying attention to the tissue tone and texture, as well as the client's responses. Palpation skills are built on a practitioner's working knowledge of the dynamic sea of bodily anatomy, plus interpersonal skills to touch another person with an attentive, therapeutic quality.

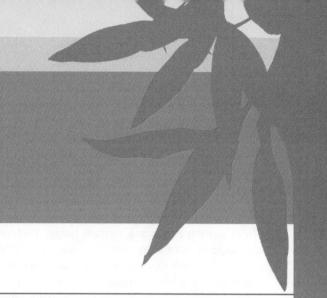

CHAPTER OBJECTIVES

1. Define palpation and name four reasons a manual therapist uses it.

2. Describe how palpation is approached as a science.

3. List six elements that are observed during palpation.

4. Describe how palpation is approached as an art.

5. Describe the interpersonal skills a practitioner uses during palpation.

6. Contrast the differences between classroom palpation and therapeutic palpation.

7. List five guidelines to keep in mind during palpation.

8. Describe the palpatory qualities of tissue layers, including skin, fascia, muscle, and bone.

9. Define an endangerment site and explain why they should be avoided in palpation.

10. Describe the palpatory quality of peripheral nerves and arteries.

KEY TERMS

Assessment

Broad-hand gliding

Classroom palpation

Cross-fiber strumming

Endangerment sites

Feedback

Fingertip palpation

Flat-finger palpation

Mindful touch

Motor response

Objective findings

Palpation

Pincher palpation

Sensory intake

Subjective findings

Therapeutic palpation

Tissue layering

Tracking

Palpation is the clinical examination of the human body through touch. Palpatory skills are fundamental tools in the practice of therapeutic massage and bodywork. The palpation of passive tissue helps us learn to identify specific muscles and joints, and to recognize what feels normal and what does not.

The palpation of tissues during active movement helps us learn to identify a normal range of motion. This is essential to prevent injury that can occur when client motion exceeds a normal range. Understanding the range of normal motion provides a ground of reference with which to compare client patterns so that you can visualize what movements caused their pain and/or injuries. This will assist you in assessing which muscles and joints to work with and how to work with them (Figure 9.1 ■).

The wide array of palpatory applications in our field matches the diversity of approaches to therapeutic massage and bodywork. For example, a visceral practitioner learns to palpate various organs; a cranialsacral therapist learns to palpate cranial rhythms and structures.

In kinesiology classes, students learn to ask their partners to move so that the muscle they are palpating contracts and bulges out, making it easier to identify. This type of palpation training also prepares you to use active techniques in a massage session.

Palpation is often practiced in therapeutic massage as a listening, centering touch—a touch that helps us to simply make contact and connect with a client. Throughout a session, palpation provides feedback on the effectiveness of the work. The process is circular: By locating tender points in the muscles, you help your client to sense which muscles need to relax. As clients become aware of muscle tension, they can relax and the muscle tone changes. You register the change of tone as a softening of the tissues. The softening allows a new layer to become palpable, and you can adjust your quality of touch accordingly.

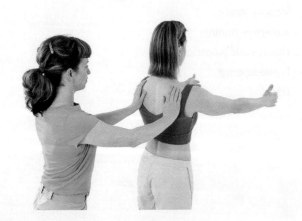

FIGURE 9.1

A practitioner makes an **active movement assessment** to check the function of the scapular muscles.

In this chapter, we examine basic palpation concepts and skills for kinesiology applications. We begin with discussions of palpation as both a science and an art. These are followed by tips for successful palpation. The second half of the chapter covers "tissue layering." This palpation exercise takes us on a palpatory journey through the anatomical landmarks of the body systems, exploring many layers of tissue including skin, connective tissues, and musculoskeletal tissues.

9.1 THE SCIENCE OF PALPATION

Palpation is both a science and an art. The science of palpation involves the ability to connect what we feel with our hands to our knowledge of joint and muscle anatomy and movement functions. In short, palpation is a knowing touch. Drawing on what we know about anatomy and kinesiology during palpation helps us to more objectively visualize the structure and function of the anatomical features that we contact.

Palpation as a science also draws on a knowledge of biological systems. We can palpate any tissue layer or body system. We can also palpate physiological rhythms, such as breathing and heart rate, as well as an array of natural movement responses, such as flexor withdrawal reflex or protective stepping reflex (see "Reciprocal Inhibition and Reflexes" in the neuromuscular chapter). In this study of kinesiology, palpation exercises focus primarily on the body systems that generate motion: the muscular, skeletal, and nervous systems.

Each body system has an intrinsic motion and rhythm to consider. In some areas of the body, it is important to follow these background rhythms while palpating the muscles and bones. For example, when applying pressure on the rib cage, it's important to follow the respiratory rhythm and ease pressure every time the client inhales.

9.1.1 Palpation As an Assessment Tool

Assessment is a body–mind process. The body experience leads during palpation. In the case of both the massage therapist and the client, the mind then processes this incoming information. For the massage therapist, the tactile experience precedes a line of thought that goes something like this: "I see this, I feel this, I hear the client say this, and all that information adds up to this." Assessment is followed by treatment. The process requires three steps:

- **Sensory intake:** Feeling what's going on during palpation.
- **Assessment:** Reflecting on and interpreting what you feel.
- **Motor response:** Adjusting your touch according to your assessment.

Although we can define these three steps, palpation is nonlinear. It is an interactive exchange between sensory and motor. All three steps occur in overlapping cycles, making palpation a fluid interchange of information that travels both ways between our hands and the client's body.

To develop a scientific approach to palpation, be aware that the brain interprets sensory information extremely fast. This means that the first impression we get during palpation is probably the most accurate. It is the "blink moment," similar to the first impression that pops up when meeting a new person, but we get this snapshot impression through touch. After this moment, the mind has a tendency to interpret and project conclusions on the experience. In addition, the fingers tend to desensitize to what they are feeling if we stay in one place too long. In fact, they may even go numb.

For these reasons, it is usually a good idea to move to another palpation site to get another impression after completing an initial palpation. If there is a need to reassess the first palpation, it helps to palpate the same area on the other side of the body, then come back to the initial palpation sight and compare the two sides. Doing this follows primary rules of thumb for holistic balancing in palpation: always palpate both sides evenly, and palpate the spine last to leave your partners or clients with a feeling of midline.

9.1.2 Palpation Goals in Therapeutic Kinesiology

The type of palpation we use for assessment depends on a client's condition and the goals for the session. Different types of treatment require different types of assessment. For example, if the treatment goal is to relieve muscle pain, palpation might be focused on finding tender points in muscles. If the treatment goal is to increase joint range of motion, palpation might be focused on finding structures that restrict the joint range of motion. We palpate to:

- Identify injured or pained areas
- Assess resting tone and symmetry
- Keep track of where we are working
- Find and treat tender points in the soft tissues
- Improve our client's body awareness and body–mind connection
- Track tissues' responses in the client
- Prepare and position a client for moving during an active technique

9.1.3 Tracking Skills

Tracking is the ability to pay attention to and follow many things that are going on at once, to closely monitor all of the details of an event. A professional tracker finds wild animals in nature by paying attention to the many details of a terrain and noticing clues and subtle markers of change. During palpation, tracking is a body-based skill. We track properties of the tissues that we notice, such as tissue and texture, noticing the client's response to our touch. Successful tracking requires the ability to maintain a roving attention. We track locally, noticing a specific area, and globally, noticing all of what is going on in the client's body and noting the client's response to touch. We even track the client's facial expression to watch for pain responses, such as a grimace or tense look.

Effective tracking is a complex, three-dimensional skill that requires an oscillation of attention between self and other. You will need to be able to track responses in your own body as well as in your clients. During palpation exercises, you learn to notice where your attention and intention travel from moment to moment. You also learn to sense your own posture, body mechanics, and hand-use patterns. At the same time, you need to track your thought processes, especially while assessing palpatory findings. It all comes together when, as a practitioner, you can seamlessly track what you just did, what you plan to do next, and where it fits in your treatment plan.

The information gained during palpation is both objective and subjective. Part of the science of palpation involves being able to discern what you actually feel (the **objective findings**) and what you imagine you are feeling (the **subjective findings**). Objective findings are the conclusions drawn from a palpatory assessment that can be confirmed by two or more people. In contrast, subjective findings are the personal interpretations that you make about what you find during a palpatory assessment. Here is a list of objective elements to track during palpation:

- Resting tone: Muscular and autonomic tone, high or low tone, irritability or flaccidity
- Tissue density
- Changes in tissue temperature
- Changes in continuity of tone
- Symmetry or asymmetry
- Organic and intrinsic movements from physiological rhythms
- Range and quality of joint motion
- Reflex responses
- Relaxation response
- Guarding responses that may indicate pain

9.2 THE ART OF PALPATION

The ability to integrate tactile sensitivity and awareness with interpersonal skills is an art. The art of palpation is a receptive, listening touch that integrates a knowledge of joint and muscle function with our ability to choose appropriate hand positions and qualities of touch. Palpation builds an important foundation for the art of massage. During massage, we must continually return to the listening quality of palpatory touch in order to gauge changes in the tissues. This, in turn, guides the choices we make and shapes the progression of the massage session.

The very act of touching another person with focused attention is therapeutic. When a client is willing to actively receive and respond to your touch, the responsive quality of the connection deepens the process. In this regard, the art of palpation could be compared with a fine dance duet.

Couples know what type of dance they like because of the overall feeling they get while doing it, although they may not understand why. They learn to pay attention to the intricate steps and rhythms of the partnership. In the same way that dance partners learn to track each other's responses, a practitioner and client also learn how to recognize and respond to each other's subtle movements and other clues. The receptive interaction between the two establishes a perceptual bridge.

The art of palpation is touch with presence. It is interpersonal in nature. During this two-person process, you and your client pay attention together to the tissues that you are contacting. The receptive, sensitive, and respectful quality of your touch will deepen over time. The process is circular. How you touch your client affects how your client responds, and how your client responds, in turn, affects how you touch.

Palpation thus becomes a therapeutic tactile dialogue. Three levels of processing occur: what goes on in you as a practitioner, what goes on in your client, and the synergetic exchange between you. Your quality of touch is greatly influenced by your focus, which needs to center on the client for a therapeutic exchange to occur (Figure 9.2a ■). Distractions do occur. If the mind does become distracted during palpation exercises, simply return your attention to your client and your work to reestablish a listening quality of touch (Figure 9.2b ■).

9.2.1 Palpation as Mindful, Body-Centered Touch

Developing palpation as an art requires a specific orientation to the body. The body is a living and breathing work in progress, a sensory-motor system that expresses consciousness in natural postures and movement responses. Body patterns, specifically muscular patterns, are in this sense psychology in motion. It is important to remember that when palpating another person, we touch more than just a part of a body—we touch the whole person. We touch our clients' aliveness and vitality as well as their fears, injuries, and muscular defenses.

Artful palpation is **mindful touch** because it is practiced with a conscious deliberation and sensitivity. Artful palpation is interactive; it involves two people paying attention together to the little things in the body, to the things we usually don't notice or know are there. As your clients sense that your hands are listening to their tissues, they learn to listen to themselves. They also learn to trust that you are paying attention to what you are doing, which helps build rapport and trust. The more the client trusts you, the more the client relaxes, which in turn makes the treatment more effective.

9.2.2 Classroom Palpation and Therapeutic Palpation Differences

Classroom palpation is somewhat different in focus from the palpation a practitioner does during a session. Classroom palpation frequently focuses on finding and assessing

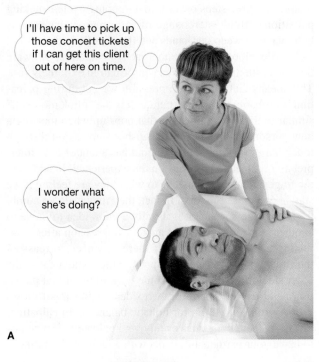

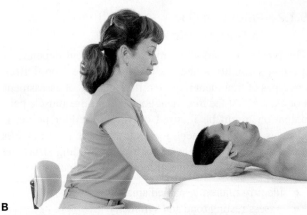

FIGURE 9.2

a) The inner dynamics between a practitioner and client can get complex. If a practitioner loses her therapeutic focus, she will break her connection with the client, which most clients are sensitive to on some level. b) The art of palpation requires the practitioner to remain focused on the client, which can help the client relax.

specific structures. This orientation changes in a professional practice. A practitioner takes a more open focus, practicing **therapeutic palpation** to feel what is actually there before looking for or assessing specific anatomical structures. The challenge lies in noticing things outside of your normal awareness.

In practice, palpation turns into treatment in a matter of seconds because of how people naturally respond to touch, in both positive and negative ways. A static, listening touch often triggers the relaxation response, which begins to change and improve the client's physical state. For example, once we locate a tender point in the client, the very act of touching it starts to change it. The information practitioners receive from our hands during palpation comes to us in a millisecond. The same is true for the client. As soon as the sensory information picked up through being palpated is perceived by the brain, the body starts to respond. These responses cause changes, meaning that palpation has turned into treatment almost instantaneously.

Given the integral role of palpation in treatment, all tactile applications presented here and throughout the rest of the text are designed with the intention of not only locating and assessing particular tissues, but improving muscular function and skeletal alignment efficiency as well.

To prepare students for success, palpation instructors can differentiate between palpation skill sets for the classroom and for a professional practice. In hands-on kinesiology studies, classroom skills begin with the palpation of anatomical structures, specifically joints and muscles. The palpation exercises in this chapter are introductory and practiced with more of an open focus. They provide a foundation for subsequent exercises and should be studied first. They also can be studied in modality class to improve the presence and quality of touch for any type of massage technique.

9.2.3   Working *With* Rather Than *On* Clients

As mentioned earlier, the minute we place our hands on our clients, their bodies start to respond. Two primary responses can occur: the tissues either move toward or away from the point of contact. The motor responses of single-celled organisms demonstrate the simplicity of direction in tissue response. A biologist gently probes an amoeba in a Petri dish using a sharp probe. The single-celled organism responds with a movement away from the stimulus. But unlike amoebas, human beings can inhibit their natural responses.

When your clients think that you are working on them and are going to fix them, they are likely to remain passive during a session. They may even restrict natural responses. But when you encourage your clients to actively participate in the session, using their attention and intentional movement to direct how their bodies change, the effects of bodywork increase exponentially. Engaging a client's active participation also empowers the client with valuable tools for changing body patterns.

9.3   PALPATION TIPS

There are many ways to palpate and build palpation skills. Practice is key to becoming skillful in palpation. Practice on yourself, on your pets, and on your friends and family. Here are some more tips to assist you in developing this foundational skill.

9.3.1   Palpate the Structure on Yourself First

Self-palpation is a great learning tool. Whenever possible, palpate a structure on yourself first before palpating it on a partner (Figure 9.3 ■). This will help you to determine the

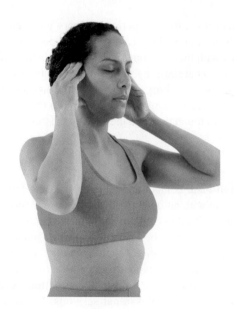

FIGURE 9.3
Self-palpation

precise location, shape, and depth of the structure. In addition, you will be able to control the speed and duration of the exploration.

Experiential learning improves memory. By learning where to locate structures through self-palpation, you will develop a log of personal experiences about sensitive or unusual structures. You will learn firsthand which areas are sensitive and need to be palpated slowly and sensitively. You will develop a personal sense of the right amount of pressure and duration of your palpation. But most importantly, you will develop sensitivity for your partner's experience.

9.3.2   Tell Your Partner What You Are Doing and Ask for Feedback

Before you begin, tell your class partner or client what you are going to do. With clients, you'll want to be general so as to avoid confusing them with too much anatomical language or technical terms: "I'm going to palpate this area to see what's going on here. Let me know if you feel any pain or anything else that is unusual." Avoid surprises, especially when palpating delicate, ticklish, or injured tissues.

The type of information you ask for will color your partner's response. When asking for **feedback**, use general questions, such as "How does this area feel?" If you ask a leading question, such as "Does this hurt?," your partner will probably focus on pain rather the general sensation of the area and may even begin to look for pain. Ask leading questions only if you want specific information, and remember that the phrasing of your question can often shape the response you'll receive.

Also make sure to tell your palpation partners directly to let you know if they feel any pain or discomfort. You can gauge the effectiveness of your communication by the response you get.

Encourage your palpation partners to listen to your touch with their bodies. Even ask your partners to touch you back with their awareness. This will help them increase their body awareness by centering their attention on the areas you are touching. Also ask your partners to notice their own body responses, which can help them learn how to relax into touch during a therapeutic massage.

9.3.3 Palpate with an Open Mind and Broad Focus

Using full-hand contact and an encompassing touch helps you palpate with an open mind and keep your focus broad. This approach allows you to sense many tissue layers and keeps your mind free of a narrow, limiting agenda.

To develop palpation as a therapeutic skill, it's helpful to remember that palpation is a client-centered skill. We want to be able to cultivate palpation skills that will work during professional sessions. Skillful palpation is noninvasive; it does not interrupt the session with its annoying demands that we "verify the results." We need to learn to move on and not get stuck on a detail or evaluation.

Never assume you know what your partner is feeling. For example, a practitioner may say, "Here's a tender spot," assuming that he or she can feel the client's pain. It is more helpful to ask, "Is this tender?" than to assume your interpretations are accurate.

9.3.4 Trust What You Feel and Avoid Second-Guessing

A lot of students worry excessively in the classroom about trying to palpate the "right" way. This can actually detract from the learning process. It is essential to trust what you feel. Learn to listen to your own touch and interpret your own palpation findings.

During class, students often want the instructor to verify what they feel. This is okay to do occasionally, but realize that it can develop into a habit of second-guessing.

Trust what you feel as you palpate. If you need feedback, turn to your own resources first. Try palpating the same

structure on the other side of the body, palpate the same area on yourself, or palpate it on another person. Better yet, ask your palpation partner for feedback.

9.3.5 Palpate Slowly—But Not Too Slowly

Palpate slowly enough to allow your hands to sink into the tissues. Moving slowly gives you time to notice what you feel, ask for feedback, and assess the tissues. It also allows your partner ample time to feel the area and the effects of your touch, and to respond. However, the trick is not to palpate so slowly that you hold up the session and even irritate your partner with a tentative quality of touch.

If palpation is too slow and you stay in one place too long, it is easy to overanalyze what you feel or second-guess your findings. When the mind starts interpreting what the hands feel, palpation shifts from a body-centered process to a mental analysis. Once you note what you have palpated, which only takes a few seconds, move on to the next area to avoid the numbing effects of staying in one place too long. This will help you move in a steady progression that is thorough but not rushed.

9.3.6 Relax Your Hands as You Sink into the Tissues

Notice which layers yield to your touch and which layers hold resistance. You may even want to call your client's attention to this, especially when palpating a muscle. Clients need to first feel their muscles in order to relax them. The tactile feedback they receive during palpation feedback is invaluable to the relaxation process.

The best way to get our clients to relax is to relax ourselves. The quality of our state of being, of our movement, translates through our hands into the quality of our touch. The palpation of each location involves a movement sequence with the hands that has a beginning, middle, and end. Pause at the end of each palpation. This provides a moment to relax your hands and to note what you feel. It also gives clients a moment to tune into their bodies and to your touch.

BRIDGE TO PRACTICE
Round-Robin Palpation

Palpating many different partners in a round-robin classroom exercise can help build your palpation skills in many ways. You get to palpate the same structure in one person after another so that you can compare different body types. It also cuts your palpation time short, which helps reduce overanalyzing the palpation findings or getting stuck trying to figure out if they are right or wrong. And it keeps you moving at the therapeutic pace that you'll need to develop to work effectively in the field.

Notice how the client responds when you reach a tissue barrier or layer of resistance. Rather then push past it, stay there. Invite your client to join in the awareness of the resistance.

9.3.7 Adapt Your Hands to the Shape and Depth of Tissues

Different types of tissues require different uses of the hands for effective palpation. The various hand positions are precursors to manual therapy techniques.

Static contact is a general palpation skill that involves holding your hands on or around an area of the body using full-hand contact in an encompassing manner. Because it is inclusive of many tissue layers, this palpation method is used to assess the overall tone and density of the tissues and is sometimes described as a listening touch. Static contact is also a great way to make initial contact with your client and start a session.

Classroom palpation, where you are looking for specific structures, usually requires more specific types of touch, such as fingertip touch, flat-finger touch, cross-fiber strumming, broad-hand gliding, and a pincher palpation.

- A **fingertip palpation** works great for locating bony landmarks or ligaments because it is a precise and targeted touch (Figure 9.4a ■). You will probably want to use fingertip palpation when applying direct pressure straight into the muscle belly or tendon, such as when you are looking for tender points in the tissues. Fingertip palpation is a precursor to massage modalities based on pressure point techniques, such as shiatsu or trigger point therapy.
- A **flat-finger palpation** is helpful for locating thin, tubular muscle bellies or tissues covered with slippery fascia, which are easy to slip off of (Figure 9.4b ■). Pressing into the center of a muscle with flat-finger pressure, in a direction that is perpendicular to its fibers, allows you to pin a slippery muscle against underlying structures.
- **Cross-fiber strumming** can be done with your fingertips or a flat-finger touch. Use it to check the general resting tone of individual muscles or tendons

(Figure 9.4c ■). It is often used to locate taut bands in muscles and is a precursor to cross-fiber friction techniques used to loosen taut bands of tissue.

- A **broad-hand gliding** is helpful for feeling the general tone of a large area. We will be using broad-hand gliding to explore the contours and tone in large muscle groups covering general areas, such as the spine. Gliding is a precursor to effleurage strokes (Figure 9.4d ■).
- A **pincher palpation** is exactly what it sounds like: you pinch the muscle belly to grasp certain muscles, such as the sternocleidomastoid in the neck and the trapezius in the upper shoulder (Figure 9.4e ■).

You can also explore the density and responsiveness of tissues by walking down the tissues with your fingertips, the way a kitten paws a pillow. Or you can trace the clear contours and outlines of bony landmarks when looking for muscular attachments.

9.3.8 Refer to Anatomical Pictures or Skeletal Models as You Palpate

The more you know and understand about the tissues and systems involved in the production of movement, the easier they are to visualize, find, and feel. When you palpate the body, visualize and conceptualize the anatomical structures that you are feeling. It is important that these visualizations be anatomically accurate, so keep a good anatomy text and skeletal model nearby to look at when you are unable to create a clear mental image of the tissues and structures you are feeling (Figure 9.5a-b ■).

9.4 TISSUE LAYERING

We can only touch the skin. Everything we feel during palpation we feel through the skin. It is impossible to directly palpate deeper structures. During palpation, we press through layers of tissue to feel underlying structures; developing palpation skills involves the ability to discern

GUIDELINES
Palpation Tips Summary

1. Palpate the structure on yourself first.
2. Tell your partner what you are doing and ask for feedback.
3. Palpate with an open mind and broad focus.
4. Trust what you feel and avoid second-guessing.
5. Palpate slowly—but not too slowly.
6. Relax your hands as you sink into the tissues.
7. Adapt hand positions and hand movements to the shape and depth of tissues.
8. Refer to pictures in an anatomy textbook and look at skeletal models as you palpate.

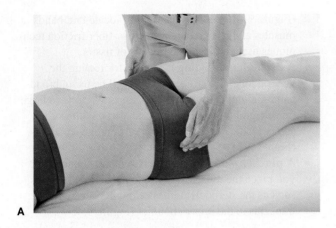

A

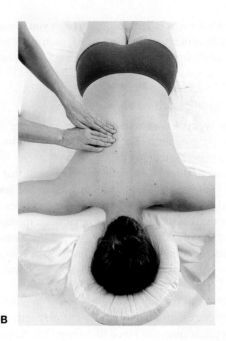

B

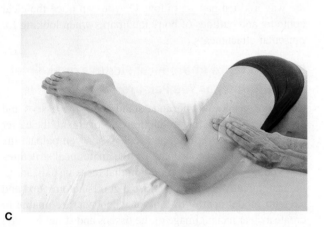

C

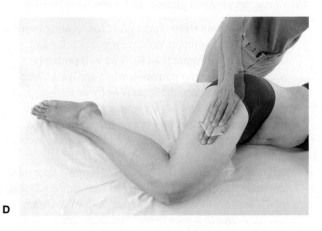

D

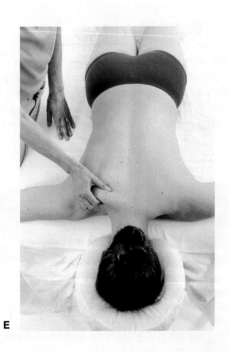

E

FIGURE 9.4

Various palpation tools: a) Fingertip touch b) Flat-finger touch
c) Cross-fiber strumming d) Broad-hand gliding e) Pincher
palpation

FIGURE 9.5

a) **Textbooks make great study aids for palpation.** b) **Skeletal models also make great study aids for palpation.**

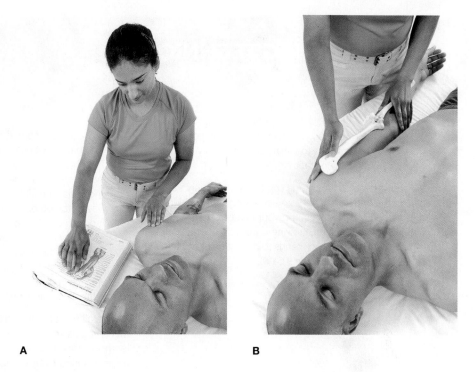

A   B

tissue layers and to adjust our touch to the properties of each layer. Touching superficial fascia, for example, is very different from touching deep fascia because of differences in the composition and depth of each tissue.

We will practice **tissue layering**—palpation exercises for each tissue layer of the body systems involved in posture and movement. These layers begin at the skin and superficial fascia, and continue down through the deeper fascias, muscle layers, nerves, and bones.

We differentiate and compare each layer in the following palpation explorations, as well as explore the various types of connective tissues. You'll find descriptive language in the exercises that give visual learners images to help them recognize what each layer feels like through the skin and how to contact each layer. In later chapters, we examine specific bones and muscles with palpation and patterning touch exercises.

9.4.1 Skin

The health of the skin is evident in its tone, texture, and responsiveness. Healthy skin is elastic; it stretches in most directions and rebounds when released. Scar tissue thickens skin over sites of old injuries, often gluing it to underlying tissues. The delicate connective tissue fibers that attach skin to underlying tissues weaken with age, causing wrinkles. Keep this in mind when pressing through overly loose skin during palpation to avoid overstretching weak skin.

Thin, dry skin can feel like parchment. Thick skin can feel like leather, either supple and smooth or scarred and tough. Skin is also very porous and secretes natural oils. Depending on a person's genetics, it can range from feeling extremely dry and papery to feeling thick and oily.

Use deep pressure when palpating through the areas of thicker skin covering the palms of the hands, the soles of the feet, and the lower back. In contrast, be careful when palpating through the thin, delicate skin over the armpits, the inner thighs, and in the anterior neck. These areas tend to be highly sensitive and can be easily irritated. In irritable or ticklish areas, palpate with a broad, firm touch.

Learning how to isolate touch to only the skin is a skill used in the technique of superficial lymph drainage. During lymph drainage, a practitioner lightly stretches the skin to pull on delicate recticular fibers attached to lymph capillaries embedded in superficial fascia. This light stretch pulls open slits in lymph capillaries, allowing intercellular fluid to drain into lymph vessels.

9.4.2 Superficial Fascia

The superficial fascia is a loose connective tissue lying directly under the skin. This spongy tangle of loose fibers serves as a basement membrane for the skin, providing a tissue bed to house subcutaneous cells, glands, fluids, and delicate circulatory vessels. Like the skin, this layer is also filled with many sensory cells and nerves, making it highly sensitive to light touch. Fibers in this layer are arranged in an open, porous weave that resembles bubble wrap except the hollow spaces are filled with adipose cells and laced with nerves and circulatory vessels.

EXPLORING TECHNIQUE
Static Contact

It is essential to learn to relax your hands while practicing massage. A good way to do this is to initiate contact with your client or palpation patterning using static contact.

1. Have your partner lie down in a comfortable position. Pick a part of the body you want to practice on. The shoulder or arm is a good place to begin. Let your hands mold around the area you are touching, cradling it front and back. Sculpt the palmar surfaces of both hands to the shape of the body part they are touching (Figure 9.6a ■).

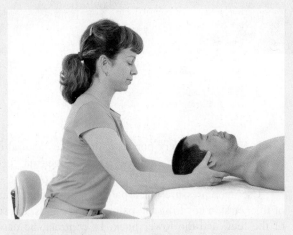

FIGURE 9.6a

2. Sense the boundaries between where your skin ends and your partner's body begins.
3. Then sink your awareness below these boundaries into the many layers of tissues within the body. Imagine your hands encompassing all the layers of tissues under the skin, all the way to the other side of the body.
4. Tune all your senses to your partner's tissues (Figure 9.6b ■). Sense any intrinsic movements you feel between your hands. Continue to hold your partner with an encompassing touch while allowing intrinsic movements to occur.
5. Practice on different areas of the body, especially in the trunk, head, and neck.

Recall from the introductory chapter that all efficient movement begins from a place of rest. This practice will help you learn how to relax your hands on the client so that you can begin working from a place of rest.

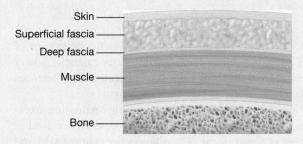

Skin ——
Superficial fascia ——
Deep fascia ——
Muscle ——
Bone ——

FIGURE 9.6b

Superficial fascia varies according to composition: adipose makes it spongier, connective tissue fibers make it denser, and fluid makes it squishier. In places where it is thick, superficial fascia provides a layer of substantial insulation and padding directly under the skin.[1] Pockets of fluid in areas that are swollen or injured will displace sideways; adipose tissue simply compresses and springs back upon release. It is not uncommon to find a pocket of fluid over the sacrum in at least one student in a large class.

9.4.3 Deep Fascia

The next layer underneath the superficial fascia is the deep fascia, a dense, irregular connective tissue made up of crosshatched layers of collagen fibers. Deep fascia is found directly under superficial fascia in white glistening sheets that envelope muscle. When we peel superficial fascia from underlying tissues, we find a milky opaque layer that resembles a mix of thin rubber and fibrous parchment. Most people recognize this filmy tissue from seeing it on raw chicken.

EXPLORING TECHNIQUE
Palpating the Skin

1. Using a gliding touch, run your hands over your partner's skin without compressing the underlying tissues.
2. Using a flat-finger touch, check for skin elasticity by lightly stretching it in one direction. Then release it and notice how it recoils. Explore stretching the skin in one area in several directions (Figure 9.7 ■).

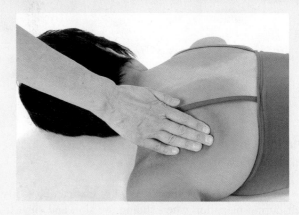

FIGURE 9.7

EXPLORING TECHNIQUE
Palpating Superficial Fascia

1. Gently press into the skin and release. Sense the springy layer underneath, which is the superficial fascia. Continue to apply light compression and release, like pressing a sponge with water in it (Figure 9.8a ■).

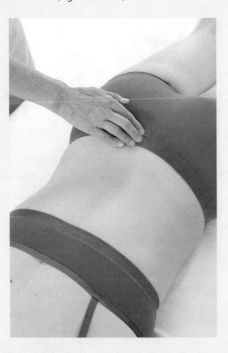

FIGURE 9.8a

2. Gently walk your fingertips around this layer the way a cat would paw a pillow. The more body fat a person has, the thicker this layer will be. It will feel dense in areas where there is more fiber, such as at the posterior base of the head or in the soles of the feet. It will feel spongy and springy in areas where there is more adipose tissue and fluid, such as on the belly or around the waist.
3. Gently lift the skin and superficial fascia from the underlying tissues, but be careful to avoid stretching overly loose skin (Figure 9.8b ■).

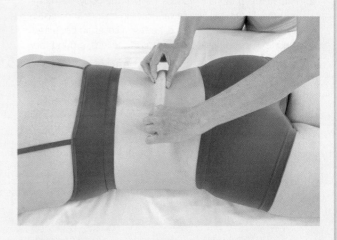

FIGURE 9.8b

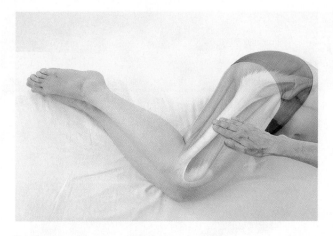

FIGURE 9.9
Palpating fascia over bone

Deep fascia has a slippery quality that can be easily felt during palpation when sliding the skin and superficial fascia over underlying muscles and superficial bones (Figure 9.9 ■). This layer of tissue has few sensory nerves. When deep fascia thickens and becomes inelastic, it can feel rubbery and difficult to penetrate, especially in areas like the lower back or directly lateral to the upper thoracic

spine. Because work on this layer can feel ineffective, many clients ask for deeper pressure when massage therapist are unable to get this layer to yield or stretch. To penetrate deep fascia during massage, focus on sinking into the muscle tissue under it. Because muscle tissue is more abundant in sensory fibers, the client is likely to be more responsive to work that makes its way into muscle tissue.

9.4.4 Muscle

The muscles play a central role in movement because they generate joint motion. The muscles are the workhorse of action; they power each and every physical activity that is humanly possible.[2] A large portion of massage education is spent studying muscular structure and function. Given their central role in both movement and manual therapy, it is essential that you become proficient at palpating muscles.

Muscle tissues vary in tone depending on a number of factors, including genetics, psychological tension, muscular strength, injuries and traumas, postural strains, and movement habits. Some people are more aware of and have better control over their muscles than other people. Because the skeletal muscles are under our conscious control, keep in mind when palpating them that you are also palpating a certain level of your partner's consciousness. The resting

EXPLORING TECHNIQUE
Palpating Deep Fascia

1. Begin by compressing skin and superficial fascia, and then slide them over the deep fascia underneath, which often feels slick, like slipping on ice. For example, you might slide off of the deep fascia when using a cross-fiber strumming across tight erector spinae muscles or muscles on the tops of the shoulders (Figure 9.10 ■).
2. Palpate deep fascia in various parts of the body, over different muscle groups. Notice variances in texture and elasticity. Contrast gliding across deep fascia covering bone and muscle. A good place to do this is in the legs, around the shins and calves.

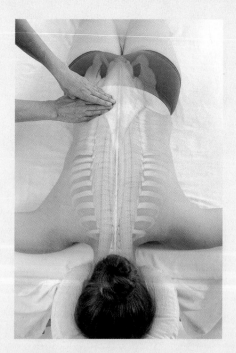

FIGURE 9.10

tone of an individual's muscle tissue is an artifact of how that person uses his or her muscles.

Muscle cells are grouped together in long, parallel bundles, and each cell is filled with fibers and fluid. Fibrous connective tissues bind and wrap muscle cells and muscle fascicles (bundles of cells) in groups. The fibers in muscles are comparable to the grain in wood, with the direction of the fibers reflecting the shape and thickness of the muscle. There are flat, tubular, spiral-shaped, and even feather-shaped muscles (see "Muscle Shapes" in the muscle chapter).

Muscles are also highly innervated with sensory nerves, so they can be sensitive and responsive to touch and have tender spots in them. Generally, muscle tissue has a distinctly firm yet fleshy and fibrous feel. Strong, conditioned muscles with a well-developed blood supply have a plump yet firm quality, similar to how the muscles feel on a horse. Chronic holding and tension make muscles fibrous, thick, and even numb. This quality is commonly reported when working on the muscles of the upper back and shoulders, where people commonly hold a lot of tension. Muscles that are weak and overstretched will tend to feel ropy and taut.

There are many ways to palpate the muscles. How we touch them affects how they respond. A strong, slow, compressive touch can help relax chronically held muscles. Deep, strong kneading and cross-fiber friction can loosen the fibrous buildup that develops in overstretched, weak muscles.

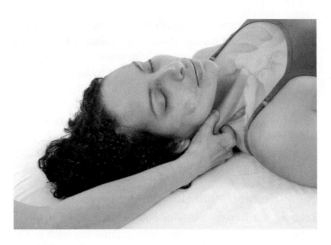

FIGURE 9.11
Pincher palpation

A pumping, kneading touch can restore local circulation to dehydrated or knotty muscles. A slow, flat, deep stroke across a muscle belly can relieve soreness and help it relax. Pinching and lifting the muscles can stretch the fascial pockets in which they are embedded and restore movement between muscle layers (Figure 9.11 ■). An easy way to differentiate muscle from other tissues during palpation is to have your palpation partner contract and relax the muscle as you palpate it.

EXPLORING TECHNIQUE
Palpating Muscle

1. Explore tracing muscles on your partner's body. Look at anatomical pictures of the muscles while you trace them. Contrast raking your fingertips along the fibers of long muscles, such as the erector spinae along the spine, then raking your fingertips back and forth across the fibers. Follow the grain of the muscle fiber. Because muscles generally hug the bones, explore squeezing or pressing down to the bone to transcend the superficial tissue layers and feel the muscle tissue.

2. Pincher palpation is a great way to feel muscles that are easy to pick up, such as the trapezius on the tops of the shoulders, or the long muscles of the limbs. Explore squeezing round muscles, such as the deltoid and triceps, and lifting the edges of flat muscles, such as the latissimus dorsi (Figure 9.12 ■).

3. Imagine the muscles as putty or dough. Explore kneading the muscle tissues on the back or in a limb as though you were kneading dough in order to loosen and warm the tissue.

4. Explore muscle elasticity by gently picking up and releasing a muscle, or pressing into muscle tissue, then making small circles. You can also approximate a muscle by pushing its two ends together, then slowly releasing it. An elastic muscle will slowly spring back out in your hands. Next, slowly pull its ends apart to elongate it.

5. Explore changes in muscle tone by having your partner first contract the muscles that you are palpating, then relax them. As the muscles contract, they bulge and shorten. As the muscles relax, they will soften and take on a melting quality.

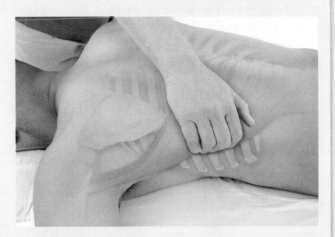

FIGURE 9.12

In this section, the palpation exercises focus on being able to distinguish muscle tissue from adjacent fascias and on making direct tactile contact with muscle tissue. In subsequent chapters, the palpation exercises focus on differentiating individual muscles and groups of muscles.

As you palpate, watch your partner's face. If you touch a pained or sensitive area, your partner will probably grimace, so adjust your touch accordingly. Also make sure to tell your partner to let you know if he or she feels any pain or discomfort, and again, adjust your palpation to meet your partner's needs.

9.4.5   Tendons and Ligaments

Tendons are fibrous bands or bundles that attach muscles to bones. The tendons of long, tubular muscles, such as the biceps brachii or the long muscles crossing the wrists and ankles, feel like cords that you can strum across. The tendons of broad, flat muscles, such as the muscles attached to the base of the skull or the gluteus maximus in the hip, are not as clearly distinguishable to the touch. They often feel like thick, fibrous bands.

Ligaments are short bands of dense connective tissue that connect bone to bone. The ligaments are easy to palpate in areas such as the sides of the wrists, knees, and ankles (Figure 9.13 ■). Because their fibers run in parallel bundles, ligaments usually feel like taut bands or flat strips of thick elastic. If a ligament is overstretched and weakened, it usually feels ropy and may even be tender. Damaged ligaments are usually tender to touch.

Many ligaments are found directly under tendons. A simple way to distinguish a tendon from a ligament is to trace the tissue from one end. If you are on a tendon, palpate along it and you will end up feeling muscle fibers. When palpating a ligament from one attachment to the other, its short span will lead you to the bony landmark at its origin.

9.4.6   Bone and Periosteum

Bone tissue is probably the most easily palpable tissue. It is dense and has easy-to-trace edges. A thin sheath of connective tissue called *periosteum* wraps the outer layer

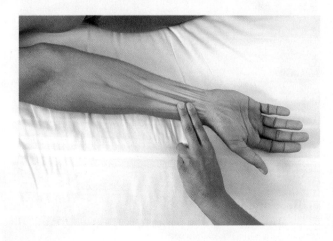

FIGURE 9.13
Palpating tendons

of bone, giving it a slippery feel. The joints are highly innervated with sensory nerve receptors to provide the brain with information about changes in joint position during movement. Muscle tendons and ligaments blend into the periosteum. When muscle tendons or ligaments have been strained, their fibers pull away from the bone creating micro-tears in the periosteum and making it tender to touch.

The skeletal system is our primary system of support. Prevertebral creatures such as jellyfish lack the structural integrity that our skeletal system provides. Given the clear shape and edges of the bones and the sensory receptors in the joints, simply tracing the bones and slowly moving the joints can go a long way toward increasing a client's awareness of bony alignment and joint motion.

People come in many shapes and sizes with many tissue variations. The anatomical structures we palpate will vary from person to person, so it is helpful to use the bony landmarks to begin palpation (see "Bony Landmarks" in the skeleton chapter). You can think of the bony tubercles, ridges, and processes as islands in a sea of tissue. When you become lost, look for the nearest bony landmark to orient yourself on dry land. It helps to have pictures or models of the bones to look at as you palpate them.

9.4.7   Endangerment Sites, Peripheral Nerves, and Arteries

Endangerment sites are locations in the body with sensitive or delicate tissues that could be damaged during massage and bodywork.[3] Examples of endangerment sites are peripheral nerves, blood vessels, the eyes, the trachea, and the xiphoid process at the tip of the sternum. During a palpatory study of bodily structures, it is helpful to gently and slowly palpate endangerment sites to learn where they are and what they feel like. This will help you to recognize them and avoid putting pressure on them during hands-on work. Throughout the text, cautions to warn of specific endangerment sites are placed in palpation exercises and other appropriate places.

In this last section, we look at two tissues to avoid putting pressure on, both of which are located throughout the body: peripheral nerves and arteries. The peripheral nerves are bundles of long, round cords. The *ulnar nerve* in the ulnar notch of the elbow is probably one of the most recognizable peripheral nerves. Most of us have felt the ulnar nerve "zing" when we bump the elbow, or "funny bone," on something hard.

Palpating nerves can irritate them and cause pain; therefore, peripheral nerve palpation is not recommended. It is helpful, however, to lightly trace the peripheral nerve pathways from the spine down the limbs to the fingers and toes to study their locations and become familiar with the continuity of nerves. As you trace them, imagine the peripheral nerves as long, white roots running between muscles and lightly comb your fingertips along their pathways.

It is important to recognize when we are pressing on nerves, especially because they can be mistaken for ropy

EXPLORING TECHNIQUE
Palpating Tendons and Ligaments

1. Lightly strum your fingertips across the tendons along the back of your hand, the top of your foot, or the front of your ankle. Be careful not to do it too long because you could irritate the sheaths around the tendons.
2. Strum your fingertips across the ligaments on the sides of your knees, ankles, and wrists (Figure 9.14 ■).
3. Trace a tendon up into the muscle belly where it is attached.
4. Trace a ligament from one bone to the next.

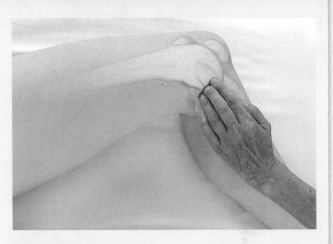

FIGURE 9.14

EXPLORING TECHNIQUE
Palpating Bone and Periosteum

1. Meticulously trace the bones in one foot. Feel the edges and shape of each *tarsal, metatarsal,* and *phalanx* in the toes (Figure 9.15 ■). After you have traced all the bones in one foot, stand up and walk around, noticing any differences in how that foot feels.
2. Trace any bony structure in a part of your partner's body where you both want to increase an awareness of structural support.
3. To feel the periosteum, pin the skin against the shin bone, then slide it around on the periosteum covering the bone. It will feel slippery, as though you were skating across the bone. Explore the periosteum of the elbow, and even of the skull.

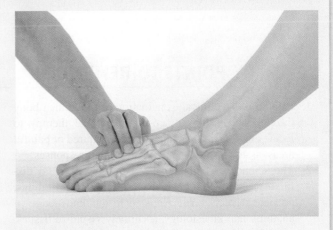

FIGURE 9.15

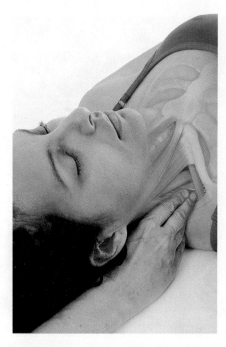

FIGURE 9.16
When palpating around peripheral nerves or blood vessels, be very careful not to compress them.

muscles or tendons (Figure 9.16 ■). We need to be careful to distinguish nerves from surrounding tissues to avoid stretching or putting compression on them during bodywork. One of the easiest and most effective ways to do this is to explain to our partners or clients how important it is that they speak up if they think we are pressing on a nerve. Your partners will know when you're on a nerve because they will feel a sharp, distinct shooting pain or a prickly, pins-and-needles sensation.

You will also want to be careful when applying deep pressure over large blood vessels to avoid damaging veins and restricting circulation. Avoid deep pressure over varicose veins—enlarged vessels caused by faulty valves and poor circulation—which are most commonly found in the calves. There are specific areas in the body in which large arteries are located. Carotid arteries supplying blood to the brain run directly medial to the sternocleidomastoid muscles in the neck. Femoral arteries run below the inguinal ligaments lateral to the iliopsoas tendons. Whenever you feel a pulse, you are pressing on an artery. It's important to avoid direct pressure on arteries because it can cut off vital blood supply to surrounding tissues.

CONCLUSION

We can draw parallels between deep-sea diving and palpation. When diving in unknown anatomy, you can visualize the inner human terrain as your touch sinks into the ocean of tissue in each part of the body. Imagine that you could shrink to a microscopic level, then dive through the skin into a palpatory adventure.

With a mindful presence, you could slowly submerge through a layer of viscous fluid in the superficial fascia, descend through a scaffolding of loose fibers, and slide between diverse cells. At the bottom, you will land on a firm, glassy surface of deep fascia covering a fleshy muscle buried beneath it. As this muscle begins to contract and bulge into a rising mound, you can inch your way off the mound, funnel down a tendinous chute, and carefully pick your way over a ligamentous bridge, crossing a joint then sliding farther down into a hard bony crevice.

While regaining some footing on the bone, perhaps you slip off a layer of slick periosteum and tumble over a peripheral nerve cord, sending a zinging sensation into the client who flinches and yelps. This jolts you out of the visualization, driving home the realization that skillful palpation involves a biologically based knowledge of the body, an ability to imagine the tissue being palpated, and the vital capacity to be responsive to the needs of the client.

SUMMARY POINTS TO REMEMBER

1. Palpation is a clinical examination of the human body through touch. It is practiced in manual therapy to locate anatomical structures, identify injured or painful areas, assess tissue tone, and track client responses.

2. The science of palpation involves the ability to distinguish between objective and subjective findings, connect what is being palpated to our knowledge of anatomy and kinesiology, accurately visualize tissues, make knowledgeable clinical assessments, and develop effective treatment plans.

3. Six elements that are observed during palpation include the tone of tissues, the density of tissues, range and quality of motion, symmetry or asymmetry, reflexes and relaxation responses, and guarding responses that indicate pain.

4. The art of palpation is the ability to integrate tactile skills with interpersonal skills, using touch to connect with clients and recognizing that the act of touching another person with focused attention is therapeutic and can initiate change.

5. Interpersonal skills that a practitioner uses during palpation involve touching with a respectful, sensitive presence; tracking both your own and the client's responses to touch; and being attentive to the interaction that occurs between you.

6. Classroom palpation is usually focused on finding and assessing specific structures in the body for the purpose of learning. Therapeutic palpation takes an open-ended focus; the practitioner feels what is there before focusing on specific structures.

7. Five guidelines for palpation are telling your partner what you are doing and asking for feedback, maintaining an open mind and broad focus, trusting what you feel, allowing ample time to sink into the tissues, and relaxing your hands and allowing them to adapt to the shape and depth of the tissues.

8. Palpation of all tissue layers occurs through the skin, which lies over a soft, spongy layer of superficial fascia. The next layer is usually deep fascia, a tough, smooth, slippery tissue. Deep fascia covers other tissues such as muscle, which has a meaty quality; bone, a hard, well-defined tissue; and ligaments and joint capsules.

9. An endangerment site is a location in the body with sensitive or delicate tissues that could be damaged during massage and bodywork and should be avoided. Examples of endangerment sites are the peripheral nerves, arteries and varicose veins, the eyes, and delicate structures such as the trachea or the xiphoid process at the tip of the sternum.

10. Peripheral nerves, which feel like bundles of long, round cords, should usually be avoided in palpation because pressure can irritate them and cause discomfort such as numbness or pain. Arteries, which feel like a thumping pulse, and varicose veins, which you can usually see, should be avoided during palpation because pressure on them can cut off circulation.

REVIEW QUESTIONS

1. Palpation is the clinical examination of the human body through _____.

2. Name three reasons that a massage and bodywork practitioner needs to learn palpation for applications of therapeutic kinesiology.

3. To approach palpation as a science, learn to
   a. distinguish between objective and subjective assessments and visualize the anatomical structures you are palpating.
   b. visualize structures you are looking for and to visualize any anatomical anomalies you intuit are in the tissues.
   c. pay attention to visceral sensation you feel in your own body as you are palpating physiological rhythms.
   d. attune to the energetic rhythms of the anatomical structures you are palpating.

4. List six elements that a practitioner tracks during palpation.

5. True or false (circle one). The very act of touching another person with focused attention is therapeutic, which is why palpation becomes treatment quite rapidly.

6. We can approach palpation as an art by recognizing and being sensitive to
   a. the client's verbal experiences and responses, to our own verbal experiences and responses, and to the dialogue and conversation that occurs between us.
   b. the client's bodily experiences and responses, to our own bodily experiences and responses, and to the interaction that occurs between us.
   c. the client's health history and level of disclosure, to our assessment of the client's diet and exercise habits, and to a mutual discussion of these topics.
   d. the client's skin and muscle tone, our own level of physical exertion and effort, and how our interaction affects the rate of our skill acquisition.

7. How are classroom palpation skills different from the therapeutic palpation skills used in a clinical practice?

8. Name four guidelines to improve the success of palpation.

9. Four ways to actively work with a partner during palpation to improve the success of the palpation process are to
   a. remain silent and move quickly, critique any feedback you receive for accuracy, track your own body responses, and coordinate your touch with your breath.
   b. look for dysfunctional areas in the body, measure joint range of motion, encourage your partner to breathe through pain, and use deep pressure.
   c. notice what your partner says, suggest ways that your partner can cope with pain responses, use only a light touch, and adjust your touch often.
   d. tell your partner what you are going to do, ask for feedback, track your partner's response, and adjust your touch accordingly.

10. True or false (circle one). We can only palpate the skin; everything else we feel through the skin.

11. During palpation, superficial fascia feels like a
    a. slippery, dense layer directly over muscle or bone.
    b. stringy, fibrous layer directly over scar tissue.
    c. springy, spongy layer directly under the skin.
    d. dense, meaty layer between the skin and bone.

12. True or false (circle one). When palpating a pocket of fluid in the superficial fascia, the fluid displaces sideways.

13. During palpation, deep fascia feels like a
    a. soft, spongy, and often fluid-filled sheath of tubular connective tissue wrapping tendons.
    b. flat, tough, and often slippery layer or sheet of dense connective tissue covering the muscles and bones.
    c. pulsating yet tough tubular sheath of dense connective tissue permeating muscles and organs.
    d. flat, tough, and short sheet of dense connective tissue crossing joints and connecting bones.

14. During palpation, ligaments feel like a
    a. soft, spongy, and often fluid-filled sheath of tubular connective tissue wrapping tendons.
    b. flat, tough, and often slippery layer or sheet of dense connective tissue wrapping muscles and bones.
    c. pulsating yet tough, tubular sheath of dense connective tissue permeating muscles and organs.
    d. flat, tough, and short sheet of dense connective tissue crossing joints and connecting bones.

15. What does muscle tissue feel like during palpation?

16. An easy way to locate a muscle and differentiate it from surrounding tissues is to have your partner
    a. identify each layer of muscle as you palpate it.
    b. breathe deeply into the muscle you are palpating.
    c. contract and relax the muscle as you palpate it.
    d. flex and extend the joint as you palpate the muscle.

17. You can tell that you are pressing on a nerve when the client reports
    a. numbness, sharp pains, or prickly pins-and-needles sensations.
    b. dull, achy pains that gradually dissipate with petrissage strokes.
    c. pointed, local pain that refers to another part of the body.
    d. numbness or tickling pain that lightly burns when stretched.

18. You can tell that you are pressing on an artery when feeling a
    a. soft, spongy, fluid-filled texture.
    b. flat, tough, and slippery layer.
    c. pulse over a round, tubular structure.
    d. tough, short sheet of dense tissue.

Notes

1. See Gil Hedley's remarkable dissection video, "The Integral Anatomy Series, Vol. 1: Skin and Superficial Fascia" (2005), in which he actually separates the superficial fascia from the body in its entirety.

2. Todd, M. (2008). *The Thinking Body*. Gouldsboro, ME: The Gestalt Journal Press.

3. Benjamin, P. (2011). *Massage Therapy: Blending Art with Science*. Upper Saddle River, NJ: Pearson.

PEARSON
myhealthprofessionskit™

Use this address to access the Companion Website created for this textbook. Simply select "Massage Therapy" from the choice of disciplines. Find this book and log in using your username and password to access interactive activities, videos, and much more.

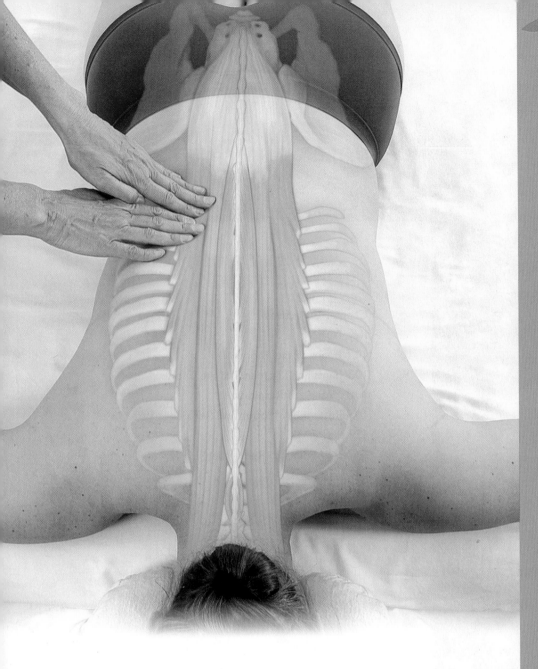

PART

2

Palpation and Practice

Chapter 10

The Thorax
and Respiration

Chapter 11

The Ankle and Foot

Chapter 12

The Knee

Chapter 13

The Hip and Pelvis

Chapter 14

The Spine

Chapter 15

The Head and Neck

Chapter 16

The Shoulder Girdle

Chapter 17

The Arm and Hand

Chapter 18

Body Mechanics
and Self-Care

CHAPTER

10   The Thorax and Respiration

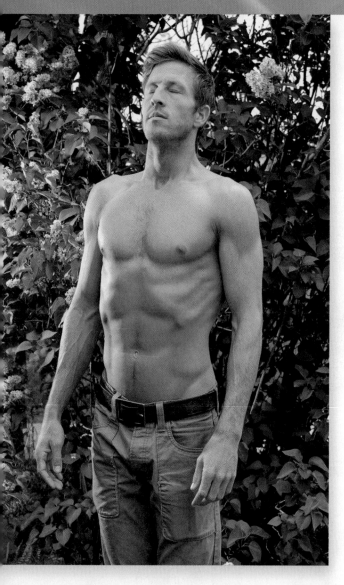

CHAPTER OUTLINE

Chapter Objectives

Key Terms

10.1 Bones of the Thorax

10.2 Joints and Ligaments of the Thorax

10.3 Muscles of Respiration

10.4 Respiratory Motion and Restrictive Patterns

Conclusion

Summary Points to Remember

Review Questions

Breathing is the most constant and obvious rhythm in the body. A focused awareness on breathing brings a person into a present-moment experience. This makes breathing practices a cornerstone of meditation and a bridge for building the body–mind connection in body-based therapies. One universal, yet simple, body meditation is to observe the breath moving in and out of the body. Whenever the mind wanders, a person brings the awareness back to the breath.

Breathing exercises are highly therapeutic and also convenient. They can be practiced anytime, anywhere. A series of deep breaths can reduce fatigue and combat drowsiness. Coordinating deep breathing with arm stretches can open the lungs and energize the body. Slow, quiet breathing for only a minute can induce a relaxation response in even the most stressful situations.

There are many therapeutic skills for working with respiratory patterns. Focused breathing can help a massage practitioner to remain centered and relaxed while giving massage and allows the practitioner to model healthy, relaxed breathing. Simple, well-timed cues can help clients establish healthy breathing patterns. Just reminding a talkative or stressed client to breathe can help bring that client into a body-centered awareness.

CHAPTER OBJECTIVES

1. Identify the three main functions of the thorax and primary function of respiration.

2. List the bones and bony landmarks of the thorax, and demonstrate how to palpate them.

3. Identify the four major joints of the thorax and describe their locations.

4. Define and describe a rib separation and a rib dislocation.

5. Identify and describe two types of rib motion.

6. Identify the two primary muscles of respiration and the motion that they generate.

7. Define intra-abdominal pressure (IAP) and describe its role in respiration.

8. Identify the origins, insertions, and actions of the primary respiratory muscles.

9. Demonstrate the active movement and palpation of each primary respiratory muscle.

10. Identify the trigger points and pain referral patterns of the primary respiratory muscles.

11. Describe and demonstrate the postural patterns of inhalation and exhalation fixations, paradoxical/upper chest breathing, and belly breathing.

12. Define chronic obstructive pulmonary disease and name three types.

13. Define hyperventilation. Describe its symptoms and what to do when it occurs.

KEY TERMS

Central tendon

Chronic obstructive
  pulmonary diseases

Costovertebral joints

Crura

Diaphragm

Exhalation fixation

False ribs

Floating ribs

Hyperventilation

Inhalation fixation

Intercostals

Intra-abdominal pressure

Manubrium

Paradoxical breathing

Respiration

Scalenes

Sternocostal joints

Sternum

Thorax

True ribs

Upper chest breathing

Xiphoid process

MUSCLES IN ACTION

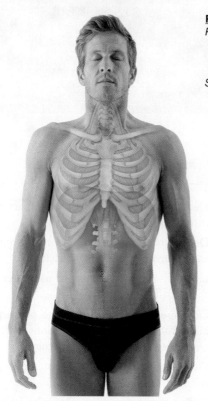

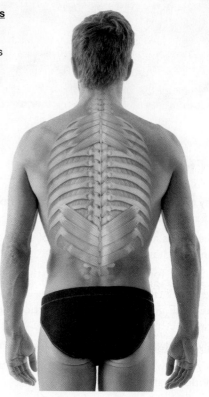

Respiratory Muscles
Primary:
  Diaphragm
  External intercostals
  Internal intercostals
Secondary:
  Scalenes
  Serratus posterior
  inferior
  Serratus posterior
  superior

Our journey through the specific parts of the body begins with the thorax and respiration because the skeletal alignment and functional efficiency of the body depend on its capacity for normal and full breathing. The first step in the process of structural integration of the body is to open and normalize respiration, which is essential for bringing the upper body into alignment over the lower body.

This chapter is strategically placed to emphasize breathing as the starting place for working with body patterns. In the same way that life begins with our first breath, addressing the thorax and respiration first has a number of benefits. **Respiration** is the intake of oxygen from external air into the body and the elimination of carbon dioxide from the body to external air. Working with the respiratory mechanism taps into a primary source of energy for the entire body. By opening up the respiratory structures first, massage and bodywork practitioners can increase the circulation of oxygen to other parts of the body, which in turn helps those areas be more responsive to touch.

The thorax forms a skeletal container of ribs with three primary functions: The rib cage houses and protects the heart and lungs, provides attachment sites for the muscles of the shoulder girdle and cervical spine, and functions as a mechanical bellows for breathing. A living being can survive for weeks without food, for days without water,

but only for a few minutes without air. The human body requires a constant supply of oxygen for survival, yet the lungs lack any direct power to pull air into the body. They rely on the respiratory system to carry out this crucial task. The respiratory system includes all the muscles, bones, and joints that work together to expand the thorax and draw air into the lungs. As the thorax expands and internal space in the lungs opens, the balance of air pressure inside and outside of the body changes, which causes an inflow of air into the lungs.

Although respiration is a reflexive movement controlled by the autonomic nervous system, the skeletal muscles involved in breathing can be consciously influenced and controlled. This has many implications in the practice of massage and bodywork. Tracking respiratory motion provides us with a great reminder that the body is always in motion, even on an intrinsic level. The respiratory rhythm provides an emotional barometer about a person's psychological and physiological state of being. When a person feels tense and guarded, respiration speeds up; when a person feels trusting and relaxed, respiration slows down.

Palpating respiratory motion can improve your quality of touch. Of all the physiological rhythms in the body, respiration is the most easily observed and palpated. Following respiratory motion with touch can help you connect more deeply with your partner's inner processes and physiological movements. During the palpation exercises on and near the thorax, let your hands literally ride the ongoing waves of respiratory motion.

Respiratory structures are a logical place to begin structural bodywork focused on improving skeletal alignment. Inhalation can lift and float the thorax like a helium balloon rising over its string. As you read through the second half of this text and practice the palpation exercises in it, you are encouraged to use a directed awareness of your own breathing to improve posture and body mechanics as you work. Inhalation provides an opportune moment for lengthening your trunk, expanding your chest and shoulders, and realigning your upper body over your pelvis. Exhalation provides another opportune moment to relax into the pelvis, which can help you with grounding and centering the body.

In this chapter, we study and palpate the structure and function of the respiratory system. We also explore ways to improve breathing that are based on principles of kinesiology. As all chapters in the second half of the book, this chapter begins with a study of the bones in the thorax, followed by a look at the ligaments, joints, and muscles involved with respiration. The chapter concludes with a look at respiratory motion and patterns. During the remainder of our trek through diverse body terrain, use the flow of your breath to keep your entire body energized and mobile while you sit and read, and relaxed and centered while you practice the many exercises yet to come.

10.1 BONES OF THE THORAX

The **thorax** is a bony cage made up of the ribs, the sternum, and the thoracic vertebrae. There are 12 pairs of ribs (24 ribs in total) that attach to the sternum via the costal cartilage (Figure 10.1 ■). The top seven ribs are called the **true ribs** because they attach posteriorly to the thoracic vertebrae and anteriorly to the sternum via costal cartilage. Ribs 8, 9, and 10 are called **false ribs** because they have indirect attachments to the costal cartilage. The bottom two ribs, 11 and 12, are called **floating ribs** because their distal ends lack any attachment to bone or cartilage; they seemingly "float" in the soft tissues over the kidneys.

Each rib is a curved, flat bone (Figure 10.2 ■). The 1st pair of ribs (top rib ring) forms a band around the uppermost aspect of the rib cage, at the junction between the cervical spine and the thoracic spine. In an optimal posture, the top rib ring orients in the horizontal plane and provides a foundation for the shoulder girdles (Figure 10.3a-b ■).

Each rib from 1 to 7 gradually increases in length and diameter, whereas each rib from 8 down the rib cage gradually decreases in length and diameter, which gives the thorax a barrel shape. Moving down the cage, each rib gradually orients along a progressively greater diagonal incline, with the

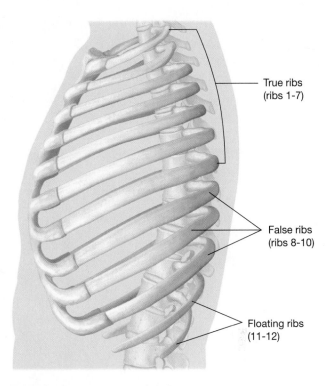

FIGURE 10.1

Rib cage: side view

floating ribs orienting along 45-degree angles at the bottom. A rim of flexible fibrocartilage connects the lower, anterior aspects of the ribs along the **costal arch** (Figure 10.4 ■).

The **sternum** is a flat, thin bone shaped like a dagger. It has three parts: a **manubrium** at the top, the **body of the sternum**, and a small bony tip called the **xiphoid process** (Figure 10.5 ■). Strong pressure on the xiphoid process could injure or break it, so avoid putting direct pressure on this vulnerable structure in the center of the costal arch. The top of the manubrium, called the **jugular notch,** has a slightly curved shape. The sternum is, in a sense, a floating bone

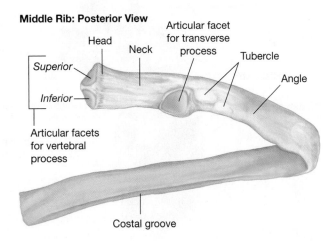

FIGURE 10.2

A rib

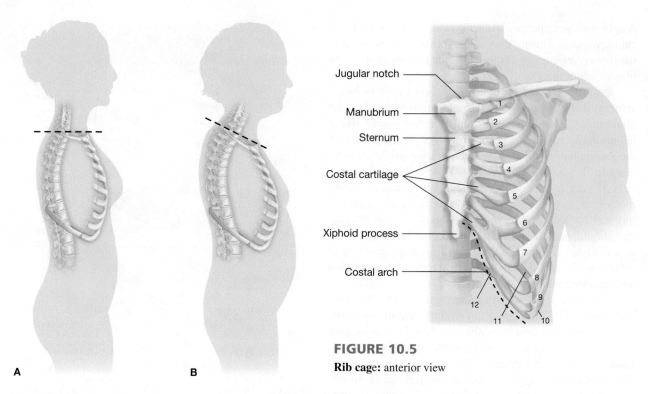

A

B

FIGURE 10.3

Position of top rib ring: a) The top rib ring is horizontal in an ideal posture. b) The top rib ring becomes anteriorly depressed in a "dowager's hump" posture.

FIGURE 10.5

Rib cage: anterior view

Jugular notch

Manubrium

Sternum

Costal cartilage

Xiphoid process

Costal arch

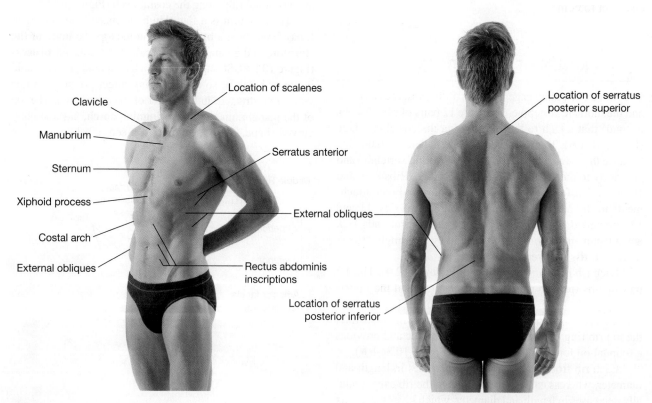

Clavicle

Manubrium

Sternum

Xiphoid process

Costal arch

External obliques

Location of scalenes

Serratus anterior

External obliques

Rectus abdominis inscriptions

Location of serratus posterior superior

Location of serratus posterior inferior

FIGURE 10.4

Surface anatomy of the thorax

BONE PALPATION
The Thorax

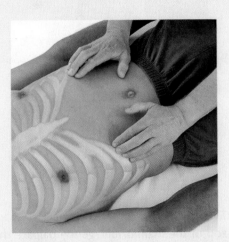

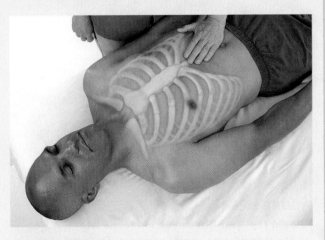

FIGURE 10.6a

Walk your fingertips out along the **costal arch** and notice where it ends along the sides of the body. Gently palpate the sides of the costal arch toward the floating ribs. (See Figure 10.6a ■) Be careful not to poke or push the lateral ends of the ribs.

FIGURE 10.6b

Carefully and gently palpate the **xiphoid process**. *Are you palpating the bottom of the sternum, in the center of the solar plexus? Does it feel like a delicate bony tip?* (See Figure 10.6b ■)

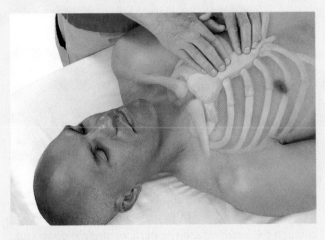

FIGURE 10.6c

Walk your fingertips along the flat **sternum**, noticing where it meets the manubrium. *Are you on the center of the chest, over the heart?* (See Figure 10.6c ■)

(continued)

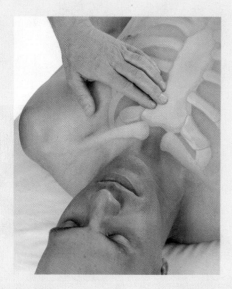

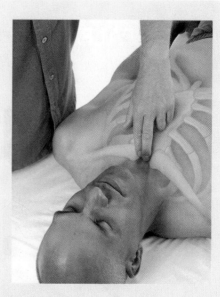

FIGURE 10.6d

Palpate the **manubrium** and feel its lateral edges where it joins with costal cartilage. *Do you feel the joint line between the manubrium and the sternum?* (See Figure 10.6d ■)

FIGURE 10.6e

At the top of the manubrium, gently palpate the **jugular arch**. *Is the jugular notch slightly curved?* (See Figure 10.6e ■)

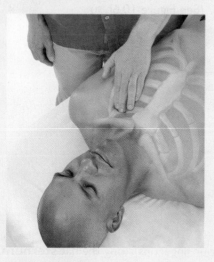

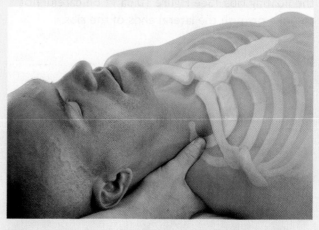

FIGURE 10.6f

Palpate the **2nd rib** directly under the clavicle. (See Figure 10.6f ■)

FIGURE 10.6g

Palpate the **lst rib** on top of the shoulder, directly in front of the edge of the trapezius. *Are you pressing through the overlying scalene muscles straight down into the lst rib?* (See Figure 10.6g ■)

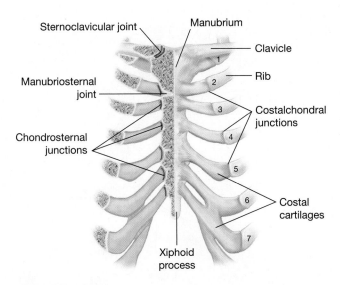

FIGURE 10.7

Sternocostal joints

because it rises and sinks with each breath cycle. It also provides a protective covering over the anterior side of the heart.

10.2 JOINTS AND LIGAMENTS OF THE THORAX

There are many small joints that connect the ribs to the sternum along the front of the rib cage and the ribs to the spine along the back of the rib cage. The joints of the thorax can be easy to remember because they are named after the bony articulations they describe.

10.2.1 Anterior Costal Joints and Intercostal Spaces

The **sternocostal joints** join the top seven ribs to the sternum (Figure 10.7 ■). They include two separate junctions on each side of the sternum:

- The *costalchondral* junction connects the rib to the costal cartilage.
- The *chondrosternal* junction connects the costal cartilage and the sternum.

Periosteum (fascia over bone) covering the ribs blends into the perichondrium (fascia over cartilage) at the costalchondral joints. The first costalchondral junction is a stiff fibrous joint; the second through seventh junctions are synovial joints that sometimes have disks and permit a small gliding motion. The sternum and manubrium have a series of lateral facets that articulate with the clavicle and the costal cartilages to allow motion of the sternum in the sagittal plane.

The sternum and manubrium join at the **manubriosternal joint.** The manubriosternal joint contains a fibrocartilage disk covered by dense connective tissue, similar to the structure of the pubic symphysis. This fibrocartilage joint is only semimovable. It allows the angle of the sternum to change as the rib cage expands during inhalation and during extension of the thoracic spine. As a person ages, the body gradually absorbs this disk, so by middle age, the manubriosternal joint becomes fibrous and immovable.

Although not true anatomical joints, the intercostal spaces between each pair of ribs serve as functional joints. The mobility of the intercostal spaces is important for the full expansion of the rib cage during deep breathing and a full range of spinal movement (Figure 10.8 ■). Several

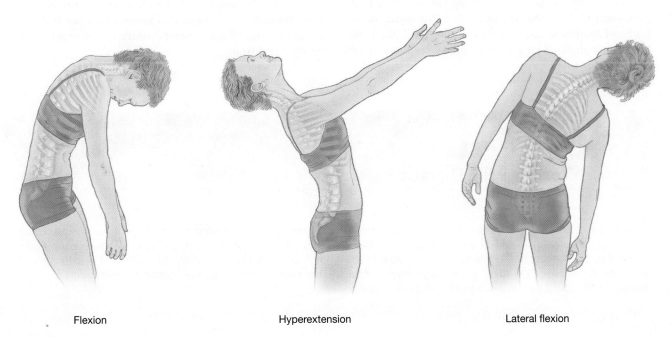

Flexion   Hyperextension   Lateral flexion

FIGURE 10.8

Flexibility of the rib cage

types of injuries to the rib cage can restrict expansion during respiration and spinal movement and can be quite painful:

- A *rib separation* is a dislocation between the ribs and the costal cartilage.
- A *rib dislocation* is a displacement of the costal cartilage from the sternum.
- A *rib fracture* is a break in the bone.

10.2.2 Posterior Costal Joints

Two types of posterior joints connect each rib to each vertebral segment:

- **Costovertebral joints**
- **Costotransverse joints** (demifacets)

The costovertebral joints are small synovial joints formed by the junction between the inferior and superior facets of one rib and the bodies and disk of two vertebrae (Figure 10.9a-b ■). A *radiate ligament* with three bands covers each costovertebral joint, attaching the facets of the rib to the vertebral bodies and disk. The costovertebral joints move with rotation and gliding motions. Each rib from the 2nd to the 9th has two costovertebral joints. The 1st rib and ribs 10 to 12 have only one costovertebral joint, which makes them more mobile than the other costovertebral joints.

The costotransverse joints attach the rib to the thoracic vertebrae at the transverse processes. There are 10 costotransverse joints along each side of the spine, from the 1st rib to the 10th. Each joint has three *costotransverse ligaments* that bind each rib to the vertebra and cover the joint capsule.

A total of 64 costovertebral and costotransverse joints flank both sides of the spine, forming two columns. Each joint facet is about the size of a small fingernail, so the range of motion in each joint is minute. Still, the combined movement of all 64 joints allows the thoracic rib

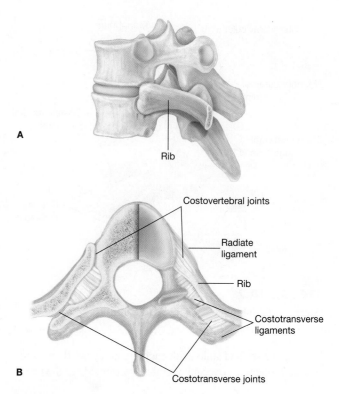

FIGURE 10.9

Costovertebral and costotransverse joints. a) Lateral view b) Superior view

cage to expand fully during inhalation. Many clients have postural strains that restrict respiratory motion. A common postural problem occurs when the thoracic spine is held in chronic flexion, rounding the upper back and shoulders, and creating stiffness in the thoracic spine. Chronic thoracic flexion and rigidity will restrict movement in the posterior costal joints, thereby restricting normal respiratory expansion.

BRIDGE TO PRACTICE
Working with Thoracic Rigidity

If your client suffers from thoracic rigidity, you can restore motion to the spine by loosening the posterior costal joints. To do this, apply direct pressure along a row of acupressure points on either side of the spine, along the bladder meridian (see Figure 10.10b-c). Press in with a pulsing, rhythmic motion to loosen tight joint capsules, improve synovial fluid circulation, and move the thoracic spine into extension. As you apply pressure, encourage your client to allow the pressure to pass through the body into the front and widen the chest and shoulders.

BONE PALPATION
Costal Joints

Caution: *Never apply deep or thrusting pressure on the rib cage or spine of a person with brittle bones from conditions like osteoporosis. Make sure your partner agrees to give you feedback if anything becomes uncomfortable or causes pain. It's your partner's job to say "stop" should the need arise.*

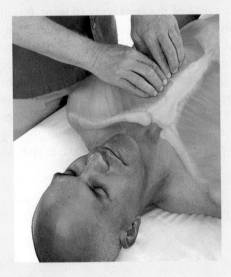

FIGURE 10.10a

With your partner supine, walk your fingertips along the **sternocostal joints**. Touch both sides at once to compare for symmetry. These joints are often stiff and slightly tender. Tender points in this area, which overlies the pericardium, could be musculoskeletal or visceral in origin. *Are any of the sternocostal joints sore?* (See Figure 10.10a ■)

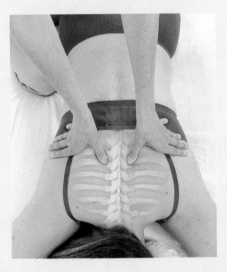

FIGURE 10.10b

It is difficult to directly palpate the posterior costal joints, but you can feel their motion or lack of motion. With your partner prone, apply direct, bilateral pressure over the **costovertebral** and **costotransverse joints** along each side of the thoracic spine. Sink in to the point of resistance. If the joint is flexible, there will be a small amount of give as you press into the tissues over the joint. *Are you about 1 inch lateral to the spinous processes along each side of the spine?* (See Figure 10.10b ■)

(continued)

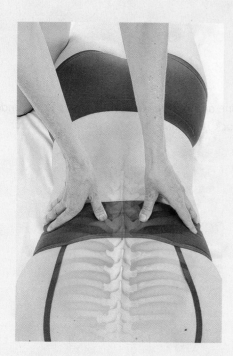

To get a sense of the continuity of **joint flexibility along the spine**, move up and down along the thoracic spine, applying direct pressure over the costovertebral and costotransverse joints on each side of the vertebrae. You will feel a small amount of give where the joints are flexible and rigidity where they are stiff. *In which parts of the thorax do these joints move and in which parts of the thorax are they rigid? How do these patterns of motion relate to your partner's posture? (See Figure 10.10c ■)*

FIGURE 10.10c

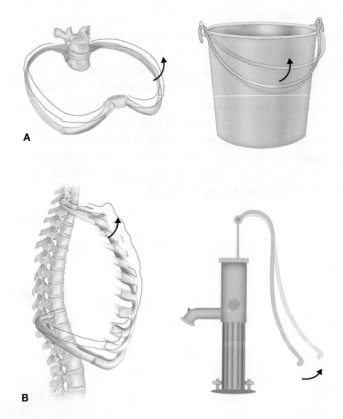

A

B

FIGURE 10.11

Rib motion: a) The lower ribs move like a bucket handle. b) The upper ribs move like a pump handle.

10.2.3 Rib Motion

The costal joints attaching the ribs to the sternum and spine allow the rib cage to expand during inhalation. The opening and closing movement of the ribs has been compared to the motion of gills on a fish. Each rib rotates on its own axis, turning like the slats of a Venetian blind. This small range of rotational motion is made possible by the posterior costal joints.

The axis of motion in each rib depends on the shape and location of that rib. The lower and middle ribs turn and lift like a bucket handle (Figure 10.11a ■). The middle ribs move in an arc along the frontal plane, increasing the lateral dimension of the rib cage as they lift in a sideways direction. The upper ribs move in a sagittal arc, like a pump handle, lifting the sternum and increasing the anterior-posterior dimension of the rib cage (Figure 10.11b ■). As the ribs turn, they lever the thoracic vertebrae into extension, which also raises the chest and lengthens the spine.

During exhalation, the motion pathway reverses. Each rib then turns and sinks toward the rib below it, decreasing the overall depth, width, and length of the rib cage and trunk.

10.3 MUSCLES OF RESPIRATION

As mentioned earlier, the lungs lack any direct mechanism for drawing air into the body. They rely entirely on the respiratory muscles for this crucial function. Both lungs are encased in a double-layered *pleural sac* made up of

EXPLORING TECHNIQUE
Following Rib Motion

1. Stand or sit behind your partner and hold both sides of his or her lower ribs (Figure 10.12a ■). Imagine your fingers molding around the ribs as though they were attached by Velcro. Follow the movement of your partner's breath with your hands. *Where do the ribs move the most? Where are they stationary?*

2. Provide light compression on the rib cage as your partner exhales (Figure 10.12b ■). Then have your partner expand his or her ribs into your hands on the next inhalation, releasing your compression near the end of the inhalation.

3. Move your hands up toward the armpits and hold your partner's ribs. Use a firm touch so it doesn't tickle, then follow the movement of the breath in this location.

4. Sit beside your partner. Place one hand on the front of the rib cage and one hand on the back, then have your partner breathe between your hands. *How do your findings relate to your partner's respiratory pattern and posture?*

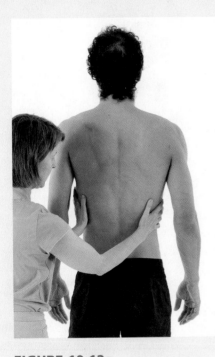

FIGURE 10.12a

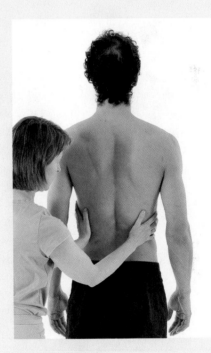

FIGURE 10.12b

SELF-CARE

Breath Support for Shoulder Girdle and Thoracic Spine

To maximize breath support for your shoulder girdle and thoracic spine as you work:

1. Breathe into a lateral expansion of your lower and middle ribs, which engages diaphragmatic breathing (Figure 10.13a ■). Imagine your shoulder girdle and arms resting on your rib cage like a coat on a hanger. As you inhale, let your breath fill and widen your shoulders and thorax from underneath.

2. Breathe into the ribs under your armpits to mobilize your upper ribs (Figure 10.13b ■). This will help keep your sternum lifted, which will prevent chronic flexion in your thoracic spine. It will also keep you from rounding your shoulders, which can interfere with full respiratory expansion. As you exhale, feel your ribs sinking and settling while keeping your neck and spine elongated. During the exhalation, imagine your rib cage like an umbrella closing around the central post, without bending or shortening your spine.

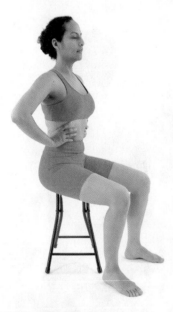

FIGURE 10.13a

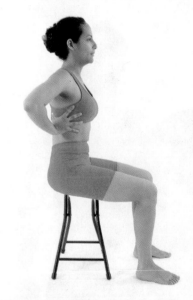

FIGURE 10.13b

serous tissues that secretes a serous fluid (Figure 10.14 ■). The fluid serves as a liquid adhesive that adheres the lungs to the inner wall of the rib cage in a vacuum seal. This bond resembles how two glass surfaces stick when there is a thin layer of fluid between them. A puncture wound to the ribs that penetrates the lung will break this seal, causing the lung to collapse and requiring surgical repair.

As the respiratory muscles contract, they expand the rib cage. This, in turn, pulls open millions of air sacs, called *alveoli,* in both lungs, causing an inflow of air. As the respiratory muscles relax, the space within the rib cage decreases and presses air out of the lungs.

Muscles that power the respiratory pump fall into two categories: primary and secondary. The primary respiratory muscles work during quiet respiration. The secondary or accessory respiratory muscles assist in the elevation and depression of the ribs during inhalation and exhalation.

They also work during deep breathing and rigorous physical activity. Respiration is a secondary function for many accessory muscles, such as the abdominal muscles that become active during forced exhalation and the cervical muscles that become active during forced inhalation. These muscles will be covered in the chapters on the spine and the head and neck.

In this chapter, the primary respiratory muscles are presented first, followed by the secondary muscles of respiration:

*   Primary muscles: *Diaphragm* and *intercostals*
*   Secondary muscles: *Scalenes, serratus posterior inferior,* and *serratus posterior superior*

10.3.1 Diaphragm

The **diaphragm** is a thin muscle situated between the visceral compartments in the upper and lower trunk; it provides a floor for the thoracic cavity and a roof for the abdominal

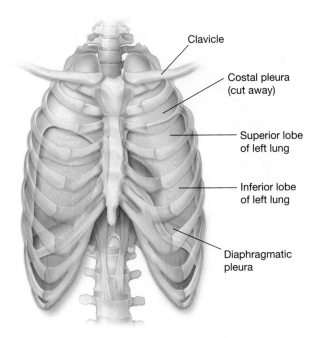

FIGURE 10.14
Pleural membranes around lungs

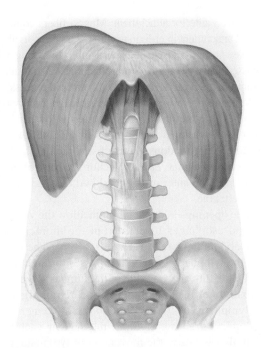

FIGURE 10.16
The **respiratory diaphragm** resembles a parachute or a jellyfish.

cavity organs (Figure 10.15 ■). The circular shape of this double-domed muscle somewhat resembles a parachute with a V cut out along the costal arch (Figure 10.16 ■). Many organs are snuggly tucked up under the bottom of the diaphragm, including the liver, pancreas, kidneys, stomach, and spleen. The heart and lungs sit on top of the diaphragm. The diaphragm is innervated by the *phrenic nerve* from cervical vertebrae three to five (C3–C5).

The diaphragm attaches along the inside of the rib cage at three attachment sites (Figure 10.17 ■):

- A *broad costal attachment*
- A *short sternal attachment*
- A *complex posterior attachment*

Along the anterior side of the rib cage, the diaphragm connects to the inside of the costal arch and the lower six ribs

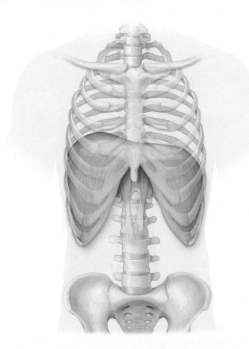

FIGURE 10.15
Respiratory diaphragm: anterior view

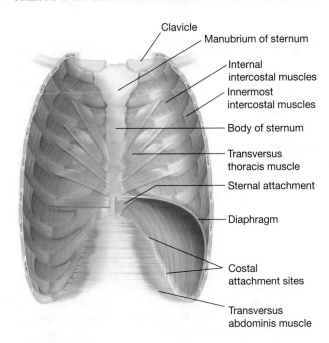

FIGURE 10.17
Costal and sternal attachments of diaphragm: posterior view of frontal section

along a broad anterior attachment. Muscle fibers coming off this broad attachment interdigitate with the transversus abdominis—a key postural muscle in diaphragmatic breathing, which is discussed shortly. A short sternal attachment also fastens the diaphragm to the posterior aspect of the xiphoid process.

Along the posterior side of the rib cage, two aponeurotic arches line the inside of the posterior lower ribs and blend into the fascias of the psoas major and quadratus lumborum. Long tendons arising from each arch, a right and left **crus** (singular: *crura*), anchor the back of the diaphragm along the anterior vertebral bodies of 2nd and 3rd lumbar vertebrae.

Three openings in the diaphragm allow the vena cava, aorta, and esophagus to pass from the thoracic cavity into the abdominal cavity (Figure 10.18 ■). The thoracic duct of the lymphatic system also passes through the diaphragm along the anterior side of the lumbar spine. Given the proximity of the diaphragm to underlying organs and major lymphatic ducts, diaphragmatic movement gives the abdominal organs a rhythmic massage on each breath cycle. It also assists in the movement of lymphatic fluid.

The diaphragm does not develop trigger points, per se, although during vigorous physical activity, diaphragmatic

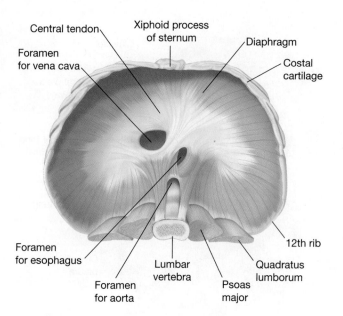

FIGURE 10.18

Openings in diaphragm: inferior view

SELF-CARE

Locating, Tracking, and Stretching the Diaphragm

When learning to palpate a complex and vulnerable muscle like the diaphragm, it helps to locate it and feel its movement in your own body first. This way you can monitor the depth and location of your touch. You can also become aware of any tightness or sensitivity you may have in your diaphragm before having a partner palpate it.

Caution: Avoid pressure directly on or below the xiphoid process, which is an endangerment site and could bruise or break under pressure. Also, avoid pressure into the gall bladder located on the right side of the xiphoid, below the costal arch, which can make a person nauseous.

1. Start in a seated position. Locate the diaphragm by slowly pressing your fingertips into your upper abdomen, about an inch or two under your costal arch and lateral to the sides of your rectus abdominis (Figure 10.19a ■). The rectus abdominis is a thick muscle, so it will be easier to locate the diaphragm if you palpate lateral to the sides of the rectus abdominis. Move your hands to different locations along your costal arch to palpate different areas of your diaphragm. *How far toward your sides are you able to palpate your diaphragm?*

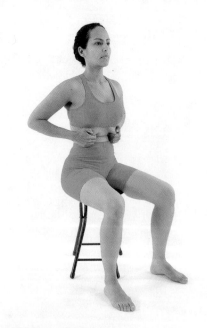

FIGURE 10.19a

2. Lean forward, then slowly jimmy your fingertips up under your costal arch to locate and stretch the diaphragm. In this position, breathe easy. On the inhalation, as your diaphragm contracts and moves down, it should push your fingers out of the costal arch. On the exhalation, as your diaphragm relaxes and moves up, you should be able to slide your fingertips farther up under the diaphragm to stretch it (Figure 10.19b ■). *Can you feel the downward movement of your diaphragm? Can you press up any deeper on the exhalation? Is your breathing any more open or freer after this exercise?*

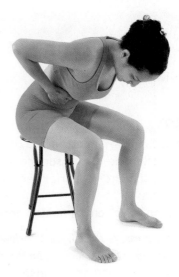

FIGURE 10.19b

tension can cause a "stitch in the side." This occurs up under the anterior and lateral regions of the costal arch, near the stomach. Spasms in the diaphragm also cause hiccups.

10.3.1.1   MOVEMENT OF THE DIAPHRAGM

The diaphragm is responsible for 70–80 percent of all respiratory movement. It contracts on the inhalation and relaxes on the exhalation. On inhalation, the diaphragm fibers shorten and draw toward the boomerang-shaped **central tendon** directly below the heart. This causes the diaphragm to flatten and move down like a piston, pressing on the underlying organs and causing distension in the abdominal wall (Figure 10.20 ■). During exhalation, as it relaxes, the uppermost portion of the diaphragm rises to the level of the middle of the sternum (Figure 10.21 ■).

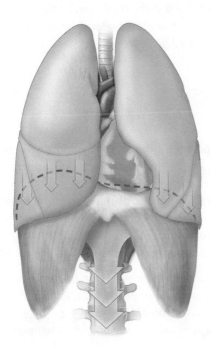

FIGURE 10.20

During inhalation, the **central tendon** pulls the diaphragm down like a piston.

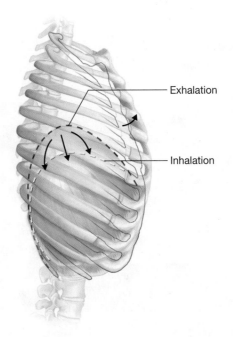

FIGURE 10.21

Range of diaphragmatic movement

MUSCLE PALPATION
The Diaphragm

Diaphragm

O–Costal attachment – Inner surface of lower six ribs
  Sternal attachment – Inner surface of xiphoid process
  Lumbar attachment – Anterior vertebral bodies of L-2 and L-3
I–Central tendon
A–On inhalation, pulls central tendon down to increase thoracic cavity volume

Caution: *Avoid pressure directly on or below the xiphoid process, which could damage the tissues. Also, avoid pressure into the gall bladder, which is located on the right side of the xiphoid, below the costal arch. This can make a person nauseous. Make sure before you begin that your partner agrees to tell you if he or she becomes uncomfortable and wants you to stop.*

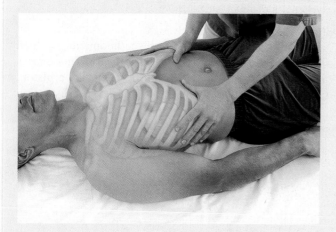

FIGURE 10.22a
Palpating the diaphragm

With your partner supine, locate the **diaphragm** by sliding your fingertips along the costal arch to the lateral sides of the rectus abdominis muscle. Have your partner raise his or her head to contract the rectus. Then place your fingertips on either side of the rectus abdominis, an inch or two below the costal arch (which provides slack in the tissues). Find the rhythm of your partner's respiration and follow for several cycles. *Which contracts first, the diaphragm or the abdominal muscles? Is your partner able to relax on the exhalation?* (See Figure 10.22a ■).

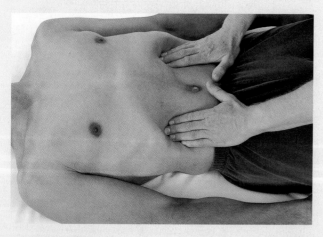

FIGURE 10.22b
Palpating the diaphragm during exhalation

As your partner exhales, gently and slowly press in and up under the costal arch. As your partner inhales, release your pressure and allow the downward movement of the diaphragm to push your fingertips out. *Can you feel the movement of the diaphragm? Does the exhalation push your hands down toward your partner's feet?* (See Figure 10.22b ■).

On the exhalation, move your fingertips along the costal arch to explore different parts of the diaphragm. *Are you able to slide your fingertips into the diaphragm more easily on the exhalation?*

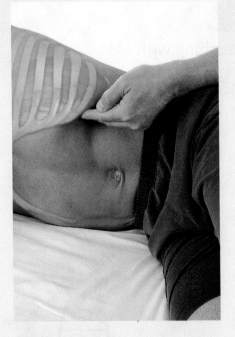

FIGURE 10.22c

Palpating the diaphragm in side-lying

The diaphragm can be easier to palpate with your partner in a side-lying position because the organs fall away from the costal arch in this position. Place a pillow between your partner's knees to raise the top thigh, which puts the sides of the abdominal tissues on slack, making it easier to palpate through this layer.

Locate the side of the costal arch. Follow the rhythm of your partner's respiration for several cycles. On the exhalation, slowly and gently press up under the costal arch. *On the inhalation, does the diaphragm push your fingertips out from under the costal arch?* (See Figure 10.22c ■). Have your partner turn over and palpate the other side.

10.3.1.2 INTRA-ABDOMINAL PRESSURE

During normal respiration, the diaphragm presses down on the upper abdominal organs, increasing **intra-abdominal pressure** (IAP) in the abdominal cavity. As mentioned earlier, the downward displacement of the organs during inhalation causes the abdominal wall to distend, but only to a degree. When the abdominal muscles are toned and the transversus abdominis is lightly contracted, they also contribute to IAP. Toned abdominal muscles provide enough IAP that as the diaphragm contracts and presses down, it can only move so far until it meets resistance of the abdominal muscles. When the diaphragm meets this counterpressure and can no longer descend, its force moves up into the lower and middle ribs and expands the rib cage. Intra-abdominal pressure from postural muscle tone transforms the trunk into a firm inflatable cylinder, which greatly reduces the compressive load on the lumbar spine and the paravertebral muscles during forward bending (Figure 10.23 ■).

Abdominal muscle tone, especially in the transversus abdominis, is crucial for normal diaphragmatic breathing. Toned abdominal muscles provide a counterpressure for the diaphragm to lever off in order to expand up into the lower and middle ribs. A hallmark of diaphragmatic breathing is the lateral expansion of the lower ribs at the beginning of the inhalation. In fact, focusing on initiating breathing by expanding and widening the lower ribs can engage and improve diaphragmatic breathing.

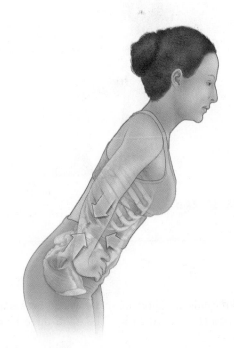

FIGURE 10.23

Intra-abdominal pressure from postural muscle tone transforms the trunk into a firm inflatable cylinder, which greatly reduces the compressive load on the lumbar spine and the paravertebral muscles during forward bending.

SELF-CARE
Coordinating Diaphragmatic Breathing with IAP

This exercise will help you coordinate diaphragmatic breathing with postural muscle support in your lower abdomen.

In a sitting position, cup the sides of your lower ribs, then close your eyes and breathe easy. Lightly contract your lower abdominals. Start each inhalation by expanding your lower ribs into your hands (see Figure 10.13a). Continue to practice breathing into your lower ribs until it feels easy and comfortable. If your diaphragm and obliques are tight, it will be difficult to breathe this way and will take practice.

1. Place your hands on your lower abdominal muscles, then allow your abdominal muscles to relax and distend your belly. With your belly distended, take several breaths, expanding your lower ribs as you inhale (Figure 10.24a ■). *Does distending the belly restrict the expansion of your ribs as you inhale?*

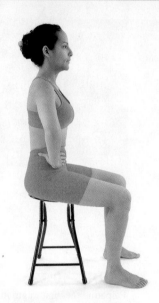

FIGURE 10.24b

2. Slowly and lightly contract your transversus abdominis by drawing your lower abdominal wall back toward your sacrum (Figure 10.24b ■). Use one-third maximum effort and hold.

Keep holding your lower abdominals and put your hands back on your lower ribs. Then breathe into the lateral expansion of the lower ribs. *Does this feel easier than trying to do diaphragmatic breathing with your abdomen distended?*

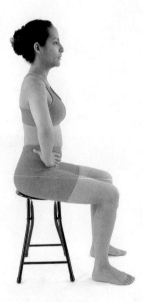

FIGURE 10.24a

10.3.2 Intercostals

The intercostals are short muscles located between each pair of ribs (Figure 10.25 ■). There are three layers of intercostals:

- External intercostals: the superficial layer
- Internal intercostals: the middle layer
- Subcostales: the deepest layer

The **external intercostals** begin lateral to the costal cartilage and extend along the sides and backs of the ribs, ending under the erector spinae muscles. They run along the same diagonal line of pull as the external obliques, perpendicular to the internal intercostals. The **internal intercostals** fill the anterior intercostal spaces directly lateral to the sternum and only extend to the sides of the body. The internal intercostals run along the

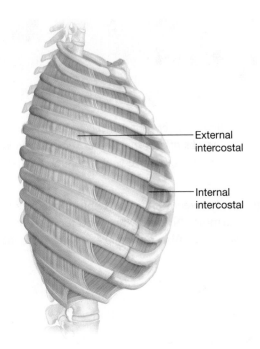

FIGURE 10.25
Intercostal muscles

same line of pull as the internal obliques. The **subcostales** lie inside the anterior lower ribs and are impossible to palpate.

The function of the internal and external intercostals is somewhat controversial. It is generally thought that the external intercostals elevate the ribs during inhalation and the internal intercostals depress the ribs during exhalation, although activity has been found in both muscles during inhalation. The subcostales assist lower rib depression during exhalation. *Intercostal nerves* from the 2nd through the 12th thoracic segments innervate the intercostals. (See TrPs for intercostals in Figure 10.26. ■)

10.3.3 Accessory Muscles of Respiration

A number of accessory muscles of respiration become active during deep breathing (Table 10.1 ■). They also work during rigorous movements that require more oxygen to fuel the increased demands of muscular activity.

Deep or forced inhalation engages accessory breathing muscles in the shoulder and neck: the *scalenes, sternocleidomastoid, pectoralis minor, serratus anterior,* and *upper trapezius.* This group of muscles elevates the

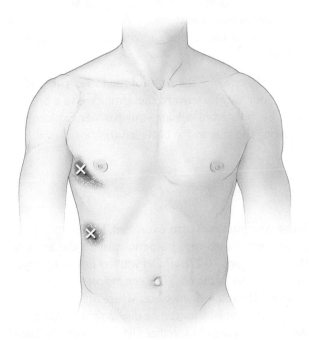
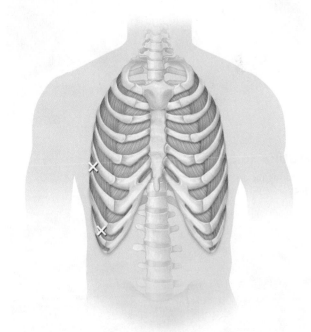

FIGURE 10.26

Trigger points develop in **intercostal muscles** in two places: several inches lateral and inferior to the nipple and several inches lateral of the costal arch between the 8th and 9th ribs. Intercostal trigger points can cause referred pain in the chest during deep breathing and pain along the sides of the ribs when rotating the spine. Tender points can be found in the intercostal muscles in abnormally narrowed spaces between the ribs, which may indicate muscular tension and fascial gluing in the intercostals.

MUSCLE PALPATION
Intercostals

Caution: Avoid direct pressure on breast tissue. To palpate the sides of the ribs safely, put your client in a side-lying so that the breasts fall away from the ribs. In addition, pressure between the ribs affects the pleural sac over the lung, so palpate carefully and avoid deep pressure over sore spots. Also, ask your partner to give your feedback if anything becomes uncomfortable.

Palpate the intercostal muscles on yourself by sliding your fingertips between your ribs. Explore the intercostal spaces on both sides of your rib cage, from your waist to your armpits. Notice where you feel respiratory movement between the ribs, which indicates the intercostals are working. Also notice areas where the intercostals feel thick and fibrous, immobile, or even sore.

External and Internal Intercostals

O–Inferior border of upper rib
I–Superior border of lower rib
A–Elevates and separates ribs on inhalation, depresses ribs on exhalation, stabilizes upper ribs

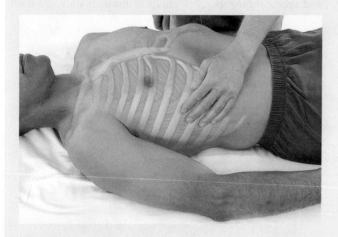

FIGURE 10.27a

Palpating the anterior intercostals

With your partner supine, begin palpating the **intercostals** between the ribs along the sides of the body (Figure 10.27a ■). Move your fingertips along the ribs toward the shoulder and armpit. Palpate across the ribs along the sides of the sternum. As you palpate the rib cage, let your hands ride on top of the respiratory motion.

Then palpate along the sides of the lower ribs and work your way up toward the armpits. Use a broad, firm touch to avoid tickling your partner. Explore tracing along the ribs and in between the ribs.

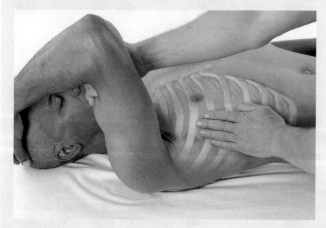

FIGURE 10.27b

Palpating the lateral intercostals

Raise your partner's arm overhead. Then explore strumming the rib cage perpendicular to the angle of the ribs (Figure 10.27b ■). *Did you feel any sharp edges along the sides of the ribs? This can indicate a rib that is turned. Did you feel any places where the intercostal spaces felt narrow? This can be due to tight myofascia that has glued the ribs together. Did you notice any fascial thickenings over the ribs? Women tend to develop tissue buildup over the sides of the ribs under the bra's elastic straps. With your partner in a prone position, palpate the back of the ribs from the shoulders to the lower back.*

TABLE 10.1 Accessory Muscles of Respiration

Muscles Active during Forced Inhalation	Action
Scalenes	Assists inspiration by elevating first three ribs
Sternocleidomastoid	Elevates anterior aspect of upper two ribs
Pectoralis minor	Elevates upper three ribs in lateral chest
Serratus anterior	Elevates lateral aspect of upper nine ribs
Upper trapezius	Elevates scapula and clavicle
Serratus posterior superior	Elevates posterior aspect of upper four ribs
Levatores costarum	Assists elevation of posterior medial aspect of all 12 ribs
Quadratus lumborum	Stabilizes lower ribs against pull of diaphragm

Muscles Active during Forced Exhalation	Action
Transversus thoracis	Depresses anterior lower ribs toward sternum
Internal intercostals	Depresses ribs
Serratus posterior inferior	Depresses lower four ribs on back
Transversus abdominis	Compresses abdominal cavity
External and internal obliques	Compress abdominal cavity
Rectus abdominis	Flexes trunk

ribs and shoulder girdle to increase lung volume (Figure 10.28a-b ■). The *quadratus lumborum* also works during inhalation to stabilize the lower ribs as the diaphragm pulls the thorax away from the pelvis.

The accessory breathing muscles will only elevate the ribs on inhalation if their cervical and scapular origins in the neck are stable. Stability requires optimal posture, specifically, symmetry and width in the shoulder girdle plus length and core alignment in the neck. When the neck is elongated and stable, the respiratory muscles connecting the neck to the ribs will lift the ribs toward the neck on inhalation. If the neck is collapsed and unstable, these same muscles will pull the neck down toward the ribs on inhalation, failing to expand the thorax. To feel the accessory muscles working during forced inhalation, take a large gasp and notice how many more muscles in your neck and upper shoulders become active.

During deep or forced exhalation, the *transversus thoracis* depresses the anterior aspect of the lower ribs toward the sternum (Figure 10.29a ■). The *serratus posterior inferior* and *internal intercostals* depress the ribs (Figure 10.29b ■). Also, the *transversus abdominis, internal* and *external obliques,* and *rectus abdominis* compress

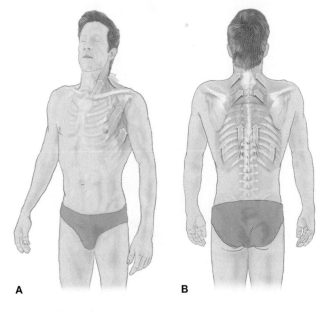

A   **B**

FIGURE 10.28

Muscles active in forced inhalation: a) sterbocleidomastoid, pectoralis minor, serratus anterior, upper trapezis b) serratus posterior inferior, and internal intercostals

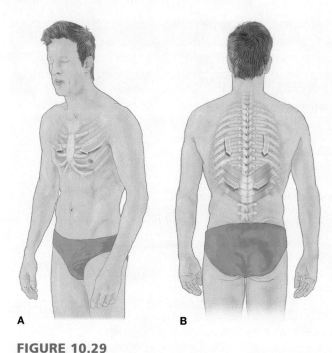

A   **B**

FIGURE 10.29

Muscles active in forced exhalation: a) Transversus thoracis
b) Serratus posterior inferior and internal intercostals

the abdominal cavity from all directions to increase intra-abdominal pressure (Figure 10.30 ■). As they compress the abdomen, they push the diaphragm upward, which helps decrease lung volume and expel air during exhalation. To feel the accessory muscles working during forced exhalation, cough and notice how your ribs depress and abdominal muscles squeeze the waist.

All of the accessory muscles also function in capacities other than breathing, including as stabilizers, synergists, prime movers, and antagonists. These muscles are covered in subsequent chapters according to their location and function.

10.3.3.1 SCALENE MUSCLE GROUP

Three **scalenes**—anterior, middle, and posterior—arise from the transverse processes of the 2nd through 6th cervical vertebrae and insert on the 1st and 2nd ribs (Figure 10.31 ■). The scalenes are innervated by the anterior branches of the *lower cervical nerves* and have multiple functions. During respiration, when the cervical origins of the scalenes are fixed, the scalenes elevate the upper ribs on inhalation. When the costal insertions of the scalenes are fixed, they work as lateral flexors of the cervical spine. The scalenes also assist in the stabilization of the lower cervical spine.

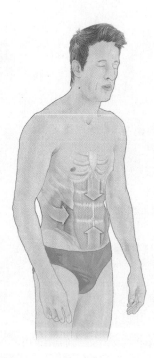

FIGURE 10.30

Abdominal muscles active in forced exhalation: rectus
abdominis and obliques

Anterior View

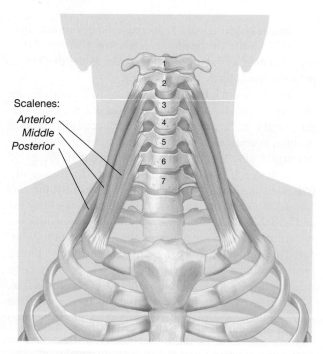

Scalenes:
Anterior
Middle
Posterior

1
2
3
4
5
6
7

FIGURE 10.31
Scalenes

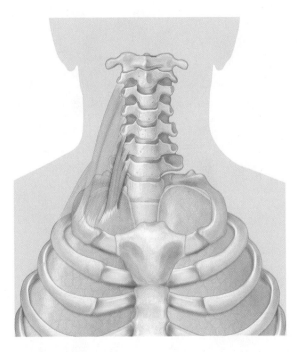

FIGURE 10.32

Fourth scalene

The scalenes can have variations in their attachments. The posterior scalene sometimes extends down to the 3rd rib. A fourth scalene muscle is also present in over half of the population.[1] This small muscle arises from the tubercles of the lower cervical vertebrae and inserts on the pleural fascia over the apex of the lungs medial to the 1st rib (Figure 10.32 ■).

When the shoulders are relaxed and resting on the rib cage and the neck is extended and upright, the scalenes literally suspend the upper ribs from the cervical spine (Figure 10.33a ■). If the shoulders are hiked or the neck collapses into an excessive curve, the scalenes tend to pull the cervical spine down toward the ribs (Figure 10.33b ■). Contractures and spasms in the scalenes elevate the 1st and 2nd ribs and can lead to both neural and vascular entrapment, a symptom of **thoracic outlet syndrome.** Clients with chronic contractures in the scalenes tend to frequently and restlessly move their head looking for relief. (See TrP for scalenes in Figure 10.34. ■)

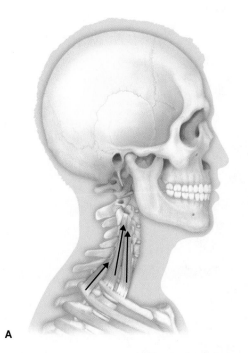

A   B

FIGURE 10.33

Action of the scalenes: a) Scalenes lifting the upper ribs b) Reverse action of the scalenes pulling the cervical spine toward the upper ribs

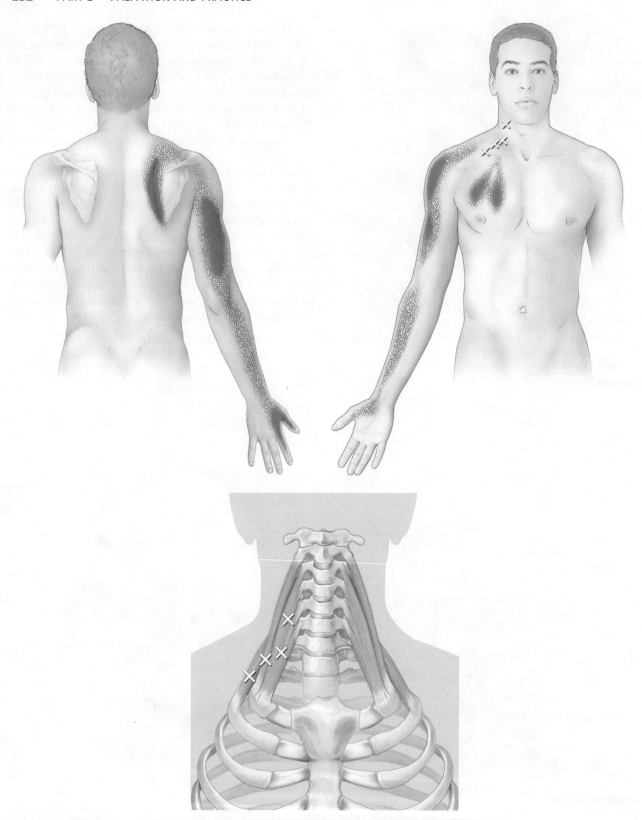

FIGURE 10.34

When dysfunctional, the **scalenes** often develop trigger points in the distal third of the muscles that are tender to touch, particularly in people with chronic neck and shoulder pain. The anterior scalene, which tends to be the most problematic, can develop two trigger points along the belly of the muscle. Taut bands usually develop in the scalenes in conjunction with trigger points, referring pain to the upper medial border of the scapula, over the top of the shoulder and into the upper arm, and into the thumb and index finger. Symptoms of scalene trigger points also include numbness and tingling in the fingers, a stiff neck, and stiffness in the fingers upon awakening.

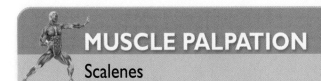

MUSCLE PALPATION
Scalenes

Palpate the scalenes on yourself by pressing into the soft tissue above your clavicle, directly posterior to the sternocleidomastoid muscle. Hold this area and take a deep breath to feel the scalenes contract. Strum across the bellies of the scalenes, then walk your fingertips up the scalenes. They usually feel ropey, and may even have tender points in them.

Hold both sides at once to see if they are symmetrical. While still holding them, lift the back of your head without lowering your chin to feel how the scalenes elevate the upper ribs. Then collapse your neck to feel how the scalenes pull the neck down in this postural aberration. Now palpate the scalenes with the head rotated to one side. Turning the head takes slack out of the scalenes and causes the sternocleidomastoid (SCM) to contract, making the scalenes easier to locate.

Note: It is easy to mistake the omohyoid muscle for the anterior scalene. The omohyoid runs diagonally across the scalenes and can be felt as a bulge when moving up and down the anterior scalene.

Caution: When palpating the scalenes, be careful not to put pressure on the subclavian artery or brachial nerves. Stop immediately if your partner reports any symptoms, such as dizziness or nerve pain.

Anterior Scalene

O–Anterior tubercles of transverse processes from
    C-3 to C-6
I–Inner border of 1st rib, anterior to subclavian artery
A–Elevates ribs on inhalation, flexes neck laterally,
    assists neck rotation

Middle Scalene

O–Posterior tubercles of transverse processes from
    C-2 to C-7
I–Below cranial surface of 1st rib, posterior to sub-
    clavian artery
A–Elevates ribs on inhalation, flexes neck laterally,
    assists neck rotation

Posterior Scalene

O–Above posterior tubercles of transverse pro-
    cesses from C-6 and C-7
I–Lateral surface of 2nd rib
A–Elevates ribs on inhalation, flexes neck laterally,
    assists neck rotation

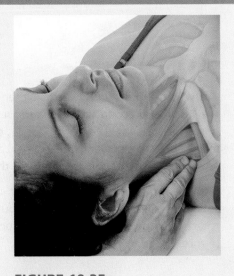

FIGURE 10.35a

Palpating the scalenes

With your partner supine, palpate the anterior scalene and middle scalene by gently but firmly pressing laterally along the distal tendons of the sternocleidomastoid (SCM), right above the upper border of the clavicle. Locate the anterior scalene directly behind the lateral edge of the clavicular head of the SCM (Figure 10.35a ■). Locate the middle scalene behind the anterior scalene and the vertebral artery (which will feel like a thumping pulse). Explore gently pressing into the muscle bellies and into the insertions on the 1st and 2nd ribs. Palpate the scalenes on both sides at once to check for muscle symmetry. *Do the scalenes feel taut and ropey?*

(continued)

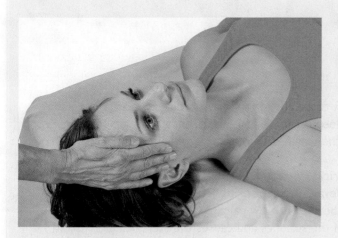

FIGURE 10.35b
Resisted movement of the scalenes

Active movement: Rest your finger pads over the scalenes, then have your partner take several short breaths. You should feel the scalenes contract and relax on each breath cycle.

Resisted movement: Have your partner resist and side-bend the neck as you lightly press against the side of the head (Figure 10.35b ■). *Can you feel the scalenes contract as your partner takes a deep breath or bends the neck to the side?*

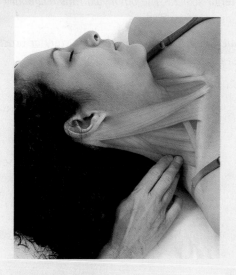

FIGURE 10.35c
Palpating the posterior scalene

The **posterior scalene** is the most difficult to palpate. The posterior scalene is usually tender. To locate it, roll your fingertips off the front edge of the trapezius, then tuck your fingertips under the trapezius to locate the levator scapulae (Figure 10.35c ■).

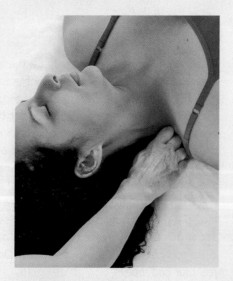

FIGURE 10.35d
Active pin and stretch of the scalenes

Active movement: Have your partner slightly elevate the shoulder to contract the levator scapulae. The posterior scalene will be right in front of it. Press the muscle belly toward its lower cervical attachments. Follow the muscle to its insertion on the 2nd rib.

Active pin and stretch: Pin the lower insertions of the scalenes against the neck, then have you partner slowly rotate the head away from your pressure to stretch (Figure 10.35d ■).

10.3.3.2 SERRATUS POSTERIOR SUPERIOR AND SERRATUS POSTERIOR INFERIOR

The serratus posterior superior and serratus posterior inferior are small muscles along the spine that assist respiration (Figure 10.36 ■). These two muscles cross the erector spinae muscles like strapping tape, anchoring the erectors to the rib cage. The serratus posterior superior and serratus posterior inferior are about the same shape and size. Both muscles are innervated by the *thoracic nerves* at the respective vertebral segments.

The **serratus posterior superior**, a serrated muscle with four fascicles, arises from fascia over the 6th cervical vertebra to the 2nd thoracic vertebra and inserts on ribs 2 to 5 under the medial border of the scapula. This small muscle lies deep to the rhomboid minor and upper half of the rhomboid major. Its diagonally oriented fibers elevate the upper thorax and ribs during inspiration. (See TrP for serratus posterior superior in Figure 10.37 ■.)

The **serratus posterior inferior** is a serrated muscle with four fascicles and is shaped like a parallelogram. It is a mirror image of the serratus posterior superior, with diagonal fibers that run in the opposite direction, upward from its origin along the spinous process of the 11th thoracic vertebra through the 2nd lumbar vertebra. Its insertions on ribs 9 to 12 allow it to stabilize the lower ribs against the upward pull of the diaphragm during inhalation. A unilateral contraction of the serratus posterior inferior on one side assists the lateral rotation of the trunk. This small muscle becomes chronically tight in an exaggerated lumbar lordosis, in which case it can be difficult to palpate because it gets buried in thick thoracolumbar fascia along with the lower ribs. (See TrP for serratus posterior superior in Figure 10.38 ■.)

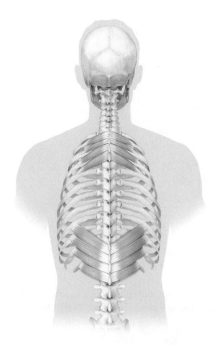

FIGURE 10.36

Serratus posterior superior and serratus posterior inferior

10.4 RESPIRATORY MOTION AND RESTRICTIVE PATTERNS

People develop restrictions to breathing for a number of reasons. They might have a belief system about how they should breathe or a postural pattern that prevents full respiration. Chronic respiratory illnesses and disease can also restrict normal respiration. Injuries, traumas, or even chronic pain patterns can limit full breathing.

Breathing is a movement sequence. Four phases of respiration occur during the sequence of one breath cycle: the inhalation, a slight pause, the exhalation, a longer pause. Normal breathing expands the anterior-posterior, the lateral, and the vertical dimension of the trunk. Every inhalation moves the spine into a subtle physiological extension. Every exhalation moves the spine into a subtle physiological flexion.

People can develop holding patterns in the respiratory muscles and become fixated along any phase of the sequence. At one extreme a person develops an **inhalation fixation,** where the intercostal and accessory inspiration muscles hold the rib cage in an inflated, barrel-chested posture. A person with this pattern has difficulty relaxing the respiratory muscles and allowing a full exhalation. At the other extreme a person develops an **exhalation fixation,** where the abdominal muscles and accessory exhalation muscles hold the rib cage in a deflated, sunken posture. A person with this pattern has trouble expanding the rib cage and breathing fully, which limits oxygen intake. To release an exhalation fixation, a person can practice diaphragmatic breathing and forced inhalation exercises that intentionally expand the rib cage and the lungs.

Massage and bodywork can be very helpful in loosening chronic muscular tensions that restrict normal respiration. You can observe and palpate respiratory motion to determine which areas of the rib cage and which phase of respiration are restricted.

Chronic tension or weakness in accessory respiratory muscles can also be addressed with either relaxation and stretching exercises or strengthening exercises to restore normal breathing.

10.4.1 Paradoxical and Upper Chest Breathing

A number of conditions cause **paradoxical breathing,** a pattern in which the chest wall constricts and moves in on the inhalation, then expands and moves out on exhalation. This reverse breathing pattern occurs in people with severe respiratory distress, chronically obstructed airways, spinal cord injuries that cause paralysis of muscles below the diaphragm, and multiple rib fractures from a crush injury.

Upper chest breathing is commonly referred to as paradoxical breathing, but this pattern is somewhat different. Upper chest breathers generally contract the abdominal muscles to lift and expand the upper chest during inhalation

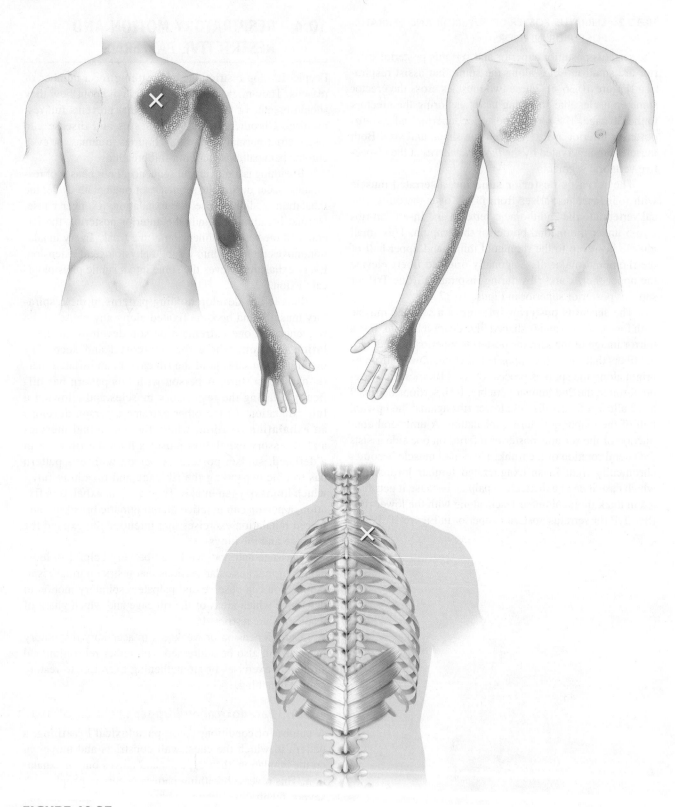

FIGURE 10.37

When dysfunctional, the **serratus posterior superior** can develop a trigger point in the scapular region that can refer deep pain and numbness over the scapula. Spillover pain can extend over the shoulder down the triceps and posterior elbow to the little finger. To access this trigger point, press under the upper medial border of the scapula.

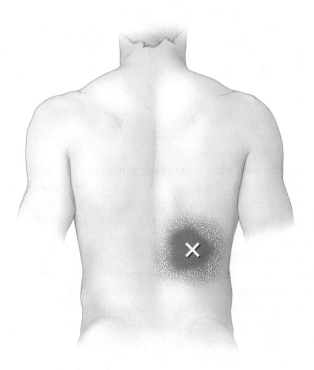
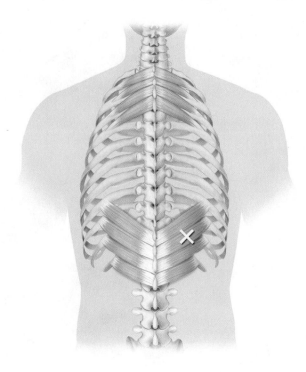

FIGURE 10.38

When dysfunctional, the **serratus posterior inferior** can develop a trigger point over the lower ribs, which can generate a nagging, aching pain around the same area.

MUSCLE PALPATION
Serratus Posterior Superior and Serratus Posterior Inferior

Because the serratus muscles along the spine lie under several layers of tissue, they can be difficult to palpate directly. Approximate the location and function of the serratus posterior superior by placing your hands over the posterior aspect of your upper four ribs, between your scapulae and spine. Breathe into your hands and feel if these ribs elevate with your inhalation.

To approximate the location and function of the serratus posterior inferior, place your hands over the posterior aspects of your lower four ribs, directly lateral to your lower thoracic vertebrae. Again, breathe into your hands to feel if these ribs move. Press into the tissue, then breathe out with a forced exhalation to feel the muscle contract. **Note:** *Both muscles are difficult to palpate because they lie under several layers of tissue.*

Serratus Posterior Superior

O–Spinous processes of C-6 to T-2
I–2nd to 5th ribs medial of the scapula
A–Assists inhalation during respiration

Serratus Posterior Inferior

O–Spinous processes of T-11 to L-2
I–9th through 12th ribs
A–Assists exhalation during respiration

(continued)

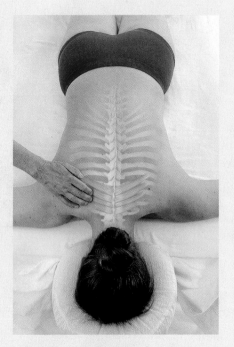

FIGURE 10.39a

Palpating the serratus posterior superior

Locate the **serratus posterior superior** on your partner in the supine position with the arms hanging off the table. Approximate its location by tracing the four fascicles of this muscle from the spinous processes of C-6 to T-2 along the 2nd to 5th ribs (Figure 10.39a ■). Sink through the overlying rhomboids using linear strokes along each fascicle. Have your partner breathe into your pressure. *Did you roll across the serrated fascicles with cross-fiber strokes? Do the ribs under the serratus posterior superior move as your partner breathes?*

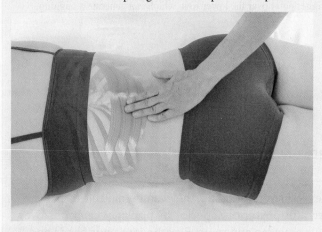

FIGURE 10.39b

Palpating the serratus posterior inferior

With your partner in the supine position, approximate the location of the **serratus posterior inferior** by tracing the diagonal fascicles of this muscle from the spinous processes of T-11 to L-2 up to ribs 9 through 12 (Figure 10.39b ■). Press into the overlying muscles and thick thoracolumbar fascia into the belly of the muscle, then have your partner do a slow, sustained exhalation to feel the muscle contract. Explore the serratus posterior inferior with both linear and cross-fiber strokes. *Are you palpating over the lower ribs?*

SELF-CARE
Breathing to Release Tension

1. If you feel yourself getting tense, focus on your own exhalation. Allow or imagine tension draining out of your body on each exhalation.
2. When you relax into an exhalation, make sure not to let your body collapse. Rather, feel your respiratory muscles and shoulders sink around the length and central support of your spine.

3. If your arms and hands get tired as you give massage, explore letting your hands relax for a moment and become heavy, sinking into your client as your client exhales. This will help you both relax together and will build rapport through a synchrony of breathing rhythms.

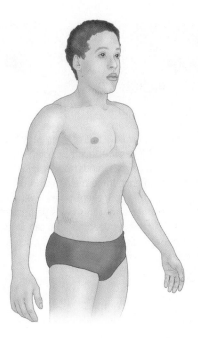

FIGURE 10.40

Person with **inhalation fixation** and inflated chest

(Figure 10.40 ■). People often develop upper chest breathing from emotional distress, breathing as though caught in a gasp. This respiratory pattern is self-perpetuating: The more effort a chest breather puts into expanding the lungs, the stronger the pattern usually becomes. Paradoxical and upper chest breathing can create or increase anxiety because they restrict air flow to the lungs and raise sympathetic tone.

10.4.2   Weak Abdominals and Belly Breathing

As discussed earlier, well-toned abdominal muscles are critical for normal diaphragmatic breathing. The abdominal muscles, particularly the transversus abdominis, maintain

intra-abdominal pressure, providing a counterpressure to the downward movement of the diaphragm. When the diaphragm can no longer move down, respiratory expansion then sequences up into the rib cage.

When the abdominal muscles are weak, the diaphragm lacks a counterpressure and keeps pushing down on the abdominal viscera, which distends the abdominal wall. This stretches the abdominal muscles, which in turn can increase any stretch weakness in them. Abdominal distension places a front load on the lumbar spine, swaying the lumbar spine into an excessive lordotic curve. It also puts a downward drag on the thorax, depressing the chest and exacerbating the lack of respiratory expansion into the rib cage. This explains why people with distended abdomens usually have a collapsed posture, a sunken chest, and a chronic thoracic curvature (Figure 10.41 ■).

Many seniors with stretch weaknesses in the abdominal muscles have stooped postural patterns and restricted respiratory expansion. As a result, they become belly breathers and develop rigidity in the rib cage and thoracic spine.

Belly breathing is advocated by many meditation and yoga instructors; however, it can lead to respiratory motion restrictions and poor posture. When a person is lying supine, belly breathing can promote relaxation and diaphragmatic breathing. In an upright position, conscious belly breathing, especially with people who have poor abdominal tone, has a detrimental effect. It disorganizes the breathing patterns and discourages the use of stabilizing muscles necessary for postural support.

10.4.3   Chronic Obstructive Pulmonary Diseases

Chronic obstructive pulmonary diseases (COPDs) cause major restrictions to respiration. Three types of COPDs are most common: asthma, bronchitis, and emphysema. All three present symptoms of inflammation, excess mucous

---

SELF-CARE
Exploring Muscle Patterns in Upper Chest Breathing

To feel the effects of upper chest breathing, explore the following exercise.

Caution: If you get dizzy or have any other symptoms, stop immediately and breathe normally.

1. Tighten your abdominal muscles and pull your solar plexus and chest up and hold them there.
2. As you hold this position, breathe into your upper chest. As you inhale, focus on lifting your diaphragm. Take several breaths this way. Notice what happens in the rest of your

body, how your posture changes and which muscles have to hold.

3. Relax and notice how your posture changes and which muscles relax. *What do you feel like when you breathe into your upper chest? Do you begin to feel anxious, or get a suffocating feeling like you cannot get enough air? Can you feel how much effort this pattern takes? What areas of the body do you think a person with this pattern would need to have loosened to restore normal breathing?*

BRIDGE TO PRACTICE
Helping Clients Relax while Breathing

If your client has trouble taking a deep breath for whatever reason, and trying to breathe better only makes the pattern worse, suggest that your client "breathe easy." You could also suggest that your client let his or her body "breathe itself." Sometimes just taking the focus away from active breathing can help a client relax.

Another way to help your client relax into breathing is to suggest that the client focus on the exhalation. Verbal cues such as "with each exhalation, let your body sink more deeply into the table and become heavier" or "with each exhalation, let your

muscles relax and tension flow out of your body" can promote a relaxation response. Make sure to speak using a relaxed tone of voice. You can also make your hands heavier on your client's body as the client exhales to encourage the relaxation.

If you do suggest that your client take a deep breath to relax, pay attention to whether or not this helps your client. Unless the client breathes slowly, taking deep breaths can actually speed up respiration, increase muscular effort, and induce a shift toward sympathetic tone.

---

production, a narrowing of the respiratory passageways, and a significant loss of flexibility in the elastic tissues of the lungs. The loss of flexibility reduces the elastic recoil of the *alveoli,* the microscopic elastic sacs that fill with air on inhalation. This loss of elasticity restricts exhalation, so air remains in the lungs. In advanced stages of COPD, a person develops hyperinflation of the lungs and a barrel chest.

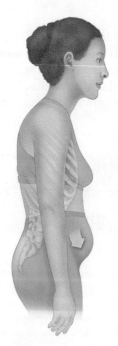

FIGURE 10.41
Person with **exhalation fixation** and collapsed posture

When working with breathing patterns, it is important to differentiate faulty respiratory patterns stemming from an illness or injury, an emotional state of shock or trauma, or habitual postural and muscular patterns to determine the best course of treatment. Be careful in prompting chest breathers to breathe deeply or consciously because in their efforts, they might go deeper into their muscular holding patterns. This is particularly true with a client suffering from shock or trauma, who might hyperventilate when feeling panicked and breathing quickly.

Hyperventilation occurs when rapid breathing creates an imbalance in gas exchange. As a result, the amount of oxygen coming in exceeds the amount of carbon dioxide going out, which causes a range of symptoms: dizziness, lightheadedness, tingling, or fainting. Prolonged hyperventilation can lead to *tetany*—a tonic muscle spasm that feels like paralysis in the hands and feet. When people hyperventilate, they become dizzy and can pass out. A simple remedy for this condition is to cover the mouth with a paper bag in order to rebreathe CO_2 and restore it to a normal level.

CONCLUSION

We have begun the second half of this kinesiology text with breathing because it is the foundation of all movement. Life begins with breathing. It is a human being's first movement after birth. Every motion a person performs relies on the ability to breathe fully and efficiently. The diaphragm functions as the prime mover in respiration; it initiates inhalation by expanding internal space in the thorax, which draws the lungs open for the inflow of air. During exhalation, the respiratory muscles relax, deflating the lungs and forcing the air to rush out, which causes the thorax to sink slightly into the pelvis in an action that can ground and center a person.

Breathing is a key element of a dynamic and upright posture. During a normal and healthy inhalation, the thorax expands and the spine lengthens, bringing the body to a more vertical posture. Because of this essential relationship between breathing and posture, the thorax and respiratory motion are a logical place to begin the study of movement in the body. Breathing is also a logical place to begin bodywork intended to improve skeletal alignment.

The coordination of breath and movement, particularly during rigorous activity, depends on a number of factors. Accessory muscles for respiration become active during deep or forced breathing and vigorous movement such as cardiovascular exercise and heavy lifting. Chronic muscular holding from respiratory illnesses and even postural patterns can affect and limit normal breathing. A person can, however, change faulty breathing patterns with awareness, focused exercises, and bodywork that releases chronically shortened muscles restricting respiratory motion.

SUMMARY POINTS TO REMEMBER

1. The three main functions of the thorax are to house and protect the heart and lungs, to provide attachment sites for muscles of the shoulder girdle and cervical spine, and to serve as a mechanical bellows in respiration. The primary function of respiration, an automatic movement controlled by the autonomic nervous system, is to provide the body with oxygen and to remove carbon dioxide.

2. The thorax is a bony rib cage made up of 24 ribs, including true, false, and floating ribs; the costal cartilage; the sternum with a manubrium and xiphoid process; and 12 thoracic vertebrae.

3. Two types of sternocostal joints—the costalchondral junctions and the chondrosternal junctions—attach ribs to costal cartilage to the sternum. Costovertebral joints connect ribs to the thoracic vertebrae, and costotransverse joints connect ribs to the transverse processes.

4. A rib separation is a dislocation between the ribs and the costal cartilage; a rib dislocation is a displacement of the costal cartilage from the sternum.

5. The rib cage expands on inhalation and deflates on exhalation; the ribs move with either a bucket-handle or a pump-handle motion; each rib rotates on its own axis.

6. The two primary muscles of respiration are the diaphragm and the intercostals. On inhalation, the diaphragm, a large double-dome-shaped muscle between the thorax and abdominal cavity, contracts and presses down to expand the thorax; the intercostals between the ribs elevate the ribs; and the scalenes elevate the 1st and 2nd ribs.

7. Intra-abdominal pressure (IAP) is an increase in pressure in the abdominal cavity due to abdominal muscle tone and the downward movement of the diaphragm.

Abdominal muscle tone provides a counterpressure to the diaphragm so that expansion sequences into the rib cage.

8. Accessory muscles of respiration increase lung volume during deep or forced inhalation and exhalation.

9. Respiration is a movement sequence that can develop muscular fixations at any phase of the sequence. In an inhalation fixation, the respiratory muscles hold the rib cage in an expanded posture; in an exhalation fixation, the respiratory muscles hold the rib cage in a deflated posture.

10. Paradoxical breathing, which occurs in severe respiratory distress from illness, injury, or paralysis, is a reversal of respiratory muscles in which the chest wall constricts and moves in on the inhalation, then expands and moves out on exhalation. Upper chest breathing, which is a holding pattern that is usually caused by anxiety, occurs when a person holds the abdominal muscles and lower ribs on inhalation while expanding the upper chest.

11. Belly breathing in a supine position can encourage diaphragmatic motion, but in a standing position, it reduces intra-abdominal pressure and disorganizes the respiratory sequence.

12. Chronic obstructive pulmonary diseases (COPDs) greatly restrict thoracic movement in respiration. The three most common COPDs are asthma, bronchitis, and emphysema.

13. Hyperventilation occurs during deep breathing when the amount of oxygen coming in exceeds the amount of carbon dioxide going out. It can lead to dizziness, tingling, lightheadedness, fainting, and even tetany—a tonic muscle spasm that feels like paralysis. A remedy for hyperventilation is to rebreathe carbon dioxide by breathing into a paper bag.

REVIEW QUESTIONS

1. The respiratory system includes
   a. all the muscles, bones, and joints that work together to expand facial bones and draw air into the sinuses.
   b. all the muscles, bones, and joints that work together to expand the diaphragm and draw air into the abdomen.
   c. all the muscles, bones, and joints that work together to expand the thorax and draw air into the lungs.
   d. all the muscles, bones, and joints that work together to expand the chest and draw blood into the heart.

2. The bones making up the thorax include the
   a. the ribs, sternum, and 12 thoracic vertebrae.
   b. the ribs, clavicle, and 12 thoracic vertebrae.
   c. the ribs, scapula, and 12 thoracic vertebrae.
   d. the ribs, manubrium, and 12 thoracic vertebrae.

3. The three primary functions of the thorax are to
   a. protect the kidneys and liver, provide attachment sites for muscles, and function as a bellows for breathing.
   b. protect the heart and lungs, provide attachment sites for muscles, and function as a bellows for breathing.
   c. protect the heart and lungs, provide attachment sites for muscles, and function as a circulatory blood pump.
   d. protect the heart and lungs, provide attachment sites for fascia, and function as a bellows for breathing.

4. Describe the differences between true, false, and floating ribs.

5. The costal arch is made up of a rim of flexible _____.

6. The three parts of the sternum are
   a. the manubrium, the body of the sternum, and the coracoid process.
   b. the manubrium, the jugular notch, and the xiphoid process.
   c. the manubrium, the costal cartilage, and the xiphoid process.
   d. the manubrium, the body of the sternum, and the xiphoid process.

7. Why would a practitioner want to avoid applying strong pressure over the center of the costal arch?

8. The joints that attach the ribs to the sternum and the spine are the
   a. sternocostal, costovertebral, and costotransverse joints.
   b. sternochondral, costovertebral, and costotransverse joints.
   c. sternocostal, chondrovertebral, and costotransverse joints.
   d. sternocostal, costovertebral, and chondrotransverse joints.

9. Describe how the ribs and sternum move during respiration.

10. The primary muscles of respiration are the
    a. diaphragm and the scalenes.
    b. diaphragm and the obliques.
    c. diaphragm and the intercostals.
    d. diaphragm and the abdominals.

11. The three insertions of the diaphragm muscle are
    a. a broad costal insertion on the inside of the posterior costal arch and floating ribs, a small insertion on the xiphoid process, and two long tendons called crura that insert along the vertebral bodies of the 2nd and 3rd lumbar vertebrae.
    b. a broad costal insertion on the inside of the anterior costal arch and lower seven ribs, a small insertion on the xiphoid process, and two long tendons called crura that insert along the vertebral bodies of the 4th and 5th lumbar vertebrae.
    c. a narrow costal insertion on the bottom of the anterior costal arch and 7th rib, a small insertion on the coracoid process, and two long tendons called crura that insert along the vertebral bodies of the 2nd and 3rd lumbar vertebrae.
    d. a broad costal insertion on the inside of the anterior costal arch and lower seven ribs, a small insertion on the xiphoid process, and two long tendons called crura that insert along the vertebral bodies of the 2nd and 3rd lumbar vertebrae.

12. True or false (circle one). During normal breathing, the diaphragm contracts and pushes down on the underlying organs, increasing intra-abdominal pressure and causing distension of the anterior abdominal wall.

13. During which phase of breathing does the diaphragm contract and what is the hallmark of diaphragmatic motion?
    a. The diaphragm contracts during the exhalation phase, and the hallmark of diaphragmatic motion is the lateral expansion of the lower ribs.
    b. The diaphragm contracts during the inhalation phase, and the hallmark of diaphragmatic motion is the lateral expansion of the upper ribs.
    c. The diaphragm contracts during the inhalation phase, and the hallmark of diaphragmatic motion is the lateral expansion of the lower ribs.
    d. The diaphragm contracts during the inhalation phase, and the hallmark of diaphragmatic motion is the anterior distension of the abdominal wall.
14. Identify which statement describes the actions of the intercostal muscles.
    a. They approximate and rotate the ribs during inhalation and depress and stabilize the ribs during exhalation.
    b. They elevate and separate the ribs during inhalation and depress and stabilize the ribs during exhalation.
    c. They flex and separate the ribs during inhalation and elevate and stabilize the ribs during exhalation.
    d. They extend and separate the ribs during inhalation and depress and stabilize the ribs during exhalation.

15. True or false (circle one). During inhalation, the thoracic spine flexes as the rib cage sinks and the sternum depresses.
16. What is the scalenes' function in respiration?
    a. The scalenes assist inhalation by fixating the upper ribs.
    b. The scalenes assist inhalation by elevating the upper ribs.
    c. The scalenes assist inhalation by depressing the upper ribs.
    d. The scalenes assist inhalation by stabilizing the upper ribs.
17. Secondary muscles of respiration work during _____ _____ (*two words*) and include all the abdominal muscles, pectoralis, sternocleidomastoid, trapezius, and the serratus muscles.
18. Describe paradoxical breathing and what causes it.
19. How is upper chest breathing different from paradoxical breathing?
20. Why is abdominal muscle tone crucial for normal diaphragmatic breathing?

Note

1. Simons, D., Travell, J., & Simons, L. (1999). *Myofascial Pain and Dysfunction: The Trigger Point Manual: Volume 1. Upper Half of Body* (2nd ed.). Baltimore: Lippincott, Williams, & Wilkins.

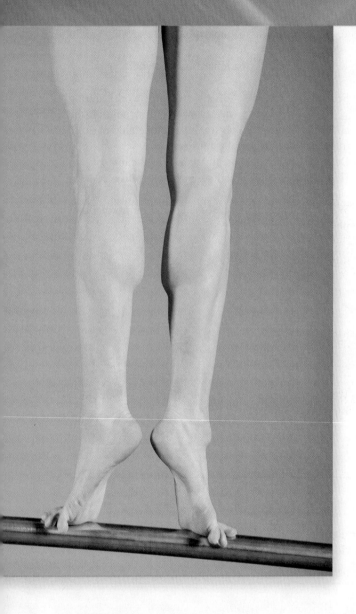

CHAPTER OUTLINE

Chapter Objectives

Key Terms

Muscles in Action

11.1 Bones of the Ankle and Foot

11.2 Joints and Ligaments of the Ankle and Foot

11.3 Muscles of the Ankle and Foot

Conclusion

Summary Points to Remember

Review Questions

The feet tell the story of the whole body. When the feet hurt, the entire body suffers. When feet are energized and springy, it can invigorate the whole body. Each part of the feet supports a corresponding kinetic chain. For example, the calcaneus supports the back of the body, and lifting the heel engages a chain of muscles from the foot and calf up the back of the leg and trunk.

Each foot is a tripod with three arches that form a sturdy yet springy osteoligamentous dome. This arched dome functions like a miniature trampoline, flattening under compression to absorb shock, then rebounding on each step with elastic and kinetic energy.

Ballet training cultivates strength and articulation in the intrinsic foot muscles, which is why ballet dancers can leap with such amazing height and agility. To increase joint mobility in the arches, which will keep them pliable, a person can explore lifting and lowering them while keeping the toes relatively straight. This will also activate the intrinsic muscles of the foot, which is a key to maintaining mobility and spring in the arches.

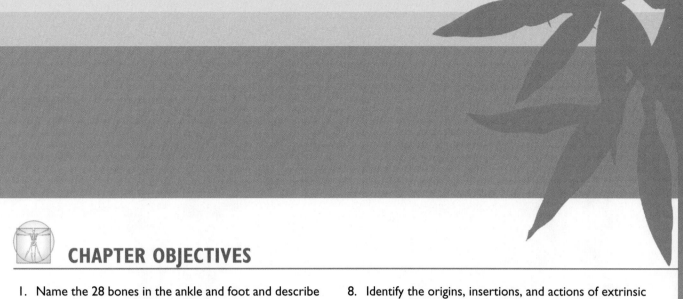

CHAPTER OBJECTIVES

1. Name the 28 bones in the ankle and foot and describe the shape and location of each one.

2. Name three functional parts of the foot and the bones in each part.

3. List and demonstrate the palpation of seven bony landmarks of the ankle and foot.

4. List the major ligaments of the ankle and foot and describe their locations and functions.

5. List the three arches of the feet, identify their functions, and describe each one.

6. Name and describe five major ligaments that support the vault of the arches.

7. List the eight major joints of the foot and describe the structure and function of each one.

8. Identify the origins, insertions, and actions of extrinsic muscles of the ankle and foot.

9. Identify trigger points and pain referral patterns of extrinsic muscles of the ankle and foot.

10. Demonstrate the active movement and palpation of each extrinsic ankle and foot muscle.

11. Identify the origins, insertions, and actions of intrinsic muscles of the ankle and foot.

12. Identify trigger points and pain referral patterns of intrinsic muscles of the ankle and foot.

13. Demonstrate the active movement and palpation of each intrinsic muscle of the foot.

KEY TERMS

Anatomical stirrup

Anterior talofibular ligament

Deltoid ligament

Hallux

Interosseous membrane

Interphalangeal joints

Intertarsal joints

Lateral longitudinal arch

Medial longitudinal arch

Metatarsophalangeal joints

Neutral position of the ankle

Plantar aponeurosis

Plantar fasciitis

Plantar plate

Retinacula

Sesamoid bones

Subtalar joint

Talocrural joint

Tarsal tunnel

Tarsometatarsal joints

Tibial torsion

Transverse arch

Transverse tarsal joint

Triceps surae

MUSCLES IN ACTION

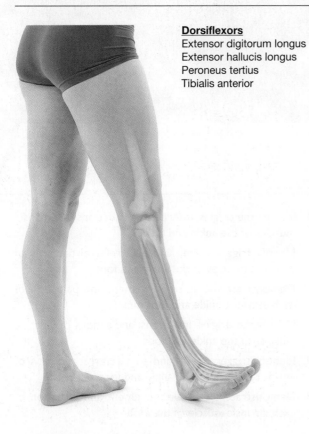

Dorsiflexors
Extensor digitorum longus
Extensor hallucis longus
Peroneus tertius
Tibialis anterior

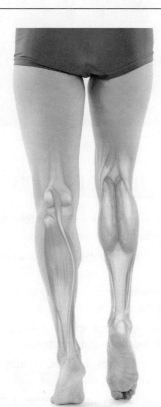

Plantarflexors
Gastrocnemius
Plantaris
Soleus

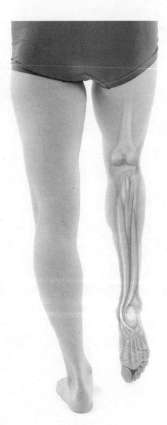

Deep Plantarflexors
Flexor digitorum longus
Flexor hallucis longus
Tibialis posterior

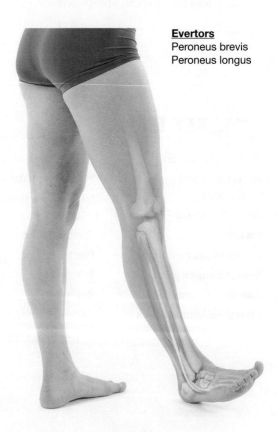

Evertors
Peroneus brevis
Peroneus longus

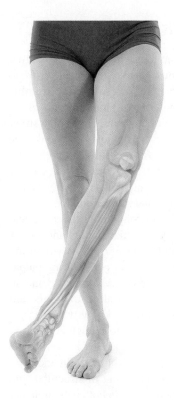

Anterior Invertors
Extensor hallucis longus
Tibialis anterior

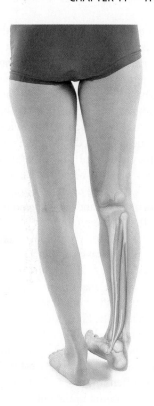

Posterior Invertors
Flexor hallucis longus
Tibialis posterior

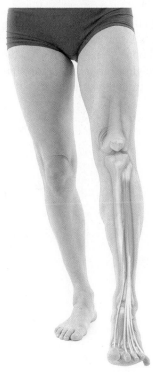

Toe Extensors
Extensor digitorum brevis
Extensor digitorum longus
Extensor hallicus brevis
Extensor hallicus longus

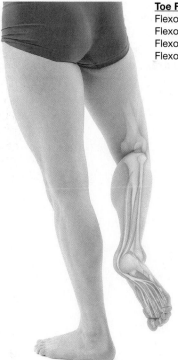

Toe Flexors
Flexor digitorum brevis
Flexor digitorum longus
Flexor hallicus brevis
Flexor hallicus longus

Now that we've established a basic understanding of the thorax and breathing as the basis of vertical posture and the energy source for all moving parts of the body, we continue our progressive journey through the musculoskeletal system by looking at the body's basis of support: the ankle and foot. We are tackling this complex part of the body before most other parts because optimal foot alignment provides the structural foundation for the entire body. The feet may be small in size, but they play a central role in weight-bearing and locomotion. They need to be sturdy enough to support the body's weight, yet strong enough to impart thrust into the body during locomotion and flexible enough to adapt to the changing contours of the ground.

When the foot is in contact with the ground, the ankle and foot move in a closed chain. Joints working in a closed chain are mechanically linked to each other; in other words, mechanical forces translate along the chain from one joint to the next. As a result, an injury or structural imbalance in the foot can affect joint alignment in the knee, hip, and even the spine. Misalignments in the feet and ankles can alter the structural balance of the entire body, affecting both posture and movement. If the feet are flat, the body loses its lift. If the feet are stiff, spinal rigidity often follows. If the feet are hurt or injured, the efficiency of motion in the entire body suffers.

In this chapter, we examine the many bones, ligaments, and muscles acting on the ankle and foot. We look at how the joints of the foot and ankle function in posture and gait, as well as trigger points and pain referral patterns in each muscle. We also use palpation exercises to locate bony landmarks, and to explore joint and muscle action and resisted movement.

11.1 BONES OF THE ANKLE AND FOOT

The ankle links the leg to the foot with a relatively similar arrangement of joints and muscles that links the forearm to the hand. Because their structures are so similar, learning the structures of the ankle and foot will make a study of the wrist and hand easier. They do, however, have some structural differences that highlight their unique functions. The hands evolved articulate joints for mobility and prehensile activities; the feet evolved rigid, sturdy joints for stability and to work as bony levers in gait. This is why the bones and joints of the feet are larger and more complex.

In observing the shapes and contours of the ankle and foot, you'll notice that many irregular bumps and ridges stand out. These topical landmarks are places where the bones rise to the surface of the soft tissues. During palpation, they are like islands in a sea, places where you can find solid ground to identify the location of joints and muscular attachments. It is helpful to know where easily palpable bony tubercles are located to recognize what is normal and avoid mistaking a bony tubercle for a soft tissue anomaly. By learning to recognize the bony landmarks, you can glimpse the underlying arrangement of structures and gather information about where to begin both palpation and hands-on work (Figure 11.1 ■).

11.1.1 Tibia and Fibula

The **tibia** and **fibula** run parallel to each other in the leg (Figure 11.2 ■). The tibia is larger than the fibula and is the most vertically oriented bone in the body. In a standing posture, it functions as a weight-bearing pillar, transferring about 90 percent of the load from the knee to the foot.

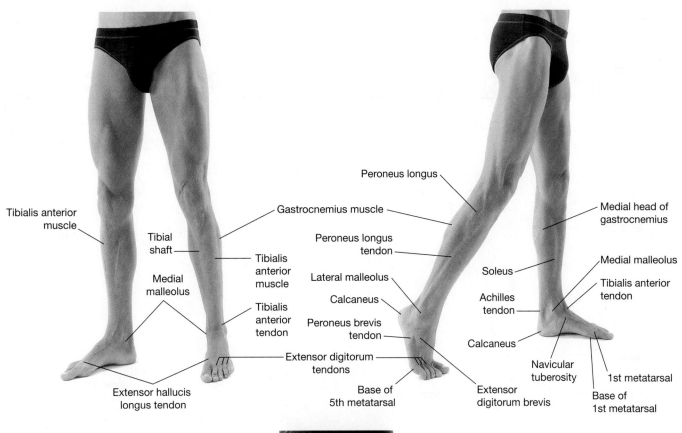

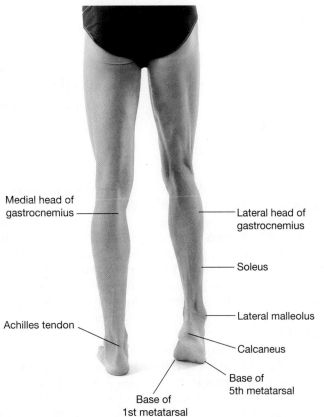

FIGURE 11.1

Surface anatomy of the foot and ankle

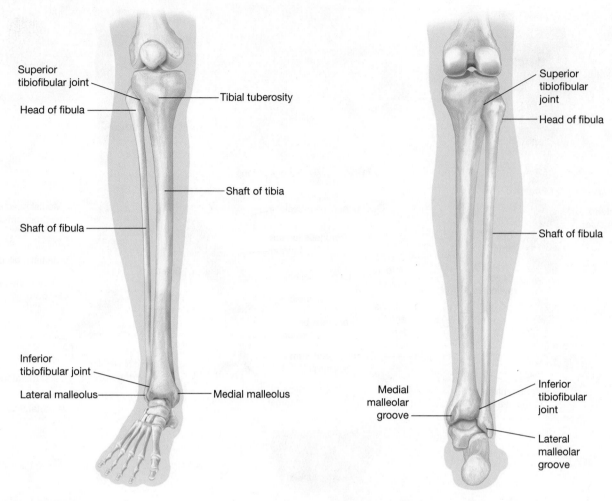

FIGURE 11.2

Tibia and fibula: anterior view

FIGURE 11.3

Bones of the foot and ankle: posterior view

You will want to become familiar with several important bony landmarks in the leg through palpation. The **shaft of the tibia** is easy to locate by its sharp anterior edge along the front of the leg. On the medial ankle, the tibia enlarges into the **medial malleolus**, a large but somewhat flat knob with a **medial malleolar groove** on its posterior edge. This groove provides a vertical notch for the tendons of posterior leg muscles—the tibialis posterior, flexor hallucis longus, and flexor digitorum longus—to pass through on their way to the sole of the foot (Figure 11.3 ■).

The long, thin fibula provides attachment sites for muscles, a pulley for tendons at the ankle, and a lateral splint for the ankle joint. The **head of the fibula** forms a small bony protuberance on the side of the leg, directly below the knee. It tapers into the shaft of the fibula, which disappears under the peroneal muscles and resurfaces at the ankle. There it enlarges into the **lateral malleolus**, which is much larger than the medial malleolus. A **lateral malleolar groove** on the posterior edge of the malleolus provides a

vertical notch for the peroneal tendons to pass through on their way to the foot.

The tibia has a torsion angle called **tibial torsion**; its distal end twists medially from 20 to 30 degrees relative to the proximal end along the long axis of the bone. Tibial torsion mirrors the torsion of the femur, which twists in the opposite direction. A flat-footed posture from chronic hyperpronation increases tibial torsion and medially rotates the tibia.

11.1.2   Bones of the Foot

Each foot is shaped like an elongated triangle with corners at the heel, first toe, and fifth toe. This triangular base forms a tripod, which is the ultimate structural compromise between a stable, four-legged structure like a table and a mobile two-legged structure like a human being.

Independent of the ankle, there are 26 bones in each foot—seven tarsal bones (talus, calcaneus, navicular, three cuneiforms, and cuboid), five metatarsals, and 14

BONE PALPATION
Tibia and Fibula

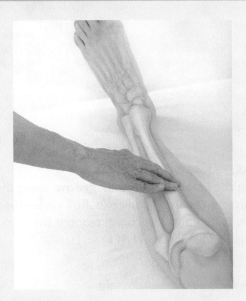

FIGURE 11.4a
Walk or slide your fingertips down the **shaft of the tibia,** exploring its length and sharp edge along the shin. (See Figure 11.4a ■). *Which side of the tibia do you feel muscle on?*

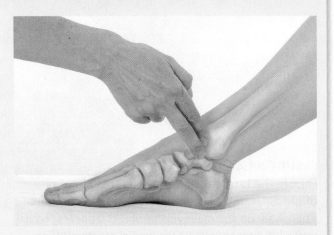

FIGURE 11.4b
Palpate the **medial malleolus** at the distal end of the tibia and find its edges (See Figure 11.4b ■). *How wide is the medial malleolus?*

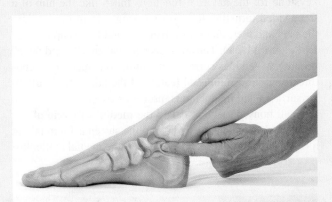

FIGURE 11.4c
Palpate the bony lip of the **medial malleolar groove** on the posterior, inferior aspect of the medial malleolus. Roll across the groove to strum the tendons that pass through it. (See Figure 11.4c ■)

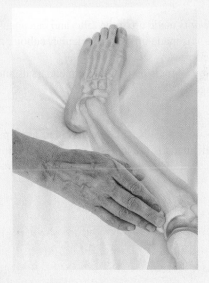

FIGURE 11.4d
To locate the **head of the fibula,** find the prominent bony knob below the side of the knee. Hold the head of the fibula with a pincher grasp, then walk down the shaft of the fibula. *Do you notice how the fibula disappears under the peroneal muscles below the head?* (See Figure 11.4d ■)

(continued)

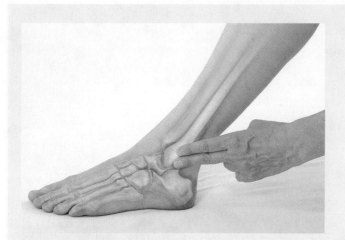

FIGURE 11.4e
Palpate the **lateral malleolus** on the lateral side of the ankle, exploring its size, edges, and contours. Then walk up the malleolus until it disappears. *Which malleolus is more anterior, the medial or lateral?* (See Figure 11.4e ■)

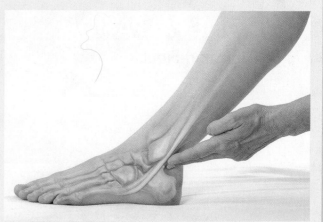

FIGURE 11.4f
Locate the **lateral malleolar groove** along the posterior edge of the malleolus. Roll across the groove to strum the peroneal tendons that pass through it. (See Figure 11.4f ■)

phalanges. They are grouped in three functional sections (Figure 11.5 ■).

- The *rearfoot* is made up of the talus and calcaneus.
- The *midfoot* is made up of the navicular, cuboid, and three cuneiforms.
- The *forefoot* is made up of the five metatarsals and the 14 phalanges.

11.1.2.1 TARSALS

The seven tarsals fit together like three-dimensional puzzle pieces. The **calcaneus** is the largest and most posterior tarsal. It provides a sturdy base for weight support. A **calcaneal tuberosity**, the flat part of the posterior heel, serves as an attachment site for the powerful Achilles tendon. A small bony ledge about 1 inch inferior to the medial malleolus, called the **sustentaculum tali**, provides an attachment site for the *spring ligament,* a primary supporting ligament of the medial arch (Figure 11.6 ■).

The **talus** sits on top of the calcaneus and serves as a keystone for the ankle. It functions much like the hub of a three-sided turnstile, transferring weight from the leg into the heel and toes, and transferring ground forces up into the leg (Figure 11.7 ■). The talus has been called a "caged bone" because 14 tendons surround it, but not one tendon attaches directly to it.[1] An unusual feature of the talus is that articular surfaces and ligamentous insertions cover it on all sides. A small bony projection called the **medial tubercle of the talus** can be found directly behind the sustentaculum tali, at a 45-degree angle off the back edge of the medial malleolus.

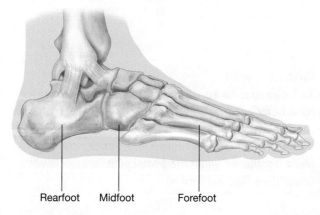

Rearfoot   Midfoot   Forefoot

FIGURE 11.5
Regions of the foot and ankle

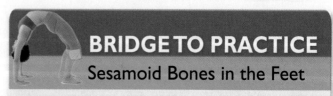

BRIDGE TO PRACTICE
Sesamoid Bones in the Feet

Avoid deep pressure directly into the sesamoid capsules of the feet during massage, which could irritate or bruise them, especially on thin clients that have little padding around the joints.

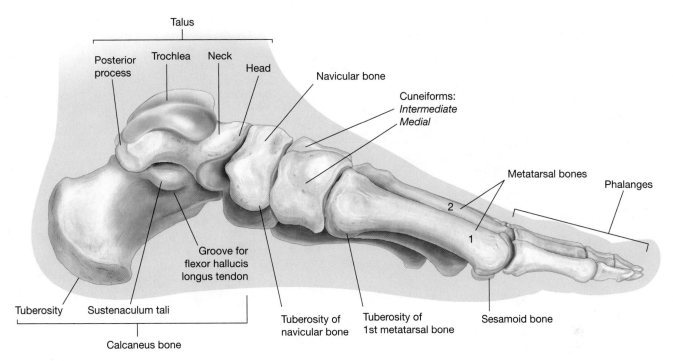

FIGURE 11.6

Bones of the foot: medial view

The **navicular** is a large cube-shaped bone that provides a keystone for the medial arch along the instep. A large **navicular tuberosity** on its medial aspect makes this tarsal easy to locate. The top of the navicular appears as a prominent bony knob that can become irritated when compressed in tight shoes (this is a common problem for people with high arches). In a pattern of hyperpronation, the navicular tends to sink and the medial arch flattens.

All three cuneiforms—the **medial cuneiform**, **intermediate cuneiform**, and **lateral cuneiform**—articulate posteriorly with the navicular and anteriorly with the first three metatarsals (Figure 11.8 ■). A large **cuboid** can be found lateral to the cuneiforms, in the depression posterior to the proximal end of the fifth metatarsal. This cube-shaped

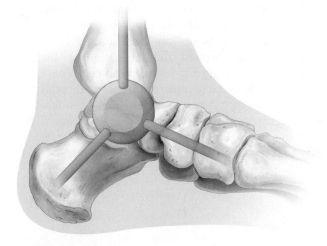

FIGURE 11.7

The **talus** is the keystone of the ankle, like a hub of a three-legged turnstile.

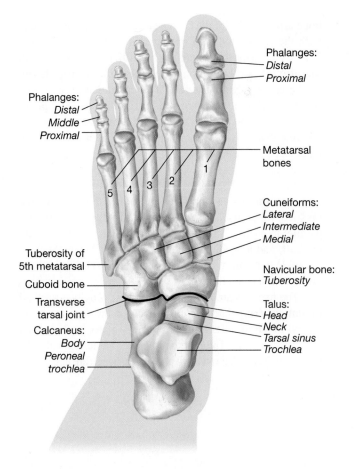

FIGURE 11.8

Bones of the foot: dorsal view

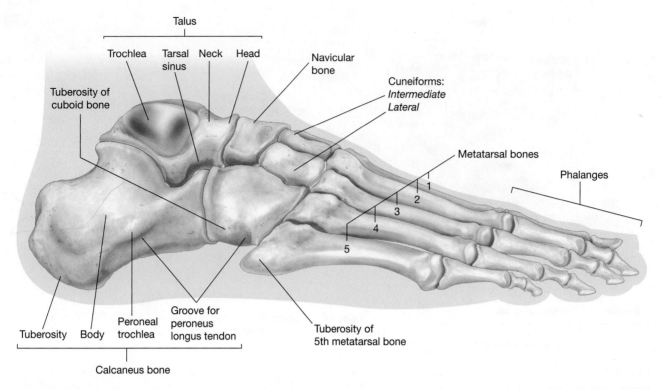

FIGURE 11.9
Bones of the foot: lateral view

bone articulates with the calcaneus on its posterior side and with the fourth and fifth metatarsals on the anterior side. Directly anterior to the cuboid, the **tuberosity of the fifth metatarsal** is a large bony prominence that projects out on the lateral edge of the foot. This prominent process can become calloused and irritated by tight shoes. The **peroneal trochlea** on the lateral side of the calcaneus is a small tubercle that provides a bony lip under which the peroneal tendons pass (Figure 11.9 ■).

11.1.2.2   METATARSALS AND PHALANGES

The **metatarsals** are the five long bones that extend like rays from the tarsals to the toes. The five metatarsals run parallel to each other. Every metatarsal has a base, a body or shaft, and a head. The metatarsals transfer weight from the ankle to the toes; the head of the metatarsals bear weight during the stance phase.

The five toes are made up of 14 small, long bones called **phalanges** (singular: *phalanx*). Each of the toes from the second to the fifth has three phalanges—a proximal, middle, and distal phalanx. The first toe is called the **hallux**. Like the thumb, the hallux has only two phalanges, which are larger than

those in the other toes. They articulate with the first metatarsal, which is also shorter and thicker than the other four, making the hallux sturdier than the other toes for weight-bearing and its function as a bony lever for pushoff in gait.

Two **sesamoid bones** about the size of small peas are located under the hallux, at the distal end of the first metatarsal (Figure 11.11 ■). Each sesamoid is encapsulated by a small synovial capsule filled with fluid that allows it to move around like a tiny marble in a fluid sac. The sesamoid bones have several functions. They create a protective tunnel for the flexor hallucis longus tendon to pass through, which prevents weight-bearing trauma. They also provide anatomical pulleys for the flexor hallucis brevis tendon and assist in weight-bearing with the large, square head of the first metatarsal.

The sesamoid bones can be fractured and their synovial capsules bruised from impact injuries such as jumping from a height and landing dead-center on them. Sesamoid injuries make it painful to bear weight through the ball of the foot. A person with such injuries develops an antalgic stance and gait, standing and walking on the heels to avoid putting pressure on or bending the hallux (first toe).

BONE PALPATION
Tarsals

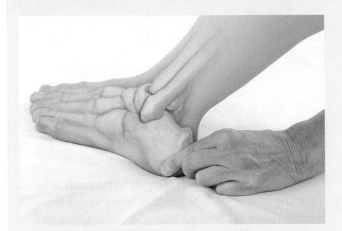

FIGURE 11.10a

To locate the **calcaneus,** grasp the sides of the heel, then palpate it along its length. Locate the **calcaneal tuberosity** on the heel at the base of the Achilles tendon. *How far does the calcaneus extend behind the ankle?* (See Figure 11.10a ■)

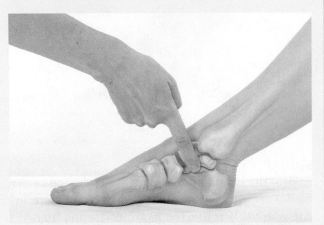

FIGURE 11.10b

Locate the **sustentaculum tali,** a small bony shelf about 1 inch below the medial malleolus. (See Figure 11.10b ■) *How far is this bony landmark from the bottom of the talus?*

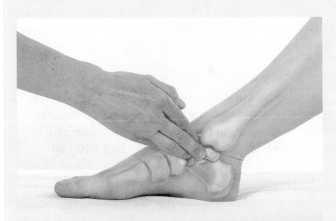

FIGURE 11.10c

To find the **medial tubercle of the talus,** a small bump under the posterior malleolus, slide your thumb on a diagonal from the medial malleolus toward the calcaneus. (See Figure 11.10c ■)

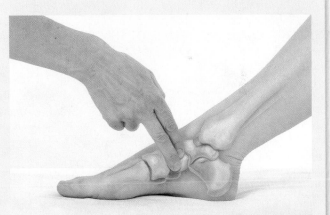

FIGURE 11.10d

To feel the **navicular tuberosity,** slide your fingertips from the medial malleolus toward the medial arch and locate the most prominent bony knob you run across. Trace from the navicular tuberosity directly medial over the smooth top of the navicular. *Do you feel the large bony bump of the navicular tuberosity along the inner side of the foot?* (See Figure 11.10d ■)

(continued)

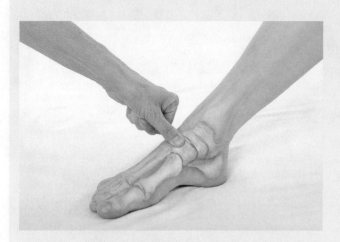

FIGURE 11.10e

Palpate the **medial cuneiform** along the top of the medial arch; it is the most prominent bump there, in line with the first toe. The intermediate and lateral cuneiforms can be found by sliding directly lateral to the medial cuneiform over the top of the foot. *Are you on the bony bump at the base of the first metatarsal?* (See Figure 11.10e ■)

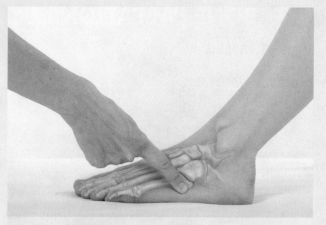

FIGURE 11.10f

To feel the **tuberosity of the fifth metatarsal,** trace the lateral edge of the foot to a sharp bony protuberance at the proximal end of the fifth metatarsal. *Are you on the lateral edge of the foot?* (See Figure 11.10f ■)

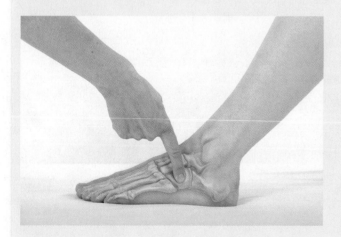

FIGURE 11.10g

Palpate the **cuboid** in the notch directly posterior and medial of the tuberosity of the fifth metatarsal. *Are you posterior to the base of the fifth metatarsal, on the lateral side of the foot?* (See Figure 11.10g ■)

FIGURE 11.11
Bones of the foot: plantar view

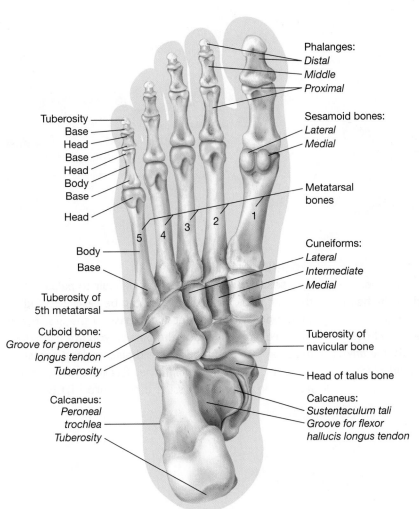

Phalanges:
Distal
Middle
Proximal

Tuberosity
Base
Head
Base
Head
Body
Base
Head

Sesamoid bones:
Lateral
Medial

Metatarsal
bones

5 4 3 2 1

Body
Base

Cuneiforms:
Lateral
Intermediate
Medial

Tuberosity of
5th metatarsal

Cuboid bone:
*Groove for peroneus
longus tendon*
Tuberosity

Tuberosity of
navicular bone

Head of talus bone

Calcaneus:
*Peroneal
trochlea*
Tuberosity

Calcaneus:
Sustentaculum tali
*Groove for flexor
hallucis longus tendon*

BONE PALPATION
Metatarsals and Phalanges

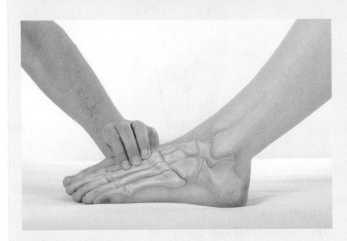

FIGURE 11.12a

Methodically trace along the length of each **metatarsal,** from its base to its head at the knuckles of the toes. Palpate the top and bottom of one metatarsal by holding the foot in a pincher hold. Locate the distal end of the metatarsals by bending the toes. *Are all five metatarsals parallel? Do you notice how the first metatarsal has a cylindrical shape that differs from the other four? Can you find the joint lines where the metatarsals articulate with the tarsals?* (See Figure 11.12a ■)

(continued)

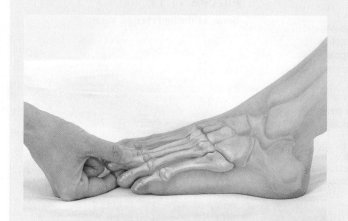

FIGURE 11.12b

Methodically palpate the **phalanges** of each toe. Notice the shape of the shaft compared to the head of each phalanx. Also notice whether the phalanges are straight, twisted, or chronically flexed, and how this affects the alignment of the metatarsals. *Are any of the metatarsals or phalanges twisted or tender?* (See Figure 11.12b ■)

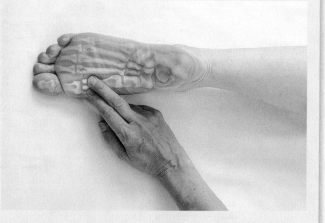

FIGURE 11.12c

The **sesamoid bones** can be difficult to palpate through thick tissue, but they can be easily located on people with thin feet at the base of the first toe. If they are easy to locate, the person you are palpating probably has thin feet, so avoid placing deep pressure on them. *Do the sesamoid bones feel like two miniature marbles in a pocket of tissue?* (See Figure 11.12c ■)

11.1.3 The Arches of the Feet

Each foot has three arches. These form a flexible curved vault that can stretch under load and rebound when the load is lifted (Figure 11.13 ■). The arches suit each foot to their position as a primary interface between the body and the ground. The main functions of the arches are to bend under weight, absorb shock from impact, and adapt the foot to uneven ground.

A **medial longitudinal arch** runs along the inside border of the foot, between the calcaneus and the hallux. Its keystone, the navicular, sits at the highest point in the arch. The medial arch is sometimes compared to a tie-rod and truss structure stretched between two bony struts, with one strut extending from the navicular to the calcaneus and the other from the navicular to the hallux (Figure 11.14 ■). The medial arch transfers compressive forces from the ankle back to the heel and forward into the toes. It also transfers tensile forces through the plantar aponeurosis by stretching under load and, during a gait cycle, recoiling to contribute elastic energy to forward thrust of the foot during pushoff.

The **lateral longitudinal arch** runs along the outside edge of the foot between the fifth metatarsal and the heel. It is more rigid and flatter than the other two arches; it normally

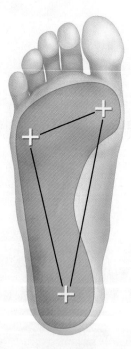

FIGURE 11.13
Three arches of the foot: plantar view

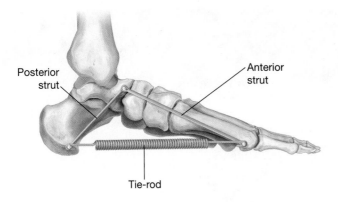

FIGURE 11.14

The **medial arch** works like a truss and tie-rod structure.

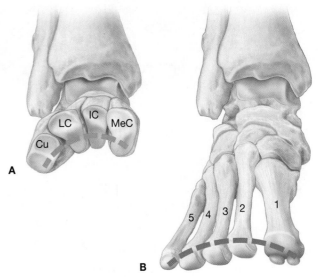

FIGURE 11.15

Transverse arch: a) Across the tarsals b) Across the ball of the foot

contacts the ground along its entire length. The rigidity of the lateral arch helps it to effectively transmit the thrust of forward propulsion through the foot during pushoff.

The **transverse arch** runs perpendicular to the longitudinal arches, across the foot between the first and fifth metatarsals and across the tarsals (Figure 11.15a-b ■). The distal, weight-bearing end of the transverse arch crosses the ball of the foot; the proximal, elevated end of this arch runs across the three cuneiforms and cuboid. The highest point of the arch is the second metatarsal, which serves as its keystone. When a client has a pronated foot that flattens the medial arch, the pronation can be due to a bony malformation or a soft tissue dysfunction. When the distal end of the second metatarsal sinks and flattens the transverse arch, a client can develop a painful callous at the base of the second toe. This callous is common among seniors or sedentary people with stiff, inflexible feet, making them reluctant to bend their toes during pushoff.

11.2 JOINTS AND LIGAMENTS OF THE ANKLE AND FOOT

Each foot alone has 25 joints and more than 100 ligaments in it (see Table 11.1 ■). The sturdy movable parts in the feet allows them the flexibility to move under many different conditions while bearing weight without collapsing. The foot can be visualized as a twisted osteoligamentous plate made of tightly packed bones strapped together by thick, strong ligamentous bands (Figure 11.17 ■).[2] In a neutral position, the proximal end of this plate at the heel and ankle has a sagittal orientation; the distal end of the plate across the ball of the

TABLE 11.1 Joints of the Ankle and Foot		
Joint	Type of Joint	Range of Motion
Proximal tibiofibular	Plane	Inferior and superior gliding Slight rotation
Distal tibiofibular	Fibrous	Inferior and superior gliding Slight rotation
Talocrural (talotibial)	Hinge	Plantarflexion and dorsiflexion
Subtalar (talocalcaneal)	Ellipsoid	Inversion and eversion Abduction and adduction
Transverse tarsal (midtarsal)	Plane	Gliding during inversion and eversion
Intertarsal (IT)	Plane	Gliding
Tarsometatarsal (TMT)	Plane	Gliding
Metatarsophalangeal (MTP)	Ellipsoid	Flexion and hyperextension Abduction and adduction
Interphalangeal (IP)	Hinge	Flexion and extension

EXPLORING TECHNIQUE
Restoring Arches in Stiff, Flat Feet

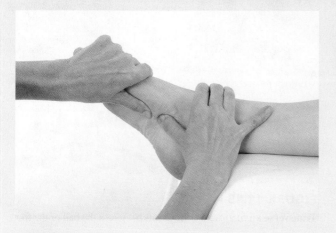

FIGURE 11.16a

1. **To loosen stiff feet:** Gently approximate the joints in each arch by slowly pressing them together until they are compressed as far as they will go (Figure 11.16a ■).

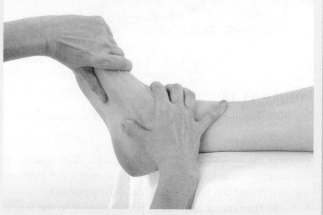

FIGURE 11.16b

2. Release the compression slowly, then apply light traction to the arch to lengthen it. (Figure 11.6b ■)

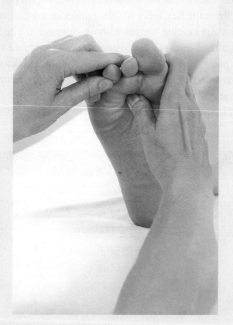

FIGURE 11.16c

3. **To restore the medial arch:** If the medial arch has fallen gently push the navicular up to lift the keystone of the arch (Figure 11.16c ■).

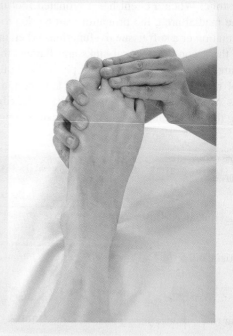

FIGURE 11.16d

4. **To restore the transverse arches:** If the transverse arch across the ball of the foot has fallen, gently lift the second metatarsal (Figure 11.16d ■). *Does the transverse arch have a callous on the dorsal surface of the second MTP joint?*

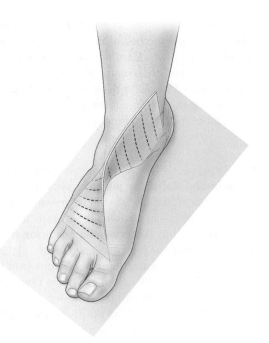

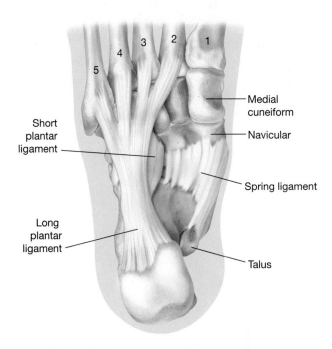

FIGURE 11.17

The foot as an osteoligamentous plate (adapted from Norkin)

FIGURE 11.18

Plantar surface of the foot

foot and the toes has a horizontal orientation. Under a weight-bearing load, the plate slightly untwists as the arches flatten. The plate twists as the forefoot and midfoot shape over and adapt to uneven ground. Four layers of dense plantar ligaments make the sole of the foot strong enough to carry the weight of the body while flexible enough to give under load.

11.2.1 Plantar Fascia and Supporting Ligaments

The structural integrity of the arches comes from a combination of plantar fascia, supporting ligaments, and muscular

forces (Figure 11.18 ■). When viewed from the medial side, the supporting fascia and ligaments of the longitudinal arches resemble four stacked decks on a ship (Figure 11.19 ■).

The top deck is a short, wide **calcaneonavicular ligament**, also called the *spring ligament,* which supports and stabilizes the center of the medial arch. The spring ligament has three parts: one part connects the sustentaculum tali to the navicular tuberosity, supporting the inside of the medial arch; the other two parts extend like small slings from the calcaneus to the underside of the navicular and talus.

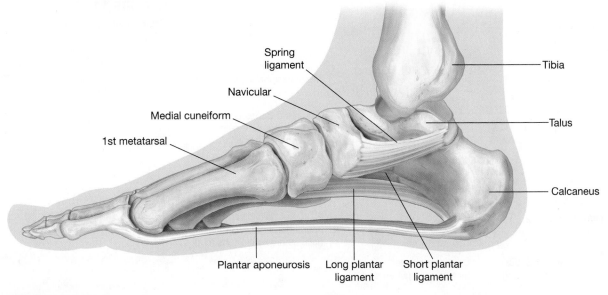

FIGURE 11.19

Plantar ligaments: medial view

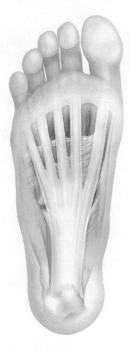

FIGURE 11.20
Planter aponeurosis

Under the spring ligament, a **short plantar ligament** connects the calcaneus to the cuboid and supports the lateral arch. Below that, a **long plantar ligament** connects from the calcaneus to the cuboid and the base of the third, fourth, and fifth metatarsals, also supporting the lateral arch. At the bottom, a long, thick **plantar aponeurosis** (fascia) connects from the calcaneal tuberosity to the base of the phalanges, cushioning and protecting the sole of the foot and stabilizing the longitudinal arches (Figure 11.20 ■). Inflammation of the plantar aponeurosis, called **plantarfasciitis,** causes this thick fascia to become stiff from scarring. As a result, it becomes inflexible and difficult to stretch, which makes walking painful.

The transverse arch is supported by a thick fibrocartilaginous pad across the ball of the foot called the **plantar plate** (Figure 11.21 ■). Cartilaginous pads and sesamoid bones embedded in the plantar plate support and cushion the metatarsal heads; a **deep transverse metatarsal ligament** across the plate binds the metatarsal heads to each other and prevents the foot from splaying sideways.

11.2.2 Tibiofibular Joints

The fibula moves with the ankle at two tibiofibular joints. The **proximal tibiofibular joint** is a synovial plane joint located inferior to the lateral side of the knee, where the head of the fibula articulates with the posterolateral aspect of the proximal tibia. **Anterior** and **posterior tibiofibular ligaments** bind the joint together (Figure 11.22 ■).

The **distal tibiofibular joint** is a fibrous joint located above the ankle, where the distal end of the fibula attaches to the distal end of the tibia. Anterior and posterior tibiofibular ligaments also bind the distal tibiofibular joint together. In the center of the joint, a small fibroadipose pad reduces friction during fibular motion. A strong **interosseous membrane** connects the tibia and fibula along the length of their shafts and stabilizes both tibiofibular joints.

Although the tibiofibular joints are structurally distinct from the talocrural joint at the ankle, they are mechanically linked to the ankle because they move with the ankle. During ankle flexion and extension, the fibula slides slightly up and down and rotates against the tibia. Injury to either tibiofibular joint will restrict ankle motion.

11.2.3 Talocrural Joint

The **talocrural joint** of the ankle is a hinge joint made up of the articulation of three bones: the tibia, fibula, and talus. This hinge joint is comparable to a mortise joint with malleolar grips on each side of the trochlear surface of the talus. It moves in a manner similar to a wrench turning around a bolt (Figure 11.23 ■).

FIGURE 11.21
Plantar plate

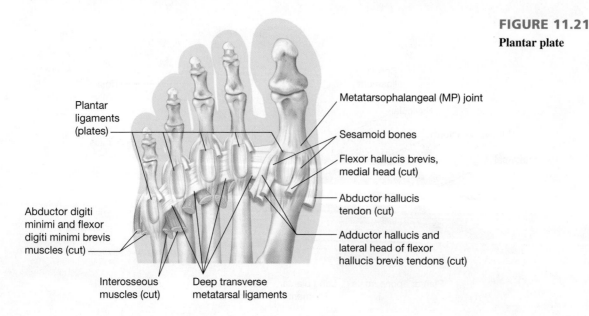

Plantar ligaments (plates)

Abductor digiti minimi and flexor digiti minimi brevis muscles (cut)

Interosseous muscles (cut)

Deep transverse metatarsal ligaments

Metatarsophalangeal (MP) joint

Sesamoid bones

Flexor hallucis brevis, medial head (cut)

Abductor hallucis tendon (cut)

Adductor hallucis and lateral head of flexor hallucis brevis tendons (cut)

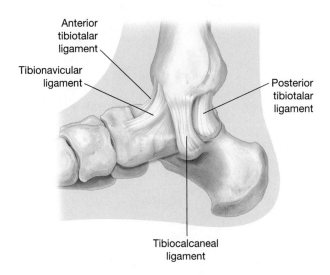

FIGURE 11.24

Deltoid ligaments of the ankle: medial view

The talocrural joint is stabilized by two strong groups of medial and lateral collateral ligaments. The **medial collateral ligament** (MCL) of the ankle is also called the **deltoid ligament** because it includes four ligaments that are collectively fan-shaped (Figure 11.24 ■). The deltoid ligament stabilizes the medial side of the ankle and limits excessive eversion.

The **lateral collateral ligament** (LCL) binds the lateral malleolus to the tarsal on the fibular side of the ankle. The LCL includes three individual ligaments that limit excessive inversion (Figure 11.25 ■). The MCL or deltoid ligament is much stronger than the LCL of the ankle because of their denser fibers and close-packed orientation. The **anterior talofibular ligament** is the most commonly injured ankle ligament; it is often damaged during inversion sprains when a person falls and rolls to the outside of the ankle.

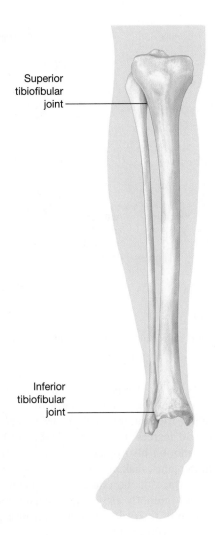

FIGURE 11.22

Tibiofibular joints

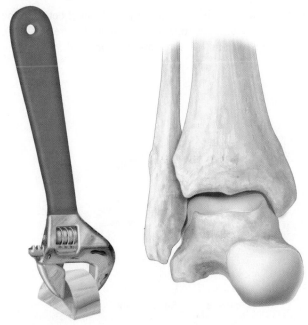

FIGURE 11.23

The **talocrural joint** resembles a mortise joint.

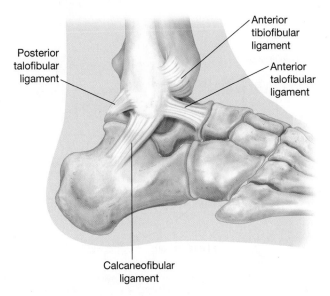

FIGURE 11.25

Lateral collateral ligaments of the ankle: lateral view

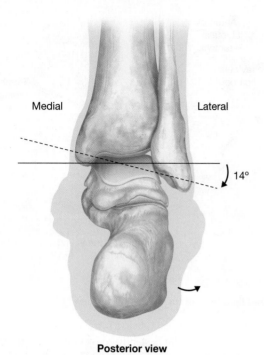

Medial   Lateral

14°

Posterior view

FIGURE 11.26

Axis of motion in the talocrural joint

The talocrural joint flexes and extends along an oblique axis that runs between the center of the medial and lateral malleolus (Figure 11.26 ■). It moves in an average range of 20 degrees of dorsiflexion (flexion) and 45 degrees of plantarflexion (extension). This range is measured from the neutral position of the talocrural, which is at a 90-degree angle in the standing position (Figure 11.27 ■). The

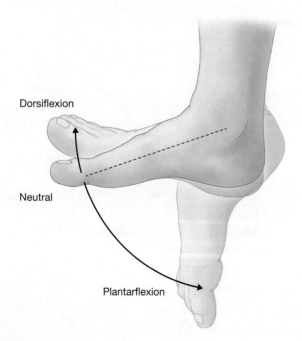

Dorsiflexion

Neutral

Plantarflexion

FIGURE 11.27

Range of motion of the ankle

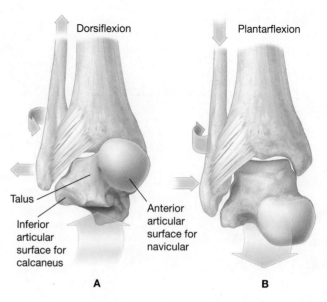

Dorsiflexion   Plantarflexion

Talus

Inferior articular surface for calcaneus

Anterior articular surface for navicular

A   B

FIGURE 11.28

a) **Dorsiflexion** with fibular motion b) **Plantarflexion** with fibular motion

talocrural reaches a close-packed position in dorsiflexion and an open-packed position in plantarflexion.

During dorsiflexion, the fibula glides up and laterally rotates about 30 degrees at the distal end (Figure 11.28a ■). This fibular motion also opens the pincher grip of the malleoli on the talus, making room for the wider anterior articulating surface of the talus. During plantarflexion, the fibula slides inferiorly and rotates medially, tightening the pincher grip of the malleoli on the narrower posterior aspect of the talus (Figure 11.28b ■).

11.2.4   Subtalar Joint

The subtalar joint is an ellipsoid joint located between the inferior talus and the superior calcaneus (Figure 11.29 ■). This complex joint has three articulations within two joint

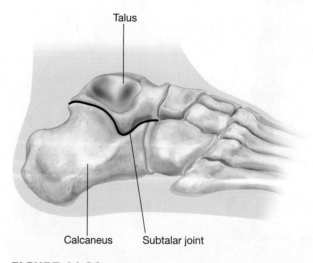

Talus

Calcaneus   Subtalar joint

FIGURE 11.29

Subtalar joint: side view

cavities. The calcaneonavicular (spring) ligament supports the subtalar joint on its inferior and medial sides; four small **talocalcaneal ligaments** anchor the talus to the calcaneus on the front, back, and sides of this joint.

The subtalar joint is also called the "lower ankle joint" because it moves with the talocrural joint during supination and pronation. It reaches a close-packed position during supination and loose-packed position during pronation. Keep in mind that supination and pronation involve the combined movement of many foot and ankle joints in all three planes (Figure 11.30 ■). The subtalar joint contributes inversion and eversion to these actions: the talocrural contributes plantarflexion and dorsiflexion. Two acronyms to remember the components of pronation and supination are SIP-ADD and PED-ABD:

Supination = **I**nversion + **P**lantarflexion + **Add**uction (SIP-ADD)

Pronation = **E**version + **D**orsiflexion + **Ab**duction (PED-ABD)

The subtalar joint moves along an oblique axis with an average range of 45 degrees of inversion and 20 degrees of eversion. Weight shifts between the outer and inner edges of the foot require subtalar motion, an action we use during tennis, skiing, or while lunging sideways. During these lateral motions, the calcaneus rocks under the talus with a unique twisting motion, moving like a small boat pitching and rolling over a large wave.[3]

The ankle and foot can become fixed in position with the medial arch lifted, called *hypersupination,* or with the medial arch fallen, called *hyperpronation* (Figure 11.31a-b ■). Both positions alter the neutral position of the ankle, which affects the range of motion in the ankle and foot (see Table 11.2 ■). When performing range of motion assessments on the ankle, make sure to start with the ankle in a neutral position, which is discussed in the next section.

TABLE 11.2 Range of Motion in the Ankle

Range of Motion	Degrees of Motion	End-Feel
Dorsiflexion	20 degrees	Firm
Plantarflexion	45 degrees	Firm
Inversion	45 degrees	Firm
Eversion	20 degrees	Firm

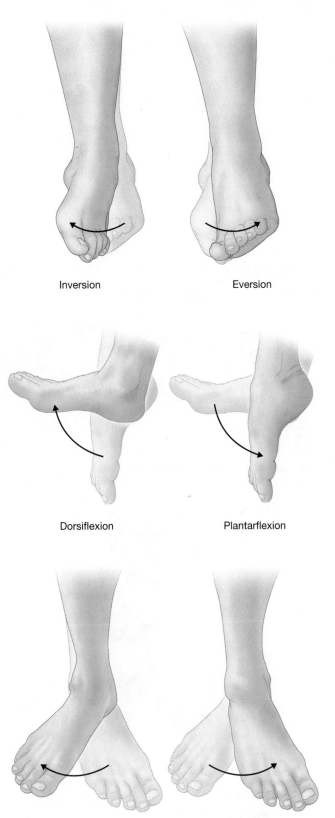

Inversion   Eversion

Dorsiflexion   Plantarflexion

Abduction   Adduction

FIGURE 11.30

Movement of the foot and ankle in three planes

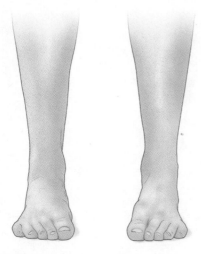

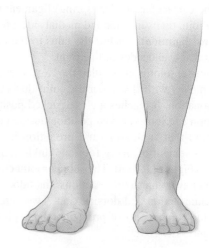

FIGURE 11.31

a) **Hypersupination** b) **Hyperpronation**

EXPLORING TECHNIQUE

Passive Range of Motion for the Ankle

Guidelines:

- Stabilize the ankle above and below the joint.
- Traction the ankle before moving it to avoid pinching joint structures.

- Slowly move the ankle along a linear pathway.
- Ask if your partner feels a stretch, which indicates you've reached end range.
- Have your partner report any pain or discomfort.
- Stop immediately if you notice any pain reactions.
- Perform all PROM tests on both ankles to make a bilateral comparison.

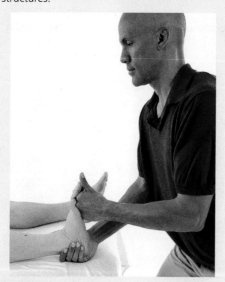

FIGURE 11.32a

a) PROM for dorsiflexion

1. **Dorsiflexion:** With your partner lying supine, hold the back of the ankle with one hand to stabilize it. Grasp the center of the foot with the other hand, traction the ankle, then flex the ankle by leaning your body weight into the foot (Figure 11.32a ■). *Does your partner feel the Achilles tendon stretching? Does the ankle dorsiflex beyond 20 degrees, which is a normal range?*

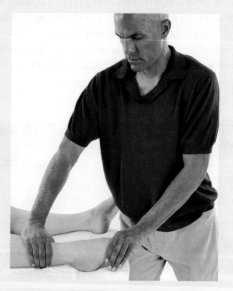

FIGURE 11.32b

b) PROM for plantarflexion

2. **Plantarflexion:** Hold the back of the ankle with one hand to stabilize it. Grasp the center of the foot with the other hand, traction the ankle, then extend the ankle by pressing the top of the foot toward the floor (Figure 11.32b ■). *Does your partner feel the dorsiflexors stretching? Does the ankle straighten?*

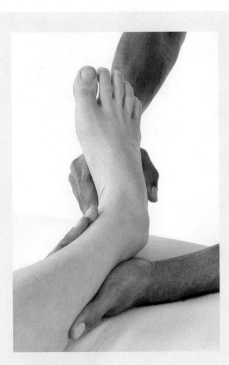

FIGURE 11.32c

c) PROM for inversion

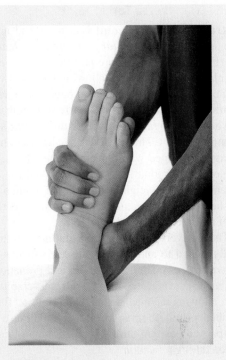

FIGURE 11.32d

d) PROM for eversion

3. **Inversion:** Hold the back of the ankle with one hand to stabilize it. Hold the bottom of rear foot and midfoot with your other hand. Traction the ankle, then turn it toward the medial arch (Figure 11.32c ■). Avoid twisting the forefoot. *Are you keeping the sole of the foot in a plane perpendicular to the sagittal plane?*

4. **Eversion:** Hold the back of the ankle with one hand to stabilize it. Hold the bottom of the rearfoot and midfoot with your other hand. Traction the ankle, then turn the foot in a lateral direction, keeping the sole of the foot in one plane (Figure 11.32d ■). Avoid twisting the forefoot. *If the ankle moves beyond a normal range in any direction, check the range of motion on the other ankle to see what is normal for your partner.*

11.2.5   Transverse Tarsal Joint

The **transverse tarsal joint** is a midtarsal articulation made up of the *talonavicular joint* and the *calcaneocuboid joint* (Figure 11.33 ■). There is little motion between the navicular and cuboid bones, allowing the talonavicular and calcaneocuboid joints to function together as one S-shaped *midtarsal joint* that divides the rearfoot from the midfoot.

The spring ligament supports the plantar side of the talonavicular joint. This highly elastic ligament has a fibrocartilage facet lined with a synovial membrane. It cradles the talonavicular joint like a hammock and functions as a shock absorber for weight coming down through the talus.[4] The short and long plantar ligaments support the plantar side of the calcaneocuboid joint.

The transverse tarsal joint is a gliding joint that is functionally linked to and moves with the subtalar joint during inversion, eversion, supination, and pronation. During midstance, the inferior side of the transverse tarsal joint opens, allowing the medial arch to depress and flatten. Like the subtalar joint, the transverse tarsal joint also reaches a close-packed position during supination and loose-packed position during pronation.

In the **neutral position of the ankle**, the talus aligns over the calcaneus between a position of inversion and eversion (Figure 11.34 ■). Ideally, in a standing posture the ankles align in a neutral position, which can be observed by the relative verticality of the Achilles tendon. The foot rolls through a pronated position during the stance phase of gait and moves into a supinated position at the end of pushoff.

Hyperpronation drops the medial arch, overstretching and weakening its supportive ligaments and tendons, which can lead to "flatfoot" or **pes planus** (see Figure 11.34). This

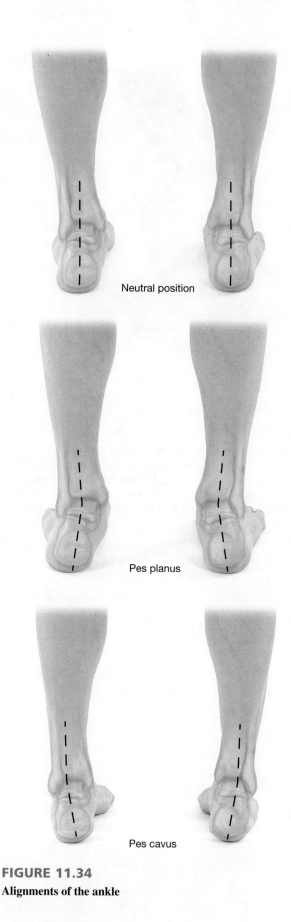

Neutral position

Pes planus

Pes cavus

FIGURE 11.34
Alignments of the ankle

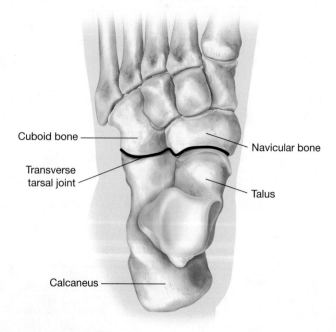

Cuboid bone

Transverse tarsal joint

Calcaneus

Navicular bone

Talus

FIGURE 11.33

Transverse tarsal joint: dorsal view

condition can be rigid and permanent, or flexible, in which case the medial arch only flattens when weight-bearing. Pes planus tips the ankle into **calcaneal valgus**, causing the distal end of the heel to turn away from midline. This creates a supination twist (see Figure 11.38b) in the forefoot and places torsion stresses on subtalar and midfoot joints.

It also causes medial rotation of the tibia, which places torsion stress on the knee. A less common condition, hypersupination, or **pes cavus**, involves excessively high arches, clawed toes, ankle rigidity, and the need for specialized shoes. Pes cavus tips the ankle into **calcaneal varus**, causing the distal end of the heel to turn toward midline.

BONE PALPATION
Subtalar and Transverse Tarsal Joints

Palpate motion in these joints on your own feet first, then on a partner.

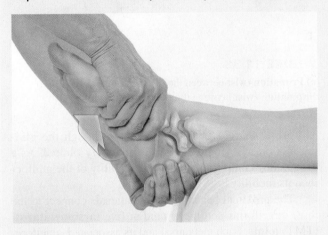

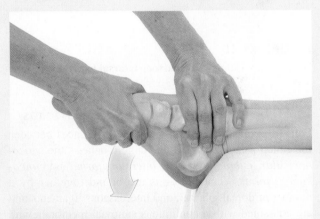

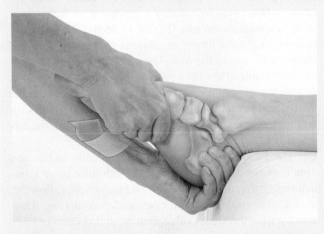

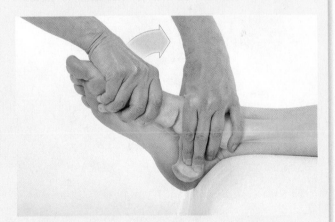

FIGURE 11.35a

Hold the sides of the **subtalar joint** with a pincher grip and passively twist the calcaneus to pronate and supinate the foot. Then actively pronate and supinate the ankle or have your partner actively pronate and supinate. *How much movement do you feel in the subtalar joint? How does the motion differ when you passively move it and actively move it?* (See Figure 11.35a ■)

FIGURE 11.35b

Hold both sides of the **transverse tarsal** joint by grasping the navicular and cuboid in one hand and holding the talus and calcaneus with the other hand. Stabilize the rearfoot and passively move the midfoot through flexion and extension, inversion and eversion, and then pronation and supination. Then actively move it through each range. *How much movement did you feel in the transverse tarsal joint? Is it different during passive and active motion?* (See Figure 11.35b ■)

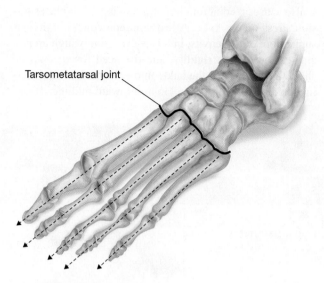

Tarsometatarsal joint

FIGURE 11.36

Weight transfers through the **tarsometatarsal joints** along five rays.

11.2.6 Intertarsal and Tarsometatarsal Joints

Four **intertarsal** (IT) **joints** occupy the spaces between the cuneiforms, navicular, and cuboid bones—the *cuneonavicular, cuboidnavicular, intercuneiform,* and *cuneocuboid joints*.[5] The IT joints are bound together by a number of dorsal, plantar, and interosseous ligaments and are contained with a continuous synovial membrane and joint capsule. They have relatively flat articular surfaces

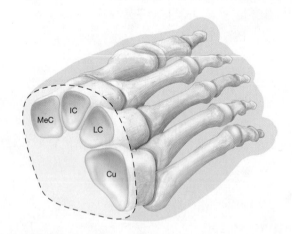

FIGURE 11.37

The triangular shape of the **cuneiforms** wedges them together, providing a stabilizing element to this bony arch.

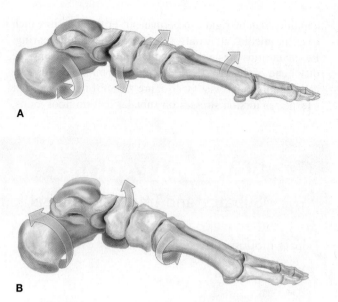

FIGURE 11.38

a) **Pronation twist** between the forefoot and midfoot b) **Supination twist** between the forefoot and midfoot

and are classified as gliding joints, although the gliding motion in a single IT joint is relatively limited. As a group, they contribute more to the stability of the midfoot than its mobility.

The proximal heads of the metatarsals connect to the three cuneiforms and the cuboid at five **tarsometatarsal** (TMT) **joints**. Each metatarsal and its associated cuneiform create a functional unit called a *ray* that transfers weight from the ankle to the toes (Figure 11.36 ■).[6] The first tarsometatarsal joint forms an obvious and easily palpable bump on the top of the foot. The second tarsometatarsal is the most stable of the TMT joints due to its setback position and the wedging of the intermediate cuneiform between the medial and lateral cuneiform (Figure 11.37 ■). The fourth and fifth metatarsals articulate with the cuboid on the lateral side of the foot.

The IT and TMT joints are mechanically linked and usually move as a group. Although each joint has a minimal range of motion, their combined movements allow the medial arch to depress and open under axial load. They also transfer the forces of supination and pronation from the rearfoot through the midfoot into the forefoot. With the calcaneus in a fixed position, they allow the forefoot to twist against the rearfoot during supination and pronation (Figure 11.38a-b ■).

BONE PALPATION
Intertarsal and Tarsometatarsal Joints

Some IT and TMT joints will be easier to move than others, depending on the feet you are palpating. Explore moving the IT and TMT joints on your own feet. Then explore moving them on the feet of several partners to feel the subtle differences in movement.

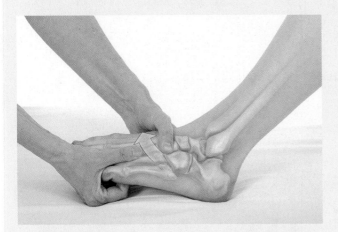

FIGURE 11.39a
To palpate general motion in the group of **IT joints** and **TMT joints,** grasp the tarsals in one hand and the metatarsals in the other. Then flex and extend the transverse arch by bending the foot in both directions. Still holding the foot in the same grasp, gently twist the forefoot and midfoot in opposite directions, in the range it moves during supination and pronation. (See Figure 11.39a ■)

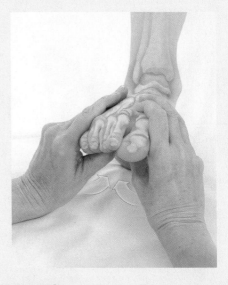

FIGURE 11.39b
To lift the **transverse arch,** hold the medial and lateral sides of the tarsals on both sides, like you would hold a burger in a bun, with your thumbs on the bottom. Lift and fold the transverse arch by pressing your thumbs up and palms medially. (See Figure 11.39b ■)

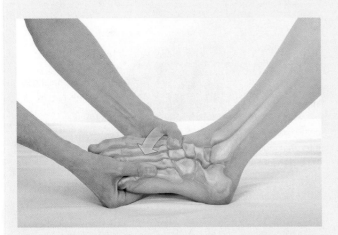

To palpate motion in a **TMT joint,** stabilize the tarsals with one hand and the metatarsal shaft with the other hand. Explore gliding the TMT joint by pressing up under the metatarsal while pressing down on the tarsals. Then reverse the movement, pressing down on the metatarsal while pressing up under the tarsals. Be aware that while moving an individual joint, the other TMT joints will move with it. *Does the first TMT joint bend more than the others? How do your partners' feet feel after having had motion palpated in these joints?* (See Figure 11.39c ■)

FIGURE 11.39c

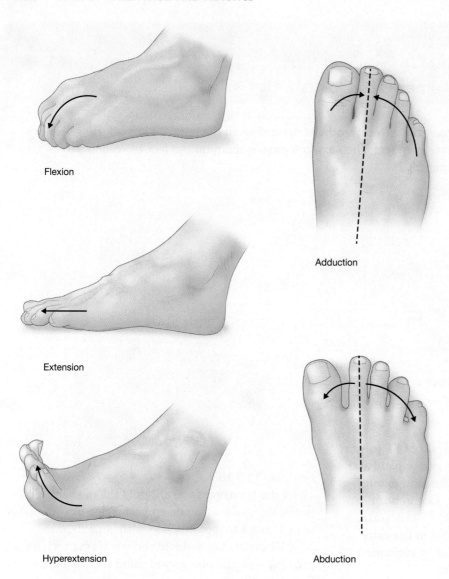

Flexion

Extension

Hyperextension

Adduction

Abduction

FIGURE 11.40

Movements at metatarsophalangeal joints

11.2.7   Metatarsophalangeal and Interphalangeal Joints

Five **metatarsophalangeal** (MTP) **joints** connect the metatarsals to the proximal phalanges. The MTPs are ellipsoid joints with two degrees of movement: flexion, extension, and hyperextension, as well as adduction and abduction (Figure 11.40 ■). The MTPs hyperextend up to 45 degrees in the pushoff phase of gait and flex slightly to grip the ground during the midstance phase. They can be actively flexed an average of 35 degrees. Flexibility in the first MTP, at the base of the first toe and the largest of the MTPs, is critical for the spring-like loading and unloading of the medial arch in gait. Abduction and adduction of the MTPs occurs relative to the second toe. The toes spread away from the second toe during adduction and draw into the second toe during abduction.

The **interphalangeal** (IP) **joints** are hinge joints between the proximal, medial, and distal phalanges. They allow flexion and extension of the toes (Figure 11.41 ■).

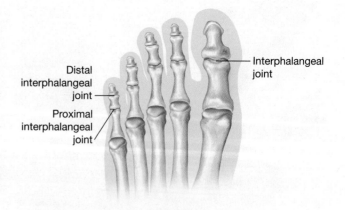

Distal interphalangeal joint

Proximal interphalangeal joint

Interphalangeal joint

FIGURE 11.41

Interphalangeal joints

BONE PALPATION
Metatarsophalangeal and Interphalangeal Joints

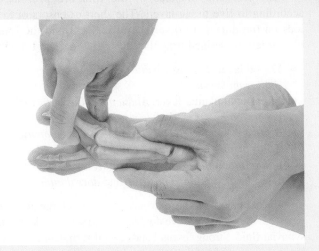

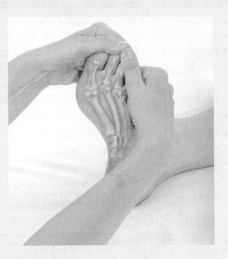

FIGURE 11.42a

To palpate motion in the **MTP joint** at the base of the first toe, hold the head of the first metatarsal in one hand and the first proximal phalanx in the other hand. To feel how the bones fit together, gently approximate the joint surfaces and release. This will also stimulate the synovial lining. Then flex and extend the joint. Avoid lateral bending or rotational movement. Systematically palpate motion in each of the second to fourth MTP joints the same way you did with the first joint. *Do you notice how the first MTP joint is larger than the other four?* (See Figure 11.42a ■)

FIGURE 11.42b

Extend the **MTP joints as a group** and stretch the ball of the foot. Slowly and carefully flex the MTP joints, which can be painful if the toe extensors are tight. *As you extend and flex the MTP joints, does your partner feel a stretch on the bottom and top of the foot?* (See Figure 11.42b ■)

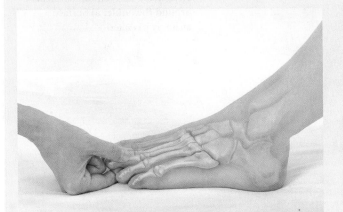

Gently approximate, then flex and extend each **IP joint** on the second through fourth toes. Then flex and extend each IP joint. *How do your partner's feet feel after having motion palpated and the approximation of each MTP and IP joint?* (See Figure 11.42c ■)

FIGURE 11.42c

Each toe from the second to the fifth has a proximal interphalangeal joint (PIP) and a distal interphalangeal joint (DIP). The hallux has one IP joint, which, along with the first MTP joint, is much larger than the other four. Although the range of active motion in the IP joints is only flexion and extension, they can be passively twisted from pressure due to tight shoes or postural aberrations. If the toes become stuck in a twisted position, the torque can pass up the chain of joints, twisting the metatarsals and affecting the alignment of the midfoot and ankle. This will lead to restrictions in foot and ankle flexibility and even chronic pain from compression between the bones and adjacent structures. To work with this pattern, massage the foot in a direction that gently untwists the bones and moves them toward normal alignment.

11.3 MUSCLES OF THE ANKLE AND FOOT

Muscles acting on the ankle and foot fall into two categories: extrinsic and intrinsic. Extrinsic muscles of the foot have origins in the leg and insertions in the foot; their tendons cross the ankle. Intrinsic muscles of the foot have both their origins and insertions in the foot. The extrinsic muscles are presented according to the compartments they occupy:

- Anterior compartment: *Tibialis anterior, extensor digitorum longus, extensor hallucis longus,* and *peroneus tertius*
- Posterior compartment: *Gastrocnemius, soleus,* and *plantaris*

- Deep posterior compartment: *Tibialis posterior, flexor digitorum longus,* and *flexor hallucis longus*
- Lateral compartment: *Peroneus longus* and *peroneus brevis*

The intrinsic muscles of the foot are presented according to five tissue layers. The short extensors of the toes on the dorsal (top) surface of the foot and the four plantar layers, defined from the superficial to deep, follow:

- Dorsal layer: *Extensor hallucis brevis* and *extensor digitorum brevis*
- Superficial plantar layer: *Abductor hallucis, flexor digitorum brevis,* and *abductor digiti minimi*
- Second plantar layer: *Quadratus plantae* and *lumbricals*
- Third plantar layer: *Flexor hallucis brevis, adductor hallucis,* and *flexor digiti minimi brevis*
- Deep layer: *Plantar interossei* and *dorsal interossei*

Each tendon of the extrinsic muscles of the foot is wrapped within a protective double-layered sheath filled with synovial fluid. Strong fascial bands called **retinacula** (singular: *retinaculum*) bind the many tendons that cross the leg and ankle (Figure 11.43a-b ▪). The tubular synovial sheaths encasing tendons allow them to slide freely inside a fluid sleeve in areas where they are strapped down by retinacula.

11.3.1 Extrinsic Muscles of the Ankle and Foot

Extrinsic muscles acting on the ankle and foot occupy four compartments in the lower leg: an anterior, posterior, deep posterior, and lateral compartment (Figure 11.44 ▪). Each compartment is formed by a thick septum, a fascial membrane with the properties of a dense rubber sheet. The septum wraps and binds muscles within that compartment

FIGURE 11.43

Retinacula and tendinous sheaths around the ankle: a) Surface anatomy b) Anterior view

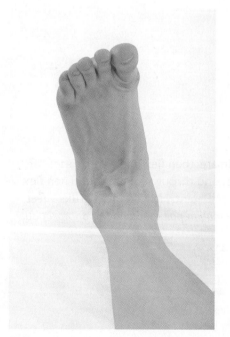

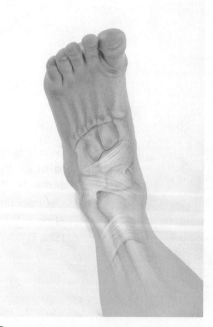

A

B

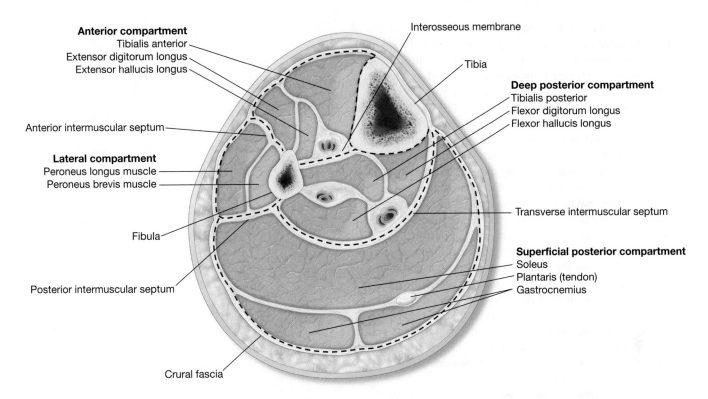

FIGURE 11.44

The four compartments of the leg: cross section

to prevent them from splaying in the lateral direction under compressive stresses.

Ideally, the fascial septum wrapping each compartment is pliable enough to allow room for occupying muscles to shorten and lengthen during movement. **Compartment syndrome** occurs when stiff, unyielding fascia around a pocket of muscles in the lower leg increases pressure within the compartment and compromises the circulation of the muscles within it. This is a serious condition because the pressure obstructs venous blood flow, causing swelling and more pressure, which can lead to necrosis of muscles and nerves within the compartment. Refer clients suspected of having compartment syndrome, with symptoms that include tight, shiny skin and relentless pain, for medical evaluation immediately.

Learning the extrinsic muscles of the foot according to which compartment they occupy can make them easier to remember. Notice how the muscles in the anterior and deep posterior compartment literally mirror each other in name and function.

11.3.1.1 MUSCLES IN THE ANTERIOR COMPARTMENT

The tibialis anterior, extensor digitorum longus, extensor hallucis longus, and peroneus tertius occupy the anterior compartment of the leg (Figure 11.45 ■). The tibialis anterior, extensor digitorum longus, and extensor hallucis longus work together as powerful dorsiflexors of the ankle. All muscles in the anterior compartment are collectively innervated by the *deep peroneal nerve.* The

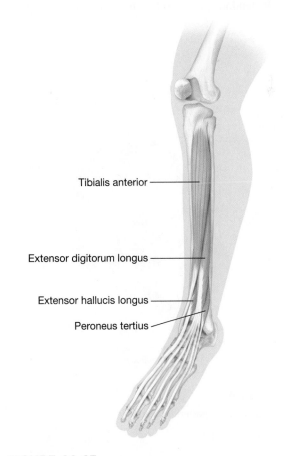

FIGURE 11.45

Anterior leg muscles: dorsiflexors in the anterior compartment peroneus tertius assists dorsiflexion, although functions with the other peroneal muscles as an evertor of the ankle, so it is discussed in the section on the lateral compartment. The superior extensor retinaculum and inferior extensor retinaculum secure the tendons of all four muscles against the lower leg and ankle.

The **tibialis anterior** is a fusiform muscle that arises from the lateral tibial condyle, the upper two-thirds of the lateral tibial surface, and the interosseous membrane. Two-thirds of the way down the shin, it tapers into a long tendon that crosses the front of the ankle. Its tendon then follows a diagonal path across the top of the foot, wrapping around the medial arch and inserting on the plantar surface of the foot at the first cuneiform and the first metatarsal head. The tibialis anterior and the peroneus longus tendon, which wraps under the foot from the lateral side and shares the same insertion site, together create an **anatomical stirrup** that lifts and supports the medial and transverse arches (Figure 11.46 ■). The tibialis anterior dorsiflexes and inverts the ankle; the peroneus longus plantarflexes and everts the ankle. They work as a team to adapt and steer the position of the foot and ankle to uneven terrain. (See TrP for tibialis anterior in Figure 11.47 ■).

The **extensor digitorum longus** is a pennate muscle that arises from the lateral tibial condyle, proximal two-thirds of the anterior fibula, and the interosseous membrane. Its tendon splits into four tendons that insert on the

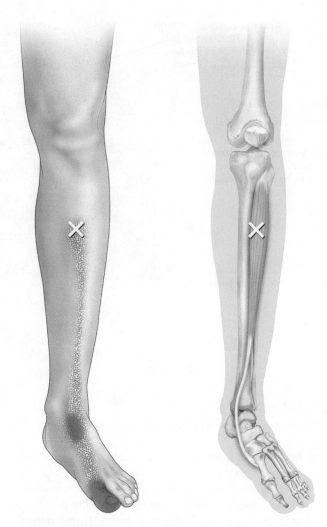

FIGURE 11.47

When tight or dysfunctional, the **tibialis anterior** often develops a trigger point in the upper third of the muscle belly, which can refer pain along the lower shin into the anterior ankle and first toe.

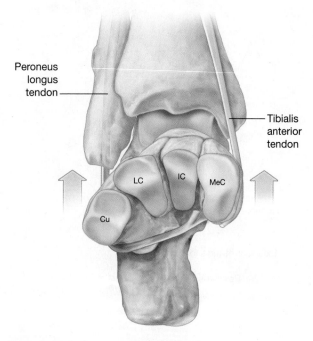

FIGURE 11.46

Anatomical stirrup: posterior view

proximal and distal phalanges of the second to fifth toes. The primary movement of the extensor digitorum longus is to extend the lateral four toes, as well as the lateral MTP four and IP joints. It also assists dorsiflexion and eversion. (See TrP for the extensor digitorum longus in Figure 11.48 ■).

The **extensor hallucis longus** lies under the tibialis anterior and extensor digitorum longus. Because it is deeper than its neighbors, it can be difficult to palpate. This thin, pennate muscle arises from the middle half of the fibula and the interosseous membrane, then crosses the anterior ankle and inserts on the distal phalanx of the hallux. Its primary action is to extend the MTP of the hallux;

it also assists dorsiflexion and inversion and is active during postural sway. (See TrP for the extensor hallicus longus in Figure 11.48 ■).

Anterior compartment syndrome is marked by a diffuse tenderness and tightness over the entire belly of the tibialis anterior. Muscles occupying the anterior compartment become tender to touch, sensitive to passive stretch, and weak. Anterior compartment syndrome can be confused with anterior **shin splints,** an irritation of the periosteum from overuse. Shin splints develop from repetitive jarring impact on foot strike, which causes excessive shear and pull in the interosseous membrane between the tibia and fibula.

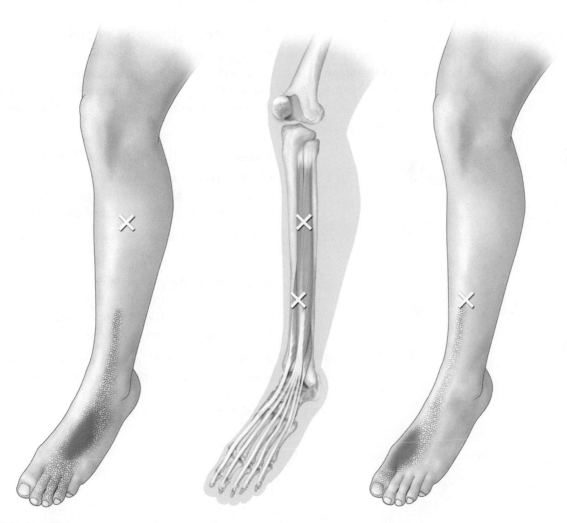

FIGURE 11.48

When dysfunctional, the **extensor digitorum longus** can develop a trigger point in the belly of the muscle, right below the tibialis anterior trigger point, which can refer pain along the dorsal side of the second through fourth metatarsals. When dysfunctional, the **extensor hallucis longus** can develop a trigger point about 4 inches above the ankle and lateral to the shin, which can refer pain along the first metatarsal.

MUSCLE PALPATION
Tibialis Anterior, Extensor Digitorum Longus, and Extensor Hallucis Longus

Begin by palpating these muscles on your own leg along the lateral side of the tibia. To locate the tibialis anterior by its contraction, dorsiflex and plantarflex your ankle; to locate the extensor digitorum hallucis, wiggle your first toe; and to locate the extensor hallucis longus, wiggle your four lateral toes. Use the same movements to locate their tendons; then trace the tendons from your ankle to their insertions.

Tibialis Anterior

O–Lateral tibial condyle, proximal two-thirds of anterior lateral tibia, interosseous membrane
I–First cuneiform, base of first metatarsal head
A–Dorsiflexes ankle and inverts foot

Extensor Digitorum Longus (EDL)

O–Lateral tibial condyle, proximal two-thirds of anterior fibula, interosseous membrane
I–Base of middle and distal phalanx of lateral four toes
A–Extends lateral four toes, assists dorsiflexion and eversion

Extensor Hallucis Longus (EHL)

O–Middle half of anterior fibula, interosseous membrane
I–Base of distal phalanx of first toe
A–Extends first toe, assists dorsiflexion and inversion

With your partner in the supine position, locate the **tibialis anterior** by pressing directly lateral along the proximal half of the tibial shaft. *Do you notice how the belly of the tibialis anterior creates a muscular mound along the lateral side of the shin?*

Active movement: Have your partner dorsiflex the ankle to contract the tibialis anterior, then palpate its contraction along the medial side of the tibia, right below the knee (Figure 11.49a ▪).

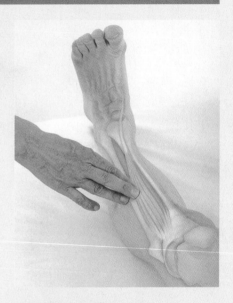

FIGURE 11.49a
Palpating the tibialis anterior contraction.

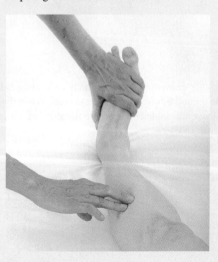

Resisted movement: Have your partner resist while you lightly press the ankle into plantarflexion and eversion (Figure 11.49b ▪).

FIGURE 11.49b
Resisted movement of the tibialis anterior.

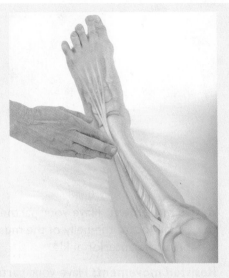

FIGURE 11.49c

Palpating the extensor digitorum longus contraction.

Locate the **extensor digitorum longus** tendon between the tibialis anterior and the peroneals. *Are you pressing between the tibialis anterior and the peroneal muscles?*

Active movement: Have your partner wiggle the lateral four toes while you locate the tendons of the extensor digitorum longus on the lateral side of the lower tibia, then follow the tendon up into the muscle belly (Figure 11.49c ■).

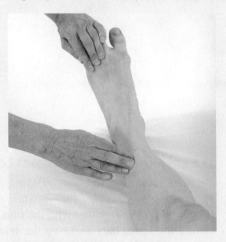

FIGURE 11.49d

Resisted movement of the extensor digitorum longus.

Resisted movement: Have your partner resist as you lightly push the lateral four toes into flexion (Figure 11.49d ■). Palpate the contraction with fingertip pressure and cross fibers strumming. *Do you feel the peroneal muscles directly lateral of this muscle?*

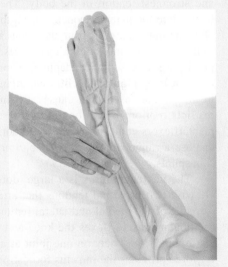

FIGURE 11.49e

Palpating the extensor hallucis longus contraction.

Locate the **extensor hallucis longus** on the lateral distal third of the tibial shaft (Figure 11.49e ■).

Separating fascial pockets: Explore sliding your fingertips between this group of muscles and the peroneal compartment. Also explore sliding your fingertips between the tibialis anterior and the tibial shaft.

(continued)

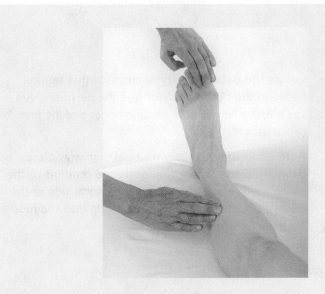

Active movement: Have your partner move the first toe as you locate the belly of the muscle and find its tendon at the anterior ankle.

Resisted movement: Have your partner resist as you lightly push your partner's first toe into flexion (Figure 11.49f ■).

FIGURE 11.49f

Resisted movement of the extensorhallucis longus.

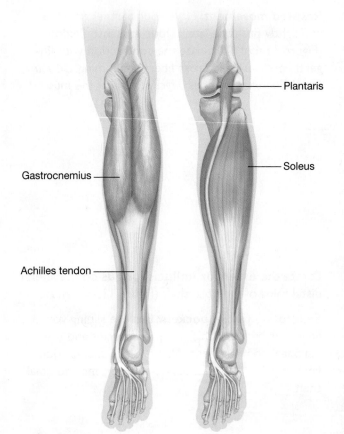

FIGURE 11.50

Posterior leg muscles: plantarflexors in the posterior compartment

11.3.1.2   MUSCLES IN THE POSTERIOR COMPARTMENT

Two large and powerful plantarflexors, the gastrocnemius and soleus, occupy the posterior compartment (Figure 11.50 ■). Together with the small plantaris located behind the knee, they make up the **triceps surae** (surae means calf). All three muscles are innervated by the *tibial nerve,* and all three insert at the Achilles tendon, the largest and strongest tendon in the body. The Achilles tendon blends into the plantar aponeurosis on the sole of the foot, allowing muscular pulls from the soleus and gastrocnemius to transfer along the longitudinal arches. This relationship predisposes a person with adaptively shortened plantarflexors to develop **plantar fasciitis,** an inflammatory condition in the plantar fascia that causes a painful tightness and restricts motion in the longitudinal arches. Tight, short plantarflexors can also overload the dorsiflexors and predispose a runner to anterior compartment syndrome and shin splints.

The **gastrocnemius** is a large, double-headed muscle with two proximal tendons that attach on the posterior side of the medial and lateral femoral condyles. This biarticular muscle flexes the knee and plantarflexes the ankle, but it only acts on one joint at a time. Its powerful force provides the impetus for a strong pushoff in rigorous activities such as race walking or running, and for sudden takeoffs in activities such as jumping or sprinting. When dysfunctional, the gastrocnemius develops trigger points in four locations. (See TrPs for the gastrocnemius in Figure 11.51 ■).

FIGURE 11.51

The most common **gastrocnemius** trigger point develops in the upper third of the medial head, which can refer pain to the instep of the foot and cause spillover pain over the calf and posterior knee. Two other gastrocnemius trigger points can develop right below the proximal tendons behind the knee, and a fourth trigger point can form in the middle of the lateral belly, all of which can refer pain locally.

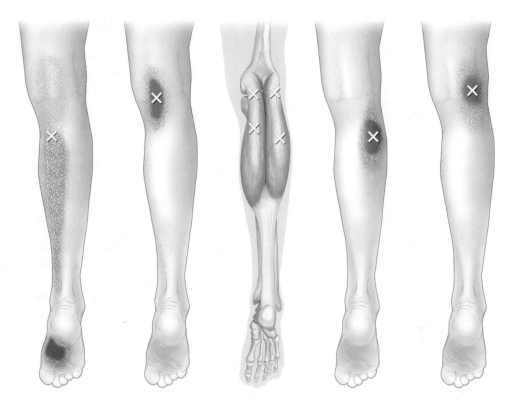

FIGURE 11.52

When tight or dysfunctional, the **soleus** can develop trigger points in three locations. The most likely soleus trigger point occurs right above the medial aspect of the Achilles tendon and refers pain into the heel. A second soleus trigger point can develop right below the proximal tendon and refer pain to the center of the calf. An uncommon trigger point in the distal lateral third of the soleus can refer pain to the sacroiliac joint on the same side. Soleus trigger points can limit dorsiflexion, making it difficult for a person to bend over to pick up things.

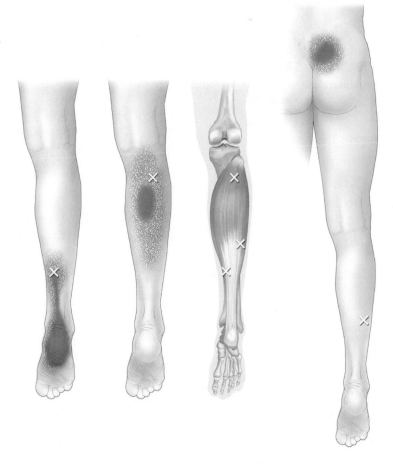

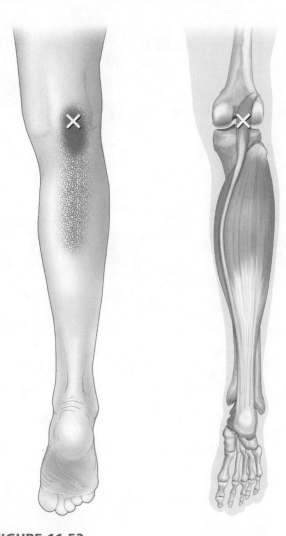

FIGURE 11.53

A **plantaris** trigger point can develop directly behind the knee, which can refer pain locally.

The **soleus** lies beneath the gastrocnemius and arises across the upper half of the posterior tibia and fibula. This bipennate muscle is remarkably resistant to fatigue due to the predominance of slow twitch fibers in it. It is continually active in postural sway, firing with slow tonic contractions. In contrast, the gastrocnemius, which has more fast fibers, fires during quick contractions. Nicknamed the "second heart" because of its rhythmic contractions during postural sway, the soleus assists in the venous return of blood to the heart. (See TrPs for the soleus in Figure 11.52 ■).

The **plantaris,** a small and somewhat weak muscle the size of a finger, crosses the posterior knee and attaches to the lateral posterior femoral epicondyle. Considered an accessory lateral head of the gastrocnemius, it assists knee flexion, although minimally. Its long distal tendon follows along the lateral edge of the soleus, blends into the medial aspect of the Achilles tendon, and inserts on the posterior surface of the calcaneus. (See TrPs for the plantaris in Figure 11.53 ■).

SELF-CARE
Stretching the Gastrocnemius and Soleus

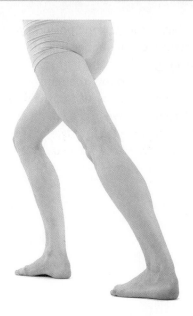

FIGURE 11.54a

1. **Gastrocnemius stretch:** Keep your knees straight to stretch the gastrocnemius because it puts tension on the muscle across both joints, both the ankle and knee (Figure 11.54a ■). To get an even stretch of both heads of the gastrocnemius, avoid lateral rotation of your hip.

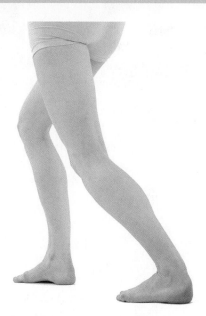

FIGURE 11.54b

2. **Soleus stretch:** Bend your knees to stretch the soleus, which puts the overlying gastrocnemius on slack (Figure 11.54b ■). The Achilles tendon is so strong and unyielding that you need to use a lot of pressure to stretch it.

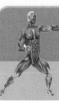

MUSCLE PALPATION
Gastrocnemius and Soleus

Begin by palpating these muscles on your own leg while sitting in a chair. Locate the double-bellied gastrocnemius by pressing into the meaty muscle covering the back of the upper calf. Follow the lateral borders of the gastrocnemius down to the Achilles tendon.

To feel both muscles contract, hold your palms against the middle calf, then raise and lower your heel. The gastrocnemius will create a superficial bulge on the upper calf as it contracts; as it contracts, the soleus bulges into a flat, wide belly under the gastrocnemius, across the middle calf.

Gastrocnemius

O–Posterior medial and lateral condyles of femur
I–Posterior calcaneus via Achilles tendon
A–Plantarflexes ankle

Soleus

O–Proximal posterior tibia and fibula, soleal line of posterior tibia
I–Posterior calcaneus via medial aspect of Achilles tendon
A–Plantarflexes ankle

(continued)

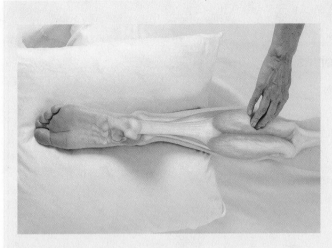

FIGURE 11.55a
Palpating the gastrocnemius

With your partner in a prone position, palpate the **gastrocnemius** on the upper half of the posterior calf (Figure 11.55a ■). Locate its proximal tendons behind the knee and follow them down into the large meaty belly on each head of the muscle. Also feel the difference between the lateral and medial heads. *Can you find the lateral edges of the gastrocnemius? How wide is the Achilles tendon?*

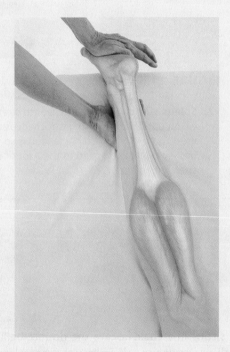

FIGURE 11.55b
Resisted movement of the gastrocnemius

Resisted movement: With the knee straight, have your partner resist as you slowly push down on the foot and dorsiflex the ankle (Figure 11.55b ■).

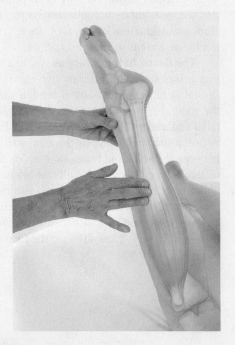

FIGURE 11.55c
Palpating the soleus contraction

Bend your partner's knee to put the overlying gastrocnemius muscle on slack while you palpate the broad and meaty **soleus** directly above Achilles tendon. Explore tracing and lifting the edges of the soleus. *Do you notice how wide the soleus is compared to the gastrocnemius?*

Active movement: With the knee bent, have your partner point the toes to contract the soleus while you palpate it (Figure 11.55c ■).

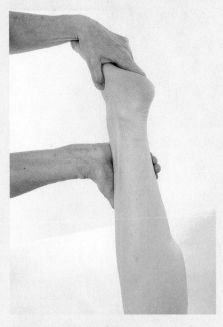

FIGURE 11.55d
Resisted movement of the soleus

Resisted movement: With the knee bent, have your partner resist as you slowly push down on the foot and dorsiflex the ankle (Figure 11.55d ■). Make sure to push against the arches and not the toes.

11.3.1.3 MUSCLES IN THE DEEP POSTERIOR COMPARTMENT

Three muscles occupy the deep posterior compartment: the tibialis posterior, flexor digitorum longus, and flexor hallucis longus. All three are sandwiched between the posterior tibia, fibula, and interosseous membrane on the front and the soleus and gastrocnemius on the back (Figure 11.56 ■).

Their tendons pass directly behind the medial malleolus, along with the tibial artery and the *tibial nerve,* which innervates all the three muscles.

The **tibialis posterior** originates along the upper two-thirds of the posterior tibia, fibula, and the interosseous membrane. The distal tendon of this bipennate muscle loops under the medial malleolus and passes through the **tarsal tunnel,** between the flexor retinaculum and talus and over the deltoid ligament. From there it dives under the medial arch, where it branches into fibrous, finger-like slips that insert posteriorly on the sustentaculum tali and inferiorly on the navicular tuberosity, cuboid, three cuneiforms, and the base of the second through fourth metatarsals. Its many tendinous slips lie directly under the spring ligament and work as a primary support and stabilizer for the medial arch. The tibialis posterior acts with the tibialis anterior to invert the ankle. It also assists dorsiflexion. (See TrP for the tibialis posterior in Figure 11.57 ■).

Another bipennate muscle, the **flexor digitorum longus,** arises from the middle posterior surface of the tibia. Its distal tendon runs between the tibialis posterior and flexor hallucis longus tendon as it passes behind the medial malleolus, then wraps under the medial arch, where it splits into four long tendons that insert on the distal phalanges of the second to fifth toes. As an antagonist

to the extensor digitorum longus, its primary function is to flex the toes, although it also assists plantarflexion, inversion, and adduction of the foot. (See TrPs for the flexor digitorum longus in Figure 11.58 ■).

The **flexor hallucis longus** is also a bipennate muscle that arises from the inferior two-thirds of the posterior fibula. It tapers into a distal tendon that passes behind the medial malleolus through a groove in the posterior talus and under the sustentaculum tali. From here, it runs between the two heads of the flexor hallucis brevis and between the sesamoid bones to insert on the distal phalanx of the hallux. The flexor hallucis longus tendon crosses under the flexor digitorum longus tendon under the midfoot, providing added support to the medial arch. It plays an important role in gait because it powers the pushoff from the first toe. (See TrPs for the flexor hallucis longus in Figure 11.59 ■).

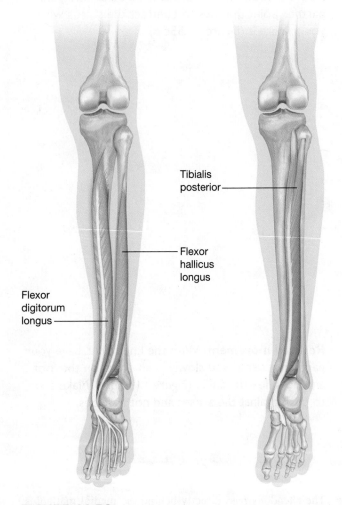

FIGURE 11.56

Posterior leg muscles: plantarflexors in the deep posterior compartment

Labels: Tibialis posterior; Flexor hallicus longus; Flexor digitorum longus

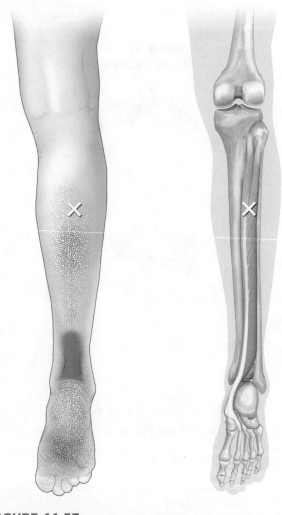

FIGURE 11.57

When dysfunctional, the **tibialis posterior** can develop a trigger point in the belly of the muscle one-third of the way down the calf, which can refer pain into the Achilles tendon and arch of the foot during walking or running.

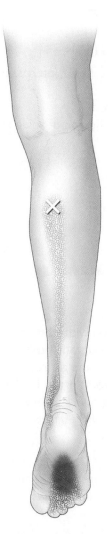
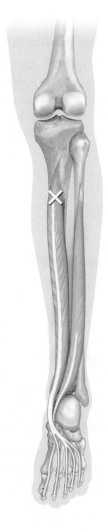
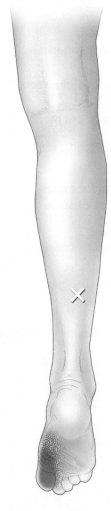
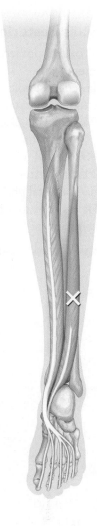

FIGURE 11.58

When dysfunctional, the **flexor digitorum longus** can develop a trigger point several inches below the knee, which can refer pain to the sole of the foot directly under the four lateral metatarsals.

FIGURE 11.59

When dysfunctional, the **flexor hallucis longus** can develop a trigger point in its belly lateral to the Achilles tendon, which can refer pain to the base of the hallux and the entire first toe.

MUSCLE PALPATION
Tibialis Posterior, Flexor Digitorum Longus, and Flexor Hallucis Longus

Palpate this group of deep muscles on yourself. Locate their tendons behind the Achilles tendon on the medial side of your lower leg. Point your toes as you palpate their tendons on the posterior side of the medial malleolus, then move up to the belly of the muscles.

To find the tibialis posterior, carefully press through the overlying gastrocnemius and soleus while you flex and extend your ankle to get the tibialis posterior to contract. Also, slip your fingertips between the soleus and the peroneals, pressing the belly of the tibialis posterior into the back of the fibula. Explore strumming across the dense, fibrous muscle as you flex and extend your ankle. Also walk your fingers down the length of the muscles.

(continued)

Tibialis Posterior

O–Proximal posterior tibia and fibula, interosseous
   membrane

I–Navicular, cuboid, cuneiforms, base of the second
   to fourth metatarsals

A–Plantarflexes ankle, inverts foot, stabilizes medial arch

Flexor Digitorum Longus (FDL)

O–Medial posterior tibia

I–Base of distal phalanges of lateral four toes

A–Flexes toes, assists plantarflexion of ankle and
   inversion of foot

Flexor Hallucis Longus (FHL)

O–Lower two-thirds of posterior fibula, interosseous membrane

I–Base of distal phalanx of first toe

A–Flexes first toe, assists plantarflexion of ankle and
   inversion of foot

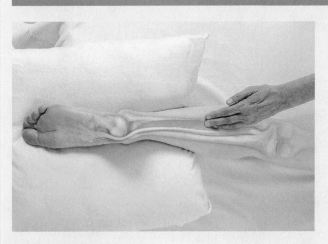

FIGURE 11.60a
Palpating the tibialis posterior

Put your partner in a prone position with a bolster or
pillow under the ankles. Locate the **tibialis posterior**
by pressing slowly into the center of the gastrocnemius
and through the flexor hallucis longus (Figure 11.60a ■).
*Are you pressing through the overlying muscles? Do you
notice how the deep posterior muscles have a denser, more
fibrous feel than the overlying muscles?*

Active movement: Have your partner invert and
dorsiflex the ankle while you palpate its belly and
locate its tendon behind the medial malleolus.

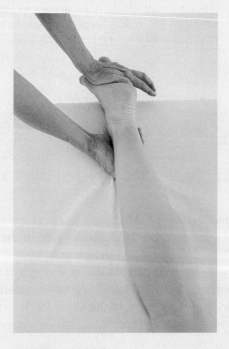

FIGURE 11.60b
Resisted movement of the tibialis posterior

Resisted movement: Have your partner resist while
you lightly press the ankle into dorsiflexion and eversion (Figure 11.60b ■). Press for a few seconds along
a diagonal line of force. To keep the FDL and FDH
relaxed, make sure your partner does not curl any of
the toes.

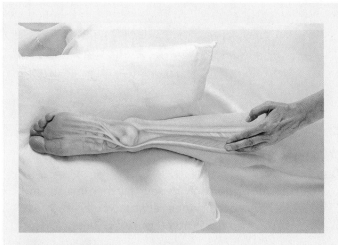

FIGURE 11.60c
Palpating the flexor digitorum longus

To locate the **flexor digitorum longus** tendon, press directly behind the tibialis posterior tendon on the medial side of the ankle (Figure 11.60c ■).

Active movement: Have your partner curl and flex toes two to five while keeping the first toe and ankle still (this is often difficult to coordinate). Locate the flexor digitorum longus contraction under the medial edge of the Achilles tendon, pressing directly into the tibia.

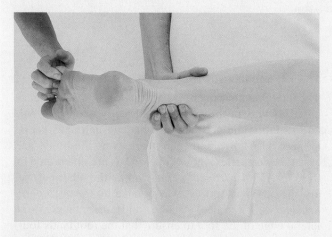

FIGURE 11.60d
Resisted movement of the flexor digitorum longus

Resisted movement: With your partner in a supine position, have your partner resist as you lightly take the lateral four toes into extension (Figure 11.60d ■).

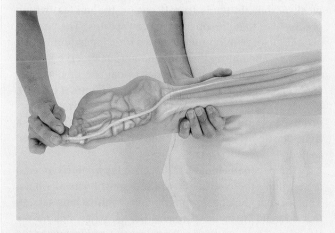

FIGURE 11.60e
Palpating the flexor hallucis longus

Have your partner curl and flex the first toe while keeping the other toes extended while you locate **flexor hallucis longus** contraction under the medial edge of the Achilles tendon, pressing directly into the tibia (Figure 11.60e ■).

(continued)

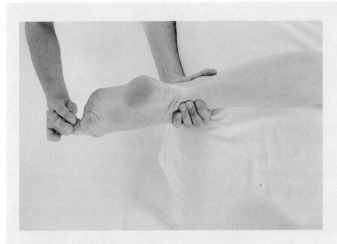

Resited movement: With your partner in a supine position, have your partner resist as you lightly press the first toe into extension (Figure 11.60f ■).

FIGURE 11.60f

Palpating the flexor hallucis longus

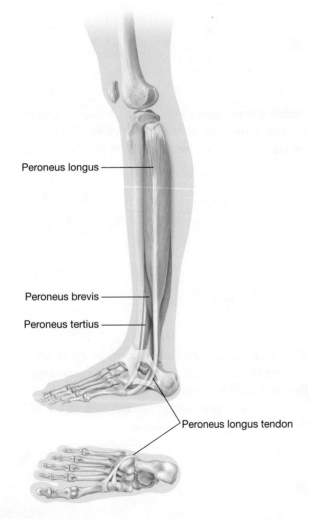

Peroneus longus

Peroneus brevis

Peroneus tertius

Peroneus longus tendon

FIGURE 11.61

Lateral leg muscles: evertors in the lateral compartment

11.3.1.4   MUSCLES IN THE LATERAL COMPARTMENT

The lateral compartment is the smallest of the four muscular pockets in the leg. It lies directly over the fibula and contains the peroneus longus and peroneus brevis (Figure 11.61 ■). Both peroneals evert the ankle and assist in plantarflexion; both peroneals are innervated by the *superficial peroneal nerve.* Unlike the other peroneals, the peroneus tertius is innervated by the *deep peroneal nerve.* From heel strike to midstance, they lift the lateral edge of the foot to ensure that the foot lands foursquare on the ground. The peroneals also pull the center of weight in the foot to its lateral edge in activities that require side-stepping, like tennis. A person with weak peroneals tends to roll out on the ankles, which predisposes that person to inversion sprains. The peroneals can also develop taut bands with trigger points that compress and entrap the common peroneal nerve against the fibula, so they can be tender to palpate or massage. (See TrPs for the peroneal muscles in Figure 11.62 ■). Peroneal tightness may lead to *lateral compartment syndrome,* a condition aggravated by high heels, flat feet, a tight elastic around the calf, and crossing the legs when seated.

The **peroneus longus** (also called the *fibularis longus*) arises along the proximal two-thirds of the lateral fibula. This slender, bipennate muscle tapers into a long tendon that descends over the peroneus brevis, wraps behind the lateral malleolus and under the calcaneus, and inserts on the sole of the foot at the medial cuneiform and base of the first metatarsal. Its distal attachment site is directly lateral to the tendon of its antagonist, the tibialis anterior. Together they create an "anatomical stirrup" that supports and lifts the transverse arch, balancing the stance foot between inversion and eversion.

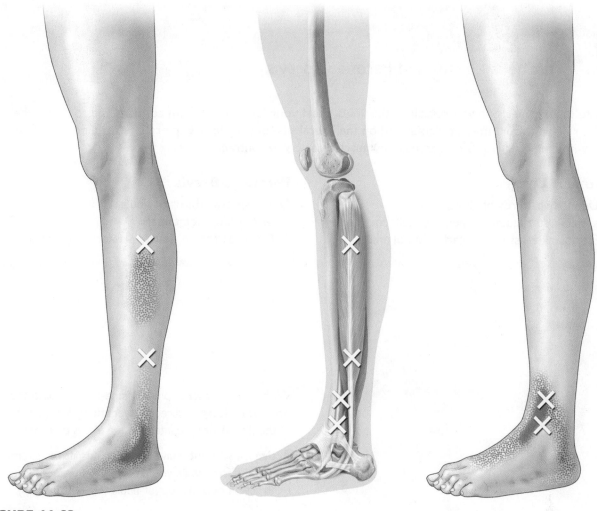

FIGURE 11.62

When dysfunctional, the **peroneus longus** often develops a trigger point below the head of the fibula, which can refer pain over and around the lateral malleolus. When dysfunctional, the **peroneus brevis** can develop a trigger point on the distal third of the muscle belly, which can refer pain over and around the lateral malleolus. The **peroneus tertius** can develop two trigger points in the belly of the muscle, staggered evenly several inches directly above the lateral malleolus, which can refer pain anterior to and over the lateral malleolus.

The smaller **peroneus brevis** (also called the *fibularis brevis*) arises below the peroneus longus along the distal two-thirds of the lateral fibula. The tendon of this bipennate muscle also loops behind the lateral malleolus. It passes under the peroneal trochlea and inserts on the tuberosity at the base of the fifth metatarsal.

The thin **peroneus tertius** (also known as the *fibularis tertius*) occupies the anterior compartment, yet is functionally grouped with the other peroneals as evertors of the ankle. It arises along the distal half of the fibula as a continuation of the extensor digitorum longus. The distal tendon of this small, pennate muscle inserts on the tubercle of the fifth metatarsal, where it assists eversion and dorsiflexion to help plant the foot squarely on the ground. The peroneus tertius is often missing on one or both sides of the body.

MUSCLE PALPATION
Peroneus Longus and Peroneus Brevis

Palpate the peroneals on yourself, along the fibula. Evert your foot to feel them contract and to locate their tendons behind your lateral malleolus and on the lateral side of your foot. Explore lifting the pocket of peroneals with a pincher grip. Strum across the muscles while you contract and relax them.

<table>
<tr><td>

Peroneus Longus

O–Upper two-thirds of fibula
I–Base of first metatarsal, medial cuneiform
A–Everts ankle, assists plantarflexion of ankle

</td><td>

Peroneus Brevis

O–Lower two-thirds of fibula
I–Base of fifth metatarsal
A–Everts the ankle, assists plantarflexion of ankle

</td></tr>
</table>

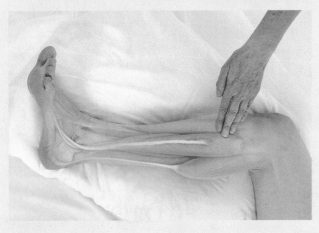

FIGURE 11.63a
Palpating the peroneus longus contraction

With your partner supine or side-lying, palpate the **peroneus longus** directly over the upper two-thirds of the fibula). *Are you lateral to the tibialis anterior?*

Active movement: Have your partner lift the lateral side of the foot while you palpate the peroneus longus contraction over the upper fibula (Figure 11.63a ■).

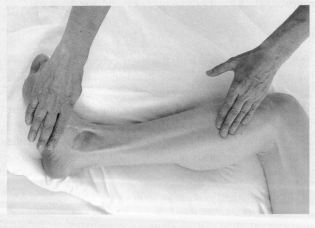

FIGURE 11.63b
Resisted movement of the peroneals

Resisted movement: Have your partner resist as you press the lateral side of the foot into inversion and dorsiflexion (Figure 11.63b ■).

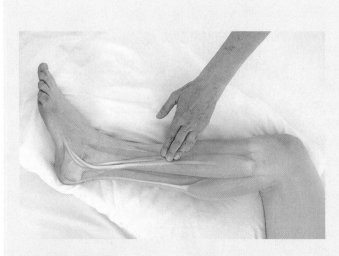

FIGURE 11.63c
Palpating the peroneus brevis.

Palpate the **peroneus brevis** directly on the lower third of the fibula (Figure 11.63c ■). *Can you differentiate the distal tendons of the peroneus longus and the peroneus brevis at their insertion sites? Can slide your fingertips between the soleus and the peroneals?*

11.3.2 Intrinsic Muscles of the Foot

The intrinsic muscles of the foot function synergistically to carry out several unique functions. They give the arches flexibility to absorb shock and to make intrinsic adjustments in the foot for balance. They also provide enough rigidity to stabilize the subtalar and transverse tarsal joints during propulsion.

There are only two intrinsic muscles located on the dorsal surface of the foot: the extensor digitorum brevis and extensor hallucis brevis (Figure 11.64 ■). Most of the intrinsic muscles of the foot are located on its plantar surface. They can be divided into four layers, from superficial to deep (Figure 11.65 ■).

In this section, we look at the intrinsic muscles on the dorsal surface first, then examine the plantar muscles from the superficial to deep layers.

11.3.2.1 SUPERFICIAL LAYER OF INTRINSIC DORSAL MUSCLES

The short extensors of the toes located on top of the foot include the extensor hallucis brevis and extensor digitorum brevis (Figure 11.66 ■). The short extensors of the toes are unique because they are the only two muscles with origins on the dorsal surface of the foot. They have no counterparts in the hand. The *deep peroneal nerve* innervates both muscles.

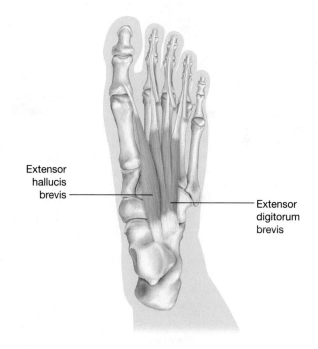

Extensor hallucis brevis

Extensor digitorum brevis

FIGURE 11.64

Short extensors of the toes: located on the dorsal surface of the foot

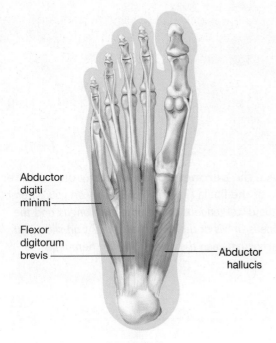

Superficial layer

Abductor digiti minimi

Flexor digitorum brevis

Abductor hallucis

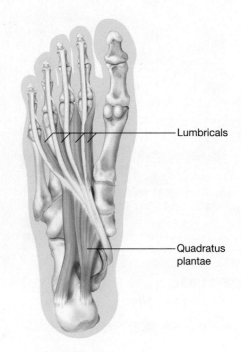

Second layer

Lumbricals

Quadratus plantae

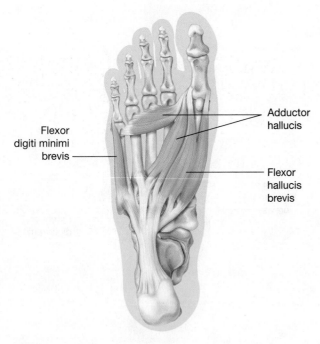

Third layer

Flexor digiti minimi brevis

Adductor hallucis

Flexor hallucis brevis

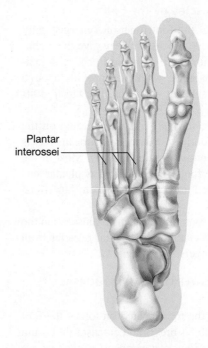

Deepest layer

Plantar interossei

FIGURE 11.65
Intrinsic muscles of the foot

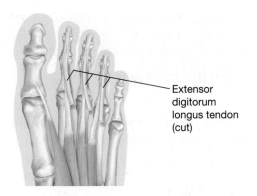

FIGURE 11.66

The bifurcation in the short extensor tendons allows the extensor digitorum longus tendons to attach over the dorsal surfaces of the middle interphalangeal joints.

Extensor
digitorum
longus tendon
(cut)

The **extensor digitorum brevis** (EDB) arises from the anterior lateral surface of the calcaneus and the inferior side of the extensor retinaculum. Three small heads of this muscle taper into three tendons that insert on the extensor digitorum longus tendons from the second to the fourth toe.

The **extensor hallucis brevis** (EHB) arises from the anterior lateral surface of the calcaneus, directly medial to the extensor digitorum brevis. It tapers into a tendon that inserts on the proximal end of the proximal phalanx of the first toe. (See TrPs for the extensor digitorum brevis and extensor hallicus brevis in Figure 11.67 ■).

Both the EDB and EHB work as the primary extensors of the metacarpophalangeal joints. The extensor digitorum brevis extends the second to fourth toes, and the extensor hallucis brevis extends the first toe. Occasionally, the EDB has a fourth belly that attaches to the fifth toe.

FIGURE 11.67

When dysfunctional, the **extensor digitorum brevis** and **extensor hallucis brevis** can each develop a trigger point in the proximal third of the muscle belly, which can refer pain locally over the center of the muscle. Trigger points in these short extensors can be aggravated by tight shoes, which usually results in a stiff manner of walking in which a person avoids bending the shoe against the muscle.

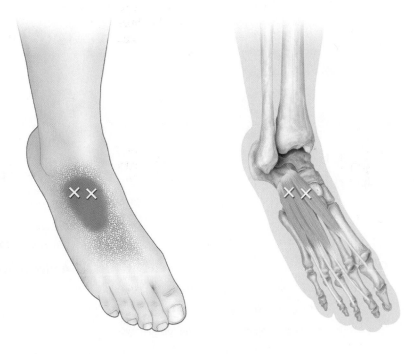

MUSCLE PALPATION
Extensor Digitorum Brevis and Extensor Hallucis Brevis

Both of these muscles are easy to palpate on the top of the foot. Palpate them on yourself first. Isolate their actions by moving your toes while keeping your ankle still. People with inversion sprains often mistake the small fleshy extensor digitorum brevis for a bruise.

Extensor Digitorum Brevis

O–Anterior lateral calcaneus, extensor retinaculum
I–Extensor digitorum longus tendons from second to fourth toes
A–Extends second to fourth toes

Extensor Hallucis Brevis

O–Anterior lateral calcaneus, extensor retinaculum
I–Proximal phalanx of first toe
A–Extends first toe

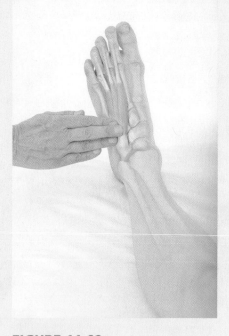

FIGURE 11.68a
Palpating the extensor digitorum brevis

With your partner sitting or supine, palpate the **extensor digitorum brevis** directly in front of the ankle on the lateral side (Figure 11.68a ■). *Do you feel the small fleshy muscle belly of the extensor digitorum brevis over the lateral dorsal surface of the tarsals?*

Active movement: Have your partner lift the lateral four toes while you feel the EDB contract.

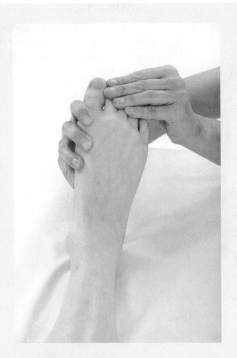

Palpate the **extensor hallucis brevis** directly medial of the EDB.

Active movement: Have your partner raise and lower the first toe while you locate the belly of the EHB.

Stretch: Stretch the extensor digitorum brevis by bending the lateral four toes into flexion (Figure 11.68b ■). Stretch the extensor hallucis longus by bending the first toe into flexion.

FIGURE 11.68b
Stretching the extensor digitorum brevis

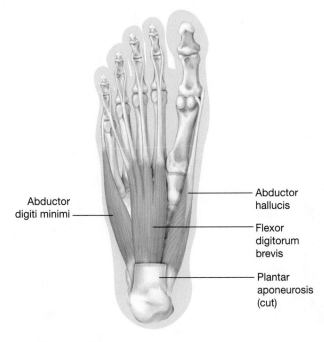

Abductor digiti minimi

Abductor hallucis

Flexor digitorum brevis

Plantar aponeurosis (cut)

FIGURE 11.69
Intrinsic muscles of the foot: superficial layer of plantar surface

11.3.2.2 SUPERFICIAL LAYER OF INTRINSIC PLANTAR MUSCLES

A layer of thick, strong aponeurosis covers the plantar surface of the foot and gives rise to three short flexors: the abductor hallucis, flexor digitorum brevis, and the abductor minimi brevis (Figure 11.69 ■). This group of muscles functions like tie-beams; their longitudinal span along the sole of the foot shores up the longitudinal arches in their weight-bearing capacity. It is interesting to note that when a person has a flat-footed pattern of hyperpronation, the foot splays into the shape of this muscle layer, which indicates a weakness in the deeper intrinsic muscles of the foot. The *medial plantar nerve* innervates both the abductor hallucis and the flexor digitorum brevis. The *lateral plantar nerve* innervates the abductor digiti minimi.

The **abductor hallucis** arises from the medial plantar aspect of the calcaneal tuberosity, the flexor retinaculum, and the plantar aponeurosis. Its long tendon runs along the medial side of the first metatarsal and inserts at the base of the proximal phalanx of the first toe on the medial side. This superficial muscle flexes and abducts the first toe. Tension in this muscle aggravates a condition called **hallux valgus**—a pattern of chronic adduction in the first

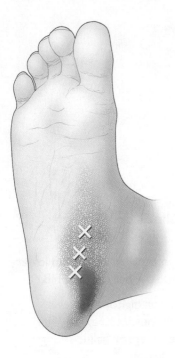

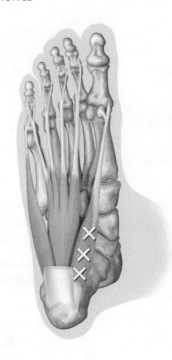

FIGURE 11.70
When dysfunctional, the **abductor hallucis** can develop three adjacent trigger points along its belly that can refer pain along the medial side of the heel.

toe that often develops into a painful bunion. (See TrPs for the abductor hallucis in Figure 11.70 ■).

The **flexor digitorum brevis** (FDB) arises from the medial aspect of the calcaneal tuberosity, directly under the plantar aponeurosis. Four heads of the FDB insert on the sides of the middle phalanges of the second to fifth toes. (See TrPs for the flexor digitorum brevis in Figure 11.71 ■).

The **abductor digiti minimi** arises from the lateral side of the calcaneal tuberosity and inserts at the base of the proximal phalanx of the fifth toe. It abducts the fifth toe and assists flexion. (See TrPs for the abductor digiti minimi in Figure 11.71 ■).

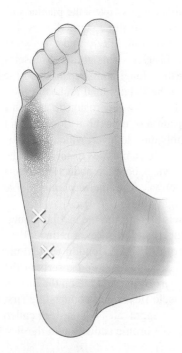

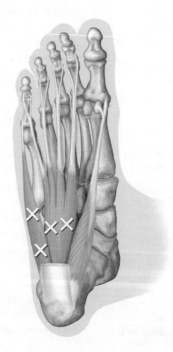

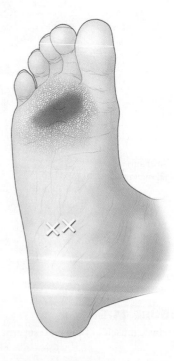

FIGURE 11.71
When dysfunctional, the **flexor digitorum brevis** can develop two trigger points next to each other in the instep, which can refer pain to the ball of the foot across the second through fourth metatarsals. Two trigger points can develop in the long belly of the **abductor digiti minimi,** which can refer pain into the base of the fifth metatarsal on the ball of the foot.

MUSCLE PALPATION
Abductor Hallucis, Flexor Digitorum Brevis, and Abductor Digiti Minimi

Muscles in this group are easy to palpate because they lie directly below the subcutaneous layer of the skin and plantar aponeurosis. Begin by palpating them on your own feet. Palpate the abductor hallucis and abductor digiti minimi along the side of the proximal half of the medial and lateral arch. Palpate the flexor digitorum by applying pressure straight into the sole of the foot, directly anterior to the calcaneal tuberosity.

Abductor Hallucis

O—Medial aspect of calcaneal tuberosity, flexor reti-
  naculum, plantar aponeurosis
I—Medial side of base of proximal phalanx of first toe
A—Flexes and abducts first toe

Flexor Digitorum Brevis (FDB)

O—Middle of calcaneal tuberosity, plantar aponeurosis
I—Sides of middle phalanges of second to fifth toes
A—Flexes PIP joints of second to fifth toes

Abductor Digiti Minimi

O—Lateral aspect of calcaneal tuberosity, plantar
  aponeurosis
I—Lateral side of proximal phalanx of fifth toe
A—Abducts fifth toe and assists flexion

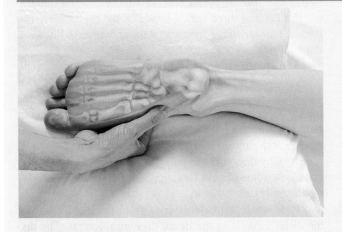

FIGURE 11.72a
Palpating the abductor hallucis

With your partner prone, palpate the **abductor hallucis** along the posterior medial edge of the foot (Figure 11.72a ■). Slowly move your partner's big toe into abduction and back. Then have your partner do the same motion. Few people can perform abduction of the first toe, although practicing this action can help people with hallux valgus (a chronic adduction of the first toe that can cause bunions). *Are you on the plantar surface of the medial arch?*

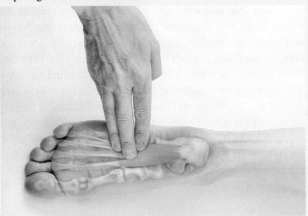

FIGURE 11.72b
Palpating the flexor digitorum brevis

With your partner prone, locate the **flexor digitorum brevis** by pressing directly into the muscle through the plantar fascia, directly distal to the plantar surface of the heel (Figure 11.72b ■). *Are you in the middle of the sole of the foot?*

Active movement: Have your partner make a fist with the toes while you locate the FDB.

Resisted movement: Have your partner resist as you slowly extend the lateral four toes.

(continued)

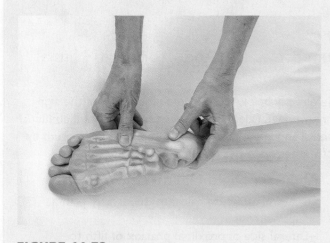

With your partner prone, locate the **abductor digiti minimi** between the heel and fifth toe (Figure 11.72c ■). It should be easy to find because it is superficial.

Resisted movement: Press lightly against the lateral side of the fifth toe and have your partner press back to get the abductor digiti minimi to contract.

FIGURE 11.72c

Palpating the abductor digiti minimi

11.3.2.3 SECOND LAYER OF INTRINSIC PLANTAR MUSCLES

The second deepest layer of muscles in the foot contains the quadratus plantae and the lumbricals (Figure 11.73 ■). Both muscles share insertions and origins along the flexor

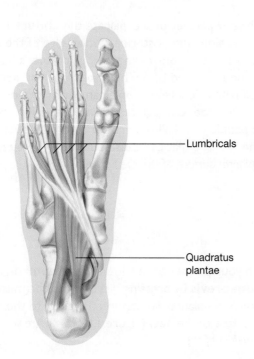

FIGURE 11.73

Intrinsic muscles of the foot: second layer of plantar surface

digitorum tendons and carry out somewhat unusual functions. The *lateral plantar nerve* innervates the quadratus plantae and three lateral heads of the lumbricals. The *medial plantar nerve* innervates the most medial head of the lumbricals.

The **quadratus plantae** is a wide flat muscle with a lateral head that arises from the middle plantar edge of the calcaneus and a larger medial head that arises from the medial aspect of the calcaneal tuberosity. Muscle fibers of both heads have a flat wide insertion on the distal tendon of the flexor digitorum longus. It assists flexion of the lateral four toes by directing the pull of the flexor digitorum longus along a line of pure flexion. (See TrP for the quadratus plantae in Figure 11.74 ■).

Four small **lumbricals** arise from the medial side of the distal tendons of the flexor digitorum longus. The distal tendons of the lumbricals insert on the proximal medial aspect of the proximal phalanges of the second through fifth toes, then split and wrap around each toe, attaching on the dorsal surface of the distal phalanx. This dual attachment and their split tendons equip the lumbricals for a unique action—they flex the MTPs while extending the PIPs and DIPs, lifting the transverse arch while flattening the toes. The lumbricals maintain the integrity of the transverse arch during toe extension and push off by preventing hyperextension of the toes. Because they work as both flexors and extensors, the lumbricals work like a two-way transistor to coordinate the chain of movement on both sides of the foot during a gait cycle.[7]

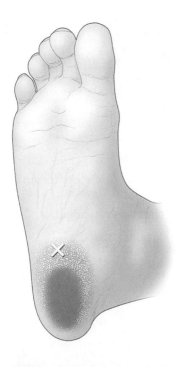
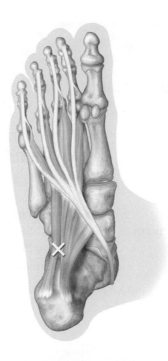

FIGURE 11.74
The **quadratus plantae** can develop a trigger point directly distal to the calcaneal origin, which may refer pain to the plantar surface of the heel.

SELF-CARE
Strengthening the Intrinsic Muscles of the Feet

This exercise will strengthen the intrinsic muscles of your feet, helping you to be able to stand for long periods without developing achiness in the soles of your feet. It will also help you develop rebound in running and elevation in jumping.

To feel the effects of these exercises, practice them on one foot first, then get up and walk around to feel the difference. Then practice on your other foot.

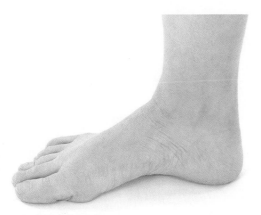

FIGURE 11.75a

1. **Lifting the arches:** To feel your lumbricals contract, push your toes flat against the ground to extend the DIPs and PIPs while flexing the MTP joints (Figure 11.75a ■). Another way to engage them is to pull the arches up while flattening the toes. This can be a difficult action to do at first, although if you practice, you'll eventually develop the coordination.

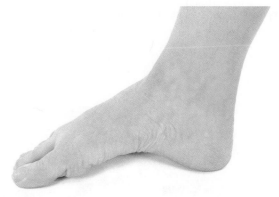

FIGURE 11.75b

2. **"Inchworm" articulation of the arches:** Practice moving your foot like an inchworm, raising your arch to pull your heel toward your toes, then extend your toes to inch your foot forward (Figure 11.75b ■). Take several steps in one direction, then reverse.

MUSCLE PALPATION
Quadratus Plantae and Lumbricals

Both of these muscles are difficult to discern during palpation.

Quadratus Plantae

O–Plantar surface of calcaneus
I–Distal tendon of flexor digitorum longus
A–Assists flexion of lateral four toes by directing pull of flexor digitorum longus along line of pure flexion

Lumbricals

O–Medial side of distal tendons of flexor digitorum longus
I–Dorsal medial surface of proximal phalanges of second to fifth toes
A–Flexes MTP joints on second to fifth toes while extending IP joints

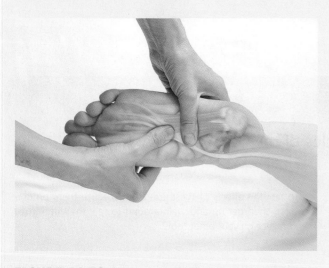

FIGURE 11.76a
Approximating the quadratus plantae

With your partner supine or prone, approximate the **quadratus plantae** by placing your thumbs on each end of the muscle, on the plantar surface of the calcaneus to the middle of the plantar surface of the foot. Press your thumbs together to shorten the muscle and hold for several seconds (Figure 11.76a ■).

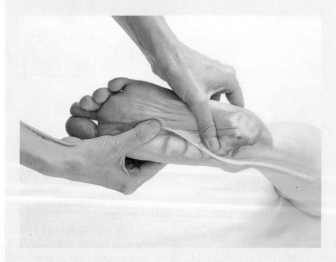

FIGURE 11.76b
Stretching the quadratus plantae and flexor digitorum brevis

Then slowly pull them apart to lengthen it (Figure 11.76b ■). Now apply deep pressure through the plantar aponeurosis straight into the belly of the muscle. *Are you able to penetrate through the thick plantar aponeurosis to locate the quadratus plantae?*

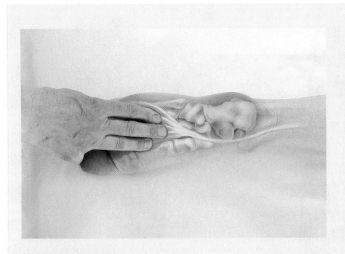

FIGURE 11.76c

Raking along the lumbricals

Locate your partner's **lumbricals** by pressing up into the spaces between the metatarsals. Rake your fingers along the lumbricals between the metatarsals to wake them up (Figure 11.76c ■). Sometimes this movement will get them to contract. When it does, your partner's transverse arch will lift as the MTPs flex and the toes extend, looking like they are spraying energy out their tips. *Did you notice any reflexive movement in the toes when you raked your fingers between the metatarsals along the lumbrical muscles?*

11.3.2.4 THIRD LAYER OF INTRINSIC PLANTAR MUSCLES

Three intrinsic muscles—the *flexor hallucis brevis, adductor hallucis,* and *flexor digiti minimi brevis*—occupy the third deepest layer of the plantar surface of the foot (Figure 11.77 ■). As a group, this layer of muscles stabilizes the foot during stance and propulsion, narrowing the foot and lifting the arches. The flexor hallucis brevis and adductor hallucis also work together to control the position of the first toe.

The **flexor hallucis brevis** has two parallel bellies that arise from the cuboid and lateral cuneiform. Each distal tendon of this small fleshy muscle encapsulates a sesamoid bone, with one inserting on the medial side and the other, the lateral side of the base of the first proximal phalanx. The flexor hallucis brevis flexes the proximal phalanx of the first toe and is innervated by the *medial plantar nerve*. (See TrPs for the flexor hallucis brevis in Figure 11.78 ■).

The **adductor hallucis** has an oblique head and a transverse head that are arranged like a number seven. The oblique head arises from the base of the second through fourth metatarsals and from the sheath of the peroneus longus tendon; the transverse head arises from the

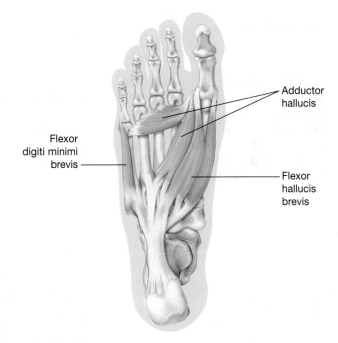

Flexor digiti minimi brevis

Adductor hallucis

Flexor hallucis brevis

FIGURE 11.77

Intrinsic muscles of the foot: third layer of plantar surface

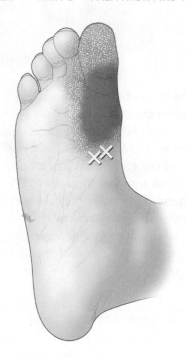
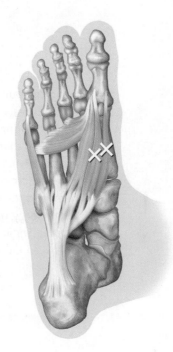
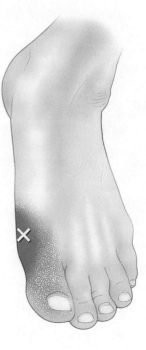

FIGURE 11.78

When dysfunctional, the **flexor hallucis brevis** can develop a trigger point in each belly, which can refer pain over the ball of the foot around the first metatarsal and along the base of the first toe.

transverse tarsal ligaments of the third, fourth, and fifth toes. Both heads insert on the lateral side of the proximal phalanx of the first toe. The adductor hallucis draws the first toe toward the second toe as it contracts. The *lateral plantar nerve* innervates both the adductor hallucis and the flexor digiti minimi. (See TrPs for the adductor hallucis in Figure 11.79 ■).

The **flexor digiti minimi brevis** arises from the base of the fifth metatarsal and the peroneus longus tendon and inserts on the proximal end of the proximal phalanx of the fifth toe. This small muscle flexes the MTP of the fifth toe and contributes to the stabilization and integrity of the lateral arch. It can develop a tender point in the center of the muscle, although no TrP or referral pattern has been identified.

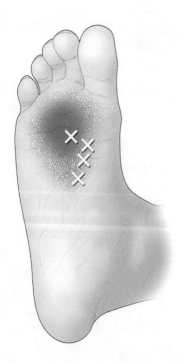
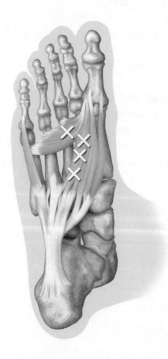

FIGURE 11.79

When dysfunctional, the **adductor hallucis** can develop three adjacent trigger points in the belly of the oblique head and one trigger point in the center of the transverse head, which can refer pain across the ball of the foot.

MUSCLE PALPATION
Flexor Hallucis Brevis, Adductor Hallucis, and Flexor Digiti Minimi Brevis

Palpate these muscles on your own foot first. The flexor hallucis brevis is easy to locate along the bottom of your first metatarsal. Curl your first toe against pressure to feel it contract. Curl your fifth toe against pressure while you palpate your flexor digiti minimi along the bottom of your fifth metatarsal. The adductor hallucis is more difficult to palpate; trace its approximate location on the bottom of your foot.

Flexor Hallucis Brevis

O–Plantar surface of cuboid and lateral cuneiform
I–Medial and lateral side of base of proximal phalanx of first toe
A–Flexes the MTP joint of first toe

Adductor Hallucis

O–Oblique head: Base of second, third, and fourth metatarsals, sheath of peroneus longus tendon
   Transverse head: Transverse tarsal ligaments of third, fourth, and fifth toes
I–Lateral side of proximal phalanx of first toe
A–Adducts first toe

Flexor Digiti Minimi Brevis

O–Base of fifth metatarsal, sheath of peroneus longus tendon
I–Proximal end of proximal phalanx of fifth toe
A–Flexes PIP joint of fifth toe

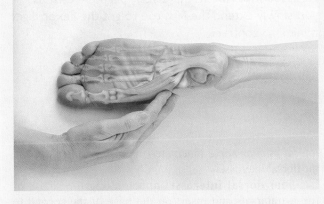

FIGURE 11.80a
Palpating the flexor hallucis brevis

With your partner supine or prone, palpate the **flexor hallucis brevis** along the plantar surface of the first metatarsal shaft to the base of the first toe (Figure 11.80a ■).

Resisted movement: Have your partner resist as you slowly extend the first toe to get the flexor hallucis to contract.

(continued)

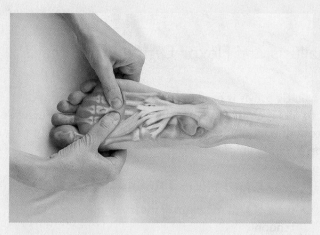

FIGURE 11.80b
Approximating the adductor hallucis

Trace the approximate location of the **adductor hallucis** like a figure 7 from the middle of the arches to the base of the first toe, then across to the base of the fifth toe (Figure 11.80b ■). Approximate both heads of the adductor hallucis by pushing the ends of the muscle belly together, then slowly stretching them apart.

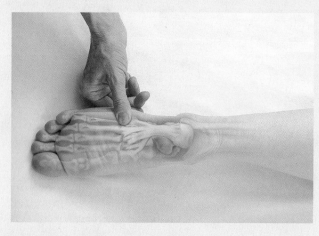

FIGURE 11.80c
Palpating the flexor digiti minimi brevis

Palpate the **flexor digiti minimi brevis** along the bottom of your partner's fifth metatarsal (Figure 11.80c ■).

Resisted movement: Have your partner resist as you slowly extend the fifth toe to get the flexor digiti minimi to contract.

11.3.2.5 DEEPEST LAYER OF INTRINSIC MUSCLES IN THE FOOT

Three **plantar interossei** attach along the medial proximal side of the third through fifth metatarsals and insert on the medial proximal aspect of the proximal phalanges of the same toes (Figure 11.81a ■). They adduct and flex the three lateral phalanges, give rise to the lateral arch, and become vigorously active from midstance to toe-off. The

lateral plantar nerve innervates the plantar interossei and the dorsal interossei.

Four **dorsal interossei** attach along the shafts of the metatarsals and insert on the base of the second to fourth phalanges as well as on the extensor digitorum longus tendons of the same toes (Figure 11.81b ■). These small bipennate muscles extend and abduct the second through fourth toes. The interossei also maintain

FIGURE 11.81

Intrinsic muscles of the foot: deepest layer a) planter interossei b) dorsal interossei

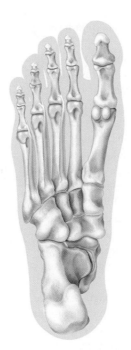

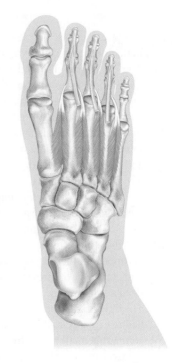

A

B

a stable, parallel alignment of the metatarsals during the stance phase and contract vigorously between midstance and pushoff to stabilize the forefoot after the heel leaves the ground.

The interossei can be located by pressing into the spaces between the metatarsals using a pincher grip, although they are difficult to discern during palpation. Gently pressing into them between the metatarsals can help to loosen and stretch them. The interossei can also be stretched by gently pulling adjacent toes apart. Trigger points in the interossei develop between the metatarsals over the belly of the muscles. They refer pain along the lateral side of the toe they act on and on the plantar surface of the metatarsal head of that same toe.

CONCLUSION

Given how many joints and intrinsic muscles there are in the foot, direct pressure on just about any point on the sole of the foot would be therapeutic. It would likely land on a trigger point location or over a ligament on one of the many joints in the feet. Many massage clients suffer from stiff and aching feet. By understanding how the joints in the foot move and how the bones fit together, a practitioner can perform subtle passive movements and joint approximations on a client's foot to restore motion to joints. In addition, a practitioner can approximate the intrinsic muscles to wake up sensory awareness in them. It is no wonder that skillful hands-on work on the feet energizes the whole body and person.

SUMMARY POINTS TO REMEMBER

1. There are 28 bones in the ankle and foot, including the tibia, fibula, seven tarsal bones, five metatarsals, and 14 phalanges.
2. Each foot can be divided into three functional parts: the rearfoot, midfoot, and forefoot.
3. The plantar surface of the foot has three arches—the medial and lateral longitudinal arches and the transverse arch—whose main functions are to bend under weight, absorb shock, and adapt the foot to uneven terrain.
4. Two tibiofibular joints are mechanically linked to the talocrural joint, a hinge joint at the ankle made up of articulations between the distal tibia, the distal fibula, and the talus.
5. The talocrural joint moves in an average range of 20 degrees of dorsiflexion and 45 degrees of plantarflexion.

6. The subtalar joint, a complex ellipsoid joint made up of the articulation between the calcaneus and talus, forms the keystone of the ankle, transferring forces in three directions. It moves in an average range of 20 degrees of eversion and 45 degrees of inversion.
7. The transverse tarsal joint, a gliding joint made up of articulations between the talus and calcaneus with the navicular and cuboid, separates the rearfoot from the midfoot and both depresses slightly and opens during midstance.
8. Chronic pronation of the foot, called pes planus, flattens the medial arch, causing a pronation twist in the forefoot, and creating torsion stresses in other joints in the foot, the ankle, and the knee. Chronic supination,

called pes cavus, is a less common condition causing high arches and rigidity in the ankle.

9. The intertarsal (IT) and tarsometatarsal (TMT) joints are gliding joints in the midfoot that depress slightly during midstance, yet maintain the vault of the arches in the middle of the foot.

10. Five metatarsophalangeal (MTP) joints are ellipsoid joints at the ball of the foot that flex and extend the toes and also allow abduction and adduction of toes.

11. The first toe, or hallux, has two phalanges and one interphalangeal (IP) joint; the four lateral toes each have three phalanges and both distal and proximal interphalangeal joints. These small hinge joints flex and extend the toes.

12. Extrinsic muscles of the foot are located in four compartments in the leg. A thick fascial sheath wraps each compartment to prevent lateral splaying of muscles from compression.

13. The tibialis anterior, extensor digitorum longus, extensor hallucis longus, and peroneus tertius occupy the anterior compartment along the front of the leg and work as dorsiflexors of the ankle and extensors of the toes.

14. Three muscles making up the triceps surae—the gastrocnemius, soleus, and plantaris—occupy the posterior compartment, work primarily as plantarflexors of the ankle and long extensors of the toes, and share a common insertion in the Achilles tendon.

15. Three muscles in the deep posterior compartment—the tibialis posterior, flexor digitorum longus, and flexor hallucis longus—work as plantarflexors and stabilizers of the ankle and long flexors of the toes.

16. Primary invertors of the ankle include the tibialis posterior and tibialis anterior.

17. The lateral compartment contains the peroneus longus and peroneus brevis muscles, which act as evertors of the ankle.

18. The extensor digitorum brevis and extensor hallucis brevis can be found on the dorsal surface of the foot; their primary function is to extend the toes.

19. The plantar surface of the foot is covered be a thick aponeurosis and four layers of intrinsic muscles that flex, abduct, and adduct the toes, as well as stabilize the vault of the arches.

REVIEW QUESTIONS

1. Identify the three functional parts of the foot and the bones in each part.
2. What is the primary function of the tibia?
3. The three arches of the foot are the
   a. medial longitudinal arch, lateral longitudinal arch, and tarsal arch.
   b. medial longitudinal arch, lateral longitudinal arch, and dorsal arch.
   c. medial longitudinal arch, lateral longitudinal arch, and transverse arch.
   d. medial longitudinal arch, lateral longitudinal arch, and plantar arch.
4. What is the function of the two sesamoid bones at the base of the proximal phalange of the first toe?
   a. They assist in mobility and provide a protective tunnel for the flexor hallucis brevis tendon.
   b. They assist in weight-bearing and provide a protective tunnel for the extensor hallucis brevis tendon.
   c. They assist in weight-bearing and provide a protective tunnel for the flexor digitorum brevis tendons.
   d. They assist in weight-bearing and provide a protective tunnel for the flexor hallucis longus tendon.
5. Of the four statements below, identify the one that is *not true*.
   a. The arches absorb shock and adapt the foot to uneven terrain.
   b. The lateral arch is the highest and most flexible arch in the foot.

   c. The keystone of the medial arch is the navicular bone.
   d. The transverse arch runs perpendicular to the longitudinal arches.
6. The three ligaments that support and stabilize the longitudinal arches are the
   a. calcaneonavicular, transverse metatarsal, and long plantar ligaments.
   b. calcaneonavicular, spring, and long plantar ligaments.
   c. calcaneonavicular, short plantar, and long plantar ligaments.
   d. calcaneonavicular, spring, and short plantar ligaments.
7. List the three bones in the talocrural joint and identify what type of joint it is.
8. The joint formed by the articulation between the talus and calcaneus, the _____ joint, is sometimes referred to as the lower ankle joint because it moves with the talocrural joint during _____ and _____ .
9. Three kinds of gliding joints that are found in the midfoot are the
   a. proximal interphalangeal joints, subtalar joint, and transverse tarsal joints.
   b. intertarsal joints, tarsometatarsal joints, and metatarsophalangeal joints.
   c. transverse tarsal joints, intertarsal joints, and tarsometatarsal joints.
   d. transverse tarsal, tarsometatarsal, and metatarsophalangeal joints.

10. True or false (circle one). The hinge joints at the base of the toes are called the metatarsophalangeal joints.

11. What is the difference between the extrinsic and intrinsic muscles acting on the foot?

12. The four muscular compartments in the leg are the
    a. anterior, posterior, lateral, and deep posterior compartments.
    b. anterior, posterior, lateral, and deep anterior compartments.
    c. anterior, superior, lateral, and deep posterior compartments.
    d. anterior, inferior, lateral, and deep posterior compartments.

13. The primary dorsiflexors of the ankle are the
    a. tibialis posterior, extensor digitorum longus, and extensor hallucis longus.
    b. tibialis anterior, extensor digitorum longus, and extensor hallucis brevis.
    c. tibialis anterior, extensor digitorum brevis, and extensor hallucis longus.
    d. tibialis anterior, extensor digitorum longus, and extensor hallucis longus.

14. If the tibialis anterior and tibialis posterior simultaneously contract, what movement of the ankle will they generate?
    a. dorsiflexion
    b. inversion
    c. plantarflexion
    d. eversion

15. The primary evertors of the ankle are the *(two words)* _____ and the _____ *(two words)*, which occupy the _____ compartment.

16. The tibialis posterior
    a. inverts and dorsiflexes the ankle.
    b. everts and dorsiflexes the ankle.
    c. inverts and plantarflexes the ankle.
    d. pronates and dorsiflexes the ankle.

17. True or false (circle one). The soleus muscle is sometimes called the second heart because it rhythmically contracts during postural sway to assist the venous return of blood to the heart.

18. How many layers of intrinsic muscles can be found in the plantar surface of the foot?

19. The collective function of the deeper layers of intrinsic foot muscles is to
    a. Stabilize the foot during the swing and pushoff phases of gait, and to narrow the foot and lift the arches.
    b. Mobilize the foot during the stance and pushoff phases of gait, and to narrow the foot and lift the arches.
    c. Stabilize the foot during the stance and pushoff phases of gait, and to widen the foot and flatten the arches.
    d. Stabilize the foot during the stance and pushoff phases of gait, and to narrow the foot and lift the arches.

20. The functional difference between the long flexors of the toes and the short flexors of the toes is that
    a. the long flexors of the toes also plantarflex the ankle.
    b. the long flexors of the toes also dorsiflex the ankle.
    c. the long flexors of the toes also stabilize the ankle.
    d. the long flexors of the toes also plantarflex the arches.

Notes

1. Kapandji, I. (1987). *The Physiology of the Joints: Lower Limb* Vol. 2, 5th ed. Edinburgh, UK: Churchill Livingstone.
2. Norkin, C., & Levangie, P. (2005). *Joint Structure and Function: A Comprehensive Analysis* (4th ed.). Philadelphia: F. A. Davis Company.
3. Kapandji, *The Physiology of the Joints.*
4. Hamilton, N., & Luttgens, K. (2002). *Kinesiology: Scientific Basis of Human Motion* (10th ed.). New York: McGraw-Hill.
5. Neumann, D. (2002). *Kinesiology of the Musculoskeletal System: Foundations for Physical Rehabilitation.* St. Louis, MO: Mosby.
6. Norkin, *Joint Structure and Function.*
7. Kapandji, *The Physiology of the Joints.*

12 The Knee

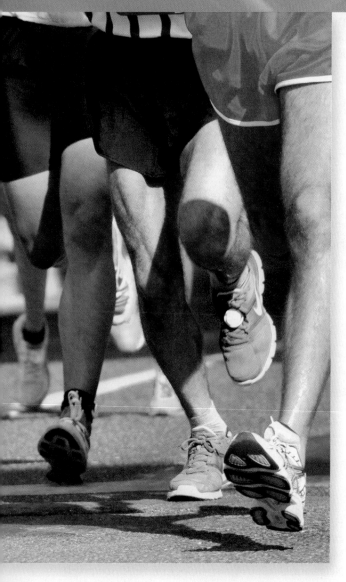

CHAPTER OUTLINE

Chapter Objectives

Key Terms

12.1 Bones and Accessory Structures of the Knee

12.2 Joints and Ligaments of the Knee

12.3 Muscles of the Knee

Conclusion

Summary Points to Remember

Review Questions

Of all the joints in the body, the knees take the worst beating. The knee is the most frequently injured joint for two reasons: It is the largest and most complex joint in the body, and it is the primary shock absorber of the lower limb. Each knee has two large fibrocartilage disks that work as shock absorbers to buffer the axial pounding the knees undergo while walking or running. The disks also cushion the joint during flexion and extension, as the bones press the disks backward and forward along a specific pathway. Even slight variance from this ideal track increases wear on joint cartilage.

One common type of injury is caused by repetitive strain from faulty joint mechanics. The knees are also frequently injured during impact sports, such as football or rugby, and during racket sports in which quick turns on the court can torque the joint structures. To prevent injury, a person can use sagittal tracking exercises to improve and help maintain optimal knee alignment during all activities, particularly sports. Any exercise to improve knee motion will be enhanced by an understanding of joint rotations during flexion and extension and the locking mechanism of the knee in extension.

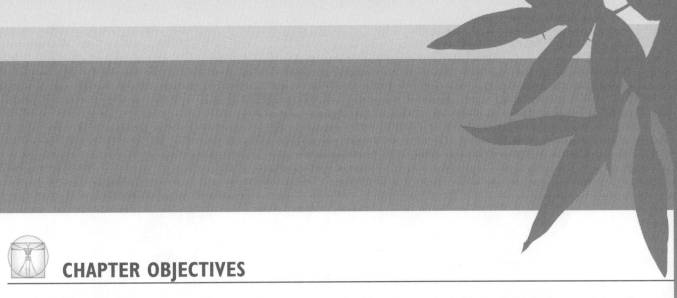

CHAPTER OBJECTIVES

1. Name the three bones of the knee.

2. List and demonstrate the palpation of 10 bony landmarks of the knee.

3. Describe the menisci and bursae in the knee.

4. Name and describe the two joints of the knee and seven supporting ligaments.

5. Describe patellar movement and problems that occur with poor patellar tracking.

6. Define the mechanical axis of the lower limb and the Q angle.

7. Describe the range of motion and joint mechanics of the tibiofemoral joint.

8. Name types of misalignments in the knee and describe the structural problems they cause.

9. Define and contrast axial rotation and terminal rotation of the knee.

10. Demonstrate the palpation of the menisci and prepatellar bursa of the knee.

11. Identify the origins, insertions, and actions of the knee flexors and extensors.

12. Identify the trigger points and pain referral patterns of the knee flexors and extensors.

13. Demonstrate the active movement and palpation of the knee flexors and extensors.

KEY TERMS

Adductor tubercle

Anterior cruciate ligament (ACL)

Chondromalacia

Drawer sign

Femoral condyles

Genu recurvatum

Iliotibial band (ITB)

Iliotibial band syndrome

Lateral collateral ligament (LCL)

Mechanical axis of the lower limb

Medial collateral ligament (MCL)

Meniscus

Patellofemoral joint

Patellofemoral pain syndrome

Popliteal fossa

Posterior cruciate ligament (PCL)

Q angle

Screw home mechanism

Terminal rotation

Tibial condyles

Tibial plateau

Tibial tubercle

Tibiofemoral joint

Translation

MUSCLES IN ACTION

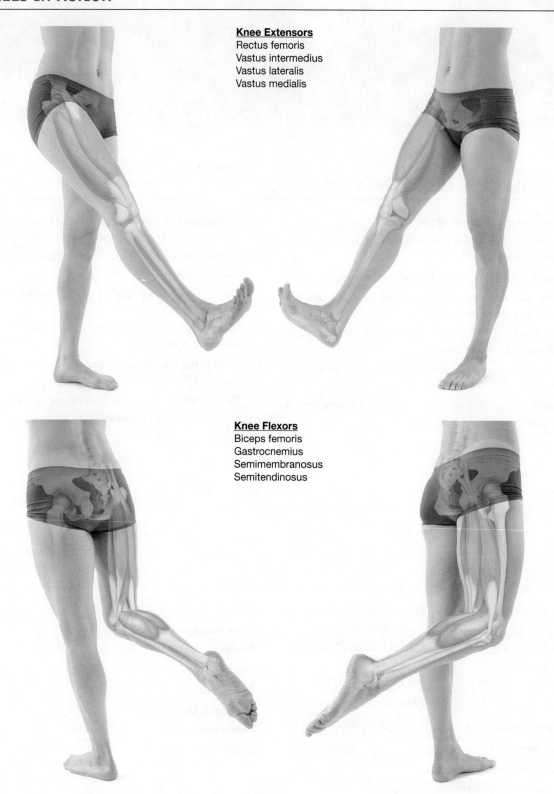

Knee Extensors
Rectus femoris
Vastus intermedius
Vastus lateralis
Vastus medialis

Knee Flexors
Biceps femoris
Gastrocnemius
Semimembranosus
Semitendinosus

In the last chapter, we explored the intricate structure and the articulate movement of the foundation of the body: the foot and ankle. From there, our exploration of kinesiology continues up the vertical axis into the knee: the largest and most complex weight-bearing joint in the body. The knee serves as a functional link between the feet and the hips. Movement of the knees allows the distance between the torso and the ground to vary. A person must bend the knees to get closer to the ground and extend the knees to lift the body away from the ground.

The functional demands on this large joint encapsulate the paradox of the human body, which is to balance vertical stability with extreme mobility. On one hand, the knees need to be stable enough to support weight in a nonmoving upright body; on the other hand, they need to be mobile enough to allow for a range of lower limb motions. Unlike other joints, the articular surfaces of the tibia and femur in the knee minimally interlock, making it one of the least stable joints in the body. Its stability comes from a complex arrangement of soft tissues: the joint capsule, tendons, ligaments, and accessory structures such as menisci and bursae.

Our knees work under a lot of mechanical stress during the course of daily activities and need to function as major shock absorbers. Walking alone routinely doubles the compressive forces of body weight on these inherently unstable joints. Going up or down stairs and running increases the compressive loads on them by up to six or seven times, creating a lot of wear and tear on the articulating surfaces. A lack of bony stability, coupled with the high functional demands we put on knees, makes them vulnerable to injuries. As a result, the knees are the most frequently damaged joints in the body.

Common knee injuries occur suddenly during strong ballistic movements. Injuries can also occur gradually from faulty movement patterns that prematurely deteriorate joint structures. Adaptive shortening in muscles and tendons on the lateral side of the knee coupled with muscular inhibitions or weakness along the inside line is a common source of knee problems. A practitioner can address this condition by freeing and lengthening myofascial tissues along the lateral line of the knee, which shifts weight and muscular engagement to the inside line of the knee.

In the following pages we explore the unique structures, finely calibrated design, and movement range of the knee. We examine the effects of muscular pulls on alignment and joint motion, with a look at common alignment issues and injuries that occur in the knee. And, as usual, specific palpation and manual therapy skills for working with the knee in a massage and bodywork practice is presented.

12.1 BONES AND ACCESSORY STRUCTURES OF THE KNEE

The knee joins the two longest and strongest levers in the body—the femur and the tibia. A large sesamoid bone—the patella—covers the anterior surface of the joint

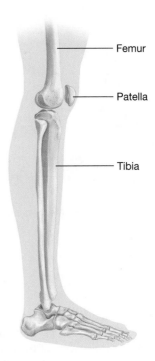

FIGURE 12.1
Bones of the knee: lateral view

(Figure 12.1 ■). Two fibrocartilage disks called menisci sit between the femur and tibia in the middle of the joint.

12.1.1 Bones of the Knee

The **femur** is the longest bone in the body; its average length is 18 inches. The bowed shape of the **shaft of the femur** allows it to slightly flex and bend under load to reduce compression forces on the knee. If the femoral shaft were completely straight and unable to flex, joint compression on the knee would increase substantially, causing premature aging and severe osteoarthritis.

The distal end of the femur flares into a triangular-shaped bone with two large knuckles on each side called **femoral condyles.** Each condyle is somewhat flat on its distal end, which maximizes the weight-bearing surfaces of the femur on the tibia. Hyaline cartilage covers the articular surfaces of both femoral condyles. The medial femoral condyle is longer than the lateral femoral condyle and about twice its size (Figure 12.2 ■). This asymmetry causes a subtle rotation in the knee as it flexes and extends, a range of motion you should be able to visualize and follow when passively moving the knee. An **intercondylar groove** separates the femoral condyles and creates a tunnel for the cruciate ligaments inside the joint. The cruciate ligaments are often injured but cannot be directly palpated or worked on.

Above each condyle is a **femoral epicondyle,** a rough lateral projection that provides attachment sites for supporting ligaments and tendons of the knee. An **adductor tubercle** located above the medial epicondyle is an insertion

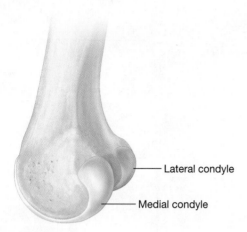

FIGURE 12.2
Femoral condyles

Lateral condyle

Medial condyle

site where the distal tendons of the adductor muscles can be easily palpated (Figure 12.3 ■). A triangular depression between the posterior aspects of the femoral condyles creates the **popliteal fossa,** where the popliteal nerve and artery descend along the back of the knee. When the knee is flexed, the popliteal fossa can be lightly palpated between the hamstring tendons, but it is important to be careful when

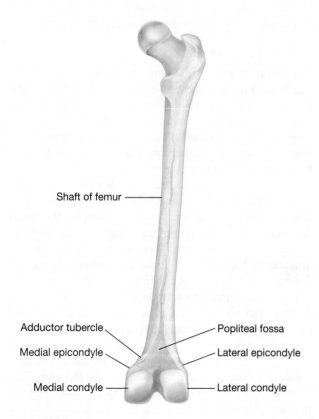

Shaft of femur

Adductor tubercle
Medial epicondyle
Medial condyle

Popliteal fossa
Lateral epicondyle
Lateral condyle

FIGURE 12.3
Femur: posterior view

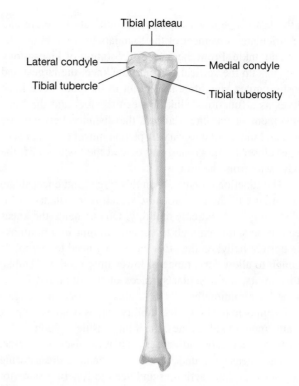

Tibial plateau

Lateral condyle
Tibial tubercle

Medial condyle
Tibial tuberosity

FIGURE 12.4
Tibia: anterior view

applying pressure to this area to avoid the nerves and blood vessels.

The **tibia,** below the knee, is a massive and strong bone with a thick vertical shaft that suits it for its primary function—to transfer weight from the femur into the ankle and foot. On its proximal end, the tibia enlarges into a broad and somewhat horizontal surface called the **tibial plateau** (Figure 12.4 ■). Below the tibial plateau, two round **tibial condyles** provide insertion sites for the distal hamstring tendons. A **tibial tubercle,** located directly below the lateral tibial condyle, provides an attachment site for the iliotibial band. Directly below the knee, a large, rough bony protuberance called the **tibial tuberosity** provides an attachment site for the patellar ligament. Once you become adept at palpating these bony landmarks, you can more easily locate the ligaments and muscular tendons attached to each one (Figure 12.5 ■).

The **patella,** a triangular-shaped bone on the front of the knee, is better known as the *kneecap.* As the largest sesamoid bone in the body, the patella lies between the quadriceps tendon and the femur. A vertical ridge on its posterior aspect is covered with a protective layer of articular cartilage that is 4-5 centimeters thick (about a quarter inch). It is the thickest articular cartilage in the body due to the tremendous pressure and friction the patella is subjected to from the powerful pull of the quadriceps during knee extension. When pressure on the patella causes pain, it is possible that the cartilage covering the underside of the patella could be damaged.

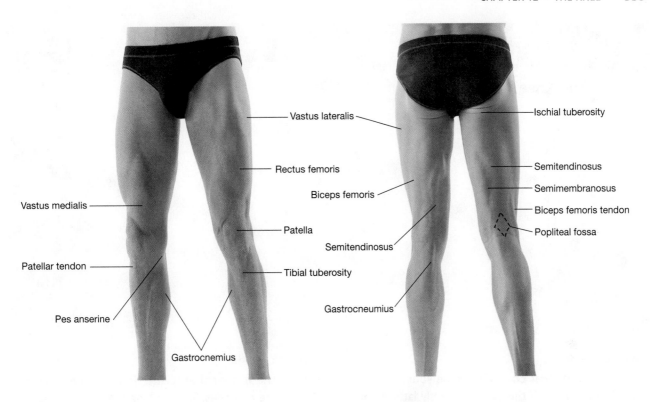

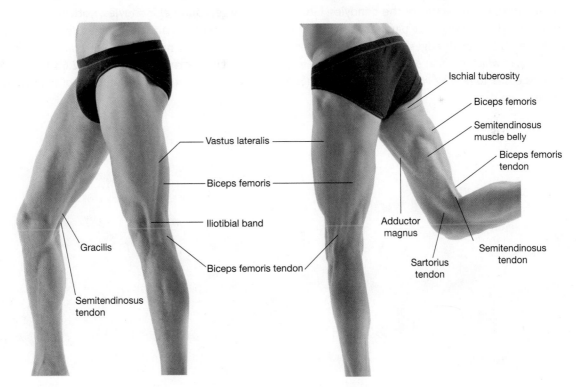

FIGURE 12.5

Surface anatomy of the knee

BONE PALPATION
The Knee

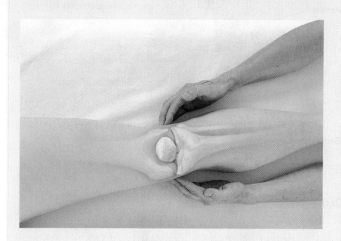

FIGURE 12.6a

To find the **femoral condyles,** slide your finger-tips off the center of the patella directly lateral until you locate the bony edges of the condyles. Hold the edges while having your partner flex and extend the knee. Follow both edges around to the sides of the knee. *In which position of the knee are the femoral condyles easier to feel? Which condyle is bigger?* (See Figure 12.6a ■)

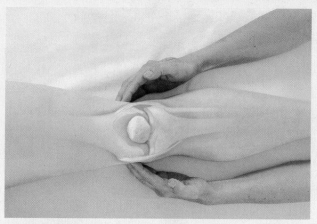

FIGURE 12.6b

Palpate the **femoral epicondyles** lateral and superior to the condyles. Strum along the sides of the large, round epicondyles, noticing where ligaments and tendons attach. Walk up the epicondyles, feeling where they narrow into the distal end of the **shaft of the femur.** (See Figure 12.6b ■) *How far up the thigh can you palpate the shaft of the femur?*

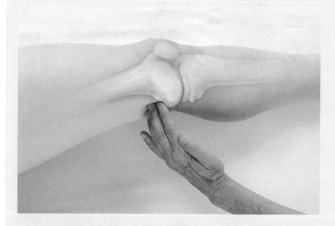

FIGURE 12.6c

Locate the **adductor tubercle** on the uppermost aspect of the medial epicondyle, at the base of the adductor tendons. (See Figure 12.6c ■) *Does it feel like a sharp ridge?*

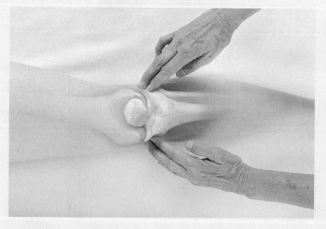

FIGURE 12.6d

Locate the distinct edge of the **tibial plateau** with the knee in flexion by palpating along the top of the tibia across the joint line. Follow it laterally to each side of the knee. *Are you palpating the uppermost edge of the tibia?* (See Figure 12.6d ■)

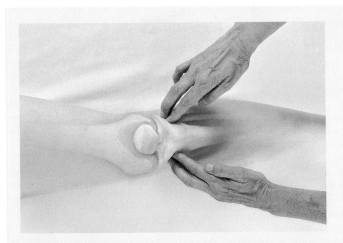

FIGURE 12.6e

To find the **tibial condyles,** drop below the tibial plateau and explore their large but somewhat flat surfaces. (See Figure 12.6e ■) *How far in the posterior direction can you palpate each condyle?*

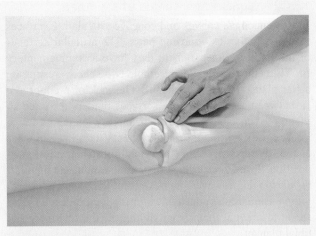

FIGURE 12.6f

Locate the small protuberance on the lateral tibia condyle called the **tibial tubercle.** It can be palpated easier with the knee in flexion. *Do you feel where the iliotibial band attaches to it?* (See Figure 12.6f ■)

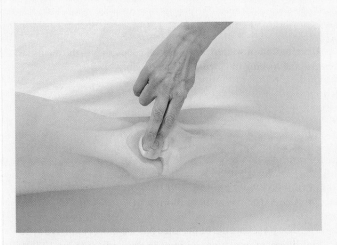

FIGURE 12.6g

Palpate the **patella** with the knee in both flexion and extension. Explore all sides of its triangular edge. With the muscles around the knee relaxed, carefully move the patella up and down. (See Figure 12.6g ■)

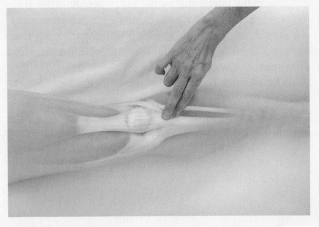

FIGURE 12.6h

Follow the ligament attached to the patella down to the **tibial tuberosity,** a large bony bump below the knee. Hold the tibial tuberosity as your partner flexes and extends the knee. *In which position of the knee do the tissues covering the patella and tibial tuberosity become taut?* (See Figure 12.6h ■)

12.1.2 Menisci and Bursae of the Knee

Most joints have convex and concave articulating surfaces that fit together as opposing pairs. The articular surfaces of the knee are mismatched; they have a complementary fit. The femoral condyles resemble two spheres resting on a flat plane (the tibial plateau). The lack of a congruent fit between convex-concave surfaces renders the knee an inherently unstable joint. This instability leads to a lot of injuries, so you may see many clients with knee injuries caused by repetitive movement in an unstable, misaligned position. Two fibrocartilage rings called **menisci** (singular: *meniscus*) do, however, improve joint congruency by providing semicircular concavities for the femoral condyles to sit on to prevent them from sliding off the relatively flat tibial plateau.

Each meniscus has a semicircular shape. The medial meniscus has an oval C-shape; the smaller lateral meniscus is shaped more like a horseshoe (Figure 12.7 ■). Several ligaments loosely anchor the open ends of the meniscus that face the center of knee to the tibia to allow slight motion in the menisci. The *semimembranosus* (a medial hamstring) attaches to the medial meniscus through capsular connections, and the *popliteus* tendon attaches to the lateral meniscus. Many people suffer from minor yet chronic knee pain caused by a meniscus shifting off center, which puts tension on its anchoring ligaments, or from tight muscular tendons pulling a meniscus off center.

The menisci function like fluid-filled shock absorbers in the knee. They transfer some weight from the femur into the tibia as an axial load and distribute some of the load around the circumference of a cartilaginous ring (Figure 12.8a-b ■). The menisci support half of the total weight on the knee, deforming under compression like a water bed distorts under body weight.

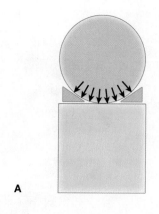

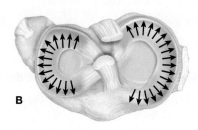

FIGURE 12.8

Distribution of weight from femoral condyles into the menisci: a) Axial loading b) Circumferential loading

The menisci have five main functions:

• Absorb shock
• Distribute load across the joint
• Reduce friction during motion
• Stabilize the joint by improving joint congruency
• Guide the pathway of motion

The joint capsule of the knee has the most extensive synovial lining of any synovial joint in the body (Figure 12.9 ■). Its lining adheres to the anterior internal surface of the joint capsule and to the sides of two cruciate ligaments inside the capsule. Like all synovial joint linings, it is a serous membrane that secretes fluid to lubricate and nourish the articular surfaces of the joint and the menisci.

Each knee has as many as 14 bursae that cushion the joint and reduce friction between moving structures. There are two types: free bursae and bursae that are *envaginations* (folds) of the synovial lining. Each bursa is sandwiched in between a number of different tissues, including ligaments, tendons, muscles, the joint capsule, bone, and skin. There are so many bursae around the knee that it is important to be aware of their general locations because deep pressure on damaged bursa can exacerbate the damage. When a client jumps with a pain response as you are working in the location of a bursa, you could be putting pressure on an injured bursa.

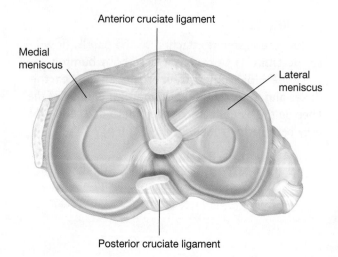

Anterior cruciate ligament

Medial meniscus

Lateral meniscus

Posterior cruciate ligament

FIGURE 12.7

Menisci in the knee: superior view

FIGURE 12.9
Bursae in the knee: side view

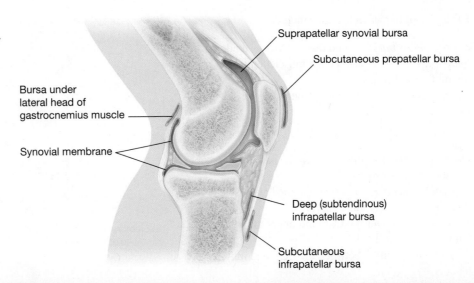

Suprapatellar synovial bursa

Subcutaneous prepatellar bursa

Bursa under
lateral head of
gastrocnemius muscle

Synovial membrane

Deep (subtendinous)
infrapatellar bursa

Subcutaneous
infrapatellar bursa

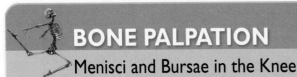

BONE PALPATION
Menisci and Bursae in the Knee

Caution: *Avoid putting pressure on a sore or painful bursa because it can increase the pain.*

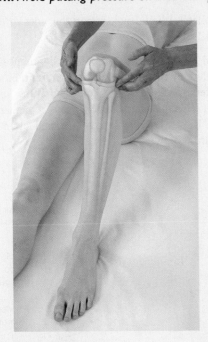

FIGURE 12.10a

Locate the **meniscus** along the joint line, between the tibial plateau and the femoral condyles. The menisci are somewhat easier to find with the knee bent, although they lack a distinct surface so you will need to use your imagination to approximate where they are located. *Are you pressing your fingertips straight into the sides of the joint space around the sides of the knee?* (See Figure 12.10a ■)

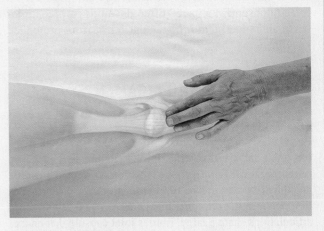

FIGURE 12.10b

Palpate the **infrapatellar bursa** with the knee in flexion by gently pressing the soft tissue below the patella. It is difficult to directly palpate this bursa, but you can feel its spongy, cushioning quality by lightly pressing and releasing several times. If the bursa is injured or inflamed, it will be sore to the touch. *Do you feel the spongy quality of the infrapatellar bursa?* (See Figure 12.10b ■)

Examples of bursae in the knee include:

- *Suprapatellar bursa* behind the quadriceps tendon
- *Subpopliteal bursa* between the muscle tendon and lateral femoral condyle
- *Subcutaneous prepatellar bursa* between the skin and the patella
- *Infrapatellar bursa* between the skin and the patellar ligament
- *Deep infrapatellar bursa* between the patellar ligament and the tibial tuberosity
- *Gastrocnemius bursa* between the medial muscle tendon and medial femoral condyle
- *Popliteal bursa* over the LCL and under the muscle tendon
- *Biceps femoris bursa* between the LCL and muscle tendon
- *Semitendinosus bursa* between the medial tibial condyle and muscle tendon
- *Gracilis bursa* between the MCL and the muscle tendon

Damage to the bursae occurs from compression injuries such as falling on the knees or from repetitive stresses to the knees from work in occupations such as tile or carpet layer or housecleaner. A bursitis referred to as "housemaid's knee" often develops in prepatellar bursa and superficial infrapatellar bursa from prolonged kneeling.

12.2 JOINTS AND LIGAMENTS OF THE KNEE

Each knee is made up of two primary joints: the patellofemoral joint and the tibiofemoral joint (Figure 12.11 ■). The **patellofemoral joint** is the articulation between the patella and the distal femur. The **tibiofemoral joint** is the articulation between the proximal tibia and the distal femur. Both articulations share a large, fibrous joint capsule that encapsulates the distal femur, the proximal tibia, and the patella.

12.2.1 Ligaments and Supporting Tendons

The absence of bony congruence in the knee requires an extensive network of ligaments and tendons to support and protect the joint. In the extended position, supporting ligaments and tendons of the knee become taut to stabilize the joint. In the flexed position of 90 degrees, most supportive ligaments of the knee become lax, which allows both rotation and the anterior and posterior **translation** of the joint (a normal yet slight backward and forward gliding motion of the tibia under the femoral condyles). **Displacement** of the knee refers to translatory motion beyond a normal physiological range, which often occurs during impact injuries such as being tackled from behind.

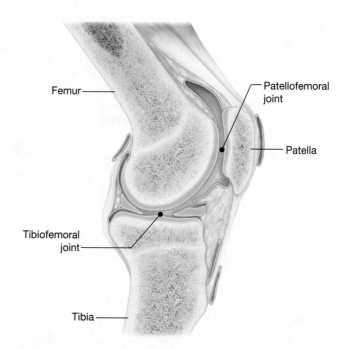

FIGURE 12.11

The patellofemoral and tibiofemoral joints

Two collateral ligaments support the sides of the knee (Figure 12.12 ■).

- A round, cordlike **lateral collateral ligament** (LCL), also called the **fibular collateral ligament,** binds the lateral femoral epicondyle to the head of the fibula, where it joins the biceps femoris (lateral hamstring) tendon. The LCL prevents excessive abduction, or genu varum (bowlegs), of the knee.

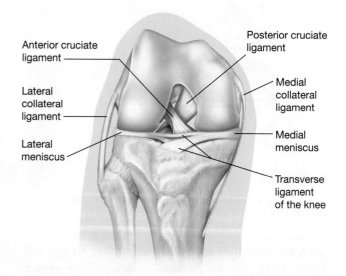

FIGURE 12.12

Collateral ligaments and cruciate ligaments: anterior view of right knee in flexion

- A flat, broad **medial collateral ligament** (MCL), also called a **tibial collateral ligament,** binds the medial epicondyle of the femur to the medial aspect of the proximal tibia. It also attaches to the medial meniscus. The MCL has a superficial and a deep layer that are separated by a bursa. This ligament prevents excessive adduction, or genu valgum (knock-knees) of the knee.

The knee has several stabilizing ligaments located inside the joint. Two cruciate (cross-shaped) ligaments in the middle of the joint orient along opposing oblique angles (see Figure 12.12). Their main function is to secure the anterior and posterior stability of the joint. They allow the knee to bend like a hinge while holding the articular surfaces together and restricting forward and backward displacement between the tibia and femur.

- The **anterior cruciate ligament** (ACL) connects the anterior intercondylar surface of the tibia to the posterior medial surface of the lateral femoral condyle. The ACL consists of two separate bands, one of which is always taut during the end range of flexion and extension. Both bands are slack at 30 degrees of flexion, where the knee is most vulnerable to anterior displacement. The ACL restricts anterior displacement of the tibia as well as hyperextension of the knee. During flexion and medial rotation, the ACL twists around the posterior cruciate ligament. The ACL also functions as a secondary restraint to varus and valgus stresses (abduction and adduction). Excessive rotation in the knee may indicate an ACL tear.

- The **posterior cruciate ligament** (PCL) connects the posterior intercondylar surface of the tibia to the lateral aspect of the medial femoral condyle (Figure 12.13 ■). The PCL is much shorter and thicker than the ACL, and about twice as strong. It also consists of two separate bands. One becomes taut in full extension and the other becomes taut at 90 degrees of flexion. Both bands stretch during deep flexion of the knee. The PCL restricts posterior displacement of the tibia, a mechanical stress that occurs in the knee on each loading step as a person walks down an incline. Repetitive loading on knees explains why they often feel sore after hiking down a mountain.

Excessive anterior or posterior translation in the knee, called a **drawer sign,** may indicate a tear or injury to a cruciate ligament.[1, 2] When a client has a drawer sign, you will feel excessive gliding of the tibia backward or forward under the femoral condyles (Figure 12.14a-b ■). Damage to the anterior cruciate often occurs when extreme valgus stress is suddenly placed on the knee, such as a football tackle from behind or a quick turn of the body that twists the knee (Figure 12.15 ■).

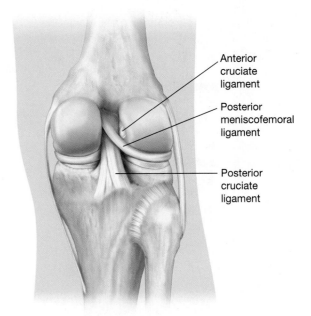

FIGURE 12.13

Posterior cruciate ligament: posterior view of right knee in extension

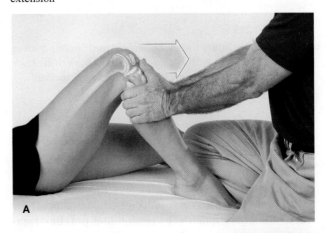

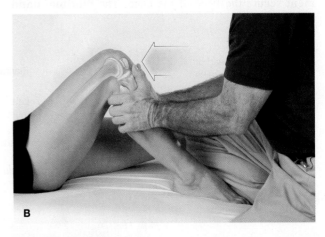

FIGURE 12.14

Drawer sign for cruciate ligaments: a) Test for anterior cruciate b) Test for posterior cruciate

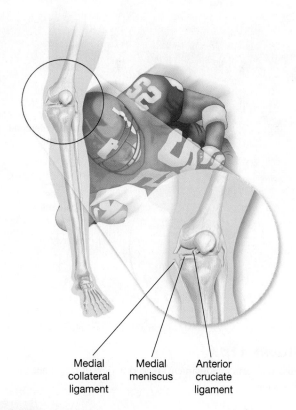

Medial collateral ligament   Medial meniscus   Anterior cruciate ligament

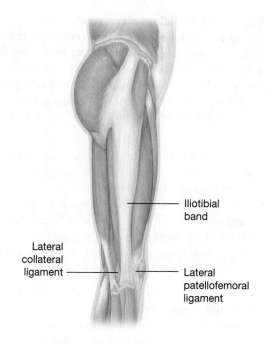

FIGURE 12.16
Iliotibial band: right knee

Iliotibial band

Lateral collateral ligament

Lateral patellofemoral ligament

FIGURE 12.15

A **common knee injury** called the "terrible triad" occurs from an extreme valgus stress, such as a posterior lateral blow to the knee, which simultaneously damages the anterior cruciate, medial meniscus, and medial collateral ligament.

The knee is also supported in extension by muscular tendons. When supportive ligaments become damaged, muscular tendons surrounding the knee provide a backup system of active restraints to stabilize the joint. Gastrocnemius and popliteus tendons shore up the back of the joint; hamstrings and adductor tendons support the sides; the strong quadriceps tendon and **patellar ligament** secure the front of the knee. The **iliotibial band**

(ITB) or **iliotibial tract** (ITT)—the long, flat, and broad tendon of the tensor fascia latae—helps to stabilize the lateral side of the knee (Figure 12.16 ■). On the back of the knee, tendons of the hamstrings and gastrocnemius define a diamond-shaped space over the popliteal fossa. A broad, flat **oblique popliteal ligament**, a tendinous expansion of the semimembranosus muscle, covers the posterior joint capsule (Figure 12.17 ■). Another popliteal ligament called the **arcuate ligament** is a thickening of the posterior joint capsule. Both popliteal ligaments become taut on knee extension to protect the joint from hyperextension. Three distal tendons of the sartorius, gracilis, and semitendinosus, collectively known as the

FIGURE 12.17
Ligaments of the knee: posterior view

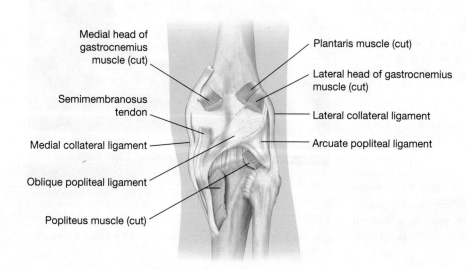

Medial head of gastrocnemius muscle (cut)

Semimembranosus tendon

Medial collateral ligament

Oblique popliteal ligament

Popliteus muscle (cut)

Plantaris muscle (cut)

Lateral head of gastrocnemius muscle (cut)

Lateral collateral ligament

Arcuate popliteal ligament

BONE PALPATION
Ligaments of the Knee

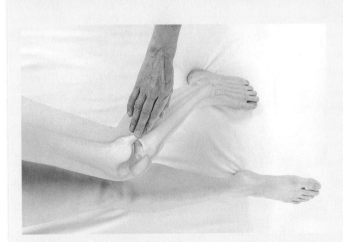

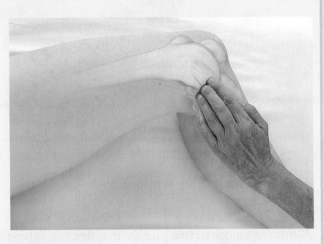

FIGURE 12.18a

Locate the **lateral collateral ligament** by palpating laterally along the joint line until you feel a short strap across the lateral side of the knee, which is the LCL. Move back and forth across it, then palpate it on the other knee. Hold the ligament while flexing and extending the knee. (See Figure 12.18a ■)

FIGURE 12.18b

Locate the **medial collateral ligament** by palpating medially along the joint line until you feel a short strap across the medial side of the knee, which is the MCL. Move back and forth across it, then palpate it on the other knee. Hold the ligament while flexing and extending the knee. (See Figure 12.18b ■)

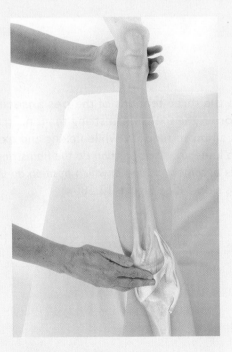

FIGURE 12.18c

Locate the **oblique popliteal ligament** by carefully pressing the crease in the back of the knee. Be careful of the popliteal nerve and artery in this area. You will be pressing into the center of this broad ligament, which crosses the joint capsule. Flex and extend the knee, noticing how tension in the ligament changes in each position. *How does tension in the ligaments change when the knee is flexed?* (See Figure 12.18c ■)

(continued)

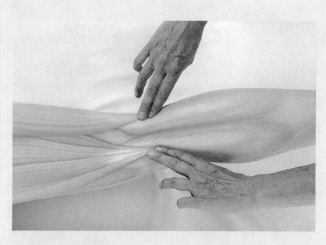

FIGURE 12.18d

Palpate the **hamstring tendons** on the back of the knee with the knee flexed. Slide your fingertips laterally along the back of the knee to hook under the hamstring tendons. Have your partner flex and extend the knee, noticing how the tendons change tension. *In which position do the hamstring tendons become taut and in which position do they become slack?* (See Figure 12.18d ■)

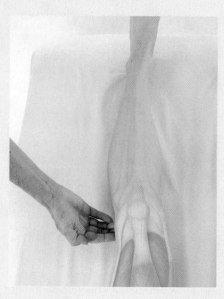

FIGURE 12.18e

Palpate the **iliotibial band** directly anterior to the lateral hamstring tendon, on the side of the knee. Hook your fingertips under the lateral edge of the ITB above the hamstring tendon and see how far up the band you can palpate. Have your partner flex and extend the knee, noticing how the ITB changes tension. (See Figure 12.18e ■)

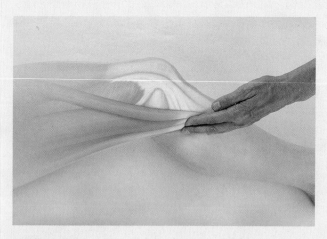

FIGURE 12.18f

Locate the three tendons of the **pes anserine** anterior to the medial hamstring tendon. Strum across all three tendons while flexing and extending the knee. *In which position do the hamstring tendons become taut and in which position do they become slack?* (See Figure 12.18f ■)

pes anserine, meaning "goose foot," insert on the proximal medial tibia and reinforce the medial aspect of the knee (Figure 12.19 ■).

12.2.2 Patellofemoral Joint

The patellofemoral joint resides within the tibiofemoral joint capsule, although it is considered a separate joint due to its unique structure and function. A number of ligaments and tendons bind the patella to the femur to secure the patellofemoral joint (see Figure 12.19). The quadriceps tendon attached to the top of the patella covers the kneecap and blends into the **patellar ligament** that anchors the bottom of the patella to the tibial tuberosity. The transverse and longitudinal fibers of the **medial** and **lateral patellar retinacula** secure the patella to surrounding structures.

The primary functions of the patellofemoral joint are to increase the mechanical advantage of the knee extensors and to protect the tibiofemoral joint. The patella serves as an anatomical pulley to deflect the pull of the powerful quadriceps tendon away from the tibiofemoral joint. This large sesamoid bone increases the mechanical advantage of the extensors by lengthening the moment arm—the perpendicular distance between the muscular line of pull and the axis of motion at the center of the joint (Figure 12.20a-b ■). The patella literally gives the quadriceps a corner to pull around.

12.2.2.1 PATELLAR MOTION AND TRACKING

The patella slides like a cable on a pulley during knee flexion and extension, gliding up and down in the intercondylar groove (Figure 12.21 ■). A changing point of contact occurs between the patella and the intercondylar groove throughout the range of motion (Figure 12.22 ■). In motions such as standing from a squat or walking up or down a hill, the pull of the quadriceps compresses the patellofemoral joint, placing 200–300 pounds of pressure on the patella. Thick

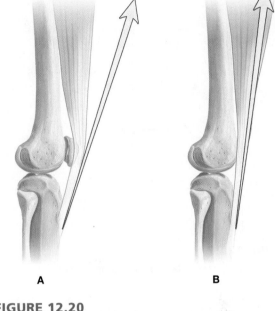

A **B**

FIGURE 12.20

Moment arm of quadriceps: a) Line of pull of quadriceps with patella b) Without patella

hyaline cartilage covering the posterior aspect of the patella lubricates the joint to reduce friction under pressure.

The patella tracks along a curved pathway that is about twice the distance of the length of the patella (Figure 12.23 ■). Each of the four quadriceps tendons pulls on the patella along a different line of pull (Figure 12.24 ■). The muscular pulls must be balanced for optimal patellar tracking along the intercondylar groove. To feel patellar tracking, lightly hold your kneecap, then slowly flex and extend your knee.

Poor patellar tracking can lead to arthritis, inflammation, recurring dislocation of the patella, and **patellofemoral pain syndrome.** Premature deterioration and

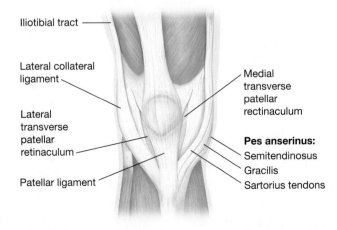

FIGURE 12.19

Patellofemoral joint: anterior view

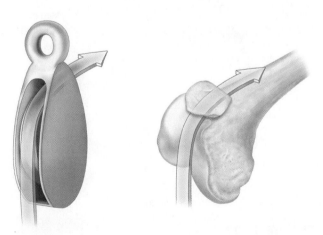

FIGURE 12.21

The **patella** functions like a cable on a pulley.

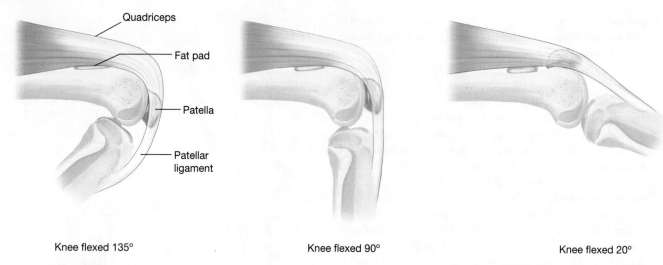

Knee flexed 135°   Knee flexed 90°   Knee flexed 20°

FIGURE 12.22

Changing points of **patellar contact** during knee motion

softening of the patellar cartilage causes a painful condition called **chondromalacia.** Inflammatory conditions in the knee damage the articular cartilage, causing the patella to adhere to the intercondylar groove, restricting its freely gliding motion and causing knee stiffness. A common muscular imbalance affecting knee alignment and patellar tracking occurs when the lateral quadriceps overpowers the medial quadriceps, pulling the patella to the lateral side of the intercondylar groove. Tracking of the patella also depends on the alignment of the hip during joint motion. Excessive lateral rotation of the hips in

a neutral position can place undue torque on the knees, causing a chronic tightness of both the iliotibial band and the vastus lateralis. This can also lead to **iliotibial band syndrome**, which is a common cause of knee pain. This inflammatory condition of the knee is caused by the continual rubbing of a tight and fibrotic ITB over the lateral femoral epicondyle. Chronic tightness in the sartorius can also torque the knee and reduce the mechanical efficiency of patellofemoral joint motion. All of these conditions underscore the importance of balanced muscular pulls on the knee.

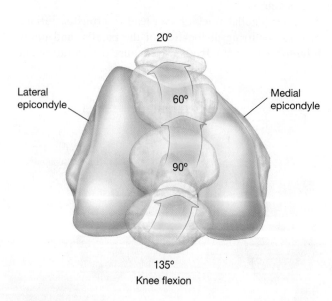

FIGURE 12.23

Patellar pathway

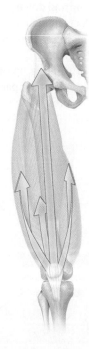

FIGURE 12.24

Lines of pull in quadricep muscles

12.2.2.2 KNEE ALIGNMENT AND THE Q ANGLE

The knee is a highly calibrated joint. When optimally aligned, the joint structures work efficiently to absorb shock and minimize wear on cartilage. When even slightly misaligned, cumulative wear on the joint structures, particularly on cartilage, leads to premature deterioration and a predisposition to overuse injury.

There are several measures of the functional alignment of the knee. The first measure is the **mechanical axis of the lower limb.** In an ideal alignment, the centers of the joints of the hip, knee, and ankle fall along a vertical line (Figure 12.25 ■). The second metatarsophalangeal joint also falls along this axis.

A second measure of knee alignment is the **Q angle:** the line of pull of the quadriceps on the knee. The Q angle is determined by two intersecting lines: one from the anterior superior ischial spine (ASIS) to the midpoint of the patella, and the other from the midpoint of the patella to the tibial tuberosity (Figure 12.26 ■). An average Q angle is 15 degrees, although it can range from 13 to 18 degrees. The Q angle tends to be greater in women because the female pelvis is wider, which increases the oblique angle of the femur.

The oblique angle of the shaft of the femur causes a medial displacement of the knee called **genu valgum**

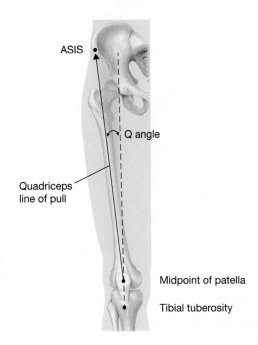

FIGURE 12.26
The Q angle

(Figure 12.27 ■). Five to 10 degrees of genu valgum is normal, although a greater degree of medial displacement results in a knock-kneed alignment. To figure out what degree of genu valgum is normal for each person, compare the right and left sides. In contrast, lateral displacement of the knee results in **genu varum**, a bowlegged alignment. Excessive genu varus or genu valgum will change the Q angle, placing undue stress on the structures of the knee. As little as 5 degrees of genu varum can increase compressive forces on the medial meniscus by 50 percent.[3]

12.2.3 Tibiofemoral Joint

The tibiofemoral joint is made up of articulations between the femoral condyles and the tibial plateau. Because it has two distinct sides, it is also considered a *double condyloid joint.* While most synovial hinge joints move in two degrees of motion—flexion and extension—the tibiofemoral joint is also classified as a *modified hinge joint* because it moves with 3 degrees of motion. It can flex and extend as well as rotate, but it can only rotate in a flexed position.

The bottom of the tibiofemoral joint consists of the tibial plateau. The smooth articular surfaces of the femoral condyles sit in the back half of the tibial plateau when the knee is extended. Because the femur meets the tibia along an oblique angle, the lateral femoral condyle sits under the center of the femoral shaft. Because the medial femoral condyle is 50 percent larger and considerably longer than

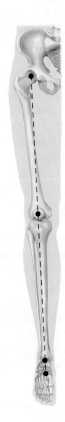

FIGURE 12.25
Mechanical axis of lower limb

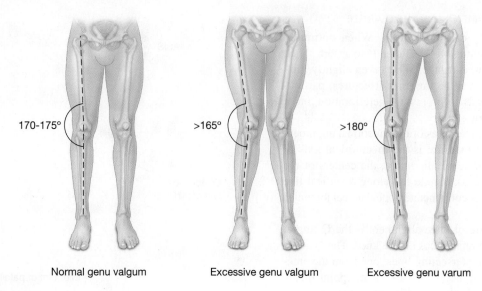

170-175°   >165°   >180°

Normal genu valgum   Excessive genu valgum   Excessive genu varum

FIGURE 12.27

Alignment patterns of the knees

the lateral condyle, it bears most of the weight of the femur when the knee is extended.

12.2.3.1 TIBIOFEMORAL JOINT RANGE OF MOTION

The primary movement of the tibiofemoral joint is flexion and extension; rotation is an accessory motion that only occurs during flexion (see Table 12.1 ■). The knee flexes and extends in the sagittal plane during gait activities, moving in the plane determined by the position of the hip. If the hip laterally rotates, the knee will follow. When assessing tibiofemoral joint motion, the first thing

TABLE 12.1	Range of Motion in the Knee	
Knee Motion	Range of Motion	End Feel
Flexion	140 degrees with hip flexed 120 degrees with hip extended 160 degrees in passive flexion	Soft
Extension	5 degrees	Firm
Medial rotation	30 degrees with knee flexed 90 degrees	Firm
Lateral rotation	30 degrees with knee flexed 90 degrees	Firm

to consider is which end of the joint is moving freely and which end remains relatively fixed. For example, the tibia moves against a fixed femur when extending the knee from a seated position, but the femur moves over a relatively fixed tibia when extending the knees to shift from sitting to standing (Figure 12.28a-b ■).

Most muscles crossing the knee are biarticular; they cross two joints. When two joints pull in opposite directions on a biarticular muscle crossing on the knee, that muscle can only stretch so far before it reaches its maximum length and restricts further motion. This explains why the position of the hip and ankle affects the range of motion in the knee. For example, the hamstrings can stretch farther when the hip is flexed than when it is extended. The knee can be actively flexed an average of 140 degrees with the hip in flexion, but only 120 degrees with the hip extended (Figure 12.29a-b ■). The knee can be passively flexed to 160 degrees, touching the heel to the buttocks, like a flexible person does when crouching.

Because the joint surfaces do not fit together in an exactly straight, complete extension of the knee actually hyperextends it in a range of 5–10 degrees (Figure 12.30a ■). Hyperextension of the knee beyond 5–10 degrees, called **genu recurvatum,** places abnormal tensions and stress on soft tissues over the back of the knee. Genu recurvatum unnaturally locks the knees, disturbing the skeletal alignment of the entire body by throwing weight back on the heels and tipping the pelvis into an anterior tilt (Figure 12.30b ■).

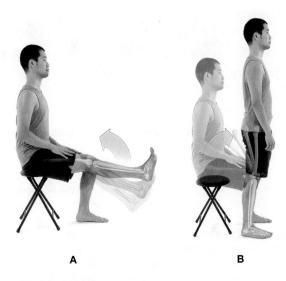

A   **B**

FIGURE 12.28

a) When extending the knee from a seated position, the femur is the fixed end of the joint. b) When standing up, the tibia is the fixed end of the joint.

When flexed at a 90-degree angle, the knee can axially rotate an average of 30 degrees medially and 40 degrees laterally (Figure 12.31a-b ■). Tibiofemoral rotations are important in sports like tennis or basketball, where quick direction changes are needed.

The range of motion in the knee varies with age, flexibility, and general health. If one knee is injured, check the range of motion in the other knee to find out what is normal for that person. Restrictions in the ankle or hip joint range of motion can also lead to restrictions in the tibiofemoral joint range of motion.

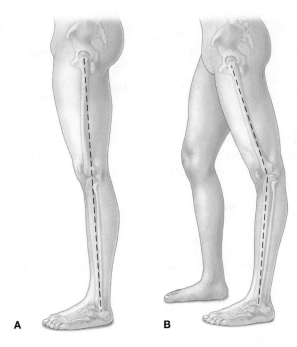

A   **B**

FIGURE 12.30

a) **Normal knee extension** b) **Genu recurvatum**

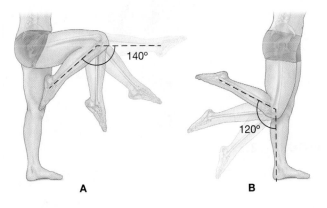

140°

120°

A   **B**

FIGURE 12.29

Range of knee motion: a) Knee flexion b) Knee extension

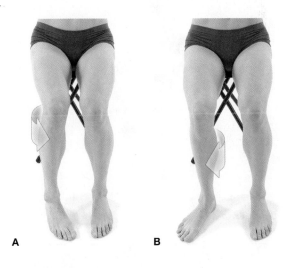

A   **B**

FIGURE 12.31

Range of tibiofemoral joint rotation in flexion: a) Internal rotation b) External rotation

SELF-CARE
Correcting Genu Recurvatum (Hyperextended Knees)

If you hyperextend your knees, you probably also hyperextend your lower back. This will break your line of force when pushing by reducing the amount of force you are able to apply. It can also lead to knee or lumbar injuries.

1. **Finding the center of the knee:** Stand with your knees straight. Then hyperextend your knees and feel what happens to the position of your hips and pelvis. If your pelvis tips, slowly bend and slowly straighten your knees, sensing support in the center of your knee when it is straight. *What happens to the alignment of your pelvis when you hyperextend your knees?*

2. **Balancing on one leg:** Stand on one leg and sense the position where your knee feels fully extended but not hyperextended, where you can feel weight passing through the center of the joint (Figure 12.32a ■). Then check in a mirror to see if your knee is actually straight. If you have a pattern of genu recurvatum, normal extension will feel slightly bent and you will need to get used to the odd feeling of this straight position. Repeat this sequence with your other knee.

3. **Flexion and extension of one knee:** Stand on one leg and slowly bend and straighten your knee (Figure 12.32b ■). To straighten your knee, push your foot into the floor. Repeat with the other knee. *Does flattening your toes on the floor improve your balance?*

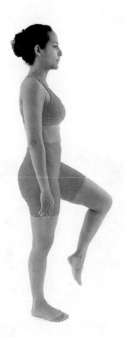

FIGURE 12.32a

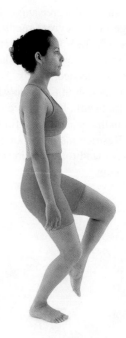

FIGURE 12.32b

12.2.3.2 FLEXION AND EXTENSION OF THE KNEE

The femur rolls, glides, and spins on the tibia during flexion and extension. If the femoral condyles were to simply roll without gliding and spinning over the smaller tibial condyles, these larger condyles would roll off the tibia (Figure 12.33a-c ■). For the longer medial condyle to move in sync with the shorter lateral condyle, the femur spins slightly on the lateral condyle during flexion. The action reverses during extension, medially rotating the distal femur. To understand the mechanics of this action, imagine how a rocking chair with uneven runners, one twice as long as the other, would turn on the shorter runner as it rocked. Similarly, during knee flexion, the difference in the size of the femoral condyles causes the femur to spin on its shorter lateral condyle (Figure 12.34 ■).

As the knee extends from a flexed position, just the opposite joint dynamic occurs. The shorter lateral condyle runs out of room and the motion transfers to a spin on the medial condyle. During the first 30 degrees of extension from flexion, the motion centers over the lateral condyle. During the next 60 degrees of extension, the motion transfers to the medial condyle of the joint.

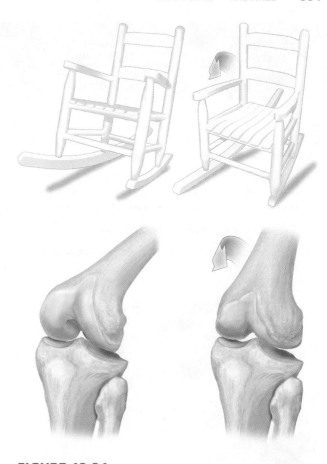

FIGURE 12.34

The condyles of the femur rock unevenly as a rocking chair would if it had uneven runners.

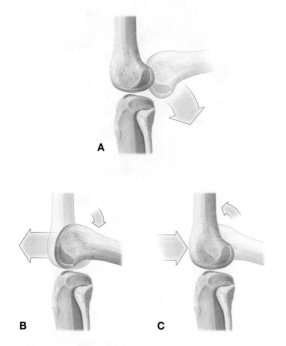

FIGURE 12.33

a) The femoral condyles would roll off the tibia if they did not also glide. b) Gliding action of the condyles during knee flexion. c) Gliding action of the condyles during knee extension.

12.2.3.3 AXIAL ROTATION OF THE KNEE

As mentioned earlier, the knee can move in a range of axial rotation in a flexed position. If the foot is free, the tibia rotates under the femur. To feel this action while sitting in a chair, rotate your foot out and in, turning it on your heel. A basketball player rotates the knee when making a quick change of direction from a low position, initiating the turn from the foot, so the tibia rotates under the femur. But if the foot is fixed, the femur rotates on the tibia. A basketball player crouched in a defensive position with both feet planted uses this motion to turn the body, rotating the femur on the tibia.

A common knee injury occurs during axial rotation when a person makes a quick turn and the sneaker sticks to the playing court, twisting the knee too far. The lateral rotation of the hip puts a valgus torque on the knee,

EXPLORING TECHNIQUE
Passive Range of Motion for the Knee

Before you perform passive range of motion tests on your partner's knee, read through these guidelines:

- Have your partner agree to report any pain or discomfort he or she feels during the motion. Watch for signs of pain or discomfort and stop if you notice any pain reactions.

- Stabilize the knee above and below the joint.

- Traction the knee before moving it to avoid pinching joint structures.

- Keep the thigh and leg in the same plane as you move the knee to avoid twisting it. Slowly move the knee along a linear pathway.

- When you feel you have reached the end range of motion, ask your partner if he or she feels a stretch, which will indicate you have reached the end range.

- Perform all the PROM tests on both knees to make a bilateral comparison.

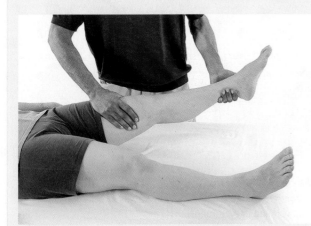

FIGURE 12.35a

a) PROM for knee extension.

1. **Knee extension:** With your partner in a supine position, place one hand above the knee to stabilize it. Grasp the underside of the ankle with your other hand. Traction the knee by pulling the ankle. Extend the knee by lifting the ankle up as you push down on the knee (Figure 12.35a ■). Five to 10 degrees of hyperextension is normal. If the knee hyperextends past this, check the range of motion on the other knee to see what is normal for your partner.

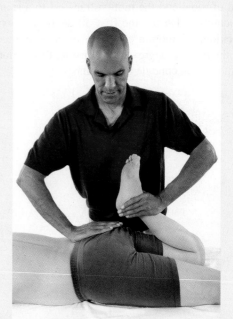

FIGURE 12.35b

b) PROM for knee flexion.

2. **Knee flexion:** With your partner in a prone position, align the knee under the hip, then pull on the lower limb to traction and open the front of the hip. This will prevent the hip from flexion and the lower back from hyperextending as you bend the knee. When the hip flexes and the lower back hyperextends during a knee flexion PROM, this indicates tightness in the quadratus femoris. Place one hand above the knee to stabilize it. Lift the ankle to 30 degrees with the other hand, then slowly move the heel toward the hip. In a normal range of passive knee flexion, the heel will touch the back of the hip (Figure 12.35b ■).

EXPLORING TECHNIQUE
Tibiofemoral Rotations

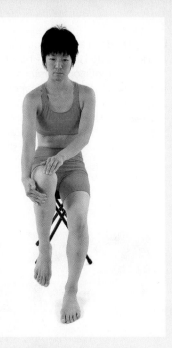

FIGURE 12.36a

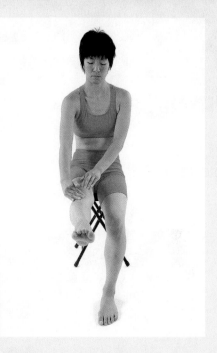

FIGURE 12.36b

1. **To explore the screw home mechanism in your own knee:** Place one hand on your tibial tuberosity and the other hand on your quadriceps tendon (Figure 12.36a ■). Notice how your hands line up vertically when your knee is bent. Slowly straighten the knee and notice how the

joint twists, causing the tibial tuberosity to shift toward the lateral side. (Figure 12.36b ■). Slowly bend and straighten your knee several times to observe changes in alignment and feel the screw home mechanism.

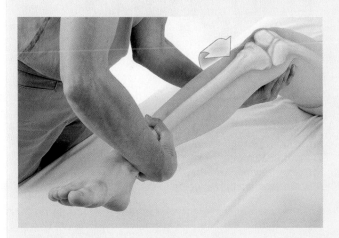

FIGURE 12.36c

2. **To track the screw home mechanism on a partner:** Begin with your partner in a supine position. Hold the lower leg with one hand while supporting the back of the knee with your other hand (Figure 12.36c ■).

   a. Lift the knee so that the hip and knee are in 30 degrees of flexion when the tibia is horizontal to the table. Hold the bones lightly so that natural joint rotations can freely occur while you move your partner's leg.

(continued)

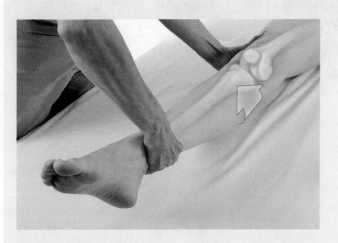

FIGURE 12.36d

b. Slowly extend and flex your partner's knee (Figure 12.36d ■). Notice how the bones rotate. *What degree of rotation do you notice or feel in the knees? Does one knee rotate differently than the other? During flexion, does the proximal tibia medially rotate while the distal femur laterally rotates? During extension, does the proximal tibia laterally rotate while the distal femur medially rotates several degrees?*

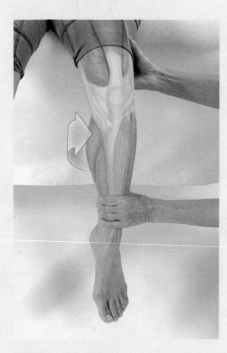

FIGURE 12.36e

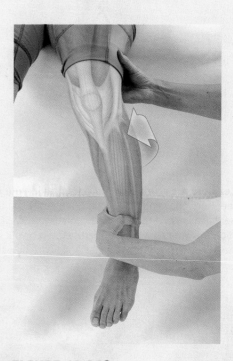

FIGURE 12.36f

3. **To check the range of axial rotation on a partner:** Have your partner sit on a massage table with the legs hanging over the side. Hold the knee under the distal femur, then turn the tibia medially and laterally

(Figure 12.36e-f ■). Move the knee slowly and gently, do not try to rotate the knee past its end-feel. *Did you notice any abnormal patterns of rotation in either knee. If so, did this exploration change this pattern?*

which can injure the "terrible triad"—the medial collateral ligament, medial meniscus, and anterior cruciate ligament. A similar injury occurs when a skier takes a quick fall on the inside edge of a ski, bending the knee into a valgus stress.

During the last 30 degrees of knee extension, the tibia and femur counterrotate into a close-packed position called **terminal rotation.** This type of rotation differs from axial rotation of the knee in flexion. Terminal rotation involves a **screw home mechanism** in which the distal femur medially rotates against the lateral rotation of the tibia. The screw home mechanism stabilizes the knee in the extended position, twisting and locking the joint structures into a tight fit. This natural stabilizing mechanism differs from hyperextending the knee past a normal range, which most people refer to as "locking the knees."

12.2.3.4 MOVEMENT OF THE MENISCI

Movement in the tibiofemoral joint occurs between the menisci and femur rather than the menisci and tibia. The menisci follow the motion of the femoral condyles on the tibia. To conform to the changing point of contact between the articular surfaces of the femur and tibia during knee motion, each meniscus moves across the tibia within a small range. Although motion of the menisci is difficult to palpate or perceive, it is helpful to understand because the chronic knee pain and injury that many people suffer often results from poor tracking in the menisci. The femoral condyles press the menisci across the tibial plateau like a pestle grinding an apricot in a mortar. The lateral meniscus moves forward and backward a distance of 12 millimeters, twice as far as the medial meniscus. During knee flexion, the menisci shift toward the back of the tibial plateau; during knee extension, they shift toward the front of the tibial plateau (Figure 12.37 ■). During lateral rotation of the knee (which laterally rotates the tibia), the lateral meniscus shifts forward and the medial meniscus shifts back; during medial rotation, they shift in the opposite direction.

A meniscus can rupture if it fails to follow the movement of the femoral condyles. This often occurs during ballistic extension of the knee that squashes and tears the fibrocartilage of the meniscus, such as kicking a ball. If the meniscus fails to shift position quickly enough, it can get crushed under the grinding load of the condyles. Tears can also occur during quick twisting movements of the knee that literally fracture the menisci. A torn meniscus can no longer follow a normal movement range and loses its ability to absorb load. The edge of a torn meniscus tends to lift and bend under pressure, which causes intense pain on the end range of both flexion and

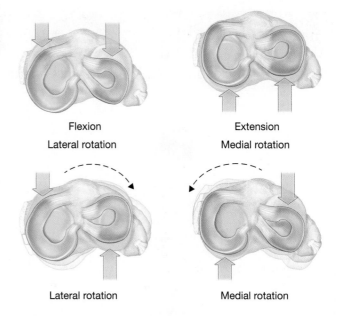

Flexion   Extension
Lateral rotation   Medial rotation

Lateral rotation   Medial rotation

FIGURE 12.37
Movement of the menisci

extension. When this occurs, a person can no longer fully bend or straighten the knee. For this reason, someone with a meniscus tear often stands and walks with the injured side in partial flexion.

12.3 MUSCLES OF THE KNEE

Muscular tendons cross and encase the knee on all sides. Some of these muscles generate motion in the tibiofemoral joint, and others function as passive restraints to stabilize the knee. Muscles that generate or assist motion at the knee include:

- Extensors: *Quadriceps*
- Flexors: *Hamstrings*
- Rotators: *Hamstrings, popliteus, gracilis,* and *sartorius*
- Synergists: *Popliteus* assists extension; *gracilis* and *sartorius* assist knee flexion

Since the primary actions of the gracilis and the sartorius occur at the hip and their actions at the knee are secondary, both of these muscles are covered in the chapter on the hip. There are three fascial compartments in the thigh housing muscle groups that act on the knee. The quadriceps compartment covers the front of the thigh and wraps around to the lateral side. The hamstrings compartment covers the back, and the adductor compartment can be found along

SELF-CARE
Tracking and Guiding Menisci Motion

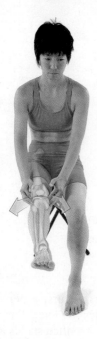

FIGURE 12.38a

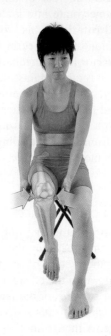

FIGURE 12.38b

The more the alignment of the knee deviates from its optimal center, the greater the risk of knee injuries due to faulty joint tracking. This exercise will help you track the menisci of the knee along their ideal path. It can also alleviate minor knee pain due to faulty tracking.

1. **Palpating the menisci:** Begin by palpating the lateral and medial menisci along the joint line on the sides of the knee, right in front of the collateral ligaments. Notice if either side is sore. *Do you feel pain along any of the meniscus during palpation?*

2. **Tracking menisci motion in flexion and extension:** Hold the sides of the menisci in one knee while slowly flexing and extending it several times. Pay attention to their pattern of motion. They should move forward as you extend the knee and move backward while you flex the knee. Keep in mind that the motion in the menisci is minimal, so it will not be very obvious. Motion of the lateral meniscus is usually easier to feel than the medial meniscus because it moves twice as far as the medial meniscus. *Do you notice the greater range of motion in the lateral menisci?*

3. **Guiding menisci motion:** To encourage the normal movement of the menisci in the sagittal plane, as you extend your knee, press the menisci forward and in as though you were turning two cogwheels together (Figure 12.38a ■) As you flex your knee, press them back and in. Track them through several movement cycles (Figure 12.38b ■).

4. After you track the menisci in one knee, get up and walk around. Notice whether that knee feels any different from the other one. *If you had pain in your knee that you thought was caused by poor tracking in a meniscus, did it change or dissipate after doing this exercise?*

5. Repeat steps 1–3 on the other knee.

the inside of the thigh (Figure 12.39 ■). Ideally, muscles in one compartment can slide freely against muscles in other compartments. If the fascial membranes wrapping the separate compartments become glued together, this will restrict or alter the line of muscular pulls on the knee. As a result, it can place undue stress on the knee joint structure.

Although the iliotibial band is not a muscular compartment, chronic shortness and inflexibility in this strong lateral tendon can also pull the knee off center and increase torsion stress on the knee. To alleviate such problems, the palpation exercises in this section encourage readers to explore palpating between compartments, which is also the technique to release fascial restrictions between muscular groups and tendons acting on the knee.

12.3.1 Knee Extensors: The Quadriceps

A group of four large quadriceps—the rectus femoris and the three muscles in the vasti muscle group (vastus lateralis, vastus intermedius, and vastus medialis)—cross the knee at the quadriceps tendon, which blends into the patellar ligament (Figure 12.40 ■). All four muscles are innervated by the *femoral nerve* and converge to share a common insertion on the tibial tuberosity. The quadriceps contract concentrically during gait to extend the knee on heel strike; they contract eccentrically to control the rate at which the knee flexes on the swing phase. Their bipennate structures make them powerful extensors of the knee; in a ballistic kick they often overpower their antagonists, leaving a person with a strain or "pull" in the hamstrings. Because the quadriceps can develop trigger points in so many places, Travell nicknamed the group the "four-faced trouble maker."[4]

The **rectus femoris,** a long bipennate muscle, originates on the anterior inferior ischial spine (AIIS), travels over the vastus intermedius directly along the anterior aspect of the

femoral shaft, and inserts on the tibial tuberosity via the quadriceps tendon and patellar ligament. This biarticular muscle crosses both the knee and hip, so it can extend the knee or flex the hip. (See TrP for the rectus femoris in Figure 12.41 ■).

The **vastus intermedius,** the smallest of the three pennate vasti, covers the upper two-thirds of the anterior and lateral surface of the femoral shaft. The vasti group generally relaxes when the knee is extended, although some parts of the muscle remain active to stabilize the knee. The deepest fibers of the vastus intermedius—the *articular genu*—attach to the upper patella and the synovial capsule. The primary function of the articular genu is to lift the joint capsule and the patella when the knee is in an extended position. (See TrP for the vastus intermedius in Figure 12.42 ■).

The **vastus lateralis** is the largest and strongest of the quadriceps. The belly of the vastus lateralis wraps the lateral side of the leg. Its long, thin origin begins below the greater trochanter and runs along the lateral edge of the linea aspera on the posterior shaft of the femur. (See TrPs for the vastus lateralis in Figure 12.43 ■).

The **vastus medialis** attaches along a thin line that runs the length of the posterior femoral shaft along the medial edge of the linea aspera, directly medial to the insertions of the adductors. Deep fibers of vastus medialis make up the vastus medialis oblique (VMO), which is an important stabilizer of the knee. When the VMO is contracted, it lifts the patella and keeps the patella tracking correctly. Chronic knee pain can occur when the vastus lateralis overpowers the vastus medialis, which is often treated with VMO isometrics and strengthening exercises. Travell describes the vastus medialis as the "buckling knee muscle" because painful trigger points in it tend, over time, to inhibit the muscle, which can lead to a sudden buckling of the knee. (Figure 12.44 ■). [5]

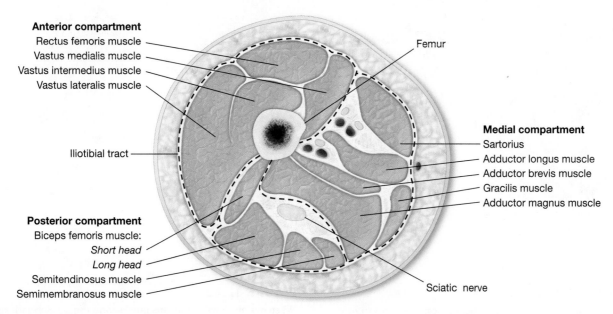

FIGURE 12.39

Cross-section of the thigh

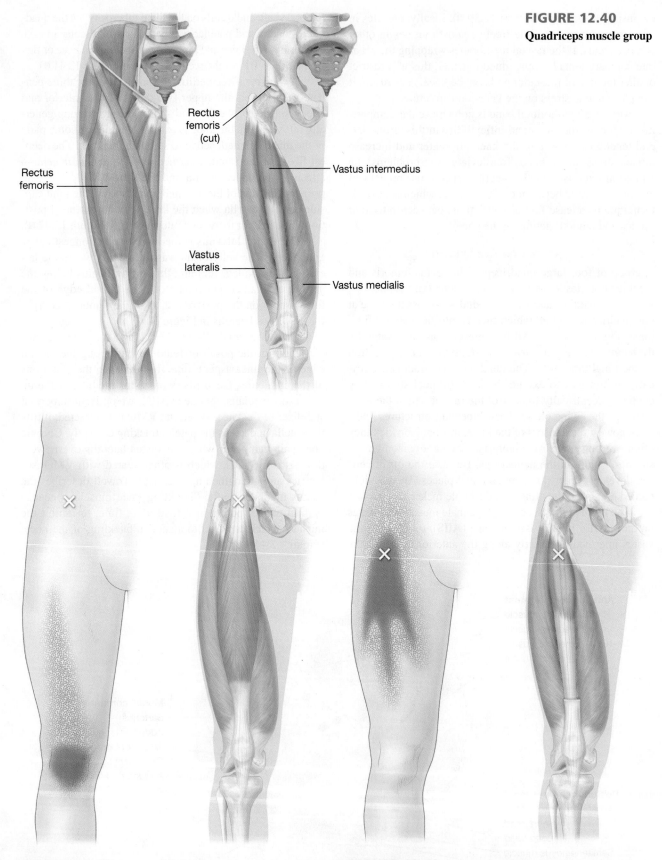

FIGURE 12.40
Quadriceps muscle group

Rectus
femoris
(cut)

Rectus
femoris

Vastus intermedius

Vastus
lateralis

Vastus medialis

FIGURE 12.41

When dysfunctional, the **rectus femoris** can develop a trigger point just below the AIIS, which can refer a deep, aching pain directly over the kneecap and can interfere with sleep.

FIGURE 12.42

When dysfunctional, the **vastus intermedius** can develop a trigger point that is difficult to palpate beneath the rectus femoris and can refer pain over a broad area of the middle thigh.

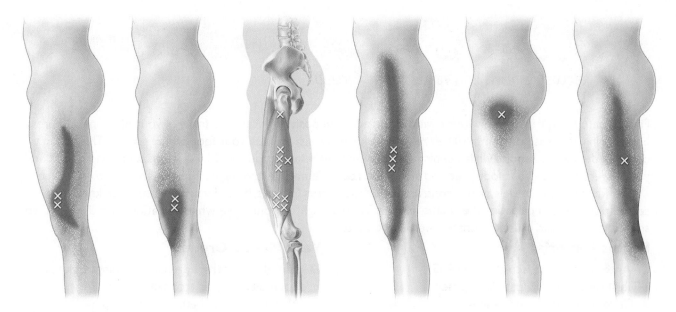

FIGURE 12.43

When dysfunctional, the **vastus lateralis** can develop a hornet's nest of trigger points in nine different locations: four in a square right above the knee, three in a column along the center of the muscle, one right below the greater trochanter, and one along the middle posterior edge of the muscle. Each trigger point or group of trigger points can refer severe pain to several locations along the muscle, from the lateral crest of the hip to the side of the knee and the patella. Trigger points in the vastus lateralis are common in children with myofascial pain syndromes; these can disturb sleep and make the side-lying position an achy, painful event. Direct pressure or bodywork on the iliotibial band can often be painful due to many trigger points in the underlying vastus lateralis.

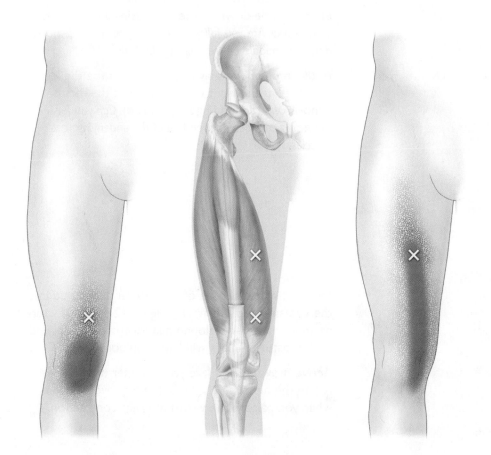

FIGURE 12.44

When dysfunctional, the **vastus medialis** develops two trigger points: one at the distal end of the muscle that can refer pain over the medial side of the knee, and the other in the middle of the muscle that can refer pain along the belly of the muscle.

MUSCLE PALPATION
Rectus Femoris and Vasti Muscle Group

First palpate the quadriceps on your own thigh. In a seated position, locate the front of your hip bone and press below it, in the crease of your hip. Then raise your knee enough to raise your foot off the ground. This action will contract the rectus femoris while keeping the vasti muscles relaxed; you should feel its proximal end bulge under your fingertips. Keep your foot lifted and strum the rectus femoris, exploring its fibers all the way to your knee.

To feel the vasti muscle group contract under the rectus femoris, begin by again lifting your knee from a seated position and palpating the rectus femoris. Then straighten your knee while palpating your thigh, and you should feel the vasti muscles contract below the rectus.

Rectus Femoris

O–Anterior inferior ischial spine (AIIS)
I–Tibial tuberosity via patellar ligament
A–Flexes hip and extends knee

Vasti Muscle Group

O–Lateralis—Lateral edge of linea aspera, gluteal tuberosity, greater trochanter
Medialis—Medial edge of linea aspera
Intermedius—Upper two-thirds of anterior and lateral femoral shaft
I–Patellar ligament and tibial tuberosity
A–Extends knee, vastus medialis oblique stabilizes the knee

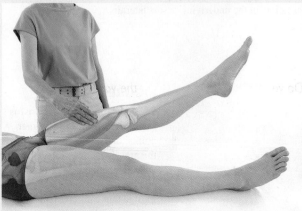

FIGURE 12.45a
Palpating the rectus femoris contraction

Palpate the proximal end of the rectus femoris below the anterior inferior iliac spine. Palpate the entire muscle down to the knee using a cross-fiber strumming. *Are you following the belly of rectus femoris down the middle of the thigh to the patella?*

Active movement: Have your partner raise the leg with the knee straight while you locate the rectus femoris contraction (Figure 12.45a ■). *Can you feel the rectus contract independent of the underlying vasti muscles.*

Follow the medial edge of the patellar tendon up into the **vastus medialis** fibers (Figure 12.45b ■). If your partner has well-developed quadriceps, the distal end of the vastus medialis will have a bulbous shape.

Active movement: Have your partner medially rotate the hip, then lift the entire leg several inches while you palpate the vastus medialis contraction.

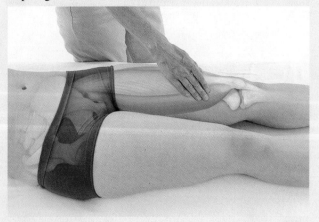

FIGURE 12.45b
Palpating the vastus medialis

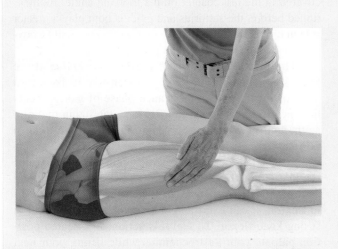

FIGURE 12.45c

Palpating the vastus lateralis

Locate the **vastus lateralis** under the iliotibial band, along the middle of the thigh (Figure 12.45c ■).

Active movement: Have your partner laterally rotate the hip, then lift the entire leg several inches while you palpate the vastus lateralis contraction. *Do you notice how wide the vastus lateralis is?*

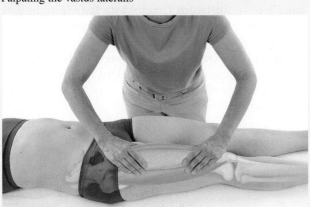

FIGURE 12.45d

Kneading and lifting the vasti muscles

With your partner still supine, explore the **vasti** by lifting, kneading, and approximating the entire muscle group. (Figure 12.45d ■) *Can you locate the medial and lateral edges of the vasti muscles? Did you notice how the vasti muscles wrap around two-thirds of the thigh? Do you feel how much meatier the vasti muscles are than the rectus femoris?*

12.3.2 Knee Flexors: The Hamstrings

The hamstrings are a group of three muscles on the back of the thigh that include the biceps femoris, semimembranosus, and semitendinosus. They connect the base of the pelvis to the tibia and fibula across the back of the knee (Figure 12.46 ■). As a group, the hamstrings work to flex the knee and extend the hip, although in this chapter focus is on their actions at the knee. The *tibial portion of the sciatic nerve* innervates all three hamstrings.

The most lateral hamstring, the **biceps femoris,** is a fibrous pennate muscle with a long head and a short head. The tubular tendon of the long head arises from the ischial tuberosity; the broad attachment of the short fleshy head originates along the middle portion of the lateral lip of the linea aspera, on the posterior shaft of the femur. Both heads insert below the knee on the lateral, posterior side of the head of the fibula. The biceps femoris generates knee flexion after pushoff to lift the knee so that the foot clears the ground. It also generates lateral rotation of the knee when it is in a flexed position. A bursa under the biceps femoris tendon below the ischial tuberosity separates it from the other hamstring tendons.

The **semitendinosus,** a fibrous pennate muscle, also arises at the ischial tuberosity. It has a long, round distal tendon that curves around the proximal medial tibia, where it inserts with the tendons of sartorius and gracilis tendons at the pes anserine.

The origin of the **semimembranosus** can be found beneath the semitendinosus on the ischial tuberosity. The belly of this broad bipennate muscle lies along the medial side of the femur; its distal tendon inserts on the proximal medial tibia posterior to the semitendinosus tendon. The semimembranosus bursa under the tendon at the knee is often a large double bursa. Both the semitendinosus and semimembranosus work as knee flexors and as medial rotators when the knee is in flexion.

Acute or repetitive overload to the hamstrings can lead to pain and trigger points. Pressure across the back of the thigh from being compressed by the edge of a chair during prolonged sitting and driving can also lead to hamstring pain and trigger points. (Figure 12.47 ▪). Prolonged sitting puts the hamstrings in a shortened position, which is why people feel so stiff upon standing. Hamstring pain usually increases when a person is sitting and walking, and it often disturbs sleep. Children suffering from "growing pains" frequently develop myofascial pain in the hamstrings.

12.3.3 Others Muscles Acting on the Knee

Other muscles acting on the knee include the gastrocnemius, gracilis, sartorius, and popliteus. The gastrocnemius functions primarily as a plantarflexor of the ankle and was covered in the last chapter on the foot and ankle. As mentioned before, the sartorius and gracilis both play a greater role in hip motion than in knee motion, so they will be covered in the next chapter on the pelvis.

The primary function of the *gastrocnemius* at the knee is as a dynamic stabilizer in extension. Its backward and downward pull in the stance phase of gait prevents the knee from dropping into flexion, stabilizing the joint as the body's weight shifts from the heel to the toes. In this stabilizing role, the gastrocnemius works as a synergist to the quadriceps. The gastrocnemius does assist knee flexion, although it is a weak knee flexor when working as a plantarflexor. However, when the knee is already in flexion, it can exert ample leverage and function as a strong knee flexor. To feel this action, in a seated position palpate your gastrocnemius while lifting your heel off the floor.

During the swing phase of gait, the *sartorius* assists the short head of the biceps femoris with knee flexion. Both the sartorius and *gracilis* assist knee flexion when the hip is also flexed. They also medially rotate the knee from a flexed position. During single-leg support, they stabilize the knee to prevent adduction (valgus angulation of the knee). To feel them working as rotators of the knee, palpate

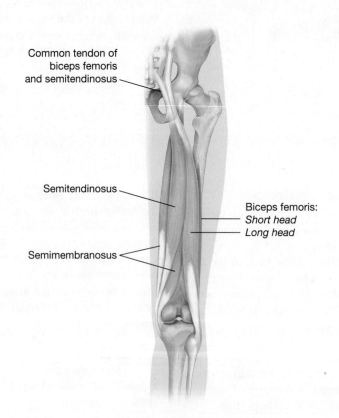

FIGURE 12.46
Hamstrings

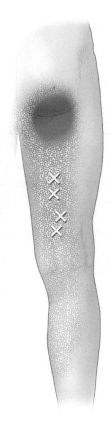
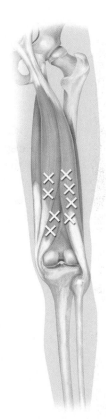
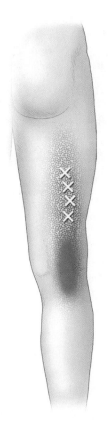

FIGURE 12.47

Dysfunction in the **biceps femoris** can lead to a cluster of four trigger points along the lower half of the belly of the muscle, which can develop referred pain over the back of the knee. When dysfunctional, the **semitendinosus** can develop several trigger points above the distal half of its belly, which can refer pain over the gluteal fold in the lower buttocks and along the posterior medial aspect of the thigh, knee, and upper calf. When dysfunctional, the **semimembranosus** can develop two or three trigger points along the distal third of its belly, along the medial aspect of the muscle. Its trigger points can refer pain over the gluteal fold in the lower buttocks, in the same area as the semitendinosus trigger points refer pain.

MUSCLE PALPATION
Biceps Femoris, Semitendinosus, and Semimembranosus

First palpate the hamstrings on the back of your own thigh. While standing, extend your leg behind your body to palpate the muscles' proximal tendons on the ischial tuberosity. Run your hand down toward the lateral side of your posterior knee to feel the biceps femoris, then down the medial side to feel the semitendinosus and semimembranosus, more popularly referred to as the "semisisters."

Next, sit down and palpate the tendons of the hamstrings on both sides of the back of your knee. Hold the tendons as you rotate your knee in and out to feel them contract. Lay your fingertips across the semimembranosus and semitendinosus tendons on the medial back side of the knee, then flex and extend your knee. You should be able to feel both tendons; the semitendinosus tendon is the more medial of the two.

Biceps Femoris

O–Long head—ischial tuberosity
    Short head—lateral lip of linea aspera
I–Lateral, posterior aspect of head of fibula
A–Flexes knee and assists lateral rotation, stabilizes knee in extension, extends hip and assists lateral rotation

Semimembranosus and Semitendinosus

O–Ischial tuberosity
I–Posterior and medial proximal aspect of medial tibial condyle
A–Flexes knee and assists medial rotation, extends hip and assists medial rotation

(continued)

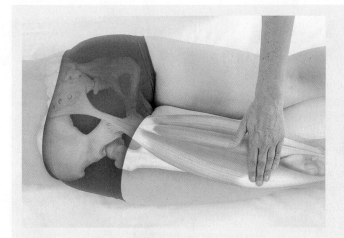

FIGURE 12.48a

Palpating the biceps femoris

With your partner in a prone position, locate the **biceps femoris** along the lateral posterior aspect of the leg (Figure 12.48a ■). Trace its distal tendon up into the belly of the muscle by strumming across its fibers. Walk up the biceps femoris to its origin on the ischial tuberosity using a pincher palpation. *Are you locating the origin in the middle of the gluteal fold?*

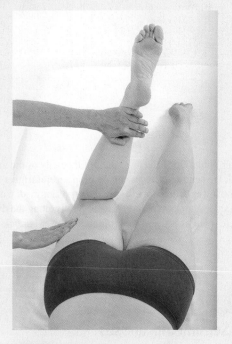

FIGURE 12.48b

Resisted motion for the biceps femoris

Resisted movement: Flex the knee and move the hip into 15 degrees of lateral rotation. Then have your partner resist while you lightly and slowly push the ankle toward the table to extend the knee (Figure 12.48b ■).

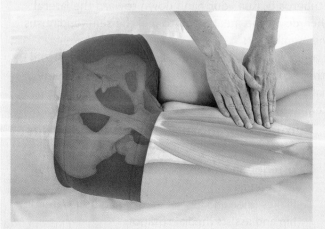

FIGURE 12.48c

Palpating the semimembranosus and semitendinosus

With your partner in a prone position, locate the **semimembranosus** and **semitendinosus** tendons along the medial side of the proximal tibia (Figure 12.48c ■). Slip your fingertips between their distal tendons and see how far you can palpate each tendon. Use a pincher palpation to walk up the tendons to the bellies of both muscles. Explore strumming across both muscles until you reach their origin. *Do you notice how hamstrings feel more fibrous than the vasti muscles?*

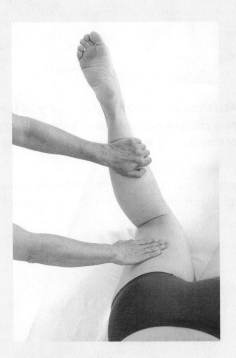

Resisted movement: Flex the knee and move the hip into 15 degrees of medial rotation. Then have your partner resist while you lightly and slowly push the ankle toward the table to extend the knee (Figure 12.48d ■). Palpate the semitendinosus and semimembranosus as they contract, then release. *How does contracting and relaxing the muscle change the quality of the tissue? Which are stronger during resisted motion: the biceps femoris or the medial hamstrings?*

FIGURE 12.48d

Resisted movement of the semimembranosus and semitendinosus

the pes anserine from a seated position, then medially rotate your leg. Chronic tightness in the sartorius can torque and abduct the knee, leading to knee pain, excessive tibial torsion, and genu varus (bowleg). Trigger points in the sartorius can cause general pain on the inside of the knee (see Figure 13.35).

The **popliteus** originates inside the articular capsule of the knee at a proximal tendon that attaches to the lateral surface of the lateral femoral condyle and to the lateral meniscus. It runs between the lateral collateral ligament and the lateral meniscus, diagonally across the back of the knee, and inserts on the proximal third of the posterior tibia, directly medial to the soleal line. The popliteus is innervated by the *popliteal nerve*. It assists knee flexion and plays a key role in unlocking the knee from terminal rotation by medially rotating the joint. (See TrP for the plantaris in Figure 12.49 ■).

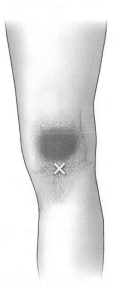
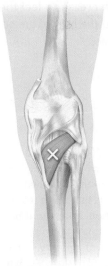

FIGURE 12.49

When dysfunctional, the **popliteus** can develop a trigger point in the belly of the muscle that can refer pain over the back of the knee. Pain from a popliteus trigger point often flares when a person is crouching, walking down stairs or an incline, or running.

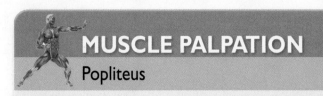

MUSCLE PALPATION
Popliteus

The attachments of the popliteus can be somewhat difficult to palpate, although the belly of the muscle is easy to locate. In a seated position with your knee flexed, press straight into the tissue below the crease on the back of the knee. As you press, medially and laterally rotate your leg several times (turning your toes in) to feel the popliteus contract.

Caution: Be careful not to put pressure on the popliteal nerve or artery, both located under the popliteus. If your palpation triggers nerve sensations or you feel a pulse, slide your fingers inferiorly off the underlying structure.

Popliteus

O–Lateral surface of lateral femoral condyle
I–Proximal posterior tibia
A–Medially rotates knee, assists knee flexion

With your partner in the prone position, locate the **popliteus** on your partner by pressing into the space below the crease on the back of the knee, right above the space between the gastrocnemius heads (Figure 12.50 ■). Strum up and down across the crease to feel the belly of the popliteus. *Do you feel the belly of the popliteus crossing the back of the knee?*

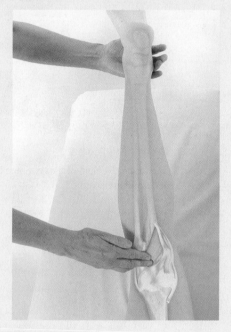

FIGURE 12.50
Palpating the popliteus

CONCLUSION

The knee's limited range of motion can create the impressions that it is a relatively simple joint. Upon closer examination, however, it becomes clear that the knee is the most complex and inherently unstable joint in the body. Its lack of stability stems from an incongruent fit between its articular surfaces, which predisposes this unique joint to injury. In addition, the knee has a number of specialized structures—supporting ligaments and tendons, a gliding patella, two shock-absorbing menisci, an extensive synovial lining, and many protective bursae—that allow it to function under high compressive loads. The act of walking puts compression on the knee that is twice the weight of the body, and a weight gain of as little as five pounds increases the load on the knees by 15 pounds. As a result of its lack of stability and the amount of compression it functions under,

the knee is the most commonly painful and injured joint in the body. Compound this instability and compression from misalignments like genu varum and genu valgus, as well as muscular imbalances, and the knee's predisposition to chronic pain, injury, and premature wear on the joint increases substantially.

The specialized structures in the knee can only provide so much protection from pain and injury. A healthy reliance on preventative measures, however, will go a long way toward limiting or preventing many of the common alignment problems and overuse injuries that occur in the knee. These measures include corrective strengthening exercises that improve joint alignment, massage and bodywork to release chronic muscular imbalances and normalize soft tissue, and neuromuscular patterning exercises that improve knee tracking along the mechanical axis of the lower limb, ensuring that the knee moves in tandem with the ankle and hip.

SUMMARY POINTS TO REMEMBER

1. The knee is made up of the junction of three bones: the patella, femur, and tibia. Its major articulating surfaces on the distal femur and proximal tibia fit together poorly, making it a highly incongruent joint that is unstable and susceptible to injury.

2. Each knee has two fibrocartilage menisci that improve joint congruency and stability, an extensive synovial lining that nourishes and pads the joint, and many bursae around the joint that reduce friction between moving parts.

3. Many supporting ligaments and tendons encase and stabilize the knee, including a medial and lateral collateral ligament on each side of the knee and two cruciate ligaments inside the joint capsule.

4. Each knee consists of two primary joints: The patellofemoral joint is an articulation between the patella and the intercondylar groove of the femur; the tibiofemoral joint is an articulation between the femoral condyles and the tibial plateau.

5. The patella slides up and down like an anatomical pulley during knee flexion and extension; its primary function is to deflect the pull of the quadriceps away from the joint to improve muscular leverage and mechanical advantage.

6. In an optimally aligned lower limb, the centers of the hip, knee, and ankle line up along a plumb that defines the mechanical axis of the lower limb and creates a Q angle (angle of pull of the quadriceps) that averages 15 degrees.

7. The tibiofemoral joint is a modified hinge joint because it can rotate when flexed. The joint has two distinct sides so it is also considered a double condyloid joint.

8. The tibiofemoral joint has three degrees of motion: an average of 140 degrees of flexion (when the hip is also flexed), 5–10 degrees of extension, and 60 degrees of axial rotation (at 90 degrees of flexion).

9. Knee extension beyond 10 degrees, called genu recurvatum, is considered abnormal, damaging to joint structures, and a source of deviation in the general skeletal alignment.

10. During flexion and extension, the knee rolls and glides so that the femoral condyles stay on top of the tibia. Because the medial femoral condyle is twice as long as the lateral femoral condyle, the knee also spins as it flexes and extends.

11. As the knee extends, it twists into terminal rotation, also called the screw home mechanism, in which the tibia and femur counterrotate into a close-packed position. During terminal rotation, the tibia laterally rotates against the medially rotating femur.

12. The menisci work like fluid-filled shock absorbers, moving with the femoral condyles and deforming under compression. They distribute weight, reduce friction, stabilize the joint, and guide the pathway of motion.

13. Two groups of muscles act as prime movers to extend and flex the knee: the quadriceps and the hamstrings. The hamstrings, popliteus, gracilis, and sartorius muscles rotate the knee.

REVIEW QUESTIONS

1. True or false (circle one). The bones in the knee include the tibia, fibula, patella, and femur.

2. Describe two unique features of the knee (not including muscles or ligaments).

3. Identify which of the following statements about the bursae is *false*.
   a. The knee has free bursae and bursae that are envaginations of the synovial lining.
   b. Bursae are located under ligaments and tendons around joints.
   c. The main function of bursae is to reduce friction between moving parts.
   d. When treating bursitis, apply deep cross-friction over the bursa.

4. The reason that the knee is the most commonly injured joint in the body is because
   a. its articulating surfaces lack congruency, making it a highly unstable joint that functions under extreme compression and torsion stresses.
   b. its articulating surfaces are highly congruent, making it a highly stable joint that functions under extreme compression and torsion stresses.
   c. its articulating surfaces lack congruency, making it a highly mobile joint that functions under extreme tensional and shearing stresses.
   d. its articulating surfaces have a lot of cartilage, making it a highly cushioned joint that functions under extreme compression and torsion stresses.

5. Name the two joints making up the knee and list their articulating surfaces.

6. True or false (circle one). The cruciate ligaments prevent the anterior and posterior displacement of the tibiofemoral joint.

7. The pes anserine is formed by the common insertion of three tendons from the
   a. sartorius, gracilis, and semimembranosus muscles.
   b. sartorius, gracilis, and semitendinosus muscles.
   c. sartorius, adductor longus, and semitendinosus muscles.
   d. sartorius, vastus medialis, and semitendinosus muscles.

8. What is the function of the patella?

9. The Q angle is
   a. the mechanical axis of the lower limb.
   b. the line of pull of the quadriceps.
   c. an axis between the tibial tuberosity and the femoral head.
   d. a vertical line providing a measure of joint alignment.

10. Why is the tibiofemoral joint a modified hinge joint rather than just a hinge joint?
    a. Because it can rotate in extension.
    b. Because it lacks rotation in flexion.
    c. Because it can rotate in flexion.
    d. Because it lacks rotation in extension.

11. The tibiofemoral joint can flex _____ degrees when the hip is also in flexion, can extend (hyperextend) _____ to _____ degrees, and can rotate _____ degrees medially and _____ laterally.

12. What is genu recurvatum and how does it affect the knee?

13. Terminal rotation of the knee
    a. is a screw home mechanism that twists the articulating structures of the knee into a close-packed position in extension.
    b. occurs as the knee moves into the flexed position.
    c. involves a range of lateral and medial rotation when the knee is flexed.
    d. occurs when rotation exceeds the normal range and becomes terminal.

14. True or false (circle one). The medial femoral condyle is twice as long as the lateral femoral condyle, causing the knee to spin on the lateral condyle during flexion and extension.

15. The five functions of the menisci are to
    a. absorb shock, distribute weight across the joint, increase friction, stabilize the joint by improving joint congruency, and guide the pathway of motion.
    b. absorb shock, distribute weight across the joint, reduce friction, mobilize the joint by improving joint congruency, and guide the pathway of motion.
    c. absorb shock, distribute weight across the joint, reduce friction, stabilize the joint by improving joint congruency, and guide the pathway of motion.
    d. absorb shock, distribute weight across the joint, reduce friction, stabilize the joint by decreasing joint congruency, and guide the pathway of motion.

16. Three structures that are simultaneously injured in the knee when it is subjected to a posterior lateral force or clipping are the
    a. medial meniscus, lateral collateral ligament, and anterior cruciate ligament.
    b. medial meniscus, medial collateral ligament, and posterior cruciate ligament.
    c. medial meniscus, lateral collateral ligament, and posterior cruciate ligament.
    d. medial meniscus, medial collateral ligament, and anterior cruciate ligament.

17. Name the primary and secondary movements that the hamstrings generate at the knee.

18. Rotators of the knee include the
    a. popliteus, hamstrings, quadriceps, and gracilis.
    b. hamstrings, sartorius, gracilis, and gastrocnemius.
    c. popliteus, sartorius, gracilis, and gastrocnemius.
    d. popliteus, hamstrings, sartorius, and gracilis.

19. Which muscle unlocks the knee from the extended position?

20. Flexors of the knee include the
    a. hamstrings, sartorius, gracilis, and gastrocnemius.
    b. hamstrings, popliteus, plantaris, and gracilis.
    c. hamstrings, popliteus, sartorius, and gracilis.
    d. hamstrings, quadriceps, sartorius, and gracilis.

Notes

1. Magee, D. (2007). *Orthopedic Physical Assessment* (5th ed.). Philadelphia: Saunders.

2. Hoppenfeld, S. (1976). *Physical Examination of the Spine and Extremities.* Norwalk, CT: Appleton-Century-Croft.

3. Neumann, D. (2002). *Kinesiology of the Musculoskeletal System: Foundation for Physical Rehabilitation.* St. Louis, MO: Mosby.

4. Simons, D., Travell, J., & Simons, L. (1999). *Myofascial Pain and Dysfunction: The Trigger Point Manual: Vol. 2. The Lower Extremities* (2nd ed.). Baltimore: Lippincott, Williams, & Wilkins.

5. Ibid.

PEARSON
myhealthprofessionskit™

Use this address to access the Companion Website created for this textbook. Simply select "Massage Therapy" from the choice of disciplines. Find this book and log in using your username and password to access interactive activities, videos, and much more.

13 The Hip and Pelvis

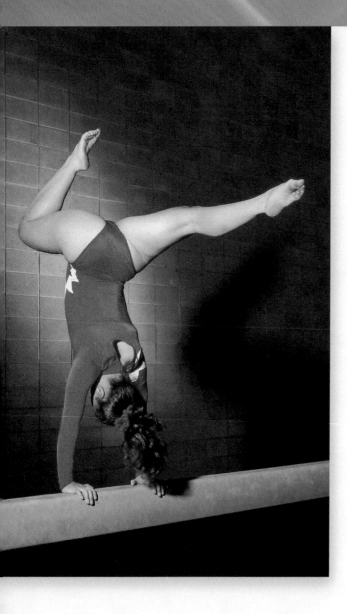

CHAPTER OUTLINE

Chapter Objectives

Key Terms

13.1 Bones of the Hip and Pelvis

13.2 Joints and Ligaments of the Hip and Pelvis

13.3 Muscles of the Hip and Pelvis

Conclusion

Summary Points to Remember

Review Questions

The highly mobile ball-and-socket joints of the hips allow dynamic motion in all three planes. The legs swing under the body in flexion and extension during walking. They also turn in or out during rotation, an action we use to make changes in direction. The full rotational capacity of the hip sockets allows an agile athlete or gymnast to make dynamic weight shifts and level changes in actions that swing the legs and lower body around the upper body. During such maneuvers, the arms support the body weight in a closed-chain, leaving the legs and feet free to move in an open chain anywhere within reach.

Unless a sport, dance, or work activity requires this range of motion, the average person probably moves the hips primarily in a sagittal plane with flexion and extension. To maintain joint health and flexibility, a person can move the hips through a broader range of motion. Movement spreads synovial fluid around the socket, lubricating and nourishing the articulating joint surfaces of the hips. A practitioner can take a client's hips through a full range of passive motion to improve freedom of movement in this large and well-muscled area of the body.

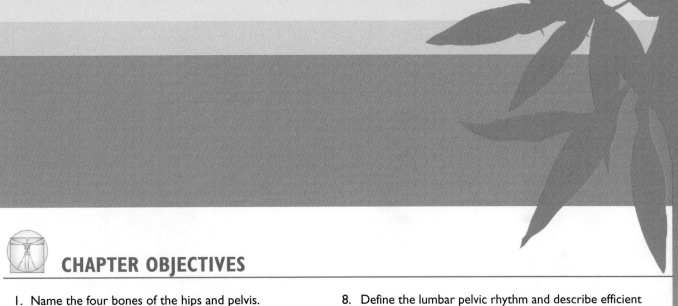

CHAPTER OBJECTIVES

1. Name the four bones of the hips and pelvis.
2. List and demonstrate the palpation of 14 bony landmarks of the hips and pelvis.
3. Describe the coxofemoral joint, its range of motion, and its supporting ligaments.
4. Describe the two femoral inclinations and how the shape of the femur creates each one.
5. Describe six ways the hip can move at the pelvis and six ways the pelvis can move on the femur.
6. Name three pelvic joints, their functions and classifications, and their ranges of motion.
7. Name and discuss four common hip problems.
8. Define the lumbar pelvic rhythm and describe efficient and inefficient rhythms.
9. Identify the origins, insertions, and actions of the muscles of the hips and pelvis.
10. Identify the trigger points and pain referral patterns of the muscles of the hips and pelvis.
11. Demonstrate the active movement and palpation of each muscle of the hips and pelvis.
12. Identify three perineal muscles and describe their general locations and functions.
13. Discuss the postural patterns that occur with chronically tight hamstrings or quadriceps.

KEY TERMS

Acetabulum

Angle of inclination

Angle of torsion

Anterior superior iliac spine (ASIS)

Counternutation

Coxofemoral joints

Crest of sacrum

Forced closure

Form closure

Greater trochanter

Head of the femur

Iliac crest

Ischial tuberosity

Lesser trochanter

Lumbar pelvic rhythm

Nutation

Pelvic girdle

Pelvic ring

Piriformis syndrome

Posterior superior iliac spine (PSIS)

Pubic symphysis

Sacral foramen

Sacroiliac joint (SIJ)

Trochanteric bursitis

MUSCLES IN ACTION

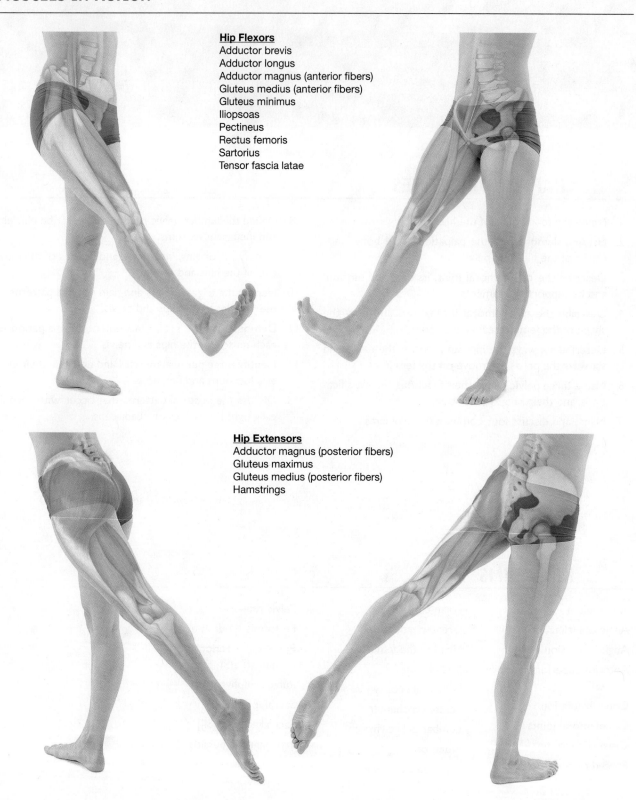

Hip Flexors
Adductor brevis
Adductor longus
Adductor magnus (anterior fibers)
Gluteus medius (anterior fibers)
Gluteus minimus
Iliopsoas
Pectineus
Rectus femoris
Sartorius
Tensor fascia latae

Hip Extensors
Adductor magnus (posterior fibers)
Gluteus maximus
Gluteus medius (posterior fibers)
Hamstrings

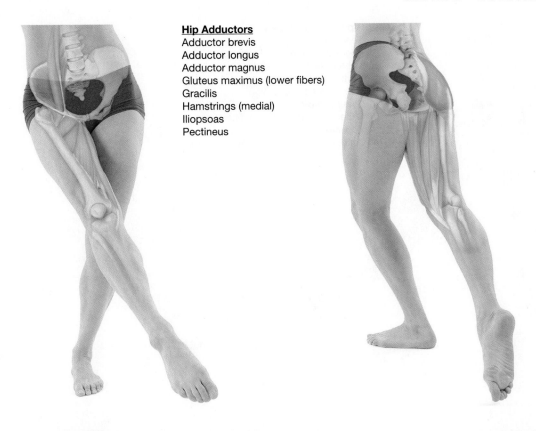

Hip Adductors
Adductor brevis
Adductor longus
Adductor magnus
Gluteus maximus (lower fibers)
Gracilis
Hamstrings (medial)
Iliopsoas
Pectineus

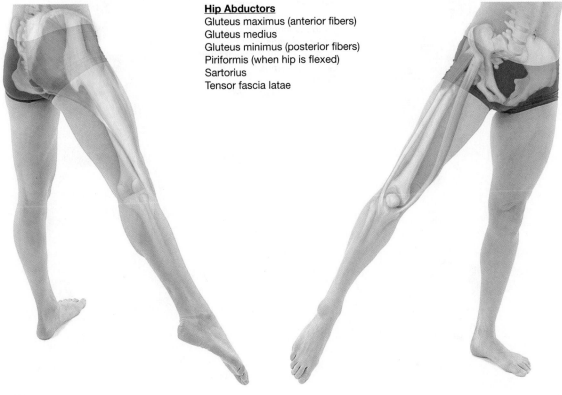

Hip Abductors
Gluteus maximus (anterior fibers)
Gluteus medius
Gluteus minimus (posterior fibers)
Piriformis (when hip is flexed)
Sartorius
Tensor fascia latae

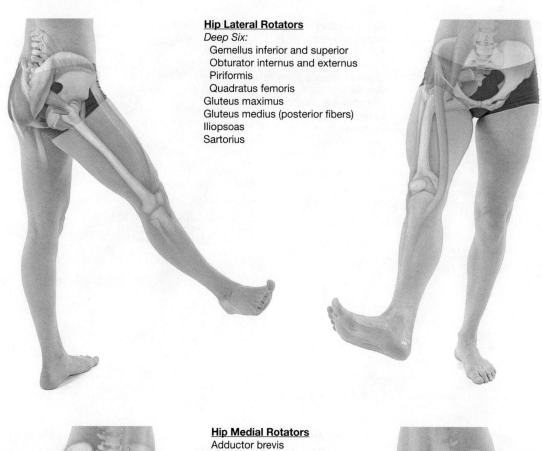

Hip Lateral Rotators
Deep Six:
  Gemellus inferior and superior
  Obturator internus and externus
  Piriformis
  Quadratus femoris
Gluteus maximus
Gluteus medius (posterior fibers)
Iliopsoas
Sartorius

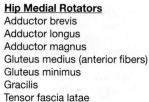

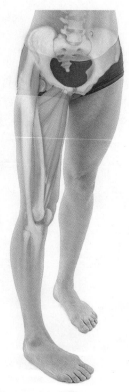

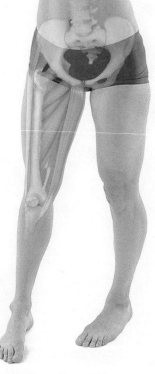

Hip Medial Rotators
Adductor brevis
Adductor longus
Adductor magnus
Gluteus medius (anterior fibers)
Gluteus minimus
Gracilis
Tensor fascia latae

After exploring the unique features of the largest and most complex joint in the body, the knee, our study travels up the femur into the hip and pelvis. The hip is the large ball-and-socket joint connecting the thigh to the pelvis. The pelvis is the bony girdle connecting the trunk to the lower limbs. The hips and pelvis provides a sturdy bony conduit through which bilateral forces from the lower limb are funneled into unilateral forces along the spine. A practitioner can enhance this line of transmission by using techniques that improve symmetry in the hips, which, in turn helps connect the inside line of the legs with core muscles of the pelvis and lumbar spine. This connection improves the weight-bearing capacity and mobility of the lower body.

The hips and pelvis are both well-balanced weight-bearing structures that support body weight while allowing for a broad range of mobility in three directions. The lower limbs swing under the body at the hip during gait activities such as walking or running. Skilled movers usually carry their bodies with their weight centered in the pelvis and hips; professional athletes and dancers usually have strong awareness of and flexibility in their hips. The body folds at the hips, bending the trunk forward so that a person can either lower the head and hands toward the ground or lift the feet toward the head.

The neutral position of the hips and pelvis affects overall posture and efficiency of movement in the body. These large ball-and-socket joints provide a major hub of motion and need to be free to move in all directions, but all too often are restricted by muscular tension. Hip position is determined by muscular tone. Ideally, intrinsic stabilizing muscles of the inner line and core support the joint neutral position during motion. The hips now have support underlying motion, which frees the extrinsic phasic muscles to generate efficient movements.

In this chapter, we look at how the hips and pelvis work in both weight-bearing and movement capacities, and how massage and bodywork can reinforce and even improve these functions. We cover the bony landmarks of the hips and pelvis that practitioners need to know, and follow this with a review of the joints and ligaments in both structures. We consider the range of motion in the hips and sacrum, and the coordination of motion between the hips, pelvis, and lumbar spine. We also examine the many muscles acting on the hips and pelvis, and explore palpation exercises for each group. Exercises are sprinkled throughout this chapter to encourage readers to explore alignment and movement patterns of their hips and pelvis in ways that can improve both posture and ease of motion in body mechanics.

13.1 BONES OF THE HIP AND PELVIS

The hip is the ball-and-socket joint located between the femur and the pelvis. The pelvis is a bony basin made up of two large pelvic bones called the **coxal** (*innominate*) **bones,** plus the **sacrum** and the **coccyx** (Figure 13.1a-b ■). To fulfill the demands of childbearing, the female pelvis tends to be rounder, wider, and shorter in height than the male pelvis.

One important structural feature to note about the pelvis is that it is where the axial skeleton meets the appendicular skeleton. The coxal bones, which are part of the appendicular skeleton, encircle and support the sacrum, which is part of the axial skeleton. The sacrum sits below the fifth lumbar vertebra where it provides a base of support for the spine. This triangular-shaped bone narrows into a smaller bone called the coccyx, which is often referred to as the "tailbone" because it is, literally, a vestigial tail.

13.1.1 Bony Landmarks of the Hip

In the knee chapter, we looked at several bony landmarks of the femur related to the knee, such as the femoral condyles, the epicondyles, and the adductor tubercle. In this chapter, we examine femoral landmarks where the hip muscles attach (Figure 13.2 ■). The **greater trochanter,** a large, irregular bony knob at the proximal end of the femur, provides a hub where the tendinous attachments of many hip muscles converge. It creates a superficial bony projection on either side of the hip that is easy to palpate in the widest part of the pelvis. A line between the greater trochanters demarks the axis of motion of hip flexion and extension.

The femur can be compared to a walking stick with a straight, cylindrical handle. The long arm of the walking stick is comparable to the shaft of the femur, which transmits weight into the knee. The handle of the stick is comparable to the **neck of the femur**—a short arm that projects medially from the greater trochanter. The neck of the femur provides a lateral overhang that projects the shaft of the femur away from the joint, which prevents impingement around the hip joint during motion and increases leverage in the abductor muscles (Figure 13.3a-b ■). Below the neck of the femur along the medial side of the shaft of the femur lies a small bony protuberance called the **lesser trochanter,** which is an attachment site for the iliopsoas tendons. The neck of the

FIGURE 13.1

Bones of the pelvis: a) Female b) Male

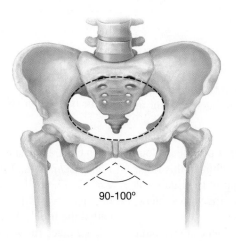
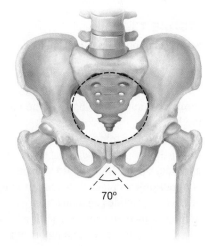

90-100°   70°

A   B

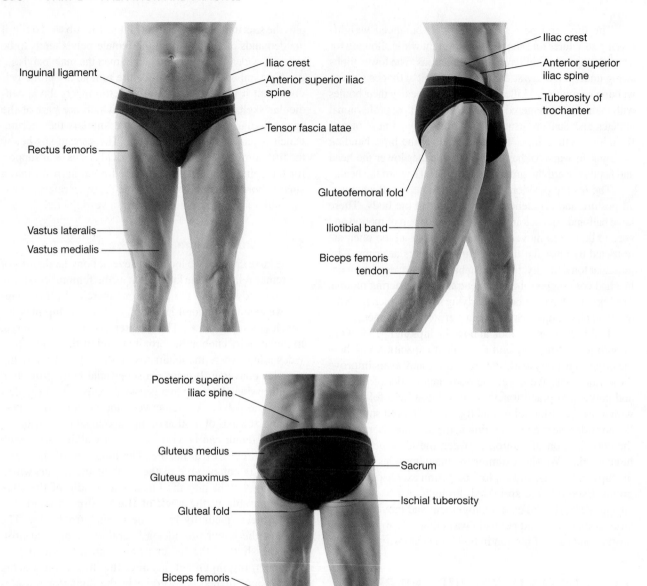

FIGURE 13.2

Surface anatomy of the hip and pelvis

femur enlarges into a round globe, called the **head of the femur,** which is the "ball" in the ball-and-socket joint of the hip.

Along the middle third of the posterior shaft of the femur, below the lesser trochanter, runs a prominent longitudinal ridge called the **linea aspera.** Although this ridge is impossible to palpate directly, it is helpful to visualize it because it provides an attachment site for the vastus lateralis, vastus medialis, and adductor muscles.

When massage clients report hip problems, they could be referring to many different places on the pelvis. For this

reason, you might want to ask your client to touch the part of the body where he or she is having trouble.

13.1.2 Bony Landmarks of the Pelvis

Each coxal bone starts as three separate bones at birth—the *ilium, ischium,* and *pubis*—that fuse into a single bone by age 25 (Figure 13.4 ■). The **ilium** (plural: *ilia*) makes up the upper two-fifths of the coxal bone. A distinct bony rim, called the **iliac crest,** defines the top of the ilium and provides a place for your hands when you rest them on the top of your hips. A smooth, fan-shaped, concave area on the

FIGURE 13.3

Femur: a) Anterior view b) Posterior view

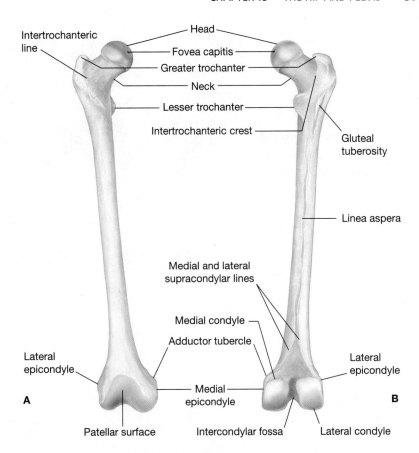

inside of each ilium, called the **iliac fossa,** provides a large attachment site for the iliacus, a hip flexor.

A sharp bony projection on the anterior end of each iliac crest, called the **anterior superior iliac spine** (ASIS), is an attachment site for the sartorius and tensor fascia latae,

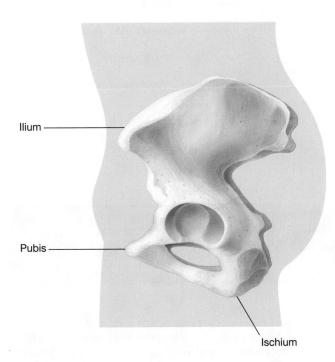

FIGURE 13.4

Coxal bone

as well as the inguinal ligament. Another bony projection, called the **anterior inferior iliac spine** (AIIS), can be found directly below the ASIS; the AIIS provides an attachment site for the rectus femoris (Figure 13.5a ■). A projection on the posterior end of the iliac crest, called the **posterior superior iliac spine** (PSIS), is directly lateral to the top of the sacrum. Below the PSIS is the **posterior inferior iliac spine** (PIIS), which is more difficult to palpate than the easily found ASIS, AIIS, and PSIS (Figure 13.5b ■). The PIIS overhangs the **sciatic notch,** a bony notch through which the large sciatic nerve passes. The sciatic notch is difficult to palpate because it is buried under the gluteus maximus and the lateral rotators.

The **ischium** makes up the bottom portion of the coxal bone. A bony bar at the bottom of the ischium is called the **ischial ramus.** It ends in a large, blunt protuberance called the **ischial tuberosity,** which is where the hamstrings and the adductor magnus attach to the pelvis. The ischial tuberosities are like the feet of the body in a sitting posture; they support the weight of the trunk. Above the tuberosities, a small bony protuberance called the **ischial spine** provides the attachment site for ligaments binding the sacrum to the pelvis. The large hole in each coxal bone is called the **obturator foramen;** it is covered front and back by the obturator externus and obturator internus.

The ischium and pubic bones connect to each other along the **pubic crest,** the bony rim across the front of the pubis. The **superior pubic ramus** is the bar-shaped part of the pubic bone that joins the ilium and provides an attachment site for the pectineus; the **inferior pubic**

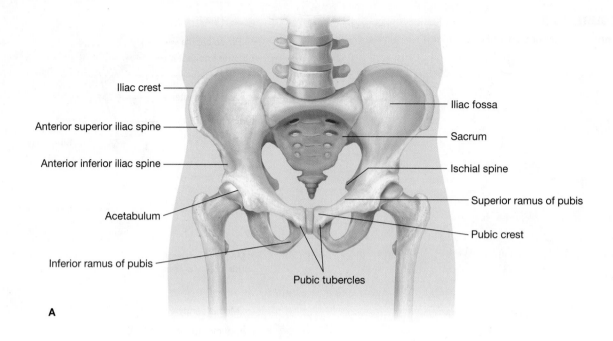

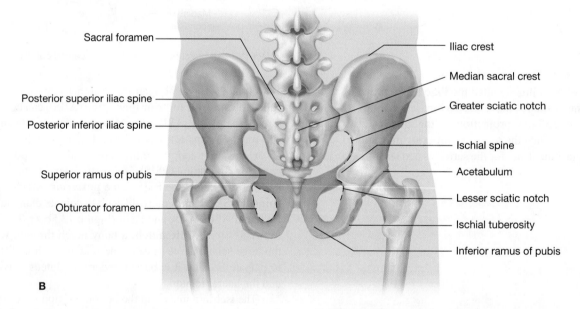

FIGURE 13.5

Pelvis: a) Anterior view b) Posterior view

BRIDGE TO PRACTICE
Assessing Pelvic Asymmetries

A lot of clients receive massage and bodywork to alleviate chronic pain caused by asymmetries from rotations that torque the pelvic girdle. To determine a general course of treatment for musculoskeletal imbalances caused by pelvic rotations, assess the symmetry of the pelvis by comparing the position of the right and left ASIS and PSIS. If one side is higher or more posterior than the other, assess which chronic muscular tensions are pulling them off center and need to be stretched.

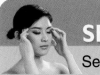

SELF-CARE
Seated Pelvic Rock

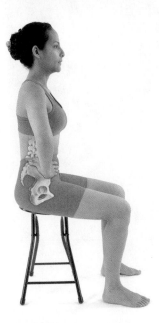

FIGURE 13.6a

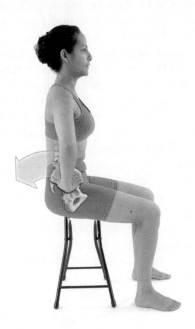

FIGURE 13.6b

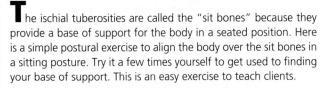

The ischial tuberosities are called the "sit bones" because they provide a base of support for the body in a seated position. Here is a simple postural exercise to align the body over the sit bones in a sitting posture. Try it a few times yourself to get used to finding your base of support. This is an easy exercise to teach clients.

1. In a seated position, place your hands on your hips to locate your pelvic bones (Figure 13.6a ■). Rock your pelvis back and forth over your ischial tuberosities (sit bones).
2. As you rock your pelvis, imagine it as a bowl filled with water. When you tip the bowl toward your tailbone, water spills out the back (Figure 13.6b ■). When you tip the bowl toward your pubic bone, water spills out the front (Figure 13.6c ■).
3. Rock back and forth several times, sensing the place in the middle where your water line would be level, where your body centers over your base of support. Whenever you find yourself slouching, rock your pelvis to adjust your position and center your pelvis.

Note: If you have back pain from habitually poor posture, shifting your base of support is the first step toward improving posture. However, sitting up straight can actually cause another level of discomfort or pain until your muscles adapt to a different position. Training the postural muscles presented in the posture chapter can help you make this transition.

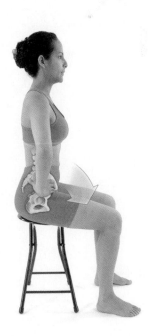

FIGURE 13.6c

ramus, also bar-shaped, attaches to the ischium and provides attachment sites for the adductors. Two small, horn-shaped **pubic tubercles,** one on either side of the superior pubic ramus, provide an attachment site for the inguinal ligament.

The sacrum and coccyx are segmented because they begin as nine separate vertebrae in the preborn, which fuse after birth (Figure 13.7 ■). Four small openings in the sacrum, called **sacral foramen,** provide passage for the sacral nerves (Figure 13.8 ■). The foramen form small indentations in two vertical rows on the posterior side of the sacrum and are acupressure points that can respond well to direct pressure. An irregular bony ridge along the midline of the sacrum is called the **median sacral crest.** A bony canal through the center of the sacrum, called the **sacral canal,** provides a protective channel for the spinal cord. It houses the cauda equina (a group of spinal nerves) and opens at the base of the sacrum into the **sacral hiatus,** where a group of small *coccygeal nerves* exit the spine. The coccyx lies directly below the sacral hiatus. You will want to be able to recognize these landmarks during palpation to know what is normal tissue tone and also to work with ligaments attached to the sacrum.

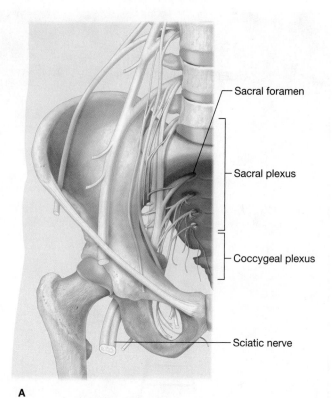

A

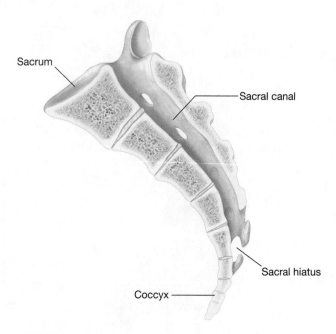

FIGURE 13.7
Sacrum: lateral view

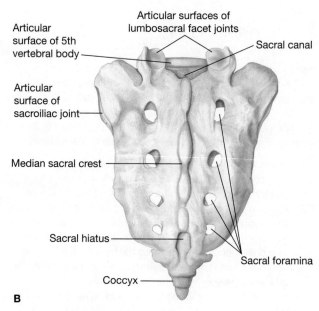

B

FIGURE 13.8
Sacrum: a) Anterior view with nerves b) Posterior view

BONE PALPATION
Hips and Pelvis

Caution: *Vulnerable areas of the pelvis can be tender or sensitive to touch, such as the iliac fossa, pubic crest, or coccyx. Palpate slowly, monitoring your partner for any signs of discomfort. Stop immediately if your partner has difficulty being touched in these areas. Also, if you are partnered with a man, you may need to ask him to move his genitals to get them out of the way to palpate some of these landmarks.*

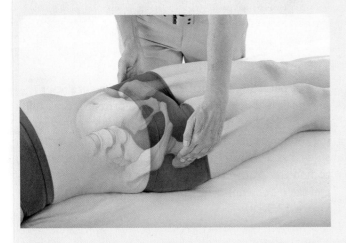

FIGURE 13.9a
Palpate the **greater trochanter** along the side of the hip by finding the most prominent bony knob at the widest part of the pelvis. Then palpate both sides at the same time to see if they are symmetrical and level with each other. *Do you notice how large the greater trochanter is?* (See Figure 13.9a ■)

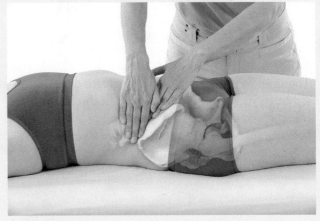

FIGURE 13.9b
Locate the **iliac crest** by placing your hand on the top and side of the coxal bone. Follow this wide bony crest in the posterior direction as far as you can, reaching under your partner. Then palpate both sides at the same time to see if they are symmetrical and level with each other. *Are you on the top of the hips? Do you notice that the iliac crest is about 8 inches long?* (See Figure 13.9b ■)

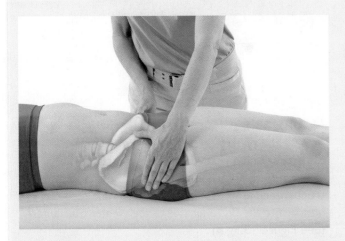

FIGURE 13.9c

Locate the **anterior superior ischial spine,** which are the sharp bony tips on the anterior end of the iliac crest. If you put your hands on your own hips, your index fingers usually land on them. Then palpate both ASISs at the same time to check for symmetry. *Are the ASISs symmetrical?* (See Figure 13.9c ■)

(continued)

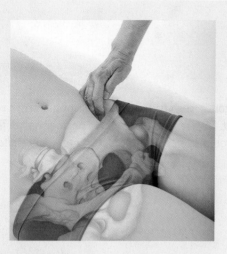

FIGURE 13.9d

The **iliac fossa** is impossible to palpate directly, although you can feel the top part of the fossa by hooking your fingertips over the top of the iliac crest and sinking down and back. Move slowly and carefully, monitoring your partner responses because this area can be highly sensitive. (See Figure 13.9d ■)

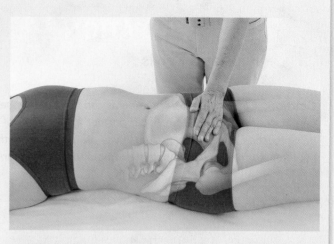

FIGURE 13.9e

Before palpating the **pubic crest,** make sure your partner's bladder is empty because pressure on a full bladder can be uncomfortable. With your thumb facing the navel, press the pubic crest with the lateral side of your hand. Then move your hands laterally to find the **pubic tubercle.** *Does the pubic crest feel like a bony rim across the front of the pelvis?* (See Figure 13.9e ■)

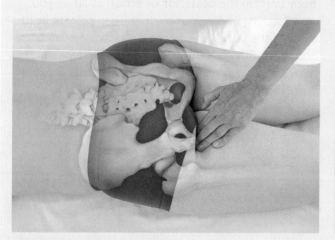

FIGURE 13.9f

Palpate the **ischial tuberosities** in the center of the gluteal fold at the bottom of the buttocks. These large bony knobs where the hamstrings attach are easy to feel. Palpate both sides at once to see if they are symmetrical. *Do you notice how large the ischial tuberosities are?* (See Figure 13.9f ■)

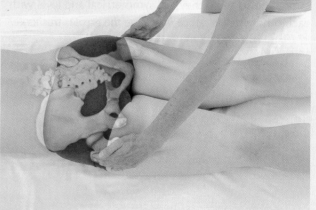

FIGURE 13.9g

Palpate the posterior side of the **greater trochanter,** which is several inches lateral of the ischial tuberosity. Explore the size and shape of the trochanter. *Do you notice that you can find tendons attached to the posterior side of the greater trochanter?* (See Figure 13.9g ■)

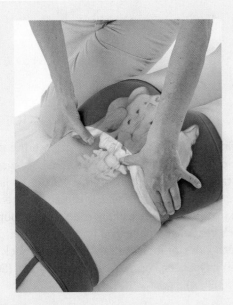

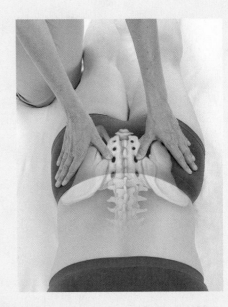

FIGURE 13.9h

Trace the iliac crest along the top of the pelvis to the small bony bump on its posterior medial end, which is the **posterior superior ischial spine** (PSIS). Then palpate both PSISs at once to see if they are symmetrical and level with each other. *Are the PSIS symmetrical? (See Figure 13.9h* ■*)*

FIGURE 13.9i

Explore the **sacrum** below the PSIS. There is often thick tissue over the sacrum, so you can press in pretty deep with your finger pads. Many people like firm pressure on the sacrum. Walk your fingertips over the surface of the sacrum, allowing them to sink into the small bony openings of the **sacral foramina.** *Can you penetrate the thick tissue over the sacrum to palpate the bone? Do the sacral foramina feel like small holes that you can easily sink into? (See Figure 13.9i* ■*)*

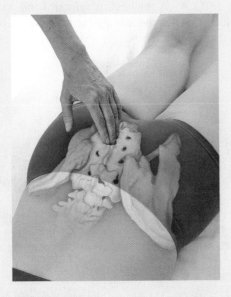

FIGURE 13.9j

Find the **median sacral crest,** which feels like a bumpy, bony ridge along the center of the sacrum. Trace its contours along its length. Occasionally, there will be a pocket of fluid over the sacrum due to excess weight and postures that compress the sacrum, or injury. Avoid deep pressure on a fluid pocket. (See Figure 13.9j ■)

(continued)

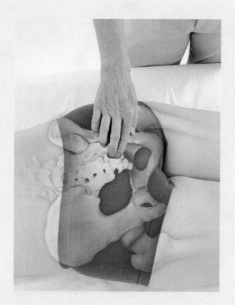

Using fingertip palpation, carefully palpate the **coccyx** below the sacrum, where five small bony segments taper into a point. It can be difficult to find if it is injured and bent forward. It can also be tender, so palpate slowly and carefully, monitoring your partner's response. Once you find the coccyx, palpate both sides of it at the same time to check for symmetry. *Does the coccyx feel like a bony tip?* (See Figure 13.9k ■)

FIGURE 13.9k

13.2 JOINTS AND LIGAMENTS OF THE HIP AND PELVIS

The true hip joint, whose anatomical name is the **coxofemoral joint,** is formed by the articulation between the head of the femur and the hip socket. The coxofemoral joints are located a hand's-width apart on either side of the pubic bone. The narrow orientation of the coxofemoral joints establishes a line of thrust from the legs into the spine that is closer to the midline of the body and therefore more stable (Figure 13.10 ■).

The **pelvic girdle,** made up of the sacrum and coxal bones, is also referred to as the **pelvic ring** because it is a somewhat circular structure. The stability of the pelvic ring depends on the integrity of the joints of the pelvis, which is discussed later in this section. The pelvic ring functions as a bidirectional compression structure that transmits mechanical forces from the trunk into the legs and from the lower limbs into the trunk. Stability in the pelvic ring is paramount for the efficient transmission of load (weight) from the body into the lower limbs and the transmission of ground reaction forces from the feet into the trunk.

The two halves of the pelvic ring join on the anterior side at a joint called the pubic symphysis, which is also discussed later in this section. A curtain of abdominal myofascias suspends the anterior side of the pelvic ring, sometimes called the *pubic arch,* from the costal arch and the lower rib cage (Figure 13.11 ■). The pelvic bowl remains level when the compressive forces from the spine into the sacrum and hips are balanced by the tensional forces of the myofascias lifting the front of the pelvic ring.

13.2.1 Coxofemoral Joint

The coxofemoral joint is a large ball-and-socket joint that evolved for weight bearing as well as movement in all three planes. It is an articulation between the head of the femur and the **acetabulum,** which is the hip socket (Figure 13.12 ■). A thick, cartilaginous band on the rim of the socket, called the **acetabular labrum,** deepens and widens the socket and holds the head of the femur securely

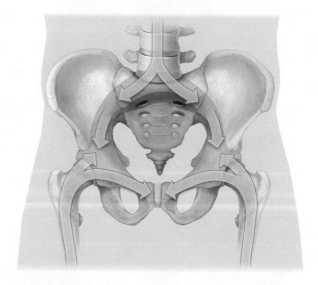

FIGURE 13.10

Lines of thrust through the pelvis

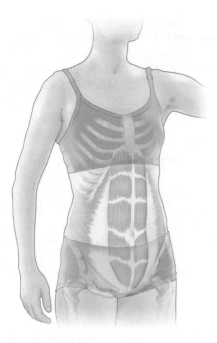

FIGURE 13.11

The **pubic arch** is suspended by a muscular wall.

in the socket. A large and sturdy joint capsule wraps the coxofemoral joint like a sleeve. This capsular sleeve has two distinct layers—a superficial layer of longitudinal fibers that encapsulates a deep layer of circular, horizontal fibers called *zona orbicularis.*

Hip dislocations are extremely rare in adults because of the depth of the socket and the fact that the socket and labrum covers three-fourths of the globe of the femur. In contrast, the glenohumeral joint of the shoulder evolved a

shallow socket that is highly mobile yet can be easily dislocated. Several ligaments also contribute to the structural integrity of the coxofemoral joint (Figure 13.13a-b ■). They are the largest ligaments in the body and become taut in the extended position.

- The **iliofemoral ligament** is also called the **Y ligament** due to its shape. It binds the ASIS to the intertrochanteric line on the neck of the femur. It limits hyperextension, abduction, and lateral rotation.
- The **pubofemoral ligament** binds the anterior pubic ramus to the anterior surface of the intertrochanteric fossa. It also limits hyperextension, abduction, and lateral rotation.

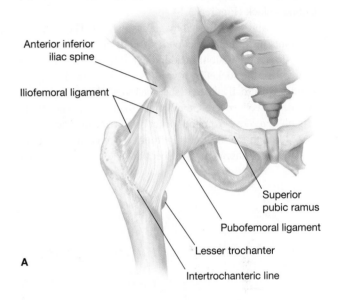

Anterior inferior iliac spine

Iliofemoral ligament

Superior pubic ramus

Pubofemoral ligament

Lesser trochanter

Intertrochanteric line

A

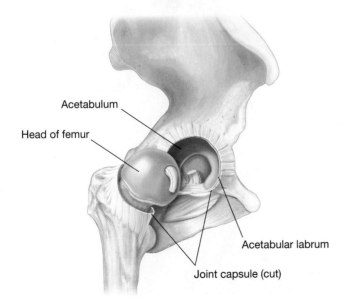

Acetabulum

Head of femur

Acetabular labrum

Joint capsule (cut)

FIGURE 13.12

Acetabulum

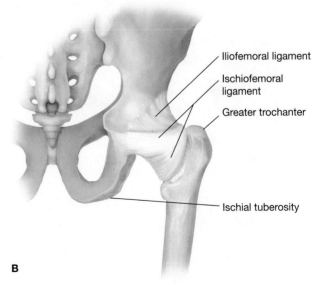

Iliofemoral ligament

Ischiofemoral ligament

Greater trochanter

Ischial tuberosity

B

FIGURE 13.13

Ligaments of the hip: a) Anterior b) Posterior

• The **ischiofemoral ligament** binds the posterior surface of the acetabular rim and labrum to the zona orbicularis and greater trochanter. It limits adduction, medial rotation, and hyperextension, which twists its fibers into a taut position.

The hip is most stable in an extended position because its ligaments are taut and its capsular fibers twist into a taut position. In the extended position of the hip, the anterior side of the head of the femur is exposed. The hip is one of the few joints to reach maximal articular contact in a position other than extension. This close-packed position of the hip occurs when it is in a combination of flexion, slight lateral rotation, and abduction, in the frog-legged position. In this position of the hip, the joint capsule untwists so that it becomes slack (Figure 13.14 ■).

Hip stability is assisted by gravity as well. The coxofemoral joints move under the load of the trunk, which creates a stabilizing compression. In addition, the head of the femur is secured into the socket by a vacuum seal generated by atmospheric pressure. If all soft tissue attachments between the ball-and-socket were severed, the head of the femur would still be difficult to remove from the socket because of the vacuum.

Although the **inguinal ligament** has no direct effect on the hip joint, it merits mention because it crosses over the hip joint and is an important anatomical landmark. This long, thin ligament runs from the anterior superior iliac spine to the pubic tubercle, crossing the iliopsoas tendon and the femoral artery and vein. It separates the thigh from the abdominal wall and is easy to palpate. Myofascial adhesions that bind the inguinal ligament to underlying or adjacent muscles can be released to enhance ease of motion in the hip.

13.2.1.1 FEMORAL ANGULATIONS

Every joint has an ideal neutral position. By assessing the position of a joint in a neutral posture, you can assess the resting tone of the muscles around the joint. If the hip flexors are tight, the joint will rest in a flexed position, indicating that the hip flexors need stretching. Because of the irregular, organic shape of the bones, joint neutrality is not always that easy to define. When observing the hip alignment in an extended position, the femurs look like two number sevens facing each other (Figure 13.15 ■).

The femur has an angle between its neck and its shaft, called the **angle of inclination.** A normal angle of inclination averages 135 degrees, which aligns the greater trochanter along the same horizontal axis as the head of the femur (Figure 13.16 ■). The hyaline cartilage on the head of the femur is the thickest in the area where it bears the most weight and friction. Abnormalities in the angle of inclination can cause premature wear to the hyaline cartilage, a lack of stability, a decreased range of motion, or degenerative changes over time. An abnormal decrease in

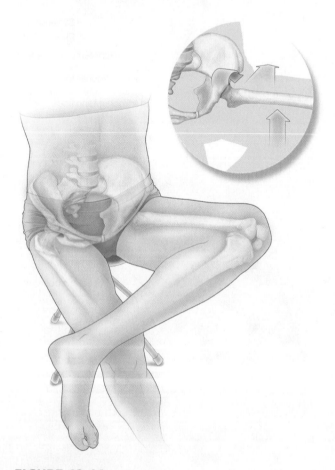

FIGURE 13.14

Close-packed position of coxofemoral joint

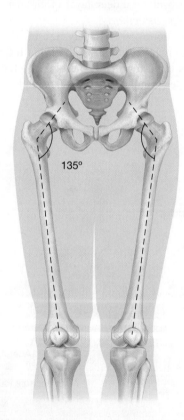

135°

FIGURE 13.15

Angle of inclination of the femur

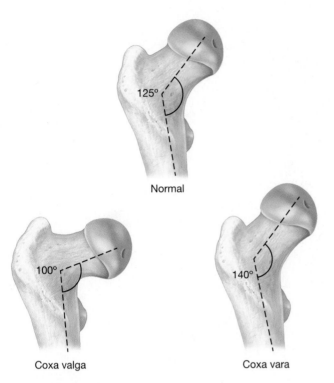

FIGURE 13.16

Variations in the angle of femoral inclination

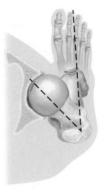
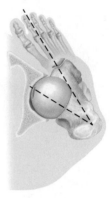

A   Anteverted hip   "Toeing-in" due to anteverted hip

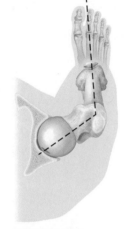
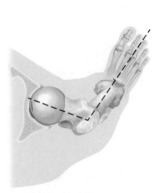

B   Retroverted hip   "Toeing-out" due to retroverted hip

FIGURE 13.17

a) **Anteversion:** an abnormal increase in the angle of torsion that causes toeing-in and restricts lateral hip rotation. b) **Retroversion:** an abnormal decrease in the angle of torsion that causes toeing-out and restricts medial hip rotation.

the angle of inclination, called *coxa valga,* straightens the femur, causing the hip to adduct when the lower limb is in a weight-bearing position (Figure 13.16). This increases joint instability, so avoid stretching or mobilizing hips with coxa valga. An abnormal increase in the angle of inclination, called *coxa vara,* bends the femur and shortens it (Figure 13.16). This causes the pelvis to drop when that side bears weight and limits the range of hip motion.

The angle between the neck of the femur and the axis through the femoral condyles is called the **angle of torsion,** which averages 15 degrees. The angle of torsion can best be seen by looking at a femur resting on a table; the neck of the femur will be raised at the angle of torsion. Pathological variances in this angle of torsion affect the biomechanics and stability of the hip joint and can lead to muscular pain from compensatory toed-in or toed-out foot patterns (Figure 13.17a-b ■).

13.2.1.2 COXOFEMORAL JOINT MOTION

Two categories of motion occur at the coxofemoral joint: movement of the hip at the pelvis and movement of the pelvis at the hip. During the swing phase of walking, the pelvis is relatively stationary while the femur swings under the pelvis, causing the head of the femur to rotate in the hip socket. Just the opposite occurs when bending over. The pelvis moves over the femur, causing the hip socket to rotate around the head of the femur.

There are six *movements of the femur at the pelvis* (Figure 13.18 ■):

1. Flexion
2. Hyperextension
3. Abduction
4. Adduction
5. Lateral rotation
6. Medial rotation

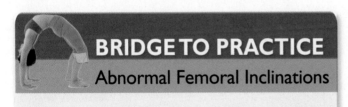

BRIDGE TO PRACTICE
Abnormal Femoral Inclinations

Although you may be able help a client with an abnormal angle of inclination or torsion by providing relief from compensatory muscular contractures, that client will still need orthopedic treatment to improve joint mechanics.

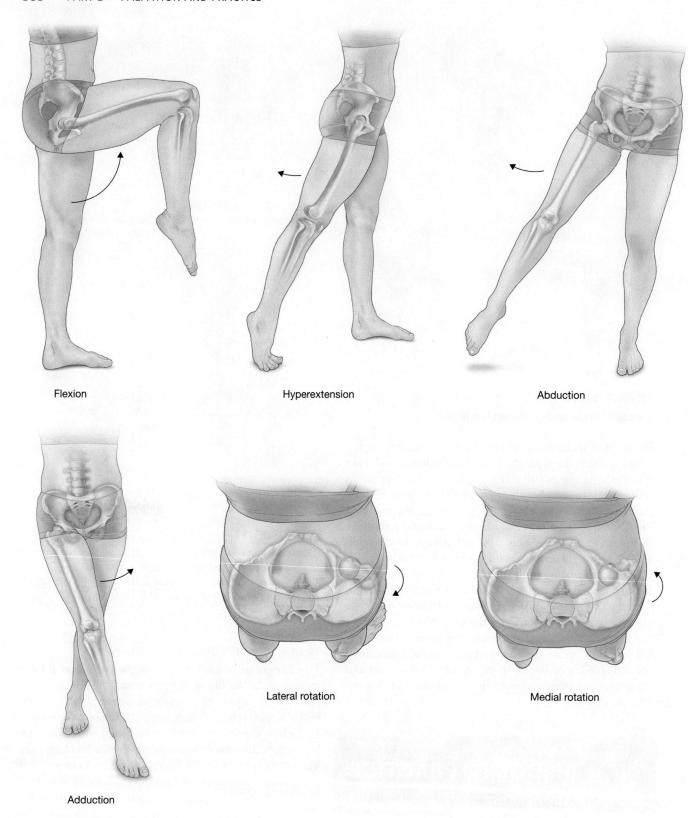

Flexion

Hyperextension

Abduction

Adduction

Lateral rotation

Medial rotation

FIGURE 13.18
Six movements of the femur at the pelvis

Although the hip rarely moves in a single plane, flexion and extension occur in the sagittal plane, abduction and adduction in the frontal plane, and rotation in the horizontal plane. The greatest range of hip movement is flexion. All other ranges of hip motion—abduction, adduction, rotation, and hyperextension—are 45 degrees or less (see Table 13.1 ■). During hip rotation at the pelvis, all movements have a firm, capsular end-feel except hip flexion, which has a soft end-feel. Recall from the joint chapter that an end-feel describes what prevents the joint from moving any farther than its end range. Hip flexion has a soft end-feel because soft tissue restricts further motion. By this definition, it could be said that there are actually seven movements of the hip, but since extension and hyperextension move in the same direction, they are considered one motion.

The difference between hip extension and hyperextension can be confusing. Extension is a return from flexion. We extend the hip when we straighten it from a bent position. Hyperextension is movement behind the frontal plane. We hyperextend the hip when we move the lower limb behind the body, like a person does while walking backward.

There are six *movements of the pelvis on the femur* (Figure 13.19 ■):

1. Posterior tilt
2. Anterior tilt
3. Right lateral tilt
4. Left lateral tilt
5. Forward rotation
6. Backward rotation

Gait involves a revolving sequence of all six movements of the femur at the pelvis and the pelvis on the femur. In the swing phase of gait, the hip moves under the pelvis in a pendular motion. As the hip swings forward, its primary motion is flexion and extension in the sagittal plane. In a normal gait pattern, the hip adducts about 5 degrees during the stance phase and abducts about 5 degrees during the swing phase. A similar degree of lateral and medial rotation also occurs. Any greater degree of hip motion would be inefficient. The pelvis moves over the femur in all three planes in a normal gait pattern. Posterior tilt and anterior tilt occur in the sagittal plane. Lateral tilt occurs in the frontal plane when the weight shifts onto the standing leg, slightly hiking the hip of the swing leg. Hip rotation turns the pelvis like a horizontal wheel each time there is forward weight shift over the standing leg.

The coxofemoral joint can move with a rolling, spinning, or gliding action between the articulating surfaces. During hip flexion or hyperextension, and hip abduction and adduction, the head of the femur rolls and glides in the socket. During lateral and medial hip rotation, only spinning occurs. The neck of the femur rotates medially and laterally like the arm of a turnstile, turning around the vertical axis.

As you study the movements of the hip, keep in mind that this joint rarely moves in a single plane. Movement in a single plane tends to be unnatural and robotic, like goose-step marching. It can even indicate a neurological disability. Still, observing hip motion in a single plane is a great assessment tool. It helps us to assess which muscles work independently of other muscles and how much control a person has over muscle actions. For example, try abducting your hip independent of lateral rotation. Doing so requires a level of muscular control that allows you to differentiate the actions of your hip abductors from your lateral hip rotators. You might find this difficult if your lateral hip rotators tend to overwork and are chronically shortened and glued to surrounding muscles.

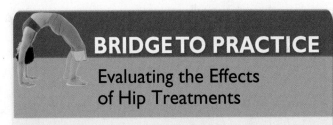

BRIDGE TO PRACTICE

Evaluating the Effects of Hip Treatments

Evaluate the effects of your hands-on techniques by assessing the range and clarity of hip motion before and after working with a group of muscles that restrict the range of motion.

TABLE 13.1	**Range of Motion in the Hips**	
Hip Motion	Range of Motion	End-Feel
Flexion	125 degrees with knee extension 140 degrees with knee flexion	Soft
Hyperextension	10–15 degrees	Firm
Abduction	45 degrees	Firm
Adduction	10 degrees	Firm
Lateral rotation	45 degrees	Firm
Medial rotation	45 degrees	Firm

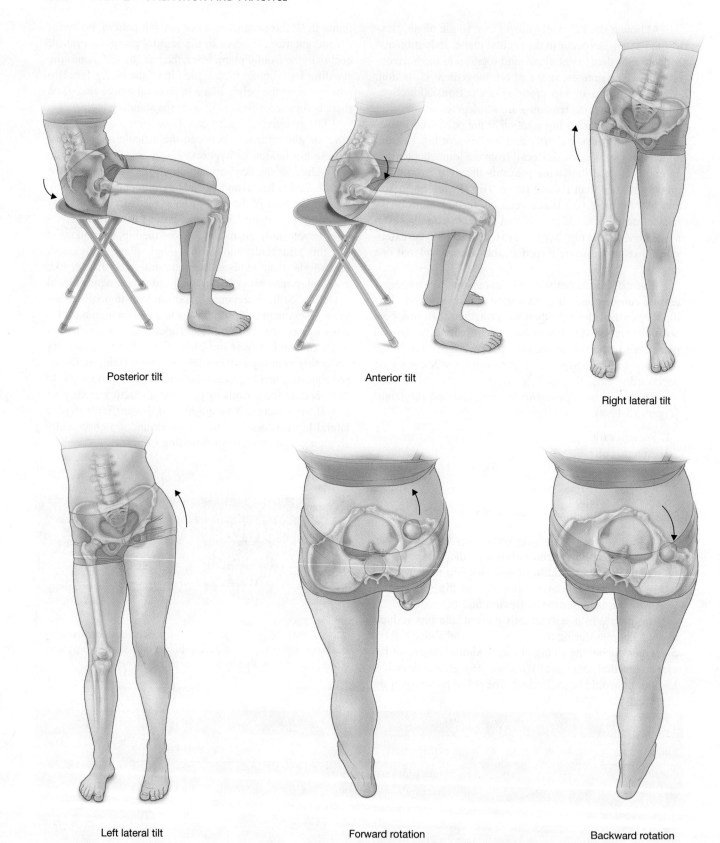

Posterior tilt

Anterior tilt

Right lateral tilt

Left lateral tilt

Forward rotation

Backward rotation

FIGURE 13.19

Six movements of the pelvis on the femur

EXPLORING TECHNIQUE
Passive Range of Motion for the Hip

Before you perform these PROM tests on the hip, read through the guidelines:

- Have your partner agree to report any pain or discomfort he or she feels during the motion. During the exercise, watch for signs of pain or discomfort and stop if you notice any pain reactions.
- To avoid impinging joint structures, always traction the hip before moving it.
- Keep the ankle, knee, and hip aligned in the same plane as you move the hip to avoid twisting the joints.

- Stabilize the pelvis before moving the hip. Also, have your partner help stabilize his or her pelvis and lumbar spine by lightly contracting the lower abdominal muscles.
- Slowly move the hip along a linear pathway. Make sure your partner does not tilt the pelvis posteriorly as you move the hip.
- When you feel you have reached end range of motion and cannot move the hip any farther, ask your partner if he or she feels a stretch, which will indicate you have reached the end range.

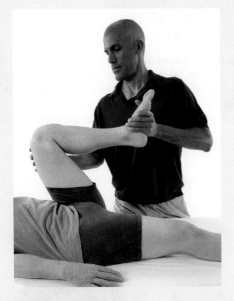

FIGURE 13.20a
a) PROM for hip flexion

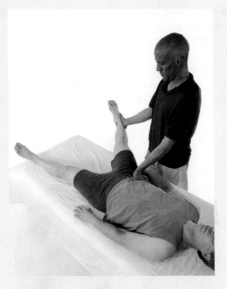

FIGURE 13.20b
b) PROM for hip abduction

1. **Hip flexion:** With your partner in the supine position, traction the hip. Then flex the hip and knee to 60 degrees. Maintain traction on the joint while you move the hip into flexion (Figure 13.20a ■). Make sure to keep the knee aligned with the hip so that you are moving the entire lower limb in the sagittal plane. End range with hip flexion is hard to reach because the pelvis tends to tilt posteriorly, which allows the hip to flex even farther.

2. **Hip abduction:** With your partner in the supine position, traction the hip. Then place one hand on the side of the coxal bone to stabilize the hip. Hold the leg with the other hand. Maintain traction as you abduct the hip. Move the limb in the same plane as the table to avoid hip flexion (Figure 13.20b ■). Avoid external hip rotation by keeping the knee facing up. *Do you notice how end range is hard to reach because the pelvis naturally tilts laterally, allowing the hip to abduct farther?*

(continued)

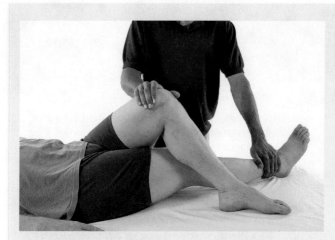

FIGURE 13.20c

c) PROM for hip adduction

3. **Hip adduction:** Stand on the side of the table opposite the hip you will be adducting. With your partner in the supine position, bend the knee closest to you and cross that foot over the other knee. Then grasp the ankle of the straight leg and traction the hip on that side. Maintain traction as you pull the foot toward you to adduct the hip (Figure 13.20c ■). *Does your partner feel a stretch along the lateral side of the hip joint?*

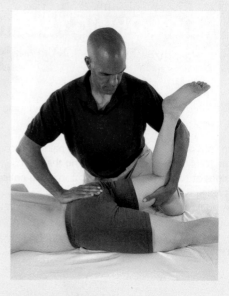

FIGURE 13.20d

d) PROM for hip hyperextension

4. **Hip hyperextension:** With your partner supine and the legs straight, reach under the thigh to traction the hip. Place one hand over the ischial tuberosity and push down to stabilize the hip. Place your other hand under the knee with the ankle resting on your shoulder. Lift the thigh directly toward the ceiling until your partner reports a stretch on the front of the hip joint (Figure 13.20d ■). *Are you moving the hip in the sagittal plane?*

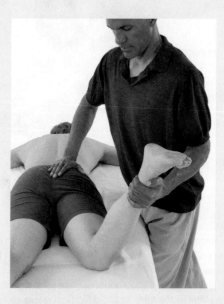

FIGURE 13.20e

e) PROM for medial hip rotation

5. **Medial rotation:** With your partner in the prone position now, traction the hip again. Stabilize the hip joint by pressing straight down above the ischial tuberosity. Bend the knee to a 60-degree angle, then slowly move the ankle away from midline to medially rotate the hip (Figure 13.20e ■). *Can you name the muscles that were stretched during each range of motion?*

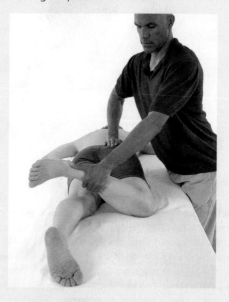

FIGURE 13.20f

f) PROM for lateral hip rotation

6. **Lateral rotation:** With your partner in the prone position, traction the hip. Stabilize the hip joint by pressing straight down above the ischial tuberosity, bend the knee to a 60-degree angle, and slowly move the ankle toward midline to laterally rotate the hip (Figure 13.20f ■). *Did the anterior side of the hip remain in contact with the table as you medially and laterally rotated the hip?*

13.2.1.3 LUMBAR PELVIC RHYTHM

Movement in hips generally occurs in coordination with motion at adjacent joints. Bending over usually involves both hip flexion and lumbar flexion because flexion of the lumbar spine allows a person to flex the hips even farther. This coordinated ratio of motion between the hips and lumbar spine is called the **lumbar pelvic rhythm.**[1] We'll look at a similar ratio of coordinated movement between the shoulder joint and the scapula, called the *scapulohumeral rhythm*, in the shoulder chapter.

In a normal lumbar pelvic rhythm in forward bending, the movement is sequential. First the lumbar spine flexes, then the hips flex (Figure 13.21 ■). As a person reverses the action and stands back up, the hips extend first, then the lumbar spine extends. The rhythm can get thrown off by postural holding patterns that take the hips or lumbar spine into chronic flexion or hyperextension in a standing posture, or by aberrant muscle firing patterns along the chain of flexor or extensor muscles. For example, a person with chronically tight lumbar muscles will usually stand with the lumbar spine in hyperextension and have restrictions to lumbar flexion in forward bending (Figure 13.22a ■). This person might even contract the lower back muscles to initiate forward bending. A person with this type of pattern needs to stretch and loosen the lumbar muscles to restore normal lumbar flexion.

You can integrate neuromuscular patterning into bodywork by stretching the client's lower back muscles while he or she bends forward. If you use this technique, you will want to encourage your client to contract the antagonists of the muscles being stretched—the abdominal flexors—by flexing the lumbar spine, which will enhance the stretch.

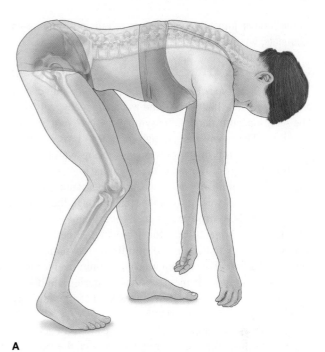

A

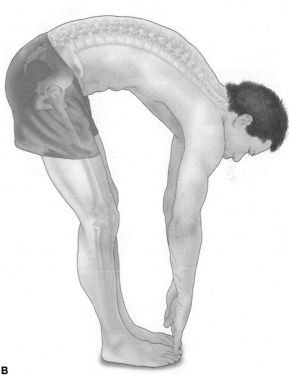

B

FIGURE 13.22

a) Deeper hip flexion compensates for chronic lumbar hyperextension. b) Excessive lumbar flexion compensates for restricted hip flexion.

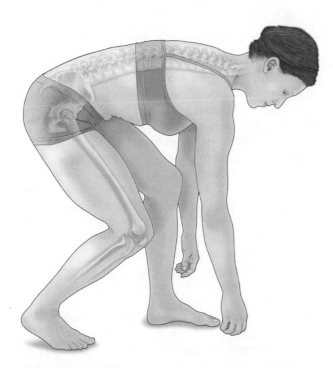

FIGURE 13.21

A normal **lumbar pelvic rhythm** in forward bending.

The lumbar pelvic rhythm can be thrown off in the opposite direction by restrictions to hip flexion. A person with chronically tight hamstrings will tend to hyperflex the lumbar spine to compensate for restricted hip flexion (Figure 13.22b). This type of pattern often occurs in people with a posterior pelvic tilt. Excessive lumbar flexion places mechanical stress on the lumbar joints and can overstretch the posterior spinal ligaments, which can lead to stability dysfunctions.

13.2.2   Joints of the Pelvis

There are three types of joints in the pelvis: the pubic symphysis, the sacroiliac joints, and the sacrococcygeal joint. The sacroiliac joints and pubic symphysis serve two primary functions. They have just enough motion to provide stress relief from torsion in the pelvic ring during walking. But because the range of motion in the sacroiliac joints and pubic symphysis is minimal, these joints provide a stable structure for the transfer of weight from the spine through the pelvis.

The **pubic symphysis** is a fibrocartilage joint joining the pubic bones along the front of the pelvic ring, which can be palpated in the middle of the pubic crest (Figure 13.23 ■). This amphiarthrotic (semimovable) joint has minimal motion. It moves primarily during childbirth, expanding to widen the pelvic bones so that the newborn can pass through the birth canal.

The **sacroiliac joints** (SIJs) are located on each side of the sacrum between the sacrum and the ilia; they are oriented in the sagittal plane (Figure 13.24a-b ■). Each SIJ is a large, unusual joint with an articulating surface the size of an ear and the shape of a boomerang. The top portion of the SIJ is classified as a synovial joint; the bottom portion of the SIJ is classified as a fibrous joint.

The **sacrococcygeal joint** is a small fibrous joint between the distal end of the sacrum and the coccyx. Although it has no active range of motion, passive motion occurs during defecation and birthing labor. Sacrococcygeal motion can amplify the SIJ motion. Many people break the sacrococcygeal joint by falling straight down on the tailbone, causing the coccyx to bend and tuck in the anterior direction.

13.2.2.1   SACRAL LIGAMENTS

The sacrum needs to be securely fastened to the base of the spine and the coxal bones in order to carry the weight of the spine. To get a picture of the thickness and strength of

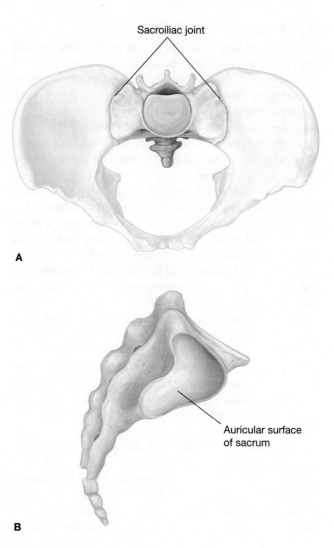

A

B

FIGURE 13.24

a) **Sacroiliac joint:** superior view b) **Sacroiliac joint surface**

the ligaments binding the sacrum to the spine and the hips, imagine the sacrum as an inverted arrowhead slung inside a form-fitting ligamentous pouch that is securely tethered to the ilium and the ischium on each side.

The **sacroiliac ligament** makes up the bulk of this imaginary ligamentous pouch. It has many ligamentous bands in two layers, an anterior and posterior layer that bind both the front and back sides of the sacrum to the ilium. This strong ligament covers most of the sacrum; its five ligamentous bands arise from each sacral segment (Figure 13.25 ■). Torsions in the sacrum can also cause asymmetries and tenderness to touch in the sacroiliac ligament.

The **sacrotuberous ligament** anchors the sacrum to the ischial tuberosity (Figure 13.26 ■). Torsions in the sacrum can cause asymmetries in the sacrotuberous ligaments—one side will be slack and the other side will be taut—and tenderness to touch.

The **sacrospinous ligament** anchors the sacrum to the ischial spine. A series of twisted bands in both the sacrotuberous and sacrospinous form a ligamentous hammock that

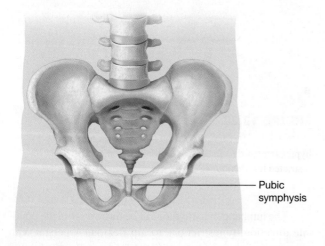

Pubic symphysis

FIGURE 13.23

Pubis symphysis

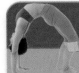

BRIDGE TO PRACTICE
Treating Chronic Lumbar Flexion

You can help a client with a pattern of chronic lumbar flexion by loosening muscles that restrict hip flexion, such as the hamstrings, the adductors, and the lateral hip rotators. Then you could show this client how to extend the lumbar spine by arching the lower back and how to sit and stand with a normal lumbar lordosis (see the "Seated Pelvic Rock" exercise in section 13.1.2). This will help your client learn how to move in a normal lumbar pelvic rhythm.

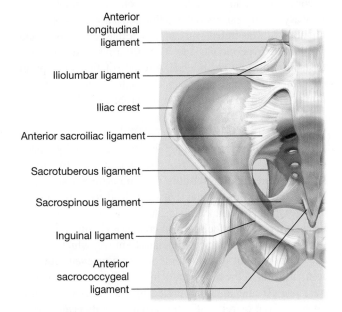

FIGURE 13.25

Sacral ligaments: anterior view

Anterior longitudinal ligament — Iliolumbar ligament — Iliac crest — Anterior sacroiliac ligament — Sacrotuberous ligament — Sacrospinous ligament — Inguinal ligament — Anterior sacrococcygeal ligament

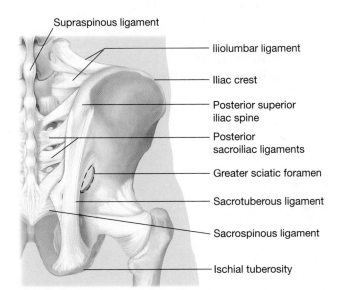

FIGURE 13.26

Sacral ligaments: posterior view

Supraspinous ligament — Iliolumbar ligament — Iliac crest — Posterior superior iliac spine — Posterior sacroiliac ligaments — Greater sciatic foramen — Sacrotuberous ligament — Sacrospinous ligament — Ischial tuberosity

suspends the lower end of the sacrum in soft tissue. The sacrospinous ligament is difficult to palpate.

Several small ligaments tether the coccyx to the sacrum, including a small segmented **sacrococcygeal ligament** that attaches the front of the coccyx to the front of the sacrum.

13.2.2.2 SACROILIAC JOINT STABILIZATION

The strength of the pelvic ring depends on the fit and stability of the sacroiliac joints (SIJs). The articulating surfaces of the SIJs are rough and irregular; the sacrum has bumps and the ilium has dimples that lock together like LEGOs and are bound together by the many thick, fibrous ligaments described earlier. Additional stabilization to the SIJs comes from the **form closure** of the sacrum wedged in between the coxal bones, which hold it in place in a close-packed position, like the blocks of an arch buttress into the keystone of the arch.

The SIJs are also stabilized by the **forced closure** of lower abdominal muscles knitting the two pelvic halves together across the front (Figure 13.27 ■). In a neutral posture, the sustained, tonic contractions of the transversus abdominis pull the anterior sides of the coxal bones closer together, which compresses the SIJs. The gluteus maximus also compresses and stabilizes the SIJs along a nearly

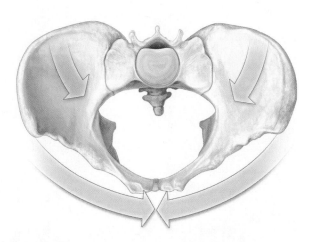

FIGURE 13.27

Forced closure of the sacroiliac joint

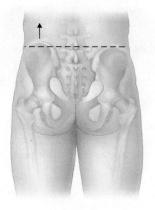
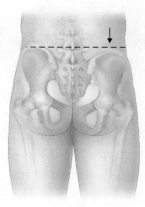

FIGURE 13.28
Upslip and downslip of pelvis

vertical line of pull. In the event that a client is suffering from SIJ pain and instability from damaged ligaments, muscles stabilizing the SIJs can be trained as a backup support system.

The SIJs are susceptible to extreme levels of mechanical stresses from both leg length discrepancies and postural asymmetries. A misalignment in an SIJ can cause joint asymmetries and instabilities that in turn lead to joint deterioration, arthritis, and low back and hip pain. A sudden force can also affect SIJ alignment, such as stepping off an unseen curb and hitting down hard on one side. This could cause an **upslip** or **downslip** in the pelvis, where one iliac crest slips up higher than the other (Figure 13.28 ■). An upslip or downslip can also occur from a leg-length discrepancy. In addition, a chronically tight quadratus lumborum or iliopsoas can torque the pelvis and pull one hip into an upslip or an anterior torque. For this reason, it is important that muscles acting on the pelvis be symmetrical.

13.2.2.3 SACROILIAC JOINT MOTION

Although their range of motion is controversial, the SIJs do allow for a small range of nutation and counternutation—a uniaxial motion in the sagittal plane. During **nutation** (L. *nutare,* meaning "to nod"), the sacrum rocks like a head nodding; the top of the sacrum tips forward as the bottom of the sacrum tips backward (Figure 13.29a ■). During **counternutation,** the sacrum rocks in the opposite direction; the top tips backward (Figure 13.29b ■). Sacral ligaments limit nutation and counternutation to a small range of motion.

Nutation takes the SIJ into a close-packed position: counternutation opens its joint space slightly. Although it is difficult to perceive, nutation is an important motion. If one SIJ becomes frozen and the other SIJ becomes hypermobile, the joint asymmetry can restrict nutation and place a torsion stress on the SIJs. This imbalance can trigger muscular spasms and pain on the hypermobile side. The piriformis tends to spasm to stabilize the hypermobile SIJ. A release of piriformis spasm can temporarily relieve the pain, although until the SIJ restriction is released on the other side, the problem will persist.

13.2.3 Hip Problems

Hyaline cartilage lining the hip joint is nourished by repetitive loading and release from joint motion. Movement literally squeezes joint fluids into the articular surfaces. Prolonged periods of inactivity can lead to degenerative changes in the hyaline cartilage. A lack of motion in the hips because a person is feeling pain creates a vicious cycle: the joint pain makes a person reluctant to move, which in turn causes more joint deterioration and pain or even arthritis. Joint arthritis in the hips occurs in 10–15 percent of people over age 55 and is compounded by increases in weight. Overuse from extreme athletic activity can also cause joint degeneration and pain. To maintain optimal joint health, a person needs to find a balance between the right amount of exercise and the right amount of rest.

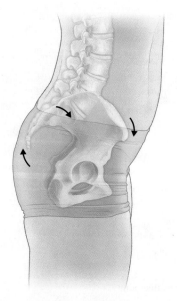
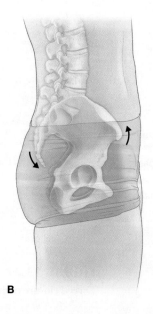

A   B

FIGURE 13.29
Sacral movement: a) Nutation b) Counternutation

BONE PALPATION
Sacral Ligaments and Sacral Motion

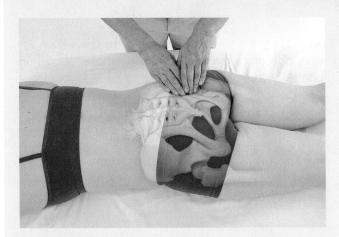

FIGURE 13.30a

With your partner prone, locate the **sacroiliac ligament** by applying broad, firm pressure over the sacrum and along the length of the sacroiliac joint. Make sure you are medial and inferior to the PSIS. The more tissue over the sacrum, the deeper you will need to press. This ligament usually feels fibrous and dense, which you can feel with cross-fiber strumming. Palpate both sides at once to check for symmetry. *Do you notice the dense and fibrous texture of the sacroiliac ligament?* (See Figure 13.30a ■)

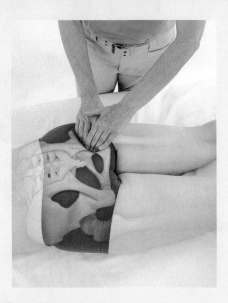

FIGURE 13.30b

With your partner prone, palpate the **sacrotuberous ligament** by locating the midpoint between the ischial tuberosity and lateral side of the sacrum. Apply deep and slow cross-fiber pressure over this area to locate this ligament. On a thin person, it feels like a thick, unyielding strap of tissue. On a large person, you will need to apply more pressure to sink through the overlying tissue. It is often tender on one side or both sides. *Does the sacrotuberous ligament feel like a taut strap stretched between the sacrum and the ischial tuberosity?* (See Figure 13.30b ■)

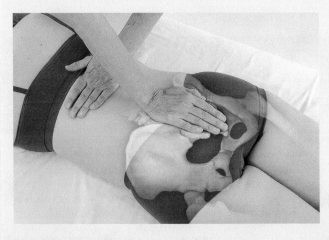

With your partner still prone, palpate **sacral motion** by placing your hand over the sacrum, cupping it with your entire hand. Tune into your partner's breathing and notice how the sacrum moves as your partner breathes. Then place one hand on the midback to pin it and apply light traction on the sacrum. *Does the traction increase the sacral motion?* (See Figure 13.30c ■)

FIGURE 13.30c

(continued)

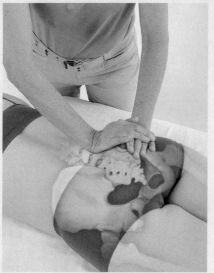

To check the amount of **flexibility in the SIJ** on each side, place the heel of your hand over the SIJ on one side along the joint line. Apply strong pressure into the joint, then release. You should feel a small amount of give and spring in the joint. If the joint is stiff, repeat several times. Each time you apply pressure, the joint should become a little suppler. Repeat the same pressure on the other sacroiliac joint. *Does the SIJ have the same amount of give on each side?* (See Figure 13.30d ■)

FIGURE 13.30d

The articular cartilage covering the head of the femur is the thickest on its superior surface, where it is under the greatest pressure in a weight-bearing position. Standing with the hips in chronic flexion places thinner areas of articular cartilage under pressure that it cannot adequately dissipate, which can lead to premature wear in the hips. Extreme degeneration of joint may require hip replacement surgery.

After the age of 50, bone density decreases approximately 2 percent per year, which can lead to osteoporosis. In addition, the trabeculae in spongy bone become thinner and eventually disappear. These skeletal changes predispose seniors to fracturing their hips from a fall. Seniors may also have poor balance from inactivity and guarding around the hips, which can restrict range of motion. Many seniors walk in a slow, careful gait to avoid falling.

One of the most common hip problems is **trochanteric bursitis.** It often develops from or is exacerbated by tight myofascias crossing the bursa, which cause too much friction during motion. Excessive friction to the bursa can create pain and inflammation, which a person will feel around the greater trochanter. Trochanteric bursitis tends to flare up and become worse after activity.

BRIDGE TO PRACTICE
Seniors with Restricted Hip Motion

To help a senior client with a restricted range of hip motion and a predisposition to falling, loosen the muscles around the hips and take the hip joint through a passive range of motion. This will help your client to relax the hip muscles during movement and it will increase joint fluid circulation. Gentle trigger point therapy on the hip can also improve range of motion by relaxing tight muscles, and it provides a great alternative for seniors with circulation problems for whom Swedish massage is contraindicated. Also, suggest that your client practice balance exercises such as holding the back of a chair and standing on one foot.

Athletes and active people sometimes tear the labrum in the hip or shoulder socket. The primary symptom of a **labral tear** is deep pain in the hip during flexion with medial rotation and adduction. Torn labrums can heal if they are minor, or they may need to be surgically repaired.

With any of these hip problems, a manual therapist can loosen chronically contracted muscles around the hips to reduce symptoms.

13.3 MUSCLES OF THE HIP AND PELVIS

Muscles acting on the hip are best understood by studying their actions and also their groups. This section is organized according to muscle groups. Before we consider these groups, it is helpful to look at an overview of the diverse actions of muscles acting on the hip and pelvis. Keep in mind that the actions of the muscles depend on the position of the hip. Most of the biarticular muscles acting on the hip and pelvis work most efficiently in midrange or when on a slight stretch. Their actions can invert depending on whether the position of the hip places the muscles in front of or behind the axis of motion. For example, an adductor that works as a hip flexor when the knee is in front of the hip joint becomes a hip extensor when the knee moves behind the hip joint. For this reason, every hip muscle performs several different joint motions.

Review the figures at the beginning of the chapter to see the six movements of the hip in three planes—flexion and hyperextension, abduction and adduction, and lateral and medial rotation. You'll want to refer back to those figures throughout this section of the chapter to help you better understand how the muscles work together to move the hip and pelvis.

The hip muscles are presented below according to their actions and groupings, as follows:

- Abductors: *Tensor fascia latae, sartorius,* and *gluteus medius*
- Adductors: *Pectineus, adductor longus, adductor brevis, adductor magnus,* and *gracilis*
- Gluteals: *Gluteus maximus, gluteus medius,* and *gluteus minimus*
- Iliopsoas: *Iliacus, psoas major,* and *psoas minor*
- "Deep six" lateral rotators: *Piriformis, gemellus superior, gemellus inferior, obturator internus, obturator externus,* and *quadratus femoris*

In addition, several muscles at the base of the pelvis or "pelvic floor," called the perineal muscles, are introduced in chapter. Techniques to stretch and balance the biarticular muscles that act on both the hip and knee—the *rectus femoris* and the *hamstrings*—are explored at the end of the chapter.

13.3.1 Hip Abductors

There are three primary abductors of the hip: the tensor fascia latae, sartorius, and gluteus medius (Figure 13.31 ■). The tensor fascia latae and gluteus medius are both innervated by the *gluteal nerve;* the sartorius is innervated by the *femoral nerve.* The tensor fascia latae and gluteus medius form a triangular muscular fan that serves as the deltoid of the hip, similar in shape and action to its counterpart, the deltoid of the shoulder. As a group, the abductors stabilize the hip during the stance phase of gait to keep the stance hip from adducting and shifting too far sideways.

The **tensor fascia latae** (TFL) is a short, thick, meaty muscle about 2 inches wide that arises below the iliac crest lateral to the anterior superior iliac spine and tapers into a long, flat tendon called the **iliotibial band** (ITB). This unusual ligament runs down the lateral line of the thigh under the side-seam of your pants, crosses the lateral side of the knee, and inserts on the proximal tibia. The tensor fascia latae abducts and medially rotates the hip; it also assists hip flexion. (See TrP for the tensor fascia latae in Figure 13.32 ■.)

BRIDGE TO PRACTICE
Anterior Hip Pain

If your client has anterior hip socket pain from a torn labrum, suggest that a client avoid the range of motion that causes pain—hip flexion with medial rotation and adduction. Explain to your client how this range of motion can increase pressure on the damaged tissue and further injure the labrum. Naturally, any passive movement of the affected hip in medial rotation and adduction is contraindicated.

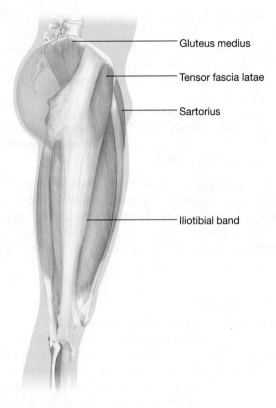

Gluteus medius

Tensor fascia latae

Sartorius

Iliotibial band

FIGURE 13.31

Hip adductors

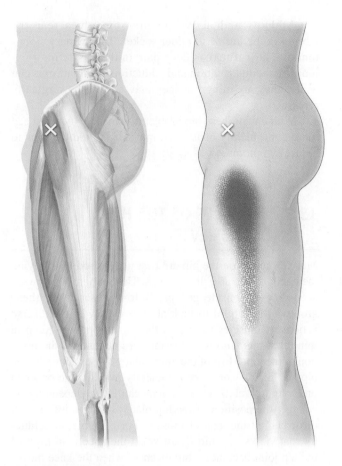

FIGURE 13.32

When dysfunctional, the **tensor fascia latae** can develop a trigger point in the upper third of the muscle, which can refer pain along the side of the leg below the greater trochanter. To practice effective trigger point therapy with the TFL, you may need to treat a nest of underlying trigger points in the gluteus minimus at the same time.

BRIDGE TO PRACTICE

TFL Pain and Trochanteric Bursitis

Myofascial pain from the TFL is often misdiagnosed as trochanteric bursitis. You can locate the source of pain by palpating the TFL and trochanteric bursa to identify which one creates symptoms. Palpate the bursa slowly and carefully. Remember that clients with TrPs in the TFL or trochanteric bursitis will have difficulty in the side-lying position because it puts painful pressure on both structures, so avoid this position. To alleviate trochanteric bursitis, loosen and separate adhered muscles and fascia around the trochanteric bursa, particularly in the tensor fascia latae and along the iliotibial band.

EXPLORING TECHNIQUE
Stretching the Iliotibial Band

ITB tightness is common among massage clients so you will want to know how to stretch it. Because the fibers are so tough, the ITB can be difficult to stretch. Here are a few techniques to help you effectively stretch it.

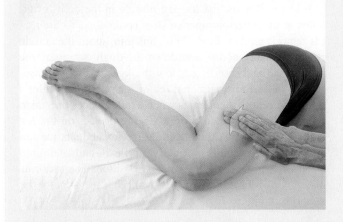

FIGURE 13.33a

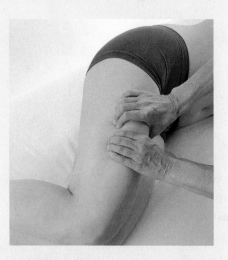

FIGURE 13.33b

1. To stretch the ITB, put your partner in a side-lying position with both hips and knees flexed and a pillow between the knees. Loosen the ITB by applying slow, deep cross-fiber strokes across the band (Figure 13.33a ■). If your partner tends to have an externally rotated hip, apply these strokes from the lateral to the medial across the band, which will move the joint toward a neutral alignment.

2. Slide your fingers under the lateral edge of the ITB above the knee to gently lift and stretch it away from underlying tissues (Figure 13.33b ■). Use this lifting technique up the length of the ITB. As you work, encourage your partner to allow the inner thigh to be heavy and sink into the other leg. Monitor your partner for pain responses because the area can be tender due to TrPs in the underlying vastus lateralis. If your partner shows muscular guarding, your pressure is too deep.

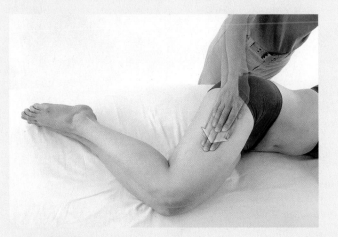

FIGURE 13.33c

3. Finish by applying several long, broad effleurage strokes down the ITB to smooth it out and stretch it longitudinally, moving from hip to knee (Figure 13.33c ■). Make sure to repeat the entire sequence on the other side.

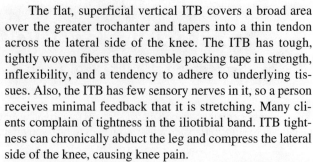

Sartorius

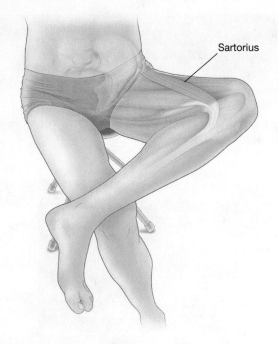

The flat, superficial vertical ITB covers a broad area over the greater trochanter and tapers into a thin tendon across the lateral side of the knee. The ITB has tough, tightly woven fibers that resemble packing tape in strength, inflexibility, and a tendency to adhere to underlying tissues. Also, the ITB has few sensory nerves in it, so a person receives minimal feedback that it is stretching. Many clients complain of tightness in the iliotibial band. ITB tightness can chronically abduct the leg and compress the lateral side of the knee, causing knee pain.

The **sartorius,** the longest muscle in the body, originates at the anterior superior iliac spine close to the rectus femoris tendon. From there, this thin, strap-like muscle runs diagonally across and down the thigh, wrapping the inner thigh and inserting below the knee at the pes anserinus. The sartorius garnered the nickname of the "tailor's muscle" because it contracts when a tailor places one ankle over the other knee to prop a sewing project on the leg (Figure 13.34 ■). Although the sartorius abducts the hip against resistance, it is a primary hip flexor and lateral hip rotator when the hip is in a flexed position. The sartorius also flexes and medially rotates the knee. (See TrPs for the sartorius in Figure 13.35 ■.)

FIGURE 13.34

Sartorius

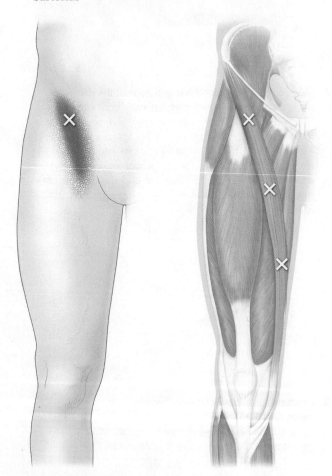

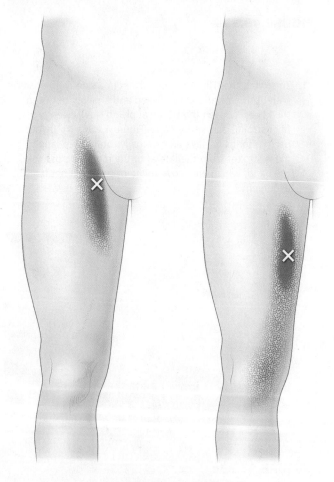

FIGURE 13.35

When dysfunctional, the **sartorius** can develop three trigger points, one in each third of the muscle, which can refer pain locally along that third of the muscle. The sartorius can also develop taut bands and cause numbness. When chronically tight, it will compress the medial side of the knee, which can cause secondary knee pain.

MUSCLE PALPATION
Sartorius and Tensor Fascia Latae

Palpate the sartorius contraction on yourself in a sitting position by laterally rotating your right hip and lifting your foot toward the other shin. To locate its distal end, strum across your inner thigh above the pes anserinus. Follow the sartorius along the medial aspect of the thigh using cross-fiber strumming all the way up to the ASIS.

Palpate the TFL while standing by pressing into its thick, meaty belly lateral to the ASIS. Alternate medially and laterally rotating your hip, and you should feel the TFL contract on medial rotation.

Palpate the iliotibial band along the outside of your thigh using cross-fiber strumming. It will feel like a flat, taut band all the way to your knee.

Sartorius

O–ASIS (anterior superior iliac spine)
I–Proximal medial tibia, superior tendon of pes anserinus
A–Flexes, abducts, and laterally rotates hip; flexes and medially rotates knee

Tensor Fascia Latae (TFL)

O–Iliac crest and posterior side of ASIS
I–Lateral condyle of tibia via iliotibial band
A–Abducts, medially rotates, and flexes hip

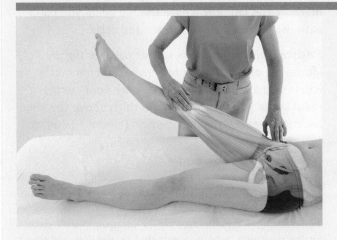

FIGURE 13.36a
Palpating the sartorius tendons during contraction

The sartorius is difficult to locate when it is relaxed, so palpate it during active movement. With your partner in a supine position, have your partner lift the leg to contract it while you locate the **sartorius tendon** below the ASIS (Figure 13.36a ■). Its tendon lies directly medial to the quadriceps femoris tendon, which will also pop out as your partner flexes the hip. Strum across the medial aspect of the quadriceps to feel the diagonal strap of the sartorius. It is about an inch wide.

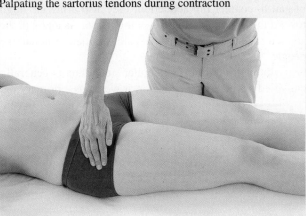

FIGURE 13.36b
Palpating the proximal sartorius

Palpate the **sartorius** along its length, from the ASIS to the pes anserinus, with cross-fiber strumming (Figure 13.36b ■). *Do you feel how narrow the diagonal strap of the sartorius is? Do you notice how difficult it is to locate the sartorius when it is relaxed?*

(continued)

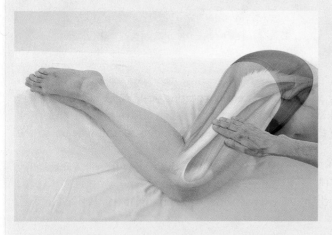

FIGURE 13.36c

Palpating the tensor fascia latae

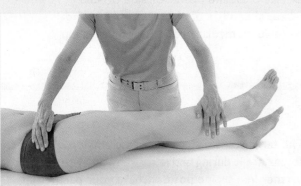

FIGURE 13.36d

Resisted movement of the tensor fascia latae

With the lower limb extended and your partner supine, locate the **tensor fascia latae** posterior to the ASIS below the iliac crest. Explore this small but thick and fleshy muscle by pressing straight into its belly and using cross-fiber strumming across its 2-inch width. Continue to strum across the TLF into its tendon, down the side of the thigh toward the knee (Figure 13.36c ■). *Can you feel where the TFL muscle belly tapers into the flat tendon of the iliotibial band?*

Active movement: Have your partner alternately medially and laterally rotate the hip while you palpate the TFL to feel it contract and relax.

Resisted movement: Have your partner slightly lift the leg off the table a few inches, then medially rotate and abduct the hip. Then have your partner resist while you lightly push the thigh above the knee back to a neutral resting position (Figure 13.36d ■).

13.3.2 Hip Adductors

The hip adductors are a fan-shaped group of muscles that include the pectineus, adductor longus, adductor brevis, adductor magnus, and gracilis. They attach along a broad area of the inferior pubic ramus and are stacked in layers, like the pages of a book (Figure 13.37a-b ■). The pectineus and adductor longus lie in the superficial, anterior layer; the adductor brevis and gracilis fill the middle layer; and the adductor magnus makes up the back, posterior layer. All of

the adductors are innervated by the *obturator nerve* except for the pectineus, which is supplied by the *femoral nerve*. The adductors stabilize the hip during the stance phase of gait to counter hip abduction; they also bring the thigh toward the midline during the swing phase. As a group, the adductors tend to be weak and undeveloped in nonactive people.

Although the flat, rectangular **pectineus** is generally classified as the lateral adductor, it works as a primary hip

BRIDGE TO PRACTICE

Adductor and Iliopsoas Trigger Points

The adductors and iliopsoas connect the inside line of the lower limb to the core line. The adductors frequently develop TrPs at the same time as the iliopsoas, creating myofascial pain and

discomfort along the inner thigh and into the core. For this reason, when you have a client with TrPs in the iliopsoas, also check the adductors for TrPs.

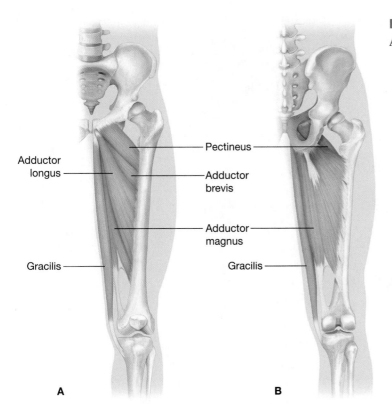

FIGURE 13.37

Adductor muscles: a) Anterior layer b) Posterior layer

A

B

flexor and medial rotator. It arises from the superior aspect of the pubic ramus lateral to the pubic tubercle and inserts below the lesser trochanter, on the back of the femur along the top of the linea aspera. The pectineus runs along an oblique angle between the distal iliopsoas tendon and the adductor longus. It provides a medial border for the **femoral triangle,** which is bordered on top by the inguinal ligament and on the lateral side by the sartorius (Figure 13.38 ■). The pectineus adducts and flexes the hip; it also laterally rotates the hip in extension and medial rotates it when the hip is flexed 90 degrees or more. (See TrP for the pectineus in Figure 13.39 ■.)

The **adductor longus** is the most superficial and prominent adductor. Its proximal tendon arises from a narrow, flat tendon along the medial, inferior aspect of the pubic ramus, right below the pubic symphysis and behind the gracilis tendon. It inserts along the middle third of the linea aspera. The adductor longus is active during free adduction whereas the adductor magnus is only active during resisted adduction. Both muscles are active during medial hip rotation. The **adductor brevis** arises along the anterior aspect of the pubic ramus behind the adductor longus tendon inferior to the pubic tubercle. It inserts on the upper third of the linea aspera behind the pectineus and adductor

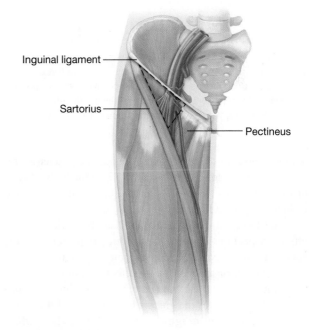

FIGURE 13.38

The pectineus creates the medial border of the **femoral triangle.**

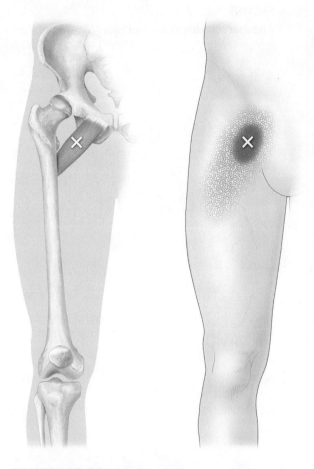

FIGURE 13.39

A trigger point often develops in the center of the **pectineus** after a fall or tripping accident, which causes discomfort during subsequent hip adduction and flexion. A pectineus trigger point creates a deep, persistent aching distal to the inguinal ligament over the hip joint, which can refer pain locally to the groin.

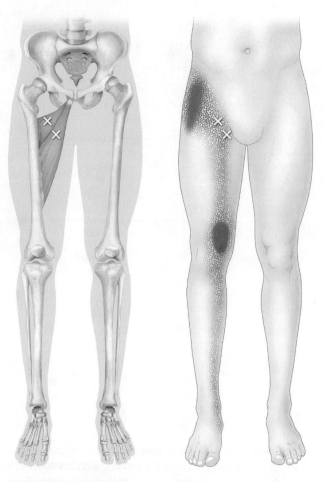

FIGURE 13.40

An **adductor brevis** trigger point can refer pain over the lateral hip area, and an **adductor longus** trigger point can refer pain in a patch above the medial knee; both trigger points can cause spillover pain along the entire inside line of the leg, from heel to groin.

longus. Vigorous activities that overload the adductor brevis and adductor longus can lead to TrPs in the belly of each of these muscles. (See TrPs for the adductor longus and adductor brevis in Figure 13.40 ■.)

The long, strapping **gracilis** arises from the medial, inferior aspect of the pubic ramus, directly posterior to the adductor longus tendon, and inserts on the proximal medial tibia at the pes anserinus. The gracilis is the only two-joint adductor; it adducts the hip and assists both hip and knee flexion. (See TrPs for the gracilis in Figure 13.41 ■.)

The **adductor magnus,** the largest of the adductor muscles, is sandwiched between the middle layer of

adductors and the medial hamstrings. Its broad, flat origin arises along the length of the inferior aspect of the ischiopubic ramus as far back as the ischial tuberosity, and its fibers fan out and attach along the entire length of the linea aspera, from just below the lesser trochanter to the adductor tubercle. The adductor magnus is a hip flexor when working in front of the joint line and a hip extensor when working behind the joint line. It adducts the hip against resistance and is quiet during free adduction. (See TrPs for the adductor magnus in Figure 13.42 ■.)

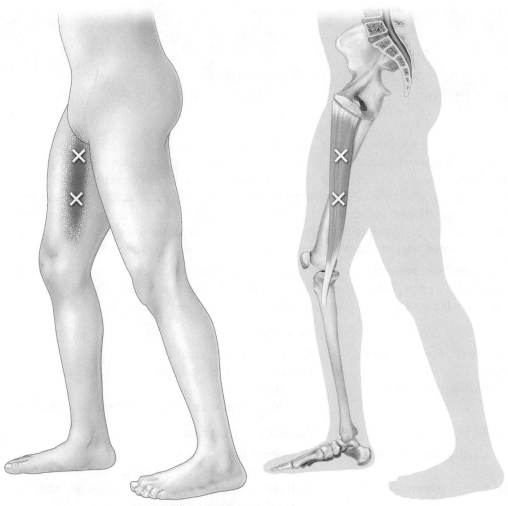

FIGURE 13.41
When dysfunctional, the **gracilis** can develop two trigger points staggered in the belly of the muscle that can produce a hot, stinging pain and refer pain along the length of the muscle.

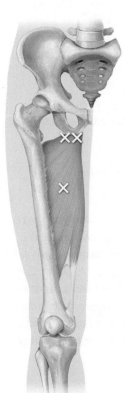
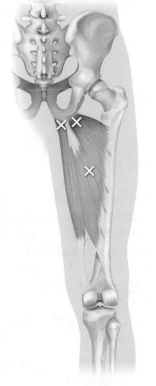
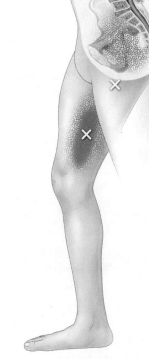
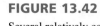

FIGURE 13.42
Several relatively common trigger points in the **adductor magnus** develop in four locations: two trigger points can develop in the middle of the muscle, one anterior and the other posterior, which can refer pain from the groin down the length of the muscle belly. Two other trigger points can develop near its proximal tendon, slightly medial and distal to the ischial tuberosity. Adductor magnus trigger points can cause deep, internal and sometimes shooting pain in the groin and pelvis.

MUSCLE PALPATION
Adductor Longus, Adductor Brevis, Pectineus, Gracilis, and Adductor Magnus

The group of adductors is easy to palpate, although differentiating individual muscles in this group is more difficult. Palpate your own adductors in a seated position, feeling their tendons along the inside of your upper thigh. The most prominent tendon there is the adductor longus tendon. The gracilis lies directly behind the longus tendon, and the pectineus lies directly medial to the adductor longus. Hold your hands across the middle of the adductors, then move your hip in adduction with your knee straight to feel the adductors contract. Use cross-fiber strumming to palpate each adductor tendon on the medial side of the knee. Find the adductor tubercle, where the adductor magnus attaches. Locate the pes anserinus, where the gracilis attaches.

Caution: The area along the upper inner adductors can be highly sensitive or ticklish. It is also close to the genitals, so palpate the adductors slowly using a flat, yet firm pressure, monitoring your partner for any signs of discomfort. If your partner is male, ask him to lift his genitals to the other side and hold them out of the way while you palpate the adductors.

Adductor Longus

O–Anterior pubic ramus, lateral to pubic tubercle
I–Middle third of linea aspera
A–Adducts hip, assists hip flexion and medial rotation

Adductor Brevis

O–Anterior pubic ramus, inferior to pubic tubercle
I–Medial lip of linea aspera
A–Adducts hip, assists hip flexion and medial rotation

Pectineus

O–Superior pubic ramus
I–Pectineal line of femur
A–Flexes and adducts hip, assists medial and lateral rotation (depending on position of hip)

Gracilis

O–Inferior pubic ramus
I–Proximal medial tibia, middle tendon of pes anserinus
A–Adducts hip, assists hip flexion and knee flexion

Adductor Magnus

O–Inferior pubic ramus
I–Linea aspera, adductor tubercle
A–Flexes, extends, and medially rotates hip; adducts hip during resisted adduction

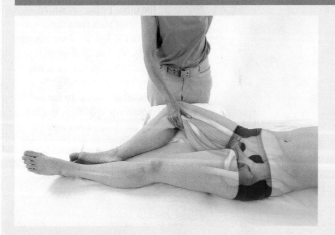

With your partner in a supine position, have your partner laterally rotate the hip, and put a pillow under the knee to flex it. Then palpate the entire **adductor muscle group** right above the knee (Figure 13.43a ■). Cup the entire muscle group with your hand and squeeze up along its length. *Are you palpating the large muscle group along the inside of the thigh? Do you notice how the adductor group tapers and narrows as it gets closer to the knee?*

FIGURE 13.43a
Palpating the adductor group

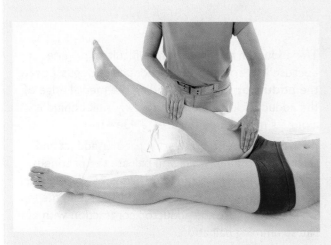

FIGURE 13.43b
Resisted movement of the adductors

Active movement: Have your partner slightly flex and adduct the hip so that you can feel the adductor group contract. Have your partner medially and laterally rotate the hip to feel different parts of the adductor group contract and relax.

Resisted movement: Have your partner extend the knee and raise the leg to flex the hip. Then have your partner resist while you lightly and slowly press the inner thigh above the knee into abduction (Figure 13.43b ▪).

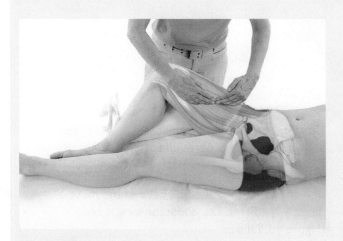

FIGURE 13.43c
Palpating between the adductors and quadriceps

Differentiating adductors and quadriceps: Have your partner lift and abduct the leg to contract the quadriceps so you can locate their medial border. You should feel the adductors relax while the quadriceps contract. With your partner relaxed, see if you can slide your fingertips between the adductor and quadriceps compartments (Figure 13.43c ▪).

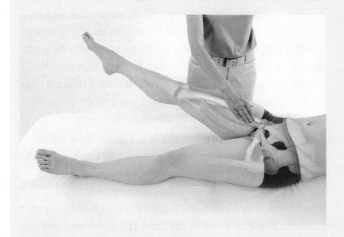

FIGURE 13.43d
Palpating the adductor longus tendon

Have your partner raise the leg to flex the hip and contract the **adductor longus,** then palpate it by locating its tendon below the lateral side of the pubic bone (Figure 13.43d ▪). *Are you on the prominent tendon of the adductor group?*

(continued)

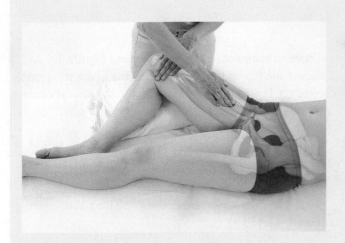

FIGURE 13.43e

Palpating the adductor brevis

The adductor brevis is more difficult to palpate because it is covered by the adductor longus. Locate the **adductor brevis** by finding the medial edge of the adductor longus tendon. Slowly sink behind it along its medial side (Figure 13.43e ■).

Active movement: Have your partner adduct and slightly flex the hip while you palpate the pectineus, adductor longus, and adductor brevis. Have your partner alternate between relaxing and adducting the hip while you explore the adductor contraction with a flat, strumming palpation.

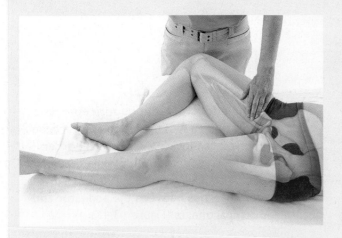

FIGURE 13.43f

Palpating the pectineus

Caution: *Be careful when palpating the pectineus because the femoral nerve and artery lie under it.*

To locate the **pectineus,** use a flat, broad palpation to slowly sink into the belly of the muscle directly medial to the adductor longus tendon (Figure 13.43f ■).

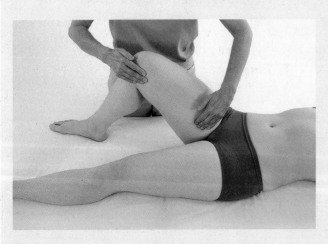

FIGURE 13.43g

Active movement of the gracilis

Use a flat palpation to locate the taut, proximal tendon of the **gracilis** directly posterior to the adductor longus tendon. Explore the length of the gracilis using a flat, strumming palpation and a pincher palpation. In a thin thigh, the slender belly of the gracilis can feel like a taut band; in a well-padded thigh, it can be difficult to find. *Can you follow the gracilis down to the pes anserinus below the inside of the knee?*

Active movement: With the knee bent, have your partner press the foot against the table while medially rotating the knee while you palpate the gracilis contraction (Figure 13.43g ■). This motion will make the gracilis contract independently of the other adductors because the gracilis acts on both the knee and the hip.

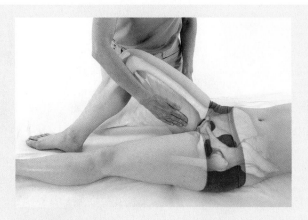

Palpate the **adductor magnus** on the most medial aspect of the inner thigh, along its broad attachment site below and anterior to the ischial tuberosity (Figure 13.43h ■). Locate its thin, distal attachment on the adductor tubercle. *Can you feel the broad adductor magnus tendon in front of the hamstring tendons on the ischial tuberosity?*

FIGURE 13.43h
Palpating the adductor magnus

13.3.3   Gluteal Muscles

Three large gluteal muscles—the gluteus maximus, gluteus medius, and gluteus minimus—cover the sides and back of the coxal bone (Figure 13.44a-b ■). All three gluteals are innervated by the *superior gluteal nerve.* As discussed in the gait chapter, the gluteus medius and gluteus maximus work as important hip stabilizers during the stance phase. Dysfunction in either one can lead to antalgic gait pattern.

The large, thick **gluteus maximus** arises from ligaments over the posterior sacrum and makes up the bulk of the buttocks' mass. Its diagonal fibers insert along the proximal half of the posterior shaft of the femur at the gluteal tuberosity and along the proximal third of the iliotibial band. The lower border of the gluteus maximus can usually be observed in the **gluteal fold,** a horizontal crease between the buttock and the posterior thigh over the ischial tuberosity. This parallelogram-shaped muscle is composed largely of slow fibers, which equip it for continuous contraction to maintain upright posture and to prevent hip flexion in the stance phase. The gluteus maximus also works as a powerful hip extensor during rigorous activity such as jumping and running, a primary hip extensor when rising from a crouched or seated position, and a lateral hip rotator. During forward bending, it eccentrically controls lowering the trunk. (See TrPs for the gluteus maximus in Figure 13.45 ■.)

The thick, fan-shaped **gluteus medius** arises from a broad origin that covers the posterior upper half of the ilium and inserts across the superior aspect of the greater trochanter. It is oriented in the sagittal plane on the side of the pelvis. The posterior part of the gluteus medius lies deep to the gluteus maximus; its anterior portion is superficial and can be easily palpated. The gluteus medius works as a primary hip abductor; its posterior fibers laterally rotate and extend the hip; its anterior fibers medially rotate and flex the hip. (See TrPs for the gluteus medius in Figure 13.46 ■.)

The smaller yet also thick and fan-shaped **gluteus minimus** lies under the gluteus medius, arising over the outer, anterior surface of the iliac bone and inserting on the superior aspect of the greater trochanter. The gluteus minimus abducts and medially rotates the hip and assists hip flexion. (See TrPs for the gluteus minimus in Figure 13.47 ■.)

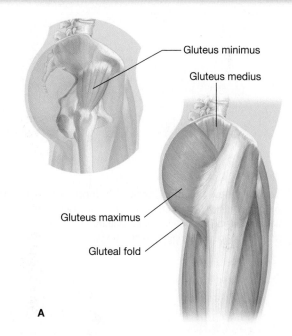

A

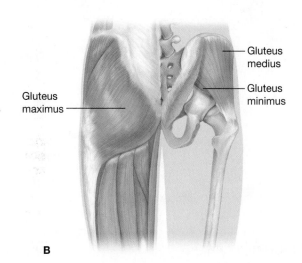

B

FIGURE 13.44

Gluteal muscles: a) Lateral view b) Posterior view

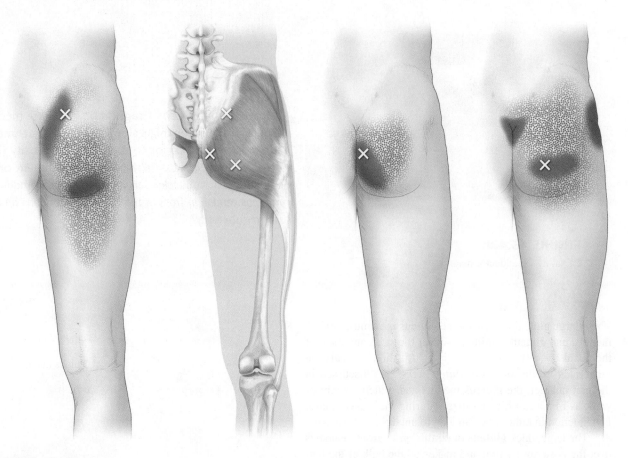

FIGURE 13.45

When the **gluteus maximus** becomes dysfunctional, it can develop three trigger points: one in the middle of the sacral attachment, another near the coccyx, and a third above the ischial tuberosity. Gluteus maximus trigger point pain can refer into the sacrum, as well as locally around the trigger points, making sitting uncomfortable. Prolonged sitting and eccentric work like walking uphill in a bent-hip posture can aggravate trigger points and pain in the gluteus maximus.

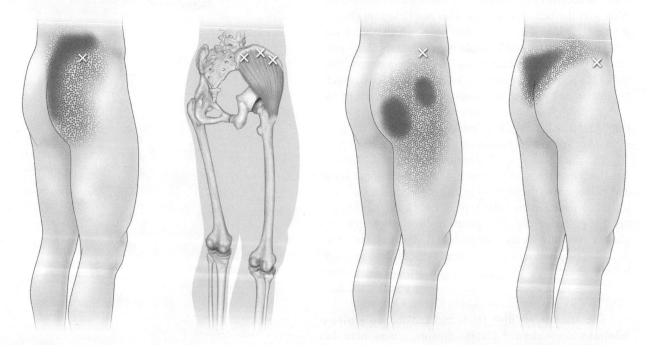

FIGURE 13.46

When dysfunctional, the **gluteus medius** can develop three adjacent trigger points directly under the crest of the hip, which can refer pain over a large area of the lower back, sacrum, and hip. The gluteus medius often develops trigger points in conjunction with the quadratus lumborum.

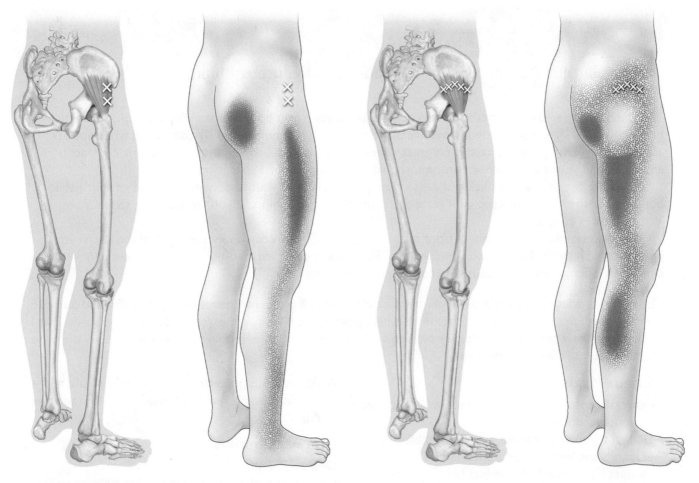

FIGURE 13.47

When dysfunctional, the **gluteus minimus** can develop a row of five trigger points under its origin and two trigger points stacked along its anterior fibers. The trigger points of this small muscle refer pain over the buttocks and along the lateral hamstrings and iliotibial band, down to the posterior lateral calf, along the peroneals, and over the lateral ankle. The gluteus minimus can refer pain over such a large area that its referral region mimics sciatic nerve pain. Constant and often excruciating pain from gluteus minimus trigger points can make both walking and sleeping in a side-lying position painful.

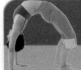

BRIDGE TO PRACTICE
Working with Gluteus Maximus Weakness or Inhibition

Many clients suffer from hip pain associated with a weak or inhibited gluteus maximus, which is evident in flat, flaccid buttocks. To check the tone in your client's gluteus maximus, have that client raise the entire lower limb from a prone position to extend the hip. The gluteus maximus should contract. If it does not, apply rigorous cross-fiber strumming across the buttocks to stimulate the muscle, then have your client raise the lower limb again. If it still does not contract, have your client extend the hip against your resistance by pressing down on the back of the thigh, right above the knee.

MUSCLE PALPATION
Gluteus Maximus, Gluteus Medius, and Gluteus Minimus

The gluteal muscles are superficial and easy to palpate on your own body. In a standing position, place your hands over the large, meaty gluteus maximus on your buttock. It should be lightly contracted when you are standing. To feel the gluteus maximus contract, squeeze your buttocks together in an isometric contraction and/or extend your hip. In both actions, you should feel it bulge and fill your hand.

To locate the smaller yet thick and dense gluteus medius, press your hands into the sides of your pelvic bones under the iliac crest. Keep your hand there and abduct your hip as if you were skating to feel your gluteus medius contract.

The gluteus minimus lies right in front of the gluteus medius, directly under the front of the iliac crest. Press straight into its fibers, which lie under the TFL. To feel it contract, medially rotate and flex the hip. It is difficult to differentiate the gluteus minimus from the overlying TFL.

Caution: The sciatic nerve, which lies under the gluteus maximus, is a common source of hip discomfort and pain due to impingement from tight overlying rotator muscles that cross over it. If your partner feels radiating nerve pain as you palpate the gluteus maximus, you could be pressing on the sciatic nerve. If this occurs, move your pressure off the nerve to another part of the gluteus maximus.

Gluteus Maximus

O–Lateral, posterior ilium, lateral sacrum and coccyx, sacrotuberous ligament
I–Gluteal tuberosity of femur and iliotibial band
A–Extends and laterally rotates hip, lateral fibers abduct hip, medial fibers adduct hip

Gluteus Medius

O–Outer surface of ilium
I–Lateral surface of greater trochanter

A–Abducts hip, posterior fibers laterally rotate and extend hip, anterior fibers medially rotate and flex hip

Gluteus Minimus

O–Lateral ilium
I–Anterior surface of greater trochanter
A–Abducts and medially rotates hip, assists hip flexion

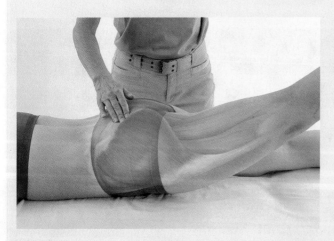

FIGURE 13.48a
Palpating the gluteus maximus contraction

With your partner prone, locate the **gluteus maximus** lateral to the sacroiliac joint using a flat palpation over the belly of the muscle. Have your partner contract the gluteus maximus by raising the lower limb while you palpate the gluteus maximus contraction (Figure 13.48a ■). Then have your partner relax and palpate it. A well-developed gluteus maximus will feel round and meaty. A poorly developed gluteus maximus can be hard to palpate because it is so thin and unsubstantial; it also gives the buttock a flat contour. Press into the buttock in several places to explore the muscle belly; strum laterally across it to feel the density of its fibers and to locate taut bands in the muscle. *Do you notice how both sides of the gluteus maximus, when well developed, have a butterfly shape?*

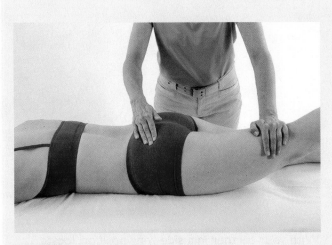

FIGURE 13.48b
Resisted movement of the gluteus maximus.

Resisted movement: Have your partner try to raise the lower limb against your resistance while you push the back of the thigh into the table (Figure 13.48b 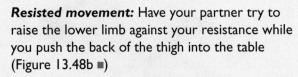)

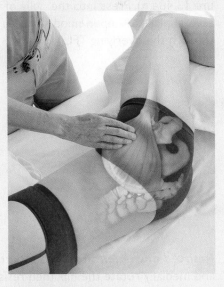

FIGURE 13.48c
Palpating the gluteus medius

With your partner in a side-lying position, locate the **gluteus medius** below the iliac crest, along the side of the hip (Figure 13.48c ■). Explore pressing into the belly of the muscle in several places to feel its thickness. Also strum laterally across it, noticing any taut bands in the muscle. *Do you feel how thick and dense the gluteal muscles are?*

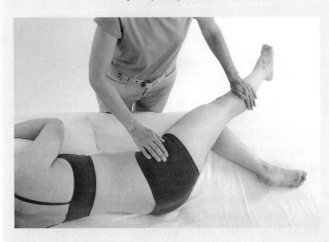

FIGURE 13.48d
Resisted movement of the gluteus medius

Resisted movement: With the limb still raised, have your partner resist as you push above the knee to press the thigh toward the table (Figure 13.48d ■).

(continued)

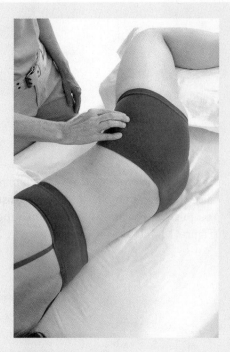

FIGURE 13.48e
Palpating the gluteus minimus

With your partner in a side-lying position, locate the **gluteus minimus** below the anterior portion of the iliac crest by using a flat palpation (Figure 13.48e ■). Press into the belly of the muscle in several places. Keep in mind that you will be pressing through the overlying TFL.

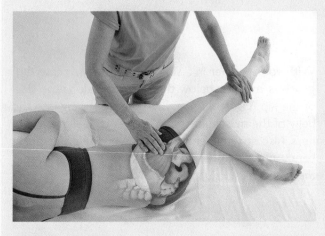

FIGURE 13.48f
Resisted movement of the gluteus minimus

Resisted movement: Have your partner abduct and medially rotate the hip, then resist as you push above the knee to press the thigh toward the table (Figure 13.48f ■).

13.3.4 Iliopsoas

The **iliopsoas** consists of three individual muscles with different locations and actions: the iliacus, psoas major, and psoas minor (Figure 13.49 ■). The iliacus is innervated by the *femoral nerve;* the psoas major and psoas minor are innervated by the *lumbar nerve plexus.* The iliopsoas is an intrinsic group of muscles in the lower torso that connects the femur to the pelvis and lumbar spine.

The largest in this muscle group is the **iliacus.** It arises from the anterior surface of the iliac fossa and inserts on the lesser trochanter. The iliacus literally lines the inside of the coxal bones and wraps around the back and sides of the pelvic organs. It works as a strong hip flexor, assists

lateral rotation and hip abduction, and stabilizes the hip in the stance phase of gait. There is a lot of controversy over whether the iliopsoas is a medial or lateral hip rotator. Also, some kinesiologists consider it a primary hip flexor, although electromyographic studies on standing subjects found the iliacus and psoas major inactive during the first 30 degrees of hip flexion.[2]

The **psoas major** is a pennate muscle that arises from the anterior bodies and transverse processes of the first to the fourth lumbar vertebrae. It joins the distal tendon of the iliacus to insert on the lesser trochanter. The psoas major is a multiarticular muscle crossing the anterior surfaces of the lumbar spine, the lumbosacral joint, the sacroiliac

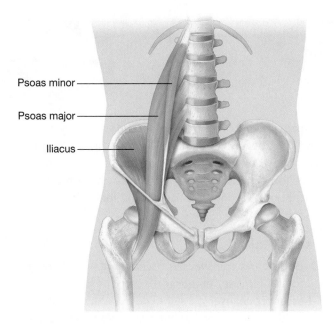

FIGURE 13.49

The iliopsoas muscle group

joints, and the hip. It is the only muscle to span the distance between the thigh and the lower back, so it is considered a key core muscle in the body. It lies behind the abdominal and pelvic viscera, in front of the lower autonomic nerve plexus. The stabilizing function of the psoas major was discussed in the posture chapter. It also assists hip flexion. Tightness in the psoas major will pull the lumbar spine into an exaggerated lordosis and tip the pelvis into an anterior tilt. This iliopsoas can be stretched with hip hyperextension and responds well to trigger point therapy (Figure 13.50 ■).

The **psoas minor** is a small, thin muscle that arises from the superior pubic ramus and attaches to the body of the first lumbar vertebra. It is absent in over half the population and its function is relatively inconsequential, although it is thought to support and level the front of the pelvic rim. Psoas minor dysfunction can create pain that is similar to appendicitis. The superficial distal tendon of the psoas minor can be easily palpated above the pubic tubercle; if this small muscle becomes overly tight it will feel taut and ropey.

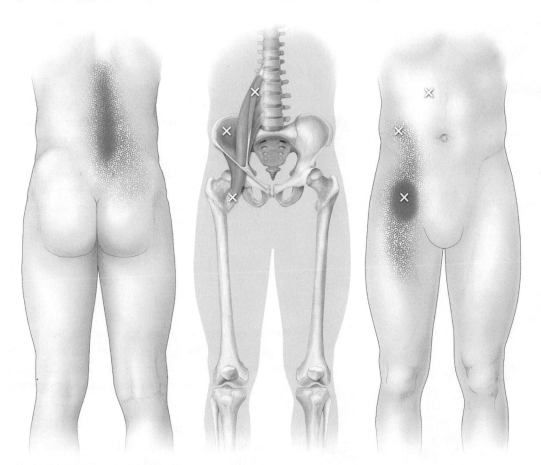

FIGURE 13.50

Because of the central location of the **iliopsoas** in the pelvic and abdominal cavities, and its location behind the abdominal viscera and anterior to the autonomic nerve plexus, dysfunction in the iliopsoas can lead to many problems. Trigger points that refer deep, unrelenting pain into the lower back and the front of the thigh can develop in three locations: the upper part of the iliacus, the distal tendon of the psoas major, and the upper belly of the psoas minor. Iliopsoas trigger points can make activities involving hip and trunk flexion and extension difficult, such as doing a sit-up or getting up out of a chair. In addition, unilateral tightness in either the iliacus or psoas major can torque the pelvis, leading to scoliosis (a lateral curvature of the spine) and causing sacroiliac dysfunction and pain.

MUSCLE PALPATION
Iliacus and Psoas Major

The iliopsoas is a deep muscle group that is difficult to self-palpate, although the distal tendon is easy to find. Palpate it in a seated position by placing your fingertips right below the inguinal ligament in the crease of the hip, directly medial to the femoral artery pulse. Then raise your knee to lift your foot off the floor. You should feel the tendon harden as the iliopsoas contracts. You can also place your hands on both tendons, then lean back from the hips (keep your spine straight) about 15 degrees. You should feel a tug in both tendons.

Iliacus

O–Iliac fossa
I–Lesser trochanter
A–Flexes and laterally rotates hip

Psoas Major

O–Bodies and transverse processes of first through fourth lumbar vertebrae
I–Lesser trochanter
A–Stabilizes anterior lumbar spine, flexes and laterally rotates hip

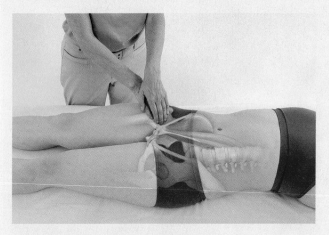

FIGURE 13.51a
Palpating the iliopsoas tendon

With your partner supine, palpate the distal iliopsoas tendon by slowly sinking your finger pads into the inguinal crease, directly lateral to the femoral artery (Figure 13.51a ■). Make sure to monitor your partner for any pain reactions because the tendon could be tender. If you feel a pulse, move your fingertips laterally. If the tendon is tender, hold it lightly until your partner reports that the tenderness has subsided.

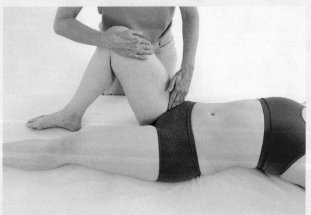

FIGURE 13.51b
Resisted movement of the iliopsoas

Active movement: Have your partner flex the hip as you palpate the tendon so that you can feel the tendon bulge as the iliopsoas contracts. *Can you feel the iliopsoas tendon harden when your partner raises the knee to contract it?*

Resisted movement: Have your partner resist as you apply light pressure against the knee to extend the hip, which will cause the iliopsoas to contract. Palpate the distal tendon as it contracts (Figure 13.51b ■).

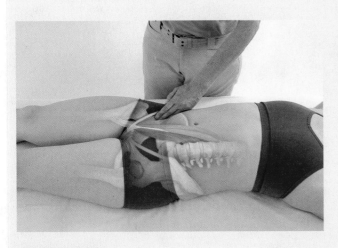

FIGURE 13.51c
Palpating the iliacus

Palpate the iliacus with your partner in a supine position with the legs extended. Curl your fingers around the anterior iliac crest and press toward the iliac fossa, into the belly of this thick, meaty muscle (Figure 13.51c ■). Make sure to monitor your partner for any pain reactions because this muscle is often tender or the area is sensitive to palpation. *Are your fingertips hooked over the top of the iliac crest?*

Active movement: Lighten your pressure. Then have your partner slide the foot toward the hip by bending the hip and knee. You should feel the iliacus contract.

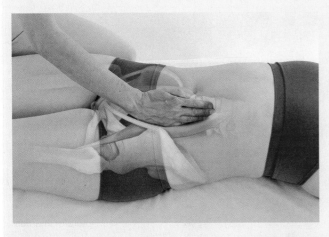

FIGURE 13.51d
Palpating the psoas major

Palpate the **psoas major** with your partner supine and a pillow under the knees. Slowly press your finger pads or the heel of your hand into the abdomen, about midway between the ASIS and the navel. Press on an angle toward the spine (Figure 13.51d ■). Make sure your partner keeps the abdominal muscles relaxed as you press in. Be mindful that you are pressing through small intestines, so press in slowly and carefully and stop at any sign of pain or discomfort. *Which is more comfortable for your partner, to palpate the psoas major with your finger pads or with a broader pressure, using the heel of your hand?*

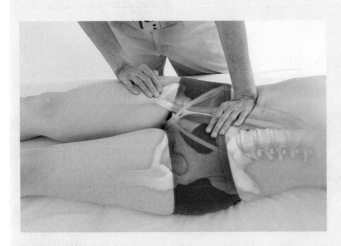

FIGURE 13.51e
Stretching the psoas major

Stretching the psoas major: Pin the belly of the psoas major with one hand, then press the abdomen toward the lower back to encourage the psoas and lumbar spine to lengthen. Apply downward traction on the upper thigh and stretch the distal attachment away from the muscle belly (Figure 13.51e ■). Because the psoas major assists lateral rotation, medially rotate the hip slightly to enhance the stretch.

(continued)

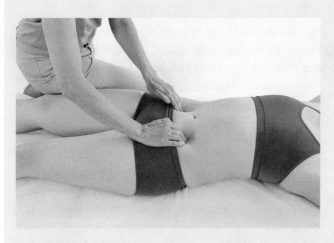

FIGURE 13.51f
Active stretch of the psoas major

Active stretch: Pin both sides of the psoas major, then instruct your partner to do a subtle posterior pelvic tilt, which will enhance the stretch (Figure 13.51f ■). *Does your partner report a stretch deep in the back of the abdominal cavity?*

13.3.5 "Deep Six" Lateral Hip Rotators

A group of six small muscles—the piriformis, the gemellus superior and gemellus inferior, the obturator internus and obturator externus, and the quadratus femoris—function as lateral hip rotators (Figure 13.52 ■). The obturator externus is innervated by the *obturator nerve;* the other five lateral rotators are innervated by the *sacral nerves.* When including the gluteal muscles, the lateral rotators of the hip are numerous and powerful. In contrast, the medial rotators of the hips are less numerous, and collectively they generate only about one-third the power of the lateral rotators. Because these six deeper lateral rotators lie under the gluteus maximus, they garnered a nickname of the "deep six." All of the deep six arise from the sacrum or coxal bone, all six run posterior to the hip joint, and all six converge on a common insertion site around the greater trochanter. Their fibers orient in a fan shape, so they are also referred to as the "rotator fan." As a group, they are analogous to the "rotator cuff" of the shoulder.

The most superior of the deep six, the **piriformis,** arises from the anterior inferior surface of the sacrum and runs diagonally out the greater sciatic foramen to its insertion site on the superior surface of the greater trochanter. This

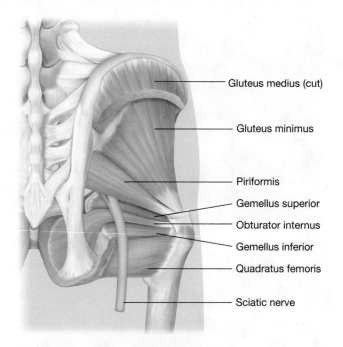

— Gluteus medius (cut)

— Gluteus minimus

— Piriformis

— Gemellus superior

— Obturator internus

— Gemellus inferior

— Quadratus femoris

— Sciatic nerve

FIGURE 13.52
"The deep six" **lateral hip rotators**

BRIDGE TO PRACTICE
Trigger Points in the Lateral Rotators

Although Travell only identifies TrP locations or pain referral patterns in the piriformis, the other five lateral rotators can also develop tender points or trigger points. A lot of clients find relief from general hip pain by having pointed pressure on tender points or TrPs in the lateral rotators. If your client has general hip pain in the buttocks region, check the belly of each lateral rotator for tender points or TrPs, then hold each point until the tenderness subsides.

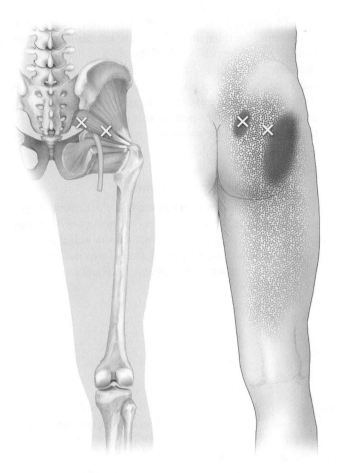

FIGURE 13.53

Myofascial pain specialist Janet Travell deemed the **piriformis** the "double devil" because spasms or chronic contractions in it can put pressure on the underlying sciatic nerve and also cause debilitating trigger points. When the piriformis becomes dysfunctional, it develops two trigger points: one directly lateral to the fifth sacral segment and the other midway between the sacrum and the greater trochanter. Both trigger points refer intense pain locally and produce spillover pain that radiates over the hamstrings and can even radiate up into the lower back.

thick, pear-shaped muscle is the only one of the deep six to arise from the axial skeleton. It passes directly over the large sciatic nerve running down the center of each buttock.

The piriformis is both a lateral rotator and abductor of the hip, although it becomes a medial hip rotator past 60 degrees of hip flexion. For this reason, sitting with the legs crossed places the piriformis in a shortened position, which can lead to piriformis syndrome. It shows up in six times as many women as men, which is not surprising given that women are more likely to sit with one knee crossed over the other.[3] **Piriformis syndrome** is a neuromuscular disorder that occurs when contractures in the piriformis muscle compress the sciatic nerve, resulting in a range of symptoms that include pain, tingling, and numbness in the posterior hip, thigh, and down the back of the leg. Piriformis syndrome usually occurs with a combination of three conditions: nerve and vascular entrapment, myofascial pain from piriformis TrPs, and sacroiliac joint dysfunction (Figure 13.53 ■). It is often aggravated by prolonged cross-legged sitting but can be effectively treated with a combination of myofascial release, trigger point therapy, and a stretching regime.

The **obturator internus** and **obturator externus** both arise from the membrane that fills the obturator foramen (Figure 13.54 ■). They sandwich the membrane on either side; the obturator externus covers the anterior side and the obturator internus covers the posterior side. The tendon of the obturator internus turns a 90-degree corner around the lateral ischium, passing below the ischial spine and inserting on the posterior lip of the greater trochanter. The tendon of the obturator externus runs up along an oblique angle across the back of the neck of the femur and inserts under the medial lip of the greater trochanter. The obturator internus works as a lateral rotator when the hip is extended and as an abductor when the hip is flexed. It also works as a medial hip rotator after 30–40 degrees of medial rotation because the greater trochanter moves in front of the vertical axis of the joint, causing an inversion of action.

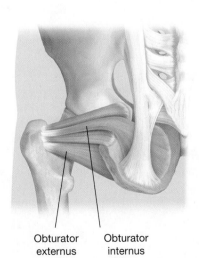

Obturator externus   Obturator internus

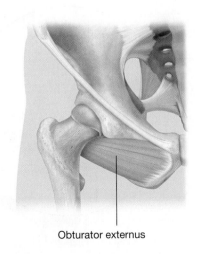

Obturator externus

FIGURE 13.54
Obturator internus and externus

The **quadratus femoris** arises from the lateral side of the ischial tuberosity and inserts on the intertrochanteric crest between the lesser trochanter and the greater trochanter. This large, fleshy muscle is oriented horizontally below the other lateral rotators. It is the most inferior of the group, is easy to palpate, and is often overlooked as a source of myofascial pain. When dysfunctional, it develops a tender point in its belly, which can be easily relieved with digital pressure.

The **gemellus superior** and **gemellus inferior** are two small muscles arising from the lateral edge of the ischial spine and the upper aspect of the ischial tuberosity, respectively. They run above and below the obturator internus and insert on the greater trochanter. All three muscles—the gemellus pair and the obturator internus—work together as a *triceps surae* (where three tendons converge) and are difficult to differentiate in palpation.

We usually think of the job of the deep six as laterally rotating the thigh under the pelvis, but during gait, they work to rotate the pelvis toward the thigh of the stance leg. Between heel strike and midstance, the pelvis makes a forward shift to come up and over the stance leg. During this shift, the lateral hip rotators on the stance side contract concentrically to rotate the pelvis toward the stance leg, and the lateral rotators on the swing side counter with an eccentric contraction (Figure 13.55 ■).

13.3.6 Perineal Muscles and the "Pelvic Floor"

The **perineal muscles** or **perineum** create a diamond-shaped muscular sling at the base of the pelvis, connecting four bony landmarks: the pubic bone, coccyx, and both ischial tuberosities. They include the **coccygeus** and the two muscles making up the **levator ani**—the *pubococcygeus* and *iliococcygeus*

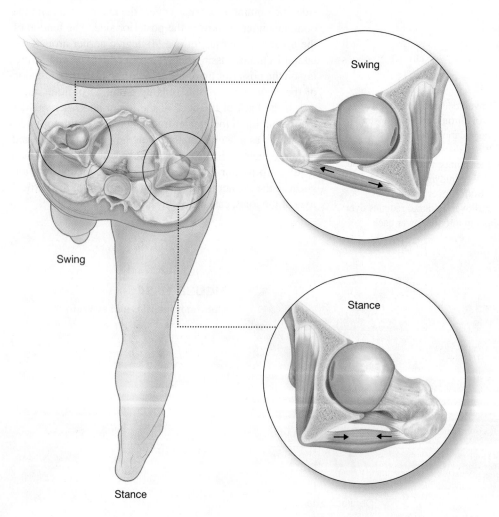

FIGURE 13.55

Lateral rotator function in gait

SELF-CARE
Stretching the Lateral Hip Rotators

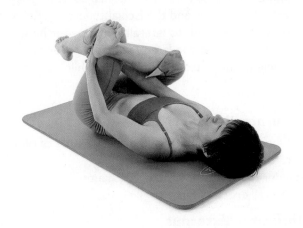

FIGURE 13.56a

1. Lie on your back in a neutral spine position with both knees bent and feet flat. To maintain a neutral spine, lightly contract your lower abdominal muscles, widen between your shoulder blades, and lengthen your neck.
2. To stretch the piriformis, place the leg of the side you want to stretch across the other knee, then pull that knee toward your chest (Figure 13.56a ■). As you stretch, make sure that both hips are touching the floor. Hold each stretch for at least 10 seconds.

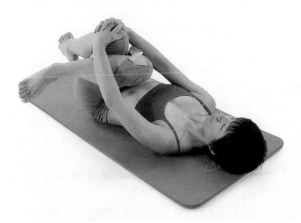

FIGURE 13.56b

3. To enhance the piriformis stretch, shift your knee to position it medial of the midline (Figure 13.56b ■).

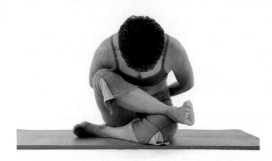

FIGURE 13.56c

4. You can also stretch the lateral hip rotators by sitting with one ankle crossed over the other knee, then leaning forward (Figure 13.56c ■).

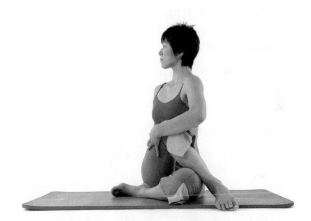

FIGURE 13.56d

5. If leaning forward is difficult, cross the foot over one knee and pull the knee toward your body (Figure 13.56d ■). Make sure to keep your spine aligned along the vertical axis as you twist. Also, keep both sit bones touching the floor.
6. Repeat every stretch you do on the other side.

MUSCLE PALPATION
"Deep Six" Lateral Hip Rotators

Self-palpation of the lateral hip rotators is easiest to feel when the muscles are contracting. In a standing position, press your fingertips into both buttocks between the greater trochanter and the ischial tuberosity. Relax the overlying gluteus maximus, then pivot on your heels and turn your feet out to laterally rotate your hips. You should feel the rotators contract under your fingertips. Explore the area the lateral rotators cover by palpating from the bottom of the greater trochanter to the middle of the buttock on one side while you are turning that foot in and out.

Piriformis

O–Anterior surface of the sacrum
I–Superior surface of the greater trochanter
A–Laterally rotates and abducts hip

Gemellus Superior

O–Ischial spine
I–Upper surface of greater trochanter
A–Laterally rotates hip

Gemellus Inferior

O–Upper aspect of ischial tuberosity
I–Upper surface of greater trochanter
A–Laterally rotates hip

Note: *It is difficult to discern individual muscles in the deep six, although you can palpate their approximate locations.*

Obturator Internus

O–Obturator membrane and posterior side of obturator foramen
I–Under medial lip of greater trochanter
A–Laterally rotates hip

Obturator Externus

O–Obturator membrane and anterior side of obturator foramen
I–Under medial lip of greater trochanter
A–Laterally rotates hip

Quadratus Femoris

O–Ischial tuberosity
I–Lower surface of greater trochanter
A–Laterally rotates hip

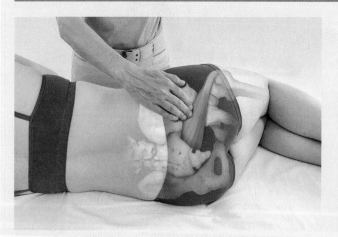

FIGURE 13.57a
Palpating the piriformis

With your partner in a side-lying position, locate the proximal attachment of the **piriformis** on the lateral side of the sacrum, midpoint between the PSIS and the coccyx. Approximate its location between this point and the middle of the sacroiliac joint, then press through the overlying gluteus maximus and strum across the belly of the piriformis (Figure 13.57a ■). Make sure the overlying gluteus maximus is relaxed.

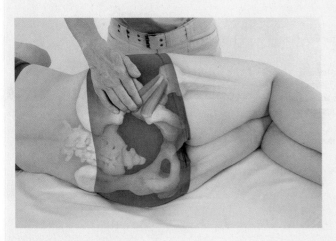

FIGURE 13.57b
Palpating the triceps surae

Palpate the **triceps surae**—the **gemellus inferior, gemellus superior,** and **obturator internus**—with your partner in a prone position. Locate the midpoint between the ischial tuberosity and the posterior side of the greater trochanter with a flat palpation, then strum across the bellies of these three rotators (Figure 13.57b ■). Use fairly deep pressure to press through the gluteus maximus. *Do you feel the fan of horizontal fibers when using cross-fiber strumming over the rotators?*

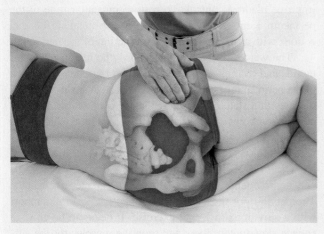

FIGURE 13.57c
Palpating the piriformis

Palpate **quadratus femoris** between the ischial tuberosity and the posterior, lower aspect of the greater trochanter (Figure 13.57c ■). Press deep to penetrate the overlying gluteal muscle. *Do you notice how the quadratus femoris is level with the gluteal fold?*

Active movement: Have your partner raise and lower the top knee while you palpate the contraction and relaxation of the rotators.

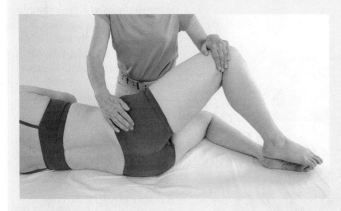

FIGURE 13.57d
Resisted movement of the lateral hip rotators

Resisted movement: In a prone position, have your partner bend the knee, then press against your hand on the inside of the ankle to contract the lateral hip rotators against resistance (Figure 13.57d ■).

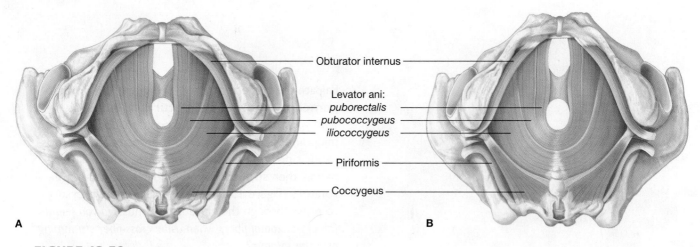

Obturator internus

Levator ani:
puborectalis
pubococcygeus
iliococcygeus

Piriformis

Coccygeus

A   B

FIGURE 13.58

The **perineal muscles:** a) Female b) Male

(Figure 13.58a-b ■). The perineum contains an anal orifice for the rectum and a vaginal opening for the vagina. The female pelvic floor is wider than the male pelvic floor to allow for childbirth. The obturator internus and piriformis form the posterior border of the perineum. Because the perineal muscles form a membrane with openings for the urethra and female genitals, this muscle group is referred to as the *urogenital diaphragm.* Because they form a muscular floor at the base of the pelvic cavity, the perineum is also known as the "pelvic floor".

There are several functional aspects of this muscle group to be aware of. The pelvic floor is also referred to as the "pelvic diaphragm" because it creates a horizontal muscular membrane across the base of the trunk that is responsive to the rhythm of respiration. As a person breathes, the pelvic floor lowers slightly to expand with inhalation, and rises slightly on exhalation. A person instinctively contracts the perineum to prevent urination, drawing this muscular hammock into the center and up. It also actively contracts during coughing, laughing, and weightlifting. A person bears down on the perineum during defecation and

childbirth. Women can lose muscular tone in the perineum after childbirth. Perineal muscle tone helps to increase intra-abdominal pressure during respiration. It can also help improve bladder control. To restore muscular tone in the perineum, Kegel exercises are often recommended. A Kegel is done with a strong rhythmic contraction of the perineum.

The weight of the pelvic organs—the rectum, bladder, uterus, and ovaries—rests on top of the muscular hammock of the perineal muscles. This constant load keeps the perineal muscles in a state of continuous tonic contraction. Perineal contraction helps stabilize the sacroiliac joints, which is an important postural response. In fact, the perineum co-contracts with the transversus abdominis as part of the postural stabilizing system. If the perineum weakens and overstretches, the pelvis girdle tends to widen between the greater trochanters. The pelvic-floor muscles can be toned for postural support with a slow-motion Kegel exercise. It needs to be slow to engage slow-twitch fibers and train the muscles for the sustained isometric contractions required to work under constant load. (See TrPs for the levator ani in Figure 13.59 ■.)

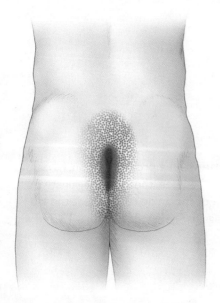

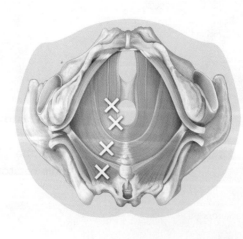

FIGURE 13.59

When dysfunctional, the **levator ani** can develop trigger points in four locations directly lateral to the anus and coccyx, which can refer pain and achiness over the sacrum and coccyx and into the vagina. Severe falls on the tailbone and prolonged slouching can activate trigger points in the perineum. *Due to the sensitive location of the perineum, treatment of perineal trigger points falls out of the scope of a massage practice.* Still, you may want to palpate the bony ridge from the pubic ramus to the ischial tuberosity and the muscles of your own pelvic floor to become familiar with this region of the body.

SELF-CARE
Exercises for the Perineal Muscles

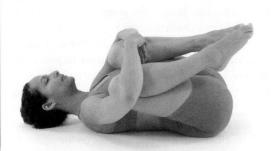

FIGURE 13.60a

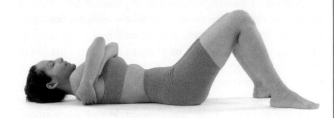

FIGURE 13.60b

Articulate movements of the pelvis performed by dancers and athletes involve coordinated movement between the pelvic floor and the trunk and the hips. Developing muscular control over the perineum can help you refine movement in the pelvis and hips and help you release muscular holding around the hips, pelvis, and lower back.

1. **Position to open pelvic floor:** Lie on your back and pull your knees to your chest (Figure 13.60a ■). Gently pull your lower abdominal wall into your lower back to lightly contract muscles in your lower abdomen. Imagine or feel your organs sinking into your lower back.
2. **Breathing:** Breathe into your sit bones and coccyx. As you breathe, imagine your coccyx and pelvic-floor muscles expanding on each inhalation, filling like a small balloon. Allow this expansion to lengthen your entire torso and lower back.
3. **Contract and relax:** Get in a supine position with your knees bent and feet flat on the floor (Figure 13.60b ■). Contract your pelvic floor by lightly drawing your sit bones closer together. This is the same contraction you would use to prevent urination. Keep your hip rotators and gluteals relaxed. If they contract, you are working too hard. Contract and relax your pelvic-floor muscles several times until you have control over these muscles.
4. **Coccygeal movements:** Stay in the same position and imagine your coccyx like a flashlight. Move the coccyx with a subtle motion to point its light toward the back of your knees, then down toward the floor, then toward one heel, then toward the other. Sense the subtle pelvic tilts and rotations that initiating motion at the coccyx creates.

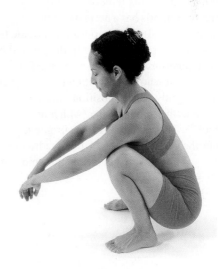

FIGURE 13.60c

5. **Squatting:** The squatting position opens the pelvic floor. Get into a squatting position that is comfortable for you (Figure 13.60c ■). You might need to use your hands to balance. Breathe into your coccyx and pelvic floor in this position.
6. **Standing:** In a standing position, slightly bend both knees. Imagine your coccyx extending to the floor like a long tail, then draw circles and figure eights on the floor. Sense the motion through your pelvic floor and in your hips. Then reverse the motion and move in the opposite direction.

Squatting stretches the area around the coccyx and opens the pelvic floor, creating an ideal position for elimination and childbirth. Women have traditionally birthed in this position, sometimes on squatting stools. A number of Asian cultures still commonly sit in a squatting position, which lengthens the lower back and may even relieve tension in it. It is also a useful position to assume occasionally to maintain flexibility in the hips and stretch the tissues around the tailbone. Squatting drops the abdominal organs into the back bottom of the pelvic bowl, giving the person more room to contract the lower abdominal muscles and hollow the lower abdomen. This can be helpful for people who have trouble sensing or controlling muscles in the area below the navel. Also, finding the subtle movements of the tail can help a person develop more articulation in the pelvic floor, which can release tension in the hips.

13.3.7   Rectus Femoris and Hamstring Balance

We covered the functions of the rectus femoris and hamstrings in the knee chapter. Now we look at how they function at the hip. The rectus femoris is a primary hip flexor. When the rectus femoris has a normal resting length, the hip can extend in a neutral standing posture. Chronic tightness in the rectus femoris pulls the hip into flexion and pulls the pelvis into an anterior tilt (Figure 13.61 ■). This pattern is evident in a person who stands with an anterior pelvic tilt, the hips in a slightly flexed position, and an exaggerated lordotic curve in the lumbar spine (which most people call a "sway back"). This pattern creates chronic tightness and shortness in the rectus femoris of the quadriceps, as well as the quadratus lumborum and the erector spinae muscles.

It is a common pattern for people who spend a lot of time sitting, who have weak hamstrings, and who have hip joint pain from arthritis that increases during hip extension. In a normal range of rectus femoris elasticity, a person should be able to kneel on both knees with the pelvis level.

Massage practitioners often develop tightness in the rectus femoris from bending over a massage table or from working in a bent-knee stance. To counter this tendency, work in an upright posture whenever possible. Also, avoid the bent-knee stance, better known as the "horse stance," for biomechanical reasons. A bent-knee stance requires sustained isometric muscular contraction, which compresses the hips and knees and contributes to adaptive shortening from isometric tension. In contrast, an upright stance places the hips and knees in a joint neutral position, which allows the muscle to lengthen and minimizes stress on the joints. In addition, an upright stance is congruent with gait mechanics.[4] Ideally, each step a person takes in walking begins from an upright posture with hips in the extended position, which places the rectus femoris in a position of ideal length.

On the back side of the hips, the hamstrings work as the hip extensors. When the hip is in the extended position, the hamstrings stabilize the hip joint and level the pelvic bowl, anchoring the ischial tuberosities down in an optimal position. The hamstrings prevent the pelvic bowl from tipping anteriorly. When the pull of the hamstrings overpowers the pull of the hip flexors and rectus femoris, the pelvic bowl will tip into a posterior tilt. Chronic tightness in the rectus abdominis often accompanies short hamstrings and contributes to a posterior pelvic tilt. (Figure 13.62 ■)

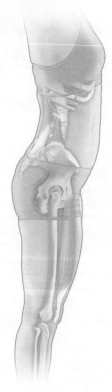

FIGURE 13.61

Rectus femoris tightness results in an anterior pelvic tilt.

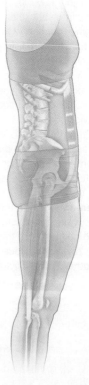

FIGURE 13.62

Hamstring tightness results in a posterior pelvic tilt.

EXPLORING TECHNIQUE
Quadriceps Length Assessment and Stretch

1. **Getting ready:** Put the quadriceps into a position of stretch, from which it can be stretched even farther. The hips should lie flat against the table with your partner in a prone position. If they do not, then hip flexors could be tight, so place traction on each thigh to open and lengthen the front of the hip joint.

2. **Quadriceps length assessment:** Stabilize the posterior hip by placing one hand above the ischial tuberosity and pressing the hip toward the table. Passively flex the knee as far as it will go (Figure 13.63a ■). If the quadriceps has normal length, the heel will touch the buttocks. The lower back and hip joint should remain still as you flex the knee. If the quadriceps is chronically tight and short, the heel will stop short of the buttocks.

   a. If the hip flexes as you bring the heel to the buttock, the rectus femoris is tight (Figure 13.63b ■).

   b. If the hip remains flat on the table but the heel does not reach the buttock, the vasti muscles are tight.

   c. If the hip flexes and the heel fails to reach the buttocks, both the rectus femoris and vasti muscles are tight.

3. **Quadriceps stretch:** Slowly bend the knee and take the heel toward the hip until your partner reports a stretch (see Figure 13.63a). When your partner reports feeling a stretch, hold it there for several seconds, then slowly release. Be careful not to stretch too far too fast.

4. **Quadriceps stretch with post-isometric relaxation:** With the knee bent, have your partner lightly press the ankle against your resistance to extend the knee and contract the quadriceps (see Figure 13.63b). Then have your partner relax. Once your partner completely relaxes, slowly take the heel toward the hip to repeat the stretch. Again, ask for feedback and be careful not to overstretch the quadriceps. The quadriceps should stretch farther due to the post-isometric relaxation response.

5. Repeat the assessment and stretch routine on the other side.

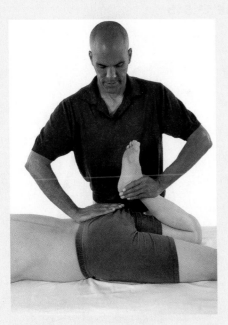

FIGURE 13.63a

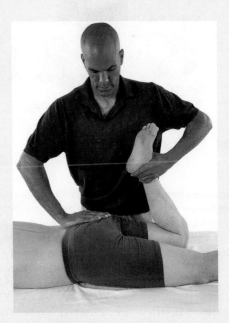

FIGURE 13.63b

EXPLORING TECHNIQUE
Hamstring Length Assessment and Stretch

1. **Getting ready:** Begin with your client in the supine position. If needed, reposition the thigh and leg so that the knee, foot, and hip align along the mechanical axis of the lower limb. Instruct your client to do a light isometric contraction in the lower abdominal muscles to stabilize the pelvis. Otherwise, your partner's pelvis may go too far into a posterior tilt as you flex the hip, which will skew the assessment by allowing the hip to flex farther than it actually can.

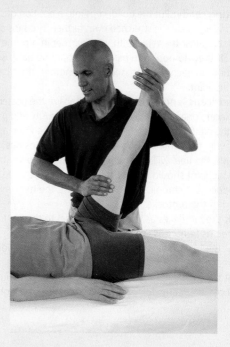

FIGURE 13.64b

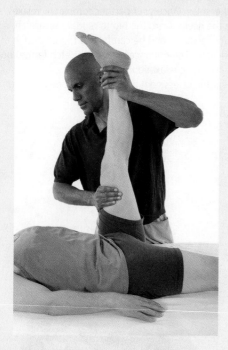

FIGURE 13.64a

2. **Hamstring length assessment:** Place one hand above the knee and the other hand below the ankle. Straighten your partner's knee. Keep the knee straight while you raise the lower limb (Figure 13.64a ■). Make sure to move the limb in the sagittal plane so that the knee stays aligned with the hip. Hip flexion to 90 degrees with an extended knee is normal. If hip flexion falls short of 90 degrees, the hamstrings are tight.

3. **Hamstring stretch with post-isometric relaxation:** Hold your partner's lower limb in the position of the hamstring stretch. Have your client press the leg lightly against your resistance to contract the hamstrings for several seconds (Figure 13.64b ■). Then have your partner relax the hamstrings. After your partner has relaxed the hamstrings for several seconds, stretch the hamstrings by taking the hip into deeper flexion.

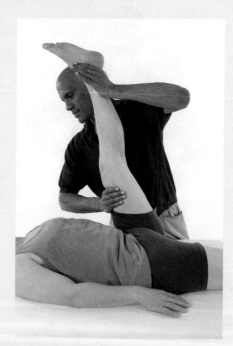

FIGURE 13.64c

4. **Hamstring stretch with reciprocal inhibition:** As you stretch the hamstrings, have your partner contract the antagonist, the quadriceps, which will enhance the stretch (Figure 13.64c ■).

5. Repeat the entire assessment and stretch on the other side.

SELF-CARE
Stretching the Hip Muscles

To effectively stretch the pelvic muscles, make sure to begin each stretch from a neutral spine position with your pelvis level. Also, contract your lower abdominals to stabilize your lumbar spine.

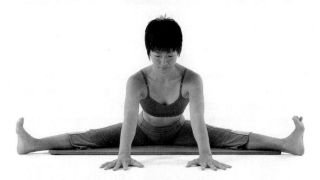

FIGURE 13.65a

1. **Adductor stretch:** Sit on the ground with your legs out at your sides in an upright neutral spine position. Make sure both ischial tuberosities are touching the ground evenly. Slowly lean forward at your hips to stretch the adductors; enhance the stretch by dorsiflexing your ankles and also contracting the quadriceps (Figure 13.65a ■). Hold until after you feel the adductors lengthen.

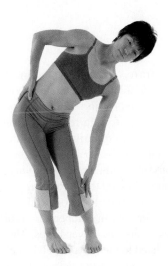

FIGURE 13.65b

2. **Gluteus medius stretch:** Stand in an upright position with your legs straight or bent, whichever is easiest for you. Push your right hip to the side and lean your trunk to the opposite side (Figure 13.65b ■). You should feel a stretch in the

muscles around the greater trochanter, especially in the gluteus medius. Hold a few seconds once you feel the gluteus medius on the right lengthen. Relax and repeat on the other side.

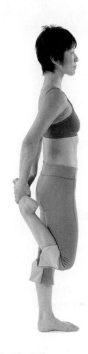

FIGURE 13.65c

3. **Vasti stretch:** Stand in an upright position, then bend one knee and pull that foot toward the back of your hip (Figure 13.65c ■). Hold until after you feel the vasti muscles above the knee lengthen, then relax and repeat on the other leg.

(continued)

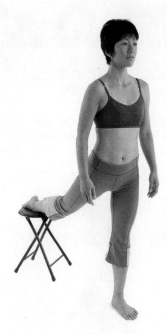

FIGURE 13.65d

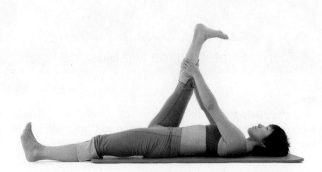

FIGURE 13.65e

5. **Hamstring stretch:** Lie on your back with your spine in neutral. Raise one leg and pull your calf toward your head. Keep the knee straight and avoid tucking the pelvis. If you cannot reach your calf, pull your pant leg, or sling a towel around your calf and use the towel to pull it toward you. To enhance the stretch, contract your quadriceps (Figure 13.65e ■). Hold until after you feel the hamstrings lengthen, then relax and repeat on the other leg.

4. **Rectus femoris stretch:** Stand in front of a stool or low chair. Place the shin of your right leg on the chair, making sure to keep your pelvis facing forward, your leg directly behind you, and your pelvis level (Figure 13.65d ■). This will allow you to stretch the rectus femoris across both the hip and the knee. Hold until after you feel the rectus femoris lengthen, then relax and repeat on the other leg.

In a normal range of hamstring elasticity, a person should be able to do a straight-leg raise to 90 degrees while maintaining a neutral spine. Hamstring weakness usually accompanies chronic tightness in the hip flexors, which pull the pelvis into an anterior tilt. The hamstrings tend to become chronically shortened and fibrous from either overuse or inactivity, which then pulls the pelvis into a posterior pelvic tilt and restricts hip flexion and forward bending As compensation to hamstring tightness, a person tends to hyperflex the lumbar spine, then has trouble extending the lumbar spine.

CONCLUSION

The ball-and-socket joint of each hip has the dual functions of supporting weight and moving freely in all three planes. The strategic location of these joints between the pelvis and the lower limb allows them to transmit ground reaction from the legs into the trunk and transfer the load of the trunk into the legs. Weight travels from the spine into the sacrum first, then into the circular arches of the pelvic girdle, and next into the coxofemoral joints of the hips. Although the bones of the pelvis form a relatively fixed and rigid bowl, the torque produced during gait as the legs swing and the spine rotates is absorbed by a slight give in both the pubic symphysis and the sacroiliac joints.

Although rarely injured thanks to their size and stability, the hips are susceptible to myofascial pain generated by muscles that overwork in compensation for bony misalignments in the trunk and lower limbs. The most common problems related to the hip and pelvis are posture and movement dysfunctions, sciatic pain and sacroiliac joint instability, chronic pelvic tilts that cause premature wear on the articular cartilage of the femoral head, and trochanteric bursitis. Fortunately, many of these functional problems can be prevented or alleviated through exercises to improve the alignment of the pelvis and hips, as well as massage and bodywork techniques for balancing the muscles in this area of the body.

SUMMARY POINTS TO REMEMBER

1. The four primary bones of the hips and pelvis are the femur, the coxal bone, the sacrum, and the coccyx. Each coxal bone is made up of three bones called the pubis, the ischium, and the ilium.

2. The femur has several important attachment sites for hip muscles, including the bony landmarks of the greater trochanter, lesser trochanter, and linea aspera. The head of the femur tapers into the neck of the femur, a lateral overhang that projects the shaft of the femur away from the hip joint.

3. Several important bony landmarks on the hips include the iliac crest, anterior superior iliac spine, anterior inferior iliac spine, posterior superior iliac spine, ischial tuberosities, pubic crest and pubic ramus, the median sacral crest, and the sacral foramen.

4. The anatomical name for the hip is the coxofemoral joint. It is a synovial ball-and-socket joint with a triaxial range of motion in all three planes.

5. Three large ligaments are attached to the coxofemoral joint. They are the iliofemoral or "Y" ligament, pubofemoral ligament, and the ischiofemoral ligament.

6. The angle between the neck and shaft of the femur is called the angle of inclination, which averages 135 degrees. The angle between the neck of the femur and the axis passing through the femoral condyles is called the angle of torsion.

7. The femur can move at the pelvis in six actions: flexion and extension, abduction and adduction, and lateral and medial rotation.

8. The pelvis can move on the femur in six actions: posterior and anterior tilt, right and left lateral tilt, and forward and backward rotation.

9. The lumbar pelvic rhythm—the coordinated movement between the lumbar spine and the hip joint—allows movement of the lumbar spine to increase the range of motion at the hip.

10. There are three joints in the pelvis: the pubic symphysis is a fibrocartilage, semimovable joint connecting the pubic bones across the pubic crest; the top half of the sacroiliac joint connecting the sacrum to the ilium is a synovial joint and the bottom half is a fibrous joint; and the sacrococcygeal joint is a fibrous, immovable joint.

11. Five sacral ligaments bind the sacrum and coccyx to the fifth lumbar vertebra and the coxal bones. These are the iliolumbar, sacroiliac, sacrotuberous, sacrospinous, and sacrococcygeal ligaments.

12. The pelvic ring is stabilized by forced closure of the sacrum wedged in between the coxal bones and the form closure of the transversus abdominis pulling the anterior ilia together.

13. The sacroiliac joints move with a small nodding motion in the sagittal plane called nutation, which rocks the top of the sacrum in the anterior direction, and counternutation, which rocks the top of the sacrum in the posterior direction.

14. Although the hip is rarely injured, it can develop these common dysfunctions: joint arthritis from premature wear on the hyaline cartilage, a loss of bone density that can lead to osteoporosis, hip fractures from falls, trochanteric bursitis, and labral tears.

15. The hip abductors are located on the lateral side of the hip. The tensor fascia latae is also a medial rotator and hip flexor; the sartorius is also a hip flexor and lateral rotator; and the gluteus medius is also a lateral and medial rotator of the hip.

16. The five adductors of the hip—the pectineus, adductor brevis, adductor longus, adductor magnus, and gracilis—are located along the inside of the thigh. Depending on the position of the joint, the adductors also work as hip flexors, extensors, and rotators.

17. There are three muscles in the iliopsoas: the iliacus, psoas major, and psoas minor. The iliacus and psoas major share a common tendon on the lesser trochanter, work as stabilizers and hip flexors, and assist lateral rotation of the hip.

18. There are three gluteal muscles. The largest, the gluteus maximus, covers the buttock and works as a powerful hip extensor, lateral rotator, and stabilizer; the gluteus medius is a primary abductor and stabilizer; the gluteus minimus is a medial rotator that assists flexion.

19. The six lateral hip rotators connecting the sacrum and coxal bones to the greater trochanter are called the "deep six" because they lie under the gluteus maximus. The only rotator attached to the sacrum, the piriformis, runs across the sciatic nerve. Piriformis spasm or contracture can cause sciatic nerve pain and develop into piriformis syndrome.

20. Perineal muscles at the base of the pelvis, including the levator ani and coccygeus, form a muscular sling that supports the pelvic organs, provides openings for the urethra and female genitals, and are collectively known as the perineum or pelvic floor.

21. The rectus femoris, a primary hip flexor, can pull the pelvis into an anterior pelvic tilt if it develops a chronic contracture. The hamstrings, primary hip extensors, can pull the pelvis into a posterior pelvic tilt if they develop chronic contractures.

REVIEW QUESTIONS

1. Name the four bones making up the pelvis.
2. The coxal bone of the pelvis is made up of the
   a. ilium, iliac fossa, and pubic symphysis.
   b. ischium, pubis, and iliac crest.
   c. ilium, ischium, and pubis.
   d. ischial spine, ilium, and pubis.
3. The superficial bony projections on the proximal third of the femur that provide attachment sites for the iliopsoas and the hip rotators are the
   a. lesser trochanter and greater trochanter.
   b. linea aspera and lesser trochanter.
   c. neck of the femur and greater trochanter.
   d. linea aspera and greater trochanter.
4. The technical name for the hip is the _____ joint.
5. The hip is made up of an articulation between the
   a. head of the femur and acetabulum.
   b. lesser trochanter and acetabular labrum.
   c. greater trochanter and the neck of the femur.
   d. head of the femur and neck of the femur.
6. The structure that deepens the hip socket is the
   a. zona orbicularis.
   b. acetabular labrum.
   c. Y ligament.
   d. joint capsule.
7. List the three main ligaments stabilizing the coxofemoral joint and name their general location.
8. Name the six movements of the pelvis on the femur.
9. True or false (circle one). The femur moves at the pelvis during forward bending of the trunk.
10. The lumbar pelvic rhythm refers to
    a. the coordinated movement between the hips and the sacroiliac joints.
    b. the coordinated movement between the hips and pubic symphysis.
    c. the coordinated movement between the hips and the knee.
    d. the coordinated movement between the hips and the lumbar spine.
11. The three types of joints in the pelvic girdle are the
    a. sacroiliac joints, the pubic symphysis, and the ischiotuberous joint.
    b. sacroiliac joint, the pubic symphysis, and the puboccoccygeal joint.
    c. sacroiliac joints, the pubic symphysis, and the sacrococcygeal joint.
    d. sacroiliac joints, the pubic tubercles, and the sacrococcygeal joint.
12. Which ligament binds the sacrum to the ischial tuberosity?
    a. sacrospinous ligament
    b. sacrotuberous ligament
    c. sacroiliac ligament
    d. sacrococcygeal ligament
13. The nodding motions of the sacrum are called _____ and _____.
14. The three primary hip abductors are the
    a. tensor fascia latae, sartorius, and gluteus maximus.
    b. tensor fascia latae, sartorius, and gluteus minimus.
    c. tensor fascia latae, sartorius, and gluteus medius.
    d. tensor fascia latae, sartorius, and gracilis.
15. What is the distal tendon of the TFL and how does tension in this tendon affect the knee?
16. Which of the four adductor muscles is a biarticular muscle acting on both the hip and the knee?
    a. the gracilis
    b. the adductor magnus
    c. the adductor longus
    d. the adductor brevis
17. True or false (circle one). The gluteus minimus is a hip abductor and medial rotator.
18. Which of the six lateral hip rotators—the piriformis, gemellus superior and gemellus inferior, obturator internus and obturator externus, and the quadratus femoris—has an origin on the axial skeleton and where does it attach?
19. When the rectus femoris overpowers the hamstrings, it can shift the pelvis into which of the following positions?
    a. a posterior pelvic tilt
    b. a forward pelvic rotation
    c. a lateral pelvic tilt
    d. an anterior pelvic tilt
20. True or false (circle one). The psoas major is a primary and powerful hip flexor.

Notes

1. Orthopedist Rene Calliet first described the lumbar pelvic rhythm in his groundbreaking text *Low Back Pain Syndrome* (published by F. A. Davis). It is also referred to as the "pelvic lumbar," "lumbopelvic," "pelvicfemoral," and "femoralpelvic" rhythm by other writers.

2. Basmajian, J., & DeLuca, C. (1985). *Muscles Alive: Their Functions Revealed by Electromyography* (5th ed.). Baltimore: Williams & Wilkins.

3. Simons, D., Travell, J., & Simons, L. (1999). *Myofascial Pain and Dysfunction: The Trigger Point Manual: Vol. 2. The Lower Extremities* (2nd ed.). Baltimore: Lippincott, Williams, & Wilkins.

4. Foster, M. (2005, April/May). A Case for the Human Stance. *Massage and Bodywork Magazine,* pp. 72–81.

CHAPTER

14   The Spine

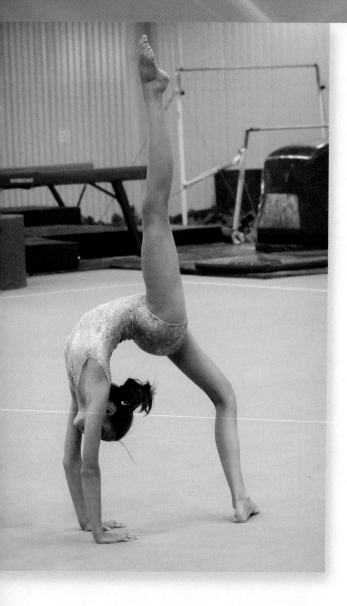

CHAPTER OUTLINE

Chapter Objectives

Key Terms

14.1 Bones of the Spine

14.2 Joints and Ligaments of the Spine

14.3 Muscles of the Spine

Conclusion

Summary Points to Remember

Review Questions

Unlike the knee, which has only two fibrocartilage disks, the spine has 24 of them. A series of long, strapping ligaments binds each disk between adjacent vertebral bodies, creating a tightly packed cylinder with 24 bendable segments. This osteoligamentous column is sturdy enough to absorb high levels of axial compression and flexible enough to bend in every direction. The incredible flexibility of the spine is most evident in the extreme backbends of gymnasts, especially during aerial jumps involving flips and weight shifts between the hands and feet.

The average person can keep the spine healthy by taking it through a full range of movement on a daily basis. The sun-salutation

from yoga moves the spine and hips through complete flexion and extension cycles. Side-bending and twisting yoga stretches take the spine through lateral motion and rotation. Or people can make up their own routines, moving the spine in each direction with dance movements or calisthenics. Whatever type of routine a person chooses, the challenge is to get movement to sequence through each vertebral segment, particularly in stiff areas. Massage and manual therapies can also improve spinal mobility by loosening joint structures and normalizing muscle tone in a way that improves muscular balance.

 CHAPTER OBJECTIVES

1. List the three parts of the spine and the number of vertebrae in each part.

2. Define and contrast kyphotic and lordotic curves and identify their locations in the spine.

3. Name and describe the typical features of a vertebra.

4. Demonstrate palpation of the spinal curves, spinous processes, and the lamina groove.

5. Name and describe the two types of spinal joints and their supporting ligaments.

6. Identify the normal range of motion in each part of the spine.

7. Identify the origins, insertions, and actions of the three layers of posterior spinal muscles.

8. Demonstrate the active movement and palpation of each posterior spinal muscle.

9. Identify the trigger points and pain referral patterns of the posterior spinal muscles.

10. Identify the origins, insertions, and actions of the abdominal muscles.

11. Demonstrate the active movement and palpation of each abdominal muscle.

12. Identify the trigger points and pain referral patterns of the abdominal muscles.

 KEY TERMS

Atlas	Facet joint	Paravertebral
Axis	Iliolumbar ligament	Prevertebral
Cervical	Interbody joint	Spinous process
Coupled motion	Intervertebral disk	Supraspinous ligament
Cranial protraction	Kyphosis	Thoracic
Cranial retraction	Lamina groove	Thoracolumbar fascia
Dens process	Lordosis	Transverse process
Erector spinae	Lumbar	Vertebral body

MUSCLES IN ACTION

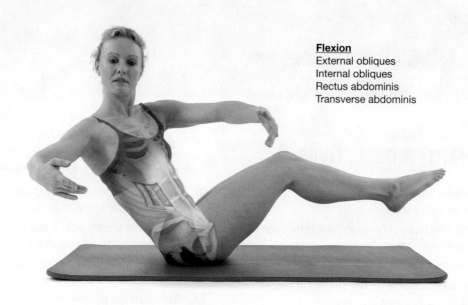

Flexion
External obliques
Internal obliques
Rectus abdominis
Transverse abdominis

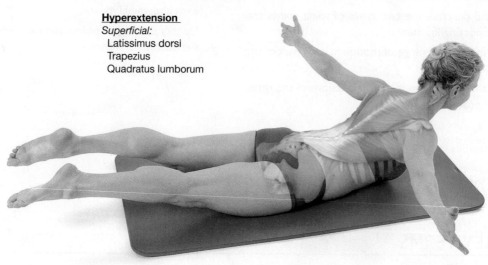

Hyperextension
Superficial:
  Latissimus dorsi
  Trapezius
  Quadratus lumborum

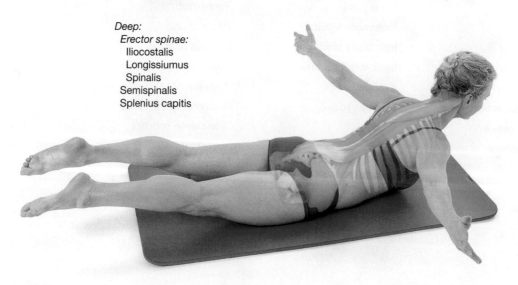

Deep:
 Erector spinae:
  Iliocostalis
  Longissiumus
  Spinalis
 Semispinalis
 Splenius capitis

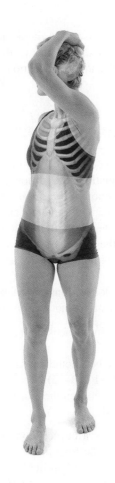

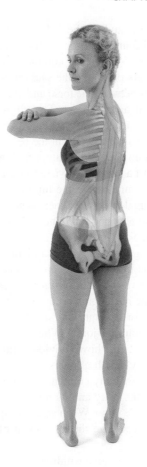

Rotation

Erector spinae:
  Iliocostalis
  Longissiumus
  Spinalis
External obliques
Internal obliques
Splenius capitis
Spelnius cervicis
Sternocleidomastoid
Transversospinalis

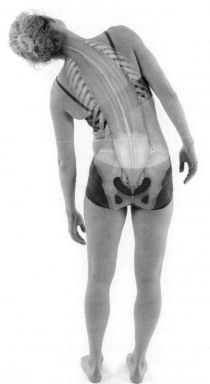

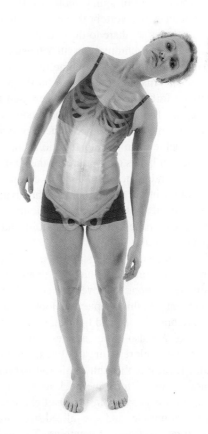

Lateral Flexion

Erector spinae:
  Iliocostalis
  Longissiumus
  Spinalis
External obliques
Internal obliques
Quadratus
  lumborum (unilateral)

In the previous chapter we studied the pelvis and hips, which provide a structural foundation for the spine. In this chapter, we look at the spine—a stacked column of vertebral segments. The spine sits on top of the sacrum, which channels mechanical forces between the torso and the lower extremities in a reciprocal arrangement. The alignment and balance of the spine is affected by the alignment of the hips and pelvis. Even a small rotation in the pelvis can transfer into the spinal column where it is amplified by the many vertebral joints that can become twisted or chronically bent. As a result, asymmetries in the hip and pelvis can cause or exacerbate spinal curvatures such as scoliosis, leading to chronic muscular tensions and joint dysfunctions throughout the torso and neck.

As we journey through the complex and intricate structures of the spine, it is important to realize its central role in the vertical support of the entire trunk and movement of the torso. The spine is complex because it consists of so many individual vertebrae, joints, and muscles. Each muscle of the spine acts on multiple joints. When looking at the muscles of the spine, consider how individual muscles can generate motion in many vertebral joints. Most people think of the spine as a narrow bony column, but in fact it extends into the middle of the body and its muscular connections fan out into the whole torso. When studying spinal movement, it is helpful to visualize the movement of the whole trunk.

Each vertebral segment can move within a small range of motion. The total range of spinal motion reflects the sum of movement in many vertebral segments. Ideally, each segment contributes its share to the overall motion of the spine. However, when chronic muscular tensions and joint dysfunctions glue groups of vertebrae together, they will move in blocks. This increases stress on the mobile segments, which are forced to move under increased load. For example, if segments in the thoracic spine become rigid, the joints that are still mobile are forced to bend or twist in a greater range to achieve an overall functional range of motion. When a person bends over or arches the spine, the mobile joints move under increased load to compensate for the lack of motion in the fixated joints. This dynamic increases the mechanical stress on the moving joints, causing cumulative tissue damage that can lead to joint stability dysfunctions, pain, and injury.

A practitioner needs to understand specific spinal structures in order to restore a continuity of motion to the spine by releasing restrictions to movement around immobile vertebral segments. In this chapter, we look at the different types of vertebrae, joints, and ligaments of the spine and how they move. We also cover muscles acting on the vertebral column and explore their structures, functions, and trigger point locations through palpation exercises. Although we are going to study the neck as part of the vertebral column in this chapter, in the head chapter, we will look at the throat muscles and specialized structures in the neck related to jaw motion and breathing. Throughout

this chapter, spinal exercises and therapeutic applications are presented, as well as discussions of the central role of posture in spinal health and the prevention of back pain and injury.

14.1   BONES OF THE SPINE

The spine is a segmented, curved column made up of 24 vertebrae. Its main functions are to house and protect the spinal cord, provide a bony core of support for the torso and head, allow movement of the torso, and provide attachment sites for soft tissues and muscles. Many of the vertebrae and muscles in the spine and torso can be identified by observing prominent landmarks in the topical anatomy (Figure 14.1 ■).

There are three major sections of vertebrae in the spine: the cervical, thoracic, and lumbar sections (Figure 14.2 ■).

- The **cervical** spine in the neck has seven vertebrae (C-1 to C-7).
- The **thoracic** spine between the neck and lower back has 12 vertebrae (T-1 to T-12).
- The **lumbar** spine between the thorax and the sacrum has five vertebrae (L-1 to L-5).

The human spine is a curved column that evolved to bend and flex under the load of axial compression. A curved column is highly resilient because it can flex and bend under stress and withstand up to 10 times as much mechanical stress and compression as a straight column. Each part of the spine curves in either the anterior or posterior direction. The degree of curvature in the spine varies among individuals and affects the position of the sacrum (Figure 14.3 ■).

As mentioned in the chapter on posture, an anterior curve is called a **lordosis** or lordotic curve; a posterior curve is called a **kyphosis** or kyphotic curve. The kyphotic curve is known as a primary curve because it develops first, in utero, from the curled position of the fetus. A newborn arrives with its spine flexed in a primary kyphotic curve (Figure 14.4 ■). The lordotic curves of the neck and lower back develop in the spine in response to gravity. As the infant lifts the head, a lordosis forms in the cervical spine; as the infant pushes up from a prone position and crawls on its way to sitting and standing, a lordosis forms in the lumbar spine (Figure 14.4).

The vertebrae are the building blocks of the spine. Understanding the basic structure of a vertebra and the differences in the cervical, thoracic, and lumbar areas builds a foundation for learning about the posture and movement functions of the spine. For example, in order to support weight, the vertebrae grow increasingly larger from the top to the bottom of the spine (Figure 14.5 ■).

All the vertebrae have an irregular shape but a similar structure. A typical vertebra has a bony projection that extends posteriorly called the **spinous process** (SP)

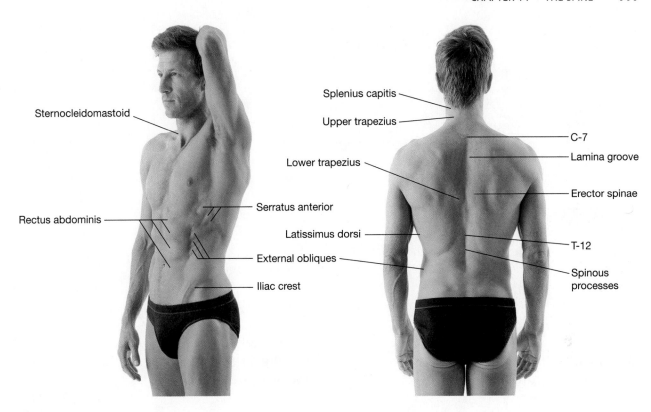

FIGURE 14.1

Surface anatomy of the spine and trunk

FIGURE 14.2

The spine

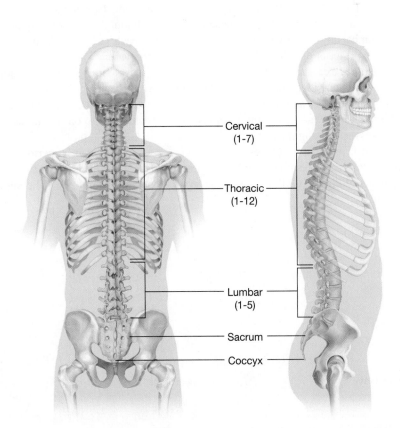

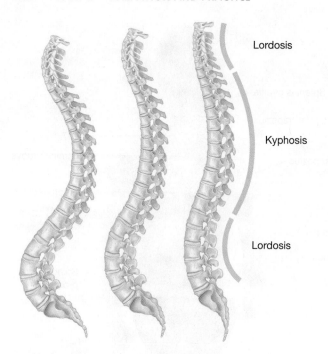

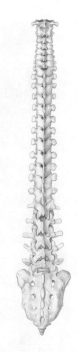

Lordosis

Kyphosis

Lordosis

FIGURE 14.3

Types of spinal curves

FIGURE 14.5

The spine: posterior view

(Figure 14.6 ■). The SPs provide attachment sites for soft tissues such as ligaments and tendons, and they also serve as lever arms for spinal motion. The shape of the spinous processes in each section of the spine varies (Figure 14.7 ■). The cervical SPs are bifurcated and slant down at a 45-degree angle. The thoracic SPs are longer, more slender, and slant down at a sharper angle than those in the cervical spine. The lumbar SPs are large, square, and project straight back in the posterior direction.

Each vertebra also has a **transverse process** (TP) that projects laterally off to each side. The TPs also provide attachment sites for soft tissues and serve as lever arms for movement. A practitioner can determine the location of a vertebra and assess spinal alignment by palpating the spinous processes and transverse processes of the vertebrae. Ideally, the spinous processes align vertically and are usually easy to palpate along the midline. The transverse

processes can be more difficult to palpate depending on their location and the thickness of overlying tissues.

Each vertebra has an oval **vertebral body** that provides a weight-bearing structure. A large opening posterior to the body of a vertebra, called a **vertebral foramen,** provides a channel for the spinal cord to pass through the vertebral column. A bony arm connecting the body of the vertebrae to each transverse process is called the **pedicle.** A bony arch connecting the TPs to the SP is called the **lamina** of the vertebra. A column of adjacent lamina creates a groove along each side of the spine called the **lamina groove.** The lamina groove is easy to palpate and apply pressure point techniques to on the thoracic spine, which can be effective in loosening tissues in the mid- and upper back.

A concave superior and inferior **articular process** (facet) projects from the pedicle of each vertebra in the posterior direction. The superior articular processes face

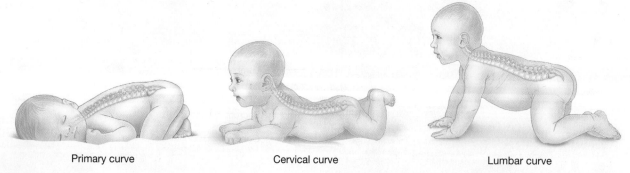

Primary curve   Cervical curve   Lumbar curve

FIGURE 14.4

Development of spinal curves

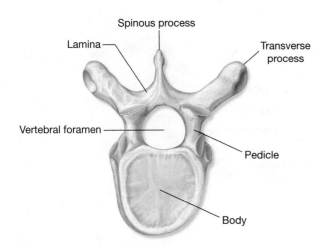

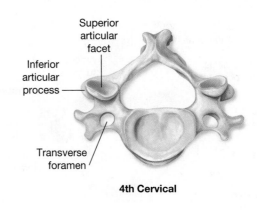

4th Cervical

FIGURE 14.6
Structure of a typical vertebra

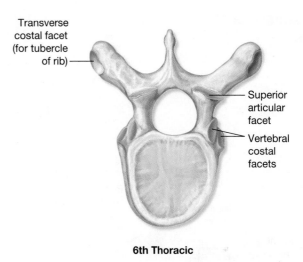

6th Thoracic

backward; the inferior articular processes face forward. The facets overlap like shingles, forming small facet joints along the posterior spine. Each thoracic vertebra also has three small **costal facets** on its transverse process that provide articulating joint surfaces for matching costal facets on the ribs. In the cervical spine, the facet joints are stacked in an arrangement that forms an **articular pillar**—a groove along either side of the spinous processes along the posterior neck.

The first cervical vertebra, the **atlas,** supports the weight of the cranium and is named after the Titan in Greek mythology who holds up Earth. The ring-shaped atlas lacks a spinous process but has two large concave depressions on its superior surface that articulate with two convex condyles on the base of the occiput (Figure 14.8 ■). The second cervical vertebra, the axis, has a unique, peg-like projection called the **dens process** or ondontoid process (Figure 14.9a ■). Like a finger in a ring, the dens process projects up into the atlas, providing a pivotal axis for rotational movement of the head (Figure 14.9b ■). Each cervical vertebra has a small opening between the pedicle and transverse process called a **transverse foramen** that provides a protective tunnel for the vertebral artery (Figure 14.10 ■).

14.2 JOINTS AND LIGAMENTS OF THE SPINE

Movement of the spine occurs in two kinds of joints: the interbody joints along the front of the spine and the facet joints along the back of the spine. Each vertebral segment has both kinds of joints. They vary in size and shape in each area of the three areas of the spine, which reflect the differences of range of motion and weight-bearing capacities in the cervical, thoracic, and lumbar vertebrae.

Spinal movement is unique in several ways. Each joint in the spine moves within a small range that contributes to the overall movement of the spine. The sum of movement in the many spinal joints allows the spine to flex, hyperextend,

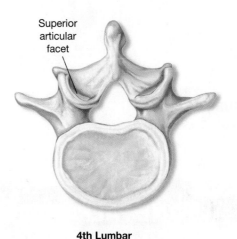

4th Lumbar

FIGURE 14.7
Types of vertebrae

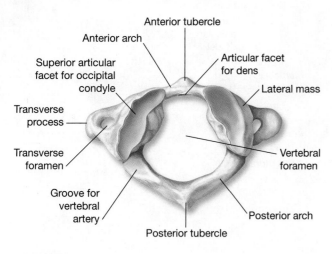

FIGURE 14.8

Atlas

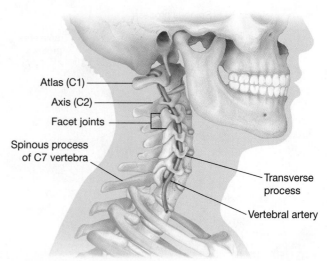

FIGURE 14.10

Transverse artery in cervical spine

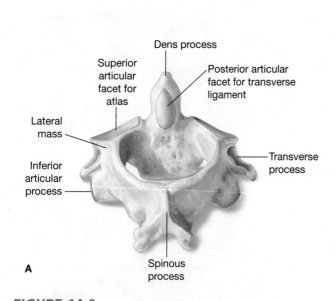

A

FIGURE 14.9

a) **Axis** b) **Dens Process**

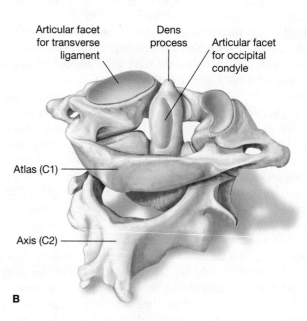

B

BONE PALPATION
The Vertebrae

Caution: *Avoid putting pressure on the transverse processes of the cervical spine because the vertebral artery passes through them via the vertebral foramen. Pressure on the artery could compromise circulation to the brain. The cervical TPs are located on the sides of the neck, on the most lateral edge of the articular pillar. Whenever working in this location, if you feel a pulse, move your touch off the pulse. If your partner reports any discomfort or pain, stop immediately.*

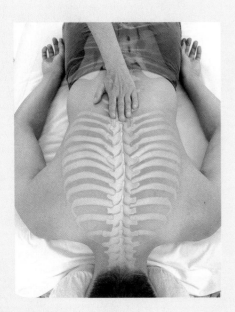

FIGURE 14.11a

With your partner in a prone position, palpate the **spinal curves** using flat, broad, general contact to slide your hand up and down your partner's spine, from the base of the neck to the sacrum. Notice the shape of the spine, where the curves change, and where they are concave and convex. Also notice where the vertebrae are prominent and easy to feel and where they disappear under tissue. *Where are the most prominent vertebrae? Do any areas of the curves deviate from normal, either sinking too far forward or sticking out too far backward? Do they align along the midline of the back or deviate in a lateral direction?* (See Figure 14.11a ■)

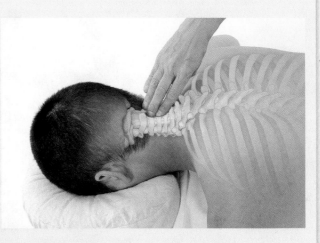

FIGURE 14.11b

With your partner still prone, palpate the **cervical spinous processes** (SPs) by carefully and gently pressing their small bony bumps along the midline of the posterior neck. The **SP of C-2** is the most prominent bump in the upper neck, about an inch below the occiput. The **SP of C-7** is the most prominent bony bump at the base of the neck. The SPs of **C-4 and C-5** are often difficult to find because they are shorter and tend to sink anteriorly. If they are hard to locate, have your partner press the back of the neck into your fingertips as you palpate them. *Do you feel two small points on the SP of C-2, which is bifurcated? Can you count down each of the seven cervical SPs? Do you feel the prominent SPs of C-6 and C-7 at the base of the neck?* (See Figure 14.11b ■)

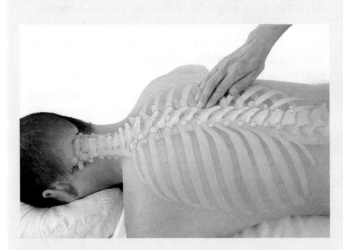

FIGURE 14.11c

From the SP of C-7, walk your fingertips down the easily observable row of small bony bumps of the **thoracic SPs.** Notice where they are prominent posteriorly and where they sink anteriorly (which could indicate areas of chronic flexion or hyperextension). Notice whether two SPs feel stuck together or feel too far apart. Also notice whether any SPs deviate in a lateral direction. *Do you notice how pointy the thoracic SPs are and how they point downward? Can you count down each of the 12 thoracic SPs? Are any of the SPs tender?* (See Figure 14.11c ■)

(continued)

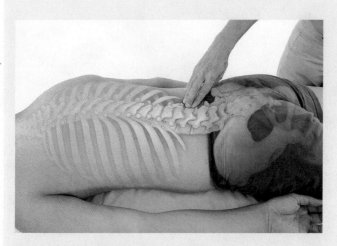

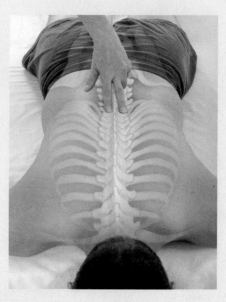

FIGURE 14.11d

Palpate the contours of the larger **lumbar SPs** in the lower back. Notice where they become buried in tissue and disappear anteriorly or where they are sore. *Do the lumbar SPs feel square? Do you count five lumbar SPs? Are they aligned in a row?* (See Figure 14.11d ■)

FIGURE 14.11e

To palpate the **lamina groove,** slide your index finger and middle fingers along the sides of the spine, between the SPs and the TPs. Move up and down as though your fingertips were skis sliding along a slope. *Does the lamina groove feel like a bony ditch? Are your fingertips between the SPs and the TPs? Do you notice areas that are sore, where there are knots, taut bands, or bumps?* (See Figure 14.11e ■)

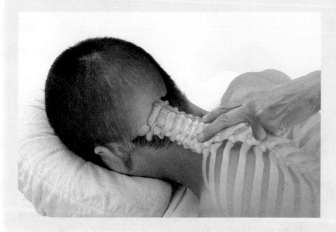

FIGURE 14.11f

With your partner first prone, then supine, palpate both sides of the **articular pillar** by placing the fingertips on a single SP, then sliding them laterally about one inch into the bony depression between the SP and the TPs. Press your fingertips straight up into the articular pillar, sinking through overlying tissue. Move down the neck one vertebral segment at a time, exploring each segment of the pillar with small, circular strokes. *Do you notice the small, ropey muscles filling the articular pillar? Do you feel any bumps in the articular pillar, which are the ligaments and joint capsules of the cervical facet joints?* (See Figure 14.11f ■)

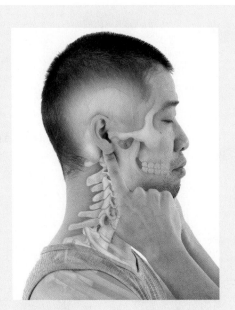

FIGURE 14.11g

Carefully and lightly palpate the **C-1 transverse process** (TP) in the hollow behind your ear, anterior to the mastoid process and behind the angle of the jaw. Avoid putting any pressure on it. If the neck is well aligned and the head can rock freely on the atlas, it feels like a small bump. *Do you feel the small bony bump in the soft spot right behind the earlobe, in front of the mastoid process? (See Figure 14.11g ■)*

and rotate in a whole body movement. Lateral flexion of the spine always occurs with some degree of rotation in a **coupled motion.**[1] As the lumbar and thoracic vertebrae laterally flex to the left, they rotate to the left; as they laterally flex to the right, they rotate to the right (Figure 14.12 ■). The pattern reverses in the cervical spine. As the neck laterally flexes to the left, the cervical vertebrae rotate to the right. As the neck laterally flexes to the right, the cervical vertebrae rotate to the left.

In a normal range of spinal motion in the sagittal plane, at end range of flexion the lumbar and cervical curves flatten and the thoracic curve increases (Figure 14.13a ■). At end range of spinal hyperextension, the lumbar and cervical curves increase and the thoracic curve flattens (Figure 14.13b ■).

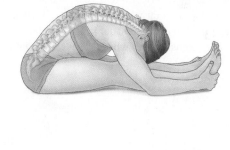

A

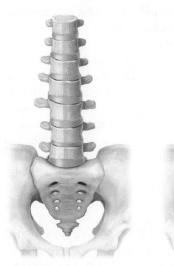

FIGURE 14.12
Coupled motion of the spine

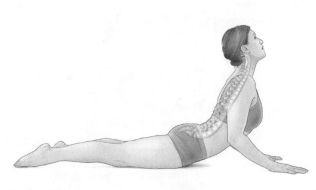

B

FIGURE 14.13
a) **Spinal flexion** b) **Spinal hyperextension**

14.2.1 Interbody Joints

The **interbody joints,** also called the **intervertebral joints,** are situated along the front of the spine (Figure 14.14 ■). These semimovable fibrocartilage joints are formed by the junction of an intervertebral disk with an adjacent vertebral body. The interbody joint surfaces are nearly flat through the lumbar and thoracic spine. In the cervical spine, interbody joint surfaces have a saddle shape. All of the interbody joints have a triaxial range of motion in all three planes and can also move in nonaxial linear motions such as forward and backward gliding (also called translation). Although the range of movement in a single interbody joint is minimal, their combined movement allows the spine to bend in long, graceful arcs.

Each **intervertebral disk** is made up of dense fibrocartilage that surrounds a spherical gelatinous core called the **nucleus pulposus** (Figure 14.15a ■). The nucleus pulposus consists of 70–90 percent water. The fibrocartilage contains **annulus fibers** organized in concentric rings, or bands, that contain 40–60 percent fluid. Over the course of a day, compression from body weight gradually squeezes fluid out of the nucleus of each disk. As a person sleeps, compressive stress is lifted and disks imbibe, reabsorbing fluid. This is why a person is an inch or two taller in the morning.

Intervertebral disks evolved to work under axial compression. They function as the shock absorbers of the spine, distributing and dissipating loads between consecutive vertebrae. The nucleus pulposus functions like a ball-bearing in the center of each disk, providing a malleable, sponge-like sphere around which the vertebral bodies can bend, swivel, and roll during spinal movement in all three planes (Figure 14.15b ■). During rotational movement of the spine, the annulus fibers in a vertebral disk twist and stretch, absorbing torsion stresses in their range of elasticity. Twisting or bending the spine beyond a normal range can tear the annulus fibers. The lumbar spine, which allows minimal rotation, is

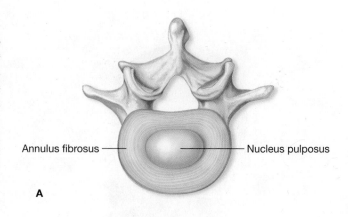

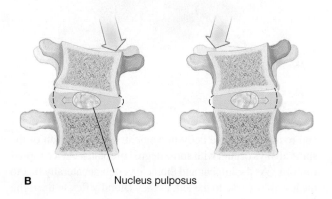

Annulus fibrosus — Nucleus pulposus

A

B — Nucleus pulposus

FIGURE 14.15

Vertebral disk: a) Superior view b) Nucleus pulposus as ball-bearing

susceptible to rotation injuries from activities such as golfing. To protect the lumbar spine from rotational injuries, a person needs to have good tone in the abdominal muscles wrapping the waist, especially in the oblique muscles.

The intervertebral disks narrow in circumference in the cervical region of the spine, become shorter in height in the thoracic region, and are the widest and tallest in the lumbar region. The cervical and lumbar disks have a wedge shape with a longer anterior side that supports the lordotic curves in the neck and lower back. The disks constitute about 25 percent of the total height of the vertebral column. Over the years, they gradually dehydrate and shrink under load, and they grow brittle. This explains why seniors lose height as they advance in age.

Axial load compresses a disk. The combination of daily compression with postural stresses and injuries can prematurely deteriorate the disks, tearing annulus fibers and squeezing fluid to one side of the disk, resulting in a **bulging disk** (Figure 14.16 ■). The annulus fibers can become so torn that the disk ruptures, resulting in a **herniated disk.** If a damaged disk presses on adjacent nerve roots, it can cause radiating pain down the hips and legs, which often occurs in the L-4 and L-5 segments of the lower back. This underscores the importance of applying massage and bodywork strokes in a direction that shifts the client's bones toward optimal alignment in every session.

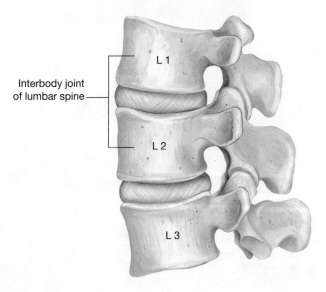

Interbody joint of lumbar spine —

L 1

L 2

L 3

FIGURE 14.14

Interbody joints

BRIDGE TO PRACTICE
Bulging Spinal Disks

If your client has a bulging disk in the lumbar spine, use lengthening strokes down the lower back, hips, and legs rather than upward strokes that could compress the lower back and exacerbate disk symptoms. You can also apply light traction to relieve minor pain coming from a bulging disk. Make sure to refer clients with persistent or unrelenting back pain for medical evaluation.

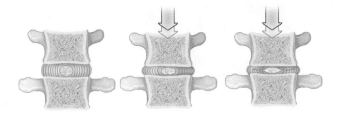

Normal disk   Normal disk under axial load   Diseased disk under axial load

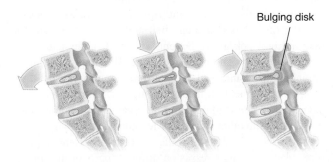

Bulging disk

Stages of disk deterioration

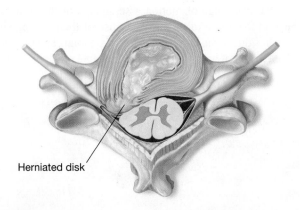

Herniated disk

FIGURE 14.16

The dynamics of **vertebral disk dysfunction and injury**

14.2.2 Facet Joints

The **facet joints,** or **apophyseal joints** (*apophysis* refers to bony "outgrowth"), are small synovial plane joints made up of articulations between vertebral facets. Each vertebral segment has two facet joints, one on each side. The articular surfaces of the facets in each section of the spine face a different direction (Figure 14.17 ■). The cervical facets orient along a 45-degree diagonal plane and are the most freely movable of all sections of the spine; the thoracic facets orient along the frontal plane and favor rotation; the lumbar facets orient along the sagittal plane and favor flexion and extension.

The cervical spine allows the greatest range of lateral flexion, an average of 45 degrees to each side (Figure 14.18 ■). Although the thoracic and lumbar sections of the spine can laterally flex to about the same degree, the 30 degrees of lateral flexion in the thoracic spine is distributed over 12 vertebral segments, which is slightly more than 2 degrees per segment. The ribs act as splints limiting the range of lateral flexion in the thoracic spine. In contrast, each lumbar segment can laterally flex twice as far as each thoracic segment, about 4 degrees. But the lumbar spine has an extremely limited range of lateral rotation because its facet joints are oriented in the sagittal plane and the joint surfaces bump into each other after 1 degree of rotation.

Ideally, spinal movement sequences through the many joints of the spine, from one end to the other. The range of each interbody joint and facet joint contributes to the overall motion of the spine. When each facet joint of the spine can move within its range during spinal movement, there will be a continuity of motion along the chain of joints.

When a client complains of back pain, a practitioner needs to make a general assessment about what tissue is generating pain: muscle and tendon, ligament, joint capsule, or disk. In the absence of a recent injury, structural abnormalities, or illness, postural patterns are suspect as a cause of back pain. Faulty postures can be assessed by observing the neutral position of the spine and determining which areas of the spine are habitually held in flexion, hyperextension, rotation, or lateral flexion. In faulty postures, some joints of the spine can become rigid and develop motion restriction,

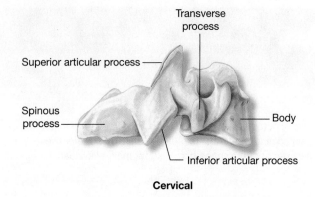

Cervical

- Superior articular process
- Transverse process
- Spinous process
- Body
- Inferior articular process

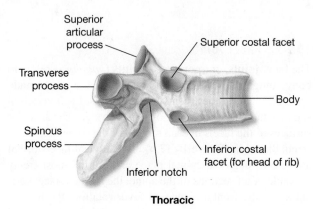

Thoracic

- Superior articular process
- Superior costal facet
- Transverse process
- Body
- Spinous process
- Inferior costal facet (for head of rib)
- Inferior notch

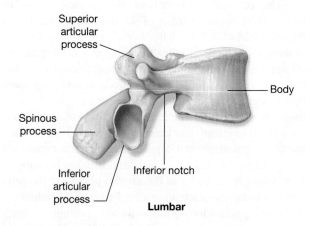

Lumbar

- Superior articular process
- Body
- Spinous process
- Inferior articular process
- Inferior notch

FIGURE 14.17

The orientation of the articular facet of each vertebra determines the movement range in that part of the spine.

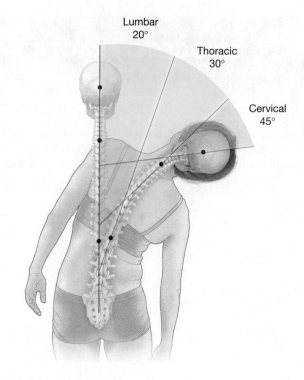

Lumbar 20°
Thoracic 30°
Cervical 45°

FIGURE 14.18

Range of lateral flexion in the spine

while others can develop stability dysfunctions from moving beyond a normal range. It is common for groups of adjacent vertebrae to become rigid and move as a block, causing the joints above and below the restricted areas to take up the slack, move beyond a normal range, and even shear (slide forward or back) or bend. Bending is the most damaging mechanical stress on a spinal joint because it tips a vertebral segment off its base of support, compressing one side of the spine while placing the ligaments, tendons, and muscles on the other side under tensional stress, which can lead to stretch weakness. Collapsed or hyperextended postures place bending stresses on different parts of the spine, usually in the center of the curves, such as the midcervical or midthoracic areas, or are at the junction of curves, such as the thoracolumbar junction.

Passive range of motion assessments of the spine are beyond the scope of this text because of their complexity, which is due to the intricacy of the spinal joints and the combined action of many facet joints in a single range of motion.

TABLE 14.1 **Range of Motion in the Spine**				
	Cervical Spine	**Thoracic Spine**	**Lumbar Spine**	*Total Range*
Flexion	40–60 degrees	30–40 degrees	50 degrees	120–150 degrees
Hyperextension	40–75 degrees	20–25 degrees	15 degrees	75–115 degrees
Lateral flexion to one side	45 degrees	30 degrees	20 degrees	95 degrees
Rotation to one side	50–80 degrees	30 degrees	5 degrees	85–115 degrees

SELF-CARE
Arcing Exercise for Spinal Movement

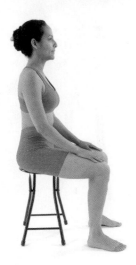

FIGURE 14.19a

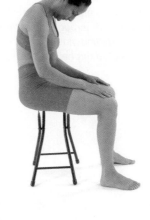

FIGURE 14.19b

(This exercise is adapted from a Rolfing Movement/Aston Patterning exercise.) Explore arcing slowly at first, moving one spinal segment at a time. Then speed it up to make the action more fluid and less controlled. For feedback, sit sideways to a mirror and watch yourself arc.

1. **Getting ready:** Begin sitting in a neutral, upright posture (Figure 14.19a ■). Stabilize your spine in neutral by lightly contracting your lower abdomen and lengthening your neck. Keep your lower abdomen contracted during the whole exercise.

2. **Flexing the spine:** Breathe in and as you exhale, rock into a posterior pelvic tilt. Let the flexion sequence up your spine one vertebra at a time, rounding it into a C-curve shape (Figure 14.19b ■). As you move, keep your shoulders wide and keep them over your hips. Avoid folding your chest or rounding your shoulders. Relax in this flexed position and take several deep breaths into the back of your waist. *Do you feel the back of your spine open sequentially from the bottom to the top? Are you moving slowly enough to flex one vertebral segment at a time?*

3. **Extending the spine:** As you inhale, rock into an anterior pelvic tilt and extend the front of your spine like a zipper unzipping into a long backward arc (Figure 14.19c ■). Keep your neck long and supported, as though an invisible hand were lifting the back of your head. Avoid dropping your head behind you (Figure 14.19d ■). Keep your shoulders over your pelvis. *Do you feel the front of your spine zip open from the bottom to the top?*

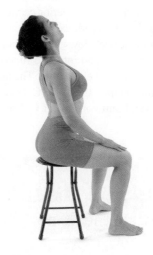

FIGURE 14.19c

(continued)

4. **Returning to neutral from extension:** Return to your starting position in three steps. First, relax your jaw and slightly flex your neck to return your head to neutral. Second, let your chest sink slightly to return your thorax to neutral. Third, tilt your pelvis and return it to neutral. You have just moved through one arcing movement.

5. Repeat arcing several times, until it feels like a fluid, smooth motion. Feel the back of your spine open as you flex, and the front of your spine open as you extend. *Which segments of your spine do you tend to skip? Which segments of your spine do you tend to move too much? Did you keep your shoulders over your hips through the entire movement? Did you focus on getting movement to sequence through rigid segments? Did this help stabilize overly loose segments?*

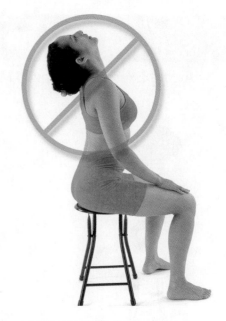

FIGURE 14.19d

Spinal motion can be assessed by observing a client's active movement and noting any areas that have a restricted range of motion and any that move beyond a normal range.

14.2.2.1 MOTION IN THE CERVICAL SPINE

Patterns of movement in the cervical vertebrae affect motion patterns in the entire spine. The reason for this is that neuromotor development begins in the head and neck and sequences down into the body. Cervical motion begins with the rooting and sucking movements of an infant. An infant comes into the world with primarily flexor tone because it has been curled into fetal flexion. The first time the newborn lifts the head to nurse, extensor tone builds in the posterior cervical muscles. Each time the infant lifts the head, extensor tone increases, gradually building from the neck down into the thoracic spine.

The cervical spine is divided into two functional units that can move independently of each other. The upper cervical unit consists of the occiput, the atlas (C-1), and the axis (C-2); the lower cervical unit consists of C-3 through C-7.

Specialized joints between the occiput, C-1, and C-2—the atlantoaxial and the atlanto-occipital joints (which are discussed in the chapter on the head and neck)—give the upper cervical spine a greater range of motion than the lower cervical spine. The cervical segments from C-2 through C-7 permit a small range of movement in each plane and linear motion in two directions: **cranial protraction,** an action of thrusting the chin forward, and **cranial retraction,** an action of pulling the chin back. The upper and lower cervical units move opposite of each other during protraction or retraction of the neck (Figure 14.20a-b ■).

A forward head posture, also called "chin-poke" or "computer neck," chronically protracts the cranium, placing the cervical joints under excessive shearing stresses. People with this pattern develop an obvious crease across the back of the neck and a tendency for the midcervical spine (especially the C-4 and C-5 vertebrae) to become unstable and glide anteriorly. A practitioner can address the pattern by stretching shortened muscles along the back of the neck,

BRIDGE TO PRACTICE
Balancing the Spine

To balance the spine, you can release restrictions to movement by loosening tissues around stiff vertebral segments. You can address unstable spinal segments by approximating overstretched soft tissues in these areas, particularly in the thoracic spine. This will provide your client with a passive education about where he

or she needs to improve muscular tone. The client will then need to learn to contract and control stabilizing muscles around unstable vertebral joints (see chapter 7 for more information about training postural muscles).

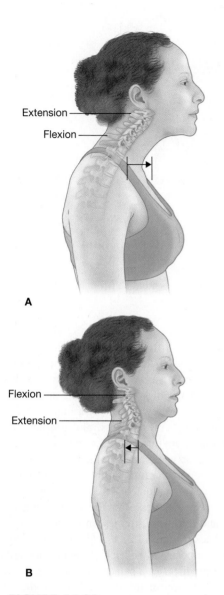

A

B

FIGURE 14.20

a) **Protraction** hyperextends the upper cervical unit and flexes the lower cervical unit. b) **Retraction** flexes the upper cervical unit and hyperextends the lower cervical unit.

although, ultimately, only the client can correct the pattern through active muscular contraction. The client will need to learn how to actively move the lower cervical spine in the posterior direction to realign the cervical vertebrae.

14.2.2.2 MOTION IN THE THORACIC SPINE

The thoracic spine can move in three planes, but the frontal plane orientation of its facet joint surfaces favors rotation and lateral flexion. The thoracic section of the spine is far more stable than the cervical and lumbar sections because its costal articulations and nearly vertical and long spinous processes restrict range of motion. As mentioned in the earlier discussion of facet joints, thoracic flexion averages 35 degrees; the upper thoracic segments have a greater range of flexion than the middle and lower segments.

Hyperextension in the thoracic spine is limited to 15 degrees because the spinous processes overlap

---

BRIDGE TO PRACTICE
Forward Head Posture

If your client has a forward head posture, you can coach your client to press the C-4 and C-5 vertebrae straight back to straighten the neck. This simple exercise, if practiced diligently, will also engage postural muscles in the neck, stabilizing the cervical spine and preventing cranial protraction.

---

like shingles and bump into each other at end range of motion. Lateral flexion of the thoracic spine averages 30 degrees to each side and is limited by the ribs, which act like splints between adjacent transverse processes. The greatest range of motion in this part of the spine relative to the rest of the spine is rotation; the thoracic spine can rotate to each side an average of 30 degrees.

The body of a typical thoracic vertebra is as wide as it is deep, with exceptions in the 1st and 12th, which serve as transitional vertebrae between the cervical and lumbar spines and possess characteristics of both. The body of the 1st thoracic vertebra is wider than most, similar to a cervical vertebra. The facet surfaces of the 12th thoracic vertebra face in lateral and posterior directions, which allows T-12 a greater range of motion than the rest of the thoracic vertebrae. As a result of this structural difference, T-12 can develop strain and pain from one-sided activities that chronically torque it, such as shoveling with the spine in flexion or carrying a baby on the right hip.

A major issue with the thoracic spine is that the line of gravity falls anterior to the thoracic vertebrae, making it susceptible to the bending stresses common in a hunched posture. The thoracic ligaments and muscles counter this tendency, keeping the thoracic spine upright, although abdominal distension and a forward head posture increase the load on the thorax and its inclination toward collapse. A distended abdomen places a downward drag on the rib cage, pulling the thoracic joints into increased flexion; a forward head posture places a front load on the thorax, increasing strain on the upper thoracic kyphosis. Problems occur when a habitually slumped posture overstretches the ligaments and muscles along the thoracic spine. Once the posterior ligaments become overstretched, a client with this pattern will usually experience chronic pain in the midthoracic region. Direct anterior pressure on the thoracic facet joints, applied one segment at a time along the lamina groove, can begin to straighten an excessive kyphotic curve (Figure 14.21 ■).

The thoracic spine is also susceptible to the chronic rotations found in spinal scoliosis. A practitioner can observe rotational fixations in the spine with a client in a flexed posture: the TPs of the rotated vertebrae will be higher on the side they rotate away from and will disappear on the side they are rotated toward (Figure 14.22 ■).[2]

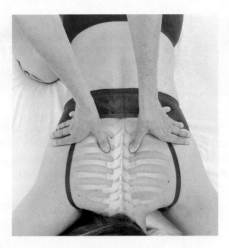

FIGURE 14.21
Acupressure along the thoracic spine

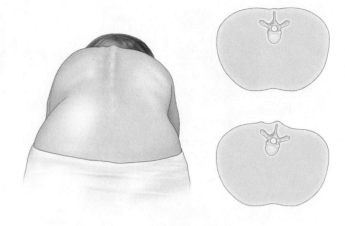

FIGURE 14.22
The rotated transverse processes protrude when the spine is flexed.

14.2.2.3 MOTION IN THE LUMBAR SPINE

The lumbar vertebrae and disks are larger than those in the rest of the spine in order to bear weight. The lumbar spine works under a heavy load; walking alone can increase the load to twice the body's weight.

The greatest range of motion in the lumbar spine is flexion and extension of 50 degrees. Although this range of flexion is comparable to flexion in the thoracic spine, 50 degrees distributed among just five lumbar segments makes this part of the spine remarkably flexible in forward bending. As the lumbar spine goes into flexion, the lordotic curve flattens; rarely does it bend into a kyphotic curve. Lumbar rotation is limited by the interlocking of articulating facet joints. Most lateral flexion in the lumbar spine occurs at the facet joints between L-5 and the sacrum, which have articulating surfaces oriented toward the frontal plane.

The most common cause of lower back pain is strain from varying combinations of muscular weakness, obesity, faulty postures, and poor lifting techniques. Bending at the waist while lifting places the lumbar spine in flexion, which requires more muscular work because it places the load farther from the center of gravity. Bending and twisting while lifting places the lower back at a high risk for damage because it compresses, shears, and torques the disks. The erector spinae are minimally active in a slumped posture, leaving the passive restraints—the ligaments and joint capsules—to support the lumbar and thoracic spine. A slumped posture places the lumbar spine in chronic flexion, increasing compressive stresses on the anterior side of the lumbar disks and tensional stresses on ligaments and muscles along the back (Figure 14.23 ■). Habitual slumping presses the nucleus pulposus to the back of the disk toward the spinal cord and predisposes a person to a bulging disk. In contrast, hyperextension of the lumbar spine reduces the size of the intervertebral foramen, narrowing the space around lumbar nerve roots, which can lead to nerve impingement and radiating pain down the hips and legs.

BRIDGE TO PRACTICE
Working with Pain from Thoracic Kyphosis

If you have a client who complains of pain associated with an excessive kyphotic curve and rounded shoulders, avoid lengthening already overstretched muscles and ligaments spanning the thoracic spine. Release chronic muscular holding in the thorax with trigger point therapy. Improve muscular tone by approximating the erector spinae muscles along your client's thoracic spine while gently pressing the thoracic curve in an anterior direction.

As you apply pressure, coach your client to widen the chest and let your pressure sink all the way into the sternum, which will help him or her to extend the thoracic spine. Encourage your client to lift the sternum when sitting or standing and recommend extending the thoracic spine by stretching backward over a physioball or pillow.

Because of the lumbar spine's key role in weight support and force transmission, it is important to maintain a neutral spine position when sitting, standing, walking, and lifting. The waiter's bow exercise is used to assess postural muscle control and to cultivate a habit of maintaining neutral spine during daily activities.

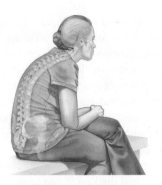

FIGURE 14.23

Chronic spinal flexion shifts the center of weight in the head, thorax, and pelvis off the vertical axis, which greatly increase mechanical stresses on the spine.

SELF-CARE
Waiter's Bow Exercise for Neutral Spine

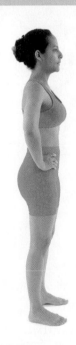

FIGURE 14.24a

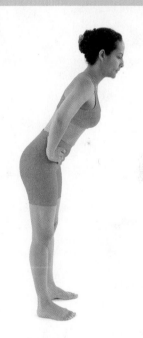

FIGURE 14.24b

1. Stand a neutral, vertical posture. Stabilize your spine in neutral by lightly pulling your lower abdomen straight back, then lightly contracting the deep muscles along the front and back of your spine (Figure 14.24a ■). Reach out the top of your head to elongate your neck and engage the cervical stabilizers. Take several breaths while maintaining this stable position. *Does your spine break or bend anywhere along the column?*

2. Keeping your spine long, straight, and stable, lean forward by bending at the hips. This is sometimes called the "waiter's bow" (Figure 14.24b ■). *Can you keep your spine neutral as you lean forward? Check your posture in a mirror or*

put a yardstick along your back and keep your spine against it as you lean forward. Come back to neutral, then slowly lean forward again. Explore this action several times while concentrating on maintaining a neutral spine (described in step 2).

To minimize stress on the spine always bend at the hips, not in the spine, especially during force application. Practice this exercise to learn this to maintain neutral spine during forward bending. You can also use it in client assessments for postural control. Get into the habit of doing simple tasks like brushing your teeth with your spine in neutral.

14.2.3   Spinal Ligaments

An extensive network of spinal ligaments stabilizes and protects the vertebral column (Figure 14.25 ■). A strong **nuchal ligament** connects the base of the skull to the upper cervical vertebra and keeps the head extended. The nuchal ligament can be up to an inch thick; its dense fibers provide an attachment site for the trapezius tendons and can be palpated easily at the base of the occiput.

Several longitudinal ligaments run up and down the spine like dense pieces of strapping tape (Figure 14.26 ■). An **anterior longitudinal ligament** runs down the front of the spine from the base of the occiput and to the anterior surface of the sacrum (Figure 14.27 ■). This thick, continuous ligament covers the vertebral bodies and disks. It limits hyperextension of the spine, particularly in the lordotic curves of the lumbar and cervical sections, and reinforces the anterior side of the interbody joints. The **supraspinous ligaments** bind one spinous process to another along the posterior spine and prevent hyperflexion. They can be palpated with cross-fiber strumming between adjacent spinous processes and are often tender in vertebral segments under excessive tensional stress from chronic spinal flexion or under compression from chronic spinal hyperextension. A series of segmented **interspinous ligaments** that lie deep to the supraspinous ligament connects adjacent spinous processes. These are the most developed and thickest in the lumbar region. A **posterior longitudinal ligament** lines the anterior surface of the vertebral foramen along the back of the vertebral disks and bodies. All the ligaments along the posterior side of the spine limit flexion.

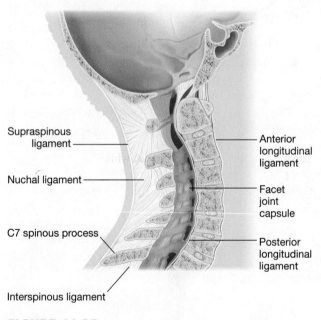

FIGURE 14.25
Spinal ligaments: lateral view

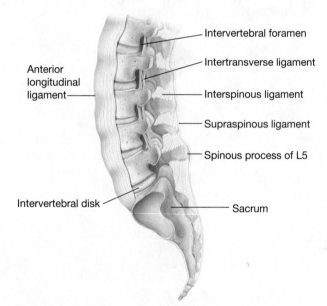

FIGURE 14.26
Longitudinal ligaments: lateral view

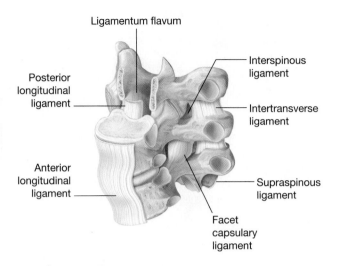

FIGURE 14.27
Spinal ligaments: anterolateral view

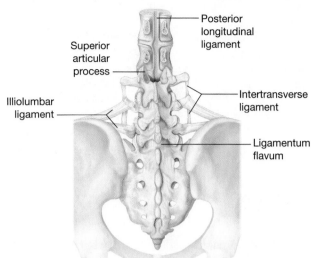

FIGURE 14.28
Spinal ligaments: posterior view

A segmented **ligamentum flavum** connects one vertebra to another along the posterior surface of the vertebral canal. The thick fibers of ligamentum flavum cover and support the anterior surfaces of the facet joints and prevent hyperflexion. The ligamentum flavum also has a high percentage of elastin fibers that make it more elastic and resilient.

A series of short **intertransverse ligaments** bind adjacent transverse processes to each other and become taut during lateral flexion of the spine (Figure 14.28 ■). A strong, short **iliolumbar ligament** arises from each of the transverse processes of the fifth lumbar vertebra and from adjacent fibers of the quadratus lumborum. It attaches along the medial aspect of the crest of the ilium. Although small, the iliolumbar ligaments fill the important function of securing the fifth lumbar vertebra to the iliac crest and the sacrum.

The lumbar spine is also supported by a thick, broad sheath of **thoracolumbar fascia,** which covers the lower back and provides attachment sites for abdominal muscles wrapping the waist. This is why abdominal muscle tone supports the lumbar spine; it transfers pull into the lower back through the thoracolumbar fascia, supporting the lordotic curve of the lumbar spine like a soft-tissue girdle.

SELF-CARE

Stretching the Posterior Spinal Ligaments

This stretch can give you a deep stretch along the posterior ligaments of the spine. It will also help you learn to move each vertebra individually.

Caution*: If your upper cervical spine is injured, in pain, or unstable, do not attempt this stretch.*

1. Begin standing in neutral spine posture with your feet under your hips. Contract your lower abdominal muscles to support you as you stretch. Lift your sternum and lengthen your neck by reaching the top of your head.

(continued)

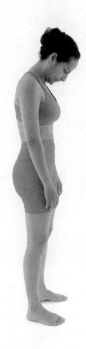

FIGURE 14.29a

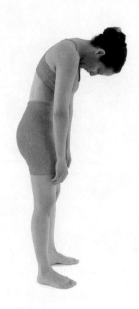

FIGURE 14.29b

2. Flex the uppermost cervical spine by tipping your head forward, isolating neck flexion to the atlanto-occipital joints (Figure 14.29a ■).

3. Continue to flex one vertebra at a time, slowly curling your neck like a seahorse until your chin is resting on your upper chest (Figure 14.29b ■). If your cervical spine is restricted at any one segment, you will not be flexible enough to stretch this far at first but should be able to with regular practice.

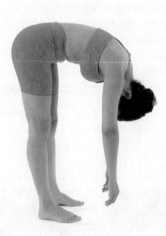

FIGURE 14.29c

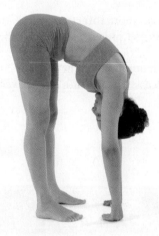

FIGURE 14.29d

4. Let your arms hang as you continue to slowly roll down through your thoracic and lumbar spine (Figure 14.29c-d ■). Make sure to flex one segment at a time.

5. Once you reach the bottom of your stretch, breathe into your spine.

6. Reverse the movement and roll back up in one smooth motion, restacking your spine as you go.

14.3 MUSCLES OF THE SPINE

The muscles of the spine are of particular importance to understand because one of the primary reasons that people receive massage is to alleviate back pain. The type of back pain that practitioners can treat the most effectively comes from muscular dysfunction associated with poor posture. There are three main layers of spinal muscles that run along the back from the head to the sacrum. These vertical spinal muscles lie under several layers of extrinsic trunk and shoulder muscles. When dysfunctional, each of the many spinal muscles can develop painful trigger points; some can develop trigger points in multiple sections.

Generally speaking, the spinal flexors are located on the front of the trunk and neck and the spinal extensors are located along the back of the neck and torso. A group of longitudinal erector spinae muscles running along the back of the spine are collectively referred to as **paravertebral** muscles. The prefix "para" is from the Greek translation and means *beyond*, so the paravertebral muscles are located beyond or behind the spine. The paravertebral muscles are arranged in several layers. The fascicles of the deepest layers span a single vertebral segment, those of the middle layers span three to four vertebral segments, and the fascicles of outer layers are almost vertical and span up to six or seven segments.

"Pre" refers to *before;* the **prevertebral** muscles—the longus colli and iliopsoas—run along the front of the cervical and lumbar spine in a single layer. Although the prevertebral muscles skip most of the thoracic spine, the *thoracis,* located along the inside of the anterior ribs and sternum, is sometimes considered a prevertebral muscle because it almost completes the myofascial pathway between the neck and lumbar regions of the torso (see Figure 10.17).

The muscular layers covering the spine are listed below from the large extrinsic muscles to the smaller intrinsic muscles:

- Superficial layer: *Trapezius, latissimus dorsi, splenius capitis,* and *splenius cervicis*
- Middle paravertebral layer: *Erector spinae muscle group* (made up of the *spinalis, longissimus,* and *iliocostalis*)
- Deep paravertebral layer: *Transversospinalis* (made up of the *multifidi* and *semispinalis capitis*), *suboccipitals,* and *rotatores*

Spinal muscles on the anterior side of the spine include:

- Cervical flexors and prevertebral muscles: *Scalenes, sternocleidomastoid, longus capitis, longus colli,* and *anterior suboccipitals*
- Extrinsic abdominal muscles: *Rectus abdominis, internal* and *external obliques,* and *transversus abdominis,* plus a small muscle along the back of the abdominal cavity known as the *quadratus lumborum*

The trapezius and latissimus dorsi attach to the shoulder girdle and are considered primary muscles of the shoulder, so they are covered in the chapter on the shoulder. They are mentioned here because in order to palpate underlying spinal muscles, a practitioner will need to press through the trapezius and latissimus dorsi. The sternocleidomastoid, suboccipitals, and longus muscles attach to the cranium, therefore they are covered in the chapter on the head and neck.

As you study the muscles in this chapter, keep in mind the relationship that their length and location have to the movement that they generate. The closer a muscle's line of pull is to the axis of motion, the less likely it is to produce flexion or extension and the more likely it is to fill a stabilizing role. When contracting bilaterally, these deep spinal muscles increase axial compression of the spine. This has been verified by EMG studies of the quadratus lumborum, multifidus, and psoas major.[3] When the longer and larger spinal muscles contract bilaterally (on both sides at once), they generate either flexion or extension of the spine. When they contract unilaterally (only on one side), they generate either rotation or lateral flexion of the spine.

14.3.1 Splenius Capitis and Splenius Cervicis

Two superficial muscles, the splenius capitis and splenius cervicis, run along the length of the posterior neck (Figure 14.30 ■). They lie under the trapezius muscle and over the erector spinae, forming a palpable muscular bulge along the length of the posterior cervical spine. The *cervical nerve* innervates both splenii muscles.

The large and broader **splenius capitis** is a meaty muscle with parallel fibers that arises along the nuchal ligament from C-3 to C-6 and spinous processes of C-7 to T-4, then ascends diagonally to an insertion on the mastoid process and the lateral third of the superior nuchal line of the occiput. The *mastoid process* is a prominent bony bump on the temporal bone that can be easily palpated behind the ear. The *superior* and *inferior nuchal lines* are two subtle

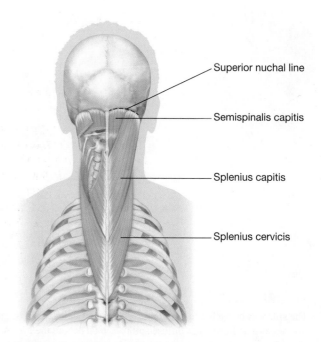

Superior nuchal line

Semispinalis capitis

Splenius capitis

Splenius cervicis

FIGURE 14.30
Splenius capitis and splenius cervicis

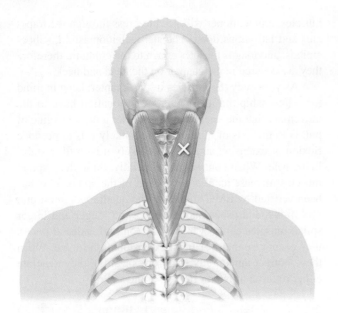

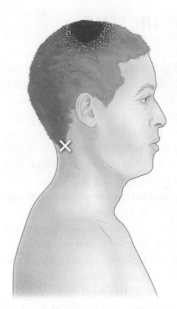

FIGURE 14.31

When dysfunctional, the **splenius capitis** can form a trigger point in the belly of the muscle that causes neck pain and refers headache pain to the top of the cranium.

bony ridges that run horizontally across the posterior aspect of the occiput bone at the base of the cranium. The splenius capitis can be easily palpated between the upper trapezius and sternocleidomastoid, where its fibers are superficial. A bilateral contraction of this large muscle extends the head and neck; a unilateral contraction laterally flexes and rotates the head and neck to the same side. (See TrP for the splenius capitis in Figure 14.31 ■).

The **splenius cervicis,** which lies deep to the splenius capitis, is a strap-like muscle that arises from the spinous processes of T-3 to T-6 and twists on its path to its insertion on the transverse processes of C-1 to C-3. A bilateral contraction of the splenius cervicis extends the cervical spine; a unilateral contraction laterally flexes and rotates the neck to the same side. Both splenius muscles usually work as synergists with the upper trapezius. (See TrPs for the splenius cervicis in Figure 14.32 ■).

14.3.2 Erector Spinae

Deep to the outer layer of spinal muscles and posterior to the spine lies another large group of spinal extensors called the **erector spinae** (ES) muscles. The large, ropey fascicles (muscle slips) of this complex group of muscles cascade along the back from the occiput to the sacrum.

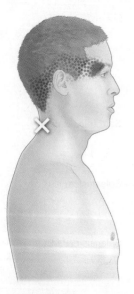

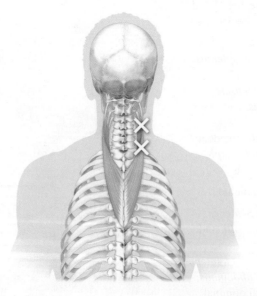

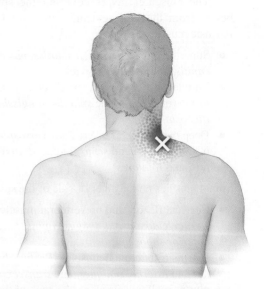

FIGURE 14.32

The **splenius cervicis** can develop several trigger points: One trigger point that develops lateral to the C-4 spinous process can refer pain over the eye and generates diffuse spillover pain behind the eye. A second trigger point that develops in the muscle belly lateral to C-7 can refer pain to the base of the neck and give a person a stiff neck. Postural stresses such as craning the neck forward to read fine print or looking through a camera viewer can overload both splenius muscles and activate trigger points.

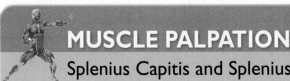

MUSCLE PALPATION
Splenius Capitis and Splenius Cervicis

Locate the splenius capitis and splenius cervicis on your neck by pressing below the occiput, behind the origin of the sternocleidomastoid and anterior to the trapezius. Then press along the belly of muscles over the lamina groove, working your way down the cervical spine. Also explore them by strumming across their fibers. To feel them contract, hold this area with a flat palpation touch, then rotate your head to that side and look up. Palpate both sides at once to check for symmetry.

Splenius Capitis

O—Nuchal ligament from C-3 to C-6 and spinous processes from C-7 to T-4

I—Mastoid process and lateral third of nuchal line of occiput

A—Bilaterally extends head and neck, unilaterally laterally flexes and rotates head and neck to same side

Splenius Cervicis

O—Spinous processes of T-3 to T-6

I—Transverse processes of C-1 to C-3

A—Bilaterally extends neck, unilaterally laterally flexes and rotates neck to same side

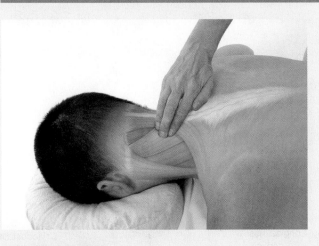

FIGURE 14.33a

Palpating the splenius capitis: prone

With your partner in the prone position, palpate the **splenius capitis** between the upper trapezius and upper sternocleidomastoid (Figure 14.33a ■). Follow its fibers up to the mastoid process and occiput. Explore its fibers down to its insertion on the upper thoracic vertebrae.

Active movement: To feel the splenius capitis contract, have your partner lift the head slightly while turning it to that side while you palpate it. Repeat on the other side. *Can you follow its fibers to its insertion on the mastoid and occiput?*

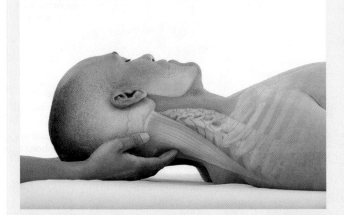

FIGURE 14.33b

Palpating the splenius capitis: supine

The **splenius cervicis** is a flatter muscle that is more difficult to isolate in palpation. With your partner supine, approximate the location of the splenius cervicis by pressing into the lamina groove from C-1 down to T-6 (Figure 14.33b ■). If you are palpating a small person, the splenius capitis will feel like a rounded mound of muscle lateral to the spinous processes that is easy to slip off. To avoid this, press slowly into the center of the muscle belly toward the center of the spine.

(continued)

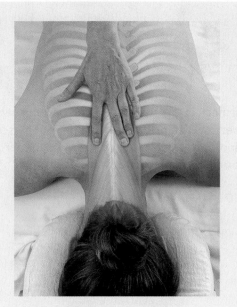

With your partner prone, palpate the **splenius muscles** along both sides of the lamina groove of the thoracic and cervical spines using a flat fingertip touch (Figure 14.33c ■).

Active movement: Have your partner tip the head to look up and to feel both sides contract at once. *Can you feel how the splenius muscles contract and fill the lamina groove when your partner rotates and extends the neck? As you palpate both sides of the lamina groove at once, do the muscles there feel symmetrical?*

FIGURE 14.33c

Palpating the splenius cervicis

Each individual fascicle spans from six to eight vertebral segments. The erector spinae group is made up of three sections that run parallel to each other—the spinalis, longissimus, and iliocostalis (Figure 14.34 ■). Each of these sections has three or four subsections named after the part of the spine they cross: the *lumborum* (lumbar), *thoracis* (thoracic), *cervicis* (cervical), and *capitis* (cranial). Each subsection is innervated by the *spinal nerves* at that respective segment.

The **spinalis** lies closest to the spine. The vertical fascicles of the thin *spinalis cervicis* arise from and attach to the spinous processes of the cervical vertebra in a curved configuration, like rings on a target. The vertical fascicles of the *spinalis thoracis* are functionally more significant. They arise from the spinous processes of the midthoracic vertebrae and attach to the spinous processes of the lower thoracic and upper lumbar vertebrae. (See TrP for the spinalis in Figure 14.35 ■.)

The **longissimus** runs along the spine lateral to the spinalis. Its nearly vertical fascicles arise from a thick, broad tendon that descends the length of its medial muscle along the lumbar spine and attaches to the sacrum and iliac crest. The *longissimus lumborum* ascends along the lower back and attaches to the lower ribs. The *longissimus thoracis* follows the same upward path to insertion sites on the middle and upper ribs. The *longissimus cervicis* runs from the upper ribs to the lower cervical transverse process. Finally, the *longissimus capitis* arises from the transverse process of the thoracic vertebra and attaches on the mastoid process. (See TrPs for the longissimus in Figure 14.36 ■.)

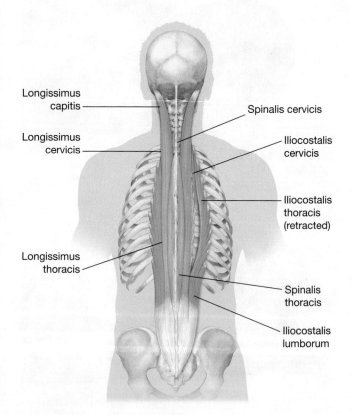

FIGURE 14.34

Erector spinae

FIGURE 14.35

The **spinalis** can develop a trigger point in the lower third of the muscle belly.

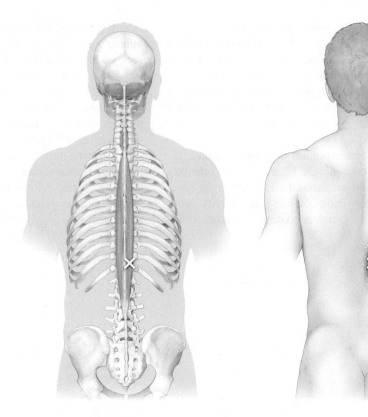

FIGURE 14.36

When dysfunctional, the **longissimus** can develop several trigger points in the lower-rib area, close to the spine: One trigger point develops lateral to the 1st lumbar vertebra and refers pain over the iliac crest and lower back, and a second trigger point develops lateral to the 10th thoracic vertebra and refers pain to the lower buttocks.

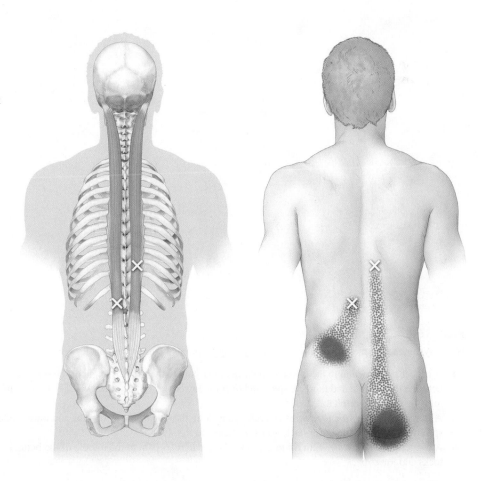

The **iliocostalis** is the most lateral portion of the erector spinae. It also arises from a thick, broad tendon, which is lateral to the longissimus tendon and attaches to the sacrum and iliac crest. The *iliocostalis lumborum* inserts on the lower six ribs; the *iliocostalis thoracis* inserts on the upper six ribs; and the *iliocostalis cervicis* inserts on transverse processes of the lower cervical vertebrae. (See TrPs for the iliocostalis in Figure 14.37 ■.)

Although their name implies that they maintain the upright position of the spine, the ES muscles are relatively quiet in a standing posture, except for fascicles in the lower thoracic region. Short bursts of muscular activity occur when the body sways forward. A bilateral contraction of the longissimus and iliocostalis hyperextend the thoracic and lumbar spine; their unilateral contractions side-bend the thoracic and lumbar spine and assist rotation. All three muscles fire during vigorous exercise performed in an upright position, the spinalis being the most active, the longissimus moderately active, and the iliocostalis minimally active. The erector spinae muscles work eccentrically during forward bending to control the lowering of the head and trunk, but relax at the end of the action, leaving the vertebrae supported by ligaments. Surprisingly, the erector spinae muscles are minimally active during the reverse action in a return to the vertical position. The entire erector spinae engages most powerfully when a person arches the spine from a prone position into the flying position.[4]

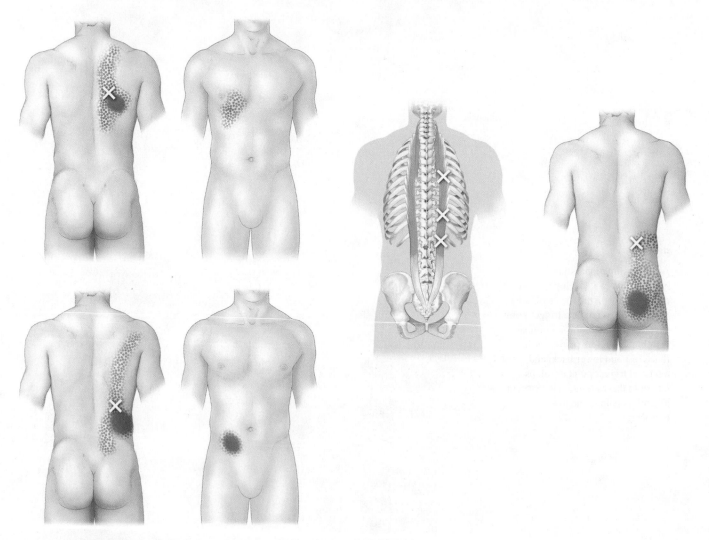

FIGURE 14.37

When dysfunctional, the **iliocostalis** can develops trigger points in three locations:

- A trigger point medial to the lower scapula can refer pain to the inferior angle of the scapula. Its spillover pain, which occurs between the scapula and thoracic spine and over the lower ribs on the chest wall, is often mistaken for visceral pain such as symptoms from angina or pleurisy.
- A trigger point over the lower ribs can refer pain along the side of the lower ribs and lower abdomen. It can send spillover pain from the lower back over the scapula to the shoulder.
- A trigger point below the 12th rib in the lower back can refer pain to the middle of the buttocks and radiate pain over the entire buttocks and lower back.

MUSCLE PALPATION
Erector Spinae: Spinalis, Longissimus, and Iliocostalis

The erector spinae muscles are difficult to palpate on yourself because of their location. If you can reach your spine, palpate them by strumming laterally across the muscles next to your spine. They will feel like ropey bands along the sides of your spine.

Feel the erector spinae contract by placing the palms of your hands across your lower or midback, then arching your back and rubbing your fingertips across them. When contracted, they feel like large muscular mounds on either side of the spine.

Spinalis

O–SPs of upper cervical and midthoracic vertebrae
I–SPs of lower cervical, lower thoracic, and upper lumbar vertebrae
A–Unilaterally assists thoracic and lower cervical extension, bilaterally assists lateral cervical and thoracic flexion and rotation

Longissimus

O–Tendon along lumbar spine, sacrum, and iliac crest
I–Lower ribs, TPs of thoracic and cervical spine, mastoid process
A–Bilaterally extends spine, unilaterally generates lateral flexion and rotation of the spine

Iliocostalis

O–Sacrum and iliac crest
I–Ribs and TPs of lower cervical vertebrae
A–Unilaterally extends the thoracic and lumbar spine, bilaterally generates lateral flexion and rotation of thoracic and lumbar spine

Note: It is difficult to differentiate the individual sections of the erector spinae during palpation, so we will palpate all three sections together.

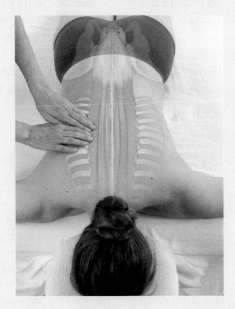

FIGURE 14.38a
Palpating the erector spinae

Locate the **erector spinae** with a cross-fiber strumming motion across the muscles next to the spine (Figure 14.38a ■). The fascicles often feel like a dense mound of muscle. They can also feel ropey, in which case your fingertips will roll across them. Explore all three sections which are the widest in the thoracic region. They are the smallest and most difficult to palpate in the cervical region, where they are buried under larger overlying muscles. *Do the vertical fascicles of the erector spinae feel ropey?*

Active movement: To feel the erector spinae contract have your partner arch the back and raise the legs and head, then relax several times. *Can you feel the erector spinae bulge and shorten as they contract?*

(continued)

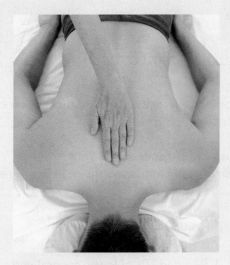

FIGURE 14.38b
Checking continuity of erector spinae tone

To **check for continuity of tone,** run your hand along the spine and note the general continuity of muscular tone in the erector spinae (Figure 14.38b ■). In areas where the erector spinae is well developed, you will feel large, elevated mounds of muscle along the sides of the spine. In areas where it is taut, weak, or overstretched, the muscle fascicles will feel thin and ropey. This usually occurs in the thoracic spine of a thin person with an exaggerated kyphosis. *Do the thoracic fascicles lie closer to the spine or the scapula than the lumbar fascicles?*

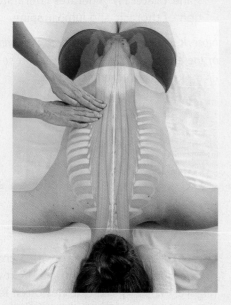

FIGURE 14.38c
Palpating the lumbar erector spinae

To palpate the lateral side of the **lumbar erector spinae,** locate the attachment along the iliac crest by hooking the top of the muscles along their lateral side, then tracing the muscles toward the spine (Figure 14.38c ■). *Do you notice how thick the erector spinae tendons are where they attach to the iliac crest?*

14.3.3 Transversospinalis

The **transversospinalis** lies medial and deep to the erector spinae from the occiput to the sacrum. It consists of three muscles: the rotatores, multifidi, and semispinalis capitis (Figure 14.39 ■). *Spinal nerves* innervate both the rotatores and the multifidi; *cervical nerves* innervate the semispinalis capitis.

The **rotatores** are small, single-segment muscles that lie deep to the multifidus and are difficult to palpate. They run diagonally up from the transverse process of one vertebra to the spinous process above it. Both the multifidi and rotatores assist extension and rotation of the spine.

The diagonal fascicles of the **multifidi** (singular: *multifidus*) run along the spine in a herringbone pattern. Each fascicle runs diagonally from the transverse process of one vertebra to the spinous process of a vertebra that is three or four segments higher. The multifidi fascicles originate on the posterior sacroiliac ligaments, the posterior superior iliac spine, and the transverse processes of L-5 to C-2 and insert on the spinous processes of L-5 to C-2. When the lumbar and cervical mulitifidi contract, their fascicles fill the lamina groove and can be easily palpated; when they relax, they are difficult to feel and the lamina groove feels soft. The fascicles are thickest over the sacrum and the lumbar spine and become thinner in

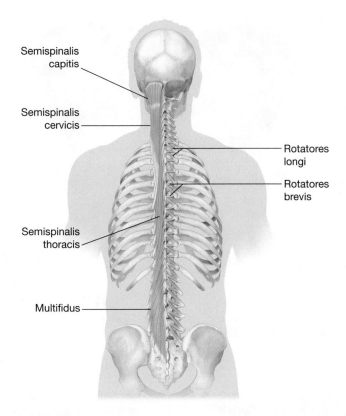

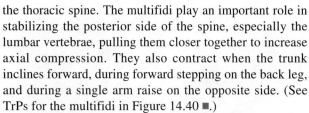

the thoracic spine. The multifidi play an important role in stabilizing the posterior side of the spine, especially the lumbar vertebrae, pulling them closer together to increase axial compression. They also contract when the trunk inclines forward, during forward stepping on the back leg, and during a single arm raise on the opposite side. (See TrPs for the multifidi in Figure 14.40 ■.)

The **semispinalis capitis, semispinalis cervicis,** and **semispinalis thoracis** lie over the upper multifidi fibers in fascicles that span five or more vertebral segments. The diagonal fibers of the semispinalis capitis arise from the transverse processes of T-6 to C-4 and insert in a broad flat attachment between the nuchal lines on the occiput. In the neck, their fibers somewhat blend with the underlying multifidi. A bilateral contraction of the semispinalis capitis extends the head and cervical spine; a unilateral contraction rotates the head and neck to the same side. This deep spinal muscle also works as a neck stabilizer to restrain flexion of the head. The semispinalis thoracis and semispinalis cervicis arise from the transverse processes of all the thoracic vertebrae and insert on the spinous processes of the T-6 to C-4. A unilateral contraction of both muscles rotates the lower cervical and upper thoracic spine, a bilateral contraction hyperextends the lower cervical and upper thoracic spine. (See TrPs for the semispinalis in Figure 14.41 ■.)

FIGURE 14.39

Transversospinalis

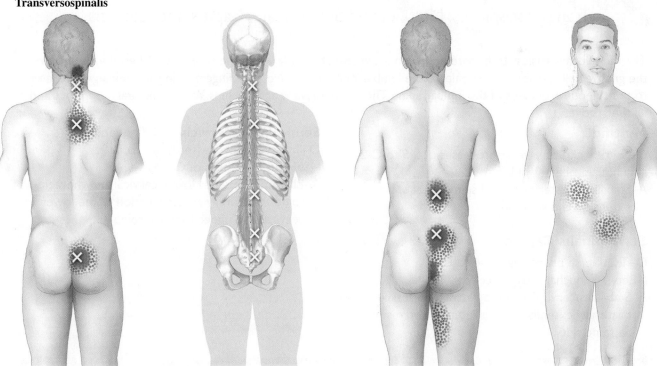

FIGURE 14.40

When dysfunctional, the **cervical multifidus** can develop a deep trigger point around the midcervical spine that can refer pain to the occiput. The **thoracic and lumbar multifidi** can develop trigger points in four locations: slightly lateral to the lower sacrum, slightly lateral to the upper sacrum, slightly lateral to the 2nd lumbar vertebra, and lateral to the 4th or 5th thoracic vertebra. All multifidi trigger points refer pain locally as well as into the abdomen, over the sacroiliac area and coccyx, and down the back of the thigh. Multifidi trigger points often develop with articular dysfunctions caused by chronic rotations in adjacent facet joints.

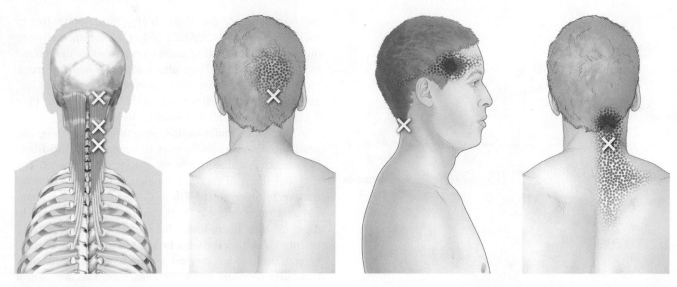

FIGURE 14.41

When dysfunctional, the **semispinalis** can develop three trigger points: one over the occiput, a second near the C-2 segment that refers pain to a band around the forehead, and a third near the C-4 segment that refers pain over the back of the head.

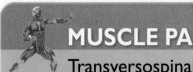

MUSCLE PALPATION

Transversospinalis: Multifidi and Semispinalis Capitis and Cervicis

The multifidi are easiest to palpate in the lamina groove, but only when they contract. When they are relaxed, the groove will feel soft. To self-palpate the lumbar multifidus, place your fingertips in the lamina groove lateral to the spinous processes of the lumbar spine. Then lean forward at your hips. You should feel it contract and fill the groove.

Multifidi

O–Sacrum and transverse processes of L-5 to C-2
I–Spinous processes of L-5 to C-2
A–Stabilizes posterior side of spine, assist spinal
   extension and rotation

Semispinalis Capitis

O–Transverse processes of T-6 to C-4
I–Between nuchal lines of occiput
A–Stabilizes cervical spine to restrain neck flexion,
   bilaterally extends neck, unilaterally rotates head
   to same side

Semispinalis Cervicis and Thoracis

O–Transverse processes of T-1 to T-12
I–Spinous processes of C-4 to T-6
A–Bilaterally extends lower cervical and thoracic
   spine, unilaterally assists rotation of the lower
   cervical and upper thoracic spine

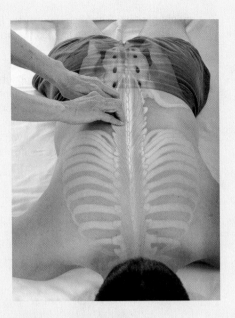

FIGURE 14.42a
Palpating the lumbar multifidus

With your partner in a prone position, palpate the **lumbar multifidus** in the lamina groove lateral to the spinous processes (Figure 14.42a ■).

Active movement: The lumbar multifidus is difficult to feel when it is relaxed. Have your partner contract it by barely lifting the head to feel its fibers fill the lamina groove. *Do you feel the lumbar multifidus contract and fill the lamina groove as your partner lifts his or her head, then relax and soften when your partner lets the head rest on the table?*

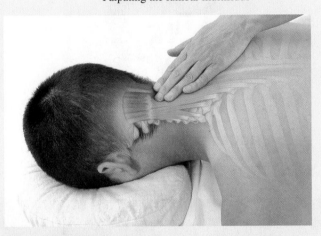

FIGURE 14.42b
Palpating the semispinalis capitis

The **semispinalis capitis** and **semispinalis cervicis muscles** are difficult to differentiate through the overlying muscles, especially when a person has a neck-forward posture that shifts the midcervical vertebrae in the anterior direction. You can approximate its location by running your fingertips along the lamina groove of the upper thoracic and lower cervical spines (Figure 14.42b ■). Feel its action by having your partner press the cervical vertebrae back into your fingertips.

SELF-CARE
Correcting a Lumbar Sway Back with Lumbar Multifidus Training

This exercise will help you correct an exaggerated lumbar curve, which most people call a "sway back." The lumbar multifidus is easy to palpate and contract. Several natural movements cause it to fire, such as raising one arm, stepping forward, or bending forward at the hips. Here is a simple exercise to engage the lumbar multifidus and correct a lumbar sway back.

1. **Getting ready:** Begin sitting in a neutral position. Rock your pelvis to level it over your sit bones. Lightly contract your lower abdominal wall to engage the transversus abdominis muscle, an important postural muscle wrapping the waist.

(continued)

2. **Checking the lumbar multifidus to see if it contracts:**
To palpate the lumbar multifidus contraction, place your fingertips right next to your spine, in the lamina groove (Figure 14.43a ■).

3. Then lean forward from your hips about 15 degrees. Keep your spine straight as you lean forward (Figure 14.43b ■). You should feel the lumbar multifidus contract and bulge under your fingertips. If it is already contracting, you will not feel any change in muscular tone. Keep your fingertips on the lumbar multifidus to monitor it as you return to an

upright position. If it softens under your fingertips, it has relaxed and you will need to keep practicing to contract it and keep it contracted.

4. **Daily practice:** Repeat this exercise until you can keep your lumbar multifidus contracted in an upright posture. This can take a lot of practice if your lumbar multifidus is chronically inhibited. Keep practicing and in time you will notice that your lumbar curve is elongating. You can also place your hands on your lower back whenever you're sitting or walking to check and see if it is contracting.

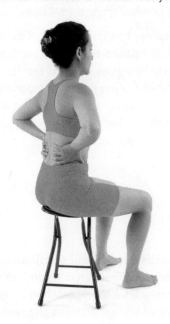

FIGURE 14.43a

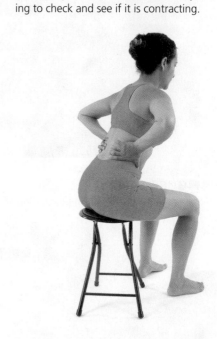

FIGURE 14.43b

SELF-CARE
Stretching and Strengthening the Spinal Extensors

As a massage therapist or bodyworker, or anyone who spends a lot of time working standing up and bending over a table, you use a lot of flexor muscles. To keep your muscular system balanced, it is important to stretch the flexors and strengthen extensors on a regular basis. Here are several simple exercises to balance your body.

1. **Stretching the flexors:** Lie over a physioball and let your body weight stretch your trunk and hip flexors (Figure 14.44a ■). Make sure the ball is large enough to support the back of your head to avoid hyperextending your neck. *Is your entire back in contact with the ball? Can you elongate your lower back to avoid hyperextension? Do you feel a stretch in the front of your hips?*
   a. Reach your arms overhead to enhance the stretch, but make sure to keep your chest wide. Avoid hiking your shoulders and laterally rotate your arms. Reach through your fingertips.

b. Slowly rock your weight from side to side and allow your trunk and head to slowly sift laterally like a sandbag. The subtle movement will loosen and relax your neck, spine, and abdominal organs during this passive stretch.

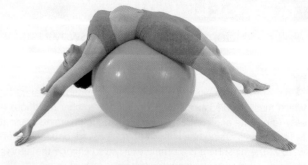

FIGURE 14.44a

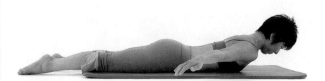

FIGURE 14.44b

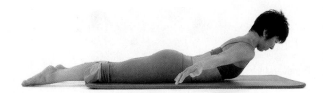

FIGURE 14.44c

2. **Strengthening the extensors:** Lie prone on the floor. Lightly contract your lower abdominals to stabilize your lumbar spine. Practice this exercise slowly, in progressive steps. This will help you contract the stabilizer muscles closest to the spine first, then contract the middle layer of muscles next, and contract the superficial muscles last. If you contract your muscles progressively, this exercise should feel easy because your stabilizers will prevent joint stress or discomfort from hyperextension.

   a. Contract the deepest layer of spinal muscles, the multifidi, by just barely lifting your head off the floor (Figure 14.44b ■). Look at the floor to keep your neck and entire spine elongated. Touch your lower back to monitor the degree to which the spinal muscles are contracting. *Can you feel the multifidus contracting next to the spinous processes, filling your lamina groove? Can you keep the erector spinae relaxed?*

   b. Contract the erector spinae by lifting your head, shoulders, and legs off the floor to arch your spine (Figure 14.44c ■). Focus on the erector spinae contraction by keeping your back as wide as you can as you arch it. Avoid lateral rotation in the hips pinching the scapulae together. *Are your lower abdominals still lightly contracted? Are you keeping the midscapular region wide? Are your legs parallel?*

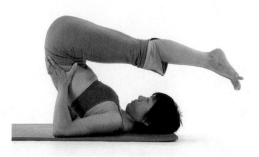

FIGURE 14.44e

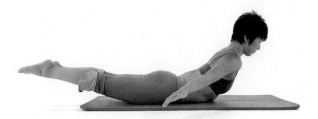

FIGURE 14.44d

   c. Contract the extrinsic muscles along your entire back side by lifting your arms, legs, and maximally arching your spine (Figure 14.44d ■). *Can you feel your trapezius, latissimus dorsi, gluteals, hamstrings, and plantarflexors working together along the back pathway? Are your toes pointed?*

   d. Relax completely. Repeat the entire exercise several times. If your back feels tight after doing this exercise, stretch your extensors afterward.

3. **Stretching the extensors:** Lie on your back. Lengthen your entire spine. Contract your lower abdominals to stabilize your lumbar spine. Lift your legs over your head into a quasi-plow position. Keep your spine and legs more horizontal than vertical to avoid hyperflexion in the neck or upper back (Figure 14.44e ■).

14.3.4 Abdominal Muscles and Quadratus Lumborum

The abdominal wall has four layers of muscles: the rectus abdominis, external oblique, internal oblique, and the transversus abdominis (Figure 14.45 ■). All four abdominals work together to flex, laterally flex, or rotate the lumbar spine and lower torso. Both the obliques and the transversus abdominis are flat, broad muscular sheaths that wrap the waist and arise from the thick thoracolumbar fascia, forming a muscular wall around the abdominal cavity and the lumbar spine. They support and stabilize the lumbar spine and torso in an extended posture, preventing both lower back pain and injury. The quadratus lumborum (QL), a small, deep muscle tucked behind the psoas major and in front of the thoracolumbar fascia, strengthens the posterior wall of the abdominal cavity (Figure 14.46 ■). The rectus abdominis, obliques, and transversus abdominis are innervated by the *thoracic nerves.* The internal oblique

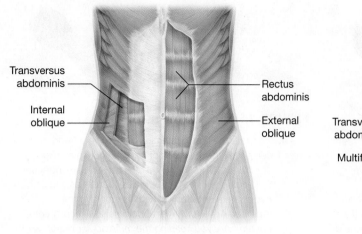

FIGURE 14.45

Abdominal muscles

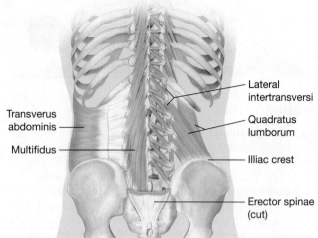

FIGURE 14.46

Quadratus lumborum

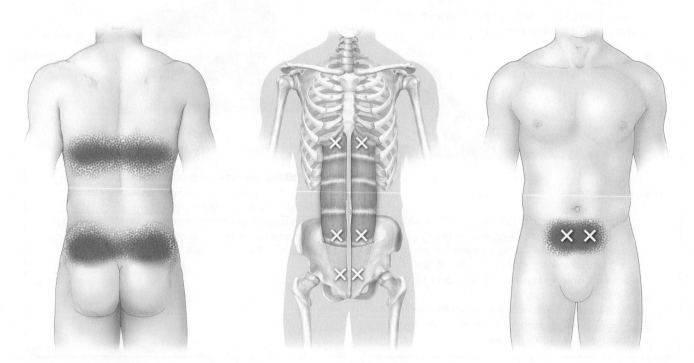

FIGURE 14.47

When overworked, the **rectus abdominis** can develop trigger points on either side of the upper and lower inscriptions of the muscle that can refer pain locally over the abdomen or cause a backache in a band across the lower thoracic region or across the sacrum and hips. It can also develop trigger points just below the navel on either side that can cause abdominal cramping in the center or near the anterior aspect of the iliac crest. Another rectus abdominis trigger point can develop just above the pubic bone and can cause diarrhea.

BRIDGE TO PRACTICE
Diastasis Recti in the Rectus Abdominis

Some people have a split in the rectus abdominis called *diastasis recti*, also called *abdominal separation*. This benign condition is common in newborns and usually self-corrects with maturation. It also occurs during pregnancy from the growing uterus stretching the rectus abdominis. It creates a ridge-like depression between the two sides of the rectus abdominis that can be easily palpated as the muscle contracts. If your client has this condition, avoid direct pressure in the center of the rectus abdominis because it could stretch already overstretched tissue there and exacerbate the split.

and transversus abdominis are also innervated by the *first lumbar nerve*. The QL is innervated by the *thoracic* and *lumbar nerves*.

The powerful **rectus abdominis** arises from the costal cartilage of the 5th, 6th, and 7th ribs and the xiphoid process. This long, strapping muscle descends along the front of the abdominal wall and inserts on the pubic crest and pubic symphysis. The rectus abdominis also attaches laterally to the abdominal aponeurosis—a thick fascial membrane covering the abdominal cavity—and attaches medially to the linea alba. When well toned, its four tendinous inscriptions (segments) take on a sculpted, well-defined shape that many people call a "six-pack." The rectus abdominis is the primary flexor of the trunk. It laterally flexes the lower spine when contracting unilaterally, and tilts the pelvis in a posterior direction when contracting in a stationary posture (See TrPs for the rectus abdominis in Figure 14.31 ■.)

The external and internal obliques wrap the waist, connecting the rib cage to the pelvis like a large muscular cuff with criss-crossed diagonal fibers. The **external oblique** is a broad flat muscle arising from muscular slips on the sides of the 5th through 12th ribs. Its diagonal fibers descend from the ribs toward the pubic bone, making a V-shape across the front of the abdomen. The external oblique connects to the pelvis via a broad insertion site along the iliac crest, blends into the abdominal aponeurosis all the way to the linea alba and the inguinal ligament, and covers the costal arch. The **internal oblique** lies deep to the external oblique. Its thick, diagonal fibers arise along the iliac crest, thoracolumbar fascia, and abdominal aponeurosis and insert on the costal cartilage of ribs 10–12.

When the external oblique contracts independently of the internal oblique, it elevates the abdominal wall. When the internal oblique contracts independently of the external oblique, it depresses the abdominal wall. The internal oblique also rotates the lower spine. When the obliques contract isometrically together, they compress the abdominal viscera and cinch the waist (Figure 14.48 ■). Together, they play an important role as secondary stabilizers of the lumbar spine, working eccentrically to control rotation of the waist during leg and trunk movement. A bilateral contraction of both obliques flexes the trunk; a unilateral contraction of either

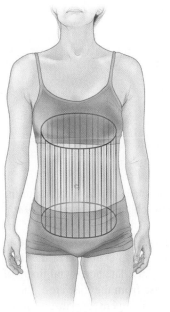
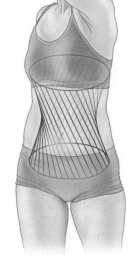

Relaxed   Contracted

FIGURE 14.48
Oblique contraction (adapted from Kapandji)

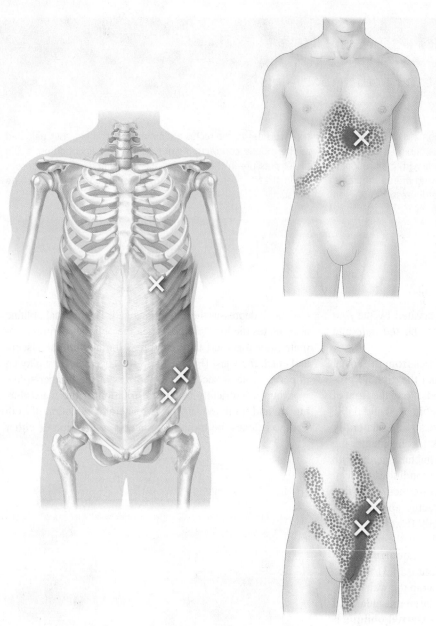

FIGURE 14.49

The **obliques** can develop trigger points in several places: One trigger point over the costal arch can produce deep epigastric pain similar to heartburn, and a second pair of trigger points in the lower lateral abdomen above the inguinal ligament can refer pain into the groin.

side bends the lower trunk or rotates the lower trunk to the opposite side. (See TrPs for the obliques in Figure 14.49 ■.)

The **transversus abdominis** is the deepest layer of the abdominal muscles (Figure 14.50 ■). It was introduced in the chapter on posture as a postural stabilizer of the lumbar spine and the sacroiliac joints. The horizontal fibers of the transversus abdominis arise from the iliac crest, thoracolumbar fascia, and inguinal ligament, and insert on the abdominal aponeurosis and linea alba. Unlike the obliques that cross the lower ribs, the transversus attaches to the internal surface of the lower ribs, where its fibers interdigitate with the costal attachments of the diaphragm fibers. The transversus abdominis wraps the waist like a built-in muscular cummerbund, compressing the abdominal cavity to support the viscera and maintain intra-abdominal pressure, which is crucial for normal diaphragmatic breathing.

As a group, the abdominal muscles flex the spine from a prone position. They also play a minor role in flexing the spine from an extended position. In an ideal recruitment pattern of spinal flexion, the abdominal muscles contract in the deepest layer first, then the middle layer, then the superficial layer (Figure 14.51 ■). Before any movement of the trunk or hips, the transversus abdominis should contract isometrically to stabilize the lumbar spine and the sacroiliac joints. As the movement begins, the obliques should contract eccentrically to stabilize the lumbar spine during hip motion and trunk rotation. The rectus abdominis contracts last, working concentrically to flex the trunk. When the rectus abdominis contracts without the support of the underlying stabilizers, it tends to shorten and bulge forward, compressing the trunk while allowing the viscera to distend.

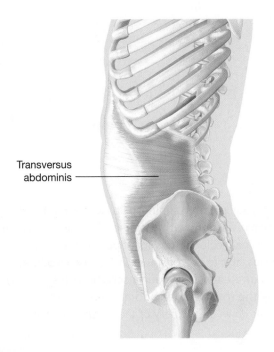

Transversus abdominis

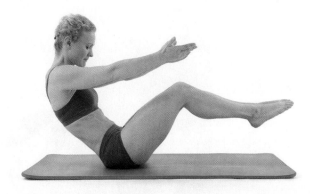

FIGURE 14.51

Sit-up with hollow from underlying stabilizer contraction

FIGURE 14.50

Transversus abdominis: side view

MUSCLE PALPATION
Rectus Abdominis, Obliques, and Transversus Abdominis

Locate the abdominal muscles on your own body by palpating their contractions. To feel the transversus abdominis contract, get in a side-lying position and place your hands over your lower abdominal wall. Let your abdomen relax so that the weight of your abdominal viscera distends your lower abdominal wall. Lightly contract the transversus by pulling it toward your lumbar spine.

To feel the obliques contract, lie in a supine position. Squeeze the sides of your waist with a pincher grip, then contract your obliques by narrowing your waist. You should feel them harden under your hands. You can also feel the obliques contract by lifting your head from a side-lying position.

To feel the rectus abdominis contract, lie in a supine position and place your hands over the midline of your abdomen. Lift your head and shoulder in a sit-up and you should feel it contract.

Rectus Abdominis

O–Costal cartilage of 5th, 6th, and 7th ribs, xiphoid process
I–Pubic crest and pubic symphysis
A–Flexes the trunk, posteriorly tilts pelvis

External Oblique

O–External surfaces of lower eight ribs
I–Anterior iliac crest, abdominal aponeurosis to linea alba
A–Compresses abdominal viscera, bilaterally flexes spine, unilaterally side bends the spine, rotates trunk to opposite side

Internal Oblique

O–Ribs 12 through 10
I–Iliac crest, thoracolumbar fascia, abdominal aponeurosis to linea alba
A–Compresses abdominal viscera, bilaterally flexes spine, unilaterally side-bends the spine, rotates trunk to same side

Transversus Abdominis

O–Iliac crest, inguinal ligament, thoracolumbar fascia, internal surface of lower ribs
I–Abdominal aponeurosis to linea alba
A–Compresses abdominal viscera, stabilizes lumbar spine and sacroiliac joints

(continued)

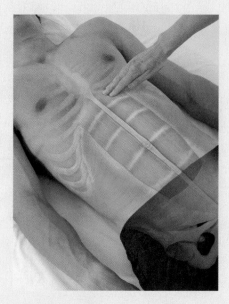

FIGURE 14.52a

Palpating the upper rectus abdominis

With your partner supine, palpate the **rectus abdominis** along either side of the midline of the abdominal region. Press its upper segment against the ribs, above the costal arch (Figure 14.52a ■). Press into each of its four inscriptions (segments) along the front of the abdomen. *Are you pressing straight down on the belly of the rectus abdominis?*

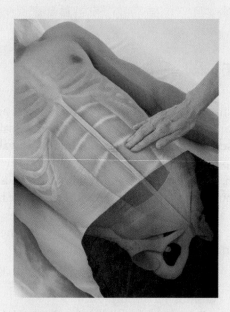

FIGURE 14.52b

Palpating the middle inscription of rectus abdominis

Active movement: Have your partner raise and lower the head several times in a partial sit-up as you palpate each inscription (segment) of the rectus abdominis (Figure 14.52b ■). Also find the lateral borders of the rectus abdominis. *As your partner contracts the rectus abdominis, are you able to feel its inscriptions and its lateral borders?*

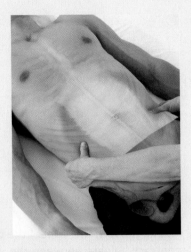

FIGURE 14.52c
Palpating the obliques to check for congruency

With your partner supine, palpate the **internal and external obliques** by grasping and squeezing the sides of the waist (Figure 14.52c ■). They are easy to feel on a well-toned, thin person, but they can be difficult to discern when they have low tone, causing the sides of the waist to feel soft. *Are you palpating the diagonal fibers of the obliques along the sides of the waist?*

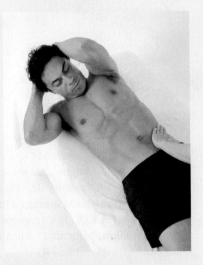

FIGURE 14.52d
Palpating an oblique contraction

Active movement: To feel the obliques contract, lay your palms flat on one side of the abdomen, then have your partner do a diagonal sit-up (Figure 14.52d ■).

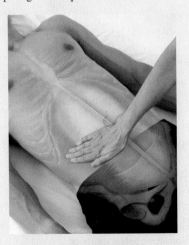

FIGURE 14.52e
Palpating the transversus abdominis

With your partner supine, locate the **transversus abdominis** using a flat palpation directly lateral to the midline of the abdomen (Figure 14.52e ■). *If the transversus abdominis has good resting tone, do you feel a flat layer of muscle over the lower abdominal wall?*

(continued)

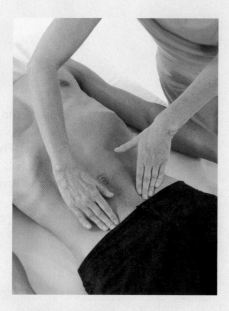

FIGURE 14.52f

Palpating the transversus abdominis during isometric contraction.

Active movement: To feel the transversus abdominis contract, palpate between the inguinal ligament and the navel while having your partner pulls the lower abdominal toward the sacrum (Figure 14.52f ■).

The **quadratus lumborum** (QL) is a small, fleshy muscle with quadrangular fibers. Its lateral fibers run between the iliac crest and the 12th rib, and its medial fascicles run diagonally from the transverse processes of the lumbar vertebrae to insertions on the posterior medial aspect of the iliac crest. The QL lies too close to the midline of the body to effectively flex or extend the spine (Figure 14.53 ■). Instead, it stabilizes the bottom rib during inhalation and assists forced exhalation in actions such as coughing or sneezing. When it contracts unilaterally, the QL laterally flexes the lumbar spine or hikes (elevates) the hip, which garnered it the nickname of the "hip hiker" muscle. The QL is a frequent source of lumbar pain and trigger points, particularly when a unilateral contracture hikes one hip (Figure 14.54 ■).

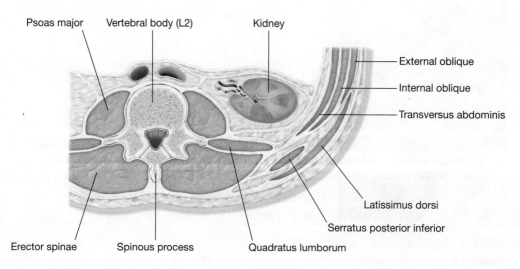

FIGURE 14.53

Quadratus lumborum: sagittal section at L-3

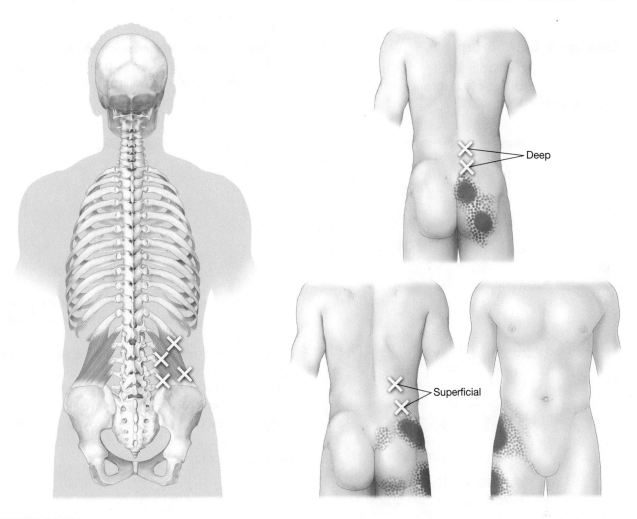

FIGURE 14.54

The **quadratus lumborum** is a frequent site of trigger point pain. When dysfunctional, it develops trigger points in four locations: Two deep trigger points lateral to the lower transverse processes can refer pain across the sacroiliac joint and into the buttocks; two superficial trigger points along the lateral edge of the QL just below the bottom rib and just above the iliac crest can refer pain over the iliac crest and greater trochanter. Quadratus lumborum trigger points can cause such severe lower back pain that simple movements such as rolling over in bed or standing up to walk become unbearable. Asymmetries in the pelvis such as an upslip can cause dysfunction in the QL on one side. Fortunately, trigger point therapy can provide immediate pain relief from a problematic QL.

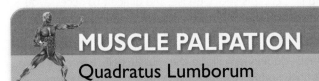

MUSCLE PALPATION
Quadratus Lumborum

The quadratus lumborum is a difficult muscle to locate with self-palpation, although you can approximate its location. Place your hands on your hips so that your thumbs point toward your lower back. Relax your waist muscles so you can palpate through them. Press your thumbs into the sides of your waist, straight toward your spine. Arch your lower back and you should feel the sides of the erector spinae contract and bulge. Straighten your spine and as you do, press your thumbs toward your spine anterior to the erector spinae into the QL, which feels like a small meaty muscle. Once you find it, rock your thumbs up and down along the sides of the QL.

(continued)

Quadratus Lumborum

O–Posterior medial iliac crest
I–Transverse processes of 1st through 4th lumbar
  vertebrae and 12th rib

A–Unilaterally side-bends the lumbar spine or hikes
the hip, assists forced exhalation during coughing,
stabilizes bottom ribs against upward pull of diaphragm during inspiration

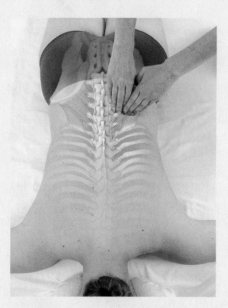

FIGURE 14.55a

Palpating the quadratus lumborum

With your partner in a prone position, palpate the
lateral edge of the **quadratus lumborum** by sliding your thumbs from the lateral top edge of the iliac
crest, under the erector spinae (Figure 14.55a ■). The
QL is usually easy to palpate with the thumbs or fingertips on a thin person with a long waist. It can be
difficult to palpate on a person with a short waist or
a larger person with thick tissue around the waist. *Are
you pressing into the QL from a lateral direction under the
overlying erector spinae?*

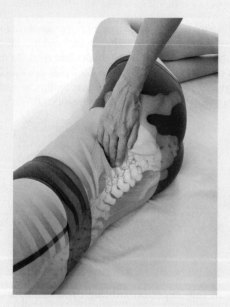

FIGURE 14.55b

Palpating the quadratus lumborum in
side-lying

Side-lying position: If the space between the lower rib
and iliac crest is short, dense, and difficult to access, you
can palpate the QL more easily with your partner in a
side-lying position (Figure 14.55b ■).

Once you find it, walk up the muscle belly toward the
12th rib and down the muscle belly toward the iliac
crest. This side-lying position is also a great position to
stretch the QL with a myofascial stripping technique.

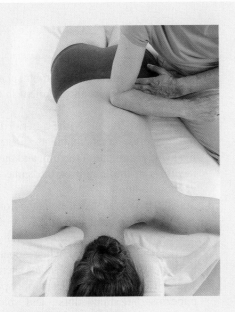

FIGURE 14.55c

Palpating the quadratus lumborum with the elbow

Active movement: Have your partner make a small, hip-hiking movement so you can feel the QL contract. Have your partner relax and sink your pressure into the muscle belly. You may need to jimmy your knuckles or elbow through the overlying fascia to locate the belly of the QL (Figure 14.55c ▪). *When your partner hikes the hip, do you feel the QL contract?*

CONCLUSION

The uniquely upright human spine comes with great assets and liabilities. During standing and walking, our backbone is balanced along the line of gravity. Our uniquely vertical posture requires less muscular effort than that of any other animal on the planet. Yet any slight deviation of our spine from vertical throws the whole structure off balance. As the human race advances in technology and increases in life span, sedentary lifestyles and obesity increase, causing a widespread propensity for poor posture, back pain, and repetitive-use injuries continues to grow among the human population. As a result, more and more people are receiving massage and bodywork for relief.

To work effectively to alleviate back pain, a practitioner needs to understand the structure and function of spinal muscles and joints. In addition, a practitioner needs to recognize how a person's posture and movement contribute to back problems. Massage and bodywork techniques such as myofascial release, passive stretching, and trigger point therapy can go a long way toward alleviating back pain, but prevention goes even further. Hands-on therapies can help clients restore vertical alignment and a continuity of muscular tone along the trunk and spine. Even more than that, a holistic practitioner treats the whole person. As holistic practitioners, we can provide a passive and active education for our clients to improve their understanding and awareness of how postural patterns affect the spine and what they can do to change faulty spinal patterns.

SUMMARY POINTS TO REMEMBER

1. The spine has 24 vertebrae—seven cervical, 12 thoracic, and five lumbar—which house and protect the spinal cord, support the trunk, allow movement, and provide attachment sites for muscles, tendons, and ligaments.

2. The three curves of the spinal column—two lordotic curves in the cervical and lumbar regions and a kyphotic curve in the thoracic region—give the spine a flexibility and shock-absorbing capacity.

3. Each vertebra is an irregular bone with a similar structure—a body to support weight, a vertebral foramen to provide a channel for the spinal cord, a spinous process and two transverse processes that serve as attachment sites for muscles and bony levers, a pedicle and lamina connecting the processes, and two articular processes for posterior facet joints.

4. The 1st and 2nd cervical vertebrae, the atlas and axis, have unique structures to support the weight of the cranium and allow free rotational movement of the head.

5. The spine has two types of joints: fibrocartilage interbody joints along the front of the spine made up of a closed column of stacked vertebral bodies and disks; and a series of small synovial plane joints called facet joints along the posterior spine.

6. The orientation of articular surfaces in the facet joints in each part of the spine allows a specific range of motion: The cervical facets orient along a 45-degree diagonal and allow free motion of the neck in all planes, the thoracic facets orient in the frontal plane and favor rotation, and the lumbar facets orient in the sagittal plane and favor flexion.

7. Five spinal ligaments—the anterior longitudinal ligament, supraspinous ligaments, posterior longitudinal ligament, ligamentum flavum, and intertransverse ligaments—run the length of the spine and stabilize the vertebral column.

8. Spinal flexors are located along the front of the spine and extensors are located along the back of the spine. When a flexor or extensor contracts bilaterally, it generates spinal flexion and extension; when it contracts unilaterally, it generates spinal rotation and/or lateral flexion.

9. There are three layers of posterior spinal muscles: the trapezius, latissimus dorsi, and splenii muscles are found in the superficial layer; the erector spinae muscles are in the middle layer; and the transversospinalis are in the deep layer. The middle and deep layers are referred to as paravertebral muscles.

10. Four abdominal muscles cover and wrap the abdominal cavity: The rectus abdominis is the primary trunk flexor, the internal and external obliques lie under the rectus abdominis, and the transversus abdominis lies deep to the obliques.

11. The quadratus lumborum runs along the back of the abdominal wall and when dysfunctional is a frequent cause of low-back pain.

REVIEW QUESTIONS

1. Name the three parts of the spine, their general locations, and the number of vertebrae in each part.

2. The four functions of the spine are to house and protect the _____ (two words), to allow spinal _____, to provide _____ (two words) for soft tissues, and to provide _____ for the trunk.

3. True or false (circle one). A normal thoracic spine has a lordotic curve and a normal cervical and lumbar spine have kyphotic curves.

4. A typical vertebra has
   a. a body, a pedicle and lamina, two transverse processes, and a spinous process.
   b. a body, a dens process, a transverse process, and two spinous processes.
   c. a body, a pedicle and lamina, two transverse processes, and two spinous processes.
   d. a body, a pedicle and lamina, a transverse process, and a spinous process.

5. Coupled motion of the thoracic and lumbar regions of the spine that occurs during side bending is
   a. a combination of either flexion or extension with gliding.
   b. a combination of flexion and extension with rotation in the same direction.
   c. a combination of flexion and extension with rotation in the opposite direction.
   d. a combination of either flexion or extension with counterrotation.

6. The interbody joints of the spine are classified as _____ joints and are made up of articulations between the _____ (two words) and _____ (two words).

7. The facet joints are small synovial plane joints along the posterior spine made up of articulations between the
   a. vertebral facets.
   b. spinous processes.
   c. transverse processes.
   d. vertebral bodies.

8. Which joints of the spine function as shock absorbers, the interbody joints or the facet joints?

9. At which joint does 80 percent of cervical rotation occur and what type of joint is it?
   a. the atlanto-occipital joint, a pivot joint
   b. the atlantoaxial joint, a condyloid joint
   c. the atlantoaxial joint, a pivot joint
   d. the atlanto-occipital joint, a condyloid joint

10. True or false (circle one). The most freely movable part of the spine is the thoracic spine.

11. Which part of the spine is the most freely movable, which part of the spine favors rotation, and which part favors flexion?

12. What determines the range of motion in each part of the spine?
    a. the muscles attached to it
    b. the size of the vertebral bodies
    c. the size of the intervertebral disks
    d. the orientation of the facet joint surfaces

13. Which of the spinal ligaments can be directly palpated and where?
    a. the anterior longitudinal ligament along the vertebral bodies
    b. the posterior longitudinal ligaments along the vertebral foramen
    c. the supraspinous ligaments between the spinous processes
    d. the ligamentum flavum along the vertebral canal

14. When a bilateral spinal muscle contracts unilaterally, it will produce
    a. flexion and rotation.
    b. lateral flexion and rotation.
    c. lateral flexion and stabilization.
    d. extension and rotation.

15. Name two superficial neck extensors located along the back of the cervical spine.

16. The erector spinae muscle group is made up of three muscles, which are the
    a. spinalis, longissimus, and transversospinalis.
    b. spinalis, transversospinalis, and iliocostalis.
    c. transversospinalis, longissimus, and iliocostalis.
    d. spinalis, longissimus, and iliocostalis.

17. Of the four abdominal muscles, which ones attach on to the thoracolumbar fascia?

18. Of the four abdominal muscles, which one is a primary trunk flexor?

19. The primary functions of the transversus abdominis are
    a. trunk extension and rotation.
    b. abdominal compression and lumbar stabilization.
    c. trunk flexion and lateral bending.
    d. rotation and lateral bending.

20. The muscle that attaches the lower rib to the iliac crest and frequently has trigger points is the
    a. rectus abdominis.
    b. quadratus lumborum.
    c. erector spinae.
    d. iliopsoas.

Notes

1. Maitland, J. (2001). *Spinal Manipulation Made Simple: A Manual of Soft Tissue Techniques.* Berkeley, CA: North Atlantic Books.
2. Maitland, G., Hengeveid, E., Banks, K., & English, K. (2001). *Maitland's Vertebral Manipulation* (6th ed.). Oxford, UK: Butterworth Heinemann.
3. Basmajian, J., & DeLuca, C. (1984). *Muscles Alive: Their Functions Revealed by Electromyography* (5th ed.). Baltimore: Williams & Wilkins.
4. Ibid.

PEARSON myhealthprofessionskit

Use this address to access the Companion Website created for this textbook. Simply select "Massage Therapy" from the choice of disciplines. Find this book and log in using your username and password to access interactive activities, videos, and much more.

15 The Head and Neck

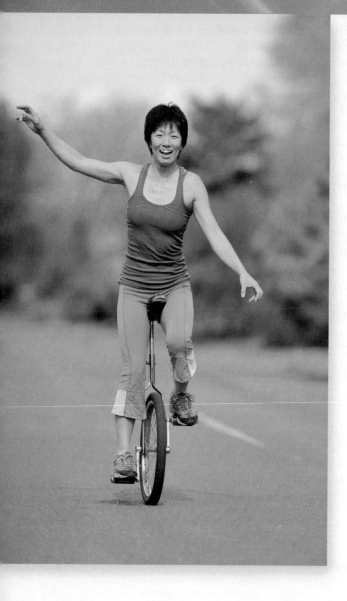

CHAPTER OUTLINE

Chapter Objectives

Key Terms

15.1 Bones of the Head and Neck

15.2 Joints of the Head and Neck

15.3 Muscles of the Head and Neck

Conclusion

Summary Points to Remember

Review Questions

It is fascinating to watch the head righting reflex of the unicycle rider. This reflex is not usually that obvious until the readjustment of the head back to a vertical position looks exaggerated. Head righting is easy to see on a horse that stands up from a lying position. Its elegant equine neck pops up first, and the rest of the body follows.

Head righting pulls the slack out of the spine, lengthening the trunk from the head to the tail. To feel this subtle reflex, a person can close the eyes and sense the small, ongoing movements that occur at the base of the head. If the suboccipital muscles are free

from chronic contractures, there will be a slight bobbing motion of the head.

A person can produce a similar lengthening effect by lifting the occiput without lowering the chin, then subtly nodding the head to activate the suboccipitals. This initiates a chain reaction along the core muscles, which elongates the spine. Most people describe the lengthening experience as a pleasant, almost magical decompression of the spine. This exercise activates intrinsic muscles of the neck, which are important joint stabilizers. It can also relieve pain and prevent neck strain and injury.

CHAPTER OBJECTIVES

1. List eight cranial bones and 14 facial bones and describe the location of each one.

2. Name and describe three cartilaginous structures of the head and neck.

3. Describe the structure and function of the hyoid bone.

4. Demonstrate palpation of cranial and facial bones and miscellaneous structures of the neck.

5. List four cranial sutures, describe their locations, and demonstrate palpation of each one.

6. Describe the structure of the temporomandibular joint (TMJ) and its range of motion.

7. Describe the atlantoaxial and atlanto-occipital joints and their range of motion.

8. Identify the origins, insertions, and actions of the muscles of the head and neck.

9. Demonstrate the active movement and palpation of each muscle of the head and neck.

10. Identify the trigger points and pain referral patterns of the muscles of the head and neck.

11. Discuss the role of the facial muscles in emotional expression and describe each one.

KEY TERMS

Atlantoaxial joint

Atlanto-occipital (AO) joint

Coronal suture

External occipital protuberance

Frontal bone

Hyoid

Mandible

Masseter

Mastoid process

Maxilla

Occipital bone

Parietal bones

Platysma

Protrusion

Pterygoids

Retrusion

Sagittal suture

Superior nuchal line

Temporal bones

Temporalis

Temporomandibular dysfunction (TMD)

Temporomandibular joint (TMJ)

Trachea

Zygomatic arch

MUSCLES IN ACTION

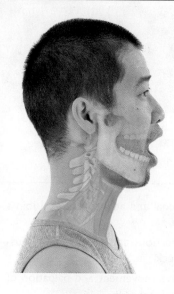

Depression
Platysma
Infrahyoid muscles:
 Omohyoid
 Sternohyoid
 Thyrohyoid

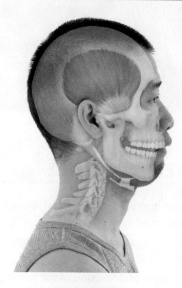

Retraction
Digastric
Temporalis

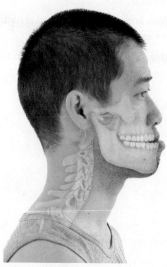

Protraction
Lateral pterygoid

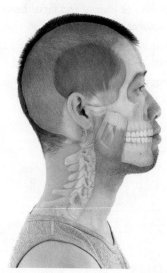

Elevation
Masseter
Medial pterygoid
Temporalis

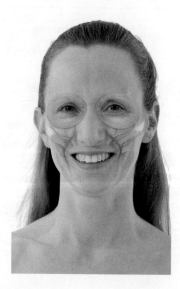

Smiling
Levator anguli oris
Levator anguli superioris
Orbicularis oculi
Risorius
Zygomatic major
Zygomatic minor

Muscles of the Head and Neck in Action

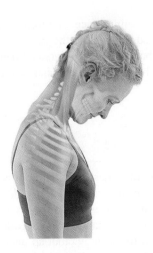

Cervical flexion
Longus capitis
Longus colli
Scalene (anterior)
Sternocleidomastoid

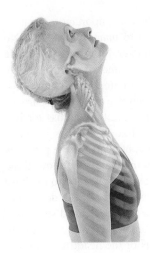

Cervical extension
Levator scapulae
Suboccipital muscles:
  Oblique capitis superior
  Oblique capitis inferior
  Rectus capitis posterior major
  Rectus capitis posterior minor
Trapezius

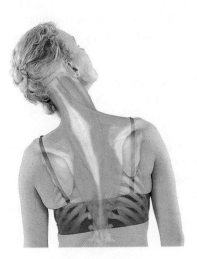

Cervical rotation
Scalenes:
  Anterior
  Middle
  Posterior
Splenius capitis
Splenius cervicis
Sternocleidomastoid
Trapezius (upper)

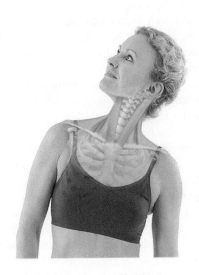

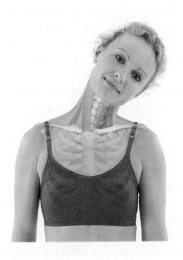

Lateral flexion
Levator scapulae
Longus capitis
Longus colli
Scalenes:
  Anterior
  Middle
  Posterior
Splenius capitis
Splenius cervicis
Sternocleidmastoid
Trapezius (upper)

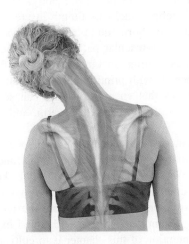

In our journey through the body, it is important to remember that every part is connected to many other parts. No one part exists in isolation. Unnatural divisions are made only to study the body one part at a time. In reality, though, many tissues in the body are contiguous and ubiquitous. The muscles, nerves, and connective tissues unite parts of the body in the same way that rivers flow across territorial boundaries, mountains rise like backbones between nations, and oceans span many continents. In the previous chapter, in order to study the entire spine, we followed the trail of bones and muscles up the cervical spine to the base of the cranium. In this chapter, we journey back down into the neck to explore the muscles and specialized structures critical to eating, talking, and breathing. We also explore bones and muscles in two areas of the head: the cranium and the face.

The head and neck house the brain, part of the spinal cord, and the major sensory organs of the ears, eyes, nose, and mouth. On a functional level, early patterns of movement in the head and neck initiate and organize movement patterns in the spine and upper body. The head also houses the specialized neurological and equilibrium structures that orient the body in space and serve as the central command post for the coordination of movement in the rest of the body. This arrangement positions the head and neck for arm movements requiring hand–eye coordination. The central role that the head and neck play in movement responses can be observed when a person balances on a unicycle or a balance beam. The righting reflexes that keep the head and neck vertical are essential for keeping the rest of the body upright as well. Simply watch a person walk around in a grocery store to notice how the head and neck lead and the body follows. A person turns a corner, for example, by first turning the head. The process is natural and innate.

The joint of most relevance in the head is the temporomandibular joint (TMJ). The TMJ is the first joint to develop in the human body, and it sets up a baseline for neuromuscular pathways in the entire body. The TMJ first moves as a preborn sucks its thumb in utero. This allows the infant to be born equipped for survival with well-established neuromuscular pathways for mouthing movements such as rooting, sucking, and crying. Motor development proceeds with primitive hand-to-mouth and hand-to-eye reflexes that ensure an infant can see and grasp food by coordinating head, neck, arm, and spinal movements.

In this chapter, we study the muscles and special features of the head that are related to the movement functions of TMJ motion. We examine the unique musculoskeletal structures of the cranial and facial bones along with their subtle movement patterns. We also explore the intricate muscles of the face and their role in emotional expression. The main intention of this chapter is to cultivate an understanding of and respect for the intricate structures of the head to provide practitioners with enough knowledge to work effectively with the cranium, face, and throat. As usual, readers are encouraged to practice the movement exercises in this chapter to build your own personal bank of experiential knowledge, which will further enhance your journey through the body.

15.1 BONES OF THE HEAD AND NECK

The head contains two types of bones: the cranial bones and the facial bones. Although the cranium seems like a unified bony vault, eight separate bones house and protect the brain. The cranial bones join at seamless joints called sutures, which can be difficult to locate without an understanding of the location and shape of the individual cranial bones.

The facial bones of the skull reside outside of the cranium. They form the many intricate and hollow cavities of the face, including the mouth and eye sockets and the respiratory sinuses. The facial bones possess numerous foramens that allow for the passage of specialized nerves and blood vessels to the sensory organs of the eyes, ears, nose, and mouth. In a study of the head, understanding the shape and location of the cranial and facial bones, as well as prominent bony landmarks in each, will help you locate the attachment sites of the muscles of the head, jaw, and throat (Figure 15.1 ■).

The neck has seven cervical vertebrae, which are discussed in detail in the chapter on the spine. Of special importance are the unique shapes of the first and second cervical vertebrae—the *atlas* and *axis*—which allow a broad range of motion in the upper cervical spine and at the base of the cranium.

15.1.1 Cranial Bones

The eight cranial bones include two parietal bones, two temporal bones, and single frontal, sphenoid, occipital, and ethmoid bones. The two large, round **parietal bones** make up a major portion of the top, sides, and back of the cranial vault (Figure 15.2 ■). The parietal bones articulate with a large **frontal bone** found across the entire forehead. The frontal bone provides attachment sites for a number of facial muscles around the eyes and brow, and its base forms the roof of the eye sockets along the **supraorbital margin.** Below center of the frontal bone resides a small irregular **ethmoid bone,** which forms the medial, inferior border of the eye sockets and cannot be directly palpated.

A large **occipital bone** makes up the base of the skull at the back of the head. A large opening in the base of the occipital bone, called the **foramen magnum,** provides a passage for the spinal cord to descend like a tail from the brain into the spine (Figure 15.3 ■). The **external occipital protuberance** is a prominent bump in the middle of the occipital bone that provides an attachment site for the

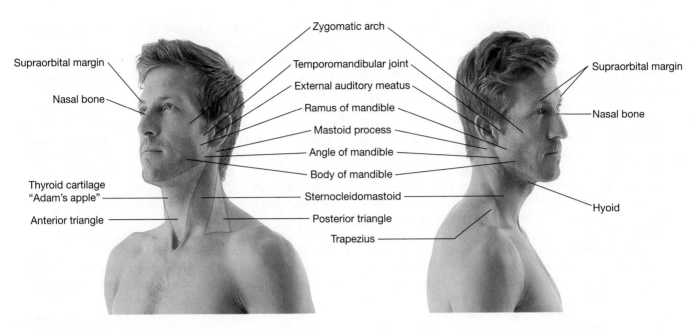

FIGURE 15.1

Surface anatomy of the head and neck

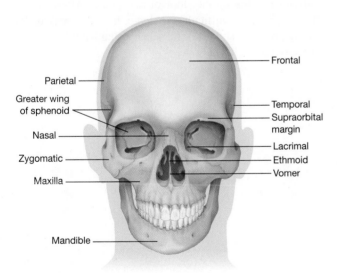

FIGURE 15.2

Cranial and facial bones: anterior view

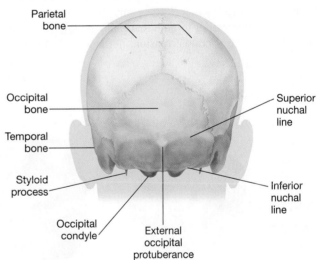

FIGURE 15.3

Cranial bones: posterior view

nuchal ligament of the spine. This protuberance is easy to palpate and provides an important bony landmark to locate when working with the suboccipital and posterior neck muscles. Two slight bony ridges—the **superior nuchal line** and **inferior nuchal line**—that run laterally across the occiput on either side of the external occipital protuberance provides attachment sites for the trapezius and splenii muscles of the neck and shoulders. The cranium rests on the cervical spine over two convex **occipital condyles** found at the base of the occipital bone. As we nod the head, the occipital condyles rock like the runners of a rocking chair in the grooves of two concave articular condyles on the superior surface of the first cervical vertebra (Figure 15.4a-b ■).

The keystone of the cranial vault is a butterfly-shaped bone called the **sphenoid,** which is the only cranial bone that articulates with all the other cranial bones (Figure 15.5a-b ■). The sphenoid articulates with the occiput directly anterior to the foramen magnum. It forms the posterior border of the eye socket and contains numerous small foramens that allow the passage of cranial nerves and blood vessels to and from the brain. The **greater wings of the sphenoid** can be directly palpated over the temples in the small bony depressions directly lateral of the eyes. Given its central location in the cranium, centering the sphenoid in the cranium is an important technique used in cranialsacral therapy that restores balance to the entire cranium. It is interesting to note that many people rub their temples to relieve cranial tension, perhaps an instinctive move to release cranial tension by adjusting the greater wings of the sphenoid.

People also instinctively massage the **temporal bones** around the ears to relieve stress, perhaps another natural tendency to address the cranial bones most directly involved with hearing, balance, and jaw motion. The temporal bones make up the sides of the cranial vault (Figure 15.6 ■). They contain a number of intricate hollow structures that house the inner ear and labyrinth—a vestibular maze of bony tunnels and chambers involved in hearing and proprioception (see "Labyrinth and Neck Proprioceptors" in the neuromuscular chapter). The **external acoustic meatus,** or ear canal, provides an opening to the inner ear. Above the ear, a broad **temporal fossa** provides a large attachment site for the temporalis, a strong jaw muscle.

Anterior to the meatus, a concave depression called the **mandibular fossa** provides a superior articular surface for the temporomandibular joint. The anterior part of the temporal bone tapers into a noticeable bar-like **zygomatic process** that extends into the cheek. A prominent bony bump on the temporal bone called the **mastoid process** provides attachment sites for the trapezius and sternocleidomastoid muscles. Below the ear canal, a slender **styloid process** projects down and anteriorly. This small, stake-like bone provides an attachment site for several ligaments and muscles making up the floor of the mouth. Although the styloid process is difficult to palpate, it could break under strong pressure, so be careful when doing hands-on palpation around this small bone.

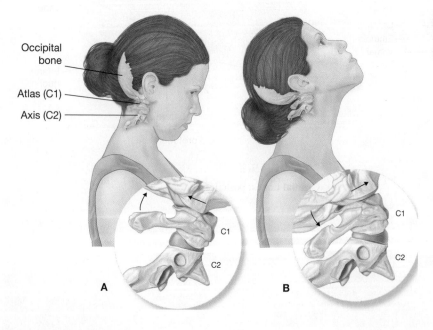

Occipital
bone

Atlas (C1)

Axis (C2)

C1

C2

C1

C2

A   B

FIGURE 15.4

Occipital condyles rocking on atlas:
a) Flexion b) Extension

FIGURE 15.5
Cranial vault: a) Superior view
b) Inferior view

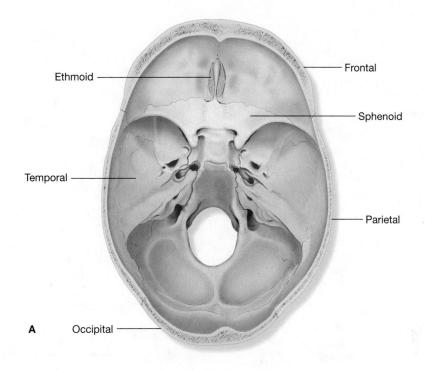

Ethmoid

Frontal

Sphenoid

Temporal

Parietal

A   Occipital

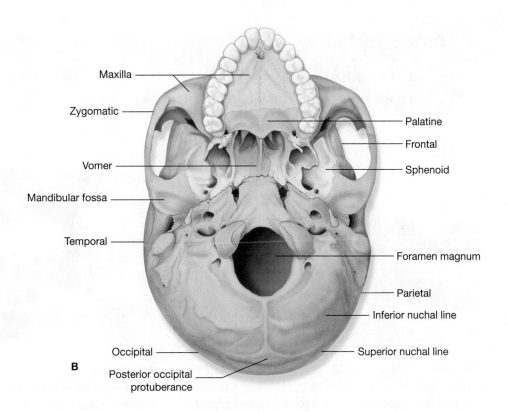

Maxilla

Zygomatic

Palatine

Frontal

Vomer

Sphenoid

Mandibular fossa

Temporal

Foramen magnum

Parietal

Inferior nuchal line

Occipital

Superior nuchal line

B

Posterior occipital
protuberance

Parietal

Temporal fossa

Occipital

Temporal

External
acoustic
meatus

Mastoid
process

Styloid
process

Zygomatic process

Frontal

Greater wing
of sphenoid

Ethmoid

Lacrimal

Nasal

Zygomatic

Maxilla

Mandible

Zygomatic arch

FIGURE 15.6

Cranial bones: lateral view

BONE PALPATION
Cranial Bones and Bony Landmarks

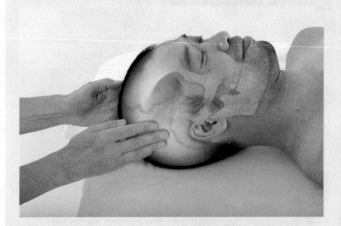

FIGURE 15.7a
Sit comfortably at the head of the table and contact the **parietal bones,** one in each hand, and explore their shape and symmetry. Gently traction the parietals in the cephalad (superior) direction. *Are your hands on the top, back aspects of the cranium? When you traction the parietals, what does your partner feel?* (See Figure 15.7a ■)

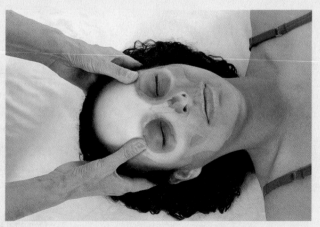

FIGURE 15.7b
Place your hands across the broad, flat **frontal bone.** Explore the shape and symmetry of the two sides of this bone across the forehead, from the eyebrows to the temples, and from the forehead to the top of the cranium. *Do you feel the lateral border of the frontal bone along a slight bony ridge over the temples?* (See Figure 15.7b ■)

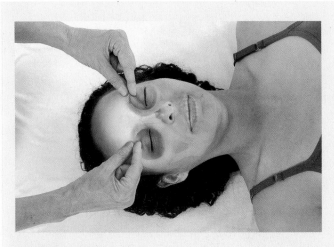

FIGURE 15.7c

Use a gentle pincher palpation to explore the bony edge of the **supraorbital margin** along the top edge of the eye socket. Use direct and light fingertip palpation to explore the infraorbital margin below the eyes. *Do you notice the curved shape of the supraorbital margin?* (See Figure 15.7c ■)

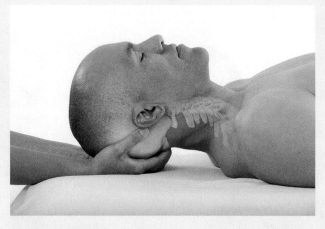

FIGURE 15.7d

Cradle the **occipital bone** on the back of the skull. Make sure your partner can relax the weight of his or her head into your hands. Press your fingertips up into the occipital bone, then explore its shape. Turn the head to one side and locate the **external occipital protuberance** in the center of the posterior occiput. *Is your partner able to give you the weight of his or her head? Are you able to feel the bump in the center of the posterior occiput?* (See Figure 15.7d ■)

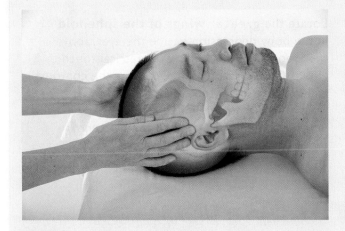

FIGURE 15.7e

Cup the **temporal bones** lightly with both of your hands. Use a symmetrical touch because asymmetrical pressure on the temporal bones can trigger a headache on some people. With the pads of your fingers, explore the shape and size of the **temporal fossa.** Gently traction the temporal fossa in the cephalad (superior) direction. *Are your hands above the ears? Are the temporal bones symmetrical?* (See Figure 15.7e ■)

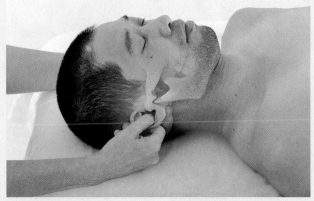

FIGURE 15.7f

Using symmetrical touch on this and all remaining steps. Grasp the ears close to the cranium between your index finger and your thumb with a gentle pincher grip. Gently palpate the **external acoustic meatus** or ear canal, then lightly traction both ears in the lateral direction. *Are the ear canals symmetrical? When you applied traction to the ear canals, how far did your partner feel the stretch inside the head?* (See Figure 15.7f ■)

(continued)

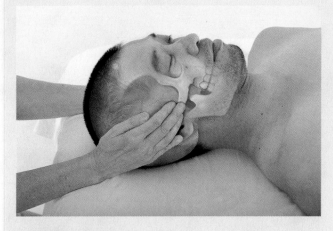

FIGURE 15.7g
Trace the **zygomatic processes** of the temporal bone from in front of the ears to the cheekbones. *Are you on the bony ridges along the sides of the cheeks? Can you find the joint line between the temporal and zygomatic bones?* (See Figure 15.7g ■)

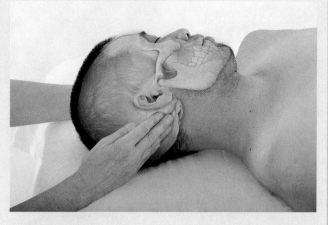

FIGURE 15.7h
Locate the **mastoid processes** behind the earlobes. Gently explore the round shape and size of the process, then strum across the tendons attached to it. *Are you on the bony bumps behind the earlobes? Are the tendons attached to the mastoid processes symmetrical in tone?* (See Figure 15.7h ■)

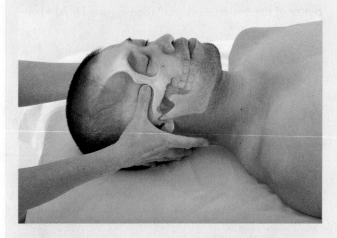

FIGURE 15.7i

Locate the **greater wings of the sphenoid** in the bony depression beside the eyes, above the zygomatic arch. Use a symmetrical touch to explore both sides at once, noticing the contours and symmetries of the sphenoid wings. Gently traction the sphenoid wings toward the ceiling. *Are you palpating about 1 inch lateral to each eye socket? Are the two sides symmetrical?* (See Figure 15.7i ■)

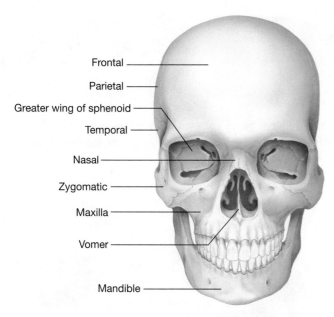

FIGURE 15.8
Facial bones

15.1.2 Facial Bones

There are 14 facial bones. All of the facial bones except the mandible and the vomer come in pairs. The nasals, lacrimals, palatines, and inferior nasal conchae—all small, thin, and irregular facial bones—form the multiplex of sinus cavities. All four of these bone pairs articulate with the paired maxilla, which make up two-thirds of the upper palate and provides a floor for the cavernous network of the sinuses.

The **maxilla** is made up of two bones (Figure 15.8 ■). The maxilla can be thought of as the keystone of the face because it articulates with so many other facial bones. Its structural articulations will be of importance later when we examine the motion of the upper palate in opening and closing the mouth. The superior border of the maxilla makes up the lower, inner portion of the eye sockets. The inferior border of the maxilla provides a bony bridge under the upper lip that contains 16 sockets for upper teeth. The bottom of the maxilla articulates with the two **palatine bones,** which together make up a hard palate ceiling in the mouth (Figure 15.9 ■). Depending on how the maxilla and palatine bones join together along the midline, the hard palate can range from a dome-shaped, cathedral ceiling to a relatively flat, horizontal ceiling. The superior edge of the maxilla articulates with two small **nasal bones** that form the bridge of the nose. The lateral borders of the maxilla articulate with the **zygomatic bones** in the middle of the cheek. The zygomatic bones make up the lower and lateral portion of the eye sockets and the prominent ridge across the top of the cheeks called the **zygomatic arch.**

The maxilla articulates with the mandible of the lower jaw through the occlusion, or fitting together, of the upper

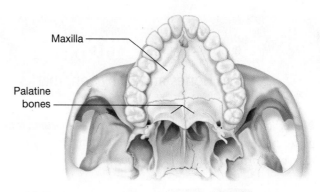

FIGURE 15.9
Palatine bones in upper palate

and lower teeth. The U-shaped **mandible** is the largest and most mobile bone in the face. It contains 16 sockets that hold the lower teeth (Figure 15.10 ■). The mandible has two major parts: the broad horizontal **body of the mandible** is what a person rests on when propping the chin on the hand; a flat and wide vertical part of the mandible called the **ramus** projects upward toward the upper jaw. The ramus has two processes along its superior border: a flat, wide **mandibular condyle** provides the lower articular surface of the temporomandibular joint; a pointed **coronoid process** provides an attachment site for the temporalis. The **angle of the mandible** forms a sharp corner at the posterior inferior corner of the lower jaw, directly anterior and inferior to the earlobe. In order to do effective work on TMJ dysfunctions, which are incredibly common, you will need to become adept at palpating the bony landmarks on the mandible to locate muscular attachments for the jaws.

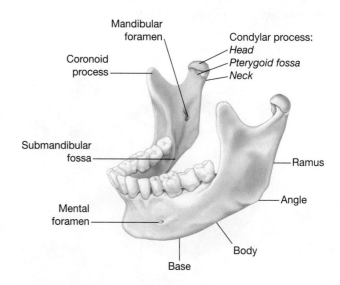

FIGURE 15.10
Mandible

BONE PALPATION
Facial Bones and Bony Landmarks

Note: *If you palpate the palatine bones on a partner, make sure to wear finger cotters or protective latex or vinyl gloves because you will need to palpate them inside your partner's mouth. If you are using latex gloves, make sure to ask your partner about latex allergies before you begin.*

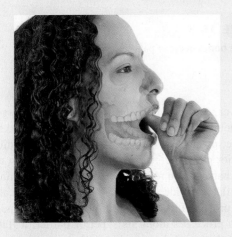

FIGURE 15.11a

After washing your hands thoroughly, locate the **palatine bones** on the back third of your upper palate by gently pressing your thumb on the roof of your mouth. Explore the contours of your palate, particularly the suture along the middle. Hook your thumb behind your front tooth and gentle traction your palate in an anterior direction. *Do you feel a suture along the middle of the upper palate? Do you feel a light stretch in your face when you gently pull your palate forward?* (See Figure 15.11a ■)

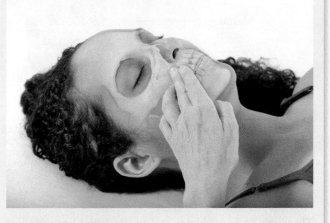

FIGURE 15.11b

Palpate the **maxilla** above the upper lip, along the top edge of the upper teeth. Walk your fingertips up the maxilla and explore the contour of your cheeks. Locate the medial edge of the maxilla along the side of the nose and follow this edge up to the inner, lower corner of the eye socket. *Do you feel the lower border of the maxilla above the upper teeth? Do you notice the rounded shape of the maxilla over the cheeks?* (See Figure 15.11b ■)

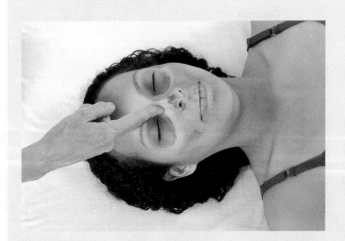

FIGURE 15.11c

Locate the small **nasal bones** between the eyes along the bridge of the nose. Move down the bridge of the nose toward the tip, noticing where nasal bones joint with nasal cartilage. Gently squeeze the nasal bones and traction them toward the ceiling. *Do you feel the bump where the nasal bones end and the cartilage of the nose begins?* (See Figure 15.11c ■)

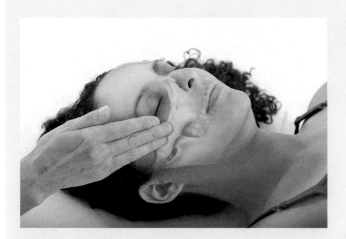

FIGURE 15.11d

Palpate the lateral half of the **zygomatic bones** of the cheeks, gently pressing both sides at once, moving in a lateral direction toward the ears. Notice where they taper into a bony ridge of the **zygomatic arch.** About an inch in front of the ear, you should feel a subtle bony ridge, where the zygomatic bone articulates with the temporal bone. *Do you notice how the zygomatic arch turns a corner on the side of the cheek? Do you feel where the zygomatic arch joins the temporal bone?* (See Figure 15.11d ■)

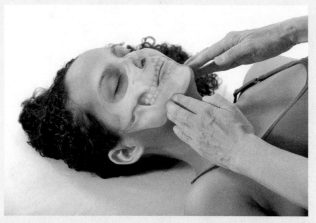

FIGURE 15.11e

Press across the **body of the mandible** along the lower half of the chin, below the lower lip. Explore the contours of the mandible using a pincher palpation along its lower edge. *Can you feel the joint lines between the lower teeth and the mandible?* (See Figure 15.11e ■)

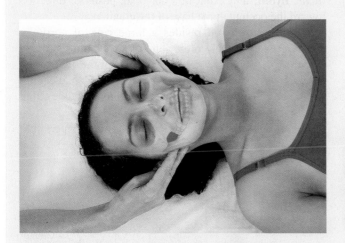

FIGURE 15.11f

Walk your fingertips along the bottom edge to the **mandibular angle,** which will feel like a right angle in the bone. *How wide is the body of the mandible from its center to its side? Do you feel the muscular attachments under the lower rib of the mandible? Did you locate the right angle at the corner of the mandible?* (See Figure 15.11f ■)

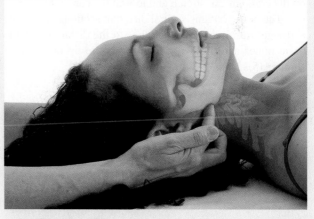

FIGURE 15.11g

Walk your fingertips up the **ramus of the mandible** toward the TMJ. Explore the posterior border of the ramus in front of the ear. Strum across the ramus toward the anterior border. (See Figure 15.11g ■)

(continued)

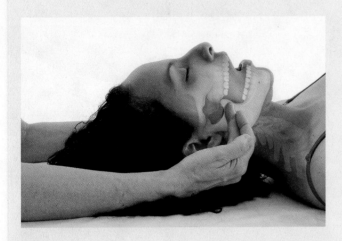

FIGURE 15.11h

Locate the **coronoid process** of the mandible with the mouth open, sliding your fingertips across the soft tissue along the cheek below the zygomatic arch. It will feel like a hard structure in the center of the cheek. Explore its shape while opening and closing the mouth. *Do you notice how far the mouth must be opened to clearly feel the coronoid process?* (See Figure 15.11h ■)

15.1.3 Miscellaneous Structures of the Head and Neck

The outer ear provides a supportive yet flexible-enough structure to allow these appendages to bend when we rest our heads on a pillow. The **auricle of the outer ear** contains strong yet flexible elastic cartilage that can usually bend and fold. Connective tissues covering the outer ear are continuous with tissues in the middle ear, which is why massaging and pulling the ears close to their attachments on the cranium can stretch and loosen the ear canal.

The nose contains several different sections of hyaline cartilage: **nasal cartilage** attaches to the distal end of the nasal bones and **alar cartilage** forms the tip of the nose (Figure 15.12 ■).

A U-shaped bone called the **hyoid** is located where the front of the neck meets the floor of the mouth (Figure 15.13 ■). The hyoid is an unusual "floating bone" because it is suspended in a sea of tissue by ligaments and the tendons of many hyoid muscles. The hyoid does not articulate with any other bone; its main function is to provide a bony attachment site for muscles of the mouth and throat. The tips of the hyoid are called the **greater horns of the hyoid;** they point in a diagonal, posterior direction toward the occiput at the base of the cranium.

Below the hyoid resides a large ring of cartilage that houses the vocal cords, called the **thyroid cartilage** (Figure 15.14 ■). It is located at the level of the 4th and 5th cervical vertebra. The thyroid cartilage and a smaller ring called the **cricoid cartilage** make a prominent bulge along the front of the neck known as the "Adam's apple," which moves up and down as a person swallows. It tapers into

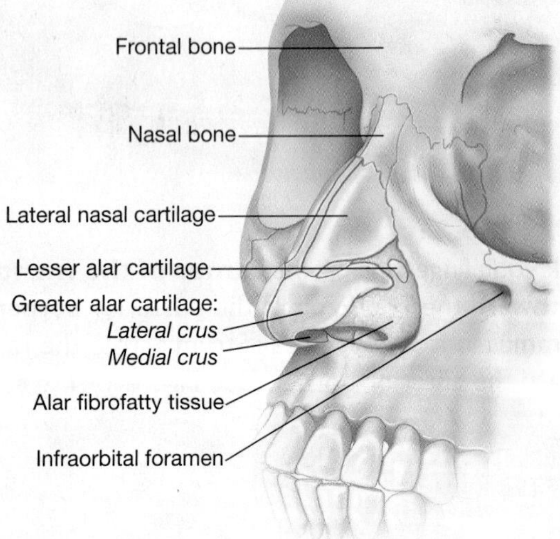

Frontal bone

Nasal bone

Lateral nasal cartilage

Lesser alar cartilage

Greater alar cartilage:
Lateral crus
Medial crus

Alar fibrofatty tissue

Infraorbital foramen

FIGURE 15.12

Nasal cartilage

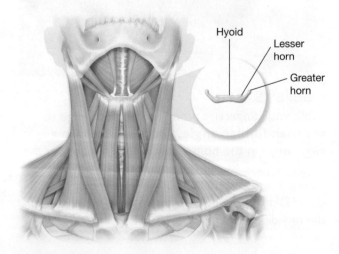

Hyoid

Lesser horn

Greater horn

FIGURE 15.13

Hyoid bone and hyoid muscles

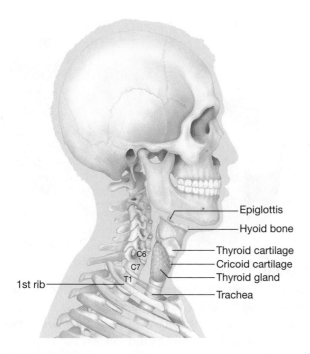

FIGURE 15.14
Miscellaneous structures of the neck

Labels: Epiglottis, Hyoid bone, Thyroid cartilage, Cricoid cartilage, Thyroid gland, Trachea, C6, C7, T1, 1st rib

the **trachea**—a long, flexible tube made of fibrocartilage rings that are better known as the "windpipe." The trachea branches into two stalk-like bronchi inside the chest where they permeate the lungs. A small, subcutaneous **thyroid gland** wraps the anterior and lateral sides of the trachea beneath the cricoid cartilage and above the jugular notch of the manubrium.

Avoid putting pressure on the thyroid cartilage, cricoid cartilage, trachea, and thyroid gland along the front of the neck, although palpating them gently will help you learn what they feel like so that you recognize them during a hands-on session.

15.2 JOINTS OF THE HEAD AND NECK

The only movable synovial joint in the head is the temporomandibular joint of the jaws. Other joints in the head include sutures, which are classified as fibrous and immovable joints, and the gomphosis peg-in-socket joints that seat the teeth into the maxilla and mandible.

The temporomandibular joint (TMJ) is a unique synovial articulation because it is the most used of all the synovial joints in the body. The TMJ moves whenever we

BONE PALPATION
Ears, Nose, Hyoid, and Throat Structures

Caution: The structures along the front of the neck can be sensitive to touch, particularly if a person has neck trauma and/or choking anxiety. Make sure to ask your partner before touching the front of the neck. Use a slow, gentle touch to palpate structures in this area.

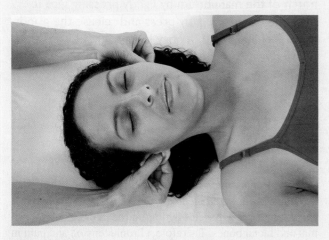

FIGURE 15.15a

With your partner in a supine position, use a pincher grasp to hold the **auricles of the ears** along the front and back, between your thumbs and forefingers. Explore their shape and flexibility, gently moving the ears. *How flexible are the ears?* (See Figure 15.15a ■)

(continued)

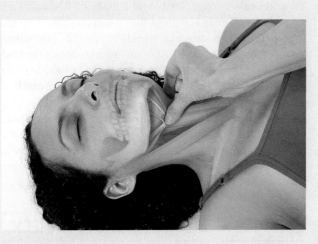

FIGURE 15.15b

Locate the **hyoid** by applying light pressure in the center of the crease under the chin, along the front of the neck. Gently walk your fingertips along the width of the hyoid. To feel how it moves, lightly hold the hyoid while your partner slowly turns and nods the head; then have your partner swallow. Gently move the hyoid through its small range of motion, in a lateral and a vertical direction. *Are you palpating the hyoid in the crease at the top of the anterior neck?* (See Figure 15.15b ■)

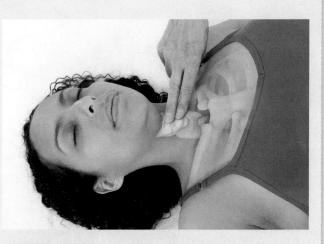

FIGURE 15.15c

Gently palpate the **thyroid cartilage, cricoid cartilage,** and **trachea** along the front of the throat, below the hyoid. Lightly touch the trachea while your partner swallows to feel its motion. *Are you palpating below the hyoid along the midline of the neck? Do you feel the ridges along the thyroid cartilage? Did you feel it move during swallowing?* (See Figure 15.15c ■)

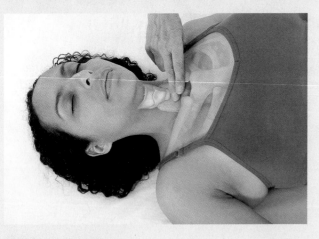

FIGURE 15.15d

Gently palpate the **thyroid gland** above the jugular notch of the manubrium by lightly pressing into it over the trachea. Lightly press and release the gland; it will feel like a thin, spongy layer over the trachea. *Are you right above the sternal notch? Does the gland feel spongy and springy?* (See Figure 15.15d ■)

talk, eat, and swallow. It is also active in subconscious stress reactions, causing a person to grind the teeth or clench the jaws in response to emotional distress. Because of its high degree of functional use and its inclination to undergo excessive wear in people experiencing emotional stress, many people suffer with chronic pain generated by TMJ dysfunction. The prevalence of TMJ problems makes it important for practitioners to understand the unique structural and functional features of the TMJ in order to provide effective treatment.

Many of the muscles acting on the TMJ attach to cranial and facial bones. Therefore, chronic tension and pain in the TMJ can broadcast throughout the head. Although the sutures of the cranium are relatively immovable, massaging them can alleviate pressure and tension in the head. Learning to locate and palpate the sutures can help you effectively

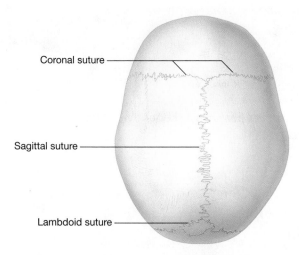

Coronal suture

Sagittal suture

Lambdoid suture

Superior

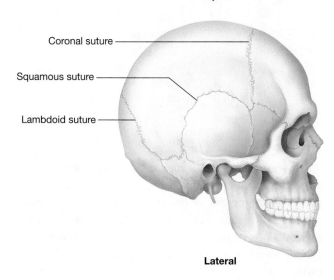

Coronal suture

Squamous suture

Lambdoid suture

Lateral

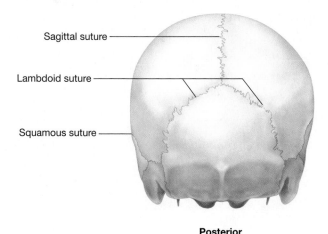

Sagittal suture

Lambdoid suture

Squamous suture

Posterior

FIGURE 15.16
Cranial sutures

treat widespread myofascial pain syndromes such as TMJ dysfunctions and chronic headaches.

Although the TMJ is the joint of greatest functional significance in the head, we cover the cranial sutures first so that you can practice palpation on them to evoke a relaxation response in the head, which makes palpating easier on the often dysfunctional and highly sensitive TMJ.

15.2.1 Cranial Sutures

Adjacent cranial bones connect to each other along fibrous joints called **sutures** (Figure 15.16 ■). The jagged tooth-like borders of the sutures interlock like interlaced fingers. Although there are many other sutures, four long sutures can be directly palpated and massaged in the cranium.

- **Coronal suture:** Between parietal and frontal bones, across the top of the head
- **Sagittal suture:** Between parietal bones, down the center of the top of the head
- **Lamboid suture:** Between occiput and parietal bones, arcs over back of skull
- **Squamous suture:** Between temporal and parietal bones, arcs over top of ear

The interdigitated and beveled structures of the sutures contain nerves, blood vessels, and connective tissues within the sutures (Figure 15.17 ■). The sutures move with a subtle and barely perceptible rhythm that is generated by the cerebrospinal fluid production and circulation in the brain. Cranialsacral therapy (CST) was developed by cranial osteopaths and is widely practiced in the massage and bodywork field. It uses a light touch to track and manipulate the subtle and slow oscillatory motion of the sutures. Cranial sutures can become immobilized or torqued as a result of head injuries, car accidents, and birthing trauma. This condition can lead to an array of symptoms including headaches, ringing in the ears, disorientation, and agitation.

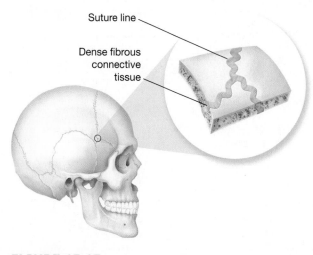

Suture line

Dense fibrous connective tissue

FIGURE 15.17
Cranial suture

BONE PALPATION
Cranial Sutures

Caution: The cranial sutures can be tender to touch if a person suffers from headaches or a head trauma. If they are tender, palpate with a light touch and avoid using deep pressure.

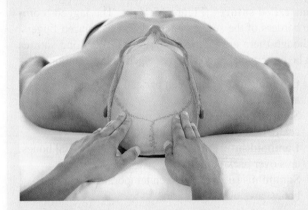

FIGURE 15.18a
With your partner in a supine position, trace the **coronal suture** across the top of the cranium, in the middle between the ears. The suture feels like a distinct, narrow bony groove with ragged edges. It connects the frontal bone to the parietal bone and usually feels like a thin depression running across the top of the head. *Does the suture feel like a thin ditch or seam along the cranium?* (See Figure 15.18a ■)

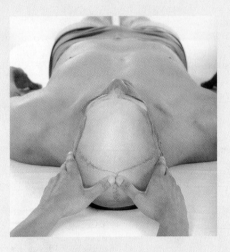

FIGURE 15.18b
With your partner in a supine position, trace the **sagittal suture** by finding the middle of the coronal suture in the center of the top of the cranium. Since the sagittal suture is over major blood vessels in the sagittal sinus of the brain, it can be tender and feel slightly swollen, in which case palpate it carefully and avoid deep pressure. *Are you in the center of the top of the skull, moving from the middle toward the back?* (See Figure 15.18b ■)

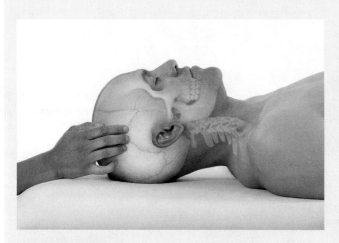

FIGURE 15.18c

With your partner in a supine position, trace the **squamous sutures** on the sides of the skull in a broad arc above the ear, along the upper border of the temporal bones. The temporalis muscle lies over this suture, so it usually feels good to palpate the suture using deep, small, circular strokes. (See Figure 15.18c ■)

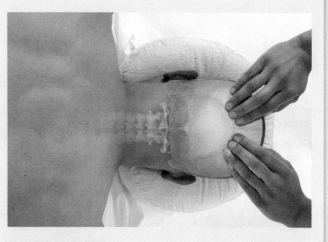

FIGURE 15.18d

With your partner in a prone position, trace the **lamboid suture** along the back of the cranium between the parietal bones and the occipital. It runs in an arc across a flat area of the posterior cranium. *Do you notice how the shape of this suture varies from one individual to the next?* (See Figure 15.18d ■)

The cranial bones provide attachment sites for connective tissue membranes—the *meninges* and *dural tube*—around the brain and the spinal cord. In CST, a practitioner lightly holds and lifts the cranial bones to stretch the connective tissues around the brain and spinal cord and restore fluid circulation to the head and base of the cranium.

Cranial mobilization has similar goals as cranialsacral therapy, but uses greater pressure to restore mobility and symmetry to the cranial bones. Cranial mobilization techniques range from cross-fiber friction on the sutures to move the bones to myofascial release on tissues covering the cranium. Learning about cranial therapies can help you understand the direction of movement of the cranial bones. These therapies provide a template for effectively massaging the head and give you confidence in treating clients who suffer from headaches, closed-head injuries, and systemic stress from high sympathetic tone. Learning how to track the subtle rhythms of the cerebrospinal fluid, which broadcasts throughout the body through the ubiquitous fascial network, can also increase your touch sensitivity.

In most approaches to CST, the cranial bones are pulled so that the cranium expands in all directions. Generally speaking, the parietal bones are lifted straight up in a cephalad direction; the frontal bone, wings of the sphenoid, and nasal bones are lifted anteriorly; the occiput is pulled back in a posterior direction; and the temporal bones are pulled out in a lateral direction.

15.2.2 Temporomandibular Joint

The **temporomandibular joint (TMJ)** is a unique and complex synovial articulation located between the mandibular condyle of the mandible and the glenoid fossa of the temporal bone on each side of the face (Figure 15.19a ■). The TMJ is usually classified as a condyloid joint, but its structure and movement are especially complex. A disk divides the joint into two compartments, each moving with different biomechanics, so the TMJ is also a compound joint. And because of the shape of its articulating surfaces and the fact that it can move in three planes, the TMJ may be considered a ball-and-socket joint as well.

To endure the wear and tear of continual use, the TMJ differs from typical synovial joints in several ways. First, the TMJ lacks hyaline cartilage on its articular surfaces. Instead, a dense, nonvascular, and fibrous connective tissue over the joint surfaces allows for continual remodeling of worn tissues. To further minimize mechanical stress on the

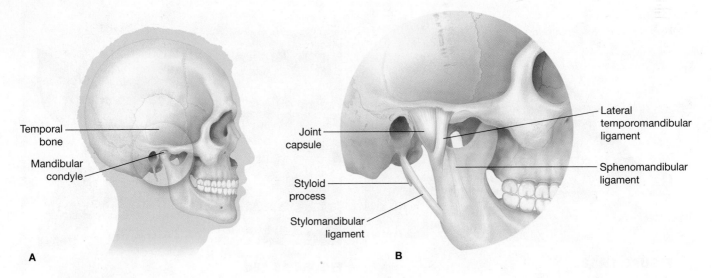

FIGURE 15.19

a) **Temporomandibular joint** b) **Temporomandibular ligaments and joint capsule**

TMJ, its thin articular disk is made up of dense nonvascular fibrous tissue that pads the joint space. In addition, a small but sturdy joint capsule surrounds the TMJ, and a **lateral temporomandibular ligament** stabilizes the joint anterior to the joint capsule (Figure 15.19b ■).

The TMJ moves in six directions (Figure 15.20 ■):

● **Lateral excursion** (lateral deviation): Jutting to the right and left
● **Protrusion** (protraction): Jutting forward
● **Retrusion** (retraction): Pulling back
● **Elevation:** Closing
● **Depression:** Opening

Chewing is a circular combination of all six movements. Grinding is a horizontal circular motion that combines lateral deviation with protrusion and retraction. TMJ motion is especially complex because the upper and lower parts move in different ways. For example, the mandibular condyle moves against the disk in a hinge-like motion during the initiation of opening the jaw; the disk and condyle move together in a forward gliding motion as the jaw continues to open. The disk divides the joint into upper and lower compartments and, as a person opens and closes the mouth, glides anteriorly and posteriorly like a pad between

two wheels (Figure 15.21 ■). In a normal range of TMJ motion, a person should be able to open the mouth far enough to place three fingers sideways between the upper and lower teeth (Figure 15.22 ■).

It is important to understand the complexity of TMJ motion every time the jaw moves. At birth, overall musculoskeletal tone is undeveloped, yet general flexor tone exists due to fetal flexion. Extensor tone begins to develop in the spine as the infant lifts its head to suckle. As the mouth opens, the mandible depresses and protracts, and the head simultaneously rocks the upper cervical joints into extension. This dynamic can be observed by watching a baby sucking its thumb. The upper palate literally rocks on the thumb, causing the head to rock on the neck. Rarely does a person open the mouth without moving the neck. If just the mandible moved when we opened the mouth, the movement would be mechanical and unnatural, engaging only one part of the joint in a hinge action without the gliding action.

Like all synovial joints, the TMJ has an ideal neutral position. To feel joint neutral in the TMJ, allow a small space to open between your upper and lower back teeth (the molars). This will relax the elevator muscles of the mandible and interrupt a habit of clenching the teeth. In neutral,

FIGURE 15.20

Temporomandibular movements

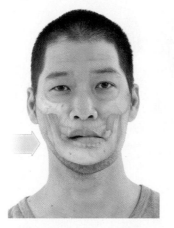

Left lateral excursion (devation)

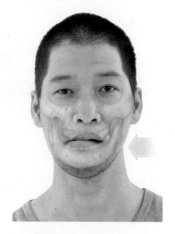

Right lateral excursion

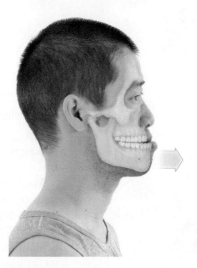

Protrusion or protraction

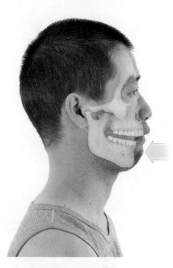

Retrusion or retraction

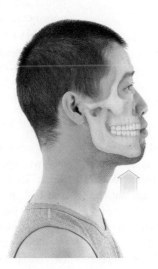

Elevation

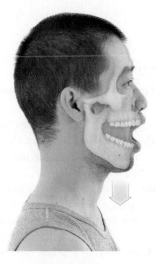

Depression

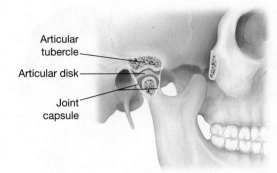

Articular
tubercle

Articular disk

Joint
capsule

Mouth closed

Mouth opened midway

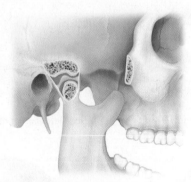

Mouth open all the way

FIGURE 15.21
Temporomandibular disk position

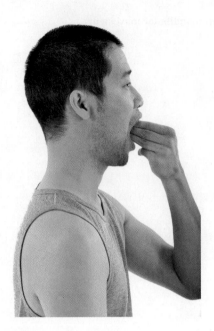

FIGURE 15.22
Normal range of TMJ depression

the tip of the tongue touches the back of the upper front teeth, although the body of the tongue should be relaxed away from the roof of the mouth. The tongue is a muscle that, like any other muscle, can hold chronic tension. When tense, the tongue tends to become plastered against the upper palate (which is why public speakers are encouraged to relax the tongue before stepping on stage). To feel how chronic tongue tension affects muscles of the head and neck, cradle your jaw and neck with both hands, then press

your tongue into the roof of your mouth and relax it several times.

Many musculoskeletal dysfunctions can develop in the jaws that fall under a broad and vague diagnosis of **temporomandibular dysfunction** (TMD). There are several causes for TMD, such as premature wear to the disk or the articulating surfaces, muscular imbalances that misalign the joint, or traumas to the head and jaws. The primary symptoms of TMD include restrictions to TMJ motion, chronic headaches, referred muscular pain in the face and neck, poor occlusion of the upper and lower teeth, and pain during TMJ motion. A person might also experience clicking while opening and closing the mouth, which occurs as a result of displacement of the disk and the impact of the disk-condyle complex against the mandibular fossa of the temporal bone.

15.2.3   Atlantoaxial and Atlanto-occipital Joints

As mentioned in the chapter on the spine, the cervical spine has two types of vertebral joints: *facet joints* and *interbody joints*. There are also specialized joints between the cranium and C-1 and C-2—the atlantoaxial joint and the atlanto-occipital joints—that allow a greater range of motion in the upper cervical spine than the lower cervical spine.

The **atlantoaxial joint** is a pivot joint that consists of two parts. The medial part of the joint complex is located

BONE PALPATION
Temporomandibular Joint Structures and Motion

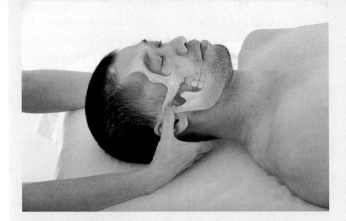

FIGURE 15.23a

To locate the **temporomandibular joint,** place your fingertips in front of the external acoustic meatus (ear canal). The small depression that surfaces when the mouth opens is the TMJ joint space. Press both sides of the TMJ while your partner slowly opens and closes the mouth, noticing how the joints move. *Are you palpating the depression directly in front of the ear canal? Are the TMJs symmetrical? Is either TMJ sore?* (See Figure 15.23a ■)

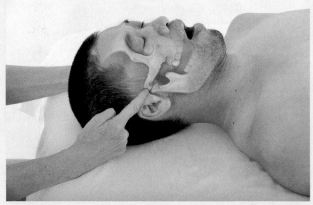

FIGURE 15.23b

With the mouth open, locate the **mandibular fossa** of the temporal bone along the top of the TMJ. It will feel like a small bony notch. *Do you feel the concave edge on the bottom of the mandibular fossa?* (See Figure 15.23b ■)

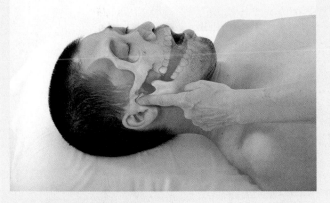

FIGURE 15.23c

Locate the **mandibular condyles** of the mandible along the bottom of the TMJ. The mouth needs to be open while palpating the mandibular condyles, which will feel like small bony knobs buried under thick tissue in the center of your cheeks. Once you locate them, hold them while your partner slowly opens and closes the mouth several times. *Do you feel the bony knob of the mandibular condyle move as the TMJ opens and closes?* (See Figure 15.23c ■)

(continued)

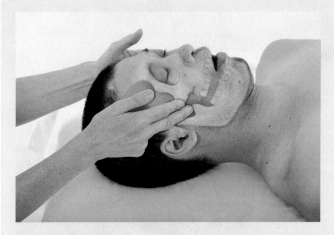

FIGURE 15.23d

To feel the **TMJ motion,** press your fingertips over the center of the TMJs. Open and close the mouth several times, noticing the slight forward movement of the disk as the mouth opens and the slight posterior motion of the disk as the mouth closes. *Is the slight gliding motion of the TMJ disks forward and backward symmetrical? If not, how is it different? Which side moves more?* (See Figure 15.23d ■)

SELF-CARE
Temporomandibular Patterning and Stretching

Use the following exercises to improve joint mechanics by slowly stretching the muscles or tracking the TMJ disk while moving the jaw. As you practice these exercises, focus on opening and closing the mouth slowly and symmetrically. Avoid quick or lateral motions that pop the jaw because they stress the joint and reinforce poor neuromuscular patterning.

You can also practice these exercises with a partner, although it helps to practice them on yourself first to get a sense of how they feel.

the tops of the ears and the hairline, along the bottom of the temporalis (see Figure 15.29). Maintain the pressure as you stretch the tissues in an upward direction (Figure 15.24a ■). Slowly open your mouth as you apply pressure to enhance the stretch. Repeat several times, moving your fingertips slightly anterior or posterior to cover the entire muscle belly.

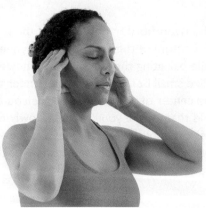

FIGURE 15.24a

1. **Temporalis stretch:** This stretch is great for alleviating headaches caused by jaw muscle tension. To stretch the temporalis, press your fingertips into the tissues between

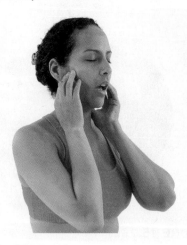

FIGURE 15.24b

2. **Masseter stretch:** Press your fingertips into the origin of the masseters below the zygomatic arch on each side of your face (see Figure 15.35). Slowly open your mouth while stretching the masseter muscles in a downward direction (Figure 15.24b ■). Repeat several times.

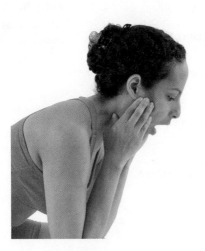

FIGURE 15.24c

3. **TMJ disk tracking:** Begin by placing your fingertips over the joint structures, which are directly in front of your ears. Slowly open and close your mouth several times (Figure 15.24c ■) . If they move asymmetrically, focus on opening and closing with symmetry. If they pop open, the disk may be snapping forward; therefore, open them slowly and evenly to allow the disc time to slide forward with ease. Apply light forward traction on your jaw as you slowly open your mouth to encourage the TMJ disks to glide forward with symmetry. Repeat several times.

between the dens process and two small synovial cavities. The lateral part of the joint complex is made up of two facet joints with nearly horizontal articulating joint surfaces (Figure 15.25a-b ■). The synovial cavities around the dens process are held in place anteriorly by a **transverse ligament** and posteriorly by two diagonally oriented **alar ligaments.** The primary motion of the atlantoaxial joint is turning the head to one side or the other. Eighty percent of axial rotation of the cervical spine occurs at the atlanto-axial joint, which also has about 15 degrees of flexion and extension.

The **atlanto-occipital** (AO) **joints** are two ellipsoid synovial joints (one on each side) between the base of the occiput and the atlas (C-1). The articulating surfaces of the AO joints are nearly horizontal; their primary action is a nodding motion that flexes and extends the head on the neck. During AO motion, the convex occipital condyles rock and glide on the concave C-1 condyles, like a mortar turning in a pestle (Figure 15.26 a-b ■). The AO joints allow for minimal rotation and lateral flexion.

Cervical rotation ranges from 50 to 80 degrees to each side (see Table 15.1 ■). Cervical flexion averages between 40 and 60 degrees. Cervical hyperextension averages between 40 and 75 degrees. Most cervical flexion and cervical extension occurs at the atlanto-occipital joints, between the occiput and C-1. Lateral cervical flexion, which averages 45 degrees, occurs in every segment of the cervical spine.

Recall that the upper cervical spine can move independently of the lower cervical spine. This is important to remember when assessing the neutral position of the neck. The upper cervical could be fixated in chronic hyperextension while the lower cervical becomes fixated in chronic flexion. To return to neutral, the upper cervical will need to move in the opposite direction of the lower cervical spine and flex while the lower cervical spine hyperextends.

15.3 MUSCLES OF THE HEAD AND NECK

As mentioned in the introduction to this chapter, the head and neck play a central role in neuromuscular development because it houses the structures that coordinate movement and balance and organize whole-body patterns. Movement of the head and jaws sequence into the spine, shoulders, and arms through the neck, so it is important to look to muscle patterns of the head and the temporomandibular joint to understand the general muscle patterns in the body.

The muscles of the face and scalp are unique because they are flat and superficial. They lie directly under the skin and attach to each other in a single, continuous plane of tissue. Rather than moving joints through space as the muscles of an arm or leg do, the facial muscles' primary function is to generate expression. They function together in a unified group as a vehicle of emotional expression, which explains why facial massage can be so effective in evoking a deep relaxation response.

The muscles of the head and neck are numerous and intricate. Several posterior neck muscles were covered in the spine chapter, such as the cervical multifidi, the semispinalis capitis, and the splenius muscles. For this study, we explore these muscles in groups based on their locations and functions. Muscles attached to the hyoid bone are included here because of their primary role in jaw and mouthing movements.

- Muscles covering the scalp: *Frontalis, occipitalis,* and *temporalis*
- Muscles of the TMJ: *Masseter, lateral* and *medial pterygoids,* and *buccinator*
- Muscles of facial expression: *Platysma, buccinator, orbicularis oris* and *orbicularis oculi, mentalis, frontalis, corrugators, procerus, nasalis, depressor septi,*

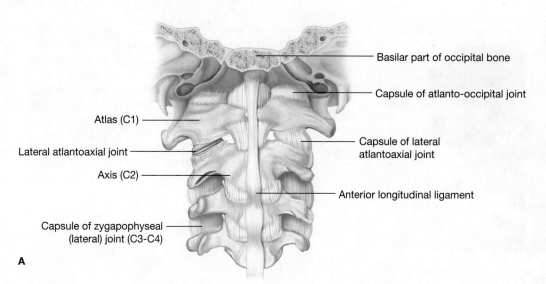

Basilar part of occipital bone

Capsule of atlanto-occipital joint

Atlas (C1)

Lateral atlantoaxial joint

Capsule of lateral
atlantoaxial joint

Axis (C2)

Anterior longitudinal ligament

Capsule of zygapophyseal
(lateral) joint (C3-C4)

A

FIGURE 15.25

**Atlantoaxial joint
complex:** a) Anterior
view b) Superior view

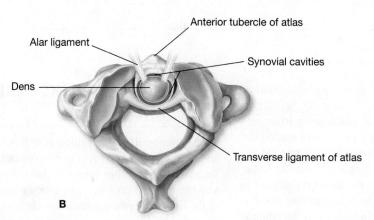

Anterior tubercle of atlas

Alar ligament

Synovial cavities

Dens

Transverse ligament of atlas

B

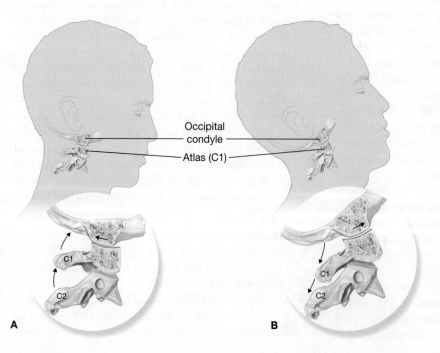

Occipital
condyle

Atlas (C1)

C1

C2

A

C1

C2

B

FIGURE 15.26

Atlanto-occipital joints: a) Flexion
b) Extension

TABLE 15.1 Range of Motion in the Cervical Spine		
Cervical Motion	Range of Motion	End Feel
Flexion	40–60 degrees	Firm
Hyperextension	40–75 degrees	Firm
Lateral flexion	45 degrees to each side	Firm
Rotation	50–80 degrees to each side	Firm

EXPLORING TECHNIQUE
Passive Range of Motion for the Neck

Before you perform these PROM tests on the neck, read through the guidelines:

- Have your partner agree to report any pain or discomfort he or she feels during the motion. During the passive motion, watch for signs of pain or discomfort and stop if you notice any pain reactions.
- To avoid impinging joint structures, lightly traction the neck and upper spine before moving it.
- Have your partner stabilize the spine by lightly contracting the lower abdominal muscles.

- As you stretch the neck, move slowly along a linear pathway.
- When you feel you have reached end range of motion and cannot move the neck any farther, ask your partner if he or she feels a stretch, which will indicate you have reached the end range.

Caution: *Do not perform these stretches on anyone with undiagnosed neck pain, dizziness, nausea, sweating, nystagmus (cross-eyed), facial parasthesia, or trouble swallowing.*

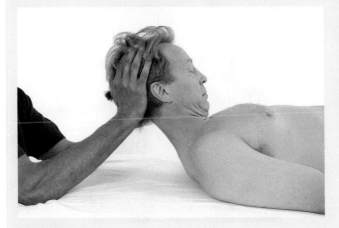

FIGURE 15.27a

a) PROM for flexion of the neck

1. **Neck flexion:** Apply light traction to the neck, then slowly lift the head to take the neck into flexion (Figure 15.27a ■). Once you have reached end range, hold it there to give your partner a sustained stretch. *Does your partner feel a stretch along the back of the neck?*

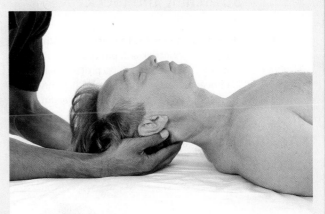

FIGURE 15.27b

b) PROM for hyperextension of the neck

2. **Neck hyperextension:** Place your hands under the upper part of the neck and slowly bend it backward (Figure 15.27b ■). *Does your partner feel a stretch along the front of the neck? Are you maintaining traction on the neck and spine as you hyperextend the neck?*

(continued)

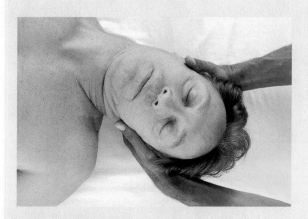

FIGURE 15.27c

c) PROM for lateral flexion of the neck

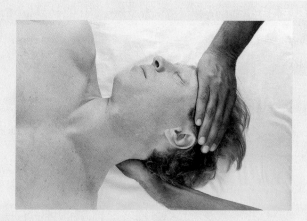

FIGURE 15.27d

d) PROM for rotation of the neck

3. **Lateral flexion:** Traction the neck and upper spine, then slowly side-bend the neck (Figure 15.27c ■). Your partner may feel the lateral flexion sequence down the back and stretch the entire spine. *Are you maintaining traction on the neck and spine? Are you keeping the face turned toward the ceiling and the head level with the table?*

4. **Neck rotation:** To rotate the head to the right, place your left hand under the base of the cranium and your right hand against the side of the upper cranium. Traction the neck and upper spine, then slowly rotate the neck by turning it toward the left while pressing the cranium toward the table (Figure 15.27d ■). Press until your partner reports a stretch. Repeat in the other direction. *Are you using leverage to rotate the neck by moving your hands in the opposite direction?*

SELF-CARE
Stretching the Neck

1. **Self-stretch in passive flexion:** To passively stretch your neck in flexion, lie on your back and put your hands behind your neck. Contract your abdominals to protect your back. Slowly lift your head up until you feel a stretch in the muscles along the back of your neck, then hold for about 10 seconds (Figure 15.28a ■).
2. **Self-stretch in rotation:** To self-stretch your neck in rotation, lie on your back and place your right hand under your neck, palm up. Hook your fingertips around the left side of

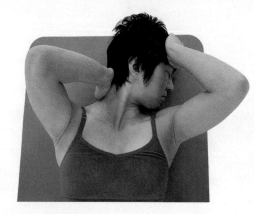

FIGURE 15.28b

your neck. Put your left palm against the right side of your forehead, then turn your head to the left. Stretch your neck by pulling the back of your neck to the right with your right hand while pressing your forehead further left with your left palm (Figure 15.28b ■).You will feel the stretch in tissues under your right hand, and may even feel the stretch in the joint structures of the cervical spine. Hold for several seconds, then repeat on the other side.

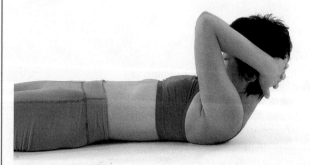

FIGURE 15.28a

depressor labii inferior and *depressor anguli oris,*
levator labii and *levator anguli oris, zygomatic major*
and *zygomatic minor,* and *risorius*
- Muscles attached to the hyoid bone:
  - Suprahyoid muscles: *Mylohyoid, geniohyoid,*
    stylohyoid, and *digastric*
  - Infrahyoid muscles: *Sternohyoid, thyrohyoid,* and
    omohyoid
- Posterior suboccipital muscles: *Posterior rectus capi-*
  tis major, posterior rectus capitis minor, oblique capi-
  tis inferior, and *oblique capitis superior*
- Anterior and prevertebral neck muscles: *Sternocleido-*
  mastoid, longus capitis, longus colli, and anterior *sub-*
  occipitals (*rectus capitis anterior* and *rectus capitis*
  lateralis)

15.3.1 Frontalis, Occipitalis, and Temporalis

Three flat muscles—the frontalis, occipitalis, and temporalis—and their associated connective tissues cover the scalp like a soft tissue cap (Figure 15.29 ■). The frontalis and occipitalis are innervated by the *facial nerve* (the seventh cranial nerve). The temporalis is innervated by the *trigeminal nerve* (the fifth cranial nerve). You will want to check these three muscles for myofascial tensions when treating chronic muscular pain in the head and jaws for a number of reasons. Relaxation of the frontalis has been associated with alpha brain wave production, which is the basis of a popular autogenic (self-hypnosis) cue used in relaxation training: "Allow your forehead to be smooth and unwrinkled." The occipitalis lies directly above the suboccipital muscles and can broadcast tension from the neck and suboccipital area into the head. Due to their interdependent function, the occipitalis and frontalis are often referred to as one muscle named the *occipito-frontalis.* The temporalis is a thick and powerful jaw muscle that frequently causes chronic headaches and TMJ problems when it becomes chronically contracted and dysfunctional.

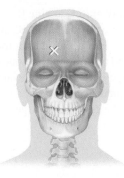
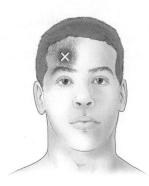

FIGURE 15.30

A habit of frowning can cause the **frontalis** to become dysfunctional and develop a trigger point over the middle of the eyebrow, which can refer localized pain over the same area and lead to tension headaches above the eyes. If the occipitalis also has trigger points, the tension headache will extend over the top of the head to the base of the skull.

The **frontalis** attaches to skin under the eyebrows and interdigitates with the orbicularis muscles of the eyelids over the supraorbital margin of the frontal bone. Its broad, vertical fibers blend into a subcutaneous musculotendinous sheath called the *galea aponeurotica,* which covers the top of the cranium. When the frontalis contracts, it raises the eyebrows or wrinkles the space between the eyebrows into a frown. (See TrP for the frontalis in Figure 15.30 ■).

The **occipitalis** is a flat, round muscle that arises on the superior attachment of the galea aponeurotica over the occiput and attaches on the inferior attachment of the galea aponeurotica and the superior nuchal line. The occipitalis fills the sole function of anchoring the galea aponeurotica to the base of the cranium against the pull of the frontalis. (See TrP for the occiptalis in Figure 15.31 ■).

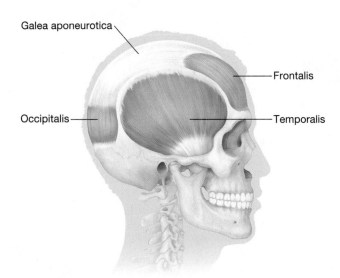

FIGURE 15.29
Frontalis, occipitalis, and temporalis

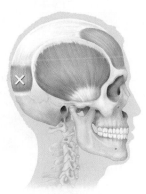
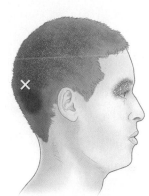

FIGURE 15.31

When dysfunctional, the **occipitalis** can develop a trigger point in the belly of the muscle that generates deep, aching pain over the occipital region and refers pain over the eyes and the upper back sides of the cranium. Chronic contractures in the occipitalis can also entrap the occipital nerve, causing superficial tingling sensations and hot prickling pain in the scalp. Occipitalis trigger point pain increases under compression pressure, causing a person extreme discomfort when trying to rest the weight of the head on a pillow.

The **temporalis** is a thick, meaty muscle arising from a broad origin covering the temporal fossa and temporal fascia. Its fan-shaped fibers converge into a flat tendon that passes under the zygomatic arch and inserts on the coronoid process of the mandible. This powerful muscle elevates and retracts the mandible during mastication; its contraction can often be observed over the temples as a person bites down. The temporalis has a high concentration of slow twitch fibers that work isometrically to maintain the elevated neutral position of the mandible, which prevents the mouth from hanging open. The temporalis can become dysfunctional from excessive gum chewing, clenching the teeth, or bruxism (teeth grinding). (See TrPs for the temporalis in Figure 15.32 ∎).

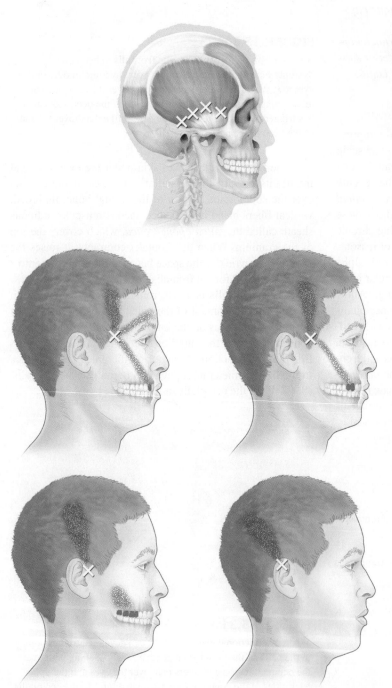

FIGURE 15.32

When dysfunctional, the **temporalis** can develop four adjacent trigger points in a row over the zygomatic arch that can refer pain to an area above each point and generate a toothache in adjacent teeth. Chronic tension headaches and jaw pain caused by the temporalis can be relieved with deep, slow circular friction over the belly of the muscle. Upward linear stripping along the fan-shaped fibers can also be effective in alleviating myofascial pain generated by this key TMJ muscle. To assist a client in releasing habitual and chronic contractures in the temporalis, suggest that he or she allow a small space to open between the upper and lower back molars.

MUSCLE PALPATION
Frontalis, Occipitalis, and Temporalis

Locate the frontalis and feel it contract and relax by resting the pads of your fingers on your forehead, then frowning while simultaneously raising and lowering your eyebrows several times to feel its range of contraction. Relax and widen your forehead to feel the frontalis relax.

Locate the occipitalis by pressing your fingertips against your occiput on either side of the midline. Again, frown while simultaneously raising and lowering your eyebrows to feel it contract to anchor the galea aponeurotica against the pull of the frontalis.

To palpate the temporalis, press your fingertips into the area from your temples to above your ears, then feel it contract by alternately opening your mouth and biting down to clench your teeth.

Frontalis

O–Supraorbital margin of frontal bone
I–Superior aspect of galea aponeurotica
A–Elevates eyebrows, furrows brow

Occipitalis

O–Galea aponeurotica over superior area of occipital bone
I–Inferior aspect of galea aponeurotica and superior nuchal line
A–Anchors galea aponeurotica against frontalis contraction

Temporalis

O–Temporal fossa and temporal fascia
I–Coronoid process of mandible
A–Elevates and protracts mandible, maintains neutral position of jaws

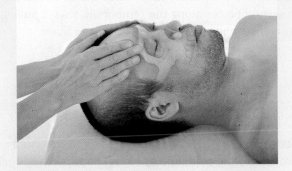

FIGURE 15.33a

Palpating the frontalis

With your partner supine, locate the **frontalis** by lightly pressing your finger pads across the forehead (Figure 15.33a ■). To feel the frontalis contract, have your partner raise and lower the eyebrows. Explore the fibers of the frontalis by applying flat, circular strokes across the frontal bone. *Are your fingertips above the eyebrows? Do you feel the frontalis wrinkle the forehead as your partner lifts the eyebrows and frowns?*

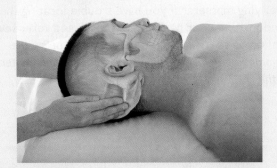

FIGURE 15.33b

Palpating the occipitalis

With your partner supine, locate the **occipitalis** by cradling the occipital bone in both hands (Figure 15.33b ■). Coach your partner to yield the weight of her or his head into your hands. Press your finger pads into the thickest part of the tissue over the occipital bone; then have your partner raise and lower the eyebrows to feel the occipitalis contract. Explore this flat, wide muscle by applying circular pressure against the occiput. *Are your fingertips palpating across the width of the occiput?*

(continued)

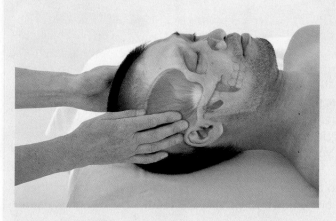

FIGURE 15.33c
Palpating the temporalis

With your partner supine, locate the **temporalis** on both sides by pressing your finger pads over the temples and above the ears (Figure 15.33c ■). See how far the temporalis fibers can stretch by pressing the muscles against the bone and pulling up with firm, linear strokes. *Where does the temporalis feel thickest: over the temples, behind the temples, or above the ears?*

Active movement: Have your partner bite down while you palpate the temporalis contraction.

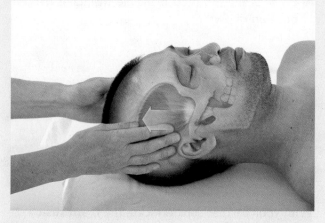

FIGURE 15.33d
Stretching the temporalis

Stretching: To stretch the temporalis, press your fingertips into the skin over the ears, then slowly pull up using deep linear friction (Figure 15.33d ■). Make sure to do both sides at once to promote symmetry. Have your partner open his or her mouth as you stretch the temporalis to enhance the effect. Stretch in several places along the temporalis, always pulling up and stripping its multiple fan-shaped fibers.

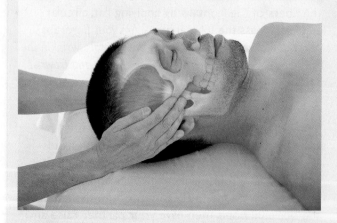

FIGURE 15.33e
Palpating the temporalis tendon

Locate the **temporalis tendon** on the coronoid process of the mandible by having your partner open her or his mouth (Figure 15.33e ■). Press into the cheek and apply gentle cross-fiber strumming across the temporalis tendon through the thick fibrous overlying masseter. If you have trouble locating the tendon, have your partner bite down and relax several times to locate it. *Are you palpating below the zygomatic arch of the cheekbone, about an inch anterior to the TMJ?*

15.3.2 Masseter, Lateral Pterygoid, and Medial Pterygoid

Muscles acting directly on the TMJ—the masseter, the lateral and medial pterygoids, and the temporalis—are some of the most active muscles in the body (Figure 15.34 ■). They work while we talk, eat, and swallow. Even when we are quiet and our jaws are seemingly at rest, this muscle group is continually active to keep the mouth closed. These muscles can become overactive in a subconscious stress reaction such as nail biting or teeth grinding. Their extreme level of activity coupled with emotional stress often leads to chronic tension in this muscle group, which can escalate into a temporomandibular disorder (TMD). Dentists often refer clients with TMD to manual therapists for specialized intraoral work (work inside the mouth) that releases tension in the powerful pterygoid and masseter muscles. The pterygoids can be difficult to palpate on a client without a clear understanding of their attachment sites. Like the temporalis, the masseter and pterygoids are innervated by the *trigeminal nerve* (fifth cranial nerve).

The powerful **masseter** is a square muscle with superficial and deep layers of fibers that give an observable definition and fullness to the posterior aspect of the check (Figure 15.35a-b ■). The superficial yet thick layer of the masseter arises from the zygomatic arch; the smaller, deeper layer arises from the coronoid process. Both layers of the masseter insert across the angle of the mandible. A bilateral contraction of the masseter closes the jaws; a unilateral contraction laterally deviates the mandible to that side. (See TrPs for the masseter in Figure 15.36 ■).

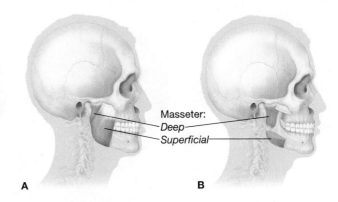

FIGURE 15.35

Masseter: a) Superficial layer b) Deep layer

Two short, thick, and powerful pterygoids lie deep to the masseter. The **lateral pterygoid,** the stronger of the two pterygoid muscles, has two heads. A superior head arises from the greater wing of the sphenoid and an inferior head arises on the lateral pterygoid plate of the sphenoid (Figure 15.37 ■). Both heads run horizontally to an insertion site on the internal surface of the mandibular condyle and the joint capsule and disc of the TMJ. A bilateral contraction of the lateral pterygoid depresses the lower jaw and a unilateral contraction laterally deviates the lower jaw. The lateral pterygoid also works as a synergist with the temporalis during grinding and chewing. Both heads work reciprocally during vertical and horizontal mandibular movement, contracting eccentrically to open the jaws and controlling the return of the mandibular condyle to its resting position while closing the jaw. (See TrPs for the lateral pterygoid in Figure 15.38 ■).

The **medial pterygoid** is a quadrangular muscle with fibers that run along the medial inner surface of the masseter (Figure 15.39a-b ■). Its wide origin arises on the lateral pterygoid plate of the sphenoid and the maxilla and inserts across the inner surface of the mandibular ramus. The medial pterygoid elevates and protrudes the lower jaw. It also works as a synergist with the masseter and temporalis during grinding and chewing. (See TrP for the medial pterygoid in Figure 15.40 ■).

15.3.3 Muscles of Facial Expression

The facial muscles serve an important role in human relationships. They allow us to read the emotional states of the people we interact with through the facial expressions they wear. The facial muscles are unique in that they are relatively flat and superficial. Rather than attaching to bones or ligaments as most muscles do, they attach to the inner surface of the skin and the subcutaneous fascia

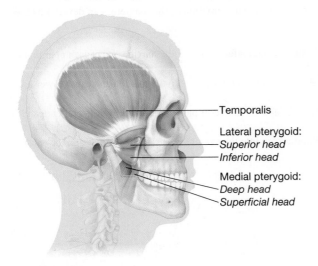

FIGURE 15.34

Lateral pterygoid, medial pterygoid, and masseter

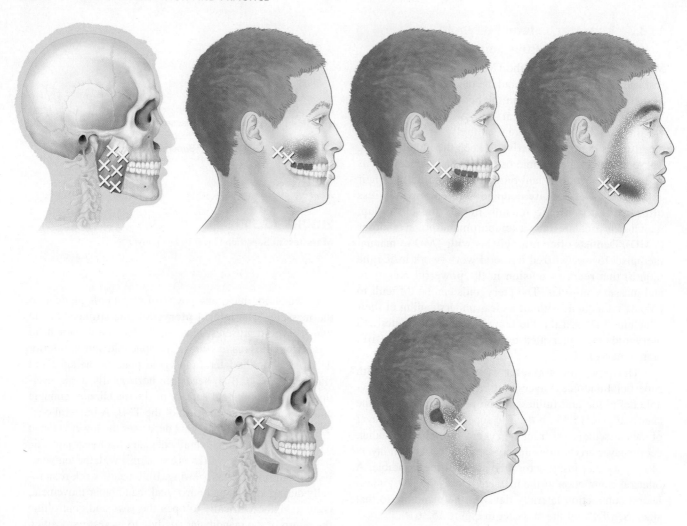

FIGURE 15.36

Because stress or emotional pain tends to trigger subconscious contractures in muscles acting on the TMJ, the **masseter** frequently develops trigger points when a person is under emotional stress. When dysfunctional, the masseter can develop trigger points in seven locations:

- Two adjacent trigger points across the top half of the superficial layer belly can refer pain over the maxilla and cause upper tooth sensitivity.
- Two adjacent trigger points across the lower half of the superficial layer belly can refer pain into the maxilla and cause lower tooth sensitivity.
- Two adjacent trigger points on the angle of the lower jaw in the superficial layer can refer pain across the lower, lateral chin and over the eyebrow.
- One trigger point directly in front of the TMJ in the deep layer can refer pain into the ear and cause tinnitus (ringing in the ears).

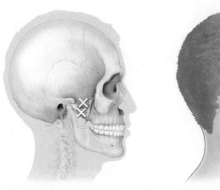

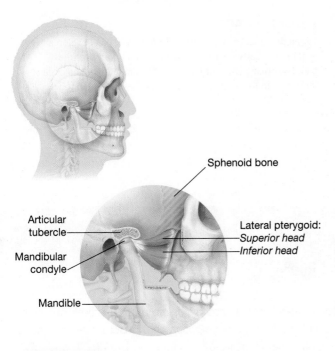

Sphenoid bone

Articular tubercle

Mandibular condyle

Mandible

Lateral pterygoid:
Superior head
Inferior head

FIGURE 15.37
Lateral pterygoid

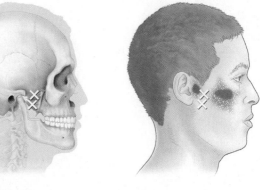

FIGURE 15.38

Dysfunction in the **lateral pterygoid** is common with clients who have temporomandibular dysfunction, creating trigger points in the belly of each head. Trigger points in the lateral pterygoid can radiate deep pain into the maxilla and the TMJ, restricting how far a person can open the jaws, making chewing painful and causing tinnitus (ringing) in the ears.

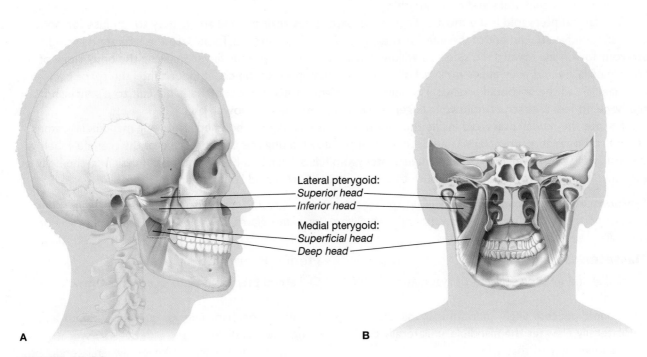

Lateral pterygoid:
Superior head
Inferior head

Medial pterygoid:
Superficial head
Deep head

A

B

FIGURE 15.39
Pterygoids: a) Lateral view b) Coronal section

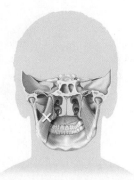
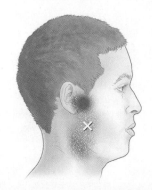

FIGURE 15.40
When dysfunctional, the **medial pterygoid** can develop a trigger point in the belly of the muscle that refers pain over the TMJ, causes diffuse pain over the side of the mandible, and creates stuffiness in the ear because it closes the eustachian tube.

MUSCLE PALPATION
Masseter, Lateral Pterygoid, and Medial Pterygoid

Note: The masseter can be palpated on the outside and inside of the cheek; the pterygoids are most effectively palpated inside the mouth. Make sure to wash your hands before practicing the following self-palpation on muscles inside your mouth.

Palpate the masseter by strumming across your cheek, perpendicular to its vertically oriented fibers anterior to the ear. It will feel like thick, meaty muscle and often has taut bands in the muscle. Then palpate the masseter by grasping the inside and outside of your cheek directly anterior to the ear and using a pincher palpation. Hold the muscle belly while you slowly open and close your mouth to feel the masseter lengthen and shorten as it contracts eccentrically and concentrically.

The lateral pterygoid is the most difficult to palpate. It lies against bone and is easy to confuse for bone. Only the medial attachment of the inferior head can be directly palpated. To palpate the lateral pterygoid, deviate your lower jaw toward the side you will be palpating. Then press your fingertip along the bony ridge of your maxilla, behind your upper molars. Follow it back and up along the cheek pouch into the space between the maxilla and the coronoid process. The muscle lies right against the bone and is difficult to distinguish from the bone. To feel it contract, hold your finger there and protrude your lower jaw.

Palpate the medial pterygoid inside the mouth by first locating the bony edge of your mandibular ramus behind and outside your molars. Then drop your finger down along the inside surface of the mandible, below the inside of your lower molars. If the medial pterygoid has a TrP, it will be quite tender. Press into the belly of the muscle, then slowly open your mouth to feel the medial pterygoid lengthen and relax.

Caution: Skillfully palpating the masseter and pterygoids requires intraoral work. When doing intraoral work with a client or partner, always wear a finger cotter or glove. Before using latex gloves, always check to see if your client has latex allergies. If they do, use vinyl gloves.

Masseter

O–Medial and inferior surfaces of zygomatic arch of maxilla
I–Coronoid process, angle and ramus of mandible
A–Bilaterally elevates the mandible, unilaterally deviates lower jaw to that side

Lateral Pterygoid

O–Superior head—Greater wing of the sphenoid
Inferior head—Lateral pterygoid plate of the sphenoid
I–Internal surface of mandibular condyle, temporomandibular joint capsule
A–Depresses and protrudes lower jaw, unilaterally deviates lower jaw to that side

Medial Pterygoid

O–Lateral pterygoid plate of sphenoid, maxilla and palatine bones
I–Internal posterior inferior surface of ramus and angle of mandible
A–Elevates and protrudes lower jaw, unilaterally deviates lower jaw to that side

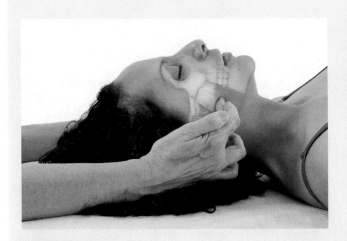

FIGURE 15.41a

Palpating the masseter

Palpate the **masseter** on both sides with your partner in a supine position by pressing along the muscle bellies from the cheekbones to the angle of the mandibles (Figure 15.41a ■). Move sideways across the masseter fibers by strumming across the sides of the cheeks right in front of the ears. *Do you feel how thick the masseters are? Do the masseters stretch as you press down along their vertical fibers? Do your fingertips fall off the medial edge of the masseters as you move toward the mouth?*

Active movement: Have your partner clench the jaw several times while you palpate the masseter contraction on the outside of the cheek.

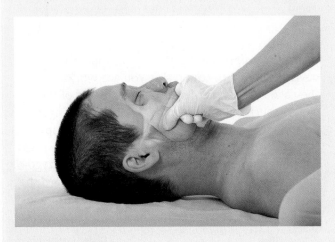

FIGURE 15.41b

Palpating the masseter interorally

Intraoral palpation: Place your index finger inside the cheek and locate the masseter with a pincher palpation, squeezing it between your index finger and thumb (Figure 15.41b ■). Explore the thickness and density of the masseter, and the length of its fibers.

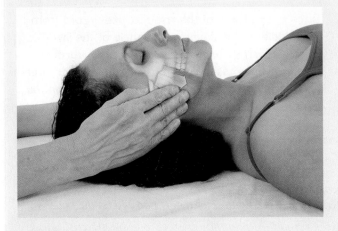

FIGURE 15.41c

Stretching the masseter

Stretching: To stretch the masseter, press your fingertips into the origin of the muscle, below the zygomatic arch. Make sure to do both sides at once to promote symmetry in TMJ motion. Slowly apply deep downward pressure to stretch the muscle and put light traction on the joint (Figure 15.41c ■). Have your partner slowly open his or her mouth as you stretch the masseter to enhance the stretch.

(continued)

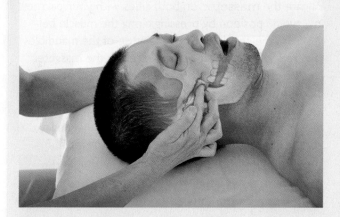

FIGURE 15.41d
Palpating the lateral pterygoid

Trace the pathway of the **lateral pterygoid** by running your fingertips below the zygomatic arch to the ear (Figure 15.41d ■). Press into the approximate location of the muscle's belly, then have your partner protract and retract the jaw to feel this muscle contract.

Active movement: Press into the belly of the lateral pterygoid below the zygomatic arch, then have you partner retract and protract the jaw.

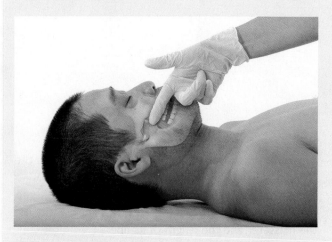

FIGURE 15.41e
Finger position for palpating the lateral pterygoid inter-orally

Intraoral palpation: Have your partner laterally deviate the mouth to the side you are working on, then slide your index finger along the roof of the cheek pouch behind the upper molars (see finger position in Figure 15.41e ■). Hold the mouth open so that your partner can relax the masseter. Then press your fingertip up under the lower edge of the zygomatic bone. Slowly slide your finger back toward the temporomandibular joint. *Is your partner able to relax and let your finger sink into the muscles?*

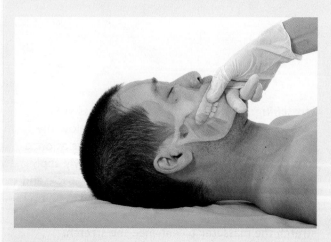

FIGURE 15.41f
Palpating the medial pterygoid

Trace the pathway of the **medial pterygoid** from the middle of the cheek to the angle of the jaw (Figure 15.41f ■). To feel it contract, press through the overlying masseter, then have your partner laterally deviate the jaw to the right and the left. *Can you feel the medial pterygoid contract during lateral deviation of the jaw?*

Intraoral palpation: Hook your fingertip over the back molars, then press into the soft tissue below the molars, along the inside of the mandible. *Does the medial pterygoid feel like a small meaty pad against the bone?*

FIGURE 15.42

Facial muscles: a) Anterior view
b) Lateral view

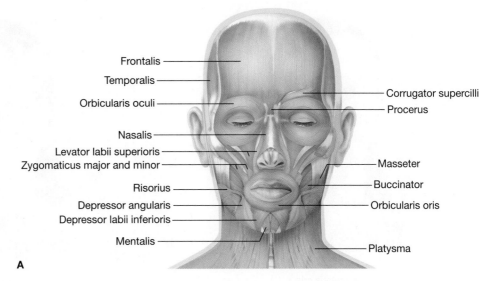

Frontalis
Temporalis
Orbicularis oculi
Corrugator supercilli
Procerus
Nasalis
Levator labii superioris
Zygomaticus major and minor
Masseter
Risorius
Buccinator
Depressor angularis
Orbicularis oris
Depressor labii inferioris
Mentalis
Platysma

A

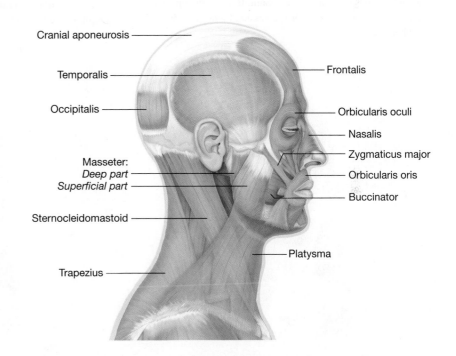

Cranial aponeurosis
Temporalis
Frontalis
Occipitalis
Orbicularis oculi
Nasalis
Zygmaticus major
Masseter:
Deep part
Orbicularis oris
Superficial part
Buccinator
Sternocleidomastoid
Platysma
Trapezius

B

(Figure 15.42a-b ■). All of these muscles connect to each other and work together as a single canvas to paint the picture of a person's inner feelings. In this sense, facial expressions are like the outer barometer of a person's inner emotional landscape.

The spectrum of facial expressions is vast and ranges from the most obvious to extremely subtle. The extent to which we can nonverbally communicate emotion through this complex group of muscles has been thoroughly documented by Paul Eckman, a noted researcher of facial expression and developer of the Microexpression Training Tool. Eckman, who trains law enforcement and security agencies how to track and interpret subtle and often fleeting facial muscle patterns in alleged criminals and terrorists, has found that only 30 facial muscles have the potential to express 3,000 different emotional states.[1] His cross-cultural investigations did, however, narrow this range down to seven universal emotions: anger, fear, disgust, surprise, sadness, happiness, and contempt. We usually think of emotions creating facial expressions, but the opposite also holds true. In the course of isolating each facial muscle and contracting it, Eckman and his colleagues made an unusual discovery. They found that an expression a person may not even know that he or she is wearing can create an emotion that the person did not choose to feel.

One great way to study the facial muscles is by isolating each one and contracting it (Figure 15.43a-p ■). This

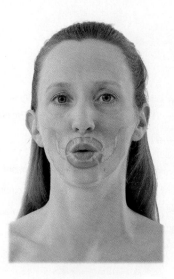

Orbicularis oris

FIGURE 15.43a

The **orbicularis oris** circles the mouth. It draws the lips into a thruster pucker for a kiss, or presses and tightens the lips together.

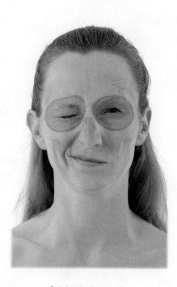

Orbicularis oculi

FIGURE 15.43b

The **orbicularis oculi** circles the eye. We use it to wink, blink, squint, or even smile with the eyes.

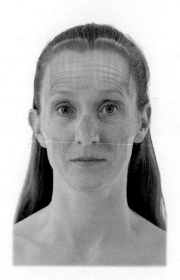

Frontalis

FIGURE 15.43c

The **frontalis,** which was discussed earlier, runs from the scalp above the hairline to the skin near the eyebrows. It raises the eyebrows and creates horizontal wrinkles across the forehead in an expression of surprise, fear, and even curiosity.

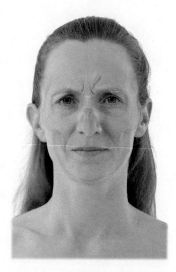

Procerus

FIGURE 15.43d

The **procerus** (also called the depresser glabellae) is a small, pyramid-shaped muscle that arises on fascia of the nasal bone and upper nasal cartilage and inserts on forehead skin between the eyebrows. It often contracts with the corrugator, a small muscle bridging the procerus with the orbicularis oculi.

FIGURE 15.43 Facial muscle actions

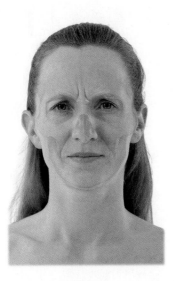

Corrugator

FIGURE 15.43e

The **corrugator** expresses confusion, concentration, or even pain from a headache. It helps us squint on a bright sunny day. Together the procerus and **corrugator** are the culprits that produce a furrow between the eyebrows and keep suppliers of products such as Botox in business. People receive Botox injections to temporarily paralyze the procerus and frontalis, which makes wrinkles less distinct.

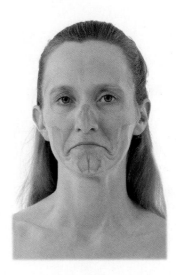

Mentalis

FIGURE 15.43f

The **mentalis** is a small muscle with vertical fibers on the chin. The mentalis wrinkles skin on the chin as a person would do when pouting, expressing doubt, or showing sadness. It also curves the lower lip into an inverted U.

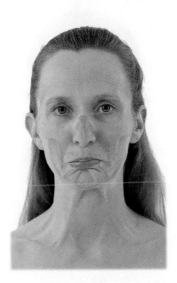

Depressor labii inferior

FIGURE 15.43g

The **depressor labii inferior** attaches to fascia on the lateral side of the lower lip and angles out to mandibular fascial insertions. It contracts when a person pouts or sulks, drawing the lower lip down and out to both sides laterally.

FIGURE 15.43 continued

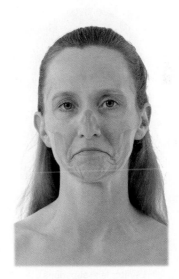

Depressor anguli oris

FIGURE 15.43h

The **depressor anguli oris** attaches to fascia on the lateral lip and fans down into the sides of the mandible. It is active when frowning, grimacing, and even grieving. All of the depressor muscles turn a smile upside down into a frown or an expression of feigned anger.

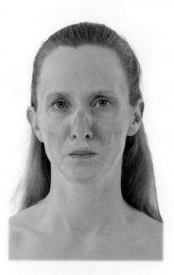

Depressor septi

FIGURE 15.43i

The **depressor septi** is a small diagonal muscle coming off the base of the nose that narrows the nostrils and pulls them down. People often contract this muscle to block noxious odors or in an expression of disgust.

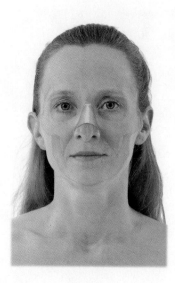

Nasalis

FIGURE 15.43j

The **nasalis** is a narrow strap muscle running across the maxilla. It widens and flares the nostrils when we are taking a deep breath to smell a fragrance such as a rose or even in the excitement of loving feelings.

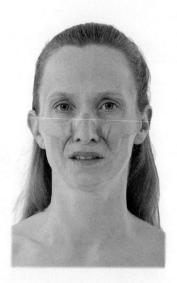

Levator labii superioris

FIGURE 15.43k

The **levator labii superioris** is shaped like a Y with two heads: one attaches to the zygomatic bone, and the other attaches to the infraorbital edge of the maxilla. Both heads converge and insert on the skin and orbicularis oris of the upper lip. The levator labii expresses disdain and contempt; it is the "something smells bad" muscle. It raises and curls the corner of the upper lip in a snarling or sneering action.

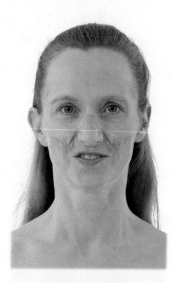

Levator anguli oris

FIGURE 15.43l

The **levator anguli oris** arises from the maxilla near the canine teeth and inserts near the corners of the mouth. It pulls the corners of the lips up into a forced, phony smile or a smirk.

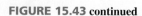

FIGURE 15.43 continued

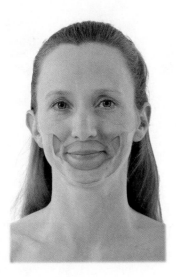

Buccinator

FIGURE 15.43m

The **buccinator** is a quadrangular muscle that arises off of the myofascia of the orbicularis muscle on the corner of the mouth and inserts on the ramus of the mandible. It compresses the cheeks when whistling, drinking out of a straw, blowing on a wind instrument, and swallowing. It also helps keeps food between the molars while chewing.

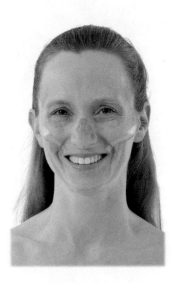

Zygomatic major

FIGURE 15.43n

The **zygomatic major** is a diagonal strap muscle that runs from the zygomatic bone to the corner of the mouth. It is a "feel-good muscle" that contracts when we smile and laugh. A genuine smile also engages the orbicularis oculi, which narrows the eyes.

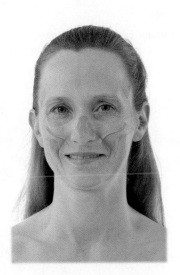

Zygomatic minor

FIGURE 15.43o

The **zygomatic minor** runs in a curve above the zygomatic major from the cheek toward the nose. It elevates the upper lip and produces the furrow lateral to the nose, creating an understated expression that can range from subtle joy to subtle fear.

FIGURE 15.43 continued

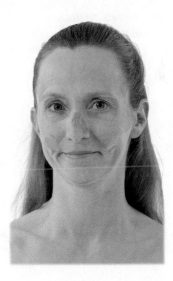

Risorius

FIGURE 15.43p

The **risorius** is a small horizontal strap muscle running from the corner of the mouth to the fascia over the middle of the masseter. It draws the lips laterally into a grin in a "yikes!" expression.

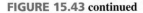

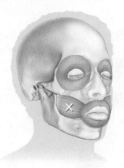
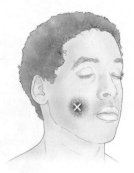

FIGURE 15.44

The **buccinator** can develop a trigger point in the center of the muscle belly from overactivity such as blowing up a lot of balloons.

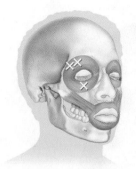
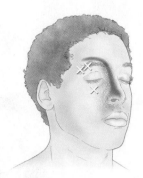

FIGURE 15.45

The **orbicularis oculi** can develop trigger points in three places, two on superior lateral points and one on the inferior, middle portion of the muscle. An orbicular oculi trigger point can refer pain along the side of the nose all the way to the tip of the nose.

experiential learning process tends to imprint the memory of each facial muscle in the motor cortex. In addition, it can be fun, relaxing, and provide deep insights into the link between emotions and muscular contractions. A short description of the action of each facial muscle is located in Figure 15.43a-p to get you started on this exploration.

Several of the facial muscles can develop trigger points from overuse. The buccinator TrP can be released with pincher palpation of the cheek inside and outside the cheek (Figure 15.44 ■). The orbicularis oculi develops superficial trigger points around the eyes from extended squinting (Figure 15.45 ■). The zygomatic major develop contractures from extended smiling (Figure 15.46 ■).

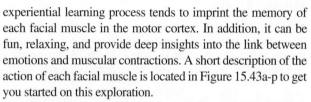
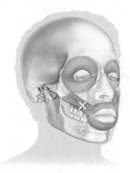
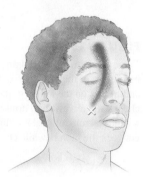

FIGURE 15.46

The **zygomatic major** can develop a trigger point in its belly, which refers pain along the medial side of the nose up to the middle of the forehead.

EXPLORING TECHNIQUE
Tracing the Facial Muscles

Palpate the facial muscles on yourself first, then on a partner who is lying in a supine position. Trace each muscle of the face in the direction of its fibers. As you trace the muscles, imagine that you are smoothing or ironing tension out of each muscle to evoke a relaxation response.

Caution: The facial muscles are superficial so it is important to use light pressure because deep pressure can bruise the face. Avoid overstretching the skin.

1. To trace the **frontalis** and **procerus** muscles, use a flat finger touch and run your fingers from the eyebrows up the forehead (Figure 15.47a ■). Then smooth the frontalis by running your fingertips from the center of the forehead in the lateral directions.

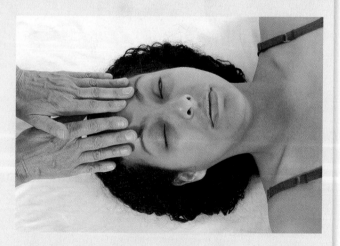

FIGURE 15.47a

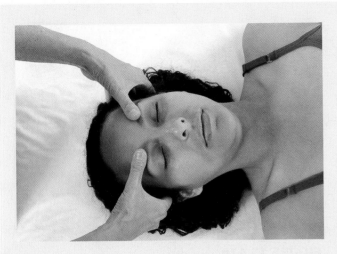

FIGURE 15.47b

2. Trace the **orbicularis oculi** across the upper rim of the eye socket, from the bridge of the nose to the corner of the eye (Figure 15.47b ■). Avoid tracing it along the lower rim of the eye socket because it's easy to overstretch the delicate tissues there.

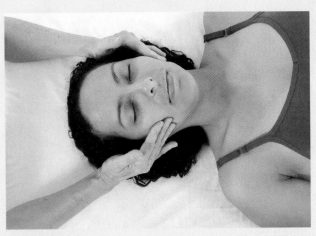

FIGURE 15.47d

4. Trace the **zygomatic** muscles along two diagonal pathways—from the corner of the mouth to the corner of the eye and the corner of the mouth to the cheekbone lateral of the eye (Figure 15.47d ■).

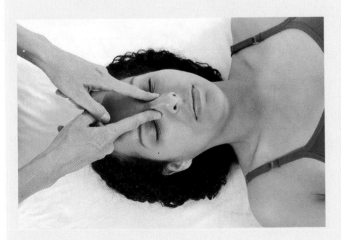

FIGURE 15.47c

3. Trace the **nasalis** and **levator labii** muscles by running your fingertips along the sides of the nose (Figure 15.47c ■).

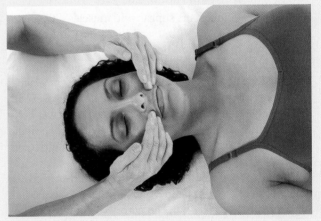

FIGURE 15.47e

5. Trace the **orbicularis oris** around the mouth by smoothing the upper lip from the center to the sides, then smoothing the bottom lip in the same manner (Figure 15.47e ■).

(continued)

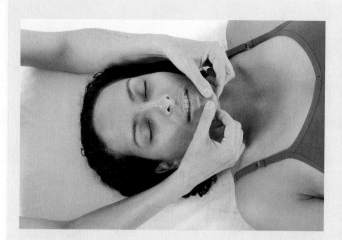

FIGURE 15.47f

6. Trace the **depressor** and **mentalis** muscles from the lower lip down to the chin (Figure 15.47f ■).

FIGURE 15.47g

7. Trace the **risorius** and **buccinator** muscles from the corner of the mouth laterally across the cheek (Figure 15.47g ■).

15.3.4 Suprahyoid and Infrahyoid Muscles

As their name implies, the **suprahyoid muscles**—the *mylohyoid, geniohyoid, stylohyoid,* and *digastric*—attach to the superior rim of the hyoid bone (Figure 15.48a-b ■). The *trigeminal nerve* (fifth cranial nerve) innervates the mylohyoid and the upper belly of the digastric. The *first cervical nerve* innervates the geniohyoid. The *facial nerve* (seventh cranial nerve) innervates the stylohyoid and the lower belly of the digastric. The suprahyoid muscles elevate the hyoid and stabilize it against the downward pull of the infrahyoid muscles.

The diagonal fibers of the **mylohyoid** arise from the inner surface of the mandible and attaches to the medial, superior rim of the hyoid. The narrower **geniohyoid** lies deep to the myolohyoid and runs from the middle inner surface of the mandible to the middle surface of the superior hyoid rim. A small, thin **stylohyoid** arises from the styloid process of the temporal bone and attaches to the greater horn of the hyoid bone. These small horizontal muscles suspend the hyoid bone from the mandible and the styloid process of the temporal bone. The mylohyoid and geniohyoid form the horizontal floor for the mouth and provides a base for the **genioglossus,** better known as the tongue (Figure 15.49 ■).

The **digastric** is a double-belly muscle. Its posterior belly runs beside the stylohyoid, from the mastoid process through a ligamentous sling attached to the superior rim of the hyoid, where it turns a corner, and its anterior belly inserts on the internal inferior mandible (Figure 15.50 ■). When both bellies contract, they elevate and stabilize the hyoid bone during swallowing and speaking. When the posterior belly contracts, it depresses the mandible to assist opening the mouth.

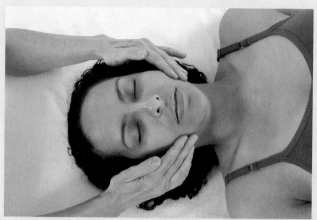

A

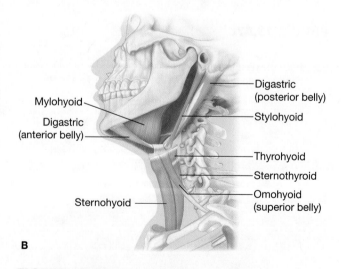

B

FIGURE 15.48

Suprahyoid and infrahyoid muscles: a) Inferior view b) Lateral view

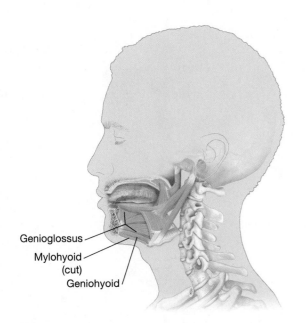

FIGURE 15.49
Geniohyoid and myolohyoid

The **infrahyoid muscles**—the *sternohyoid, thyrohyoid,* and *omohyoid*—are innervated by the *hypoglossal nerve* (12th cranial nerve). The infrahyoid muscles depress the hyoid and stabilize it against the upward pull of the suprahyoid muscles. They also cover and protect the organs situated along the front of the neck: the trachea, esophagus, thyroid gland, and larynx. The infrahyoid and suprahyoid muscles lie under a complex network of lymph nodes in the neck and can be lightly massaged with lymph drainage

techniques. Avoid placing deep pressure on the infrahyoid muscles because it could trigger choking anxiety in a client and could damage vulnerable adjacent tissues such as the trachea and thyroid gland.

The **sternohyoid** is a small narrow muscle that runs vertically from the inferior hyoid rim to its insertion on the medial clavicle, superior manubrium, and the medial end of the first rib. As its name implies, the **thyrohyoid** covers the thyroid gland. It also runs vertically from the inferior hyoid rim to its insertion sites deep to the sternohyoid on the medial clavicle and superior manubrium. Both the sternohyoid and thyrohyoid attach to the thyroid cartilage. The thyrohyoid depresses the larynx when a person swallows, closing the laryngeal opening to prevent food from entering.

The **omohyoid** is an unusual double-belly muscle connecting the hyoid bone to the clavicle and the scapula. Its small, thin vertical belly arises from the inferior hyoid, descends lateral to the sternohyoid, and tapers into a tendon that runs through a ligamentous sling attached to the superior edge of the medial clavicle. From here, its tendon turns a corner and expands into a second muscle belly that crosses the top of the shoulder and inserts on the lateral, superior scapula. The omohyoid also depresses the hyoid and assists in a combination of cervical rotation with side-bending (Figure 15.51 ■).

The **platsyma** is a thin, broad subcutaneous muscle draping from the lower jaw over the front and side of the neck, covering the clavicle, and blending into the fascia of the upper chest. This unusual muscle is innervated by the *facial nerve* (seventh cranial nerve) and is a remnant of the subcutaneous layer of muscle that horses use to twitch and

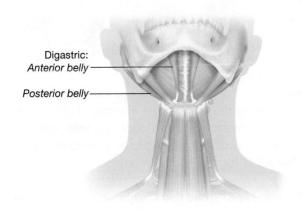

FIGURE 15.50
Digastric

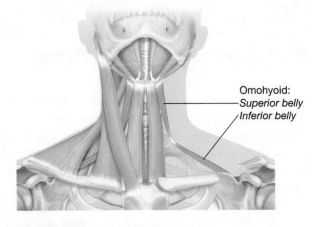

FIGURE 15.51
Omohyoid

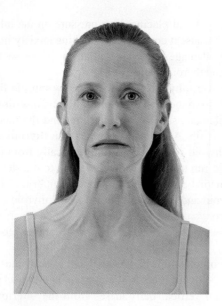

FIGURE 15.52

Platysma contraction

flick insects off their skin. The single fibers of the platysma pop out like strings under the skin when a person contracts the platysma by widening the lower jaw while pulling down the lower lip (Figure 15.52 ■). (See TrPs for the platysma in Figure 15.53 ■.)

15.3.5 Suboccipitals

Four small and deep **suboccipitals**—the rectus capitis posterior minor, rectus capitis posterior major, oblique capitis inferior, and oblique capitis superior—connect the posterior

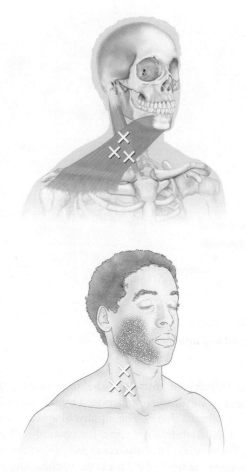

FIGURE 15.53

Three superficial trigger points can develop in the **platysma** that refer a prickling sensation over the chin.

MUSCLE PALPATION
Suprahyoids and Infrahyoid Muscles

Gently self-palpate the suprahyoid muscles by lightly pressing up into the underside of your lower jaw along the inner edge of your mandible from the center of your lower jaw to the angle of the mandible. Lightly press into the muscle bellies to feel their sling-like shape. To feel how they work when they contract, hold your fingertips on their muscle bellies under your chin, then explore moving your tongue, swallowing, protracting and retracting your neck, and slowly flexing and extending your head. *Can you feel how neck protraction and extension place the suprahyoids on slack?*

Gently self-palpate the infrahyoid muscles by gently and lightly pressing the thin muscles over the trachea. Hold the infrahyoids and explore swallowing and then flexing and extending your neck to feel them contract.

Caution: Some people have choking anxiety and do not like to be touched along the front of the neck. Before palpating, ask your partner if it is okay to touch this area of the neck. While palpating, stop if your partner shows any signs of discomfort.

Mylohyoid

O–Inner surface of mandible
I–Middle part of anterior hyoid bone
A–Elevates hyoid bone

Geniohyoid

O–Inner surface of mandible
I–Anterior surface of hyoid bone
A–Elevates hyoid bone

Stylohyoid

O—Styloid process of temporal bone

I—Hyoid bone

A—Elevate and retracts hyoid when lifting tongue and swallowing

Digastric

O—Posterior belly—Mastoid process
   Anterior belly—Internal inferior mandible

I—Ligamentous sling on superior rim of hyoid

A—Bilateral action elevates and stabilizes hyoid during swallowing and speaking, posterior belly depresses mandible

Sternohyoid

O—Inferior rim of hyoid

I—Top of manubrium

A—Depresses and stabilizes hyoid, protects organs along anterior neck

Thyrohyoid

O—Along thyroid cartilage

I—Inferior rim of hyoid

A—Depresses and stabilizes hyoid, protects organs along anterior neck

Omohyoid

O—Inferior rim of hyoid

I—Ligamentous sling on medial clavicle, lateral side of superior, anterior scapular border

A—Depresses hyoid, assists cervical rotation with side bending

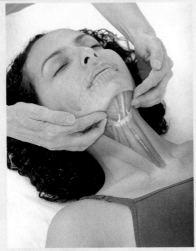

FIGURE 15.54a

Palpating the suprahyoids

Palpate the **suprahyoid muscles** by gently pressing up into the soft tissue attached to the inner edge of the mandible (Figure 15.54a ■).

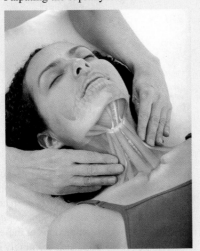

FIGURE 15.54b

Palpating the infrahyoids

Palpate the **infrahyoid muscles** with your finger pads by gently and lightly exploring the thin muscle layers over the trachea (Figure 15.54b ■)

aspect of the occiput to the first and second cervical vertebrae (Figure 15.55 ■). These small muscles lie deep to the semispinalis and are collectively innervated by the *first cervical nerve* and the *suboccipital nerve*.

The suboccipitals fill the same tissue layer as the cervical multifidus. Each suboccipital muscle is a short muscle running from the SP or TP of either C-1 or C-2 to the occiput.

- The **rectus capitis posterior minor** attaches the posterior tubercle of the atlas to the medial side of the inferior nuchal line of the occipital bone.
- The **rectus capitis posterior major** attaches the spinous process of the atlas (C-2) to the lateral side of the inferior nuchal line of the occipital bone.
- The **oblique capitis inferior** has almost horizontal fibers that run from the spinous process and the upper lamina of the axis (C-2) to the transverse process of the atlas (C-1).
- The **oblique capitis superior** attaches the transverse process of the atlas (C-1) to the occipital bone between the nuchal lines.

The suboccipitals work with the semispinalis capitis to restrain flexion of the head. They are continually active during small adjustments that people make with the head as they turn it to look or listen, or subtly nod to talk or swallow. Faulty postures that tilt the head off-center overwork and

strain the suboccipitals and the semispinalis capitis (Figure 15.56 ■). This occurs when a person has to look down at a workstation; compensates for poor eyesight or poorly fitted glasses by tipping the head to an awkward position; or holds the head in an off-center position in activities such as holding a phone to the ear with the shoulder, watching a movie from an angled position, or turning the head to one side to have a conversation on an airplane.

To improve workplace ergonomics, Travell recommends tilting the position of reading glasses so that the lower rim of the glasses rests on the cheeks (Figure 15.57a-b ■). This allows the reader to turn the eyes downward rather than tilting the head down and bending the neck into flexion, which reduces eccentric stress on muscles in the suboccipital region.[2]

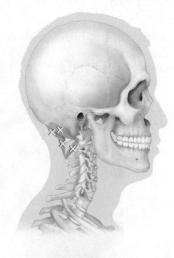

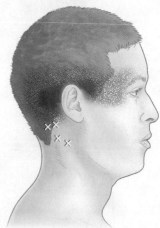

FIGURE 15.56

When dysfunctional, each **suboccipital** can develop a trigger point in its belly. Suboccipital trigger points create sore spots at the base of the skull that radiate a deep headache pain over the ear and to the back of the eye. Suboccipital trigger points can easily flare up when contractions of these muscles are triggered, which might occur from such seemingly innocuous activities as propping the head on a pillow to read in bed, wearing a hat that is too tight, or getting a neck chill from a strong wind.

Rectus capitis posterior major

Rectus capitis posterior minor

Oblique capitis superior

Oblique capitis inferior

C1
C2
C3
C4

FIGURE 15.55
Suboccipitals

FIGURE 15.57

a) Tilting the head down to read places the suboccipitals under eccentric stress. b) Tilting the glasses down to read instead of the head minimizes mechanical loading stress on the suboccipitals.

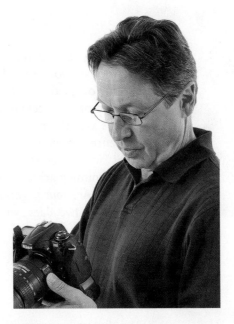
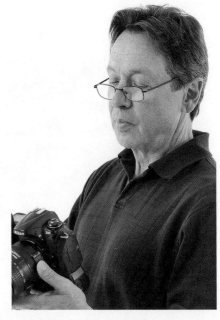

A

B

MUSCLE PALPATION
Suboccipitals

Palpate the rectus capitis posterior muscles by pressing your fingertips into the base of your occiput. Notice if they are symmetrical. Rock your head with a nodding motion to feel them contract and relax. Tip your head right and then left to feel one side contract at a time.

Caution: *The suboccipitals are often sore, particularly on people who suffer from chronic headaches, poor posture, or whiplash. Palpate them slowly and gently at first, watching and/or asking your partner for feedback. If your partner feels any pain or discomfort as you palpate, lighten the pressure on the suboccipital region until your partner can relax.*

Note: *It can be difficult to differentiate individual muscles in the suboccipitals during palpation because of the thickness of overlying tendons and fascia, although you can approximate their location by placing your fingertips between their origins and insertions.*

Rectus Capitis Posterior Minor
O–Posterior tubercle of atlas (C-1)
I–Medial part of inferior nuchal line of occipital bone
A–Bilaterally extends head, unilaterally assists rotation of head to same side

Rectus Capitis Posterior Major
O–Spinous process of axis (C-2)
I–Lateral part of inferior nuchal line of occipital bone
A–Bilaterally extends head, unilaterally assists rotation of head to same side

Capitis Inferior
O–Spinous process and upper lamina of axis (C-2)
I–Transverse process of atlas (C-1)
A–Rotates head to same side

Oblique Capitis Superior
O–Transverse process of atlas (C-1)
I–Occipital bone between nuchal lines
A–Extends head, assists rotation to same side

(continued)

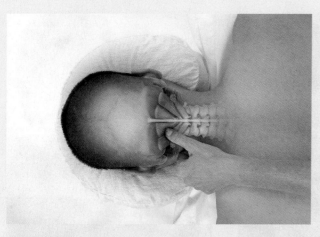

FIGURE 15.58a

Palpating the rectus capitis posterior minor

With your partner in a prone position, approximate the location of the **rectus capitis posterior minor** by tracing between the SP of C-1 and the base of the occiput. Then slowly press your fingertips into the nuchal line of the occiput along the center of the skull (Fiure 15.58a ■). Press both sides at once to check for symmetry. Use a cross-fiber strumming across the occiput to feel the muscle belly. *Are your fingertips on the center of the occiput? Are the two sides symmetrical?*

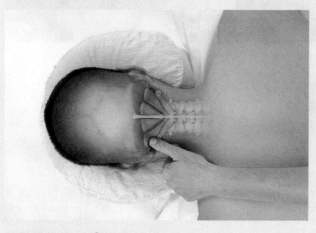

FIGURE 15.58b

Palpating the rectus capitis posterior major

With your partner in a prone position, approximate the location of the **rectus capitis posterior major** by slowly pressing into the space between the SP of C-2 and the suboccipital area slightly lateral of midline (Figure 15.58b ■). Then slowly press your fingertips into the occiput about an inch lateral of the midline. Press both sides at once to check for symmetry. Use a cross-fiber strumming across the occiput to feel the muscle belly. *Are your fingertips slightly lateral to the center of the occiput? Are the two sides symmetrical?*

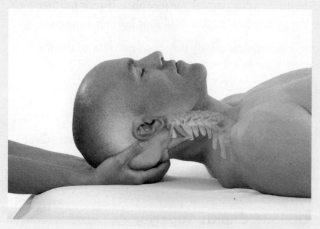

FIGURE 15.58c

Supine wedge release of suboccipitals

With your partner in a supine position, palpate the **suboccipitals** by cradling the occiput, then aligning your fingertips right below the nuchal line and slowly pressing straight up into the muscle bellies, until the weight of your partner's head and neck is resting on

your fingertips (Figure 15.58c ■). Make sure your partner can relax into your fingertips. Only press as deeply as the tissues will yield. *Are you sinking your fingertips into the suboccipital muscles? Do you feel them soften?*

With your partner in the supine position, approximate the location of both **oblique capitis inferior** muscles at the same time by tracing between the SP of C-2 and the TP of C-1 in the hollow space behind the ear. Starting at C-2, apply light pressure along the fibers of both muscles, which run horizontally across the neck. Then use a cross-fiber strumming along the sides of the neck across the bellies of the muscles.

With your partner in the supine position, approximate the location of the **oblique capitis superior** by gently tracing from the TP of C-1 straight up toward the temporal bone anterior to the mastoid process. Palpate 'both sides at once to check for symmetry. *Are your fingertips directly behind the earlobes and anterior to the mastoid processes? Are the two sides symmetrical?*

15.3.6 Sternocleidomastoid and Prevertebral Neck Muscles

The sternocleidomastoid is the most powerful neck flexor, rotator, and lateral flexor, although the scalene muscle group assists all three actions (Figure 15.59 ■). The scalenes connect the transverse processes of the cervical vertebrae to the two upper ribs and work as lateral neck flexors and neck rotators. Although the scalenes are important neck muscles, they were covered in the chapter on breathing because they attach to the upper ribs and assist rib elevation during respiration. The prevertebral muscles of the neck (anterior to the spine) that attach along the anterior side of the cervical spine, behind the esophagus, are the longus capitis and longus colli, rectus capitis anterior, and rectus capitis lateralis. These muscles work as cervical stabilizers and assist neck flexion. The sternocleidomastoid is innervated by the *spinal accessory nerve* (11th cranial nerve) and *cervical nerves;* the prevertebral muscles are innervated by the *cervical nerves.*

The powerful, diagonally oriented **sternocleidomastoid** (SCM) is a two-headed muscle named after its origin on the mastoid process (and the lateral half of the superior nuchal line) and insertions along the clavicle and sternum. A sternal head of the SCM tapers into a cord-like tendon that inserts on the lateral side of the sternal notch. A flat, strap-shaped clavicular head lies directly behind the sternal head and inserts along the top medial third of the clavicle. When contracting unilaterally, the SCM rotates the neck to the opposite side and side-bends the neck to the same side; when contracting bilaterally, it flexes the neck (Figure 15.60 ■). It divides the neck into an anterior triangle

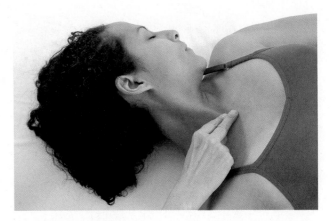

FIGURE 15.60
Sternocleidomastoid contraction

and a posterior triangle and protects large vascular and nerve trunks that it overlies (Figure 15.61 ■). (See TrPs for the sternocleidomastoid in Figure 15.62 ■.)

Two longus muscles located behind the throat and esophagus run along the front of the cervical and upper thoracic vertebra. The **longus capitis** attaches to the occipital bone anterior to the foramen magnum and inserts on the anterior tubercles of the C-3 to C-6 transverse processes (Figure 15.63 ■). The **longus colli,** a complex muscle with a superior, medial, and inferior section, continues along the path of the longus capitis down the front of the spine. Its superior section attaches at the anterior arch of the atlas (C-1) and inserts on the anterior tubercles of the C-3 to C-5 transverse processes, the medial section is plastered against the vertebral bodies of C-3 to T-3, and the inferior section attaches at the C-5 and C-6 transverse processes and inserts

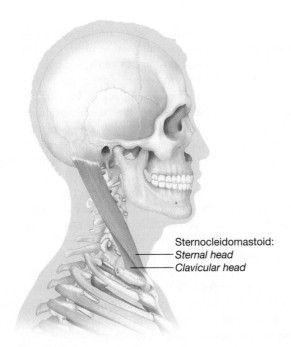

FIGURE 15.59
Sternocleidomastoid

Sternocleidomastoid:
Sternal head
Clavicular head

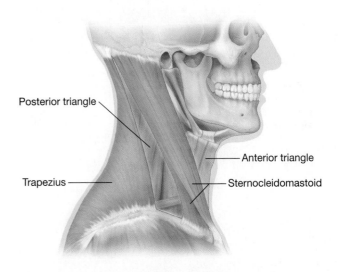

Posterior triangle
Trapezius
Anterior triangle
Sternocleidomastoid

FIGURE 15.61
The SCM divides the neck into **anterior and posterior triangles.**

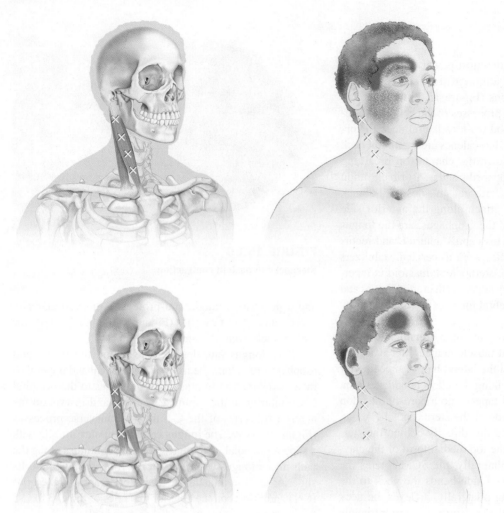

FIGURE 15.62

The **sternocleidomastoid** frequently becomes tight, short, and dysfunctional from prolonged contraction, which occurs in the forward head posture. It can develop numerous trigger points along both bellies, which can often cause tension headaches and refer pain over the eye, ear, and occiput. Because of its proprioceptive role in the postural positioning of the head, SCM dysfunction can lead to dizziness and loss of balance. Spasms on one side of the SCM cause "wryneck" or torticollis, locking the head into a fixed, off-center posture that twists the head and neck to one side.

on the T-1 to T-3 vertebral bodies. Both longus muscles run so close to the axis of joint motion in the cervical spine that they lack enough leverage to generate cervical flexion. Their main function is to compress and support the anterior side of the cervical spine, stabilizing its lordotic curve in a lengthened position similar to how the multifidus supports the lumbar lordosis. The tonic contractions of the longus muscles counter the upward pull of the trapezius, allowing the trapezius to upwardly rotate the scapula rather than pull the neck down.

The **rectus capitis anterior** and **rectus capitis lateralis** arise from the anterior aspect of the occiput and insert on the transverse processes of the atlas and axis (C-1 and C-2), mirroring their suboccipital counterparts on the posterior side of the occiput. Although their pull is limited to small movements at the base of the skull, these short muscles produce slight flexion of the head on the upper cervical spine when contracting bilaterally and slight rotation and side-bending when contracting unilaterally. The rectus capitis muscles are too deep to palpate.

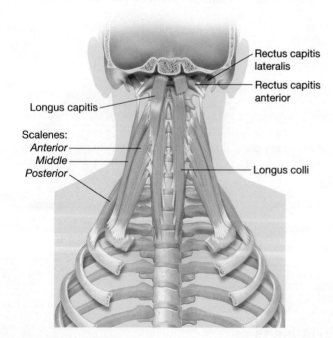

Rectus capitis lateralis

Rectus capitis anterior

Longus capitis

Scalenes:
Anterior
Middle
Posterior

Longus colli

FIGURE 15.63

Prevertebral muscles of the cervical spine

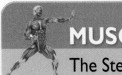

MUSCLE PALPATION
The Sternocleidomastoid

The SCM is easy to palpate on yourself and others. To locate the SCM, press into its origin below the mastoid process. Follow the sternal head of the SCM toward the sternum using a pincher palpation to squeeze the muscle belly along its length. Palpate its insertions on the sternum and the medial clavicle using cross-fiber strumming.

Sternocleidomastoid

O–Clavicular head—Medial third of superior border of clavicle
    Sternal head—Lateral side of sternal notch of manubrium

I–Mastoid process and lateral half of superior nuchal line
A–Bilaterally flexes the neck, unilaterally—side-bends the neck to same side, rotates the neck to opposite side

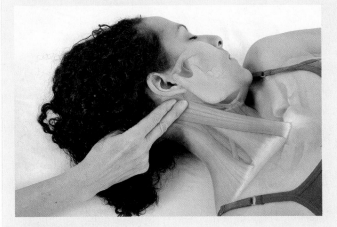

FIGURE 15.64a
Palpating the SCM origin

Palpate the **sternocleidomastoid** by locating its tendinous origin below the mastoid process, behind the ear. Apply a cross-fiber strumming below the mastoid to feel the upper end of the muscle (Figure 15.64a ■). It will feel like a thick, fibrous strap. Palpate both sides at once to check the symmetry of the SCMs. From here, walk your fingertips down the bellies of the SCMs

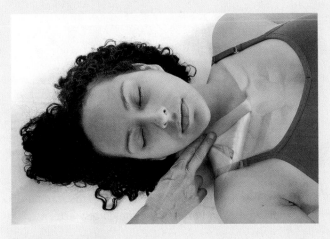

FIGURE 15.64b
Active movement of the SCM

Active movement: Have your partner lift his or her head off the table for the SCMs to contract bilaterally (Figure 15.64b ■). Have your partner turn the head to observe the SCM contract on one side. As your partner moves, notice where the SCM tendons pop out on its sternal and clavicular insertion points. Use a light pincher palpation to squeeze along the length of the muscle. Move gently and slowly, noticing the edges of the muscle. *Can you slightly lift the sternal belly of the SCM?*

(continued)

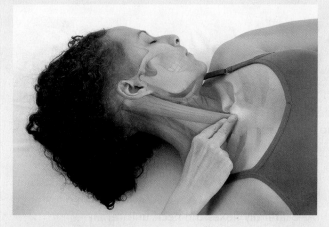

FIGURE 15.64c
Palpating the SCM sternal insertion

To differentiate the two heads of the SCM, slowly slide your fingertips across its distal tendons on the top of the manubrium and clavicle. The sternal insertion will feel like a cord (Figure 15.64c ■).

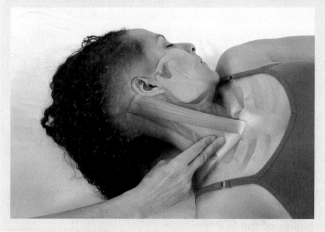

FIGURE 15.64d
Palpating the SCM clavicular insertion

The clavicular insertion will feel like a flat strap directly lateral to the sternal tendon (Figure 15.64d ■). Continue to slide across the tissues above the clavicle to feel the anterior edge of the trapezius muscle. *Do you feel the scalenes under the SCM insertions?*

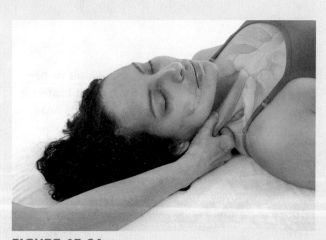

FIGURE 15.64e
Active stretch of the SCM

Stretching the sternocleidomastoid: To stretch the SCM, push the muscle belly in a posterior direction as your partner slowly turns his or her head toward that same side (Figure 15.64e ■).

Caution: *Gently hook your fingers around the muscle belly, making sure to not press on the carotid artery.*

The movement of the head and neck coordinates and organizes patterns of the entire spine. This foundational sequence is best observed in a baby, who lifts its head to look around, lengthening the entire spine. Rarely do we see a baby or small child with poor posture in the head and neck. In contrast, many adults collapse the neck into an exaggerated cervical lordosis, bending the cervical spine like a hinge and causing an anterior shear of C-4 and C-5 at the apex of the bend (Figure 15.65 ■). This pattern can be corrected with exercises that engage the prevertebral muscles. It is important to correct this pattern because a collapsed neck not only compresses cervical vertebrae and discs, it can entrap nerves, disturb the balance of the shoulder girdle, and compromise circulation to the brain.

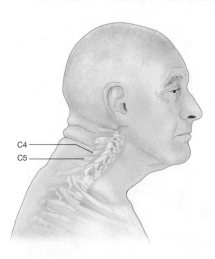

FIGURE 15.65
Cervical hyperextension

SELF-CARE
Neuromuscular Patterning to Engage the Neck Stabilizers

If you or a client has a pattern of cervical hyperextension, this exercise will help to lengthen the neck and shift the midcervical vertebrae in a posterior direction.

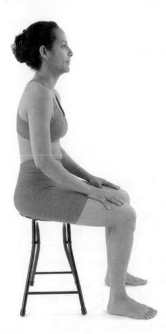

FIGURE 15.66a

1. **Preparatory position:** Sit in an upright position. Engage your postural muscles by lightly contracting your lower abdominals (Figure 15.66a ■). Widen your shoulders front and back to lengthen neck and shoulder muscles whose tensions can pull on and shorten the neck.

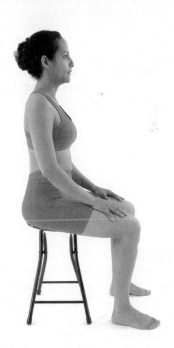

FIGURE 15.66b

2. **The atlanto-occiput (AO) lift:** Slightly lift your occiput without lowering your chin to lengthen your cervical spine (Figure 15.66b ■). You will probably feel a stretch down the back of your spine. Use only as much effort as it takes to initiate the stretch, which should engage the longus muscles.

(continued)

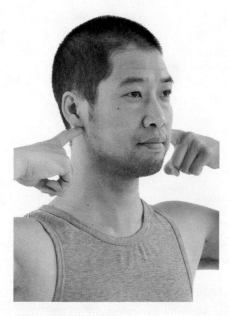

FIGURE 15.66c

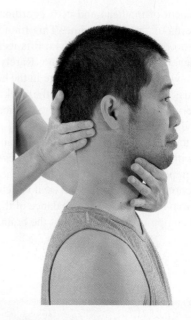

FIGURE 15.66d

3. **The atlanto-occiput (AO) rock:** Locate the axis of movement at the AO joints by lightly placing your index fingers in the hollow spot behind your ears, anterior to the mastoid process (Figure 15.66c ■). Subtly rock your head along this axis, at the AO joints. Keep your occiput lifted and your neck long as you do this movement. This subtle rocking will help you learn how to make small movements at the AO joints by engaging the intrinsic muscles. Rock for about 10 seconds, then release.

4. **AO lift and rock with a partner:** Have your partner sit or stand in a neutral position. Gently cradle your partner's occiput and the hyoid area under the chin. Be careful not to compress the throat. Gently lift your partner's occiput while gently supporting the chin to keep the head centered and prevent AO flexion and hyperextension (Figure 15.66d ■). Then have your partner subtly rock at the AO joints.

Practice the AO lift and rock whenever you can during the day. You can also do the AO lift and rock standing with your head and back against a wall, with your head against the head rest in your car, or lying down.

CONCLUSION

The muscles of the face and head provide a barometer of client's emotional states and how they use their sensory organs. The jaw muscles tend to hold emotional tension and can be dysfunctional in many clients. Given the central role of the head and the temporomandibular joint in neuromuscular development, when a practitioner can get a client to relax and yield the muscles of the head to an educated touch, a general relaxation response in the entire body usually follows. Massaging the face can help a person relax the muscles that can form a mask of tension. Releasing tension in the muscles of the forehead, around the jaws and ears, and at the base of the occiput can also help a tense client sink into a wave of deep systemic (autonomic) and somatic relaxation. For these reasons, the head can be a great place to begin a massage.

The muscles of the neck connect the head to the spine, throat, and trachea. The neck contains several vulnerable structures, such as the trachea and hyoid bone. Cervical muscles such as the suboccipitals and the sternocleidomastoid are susceptible to stresses from faulty postures such as the forward head posture, jaw tension, headaches, and injuries. In addition, the shoulder girdle is suspended from muscles of the cervical spine, so the alignment of the head, neck, and shoulder girdle all affect one another. Any work a practitioner can do to lengthen and realign the neck and release cervical muscles can greatly help to alleviate headaches, reduce jaw and neck tension, and realign the entire spine.

SUMMARY POINTS TO REMEMBER

1. Eight bones—two parietal bones; two temporal bones; and the frontal, sphenoid, occipital, and ethmoid bones—form a cranial vault that encases and protects the brain.

2. There are 14 facial bones—the mandible and vomer and the following paired bones: maxilla, nasal, lacrimal, palatine, inferior nasal conchae, and zygomatic bones.

3. The mandible of the lower jaw is the largest and most mobile bone in the head.

4. A U-shaped hyoid is called the "floating bone" because it does not articulate with any other bone. It provides attachment sites for the hyoid muscles of the mouth and throat.

5. The auricle of the outer ear is made up of elastic cartilage, and the nasal and alar portions of the nose are made up of hyaline cartilage.

6. The throat is made up of a series of cartilaginous rings called the thyroid cartilage, the cricoid cartilage, and the trachea.

7. The cranial bones are connected by fibrous joints called sutures, which have jagged, tooth-like edges that interdigitate with each other like interlaced fingers. Four large sutures that can be easily palpated are the coronal, sagittal, squamous, and lamboid sutures.

8. Cranialsacral therapy is based on the premise of a subtle motion in the sutures that occurs in response to cerebrospinal fluid rhythms.

9. The temporomandibular joint (TMJ), located between the mandibular condyle of the mandible and the glenoid fossa of the temporal bone, is a complex synovial joint with an articulating disk that slides back and forth during motion of the jaws.

10. The TMJ, the most active and often-used joint in the body, can move in six directions: lateral excursion to the right or left, protrusion and retrusion, and elevation and depression. Chewing is a combination of these six movements.

11. Eighty percent of cervical rotation occurs at the pivot joint in the atlantoaxial joint. The atlanto-occipital joints (ellipsoid joints) allow for cervical flexion and extension. Lateral cervical flexion occurs in every segment of the cervical spine.

12. The frontalis on the forehead and the occipitalis on the occiput are sometimes referred to as the occipitofrontalis because the two blend into a subcutaneous musculotendinous sheath called the galea aponeurotica, which covers the top of the cranium.

13. The temporalis, which attaches on the temporal fossa above the ear and the coronoid process of the mandible, is a powerful jaw muscle that elevates and retracts the mandible.

14. Three powerful jaw muscles—the masseter, lateral pterygoid, and medial pterygoid—connect the mandible to the zygomatic and sphenoid bones. These muscles tend to develop trigger points in temporomandibular dysfunctions (TMD) and are usually palpated intraorally (inside the mouth).

15. The hyoid bone provides attachment sites for the suprahyoid muscles of the lower jaw—the mylohyoid, geniohyoid, stylohyoid, and digastric—and the infrahyoid muscles of the throat—the sternohyoid, thyrohyoid, and omohyoid.

16. The subcutaneous platysma covering the lower jaw, neck, and clavicle is a remnant of a muscle that quadrupeds such as horses retain to twitch flies off the skin.

17. The face is covered with subcutaneous muscles that generate minimal joint motion but are highly active in the expression of emotion.

18. The sternocleidomastoid is a primary flexor of the neck.

19. The longus muscles and anterior suboccipitals run along the front of the cervical vertebrae and are referred to as prevertebral muscles.

REVIEW QUESTIONS

1. Name the eight bones of the cranium.
2. There are 14 facial bones including two single bones and six paired bones. Which of the following facial bones are the single bones?
   a. the mandible and maxilla
   b. the mandible and vomer
   c. the maxilla and vomer
   d. the mandible and zygomatic
3. True or false (circle one). The mandible is the largest and most mobile bone in the head.
4. The _____ gland covers the anterior portion of the trachea directly above the jugular notch.
5. The auricle of the ear is made up of (type) cartilage and the nasal and alar portions of the nose are made up of (type) cartilage.
6. Describe the cartilaginous structures in the throat.
7. Describe the structure and function of the hyoid bone and explain why it is unique.
8. The cranial sutures are
   a. fibrous joints between the cranial bones.
   b. cartilaginous joints between the cranial bones.
   c. synovial joints between the cranial bones.
   d. uniaxial joints between the cranial bones.
9. The suture between the frontal and parietal bones is the
   a. squamous suture.
   b. lamboid suture.
   c. sagittal suture.
   d. coronal suture.
10. The temporomandibular joint has an articular disc that
    a. cushions the joint from axial compression.
    b. slides sideways while chewing.
    c. slides forward and back to minimize stress on the joint.
    d. pops in and out of the socket during TMJ protrusion and retrusion.
11. Name the six movements of the temporomandibular joint and the direction of motion.
12. Eighty percent of cervical rotation occurs at the
    a. atlantoaxial joint.
    b. atlanto-occipital (AO) joint.
    c. upper cervical facet joints.
    d. lower cervical facet joints.
13. Describe the atlantoaxial joint.
14. The muscle that raises the eyebrows is
    a. the occipitalis.
    b. the frontalis.
    c. the temporalis.
    d. the risorius.
15. Identify which jaws muscle attaches the zygomatic arch and coronoid process to the angle of the cheek and has both superficial and deep fibers.
    a. the medial pterygoid
    b. the lateral pterygoid
    c. the masseter
    d. the buccinator
16. The two muscle groups attached to the hyoid bone that are active during swallowing, talking, and chewing are the
    a. infrahyoid and sternohyoid muscles.
    b. suprahyoid and sternohyoid muscles.
    c. infrahyoid and mylohyoid muscles.
    d. suprahyoid and infrahyoid muscles.
17. The primary function of the muscles covering the face is
    a. chewing.
    b. emotional expression.
    c. proprioception.
    d. perception.
18. The lateral pterygoid is a jaw muscle that
    a. arises from the sphenoid and the pterygoid plate of the sphenoid and inserts on the mandibular condyle and joint capsule and disc of the TMJ.
    b. arises on the pterygoid plate of the sphenoid and the maxilla and inserts across the inner surface of the mandibular ramus.
    c. arises from the zygomatic arch and the coronoid process and inserts across the angle of the mandible.
    d. arises from the zygomatic arch and the coronoid process and inserts on the mandibular condyle and the joint capsule and disc of the TMJ.
19. True or false (circle one). When the sternocleidomastoid contracts on one side, it rotates the head toward that side.
20. Which muscles connect the atlas and axis to the cranium and are continually active, making small adjustments of the head on the neck?

Notes

1. Eckman, P. (2009). *Telling Lies: Clues to Deceit in Marketplace, Politics, and Marriage* (3rd ed.). New York: W. W. Norton.

2. Simons, D., Travell, J., & Simons, L. (1999). *Myofascial Pain and Dysfunction: The Trigger Point Manual: Vol. 2. Upper Half of the Body* (2nd ed.). Baltimore: Lippincott, Williams, & Wilkins.

PEARSON
myhealthprofessionskit™

Use this address to access the Companion Website created for this textbook. Simply select "Massage Therapy" from the choice of disciplines. Find this book and log in using your username and password to access interactive activities, videos, and much more.

CHAPTER

16 The Shoulder Girdle

CHAPTER OUTLINE

Chapter Objectives

Key Terms

16.1 Bones of the Shoulder Girdle

16.2 Joints and Ligaments of the Shoulder Girdle

16.3 Muscles of the Shoulder Girdle

Conclusion

Summary Points to Remember

Review Questions

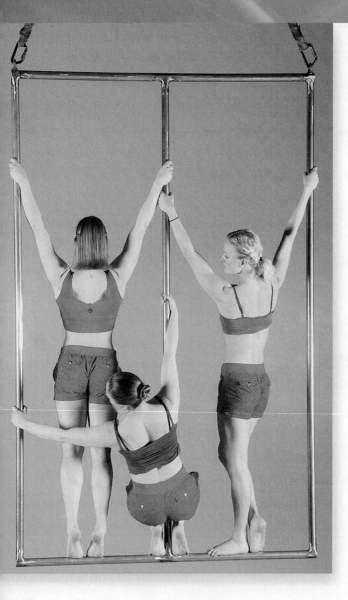

Dancers have a saying that reminds them how to use their arms: "Move your arms from your back." Nowhere is this connection between the arms and back clearer than in brachiation patterns of monkeys swinging from branch to branch, using a reach-grasp-pull sequence.

Doing a handstand compresses the shoulders along lines of force through the skeleton. In contrast, doing a pull-up extends the arms as they pull the body up, and, on the release, stretches the shoulders and trunk muscles along many lines of tension. The shoulders are the conduits between the arms and the body. Muscular

pulls pass through two layers in the shoulders: four deeper rotator cuff muscles and the broad, overlying pectoralis, trapezius, and latissimus muscles.

It's easy to think of the shoulders as being located on top of the trunk because that's where most people feel shoulder tension, but they actually attach on the sides of the trunk via an overlying cuff and broad jacket of many strong muscles. They seat the arm in the shallow yet highly mobile ball-and-socket shoulder joint and pull down to raise the arms up, which gives rise to the dancers' reminder to move the arms from the back.

CHAPTER OBJECTIVES

1. List and describe the bony landmarks on the four bones making up the shoulder girdle.

2. Demonstrate the palpation of the bony landmarks of the shoulder girdle.

3. List four joints in the shoulder girdle and their classifications and range of motion.

4. Name the major ligaments of the shoulder girdle and the location and function of each one.

5. Describe and contrast two injuries: a shoulder dislocation and a shoulder separation.

6. Describe the structure and function of the coracoacromial arch.

7. Describe the neutral position of the shoulder girdle and the criteria for scapula neutral.

8. Define scaption and describe how it relates to efficient arm movement.

9. Define and describe the scapulohumeral rhythm.

10. Identify the origins, insertions, and actions of the muscles of the scapula and shoulder.

11. Identify trigger point locations and pain referral patterns for scapula and shoulder muscles.

12. Demonstrate the active movement and palpation of each scapula and shoulder muscle.

KEY TERMS

Acromioclavicular (AC) joint

Acromion process

Clavicle

Coracoid process

Glenohumeral (GH) joint

Glenoid fossa

Head of humerus

Humerus

Inferior angle of scapula

Infraspinous fossa

Manubrium

Rotator cuff

Scaption

Scapula

Scapula neutral

Scapular winging

Scapulohumeral rhythm

Scapulothoracic joint

Shoulder dislocation

Shoulder girdle

Spine of the scapula

Sternoclavicular (SC) joint

Subscapular fossa

Supraspinous fossa

MUSCLES IN ACTION

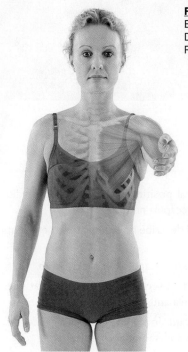

Flexion
Biceps brachii
Deltoid
Pectoralis major (upper)

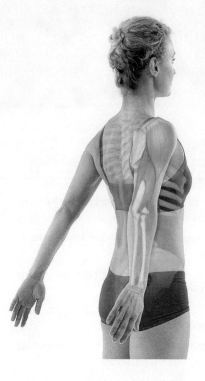

Extension
Deltoid
Latissimus dorsi
Pectoralis major (lower)
Teres major
Triceps

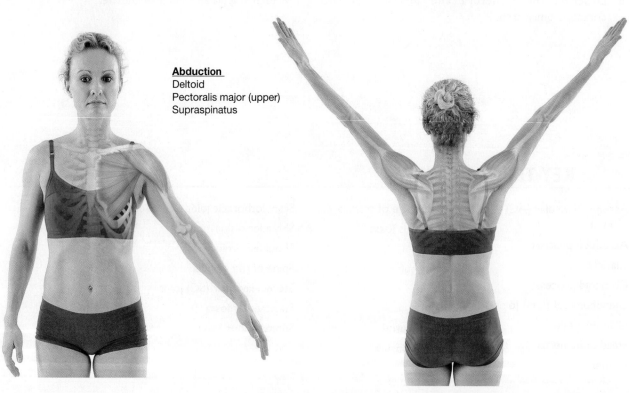

Abduction
Deltoid
Pectoralis major (upper)
Supraspinatus

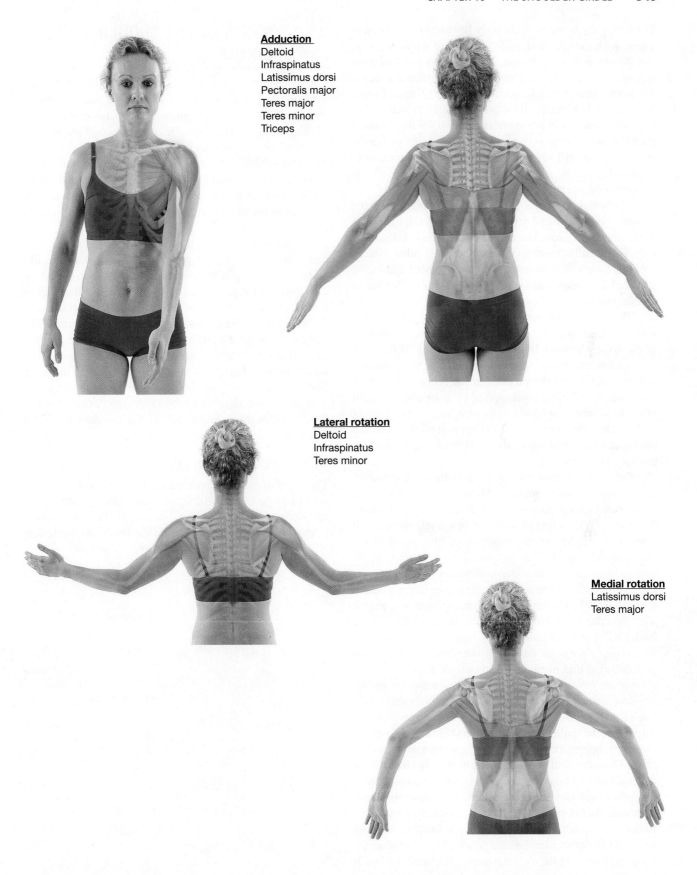

Adduction
Deltoid
Infraspinatus
Latissimus dorsi
Pectoralis major
Teres major
Teres minor
Triceps

Lateral rotation
Deltoid
Infraspinatus
Teres minor

Medial rotation
Latissimus dorsi
Teres major

The tensegrity features of the body have been compared to a tent, with muscles and tendons as guide wires, myofascial sheaths as tent fabric, and bones as struts and structural supports. The analogy of a round circus tent fits the shoulder girdle because it is suspended from the spine and trunk by a network of head, neck, and shoulder muscles. The head and spine serve as the central support for the shoulder girdle. If the central post of a circus tent leans or bends, the entire tent will sag and buckle. This point is made to emphasize how the alignment of the head and spine affects the structural integrity of the shoulder girdle.

The shoulder girdle is a bony yoke made up of the humeri (singular: *humerus*), clavicles, and scapulae. The entire shoulder girdle is tethered to the axial skeleton by only two small sternoclavicular joints. All other attachments are musculotendinous. This arrangement allows the arms to be far more mobile than the legs, yet such gains in mobility require sacrifices in stability.

The balance and stability of the shoulder girdle, more than any other body part, depends on the structural integrity of the spine, particularly of the head and neck. If the neck is elongated and the head is centered on top, the shoulders will balance across the thorax and the arms will hang in an optimally balanced position. Yet even the slightest shift of the head, neck, and spine away from centered alignment will be amplified in the tensional support of the shoulder girdle, causing some muscles to work overtime to shore up the tipsy structure.

Every movement of the arms requires a complex coordination of many muscles. Shoulder muscles work in coordinated groups to move the arms, pulling from many directions. Dysfunction or weakness in a single muscle will disturb the alignment and sequence of movement in the entire shoulder girdle. The opposite also holds true. Chronic contractures in any shoulder muscle can pull the cervical and thoracic vertebrae out of alignment like a snagged thread bunches a woven tapestry. This explains why people with shoulder problems almost always suffer from neck and back pain, and vice versa.

The challenge in balancing the shoulder girdle lies in cultivating and maintaining an optimal position so that subsequent movements begin from a centered posture. The shoulder girdle is such a mobile part of the body that establishing and maintaining its neutral position can be difficult. To address the challenge of keeping this highly mobile girdle in neutral, information on the joints, ligaments, and muscles of the shoulder girdle are presented in this chapter with an emphasis on neutral positioning and coordinated movement. Palpation exercises for bony landmarks, ligaments of the shoulder, and the many shoulder muscles are also presented. Because the hands and arms are primary working tools for a manual therapist, exercises are provided for exploring the body mechanics of the shoulder girdle. This material builds on self-care and body mechanics exercises presented in previous chapters and provides a foundation for the arm and hand exercises in the next chapter.

16.1 BONES OF THE SHOULDER GIRDLE

The rib cage is cone-shaped and far too narrow to allow the arms to hang along the sides of the body, so the broader shoulder girdle serves this purpose. The term **shoulder girdle** describes the appendicular bony structure made up of the humerus, scapula, and clavicle bones that moves with the arms (Figure 16.1 ■). To a lesser degree, the manubrium of the sternum is included as part of the shoulder girdle, although it provides a site where the shoulder girdle attaches to the axial skeleton and does not move with the arms.

The shoulder girdle positions the arms and hands to carry out a broad range of prehensile tasks. It functions like a bony yoke, suspending the arms far enough in the lateral direction that the hands can swing freely along the sides of the body without hitting the pelvis. Unlike the pelvic girdle, the shoulder girdle forms an incomplete bony ring. The posterior side of the girdle between the scapulae is open. This allows the scapulae to slide freely across the rib cage, which, in turn, increases the range of mobility in the arms. The anterior side of the shoulder girdle is anchored to the manubrium and the first rib by the sternoclavicular joints, which makes the anterior side of the shoulder girdle far more stable than the posterior side.

16.1.1 Humerus and Clavicle

The shoulder girdle has many bony landmarks that are easy to palpate. Many of these bony markings are visible and easy to observe (Figure 16.2a-b ■). The **humerus** is a long bone with a shape somewhat similar to the femur.

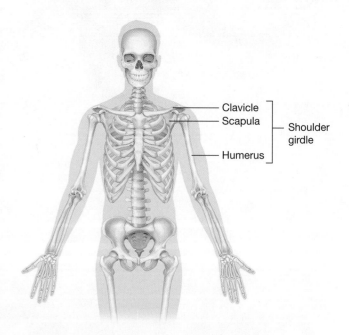

FIGURE 16.1
Shoulder girdle

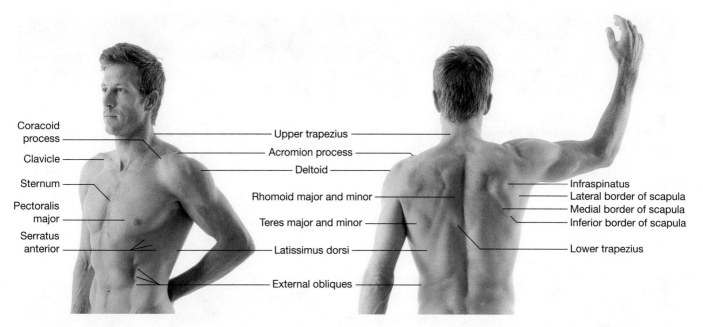

FIGURE 16.2

Surface anatomy of the shoulder girdle

It has a long, cylindrical shaft that tapers into a spherical head called the **head of humerus** (Figure 16.3 ■). The head of the humerus is the "ball" in the ball-and-socket joint of the shoulder joint. A rough, bony mound called the **greater tubercle** can be found on the lateral side of the proximal humerus. This large tubercle is surrounded by tendons of the supraspinatus, infraspinatus, and teres minor, all muscles of the rotator cuff. A smaller bony knob anterior to the greater tubercle, the **lesser tubercle,** provides an attachment site for the subscapularis. The greater and lesser tubercles are separated by a **bicipital groove** (intertubercular groove), a long yet shallow bony ditch that cradles the tendon of the long head of the biceps brachii. Both the latissimus dorsi and teres major attach along the medial lip of the bicipital groove; the pectoralis major attaches to its lateral lip. On the lateral side of the midhumeral shaft, a long, rough bump called the **deltoid tuberosity** serves as an attachment site for the large deltoid.

The **clavicle** is a round, S-shaped bone on the anterior side of the shoulder girdle. The clavicles function like horizontal struts across a yoke, balancing the shoulder girdle across the front of the upper thorax. They provide attachment sites for a number of shoulder and neck muscles, including the deltoid, upper trapezius, pectoralis major, subclavius, and sternocleidomastoid muscles. At the bottom of the medial end of each clavicle a small, saddle-shaped joint surface articulates with the manubrium at the sternoclavicular joint. The clavicle is the most frequently broken bone in the body; it often fractures in the middle when a person takes a hard fall on an outstretched hand. Clavicular fractures can disturb the horizontal balance of the shoulder girdle and result in scar tissues that restrict the function of adjacent muscles.

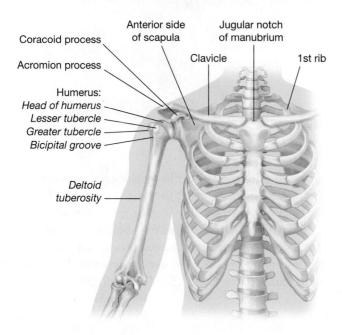

FIGURE 16.3

Bones of the shoulder girdle: anterior view

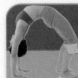

BRIDGE TO PRACTICE
Clavicular Fractures

If you get a new client with chronic neck and shoulder problems, check their health histories for clavicular fractures. If they have old fractures, you can release myofascial adhesions over fracture sites and around clavicular muscle attachments.

BONE PALPATION
Bony Landmarks of the Shoulder Girdle

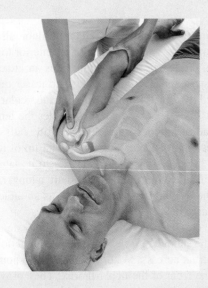

FIGURE 16.4a
Locate the **greater tubercle** on the side of the shoulder. It will feel like a bony bump on the side of the shoulder directly lateral and slightly anterior to the acromion process. Lightly hold the greater tubercle, then have your partner rotate the shoulder by rolling the arm to turn the palm up and the palm down. *Do you feel the greater tubercle move anteriorly and posteriorly as your partner rotates the humerus?* (See Figure 16.4a ■)

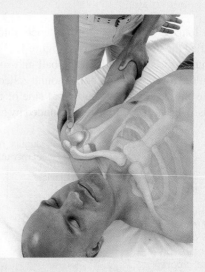

FIGURE 16.4b
Locate the **lesser tubercle** by placing your fingertips about 1 inch anterior to the greater tubercle, then having your partner laterally rotate the shoulder. As your partner rotates the shoulder, you will feel a small bump roll under your fingertips, which is the lesser tubercle. *Are you directly lateral to the upper, inside corner of the chest?* (See Figures 16.4b ■)

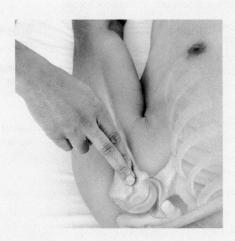

FIGURE 16.4c
Palpate the **bicipital groove** by sinking your fingertips into the area between the lesser tubercle and
the greater tubercle. To tell if you are in the bicipital
groove, have your partner bend the elbow to contract the biceps. You should feel its tendon slide in
the groove. *Do you feel a bony ditch between two bony
bumps?* (See Figure 16.4c ■)

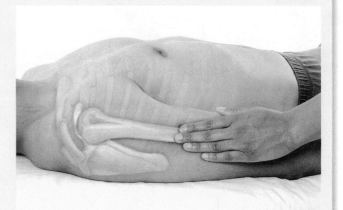

FIGURE 16.4d
To palpate the **deltoid tuberosity,** run your hand
along the lateral side of the humerus, where the
muscular contour shifts from a mound to a flat
surface at the insertion site of the deltoid muscle.
The deltoid tuberosity can be difficult to distinguish
from other bony tuberosities because it feels more
like a rise and bend along the shaft of the bone. (See
Figure 16.4d ■)

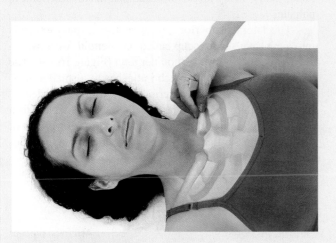

FIGURE 16.4e
Palpate the **clavicle** out to its lateral end, feeling the
joint line where it meets the acromion process of
the scapula. Explore the upper and lower surfaces
of each clavicle, noticing muscle and ligament attachments in these areas. If the clavicle has been previously fractured, you may find a large, irregular knob
of scar tissue over the break site in the middle of the
bone. *Can you trace the S-shape of each clavicle?* (See
Figure 16.4e ■)

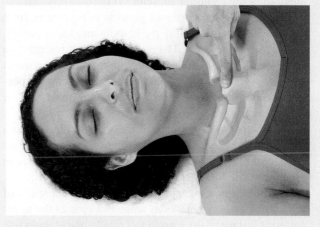

FIGURE 16.4f
Palpate the flat surface of the **manubrium** between
the medial ends of the clavicles. *Are you palpating the flat bony surface between and slightly lower
than the medial ends of the clavicles? Do you feel the
U-shaped curve that the jugular notch and medial clavicles form at the upper border of the manubrium?* (See
Figure 16.4f ■)

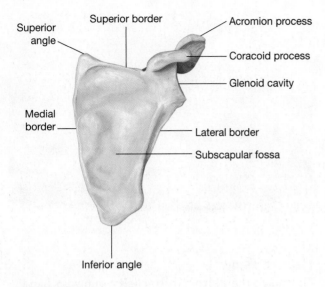

FIGURE 16.5
Scapula: anterior view

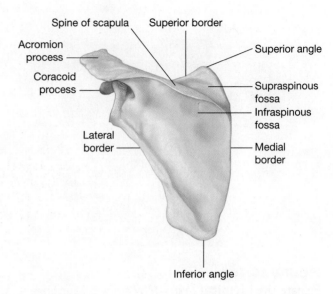

FIGURE 16.6
Scapula: posterior view

16.1.2   Scapula

The **scapula** (plural: *scapulae*), or "shoulder blade," is a flat irregular bone that lies along the back of the shoulder (Figure 16.5 ■). The triangular-shaped scapula has a number of landmarks and projections that provide attachment sites for shoulder muscles. One such landmark is a stubby, hook-like **coracoid process** that projects from the anterior, lateral point of the scapula into the upper lateral corner of the chest. The coracoid process resembles a crow's beak or a small bent finger. It provides attachment sites for several ligaments and muscles including the pectoralis minor, the coracobrachialis, and the short head of the biceps.

The superior lateral end of the scapula tapers into a broad flat surface called the **acromion process,** which juts out over the shoulder joint like a protective ledge and is an attachment site for the upper trapezius and deltoid muscles. The acromion process tapers into the prominent **spine of the scapula,** a horizontal bony ledge that crosses the upper posterior surface of the scapula and divides the scapula into two areas. Below the scapular spine, a flat and triangular **infraspinous fossa** provides a broad attachment site for the infraspinatus of the rotator cuff. Above the scapula spine, a rounded canoe-shaped depression called the **supraspinous fossa** provides an attachment site for the supraspinatus of the rotator cuff. A **subscapular fossa** covers the anterior surface of the scapula.

Like all triangles, the scapula has three corners and three borders. It tapers into a pointed, palpable **inferior angle** on the bottom corner. The levator scapula muscle attaches around the **superior angle** on the upper, inner corner of the scapula (Figure 16.6 ■). The **lateral border** (axillary border) runs below the armpit; it provides attachment sites for both the teres major and teres minor

muscles. The **medial border** is referred to as the *vertebral border* because of its proximity to the spine; it provides attachment sites for the rhomboid and serratus anterior muscles. The **superior border** of the scapula runs across its top under many layers of tissue that make it difficult to palpate.

The lateral, superior corner of the scapula expands into a concave shallow cup called the **glenoid fossa,** which serves as a socket for the shoulder joint (Figure 16.7 ■). The long head of the biceps brachii attaches to a small **supraglenoid tubercle** on the anterior, upper rim of the glenoid fossa. The long head of the triceps brachii attaches to a small **infraglenoid tubercle** on the posterior, lower rim of the glenoid fossa. Because of their locations, both tubercles are difficult to palpate.

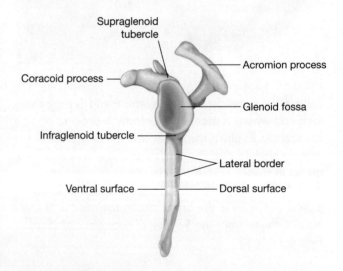

FIGURE 16.7
Glenoid fossa of scapula

BRIDGE TO PRACTICE
Slang Terms for the Shoulder Girdle

People generally refer to the clavicles as the "collar bones" and the scapulae as the "shoulder blades." In order not to confuse clients with anatomical terms, you might want to use these more familiar terms when conversing with them about the shoulder girdle. Make sure to use the anatomically correct terms when conversing with other health professionals.

BONE PALPATION
Scapula

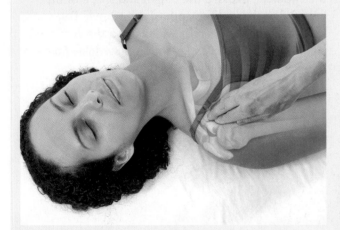

FIGURE 16.8a

Palpate the **coracoid process** below and under the lateral end of the clavicle. Use circular pressure to locate the coracoid process, which will feel like a bony bump in the center of surrounding tissues. *Do you notice how the coracoid process is easier to locate when your partner laterally rotates the arm? (See Figure 16.8a ■)*

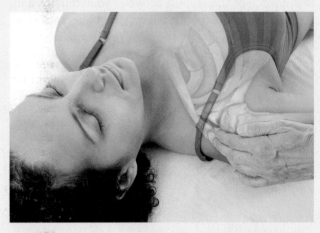

FIGURE 16.8b

Locate the **acromion process** beside the lateral end of the clavicle. It will feel like a flat bony ledge. Explore the contours of the acromion process, tracing its lateral edge, which feel like a bony shelf over the shoulder. *Are you on the bone posterior to the lateral end of the clavicle, at its highest point on top of the shoulder? (See Figure 16.8b ■)*

(continued)

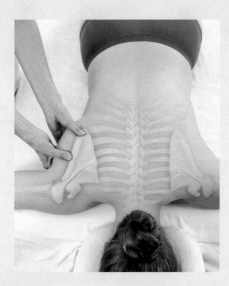

FIGURE 16.8c

Palpate the **subscapular fossa** with your partner's arm hanging over the side of the table. Grasp the lateral border of the scapula between your thumbs and fingers. Slowly press your fingertips up into the subscapular fossa, sinking through the subscapularis muscle. *Are your fingertips as medial as you can get them, along the side of the rib cage?* (See Figure 16.8c ■)

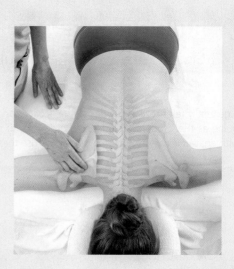

FIGURE 16.8d

To raise the scapula and make it easier to palpate, place your partner's arm behind the lower back. Locate the **spine of the scapula** on the back of the shoulder. Explore the length and shape of this bony ridge across the width of the scapula. Palpate its lateral end to where it widens into the acromion. *How far is the medial end of the scapular spine from the superior angle?* (See Figure 16.8d ■)

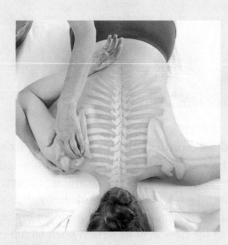

FIGURE 16.8e

Press your fingertips into the **supraspinous fossa** above the spine of the scapula. To raise the scapula and make it easier to palpate, place your partner's arm behind the lower back. Press through overlying muscles to explore the curved contours of the fossa, from the tip of the shoulder to the medial end of the scapula. *Are you above the spine of the scapula?* (See Figure 16.8e ■)

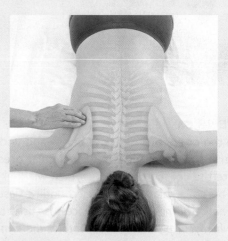

FIGURE 16.8f

Press your fingertips over the triangular surface of the **infraspinous fossa** below the spine of the scapula. Explore its broad surface to the medial and lateral edges of the scapula. *Are you below the spine of the scapula?* (See Figure 16.8f ■)

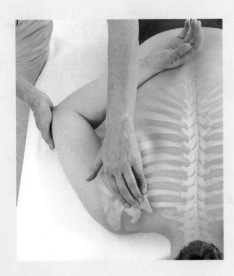

FIGURE 16.8g
Palpate the **superior angle** of the scapula by strumming your fingertips across the upper medial corner of the scapula. If overlying tissues make it difficult to find, elevate the shoulder to make it more accessible. *Are you on the medial side of the scapula, above the spine of the scapula?* (See Figure 16.8g ■)

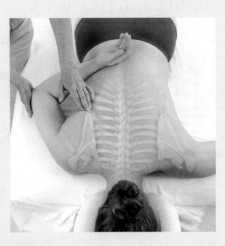

FIGURE 16.8h
Locate the sharp **inferior angle** at the bottom of the scapula. Trace around its edges on both sides. *Does the inferior angle of the scapula stick out or lie flat against the ribs?* (See Figure 16.8h ■)

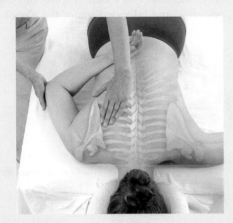

FIGURE 16.8i
Trace along the **medial border** from the inferior angle up along the inner edge of the scapula. This border is usually the length of a hand. *Are you on the medial side of the scapula?* (See Figure 16.8i ■)

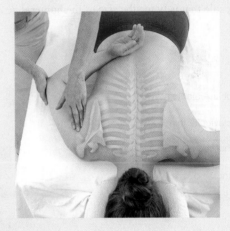

FIGURE 16.8j
Trace along the **lateral border** from the inferior angle up along the outer edge of the scapula to the armpit. *Are you on the lateral side of the scapula, below the armpit? Do you feel the fleshy muscles attached to the lateral border of the scapula?* (See Figure 16.8j ■)

16.2 JOINTS AND LIGAMENTS OF THE SHOULDER GIRDLE

There are four main joints of the shoulder girdle: the *glenohumeral, acromioclavicular, sternoclavicular,* and *scapulothoracic* joints (Figure 16.9 ■). The great mobility of the arms and hands can be attributed to the linked movement of these four joints, particularly the glenohumeral joint, the most mobile joint in the body. The shoulder girdle is a hanging structure suspended from the head and neck by a network of tensional supports that include ligaments, tendons, muscles, and fascias. It is attached to the axial skeleton by only two small sternoclavicular joints.

16.2.1 Glenohumeral Joint

The **glenohumeral (GH) joint** is a ball-and-socket joint made up of an articulation between the *glenoid fossa* of the scapula and the *humeral head* (Figure 16.10 ■). Smooth, hyaline cartilage coats the humeral head, which has a surface area three times the size of the glenoid fossa that allows tremendous flexibility in the shoulder joint. To compensate for the size difference, a fibrocartilage ring called the **glenoid labrum** attaches around the rim of the glenoid fossa like a washer, deepening the socket and stabilizing the joint. The entire GH joint is encapsulated by a large, loose joint capsule that is twice the size of the humeral head. This

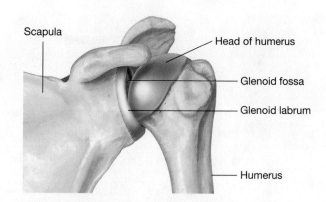

FIGURE 16.10
Glenohumeral joint

lax capsule allows for a broad range of movement in the shoulder (see Table 16.1 ■).

16.2.1.1 GLENOHUMERAL JOINT LIGAMENTS AND BURSAE

A large capsular ligament, the **glenohumeral ligament,** which is actually an outer layer of the joint capsule, covers and reinforces the joint like a cuff (Figure 16.11 ■). The anterior, posterior, and inferior parts of the glenohumeral

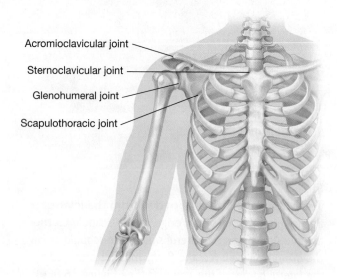

FIGURE 16.9
Joints of the shoulder girdle

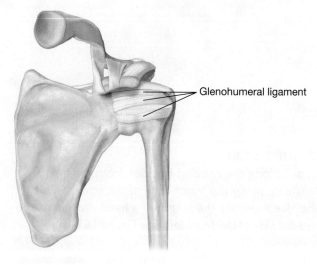

FIGURE 16.11
Ligaments of the glenohumeral joint

TABLE 16.1 **Range of Motion in the Shoulder**

Shoulder Motion	Range of Motion	End-Feel
Flexion	180 degrees	Firm
Hyperextension	45 degrees	Firm
Abduction	180 degrees	Firm
Adduction	10 degrees	Firm
Lateral rotation	45 degrees	Firm
Medial rotation	45 degrees	Firm

ligament and the joint capsule are lax in a neutral posture, when the arm is hanging beside the body. They twist and are pulled taut during abduction, drawing the joint into a close-packed position (Figure 16.12 ■).

Several bursae can be found above the glenohumeral ligament. The **subdeltoid bursa** and **subacromial bursa** reduce friction between tendons and the underside of the acromion process and are the most common sites of bursitis in the shoulder (Figure 16.13 ■). The subdeltoid bursa and subacromial bursa tend to be continuous with each other,

although sometimes they have separate bursa sacs.[1] A **subdeltoid space** exists between the top of the humerus and the subdeltoid and subacromial bursa. This space cushions the underlying supraspinatus and biceps tendons from the overlying underside of the acromion process. During arm motion, the subdeltoid space provides room for these tendons to slide above the GH joint capsule.[2]

A **coracohumeral ligament** crosses the anterior side of the subdeltoid space, attaching the coracoid process to the greater tubercle. The coracohumeral ligament has two heads that run horizontally across the top of the shoulder, blending into the top of the glenohumeral ligament. The main stabilizing function of this ligament is to prevent the inferior dislocation of the GH joint; it also limits GH hyperextension and lateral rotation. Four tendons from the rotator cuff muscles also reinforce the GH joint on the front, top, and back sides. The rotator cuff tendons seat the head of the humerus squarely in its socket and provide

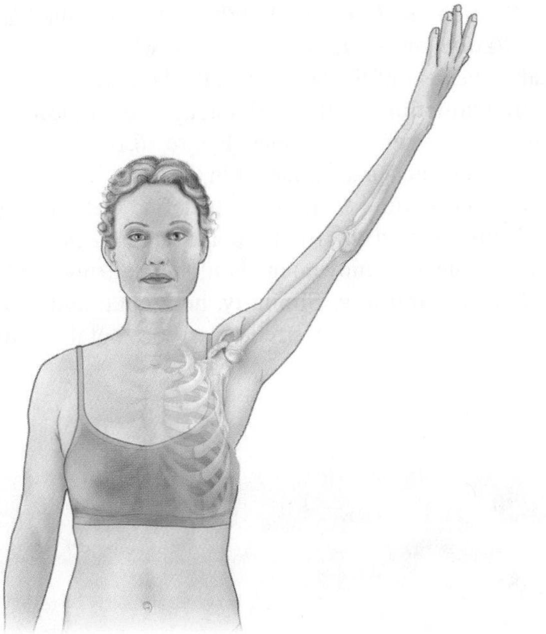

FIGURE 16.12
Close-packed position of the glenohumeral joint

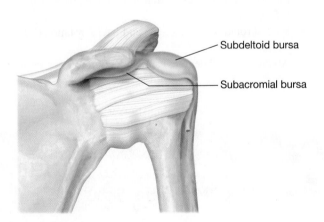

FIGURE 16.13
Bursae of the glenohumeral joint

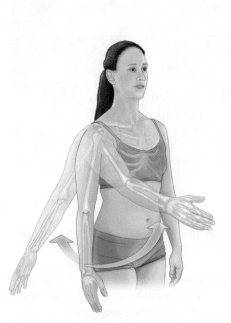
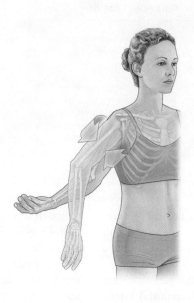
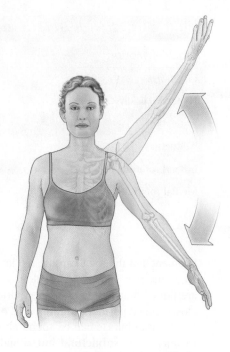

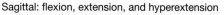

| Sagittal: flexion, extension, and hyperextension | Horizontal: medial and lateral rotation | Frontal: abduction and adduction |

FIGURE 16.14

Glenohumeral joint motion in three planes

an outer layer of protective tissues to stabilize this highly mobile joint.

16.2.1.2 GLENOHUMERAL JOINT MOTION

The GH joint moves with the three degrees of motion listed below (Figure 16.14 ■):

- Flexion (180 degrees), extension, and hyperextension (45 degrees)
- Medial rotation (70 degrees) and lateral rotation (90 degrees)
- Abduction (180 degrees) and adduction (30 degrees)

The GH joint can also move through **horizontal adduction** and **horizontal abduction,** also called *horizontal flexion* and *horizontal extension,* which is the horizontal movement of the arm across the body (Figure 16.15 ■). Circumduction at the GH engages a combination of movement in all three planes (Figure 16.16 ■).

There are some variances in the terms used to describe GH joint motion. Some schools define GH movement of the joint behind the frontal plane as *GH extension.* Others define GH movement behind the frontal plane as *GH hyperextension.* Similarly, horizontal abduction and adduction are also referred to as horizontal flexion and

BRIDGE TO PRACTICE
PROMs on the Shoulder

Unless your client demonstrates a restricted range of shoulder motion, rarely will you need to check the range of motion or apply passive range of motion (PROM) on the shoulder because it is a hypermobile joint.

On the other hand, if the joint ROM is restricted, you can use PROMs to stretch muscles and connective tissues that restrict

shoulder movement. It's important to use minimal traction when performing PROMs on the shoulder to avoid overstretching this already hypermobile joint, especially if your client has a history of shoulder injuries or dislocations. Even medium traction on an unstable shoulder joint could flare up the symptoms of an old injury.

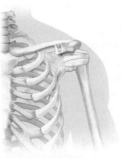
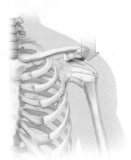

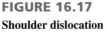

FIGURE 16.17
Shoulder dislocation

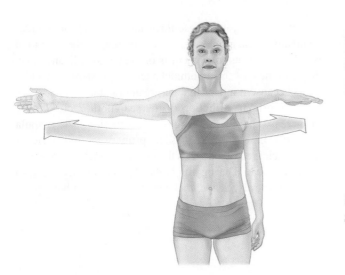

FIGURE 16.15
Horizontal abduction and adduction

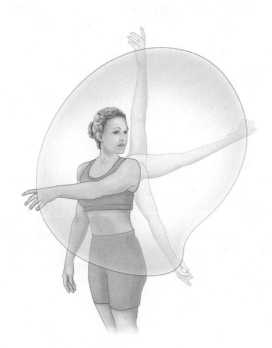

FIGURE 16.16
Circumduction of the glenohumeral joint

extension, although abduction and adduction are more widely used.

The mobility of the GH joint and the size variance of its articulating surfaces necessitates that the humeral head continually reposition to remain centered in the socket. To prevent the large humeral head from rolling off the much smaller glenoid fossa during shoulder movement, the humeral head continually changes the point of contact and axis of rotation in the socket. During lateral and medial rotation, the humeral head spins and glides either anteriorly or posteriorly. During abduction, the head of the humerus glides inferiorly, which prevents it from jamming against the acromion process and impinging structures that pass under the acromion.

The GH joint is more likely to move with efficient arthrokinematics if the shoulder girdle is in a neutral position at the initiation of a movement. If the shoulder girdle tends to sit in an off-centered position, this increases the mechanical stresses on the GH joint once the arm begins moving. For this reason, it's important to maintain an optimal neutral position of the shoulder girdle in a stationary posture while giving massage or during any activities that require repetitive movement and force applications (such as pushing or pulling).

Because the GH joint is the most mobile and least stable joint in the body, it is highly susceptible to **shoulder dislocation.** When the shoulder dislocates, the humeral head is pulled out of the socket. Severe overstretching, falls, or ballistic movements can readily dislocate the GH joint (Figure 16.17 ■). The most common dislocation occurs in the inferior direction, although the shoulder can also become dislocated in a posterior or anterior direction. Once a shoulder has been dislocated, it is easy to reinjure.

16.2.2 Scapulothoracic Joint

The glenohumeral joint can only move so far before it pulls the scapula along. The primary function of the scapula is to orient the glenoid fossa for optimal contact with the humeral head when maneuvering the arm. When the arm moves, the scapula moves at the **scapulothoracic joint**—the articulating space between the scapula and the ribs. The scapulothoracic joint is not a true anatomical joint because it does not have a joint capsule and synovial fluid. It is mechanically linked to the smaller and less-mobile acromioclavicular and sternoclavicular joints, which always move with the

scapulothoracic joint; these three joints cannot move independently of each other. Although the scapulothoracic joint is a false joint, its movement is of greater significance than the movement of the acromioclavicular and sternoclavicular joints because it moves in a far greater range.

The primary function of the scapulothoracic joint is to increase the overall range of arm motion. The scapula can move in all three planes. Its primary motion is elevation, which greatly increases the range in which a person can reach overhead. During an overhead reach, the scapula also rotates upwardly. Scapular elevation and rotation both occur

---

EXPLORING TECHNIQUE
Passive Range of Motion for the Shoulder

Before you perform these PROM on the shoulder, read through the guidelines:

- Have your partner agree to report any pain or discomfort that he or she feels during the motion. During the passive motion, watch for signs of pain or discomfort and stop if you notice any reactions.
- Check for contraindications such as a history of shoulder dislocations or separations.
- Identify why you need to perform PROMs on the shoulder. Reasons could include stretching shoulder muscles, stretching passive restraints (ligaments or joint capsule), to improve your client's awareness of movement, or to check for symptom provocation (to recreate symptoms) in order to determine which tissues are causing the symptoms.

- Stabilize the scapula before and while moving the humerus. Have your partner help stabilize by lightly contracting the lower abdominal muscles and elongating the neck.
- Apply only light traction to the joint. Avoid medium or strong traction.
- Slowly move the shoulder along a linear pathway.
- When you feel you have reached the end range of motion and cannot move the shoulder any farther, ask your partner if he or she feels a stretch. A stretch will indicate you have reached the end range of joint motion.

1. **Medial rotation of the shoulder:** With your partner in the supine position, abduct the shoulder to 45 degrees and bend the elbow to 90 degrees. Cradle the top of the shoulder to stabilize the scapula at the coracoid process and the spine of the scapula. Apply light traction on the humerus in a lateral direction. Then slowly move the hand toward the table to medially rotate the shoulder (Figure 16.18a ■). *Did you make sure the shoulder did not rise off the table? Did you maintain traction on the joint while you medially rotated the shoulder?*

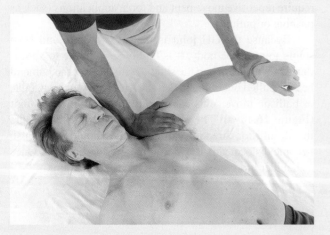

FIGURE 16.18a

a) PROM for medial rotation of the shoulder

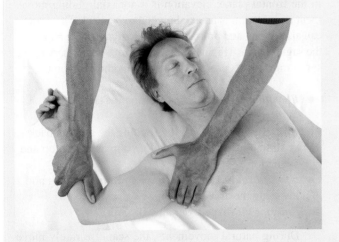

FIGURE 16.18b

b) PROM for lateral rotation of the shoulder

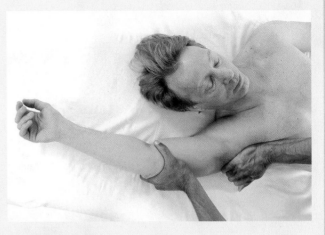

FIGURE 16.18c

c) PROM for flexion of the shoulder

2. **Lateral rotation of the shoulder:** With your partner in a supine position, abduct the shoulder to 45 degrees and bend the elbow to 90 degrees. Cradle the top of the shoulder to stabilize the scapula at the coracoid process and the spine of the scapula. Apply light traction on the humerus in a lateral direction. Then slowly move the hand toward the table in an upward direction (Figure 16.18b ■). *Did you make sure the shoulder did not rise off the table? Did you maintain traction on the joint while you medially rotated the shoulder?*

3. **Shoulder flexion:** With your partner supine and his or her arm at the side of the body, hold your partner's arm at the wrist and above the elbow. Slowly raise the arm in an arc toward the ceiling and overhead. As you move the arm overhead, make sure to laterally rotate the shoulder so that the greater tubercle does not bump into the acromion process and hike the shoulder girdle. Once the arm is overhead, press down on the subscapular fossa to stabilize the scapula. Take the humerus to end range, checking with your partner about whether he or she feels a stretch (Figure 16.18c ■).

4. **Shoulder hyperextension:** With your partner in a side-lying position, place the scapula in a neutral position. Grasp the elbow in one hand and stabilize the scapula in neutral, then slowly hyperextend the shoulder until your partner

reports a stretch (Figure 16.18d ■). Women can often hyperextend the shoulder to 90 degrees. In a female client with this degree of shoulder flexibility, you may want to skip extension on the shoulder because it will only stretch already hypermobile joint structures.

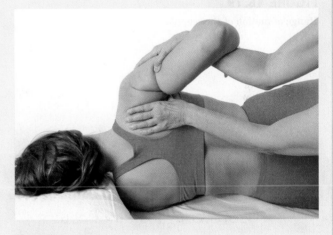

FIGURE 16.18d

d) PROM for hyperextension of the shoulder

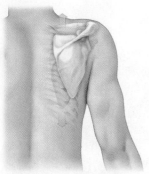

Elevation and depression

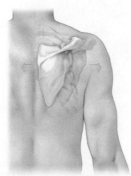

Protraction and retraction

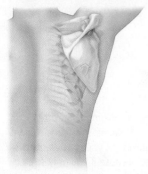

Upward and downward rotation

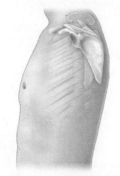

Anterior and posterior tilt

FIGURE 16.19

Range of motion of the scapula

in the frontal plane; elevation is a nonaxial gliding movement and rotation is an axial pivotal movement. The scapula can also retract and protract in the horizontal plane and tilt in the sagittal plane (Figure 16.19 ■). Here is a summary of the seven movements possible at the scapulothoracic joint:

- *Elevation* and *depression* (raising the shoulder or pulling it down)
- *Protraction* and *retraction* (pulling the scapula back or sliding it forward, also referred to as abduction and adduction)
- *Upward rotation* and *downward rotation* (lifting and lowering the arm)
- *Anterior tilt* (hyperextending the arm)

During natural movements, the scapulae rarely move in a single plane. To feel how difficult single-plane motion is, try protracting and retracting your shoulder blades without tilting or elevating them. You'll discover that this is anatomically impossible. The scapulae usually tilt with protraction. Anterior tilting occurs during shoulder hyperextension, such as when a swimmer hyperextends the arms in preparation for a dive. In all other motions, the scapula slides against the ribs. When the scapula anteriorly tilts, the inferior angle raises away from the ribs. Anterior tilting is considered a secondary motion.

The scapulae can become fixed in any off-centered position. Elevation and protraction anteriorly tilt the scapulae, which is a common pattern in a slouched posture that

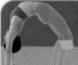

BRIDGE TO PRACTICE
Correcting Military Posture

When a person who stands in a military posture relaxes the rhomboids, the chest tends to collapse and the shoulders to round. When this occurs with a client, you'll want to help your client learn how to correct this by using

spinal muscles rather than shoulder muscles to extend the thoracic spine. Encourage your client to find an upright posture by lengthening the neck and lifting the chest to elongate the thoracic spine rather than retracting the shoulders.

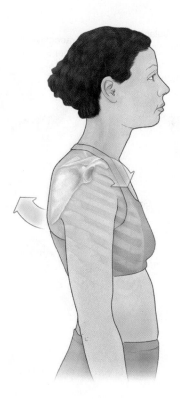

FIGURE 16.20

A collapsed posture can cause the scapula to anteriorly tilt.

rounds the shoulders (Figure 16.20 ■). In contrast, the military posture in which a person pinches the shoulder blades together in an effort to stand up straight elevates and retracts the scapulae. This postural holding pattern usually throws the elbows behind the body and overworks the rhomboids, which then chronically contract to hold the thorax upright, a supportive function much better suited for paravertebral muscles.

16.2.3 Acromioclavicular Joint

The **acromioclavicular** (AC) **joint** is a plane synovial joint connecting the lateral end of the clavicle to the acromion process (Figure 16.21 ■). This joint varies in size and may

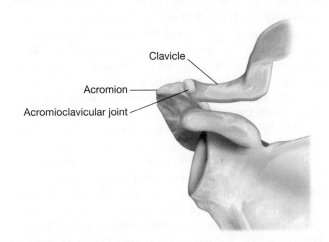

Clavicle

Acromion

Acromioclavicular joint

FIGURE 16.21

Acromioclavicular joint

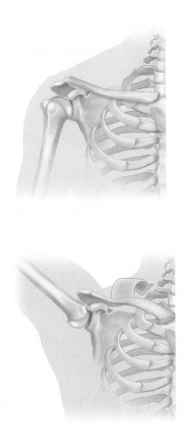

FIGURE 16.22

Lateral rotation of clavicle during shoulder elevation

or may not have an articulating disc. It allows independent movement to occur between the scapula and clavicle. During elevation of the shoulders, the clavicle laterally rotates at the AC joint and moves in the posterior direction (Figure 16.22 ■).

A primary function of the AC joint is the horizontal stabilization of the shoulder. It has a weak joint capsule that is always under tensional stress from the weight of the arms. A **superior acromioclavicular ligament** and an **inferior acromioclavicular ligament** reinforce the top and the bottom of the joint capsule (Figure 16.23 ■). Several other ligaments that are not part of the AC joint stabilize it by firmly anchoring the clavicle to the coracoid process. A **coracoclavicular ligament** secures the underside of the lateral clavicle to the top of the coracoid process. This wide ligament has two parts, a lateral portion called the **trapezoid ligament** and a medial portion called the **conoid ligament.**

The ligaments that stabilize the AC joint also maintain the integrity of the **coracoacromial (suprahumeral) arch**— a space formed by the **coracoacromial ligament** bridging the coracoid process and acromion process. This osteoligamentous arch, which is continuous with the subdeltoid space, provides a protective tunnel from compression traumas from above. Compression traumas can cause painful impingements to shoulder structures passing under the tunnel—the

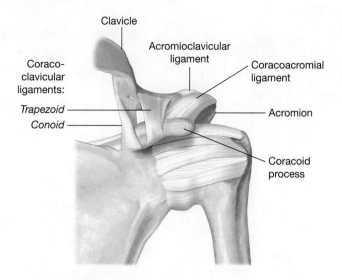

FIGURE 16.23

Acromioclavicular ligaments

subdeltoid bursa, the supraspinatus tendons, and the long tendon of the biceps brachii (Figure 16.24 ■). Such traumas are often caused by repetitive stress to the shoulder, such as carrying a heavy purse or carrying heavy equipment on the shoulder. Chronic elevation of the shoulders also decreases the space of the coracoacromial arch by half, predisposing a person to shoulder impingement.[3] Shoulder elevation requires lateral rotation in the lateral ends of the clavicles, which throws off the horizontal balance of the shoulder girdle and places mechanical stresses on all of its joints.

The most common injury that occurs at the AC joint is **shoulder separation.** People tend to separate the shoulder during impact accidents that thrust the shoulder into elevation, such as falling on an outstretched hand (sometimes called a *FOOSH injury*). This injury pulls the joint surfaces apart and can occur in varying degrees, depending on the direction of impact and the degree of separation (Figure 16.25 ■). The degree of tissue trauma in a shoulder separation is graded, ranging from a grade 1 minor ligamentous strain, to a grade

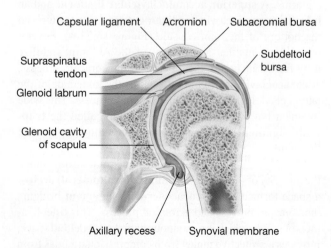

FIGURE 16.24

Coracoacromial arch: coronal section

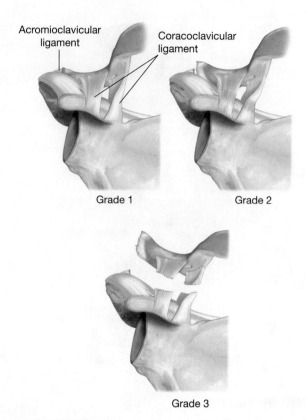

FIGURE 16.25

Shoulder separation

2 partial tear, to a grade 3 complete rupture of ligaments and separation of the AC joint surfaces. When the ligaments completely rupture and the joint surfaces totally disconnect, treatment for a shoulder separation requires surgery.

16.2.4 Sternoclavicular Joint

The **sternoclavicular** (SC) **joint** consists of the articulation of the medial end of the clavicle with the 1st rib and the manubrium (Figure 16.26 ■). Because the SC joint is the only bony articulation connecting the shoulder girdle to the axial skeleton, it needs to be stable and resilient. The SC joint has an articular disc between its saddle-shaped joint surfaces that protects the joint by absorbing impact and reducing friction during motion. The disc rides the articulating surfaces like a saddle between a rider and a horse. This small but important joint is stabilized by a **sternoclavicular ligament** covering the joint capsule and a two-headed **costoclavicular ligament** that connects the underside of the clavicle to the 1st rib.

The SC joint is a plane synovial joint that moves with two degrees of motion, one in the frontal plane and the other in the horizontal plane. Although its range of movement is limited, this small but complex joint allows us to shrug the shoulders up and down and to move the shoulders forward and back. Sometimes the SC joint is classified as a saddle joint due to its saddle-shaped articulations and its biaxial range of motion. It is mechanically linked to the AC and the scapulothoracic joints, so if it becomes injured or frozen, movement of the other two joints will also be restricted.

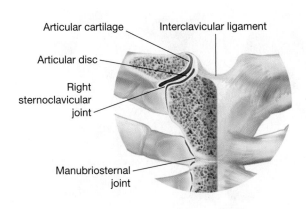

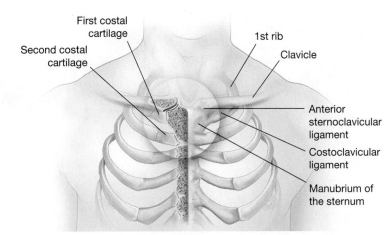

FIGURE 16.26

Sternoclavicular joint

BONE PALPATION

Acromioclavicular and Sternoclavicular Joints

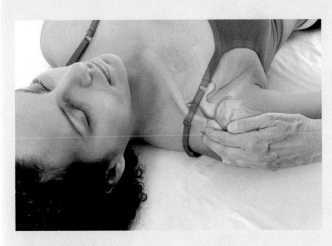

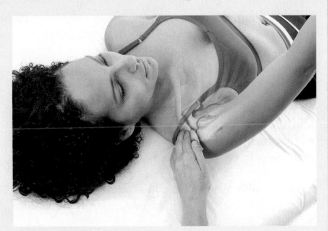

FIGURE 16.27a

To palpate the **acromioclavicular joint,** walk your fingertips laterally along the top of the clavicle out to the most lateral point of the shoulder. Look for the joint line between the clavicle and the acromion process, which will land you right on top of the AC joint. *Is the lateral end of the clavicle slightly higher than the acromion, which is normal?* (See Figure 16.27a ■)

FIGURE 16.27b

Once you have found the AC joint, hold your fingertips over the joint line (where the articulating bones meet), then palpate **AC joint motion** by slowly moving the arm. Keep in mind that as the AC moves in different planes, it continues to provide a horizontal stabilizing force to the shoulder, so there will be minimal movement at the joint. *Do you notice the small amount of AC joint motion?* (See Figure 16.27b ■)

(continued)

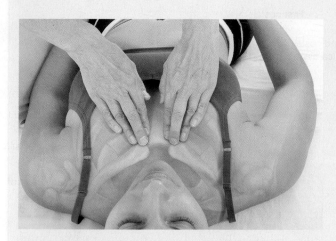

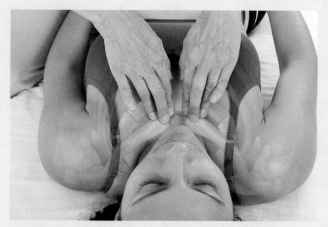

FIGURE 16.27c

The SC joint is a difficult joint to palpate because of its irregular shape. To palpate the **sternoclavicular joint,** walk your fingertips along the top of the clavicle toward the sternum. When you reach the end of the bone, locate the medial, inferior surface of the clavicle, touching the 1st rib and manubrium where they join the clavicle. Explore how these three bones fit together. *Are your SC joints symmetrical? If the SC joints are asymmetrical, which often occurs when one clavicle has been fractured, is one side sore to the touch?* (See Figure 16.27c ■)

FIGURE 16.27d

To palpate **SC joint motion,** continue to hold your fingertips over the joint as you shrug your shoulders to elevate and depress them. Then palpate the SC joints as you protract and retract your shoulders, and flex and hyperextend your arm. *Do you feel the medial end of the clavicle move with your shoulders? Does the SC joint pop or grind as is moves? Do the two sides move symmetrically? If not, what do you think creates the asymmetry, one-handed dominance, clavicular fractures, or muscular imbalances? How can you correct it?* (See Figure 16.27d ■)

In an optimal alignment, the clavicles rest in a horizontal neutral position. As the shoulders elevate, the clavicle externally rotates, twisting the SC joint. From neutral, each clavicle can be elevated to a range of 45 degrees and depressed 15 degrees. Postural aberrations in which a person holds the shoulders in an elevated position will unnaturally rotate the clavicles, putting stress on both the SC and AC joints.

16.2.5 Neutral Position of the Shoulder Girdle

Moving the shoulders toward a balanced position requires an understanding of the neutral position of the shoulder girdle. In an ideal neutral position, this bony girdle sits upon the thorax like a well-tailored suit drapes over a sturdy hanger. The clavicles align horizontally across the top of the thorax and the upper arms hang vertically along the sides of the trunk. And, as previously mentioned, the scapulae rest in the scapular plane, a vertical plane turned an average of 30 degrees diagonal to the frontal plane (Figure 16.28 ■).

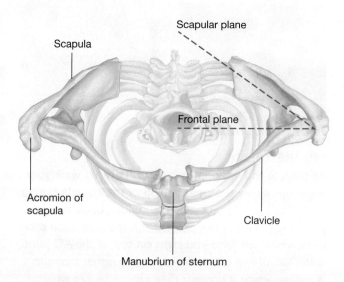

FIGURE 16.28
Scapular plane

Many people think the shoulder blades should lie flat and will unnaturally retract their shoulders in an attempt to get them to lie flat against a wall, which is unnatural and creates a muscular holding pattern.

The scapula does, however, have a neutral position called **scapula neutral.** Scapula neutral provides an important benchmark for the postural balance of the shoulder girdle and the upper half of the spine (Figure 16.29 ■). When the scapula is in neutral, it meets the following criteria:

- The medial border of the scapula runs parallel to the thoracic spine.
- The medial border of the scapula lays 5-6 centimeters lateral of the thoracic spine.
- The scapula rests flat against the thorax.
- The superior angle of the scapula is higher than the acromion and level with T-1.
- The medial spine of the scapula is level with T-3.
- The inferior angle of the scapula is level with T-7 or T-8.

Muscular forces provide the primary mechanism for securing a stable position of the shoulder and scapula neutral. The lower trapezius, which has a high percentage of slow fibers, anchors the scapula in an optimal neutral position. The arms move more efficiently when movement begins from a position of scapula neutral. Any shoulder muscle locked up in a chronic contraction will throw off the dynamic stability of the entire shoulder girdle. When a person has poor posture, the scapulae tend to rest in an off-neutral position, which is usually maintained by chronic muscular contractures. Such postural problems can be partially corrected by strengthening and stretching the shoulder muscles. Ultimately, though, a person needs to learn muscular control to maintain scapula neutral.

16.2.5.1 SCAPTION AND SHOULDER ABDUCTION

It is natural to abduct the arms in the plane of the scapula, called **scaption.**[4] This plane of scaption is determined by the direction the glenoid fossa faces, which

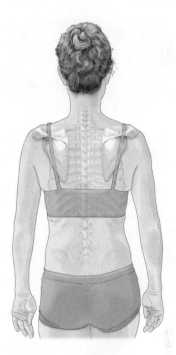

FIGURE 16.29
Benchmarks of scapula neutral

varies with individual bone structure. Raising the arm in the scapular plane is a more functional movement than raising the arm directly at the side of the body in the frontal plane.

True abduction of the arms is a complex movement requiring the following actions:

- The arms need to move in the scapular plane.
- The GH joint laterally rotates.
- The scapula upwardly rotates.
- The clavicle laterally rotates and elevates.

Abducting the arm in the frontal plane requires scapular retraction, which places more mechanical stress on the joint capsule and ligaments and can impinge space in the

EXPLORING TECHNIQUE

Assessing the Neutral Position of the Shoulder Girdle

Have your partner stand in a relaxed upright posture, then observe and trace the bony landmarks of the scapula to answer the following questions:

1. Are the clavicles horizontal? If not, are they depressed or elevated? How many degrees? Are the clavicles symmetrical?
2. Do the scapulae lie flat against the rib cage? If not, what part of each scapula is raised and to what degree is it raised?
3. Are the medial borders of the scapulae parallel to the spine? If not, guide your partner to move them so that they realign correctly.

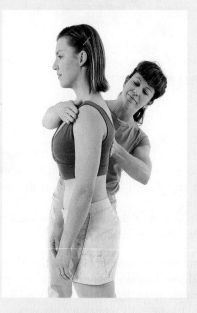

FIGURE 16.30a

4. Are the scapulae chronically protracted or retracted? When they protract, the shoulders round and the thoracic spine sinks into flexion. When they retract, the shoulder blades pinch together.

To help correct for any off-neutral position, move the scapulae toward the neutral position.

● **If the shoulders are retracted:** Encourage your partner to relax the rhomboid muscles and engage the serratus anterior.

● **If the shoulders are protracted:** With your partner standing, encourage your partner to lift the coracoid process slightly and lower the inferior angle of the scapula, which will engage the lower trapezius (Figure 16.30a ■).

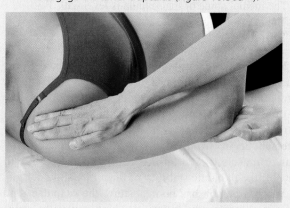

FIGURE 16.30b

● **With your partner lying supine:** Place one hand under the lower scapula and the other hand over the coracoid process and shift the scapula into a neutral position. Then drop the shoulder back by levering the head of the humerus back into the socket, gently pressing down on the proximal humerus while lifting the elbow (Figure 16.30b ■).

coracoacromial arch (Figure 16.31a-b ■). Laterally rotating the GH joint during abduction in the scapular plane drops the greater tubercle behind the acromion process so that the scapula does not elevate and hike the shoulder. In contrast, raising the arm without lateral rotation presses the greater tubercle into the acromion process, closing and impinging the subacromial space. To feel this difference, compare raising your arms right beside your body (as though you were moving them flat against a wall), then raising your arms slightly in front of your body (as though your hands were 2 feet away from the wall). Then contrast raising your arms to the side with your palms facing up (which laterally rotates the GH joint) and your palms facing down (which medially rotates the GH joint). Notice how the shoulder hikes when raising the arm with the palm down. Without lateral rotation, the head of the humerus fails to glide down in the socket (see Figure 3.19).

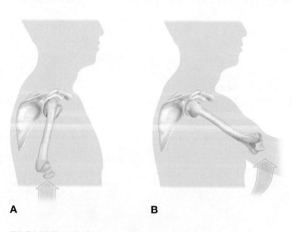

A   B

FIGURE 16.31

Abduction: a) In the frontal plane b) In the scapular plane

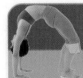

16.2.5.2 SCAPULOHUMERAL RHYTHM

The ratio of movement between the glenohumeral and scapulothoracic joints is called the **scapulohumeral rhythm.** In an ideal scapulohumeral rhythm, the scapula remains stable until 90 degrees of GH joint flexion or 60 degrees of GH joint abduction (Figure 16.32 ■). After this, the scapula moves with the humerus in approximately a 1-to-2 ratio. The ratio changes during the entire motion. By the time the GH joint has reached 180 degrees of abduction, the scapula will have upwardly rotated about 23 degrees.[5]

The scapulohumeral rhythm provides a good measure of stability in the shoulder girdle. If the scapula moves too early, it is unstable. Scapular instability reflects a lack of muscular control, which can lead to shoulder pain from postural holding and shoulder injuries from poorly coordinated movements. The scapula can also become unstable to counterbalance movement restrictions in the GH joint. In severe cases of GH immobility, a reverse scapulohumeral rhythm where the scapula moves before the GH joint can also occur. The rhythm reverses in conditions such as adhesive capsulitis, or "frozen shoulder" (Figure 16.33 ■).

Adhesive capsulitis is a condition of abnormal thickening of the joint capsule, which adheres to overlying ligaments and tendons around the shoulder. This condition restricts movement, inflames the shoulder, and causes pain during abduction and lateral rotation, making it difficult for people to brush their hair or raise their arm to put on a shirt. Adhesive capsulitis is more prevalent in women than men. The cause is unknown; it can occur after a shoulder injury or for no known reason and tends to have an emotional component. Without treatment, symptoms usually subside within 2 years.

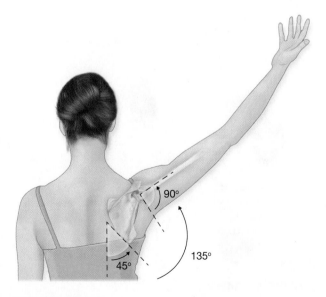

FIGURE 16.32
Scapulohumeral rhythm

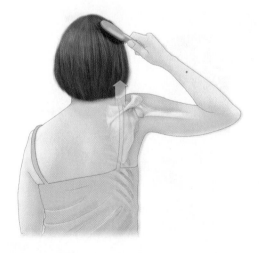

FIGURE 16.33
People with **frozen shoulder** will hike the shoulder to brush their hair.

BRIDGE TO PRACTICE
Working with Adhesive Capsulitis

Adhesive capsulitis is a frequently occurring condition that you may encounter in your practice. To treat it, you can apply trigger point therapy to the shoulder muscles that restrict motion, particularly the rotator cuff muscles; use cross-fiber friction across joint ligaments to loosen them; apply myofascial release on restricted tissues around the shoulder; then passively stretch the joint structures to restore motion. Since adhesive capsulitis usually involves movement dysfunction, you can also teach your client neuromuscular patterning exercises to improve the scapulohumeral rhythm, restoring efficient movement to the shoulders and arms.

SELF-CARE
Neuromuscular Patterning for the Scapulohumeral Rhythm

Moving your arms with an efficient scapulothoracic rhythm will reduce muscular tension and stress on your shoulders and upper spine, particularly while you give massage. Here is an exercise to improve your scapulohumeral rhythm. You will need a partner to do it.

1. **Arm flexion with a partner:** Begin standing with your arms hanging at your sides. Have your partner stand behind and rest his or her hands on your scapulae, one on each side (Figure 16.34a ■). Have your partner keep his or her hands on your scapulae and track when they begin to move while you slowly flex your arms (Figure 16.34b ■). Do the movement several times, raising and lowering your arms, and have your partner tell you at what degree of arm flexion your scapulae begin to slide. Your scapulae should remain relatively stable until 90 degrees of arm flexion, then they start to protract. *Do your scapulae move prematurely, before 90 degrees? It they do, how do they move? Do they retract, protract, elevate, depress, anteriorly tilt, or upwardly rotate?*

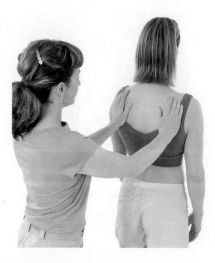

FIGURE 16.34a

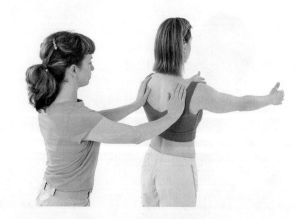

FIGURE 16.34b

2. **Arm abduction with a partner:** Have your partner track your scapulae as you slowly abduct your arms, raising them to the side of the body (Figure 16.34c ■). Make sure to move them in the plane of scaption, 30 degrees anterior to the frontal plane. The scapula should remain stable until 60 degrees of abduction, then they start to upwardly rotate, elevate, and slightly protract. *At what degree do your scapulae begin to move? How do the scapulae move? Do they retract, protract, elevate, depress, anteriorly tilt, or upwardly rotate?*

3. **Range of massage with a partner:** Move your arms in front of you as though you were giving a massage. Have your partner give you feedback about the position of your scapulae as you move. Focus on moving at the glenohumeral joint while keeping the scapulae stable but not rigid. Make sure not to retract your scapulae.

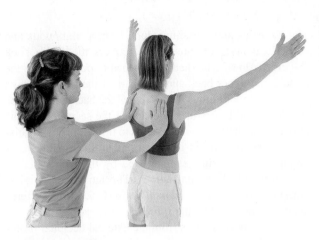

FIGURE 16.34c

16.3 MUSCLES OF THE SHOULDER GIRDLE

The muscles of the shoulder girdle work together in coordinated groups to move the shoulders and arms. Muscles encircle the shoulder like spokes on a wheel and can pull on the joint from many directions (Figure 16.35 ■). Opposing spokes work as coupled pairs; when one pulls down, the other pulls up. Coupled muscular pulls are akin to the reins on a harness; they keep the horse's head centered in the direction of movement and turn the horse with opposing pulls. Likewise, coupled pulls in the shoulder muscles keep the humerus centered in the socket as the arm moves. If a single muscle becomes chronically shortened or slack, this will disrupt the coordinated chain of action in the entire group of arms and shoulder muscles. For this reason, a practitioner needs to be able to identify and lengthen chronically shortened shoulder muscles and help a client contract chronically inhibited muscles in order to return the shoulder girdle to a balanced, neutral position.

The shoulder muscles presented in this section are organized by location and function, as follows:

- Extrinsic muscles of the posterior shoulder: *Trapezius, latissimus dorsi,* and *teres major*
- Rotator cuff muscles: *Supraspinatus, infraspinatus, subscapularis,* and *teres minor*
- Scapular muscles: *Rhomboid major* and *minor, serratus anterior,* and *levator scapula*
- Primary shoulder flexors and adductors: *Pectoralis major, pectoralis minor,* and *subclavius*
- Primary shoulder abductors: *Deltoid* and *coracobrachialis*

The biceps brachii and triceps brachii are biarticular muscles that cross both the shoulder and elbow. They work as primary elbow flexors and extensors, although they are both double-bellied muscles with a long head that assists shoulder flexion and extension. Since their actions at the elbow are of greater significance than their actions at the shoulder, the biceps brachii and triceps brachii will be covered in the arm and hand chapter.

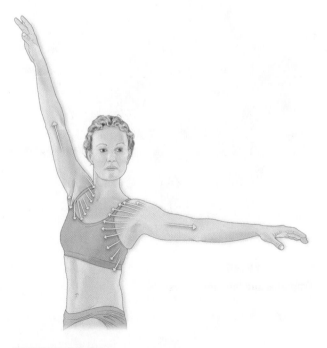

FIGURE 16.35
Tensional pulls of shoulder muscles

16.3.1 Trapezius, Latissimus Dorsi, and Teres Major

The trapezius and latissimus dorsi form a continuous and superficial layer of muscle that covers the entire back (Figure 16.36 ■). The diamond-shaped trapezius covers the middle and upper back and drapes over the shoulders like a shawl. The latissimus dorsi crosses the back between the shoulders and tapers in a V-shape at the sacrum. It is the only muscle that connects the arms to the sacrum. The latissimus dorsi is assisted in its actions by the smaller teres major. The trapezius is innervated by the *spinal accessory nerve* (11th cranial nerve). The latissimus dorsi is innervated by the *thoracodorsal nerve* (C-5, C-6). The teres major is innervated by the *subscapular nerve.*

The **trapezius** arises from the external occipital protuberance, the superior nuchal line and nuchal ligament, and the spinous process from C7 to T12. It inserts on the lateral third of the clavicle, the acromion process, and along the spine of the scapula. The trapezius divides into three functional segments. The upper fibers extend the neck in a bilateral contraction and laterally flex, rotate, or side-bend the neck and head in a unilateral contraction. The middle fibers stabilize and retract the scapula. The lower fibers have a large percentage of slow fibers that maintain scapula neutral and also depress and upwardly rotate the scapula. Postural problems

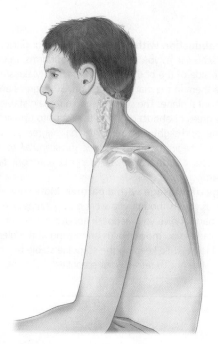

FIGURE 16.37

Trapezius imbalance in forward head posture

occur when the upper fibers become shortened and the lower fibers become overstretched, a common muscular pattern in the forward head posture (Figure 16.37 ■). (See TrPs for the trapezius in Figure 16.38 ■).

The **latissimus dorsi** is a flat, V-shaped muscle with horizontal fibers that arises from a broad origin along the spinous processes of the lower six thoracic vertebrae and the lumbar vertebrae, over the sacrum, on the posterior iliac crest, and along the bottom four ribs. This broad muscle covers most of the lower and middle back and

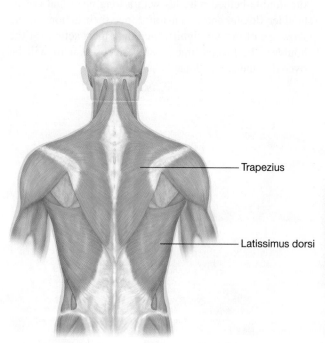

Trapezius

Latissimus dorsi

FIGURE 16.36

Trapezius and latissimus dorsi

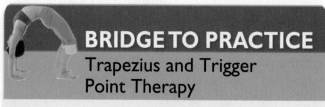

BRIDGE TO PRACTICE
Trapezius and Trigger Point Therapy

Trapezius TrPs often develop with simultaneous TrPs in the temporalis, masseter, splenius, semispinalis, levator scapula, and rhomboids. If you are working with a client who reports trapezius pain, you might want to check and treat these adjacent muscles for myofascial pain and TrPs in the same session.

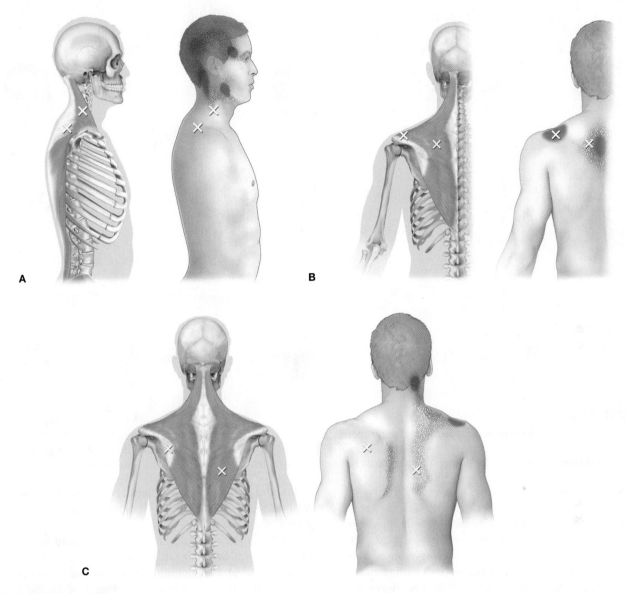

FIGURE 16.38

Many clients develop pain and dysfunction in the trapezius muscle from overuse or faulty postures such as forward head posture, hiking the shoulders, holding a phone to the ear with the shoulder, carrying a heavy purse, backpack, or briefcase on one shoulder, or grinding the teeth. When dysfunctional, the **trapezius** generates problems that many clients seek massage to alleviate, such as tension headaches, burning between the shoulder blades, a stiff or aching neck, and jaw pain. The trapezius can develop trigger points in seven different locations.

a) Dysfunction in the **upper trapezius** can result in two commonly found trigger points in the middle of its mostly vertical fibers, one slightly behind the other. These trigger points are a frequent source of tension headaches, dizziness, and vertigo (loss of balance). They can refer pain to the temples, the angle of the jaws, behind the ears, and an area from the base of the skull down the sides of the neck.

b) Dysfunction in the **middle trapezius** can lead to trigger points in two locations: one trigger point at the upper medial border of the scapula can cause a burning sensation and aching pain close to the upper thoracic spine; a second trigger point on the acromion process can refer aching pain over the lateral area of the shoulder.

c) Dysfunction in the **lower trapezius** can cause two trigger points: one often overlooked trigger point in the lower part of the trapezius medial to the inferior scapula can refer intense pain to the mastoid area of the occiput and aching spillover pain along the erector spinae in the thoracic area; a second trigger point below the medial part of the spine of the scapula can cause burning pain along the medial border of the scapula.

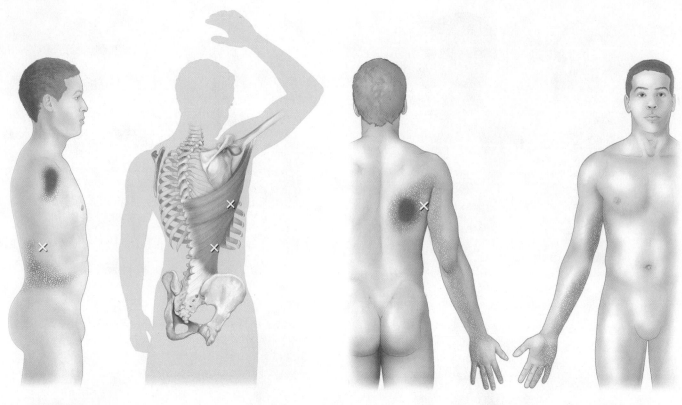

FIGURE 16.39

When dysfunctional, the **latissimus dorsi** can develop trigger points in two locations: one lateral to the inferior angle of the scapula and the other over the lower ribs that can refer constant aching pain in the midthoracic area, medial to the inferior angle of the scapula. Spillover pain from the latissimus dorsi trigger points can travel down the back of the arm into the fourth and fifth fingers.

tapers into a single insertion on the bicipital groove of the humerus, next to the teres major tendon. The latissimus dorsi is called the "swimmer's muscle" because of its powerful action in a downward stroke; it extends, adducts, and medially rotates the shoulder—movements we use in actions such as chopping wood or pulling an oar back when rowing. The latissimus dorsi also depresses

the shoulder girdle, which can indirectly affect the posture of the neck. (See TrPs for the latissumus dorsi in Figure 16.39 ■).

The **teres major** arises from the lower third of the posterior lateral border of the scapula and inserts on the medial lip of the bicipital groove of the humerus (see Figure 16.40 ■). It garnered the nickname of the "lat's

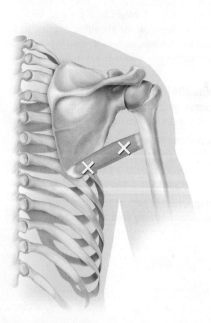

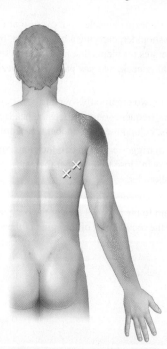

FIGURE 16.40

Dysfunction in the **teres major** can lead to three trigger points, one near its scapular tendon (which is on the anterior side of the humerus and is not shown in the figure) and two in the muscle belly, which can all refer pain over the posterior deltoid.

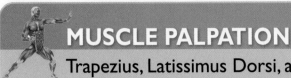

MUSCLE PALPATION
Trapezius, Latissimus Dorsi, and Teres Major

Locate the clavicular attachment of the trapezius by hooking the fingertips of your right hand over the left clavicle, in the middle of the bone. Then slide your fingertips sideways; the first pronounced muscular bump you encounter is the anterior border of the trapezius. To palpate the top of the trapezius, slide your fingertips from the scalenes backward into the superior edge of the trapezius. Elevate your shoulder to feel the trapezius contract. Follow the edge of the trapezius along the top of the shoulder up the side of the neck.

To contract the latissimus dorsi and teres major together, put one hand behind your sacrum as though you were being handcuffed. Then push down against the chair, which will contract both muscles. Palpate the lateral edge of the latissimus dorsi by reaching across the front of your body to the sides of your middle ribs. You should feel a muscular bulge along the edge of the latissimus.

Trapezius

O–External occipital protuberance, superior nuchal
   line, nuchal ligament, SPs of C7 to T12
I–Lateral third of clavicle, acromion process, and
   spine of scapula
A–Elevates, depresses, retracts, and upwardly rotates
   scapula; bilaterally extends head; unilaterally side-
   bends head and neck to same side; rotates head
   and neck to opposite side

Latissimus Dorsi

O–Spinous processes of T-7 to L-5, sacrum, posterior
   iliac crest, and bottom ribs
I–Medial lip of bicipital groove
A–Adducts, extends, and medially rotates shoulder;
   depresses shoulder girdle and retracts scapula

Teres Major

O–Lower third of posterior, lateral border of scapula
I–Medial lip of bicipital groove
A–Assists adduction, medial rotation, and extension
   of shoulder

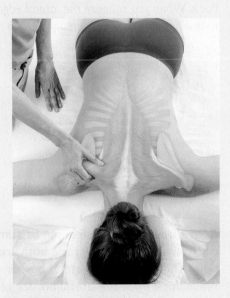

FIGURE 16.41a
Palpating the upper trapezius.

With your partner supine, palpate the upper **trapezius** along the top of the shoulder using a pincher palpation to lift it off of the underlying supraspinatus (Figure 16.41a ■). Locate the upper border of the trapezius by running your fingertips across the top of the shoulder along the side of the neck, from the front to the back. *Do you feel the distinct edge of the trapezius across the top of the shoulder?*

(continued)

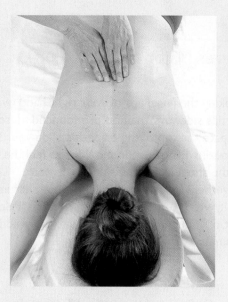

FIGURE 16.41b

Palpating the lower trapezius contraction

Active movement: With your partner prone, have your partner raise the arm over the head. Palpate the contraction of the **middle** and **lower trapezius** along the sides of the thoracic spine (Figure 16.41b ■). *Do you feel how the lower trapezius tapers into a prominent angle of tendinous tissue at T-12?*

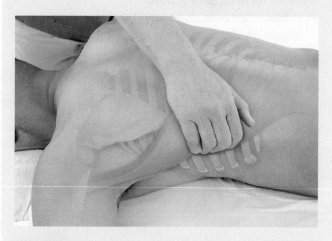

FIGURE 16.41c

Palpating the latissimus dorsi

With your partner prone, locate the lateral edge of the **latissimus dorsi** by sliding your fingertips along the sides of the ribs, from front to back (Figure 16.41c ■). Lift the edge of the latissimus with pincher palpation and slowly work your way down the lateral edge of the muscle toward the lower back. *When you squeeze the lateral edge of the latissimus dorsi, do you feel its meaty yet thin muscle fibers?*

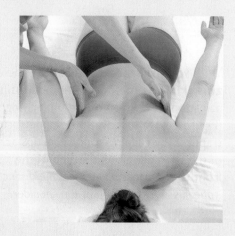

FIGURE 16.41d

Palpating the latissimus dorsi contraction

Active movement: To feel the latissimus dorsi contract, have your partner raise both arms behind the body. Then palpate the lateral border of the latissimus dorsi from the lateral border of the scapula to the medial aspect of the iliac crest (Figure 16.41d ■).

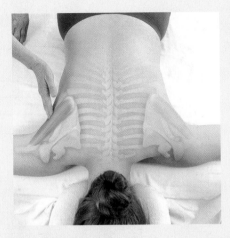

FIGURE 16.41e

Palpating the teres major

With your partner prone, locate the **teres major** by pressing along the dorsal side of the scapula, directly medial of the lateral border. Use a pincher palpation on the lower, lateral border of the scapula to grasp the teres major and latissimus dorsi together (Figure 16.41e ■).

Active movement: Palpate the teres major contraction by having your partner lift the hand toward the hips to medially rotate the shoulder.

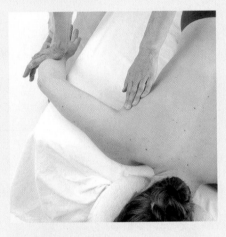

FIGURE 16.41f

Resisted movement of the teres major

Resisted movement: Differentiate the teres major from the teres minor by palpating them as they contract against resistance. To contract the teres major against resistance, have your partner lift his hand toward the hip to medially rotate the shoulder, then press against your resistance (Figure 16.41f ■).

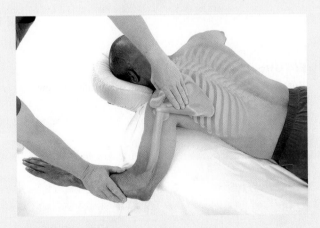

FIGURE 16.41g

Resisted movement of the teres minor

To contract the teres minor against resistance, have your partner lift his hand toward his head to laterally rotate the shoulder, then press against your resistance (Figure 16.41g ■). *Do you feel the teres major contract with medial rotation, as your partner lifts the hand toward the hips? Do you feel the teres minor contract with lateral rotation, as your partner lifts the hand toward the head?*

little helper" because it works with the latissimus dorsi in a wood-chopping action, assisting adduction, medial rotation, and extension of the arm from a flexed position.

16.3.2   The Rotator Cuff

The tendons of four muscles—the subscapularis, infraspinatus, supraspinatus, and teres minor—encircle the front, top, and back of the glenohumeral joint like a cuff, which is why they are called the **rotator cuff** muscles (Figure 16.42a-b ■). They work as a group to stabilize the head of the humerus in its shallow socket. The subscapularis, infraspinatus, and supraspinatus are innervated by the *subscapular nerve*. The teres minor is innervated by the *axillary nerve.* You can use the acronym "SITS" to remember the rotator cuff muscles, which is the first letter of each muscle in this group.

The origin of the **supraspinatus** fills the supraspinous fossa on the top of the shoulder, then tapers into a tendon that crosses laterally under the acromion process and inserts on top of the greater tubercle. This small horizontal muscle is always under load from the weight of the arm; its primary function is to prevent the downward displacement of the shoulder. It also abducts the arm and pulls the head of the humerus into its socket. (See TrPs for the supraspinatus in Figure 16.43 ■).

The **infraspinatus** arises from the infraspinous fossa of the scapula and inserts on the greater tubercle of the humerus. Like the subscapularis, the infraspinatus is also a fibrous multipennate muscle. It works with the teres minor to laterally rotate the shoulder and also stabilizes the humeral head in its socket. (See TrPs for the infraspinatus in Figure 16.44 ■).

The **teres minor** arises from the upper two-thirds of the lateral, posterior surface of the scapula and inserts on the greater tubercle below the infraspinatus tendon. Like the other rotator cuff muscles, the teres minor stabilizes the humeral head in the glenoid fossa. It works with the infraspinatus and the posterior part of the deltoid to laterally rotate the glenohumeral joint. (See TrP for the teres minor in Figure 16.45 ■).

The **subscapularis** is the most anterior of the rotator cuff muscles. It arises on the medial surface of the scapula, covering the subscapular fossa with it fibrous multipennate fascicles, and inserts on the lesser tubercle of the humerus. The subscapularis medially rotates and adducts the arm along with the teres major, and prevents the anterior displacement of the shoulder. During abduction, the subscapularis depresses the humeral head to counter the upward displacement of the shoulder by the deltoid. (See TrPs for the subscapularis in Figure 16.46 ■).

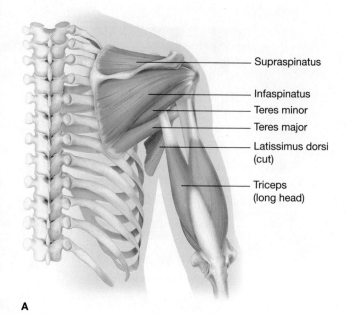

Supraspinatus
Infaspinatus
Teres minor
Teres major
Latissimus dorsi (cut)
Triceps (long head)

A

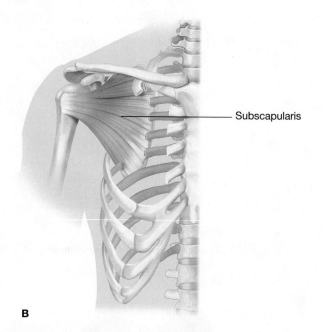

Subscapularis

B

FIGURE 16.42

Rotator cuff muscles: a) Posterior view b) Anterior view

FIGURE 16.43

When dysfunctional, the **supraspinatus** can develop two trigger points in its belly and a trigger point over its tendon, which can be palpated easily by pressing down on the top of the shoulder. Supraspinatus trigger points can cause a dull ache over the side of the shoulder, as well as restricted movement during daily activities that require arm elevation, such as brushing your hair or teeth.

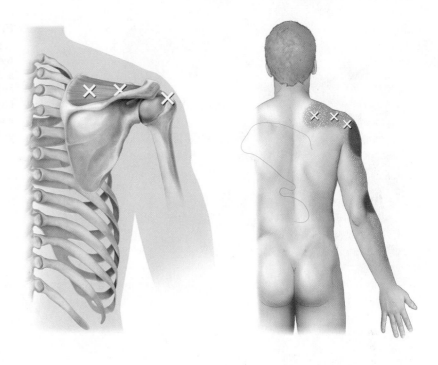

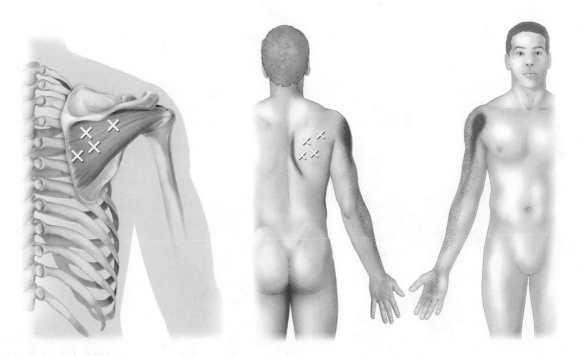

FIGURE 16.44

When dysfunctional, the **infraspinatus** develops trigger points in four locations scattered over the muscle belly, which can refer intense pain into the shoulder joint, down the biceps, and inside the medial border of the scapula. Infraspinatus trigger points can restrict medial rotation and adduction of the arm and make simple tasks like reaching back to scratch the middle of the back or sleeping on the side difficult.

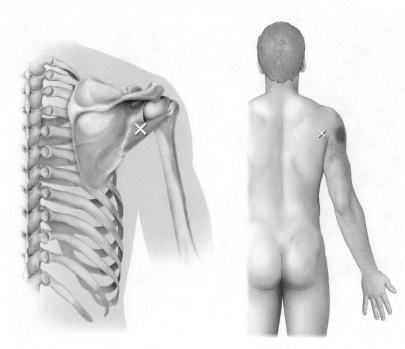

FIGURE 16.45

A trigger point can develop in the belly of the **teres minor** from overworking it with repetitive activities that involve reaching behind the body or overhead, such as painting a ceiling or pulling heavy luggage. This trigger point can refer pain locally and radiate down the lateral, posterior side of the arm.

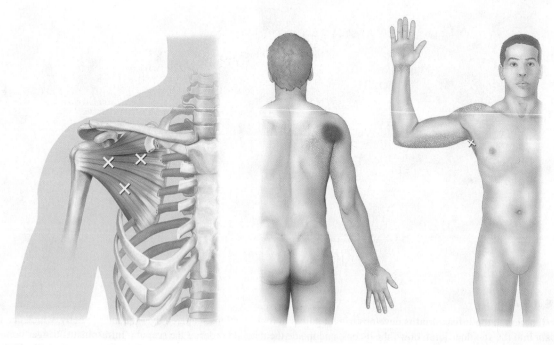

FIGURE 16.46

Trigger points in the **subscapularis** can cause severe pain both at rest and during movement, can restrict abduction, and often develop in cases of adhesive capsulitis. They can send referred pain over the posterior shoulder and triceps area, and sometimes in a strap-like ring around the wrist.

MUSCLE PALPATION

Rotator Cuff Muscles: Supraspinatus, Infraspinatus, Subscapularis, and Teres Minor

If you have short arms and lack flexibility, the rotator cuff muscles can be difficult to self-palpate. Locate your subscapularis by reaching your left hand across your body to the other armpit. Press your thumb or fingertips into the muscle belly on the anterior side of the scapula. Feel it contract by medially rotating your arm.

Locate the supraspinatus by reaching across your body and hooking your fingertips over the top of your shoulder above the spine of the scapula. Press down through the trapezius muscle into the fleshy belly of the supraspinatus.

To palpate the infraspinatus, press into the posterior side of your scapula. Press the muscle against the scapula. Move your fingertips across its fibrous muscle belly, which often has tender points or TrPs.

To palpate the teres minor, bend your elbow at a right angle and press into the muscle belly on the upper half of the lateral border of the scapula. Feel it contract by laterally rotating your arm.

Supraspinatus

O–Supraspinous fossa
I–Greater tubercle of humerus
A–Abducts GH joint, stabilizes head of humerus in glenoid fossa

Infraspinatus

O–Infraspinous fossa
I–Middle facet of greater tubercle of the humerus
A–Laterally rotates and adducts GH joint, stabilizes head of humerus in glenoid fossa

Subscapularis

O–Subscapular fossa
I–Lesser tubercle of humerus
A–Medially rotates GH joint, stabilizes head of humerus in glenoid fossa

Teres Minor

O–Upper two-thirds of lateral, posterior surface of scapula
I–Greater tubercle of humerus
A–Laterally rotates and adducts GH joint, stabilizes head of humerus in glenoid fossa

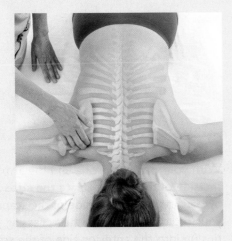

FIGURE 16.47a
Palpating the supraspinatus

With your partner prone, palpate the **supraspinatus** by pressing into the tissue in the supraspinous fossa, above the spine of the scapula (Figure 16.47a ■).

Active movement: To feel the supraspinatus contract, have your partner abduct the arm as you lightly press into the supraspinous fossa.

Resisted movement: Have your partner slowly abduct the arm against your resistance.

(continued)

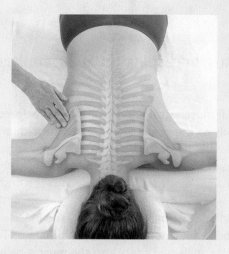

FIGURE 16.47b

Palpating the infraspinatus

With your partner prone, locate the **infraspinatus** by pressing straight into the infraspinous fossa, below the spine of the scapula (Figure 16.47b ■). *When palpating with a cross-fiber motion, do you feel the fibrous fascicles of the infraspinatus?*

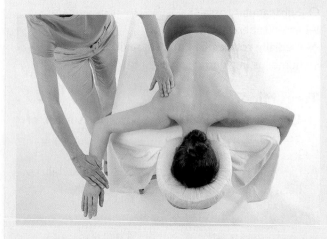

FIGURE 16.47c

Resisted movement of the infraspinatus

Active movement: To feel the infraspinatus contract, have your partner laterally rotate the shoulder by raising the hand toward the head.

Resisted movement: Have your partner press his or her palm against your resistance to laterally rotate the shoulder and contract the infraspinatus (Figure 16.47c ■).

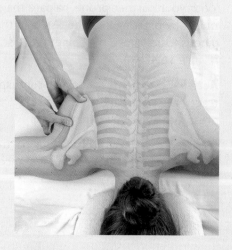

FIGURE 16.47d

Palpating the subscapularis

With your partner prone and the arm hanging off the side of the table, palpate the **subscapularis** by grasping the lateral side of the scapula between your thumb and fingers, then pressing your fingertips up into the anterior side of the scapula (Figure 16.47d ■). Use broad, firm pressure because this area can be ticklish. *Are you medial to the teres minor and teres major muscles?*

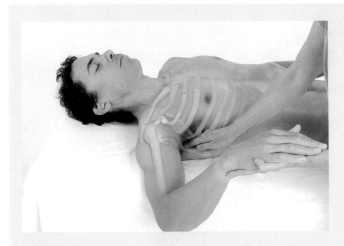

FIGURE 16.47e

Resisted movement of subscapularis

Active movement: To feel the subscapularis contract with your partner prone, have your partner medially rotate the shoulder by raising the hand toward the hip.

Resisted movement: With your partner supine, have your partner press his or her hand lightly against your resistance to medially rotate the shoulder (Figure 16.47e ■).

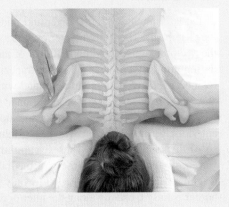

FIGURE 16.47f

Palpating the teres minor

With your partner prone, palpate the **teres minor** by pressing into the meaty tissue along the upper, lateral border of the scapula (Figure 16.47f ■).

Active movement: To feel the teres minor contract, have your partner raise the hand toward the head as you palpate it.

Resisted movement: Have your partner press against your resistance to laterally rotate the shoulder (see Figure 16.47c).

16.3.3 Rhomboids, Serratus Anterior, and Levator Scapula

The rhomboids (major and minor), serratus anterior, and levator scapula muscles attach to the three sides of the scapula (Figure 16.48 ■). They work synergistically, rotating the scapula in a manner similar to a group of children pulling a merry-go-round in a circle from different sides (Figure 16.49 ■). The opposing pulls of the serratus anterior and rhomboid muscles keep the scapula centered between excessive protraction and excessive retraction. All three muscles lie under the trapezius. The levator scapula is innervated by the *cervical nerve,* the rhomboids by the *dorsal scapular nerve,* and the serratus anterior by the *long thoracic nerve.*

The **rhomboid major** and **rhomboid minor** are parallelogram-shaped muscles with diagonal fibers that arise from the spinous processes of C-7 to T-5 and insert on the anterior side of the medial border of the scapula. Although these two muscles differ in structure, they are inseparable in function and work together to retract the scapula. (See TrPs for the rhomboids in Figure 16.50 ■).

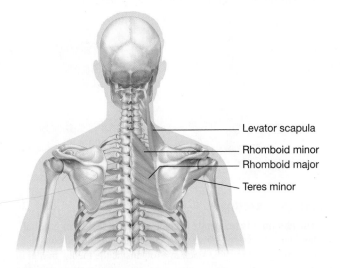

Levator scapula
Rhomboid minor
Rhomboid major
Teres minor

FIGURE 16.48

Rhomboids and levator scapula

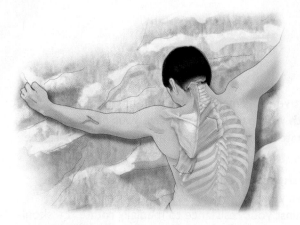

FIGURE 16.49
Coupled pulls of muscles turning the scapula

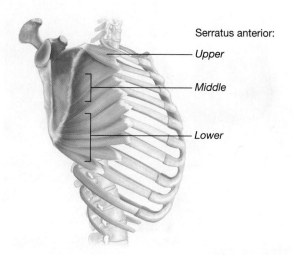

FIGURE 16.51
Serratus anterior

The **serratus anterior** is called the "finger muscle" when it is well developed because its serrated fascicles look like fingers grasping the ribs under the armpit along the side of the body. The serratus anterior has three parts: the superior, middle, and inferior sections (Figure 16.51 ■). The *superior section* is the smallest and most difficult to palpate; it has two short muscle slips that run from the superior angle of the scapula to the first and second ribs. The *middle section* is the largest; it has two broad fascicles oriented at a 45-degree angle that arise from half the length of the 2nd and 3rd ribs and insert along the entire vertebral border of the scapula. The *inferior section* is the strongest; it has about six fascicles arranged like a fan, with fingers that converge on an insertion site on the inferior angle of the scapula. It fans out in a quarter-circle to attachment sites along ribs 4–9.

Due to its multiple attachment sites, the serratus anterior has a complex movement role. It protracts the scapula against its antagonists, the rhomboids, which retract the scapula (Figure 16.52 ■). The serratus anterior also works as a stabilizer to hold the scapula flat against the thorax and begins to fire only after the arm is lifted to 30 degrees. Its horizontal line of pull on the scapula is countered by the horizontal fibers

of the latissimus dorsi, the lower and middle trapezius, and the rhomboids. The serratus anterior works as a synergist with the pectoralis minor and upper fibers of the pectoralis major during arm flexion, with the upper trapezius during upward rotation of the glenohumeral joint, and with the upper trapezius and levator scapula during elevation of the scapula. When the scapula is fixed, it also assists respiration by elevating the anterior ribs on inhalation. Weakness, inhibition, or paralysis of the serratus anterior causes **scapular winging.** In *true winging* of the scapula, the entire medial border is raised (Figure 16.53 ■). In *pseudo-winging,* only part of the medial border is raised, usually along the inferior half of the scapula. (See TrPs for the serratus anterior in Figure 16.54 ■).

The **levator scapula** arises from the medial border of the scapula above the spine of the scapula and inserts on the transverse processes of the first four cervical vertebrae. It elevates and upwardly rotates the scapula, and assists neck rotation to the same side and neck extension. (See TrPs for the levator scapula in Figure 16.55 ■).

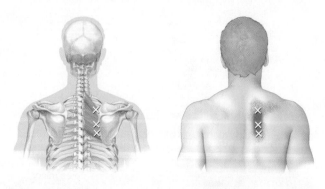

FIGURE 16.50

The **rhomboids** frequently become dysfunctional from postural holding patterns or overworking and develop taut bands with three trigger points that stack in a row inside the medial border of the scapula. Rhomboid trigger points can generate deep, aching pain in between the shoulder blades that can wake a person up at night and create crunching noises during scapular motion.

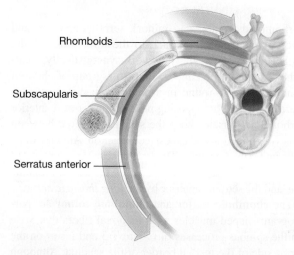

FIGURE 16.52

Agonist/antagonist relationships of serratus anterior and rhomboid

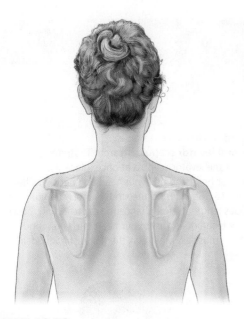

FIGURE 16.53

True winging of the scapulae

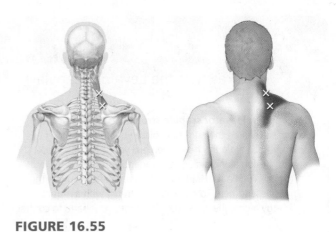

FIGURE 16.55

The **levator scapula** tends to develop trigger points in two locations along its belly that can refer intense pain locally and diffuse pain inside the medial border of the scapula and over the posterior shoulder. This muscle is usually involved in cases of neck or shoulder pain and is often the cause of a stiff neck.

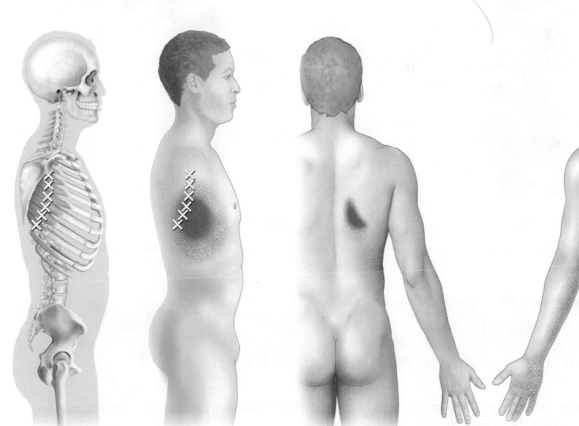

FIGURE 16.54

When dysfunctional, the **serratus anterior** can develop trigger points in each of the serrated segments, which can generate local pain, refer pain down the arm into the palm and ring finger, and contribute to abnormal breast sensitivity. Trigger points in the serratus anterior can also restrict expansion of the lower rib cage during respiration, causing an overuse of accessory breathing muscles such as the scalenes and SCM, and can cause the lower rib cage to become adhered to the subscapularis. In a barrel-chested posture, the serratus anterior tends to become overstretched. It is also vulnerable to torsion stress from situations such as gripping a steering wheel during an accident and having to turn it very fast. Women often develop fibrous buildup in the serratus anterior under the area an elastic bra strap goes around, which can be highly sensitive to palpation.

SELF-CARE
Stretching the Levator Scapula

1. **Unilateral levator scapula stretch:** To stretch the levator scapula on the right side, place your left hand over your head from the front, then pull your head and neck into flexion along a diagonal plane toward your left hip (Figure 16.56a ■). Hold the stretch until after you feel the muscle lengthen. To enhance the stretch with a muscle energy technique, press your head into your hand to contract the muscle, then relax it and stretch it again. When you are finished, stretch the other side.

2. **Bilateral levator scapula stretch:** To stretch both sides of the levator scapula at once, place your hands over your head and pull your head and neck into flexion (Figure 16.56b ■). Hold the stretch until after you feel the muscles lengthen. To enhance the stretch using muscle energy techniques, press your head into your hands to contract the muscles, then relax them and stretch again.

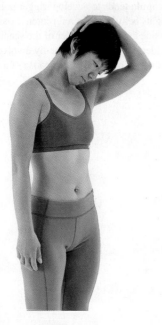

FIGURE 16.56a

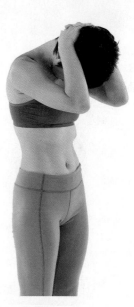

FIGURE 16.56b

MUSCLE PALPATION
Rhomboids, Serratus Anterior, and Levator Scapula

The rhomboids are difficult to self-palpate because of their location. To locate your serratus anterior, palpate the muscular slips over the sides of the ribs, under your armpit. To feel the levator scapula, reach one hand over your other shoulder to the superior angle of your scapula, then strum across the large bump of muscle fibers attached here. Raise and lower your shoulder to feel it contract and relax.

Rhomboid Minor and Major

O–Minor on spinous processes of C-7–T-1, major on SPs of T-2–T-5
I–Medial border of scapula
A–Retracts and downwardly rotates scapula

Serratus Anterior

O–Lateral surfaces of ribs 1–9
I–Anterior side of superior angle, medial border, and inferior angle of scapula

A–Protracts and stabilizes scapula, assists GH joint flexion and adduction, assists upward scapular rotation, lower fibers depress scapula, upper fibers elevate scapula

Levator Scapula

O–Transverse processes of C-1 to C-4
I–Superior angle of scapula (medial aspect)
A–Elevates scapula when neck is fixed, side-bends neck when scapula is fixed

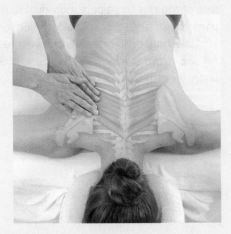

FIGURE 16.57a

Palpating the rhomboids

With your partner prone, locate the **rhomboids** using a broad, flat strumming palpation between the medial border of the scapula and the C-7 to T-5 vertebrae (Figure 16.57a ▪). *Can you feel the distinct muscular edge on the inferior border of the rhomboid major, lateral to T-5? Can you feel the distinct muscular strap of the rhomboid minor lateral to the C-7, T-1, and T-2 vertebrae? Do you feel taut bands in the rhomboids?*

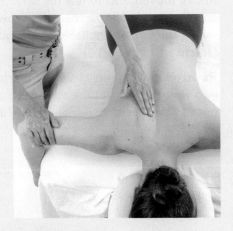

FIGURE 16.57b

Resisted movement of the rhomboids

Active movement: Have your partner retract the scapula and pull it toward the spine while you palpate the rhomboids.

Resisted movement: Have your partner gently push his or her elbow up against your hand to get the rhomboids to contract against resistance (Figure 16.57b ▪).

(continued)

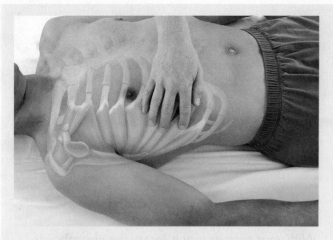

FIGURE 16.57c

Palpating the serratus anterior

With your partner supine, use a flat, broad palpation to locate the **serratus anterior** along the side of the ribs anterior to the scapula (Figure 16.57c ■). Because this area can be ticklish, press slowly and firmly along the side of the ribs to palpate individual muscle slips. If your partner has large breasts, palpate her serratus anterior in a side-lying position, which allows the breast tissue to fall away from the muscle. *Are you palpating over the ribs under the armpit?*

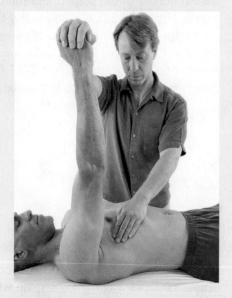

FIGURE 16.57d

Resisted movement of the serratus anterior

Active movement: To feel the serratus anterior contract, have your partner reach toward the ceiling, raising the arm off the table while you palpate the muscle.

Resisted movement: Have your partner push a fist into your hand to get the serratus anterior to contract against resistance (Figure 16.57d ■).

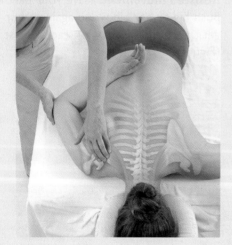

FIGURE 16.57e

Palpating the levator scapula

With your partner prone, place his or her arm behind the back to raise the medial border of the scapula, then locate the **levator scapula** using a cross-fiber strumming medial to and slightly above the superior angle of the scapula (Figure 16.57e ■). *Does the levator scapula feel like a thick, ropey strap as you move across the distal end of the muscle?*

Active movement: To palpate the levator scapula as it contracts, have your partner elevate the scapula toward the neck while you press into the muscle belly.

EXPLORING TECHNIQUE
Treating the Levator Scapula

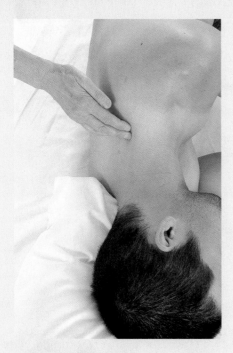

FIGURE 16.58a

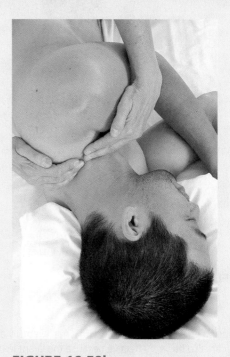

FIGURE 16.58b

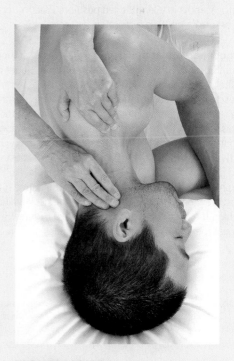

FIGURE 16.58c

Because the levator scapula is frequently the source of shoulder and neck pain, you will want to have effective techniques to work with it. Releasing tension in the levator scapula can be difficult; therefore, you may want to use a combination of techniques, such as the ones offered here.

1. **Trigger point therapy:** With your client in a side-lying position (the prone or supine positions will also work), locate any painful or tender points in the levator scapula (Figure 16.58a ■). Apply pressure on these points until your client reports that the pain has released.
2. **Muscle energy technique:** Have your client lightly press his or her shoulder up against your resistance to contract the levator scapula (Figure 16.58b ■).
3. Have your client relax then stretch the muscles by pulling the shoulder down while applying linear stripping along the belly of the muscle (Figure 16.58c ■). Repeat the entire routine on the other side.

(continued)

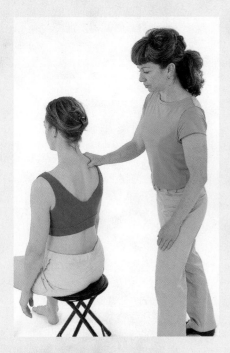

FIGURE 16.58d

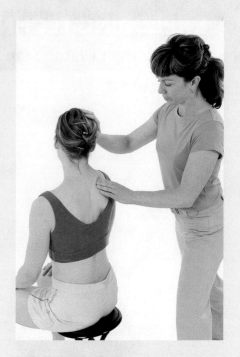

FIGURE 16.58e

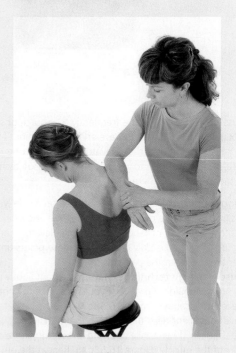

FIGURE 16.58f

Releasing the levator scapula with your client in a seated position can also be very effective because the client learns how to actively stretch it, and how to sense the posture that places the levator scapula in a lengthened position. Practice this with a partner before using it on a client.

4. **Trigger point therapy:** Have your client sit in an upright, neutral posture. Then find and release active trigger points in the levator scapula (Figure 16.58d ■).

5. **Muscle energy technique:** Have your partner contract the levator scapula by lightly pressing the back of the head and shoulder toward each other against your resistance (Figure 16.58e ■). Hold for several seconds.

6. **Active assisted pin and stretch:** Release the resistance and have your partner relax the levator scapula. Pin the origin of the muscle. Then have your partner stretch the muscle away from its origin by flexing the neck while also turning the head toward the opposite hip (Figure 16.58f ■). Repeat the entire routine on the other side.

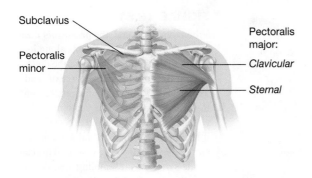

FIGURE 16.59

Pectoralis major, pectoralis minor, and subclavius

16.3.4 Pectoralis Major, Pectoralis Minor, and Subclavius

An anterior group of shoulder muscles—the pectoralis major, subclavius, and pectoralis minor—connect the scapula and humerus to the chest (Figure 16.59 ■). Chronic contractions in this muscle group contribute to faulty postures that stoop and round the shoulders and pull the head forward, disturbing the alignment of the whole shoulder girdle and upper body. Both the pectoralis major and pectoralis minor are innervated by the *pectoral nerve*. The subclavius is innervated by the *C-5 spinal nerve*.

The **pectoralis major** is a complex muscle with three sections that overlap in a fan-like arrangement. A clavicular head of the pectoralis major arises along the medial half of the clavicle, a sternal head arises from the sternum and the costal cartilages of ribs 2–7, and an abdominal head arises along the aponeurosis of the external oblique and the medial portion of the costal arch. All three heads insert along the lateral lip of the bicipital groove of the humerus. The pectoralis major covers the chest like a breastplate and is active in pushing activities. When the rib cage is fixed, it can flex, medially rotate, and horizontally adduct the humerus. The upper fibers of the pectoralis major depress the shoulder, the lower fibers assist forced exhalation, and all of the fibers protract the shoulders. (See TrPs for the pectoralis major in Figure 16.60 ■).

The **pectoralis minor** is a flat, triangular-shaped muscle that lies deep to the pectoralis major. Its three fascicles arise from the anterior surfaces of the 3rd, 4th, and 5th ribs and insert on the coracoid process of the scapula. This small muscle elevates the upper ribs if the scapula is in a stable, neutral position. If the upper ribs are depressed, it will draw the scapula forward and down, contributing to a rounded-shoulder posture. (See TrPs for the pectoralis minor in Figure 16.61 ■).

A small, triangular muscle called the **subclavius** connects the inferior surface of the middle clavicle to the medial aspect of the 1st rib. It stabilizes the sternoclavicular joint and prevents the upward displacement of the medial clavicle, although it also depresses the clavicle. To palpate this deep, fleshy muscle, sink the fingertips through the overlying clavicular fibers of the pectoralis major, which completely overlay the subclavius. (See TrP for subclavius in Figure 16.62 ■).

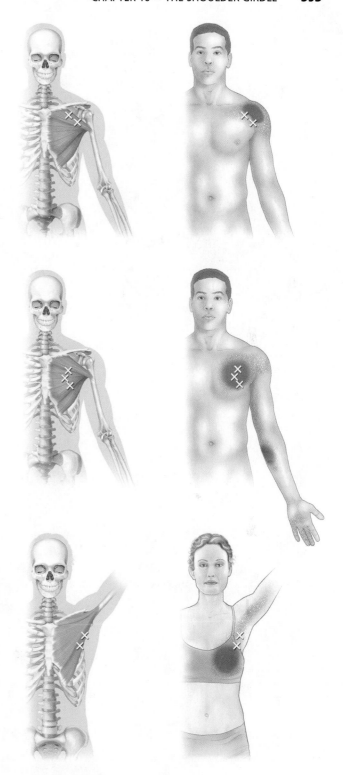

FIGURE 16.60

When dysfunctional, the **pectoralis major** can develop trigger points in seven locations: two trigger points in the clavicular head that can refer pain over the shoulder; three trigger points stacked along the lateral side of the chest that can refer pain to the middle of the anterior chest and the upper, anterior ulnar side of the forearm; and two trigger points in the lateral third of the abdominal head that can refer pain over the lower part of the anterior chest. Pain from pectoralis major trigger points often resembles and can be mistaken for heart diseases like myocardial infarction. These trigger points also cause aching pain between the scapulae.

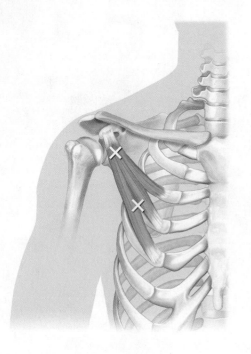

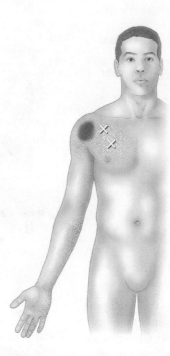

FIGURE 16.61

When dysfunctional, the **pectoralis minor** can develop two trigger points along its length that can refer pain over the deltoid region. Because the brachial plexus and axillary artery supplying the arm run under the bridge formed by the pectoralis minor attachment to the coracoid process, when it becomes taut, the pectoralis minor can entrap these underlying vessels. This can create symptoms resembling angina (chest pain due to lack of blood to the heart), causing intense pain on the anterior chest and down the ulnar side of the arm.

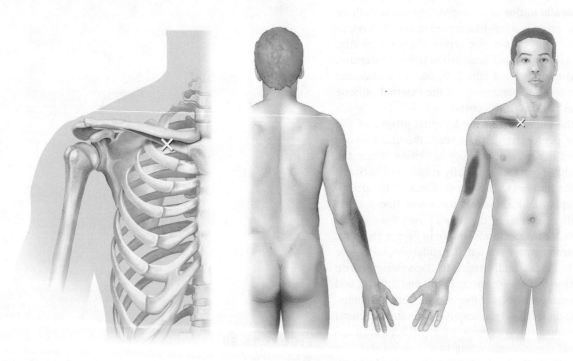

FIGURE 16.62

When dysfunctional, the **subclavius** can develop a trigger point along its medial end that can refer pain across its belly, down the biceps, over the ulnar side of the forearm, and into the thumb and first two fingers.

MUSCLE PALPATION
Pectoralis Major, Pectoralis Minor, and Subclavius

To self-palpate the pectoralis major as it contracts, press into the anterior, lateral side of your chest while adducting the arm on that side across the front of your chest.

Palpate the pectoralis minor using a cross-fiber strumming below and slightly medial to the coracoid process. Then press along its belly to feel its flat, somewhat ropy fibers.

The subclavius is difficult to palpate directly. Approximate its location by pressing up under the middle of your clavicle, through the thick and meaty muscle fibers of the upper pectoralis major into the underlying subclavius.

Pectoralis Major

O–Clavicular head–Medial half of clavicle
   Sternal head–Sternum and cartilage of ribs 2–7
   Abdominal head–Aponeurosis of external oblique
   and medial portion of costal arch
I–Lateral lip of bicipital groove
A–Adducts and medially rotates glenohumeral (GH) joint; clavicular head flexes GH joint; sternal head extends GH joint, assists elevation of thorax when shoulder is fixed

Pectoralis Minor

O–Anterior surfaces of 3rd, 4th, and 5th ribs
I–Coracoid process of scapula
A–Elevates upper ribs when scapula is fixed, tilts scapula when ribs are depressed

Subclavius

O–Inferior surface of middle clavicle
I–Medial aspect of 1st rib
A–Stabilizes sternoclavicular joint, depresses clavicle

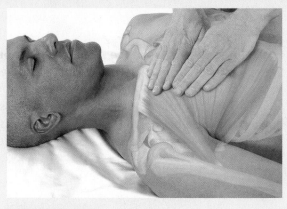

FIGURE 16.63a
Palpating the pectoralis major

Locate the **pectoralis major** using a flat, circular touch across the upper ribs, over the ribs along the medial side of the sternum, and above the medial side of the costal arch (Figure 16.63a ■). Follow its superior fibers across the top of the chest to its broad insertion on the bicipital groove of the humerus.

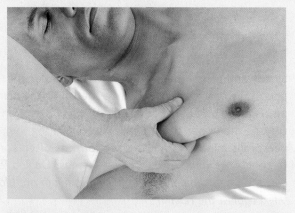

FIGURE 16.63b
Pincher palpation of the pectoralis major

Palpate the pectoralis major with a pincher palpation by grasping it under the anterior armpit (Figure 16.63b ■). *Do you feel how thick the horizontal fibers of the pectoralis major are where they cross the front of the armpit?*

(continued)

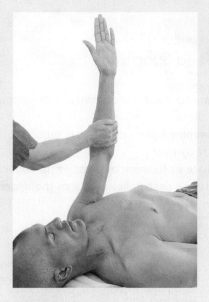

FIGURE 16.63c

Resisted movement of the pectoralis major

Active movement: Feel the pectoralis major contract by having your partner raise the arm toward the ceiling and moving it across the body.

Resisted movement: Have your partner raise his or her arm toward the ceiling, then resist as you press the humerus laterally to contract the pectoralis major (Figure 16.63c ■).

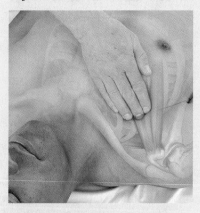

FIGURE 16.63d

Palpating the pectoralis minor

Locate the upper fibers of the **pectoralis minor** with cross-fiber strumming below and slightly medial to the coracoid process (Figure 16.63d ■). Run your fingers diagonally from the coracoid process down the muscle belly along the upper ribs, pressing through the overlying pectoralis major against the pectoralis minor.

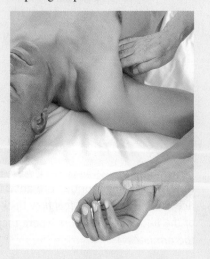

FIGURE 16.63e

Palpating the pectoralis minor from the side

Slowly and gently press your fingertips under the pectoralis major, against the ribs medial to the armpit (Figure 16.63e ■). Press in an upward direction toward the upper three ribs. When palpating the pectoralis minor from this direction, it is often sore to touch. *Are you pressing against the ribs? Do you feel how the diagonal fibers of the pectoralis minor are plastered against the ribs?*

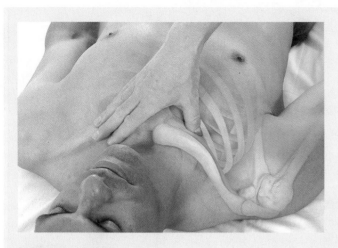

FIGURE 16.63f

Palpating the subclavius

Locate the **subclavius** by pressing your thumb up under the middle of the clavicle (Figure 16.63f ■). You will need to press through the upper pectoralis major fibers to feel the meaty fibers of the subclavius, which is often tender. *Do you feel the small mound of subclavius fibers under the clavicle?*

SELF-CARE

Stretching the Pectoralis Muscles

As you practice these stretches, make sure to maintain a neutral spinal alignment by lightly contracting your lower abdominal muscles and keeping your lower back and neck long.

1. **Pectoralis wall stretch:** Stand sideways to a wall. Externally rotate the shoulder closest to the wall and place that hand flat on the wall behind you (Figure 16.64a ■). You should feel a stretch in your chest.

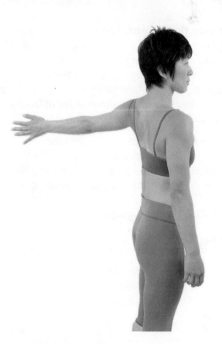

FIGURE 16.64a

(continued)

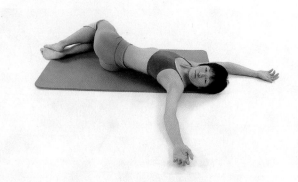

FIGURE 16.64c

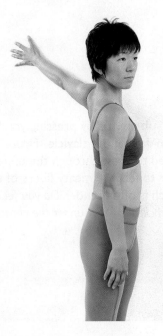

FIGURE 16.64b

2. Look for the position of stretch by moving your arm to different heights against the wall. It can be at shoulder height, hip height, or above you on a back diagonal (Figure 16.64b ■). By varying your hand position, you stretch different parts of the pectoralis muscles and different shoulder muscles, such as the anterior deltoid and biceps brachii. If you still do not feel a stretch, turn your body to face away from the wall until you do. Repeat on the other side.

3. **Pectoralis floor stretch:** Lie on the floor in a side-lying position. Raise your top arm above you, then slowly lower it behind you with your palm facing the ceiling. You can keep your trunk in a side-lying position or twist your trunk to turn your chest to face the ceiling. Look for the position of stretch by moving your arm to different locations behind you (Figure 16.64c ■).

4. Enhance the stretch by crossing your lower leg across your body (Figure 16.64d ■). Make sure to contract your abdominal muscles and keep your lumbar spine lengthened in order to avoid arching and straining your lumbar spine.

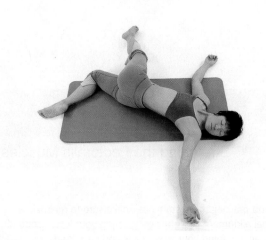

FIGURE 16.64d

Deltoid   Coracobrachialis

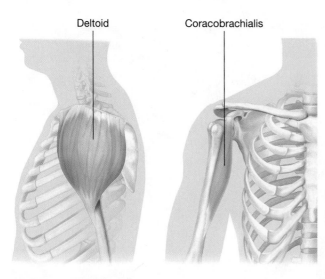

FIGURE 16.65
Deltoid and coracobrachialis

16.3.5   Deltoid and Coracobrachialis

The deltoid is a thick, fleshy muscle that caps the entire shoulder (Figure 16.65 ■). A smaller coracobrachialis muscle runs along the anterior side of the deltoid. Both muscles work together as the primary abductors of the shoulder and can be easily palpated on top of the shoulder. The deltoid is innervated by the *axillary nerve* and the coracobrachialis is innervated by the *musculocutaneous nerve.*

The superficial **deltoid** is a fibrous, multipennate muscle with three sections. The anterior section arises from the lateral third of the clavicle; a medial section arises from the lateral edge of the acromion process; and a posterior section arises from the lateral half of the spine of the scapula. All three sections of the deltoid converge into a broad insertion site on the deltoid tuberosity of the humerus. Each part of the deltoid performs a different function. The anterior deltoid works as an antagonist to the posterior deltoid and vice versa. The anterior deltoid horizontally adducts and flexes the arm, the medial deltoid works as a synergist with the supraspinatus to abduct the shoulder, and the posterior deltoid extends and laterally rotates the arm. The middle fibers of the deltoid draw the head of the humerus into the socket and prevent downward dislocation. The deltoid is a frequent source of myofascial pain from overuse in sports activities requiring arm abduction or from repetitive strain in activities that require prolonged lifting such as cutting hair or sorting mail (Figure 16.66 ■).

The **coracobrachialis** is a small, thin muscle that runs from the coracoid process to the anteromedial shaft of the humerus beside the short head of the biceps brachii. It forms the lateral, anterior border of the armpit and works as a synergist to the anterior deltoid and biceps brachii, assisting shoulder flexion and adduction. The coracobrachialis also helps to draw the head of the humerus into its socket. (See TrP for the coracobrachialis in Figure 16.67 ■).

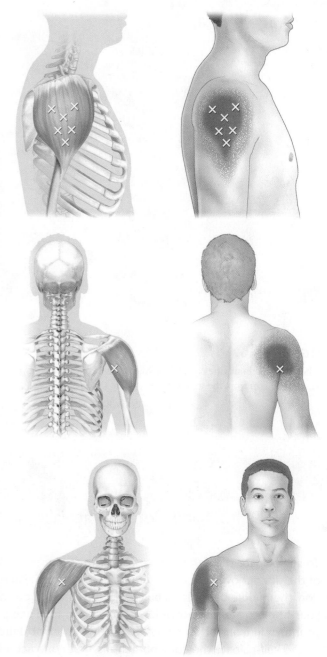

FIGURE 16.66

When dysfunctional, the **deltoid** can develop multiple trigger points throughout its many fibers, which can generate achy pain in the area around the trigger point and restrict shoulder movement. Clients usually describe movement restrictions caused by deltoid trigger points as a "catch in the shoulder" when they attempt to raise the arm.

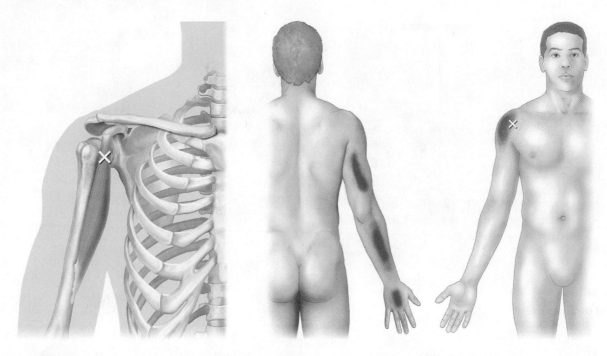

FIGURE 16.67

When dysfunctional, the **coracobrachialis** can develop a trigger point in the center of its belly, which can refer pain in a line down the back of the arm from the triceps to the middle finger.

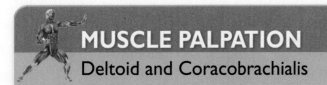

MUSCLE PALPATION
Deltoid and Coracobrachialis

To self-palpate the deltoid, raise your arm to the side, which will contract the deltoid. Explore the fleshy fibers of the deltoid over the glenohumeral joint, from the acromion process to the deltoid tuberosity. In this position, the middle deltoid will bulge. Place your hand on the back of the GH joint and move your arm behind your body to feel the posterior deltoid contract. Then place your hand on the front of the GH joint and move your arm in front of your body to feel the anterior deltoid contract.

To self-palpate the coracobrachialis, first contract it by abducting your arm to shoulder height and extending your elbow to relax the biceps tendon. Use a cross-fiber strumming under the anterior border of the armpit, below the anterior deltoid, to locate the slim muscle belly of the coracobrachialis. Adduct your arm to feel it contract and abduct your arm to feel it relax.

Deltoid
O–Lateral third of clavicle, lateral edge of acromion
   process, lateral half of scapular spine
I–Deltoid tuberosity
A–Abducts, adducts, flexes, and extends shoulder

Coracobrachialis
O–Coracoid process of scapula
I–Anteromedial shaft of humerus
A–Assists shoulder flexion and adduction

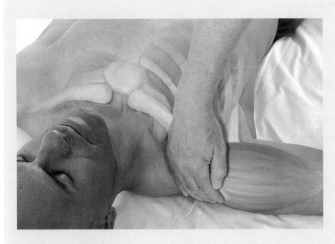

FIGURE 16.68a
Palpating the deltoid

With your partner in a seated position, locate the large, fleshy **deltoid** on the top of the shoulder (Figure 16.68a ■). Follow the deltoid fibers to the muscle's tendinous insertion site on the deltoid tuberosity. *Are you palpating the deltoid tendon on the lateral side of the arm, midway down the humerus?*

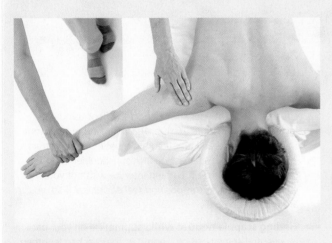

FIGURE 16.68b
Resisted movement of the posterior deltoid

Resisted movement: Have your partner raise the arm to the side, then resist as you press down right above the elbow to get the middle fibers of the deltoid to contract against resistance (Figure 16.68b ■). *In which direction would you press the arm to get the anterior fibers to contract?*

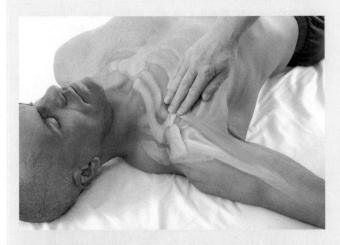

FIGURE 16.68c
Palpating the coracobrachialis

With your partner in a supine position, prepare to palpate the **coracobrachialis** by placing your partner's arm in an abducted, laterally rotated position (Figure 16.68c ■). Locate it by strumming across its slim muscular belly on the anterior edge of the armpit.

(continued)

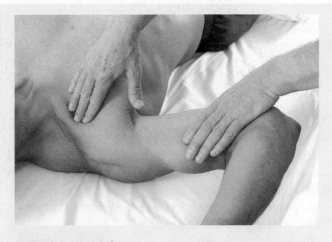

Resisted movement: Have your partner horizontally adduct the arm against your resistance to get the coracobrachialis to contract against resistance (Figure 16.68d ■). *As it contracts, do you feel the thin belly of the coracobrachialis bulge under the anterior deltoid?*

FIGURE 16.68d
Resisted movement of the coracobrachialis

SELF-CARE
Finding Scapula Neutral

It is important for you to monitor the position of your shoulder girdle and neck while you are working to avoid off-centered postures that can lead to stiffness and pain. One way to do this is to maintain the scapula-neutral posture. Since chronically tight pectoralis and shoulder muscles often pull the scapula off its neutral position, it is recommended that you stretch the pectoralis and shoulder muscles before doing this exercise.

Placing your shoulder in a scapula neutral position can be somewhat difficult to feel because it is so subtle and effortless. Make sure to keep your spine in a neutral alignment by lightly contracting your lower abdominals and lengthening the spine.

1. **Finding scapula neutral while prone:** Lie in a prone position with your arms extended by your sides along a low diagonal axis. Laterally rotate your shoulders by contracting the infraspinatus (Figure 16.69a ■). Elongate your neck to lengthen the upper trapezius.

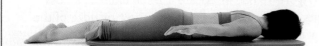

FIGURE 16.69a

FIGURE 16.69b

2. Lift the corners of your shoulder off the floor using your lower trapezius (Figure 16.69b ■). Widen and ground your upper chest to relax your pectoralis muscles. Avoid retracting the shoulder blades as you lift your shoulder. Hold for several seconds while breathing into the width of your chest. *Does holding this position feel effortless?* If so, you are doing it correctly.

3. **Finding scapula neutral while supine:** Lie on your back in a neutral-spine position. Lengthen your neck to lengthen your upper trapezius. Raise your arms above you and find the place where they are vertical, where you can feel the weight of the arms sinking into your shoulders and scapulae. Feel your scapulae against the floor, then explore doing small movements with your arms while keeping them connected to the floor (Figure 16.69c ■). *Can you feel your midscapular region touching the floor? If so, you are doing it correctly.*

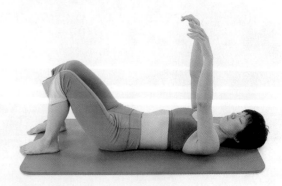

FIGURE 16.69c

4. Slowly open your arms to your sides, keeping your scapulae stable and weighted. Pause occasionally to breathe into the width of your chest and your midscapular region, which will keep your thorax open and relaxed (Figure 16.69d ■). As you open your arms, make the small adjustments needed to use your muscles symmetrically.

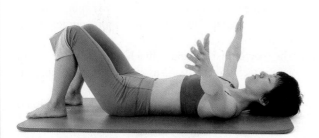

FIGURE 16.69d

5. Once your arms touch the ground, laterally rotate your shoulders by turning your palms toward the ceiling to widen your chest. Lightly press the spines of both scapulae into the floor (Figure 16.69e ■). Slowly return your arms to their starting position overhead while keeping the chest wide.

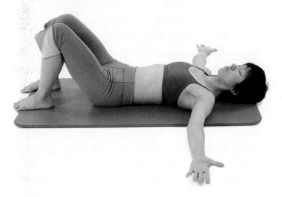

FIGURE 16.69e

CONCLUSION

The shoulder is the most mobile joint in the body. The range of mobility in the shoulders reduces the stability of the shoulder girdle. A single small joint on each side of the body, the sternoclavicular joints, attach the shoulder girdle to the axial skeleton. All other attachments are muscular and ligamentous. For this reason, muscles acting on the shoulder girdle tend to become a frequent source of myofascial pain. The prevalence of shoulder pain and dysfunction is complicated by repetitive arm movements on the job, overuse in sports activities, and faulty postures that disturb the alignment of the shoulder girdle.

Learning to maintain the neutral position of the shoulder girdle and scapulae can go a long way toward alleviating muscular imbalances and postural problems that cause chronic shoulder, neck, and back pain. The challenge lies in learning to control the muscles that place the shoulder girdle in an optimal posture and then learning to move the arms in a coordinated and efficient manner. Whatever direction a work task moves the shoulders can be countered by exercises that reverse the pattern. For example, a massage and bodywork practitioner does a lot of pushing that requires shoulder flexion and protraction. To balance the shoulder girdle by moving it in the opposite direction, a practitioner could practice pulling back on a rowing machine or on cables to strengthen muscles on the back of the shoulders. Stretching, range of motion exercises, and trigger point therapy are also very effective in alleviating myofascial pain in the shoulder muscles.

SUMMARY POINTS TO REMEMBER

1. The shoulder girdle is made up of the humeri, clavicles, and scapulae. The main function of the shoulder girdle is to suspend the arms far enough in the lateral direction that they can move freely along the sides of the torso.

2. The shoulder girdle is supported by the tensional pulls of myofascias that suspend the shoulder girdle from the head, neck, and thorax.

3. The shoulder girdle has four joints: the glenohumeral joint (a ball-and-socket joint), the acromioclavicular joint (a gliding joint), the sternoclavicular joint (an ellipsoid joint), and the scapulothoracic joint (not a true anatomical joint).

4. Only one small joint on each side connects the shoulder girdle to the axial skeleton—the sternoclavicular joint.

5. The glenohumeral joint is the most mobile joint in the body. The mobility of the scapula at the scapulothoracic joint increases the range of the glenohumeral joint.

6. Two common shoulder injuries are a shoulder dislocation, which occurs at the glenohumeral joint, and a shoulder separation, which occurs at the acromioclavicular joint. The most frequently broken bone in the body is the clavicle.

7. In the neutral position of the shoulder girdle, the clavicles are horizontal, the humeri hang vertically beside the body, and the scapulae lie in a vertical plane turned 30 degrees diagonal to the frontal plane.

8. Several benchmarks of the neutral position of the scapula, called scapula neutral, are that the medial border of the scapula runs parallel to the thoracic spine, the medial border lies 5–6 centimeters from the spine, and the scapula rests flat against the thorax.

9. Scaption is the plane of the scapula, which is determined by the direction the glenoid fossa faces. Abducting the arm in scaption places less mechanical stress on the joint structures than abducting the arm in the frontal plane.

10. The scapulohumeral rhythm is the ratio of movement of the glenohumeral and scapulothoracic joints. In a coordinated rhythm, the GH joint can flex to 90 degrees and abduct to 60 degrees before the scapulothoracic joint moves, after which the humerus and scapula move in approximately a 1-to-2 ratio.

11. The trapezius and latissimus dorsi form an extrinsic layer of musculature that covers the neck, back, and shoulders and attaches the shoulders to the spine. Their broad attachment sites along the spine result in multiple lines of pulls and multiple movement functions.

12. Four rotator cuff muscles stabilize the humerus in the glenoid fossa of the scapula and function as abductors, lateral rotators, and medial rotators of the glenohumeral joint.

13. The rhomboids, serratus anterior, and levator scapula attach the scapula to the ribs and upper spine and function as scapular stabilizers, protractors, retractors, elevators, and rotators.

14. The pectoralis muscles attach the shoulder to the anterior chest and work as primary arm flexors and adductors.

15. The deltoid and coracobrachialis muscles function as the primary abductors of the shoulder.

REVIEW QUESTIONS

1. Name the three main bones making up the shoulder girdle.
2. The four joints of the shoulder girdle are the
   a. glenohumeral, acromioclavicular, sternocostal, and scapulothoracic joints.
   b. glenohumeral, acromioclavicular, sternomanubrial, and scapulothoracic joints.
   c. glenohumeral, costoclavicular, sternoclavicular, and scapulothoracic joints.
   d. glenohumeral, acromioclavicular, sternoclavicular, and scapulothoracic joints.
3. The finger-like bony knob that projects anteriorly from the upper lateral corner of the scapula and provides attachment sites for numerous muscles and ligaments is
   a. the acromion process.
   b. the coracoid process.
   c. the greater tubercle.
   d. the lesser tubercle.
4. The _____ joint is the most mobile joint in the entire body; the _____ joint is the only joint in the body connecting the shoulder girdle to the axial skeleton; and the _____ joint of the shoulder girdle is not a true anatomical joint.
5. Which ligament covers the joint capsule of the shoulder?
6. True or false (circle one). The sternoclavicular joint has an articulating disc.
7. The range motion of the scapula includes
   a. protraction, retraction, elevation, depression, tilting, and rotation.
   b. abduction, adduction, flexion, hyperextension, and rotation.
   c. protraction, retraction, abduction, adduction, flexion, and extension.
   d. protraction, retraction, lateral rotation, medial rotation, and circumduction.
8. Match the following terms—adhesive capsulitis, shoulder dislocation, shoulder separation, and clavicular fracture—with their definitions.
   a. An injury at the acromioclavicular joint that pulls the articulating surfaces apart and can partially tear or completely tear joint structures.
   b. An injury at the glenohumeral joint that displaces the humeral head from the socket.
   c. The most common bony break in the shoulder girdle that usually occurs from a fall on an outstretched arm.
   d. Abnormal thickening and adhesions in the joint capsule of the shoulder that restricts motion, causes inflammation, and generates pain.
9. True or false (circle one). The scapula aligns along a vertical axis in the frontal plane.
10. The scapulohumeral rhythm is the ratio of movement between
   a. the clavicle and scapula.
   b. the glenohumeral and scapulothoracic joints.
   c. the humeral head and glenoid fossa.
   d. the scapula and thorax.

11. The only muscle connecting the shoulders to the pelvic girdle is the _____.

12. The four muscles of the rotator cuff are the
    a. supraspinatus, infraspinatus, teres major, and subscapularis.
    b. supraspinatus, infraspinatus, rhomboids, and suprascapularis.
    c. supraspinatus, infraspinatus, teres minor, and serratus anterior.
    d. supraspinatus, infraspinatus, teres minor, and subscapularis.

13. The _____ muscles, which attach the medial border of the scapula to the spinous process of the lower cervical and upper thoracic vertebra, retract the scapula.

14. A primary elevator of the scapula that is also a common source of intense myofascial pain in the upper back and frequently the cause of a stiff neck is the
    a. upper trapezius.
    b. levator scapula.
    c. middle trapezius.
    d. rhomboid minor.

15. Scapular winging, a condition in which the medial border of the scapula is raised off of the thorax, is caused by
    a. contracture in the rhomboids.
    b. weakness or inhibition in the rhomboids.
    c. contracture in the serratus anterior.
    d. weakness or inhibition in the serratus anterior.

16. The horizontal stability of the shoulder is maintained by the _____ muscle, which is always under tension from the weight of the arm.

17. A common postural dysfunction that occurs when the upper trapezius becomes chronically contracted and shortened while the lower trapezius becomes overstretched and weakened is when the
    a. neck hyperextends causing forward head posture and rounded shoulders.
    b. neck hyperextends causing forward head posture and retracted shoulders.
    c. neck hyperflexes causing forward head posture and rounded shoulders.
    d. neck hyperextends causing a flattened cervical curve and rounded shoulders.

18. The function of the lower trapezius is to
    a. elevate, tilt, and retract the scapula.
    b. stabilize, upwardly rotate, and retract the scapula.
    c. stabilize, upwardly rotate, and depress the scapula.
    d. depress, protract, and stabilize the scapula.

19. True or false (circle one). Trigger points in the pectoralis muscles can cause symptoms that are often mistaken for heart diseases such as myocardial infarction or angina.

20. Which group of muscles works synergistically to flex and adduct the arm?
    a. the posterior deltoid, subscapularis, and pectoralis minor
    b. the anterior deltoid, coracobrachialis, and pectoralis major
    c. the middle deltoid, subclavius, and pectoralis major
    d. the anterior deltoid, coracobrachialis, and pectoralis minor

Notes

1. Levangie, P., & Norkin, C. (2005). *Joint Structure and Function: A Comprehensive Analysis* (4th ed.). Philadelphi: F. A. Davis.
2. Kapandji, I. A. (1982). *The Physiology of Joints: Upper Limb* (5th ed., Vol. 1). Edinburgh, UK: Churchill Livingstone.
3. Ibid.
4. Magee, D. (2002). *Orthopedic Physical Assessment* (4th ed.). Philadelphia: Saunders.
5. Kapandji, *The Physiology of Joints*.

17 The Arm and Hand

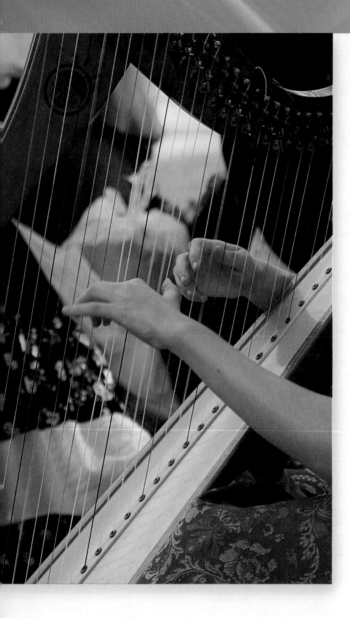

CHAPTER OUTLINE

Chapter Objectives

Key Terms

17.1 Bones of the Arm and Hand

17.2 Joints and Ligaments of the Arm and Hand

17.3 Muscles of the Arm and Hand

Conclusion

Summary Points to Remember

Review Questions

There are a number of parallels between the hand dexterity and form of a harpist and those of a massage practitioner. Upright posture allows both to work effectively and comfortably, so both need to pay close attention to body as well as hand position. Form is also essential to the success of both activities. To avoid injury, the harpist and massage practitioner must be able to sit or stand up straight to reach all the harp strings or the client's entire body without twisting or hunching. They must also work with the hands square, the fingers parallel to the forearm, and thumbs at a right angle.

A harpist produces various tones from different places on the strings; a massage practitioner evokes changes in muscular tone by working just the right tissues in the right way for the right amount of time. In both activities, force is generated with the movement of the arms and trunk, and each finger fully articulates. In massage, the fingers literally play the tissues in a rhythmic composition, which, like the harp, has a soothing and healing effect on both the body and the mind.

CHAPTER OBJECTIVES

1. Name and describe the three bones in the arm and the eight carpals, five metacarpals, and 14 phalanges of the wrist and hand.

2. Demonstrate the palpation of bony landmarks and primary movements of the arm and hand.

3. Name the origins, insertions, and actions of the major ligaments of the elbow, wrist, and hand.

4. List the four joints of the elbow and describe the structure and function of each one.

5. List the seven types of joints in the wrist and hand and describe the structure and function of each one.

6. Define supination and pronation and name the muscles that generate each action.

7. Demonstrate the four passive movement ranges for the wrist.

8. Describe the three arches and two general types of grips of the hand.

9. Define the carpal tunnel and list the structures passing through it.

10. Identify the origins, insertions, and actions of the muscles acting on the elbow and their trigger points. Demonstrate the palpation of and resisted movement for each one.

11. Identify the origins, insertions, and actions of the muscles acting on the wrist and hand and their trigger points. Demonstrate the active movement of and palpation of each one.

KEY TERMS

Carpal tunnel	Lateral epicondyle	Radiocarpal joint
Carpals	Medial epicondyle	Radioulnar joint
Carrying angle	Metacarpals	Radius
Humeroulnar joint	Metacarpophalangeal joint	Reposition
Humerus	Olecranon	Supinator
Hypothenar eminence	Opposition	Thenar eminence
Interosseous membrane	Phalanges	Transverse carpal ligament
Interphalangeal joint	Pronator	Ulna

MUSCLES IN ACTION

Elbow flexion
Biceps brachii
Brachialis
Bracioradialis

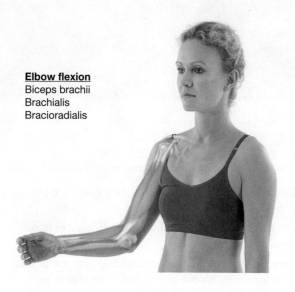

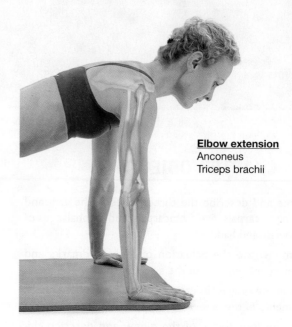

Elbow extension
Anconeus
Triceps brachii

Supination
Biceps brachii
Supinator

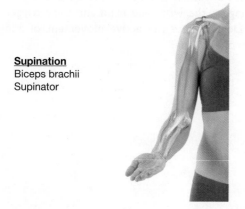

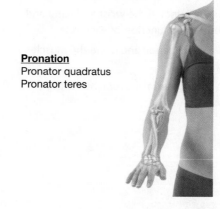

Pronation
Pronator quadratus
Pronator teres

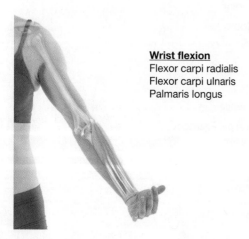

Wrist flexion
Flexor carpi radialis
Flexor carpi ulnaris
Palmaris longus

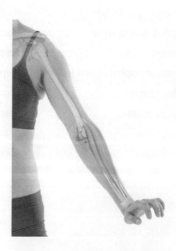

Wrist extension
Extensor carpi radialis brevis
Extensor carpi radialis longus
Extensor carpi ulnaris

Muscles of the Arm and Hand in Action

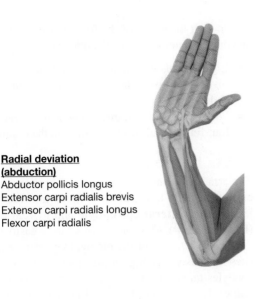

Radial deviation (abduction)
Abductor pollicis longus
Extensor carpi radialis brevis
Extensor carpi radialis longus
Flexor carpi radialis

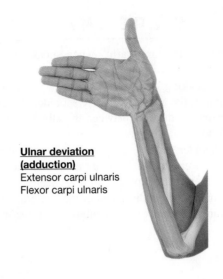

Ulnar deviation (adduction)
Extensor carpi ulnaris
Flexor carpi ulnaris

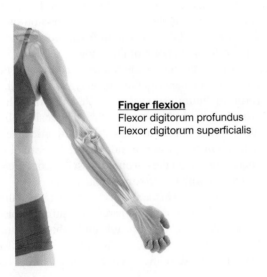

Finger flexion
Flexor digitorum profundus
Flexor digitorum superficialis

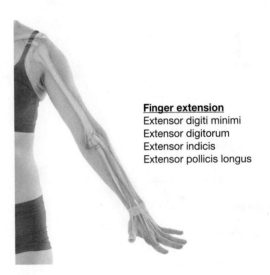

Finger extension
Extensor digiti minimi
Extensor digitorum
Extensor indicis
Extensor pollicis longus

From packing a suitcase to opening a door to reaching for a book, the extremely dexterous arm and hand allow us a broad range of prehensile capacities. The highly mobile shoulder is a servant to the hand. The shoulder allows us to position the arm and hand in just the right way for myriad specific and sophisticated tasks.

The feet evolved for weight bearing and locomotion in the closed-chain movement of the body against the ground. In contrast, the hands evolved for open-chain movement that allows us to manipulate the environment around us in infinite ways. With our hands, we can reach in every direction. Our capacity for sophisticated hand movement reflects the evolved cognitive abilities of the human brain. The area of the brain devoted to the control of the thumb alone is a marvel of neuromotor development. On a musculoskeletal level, the forearm and hand often require extra study because of their complexity, including many intricate joints and muscles.

Given the central role of the hands in work-related tasks, many people are required to perform repetitive movements of the hands, such as typing, grasping tools, and scanning products. As a result, repetitive-strain injuries in the hands and wrists tend to be prevalent among the working population. People working in the service industry averaged a 40 percent rate of injuries from overexertion on the job in 2002.[1] As a massage and bodywork practitioner, you will need to understand the intricacies of kinesiology in the arm and hand to avoid developing repetitive-strain injuries and to work effectively with clients who have such injuries.

Because the hands are the primary tools of the manual therapist, in this chapter we consider ways to use the hands that minimize stress and maximize efficiency of motion. An emphasis is placed on maintaining neutral joint positions while you work, especially during force applications. Also, you are encouraged to integrate hand movements with full-body motion to distribute and dissipate the mechanical stresses of pushing and pulling through your entire body. As with previous chapters, we systematically look at the bones, ligaments, joints, and muscles of the arm and hand. Particular attention will be paid to skeletal alignment as a key to preventing wrist and hand injuries.

17.1   BONES OF THE ARM AND HAND

People often use the term "arm" when speaking of the entire upper limb in the same way that they use the term "leg" when speaking of the lower limb. In anatomical terms, the **arm** is the area between the shoulder and elbow and the **forearm** is the area between the elbow and wrist (Figure 17.1 ■).

In the shoulder chapter, we looked at bony landmarks on the proximal end of the humerus related to the structure and function of the shoulder. In this chapter, we look at bony landmarks on the distal end of the humerus related to the structure and function of the elbow and forearm. We

also look at the bones of the forearm (the radius and ulna) and the 27 bones of the hand, which are:

- Eight carpals: the small irregular bones in the wrist
- Five metacarpals: the long bones between the carpals and the fingers
- Fourteen phalanges: three long bones in each of the four fingers and two long bones in the thumb

17.1.1   Humerus

The arm has a single bone in it: the **humerus.** The distal end of the long humeral shaft flares into two bony projections: the **lateral epicondyle** and **medial epicondyle** (Figure 17.2a ■). The epicondyles can be easily palpated at the broadest aspect of the elbow; they provide attachment sites for muscles acting on the elbow and wrist. Both epicondyles taper into bony edges called the **supracondylar ridges,** located along the distal humerus where its round shaft flattens into a wider surface (Figure 17.2b ■). Directly between the epicondyles, a deep depression on the distal humerus called the **olecranon fossa** provides an articulating notch for the point of the elbow.

The distal end of the humerus consists of three bony knobs that lie between the epicondyles. Two of these knobs form an hourglass surface called the **trochlea,** which articulates with the ulna. A third spherical knob lateral to the trochlea, known as the **capitulum,** articulates with the radius. On the posterior side of the humerus lies a bony depression called the **coronoid fossa**—a concave notch that articulates with the proximal ulna.

As discussed in the shoulder chapter, two small bumps on the glenoid fossa of the humerus—the **infraglenoid tubercle** at the bottom and the **supraglenoid tubercle** at the top (see Figure 16.7)—provide respective attachment sites for tendons of the long heads of the triceps brachii and biceps brachii.

17.1.2   Radius and Ulna

Two long bones—the radius and ulna—run parallel to each other in the forearm (Figure 17.3a ■). The **radius** runs along the medial side of the forearm and grows more prominent at the wrist, which is the location of its more important movement functions. The **ulna** runs along the lateral side of the forearm. It grows larger and more complex at the elbow, which is the location of its more important movement functions.

At the elbow, the radius narrows into a disk-like shape called the **radial head,** which fits into the radial notch of the ulna. A concave surface on the proximal end of the radial head rests against the rounded capitulum of the humerus. The radial shaft is bowed and can be palpated between the crease of the elbow and the thumb side of the wrist. As it approaches the wrist, the radial shaft enlarges and widens into the blunt **styloid process of radius** and an **ulnar notch** that rests against the ulnar head. Medial to the styloid process of the radius, an oblong-shaped **posterior tubercle** (also called Lister's tubercle) rises on the posterior surface of the radius between the extensor pollicis longus tendon and the extensor carpi radialis tendons.

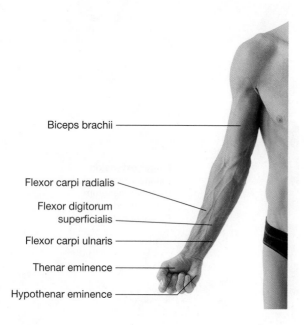

Biceps brachii

Flexor carpi radialis

Flexor digitorum superficialis

Flexor carpi ulnaris

Thenar eminence

Hypothenar eminence

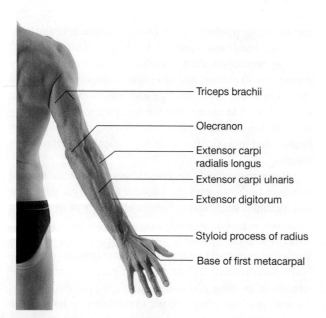

Triceps brachii

Olecranon

Extensor carpi radialis longus

Extensor carpi ulnaris

Extensor digitorum

Styloid process of radius

Base of first metacarpal

FIGURE 17.1

Surface anatomy of arm and hand

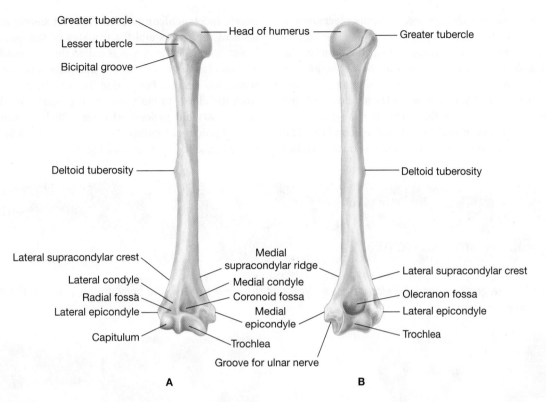

FIGURE 17.2

Humerus: a) Anterior view b) Posterior view

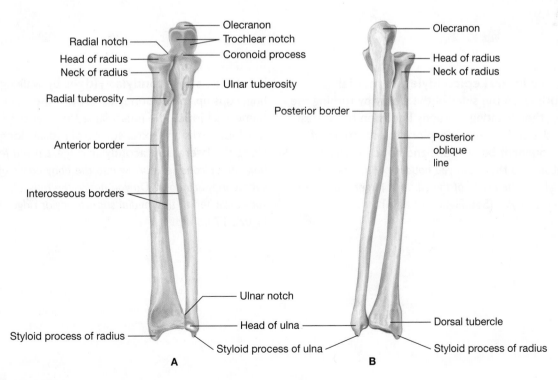

FIGURE 17.3

Radius and ulna: a) Anterior view b) Posterior view

At the elbow, the ulna enlarges into the **olecranon**—a large, curved structure shaped like a jaw. The olecranon forms the prominent and easily palpable point of the elbow, that spot we prop on when we lean on the elbows (Figure 17.3b ■). Have you ever felt a zinging sensation when you've bumped your elbow, or "funny bone"? What you actually bumped was the ulnar nerve, which runs between the olecranon and the medial epicondyle. The olecranon has two concavities on its inner surface, a **radial**

notch and **trochlear notch**, which fit snugly against the head of the radius and the trochlea of the humerus. The lower lip of the olecranon is called the **coronoid process**. The olecranon tapers into the triangular shaft of the ulna, which has a sharp bony edge that can be easily palpated from the elbow to the wrist. At the wrist, the ulna tapers into the **styloid process of ulna**, which is blunt like the styloid process of radius but smaller. It has a small, disk-shaped head that rests against the distal radius.

BONE PALPATION
Elbow and Forearm

Caution: Palpate gently around the elbow to avoid irritating the ulnar nerve in the bony groove between the medial epicondyle and the olecranon.

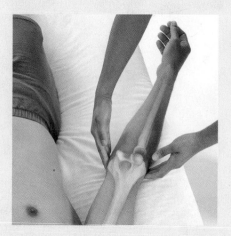

FIGURE 17.4a

Palpate the **lateral epicondyle** and **medial epicondyle** on the sides of the elbow by turning the palm up, then locating the bony knobs on the widest part of the elbow. Gently explore the contours of these prominent bony knobs and notice where tendons attach to them. *Do you notice how the medial epicondyle on the inside of the elbow is larger than the lateral epicondyle?* (See Figure 17.4a ■)

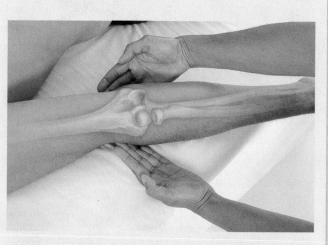

FIGURE 17.4b

Locate the **supracondylar ridges** by walking your fingertips up the epicondyles toward the shaft of the humerus. Notice the muscular attachments of the brachioradialis and extensor carpi radialis longus along the lateral supracondylar ridge. *Do you feel how the epicondyles narrow into the bony edges of the supracondylar ridges? Do you notice the muscular tissues attached to the medial supracondylar ridge?* (See Figure 17.4b ■)

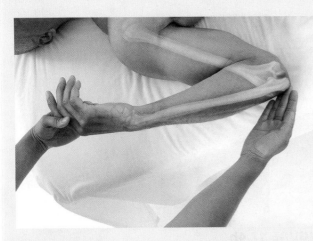

FIGURE 17.4c
Locate the **olecranon** on the point of the elbow. Palpate the sides of the olecranon. Carefully palpate the bony groove between this large process and the medial epicondyle, where the ulnar nerve passes. *Do you feel the ulnar nerve between the olecranon and the medial epicondyle? Have you ever felt a zinging sensation when you've bumped your elbow, or "funny bone"? What you actually bumped was the ulnar nerve.* (See Figure 17.4c ■)

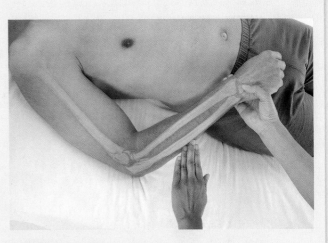

FIGURE 17.4d
Walk your fingers along the **shaft of the ulna,** from the elbow toward the lateral side wrist. Squeeze the sides of this sharp bony ridge and explore its shape. *Do you notice how the anterior side of the ulnar shaft has fleshier muscular attachments than the posterior side?* (See Figure 17.4d ■)

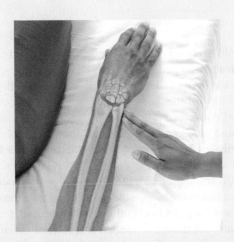

FIGURE 17.4e
Locate the **styloid process of the ulna** on the little finger side of the wrist. Use a pincher grip to explore the sides of this sharp bony process and the **head of the ulna.** *Do you feel the narrow and pointed shape of the styloid process of the ulna?* (See Figure 17.4e ■)

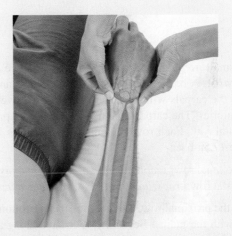

FIGURE 17.4f
Use a pincher grip to explore the **styloid process of the radius** on the thumb side of the wrist. *Do you notice how much larger the styloid process of the radius is than the styloid process of the ulna?* (See Figure 17.4f ■)

(continued)

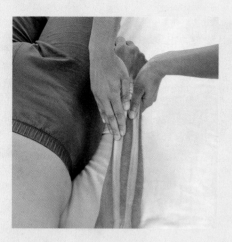

FIGURE 17.4g
From the wrist, use a pincher grip to walk your fingers up the **shaft of the radius** toward the elbow. Notice how easy it is to palpate the radial shaft in the distal forearm. *Do you notice how the shaft of the radius disappears under tissue as you approach the elbow?* (See Figure 17.4g ■)

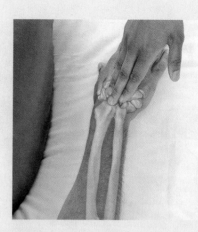

FIGURE 17.4h
Locate the large, oblong **dorsal tubercle** at the distal end of the radius in the middle of the wrist, then explore the contours of the radius around it. *Are you palpating the middle of the wrist on the posterior side? Do you notice how much larger and wider the distal end of the radius is than the distal end of the ulna?* (See Figure 17.4h ■)

17.1.3 Carpals

Eight small irregular bones called the **carpals** are located in the wrist. A basic understanding of the shape and position of the carpals will help you to work effectively with wrist injuries. The carpals line up in two rows, a proximal and distal row. Each row contains four bones, as follows (Figure 17.5a-b ■):

- Proximal row: *scaphoid, lunate, triquetrum, pisiform*
- Distal row: *trapezium, trapezoid, capitate, hamate*

In the proximal row, a large, L-shaped **scaphoid** articulates with the radius. Because it is located along a direct path of force transmission from the hand into the forearm,

the scaphoid tends to be the most frequently fractured carpal in a fall on an outstretched hand (Figure 17.6 ■). The scaphoid forms the floor of the "anatomical snuffbox," a depression at the base of the thumb between the extensor pollicis longus and adductor pollicis longus tendons. It is named such because people used to put snuff (powdered tobacco) there to inhale (Figure 17.7 ■). The **lunate,** named for it moon-like crescent shape, sits directly lateral to the scaphoid and also articulates with the radius. Its central location in the wrist makes the lunate susceptible to dislocation from falls, and it is the most frequently dislocated carpal. Lateral to the lunate, the triangular-shaped **triquetrum** articulates with the ulna. The small pea-shaped **pisiform** rests against

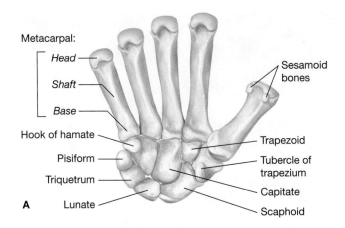

Metacarpal:

[*Head*

  Shaft

  Base

Hook of hamate

Pisiform

Triquetrum

A   Lunate

Sesamoid bones

Trapezoid

Tubercle of trapezium

Capitate

Scaphoid

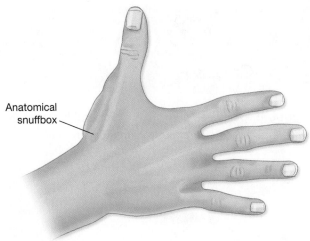

Anatomical snuffbox

FIGURE 17.7

Anatomical snuffbox

Metacarpal:

  — *Head*

  — *Shaft*

  — *Base*

  — Capitate

  — Hamate

  — Triquetrum

  — Lunate

Trapezoid

Trapezium

Scaphoid

B

FIGURE 17.5

Carpals: a) Anterior view b) Posterior view

the concave anterior surface of the triquetrum, forming a small but prominent bump in the wrist. The pisiform is often used as a fulcrum for applying pointed pressure with the wrist (Figure 17.8 ■).

In the distal row of carpals, a pyramid-shaped **hamate** sits at the base of the fourth and fifth metacarpals. The

pisiform and a hook-like projection on the anterior surface of the hamate provide attachment sites for the transverse carpal ligament over the carpal tunnel. You will need to be able to locate this ligament when treating carpal tunnel problems. The largest carpal, the **capitate** (L. *capitate:* head), resides in a longitudinally stable position in the center of the wrist, at the base of the third metacarpal. The capitate has two heads that form an hourglass shape. A small, square **trapezoid** sits wedged between the capitate and the trapezium at the base of the second metacarpal. The saddle-shaped surface of the **trapezium** articulates with the base of the first metacarpal, which forms the saddle joint of the thumb. Two small tubercles, one on the posterior surface of the trapezium (trapezium tubercle) at the base of the thumb and one on the posterior surface of the scaphoid (scaphoid tubercle), provide a broad attachment site for the flexor retinaculum crossing the carpal tunnel.

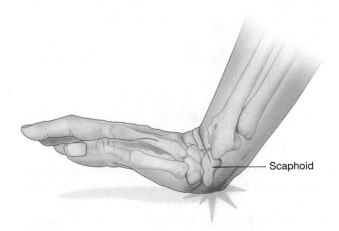

— Scaphoid

FIGURE 17.6

Scaphoid fracture

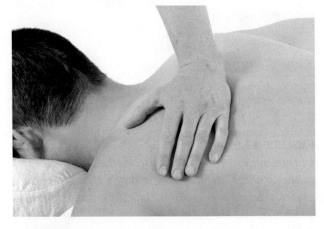

FIGURE 17.8

Pisiform as fulcrum

BONE PALPATION
Carpals

Caution: *Avoid deep pressure over vulnerable tissues (nerves, blood vessels, and tendinous sheaths) that cross the wrist, especially over previously injured or sore areas.*

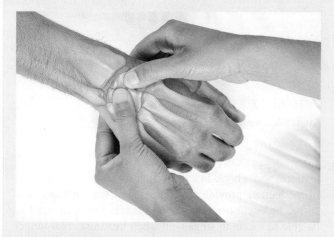

FIGURE 17.9a

Locate the **proximal row of carpals**—the scaphoid, lunate, triquetrum, pisiform—on the posterior side of the wrist by lightly pressing distal to the end of the radius and ulna. Press the carpals with the wrist flexed and then extended. *Did you notice how much easier it is to feel the carpals with the wrist flexed?* (See Figure 17.9a ■)

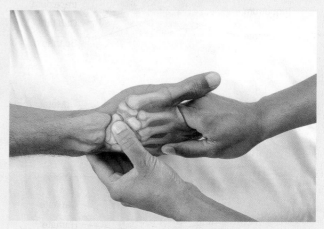

FIGURE 17.9b

To locate the **scaphoid,** press your thumb into the depression called the "anatomical snuffbox" at the distal end of the styloid process of the radius. Hold the scaphoid while you adduct the wrist by side-bending it toward the little finger. *Do you feel how the scaphoid surfaces when you adduct the wrist?* (See Figure 17.9b ■)

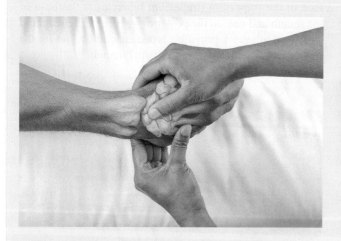

FIGURE 17.9c

Locate the **lunate** by sliding from the posterior tubercle of the radius into the depression over the carpals. To feel the lunate surface, flex the wrist. *Do you notice how the lunate disappears when you extend the wrist?* (See Figure 17.9c ■)

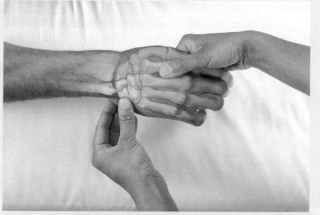

FIGURE 17.9d

Locate the **triquetrum** on the posterior, lateral side of the lunate. It will feel like a small depression. Take the wrist into flexion to feel the surface of the triquetrum. *Do you notice how difficult it is to differentiate the triquetrum from the lunate?* (See Figure 17.9d ■)

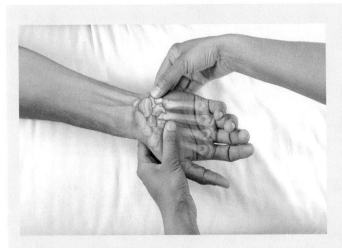

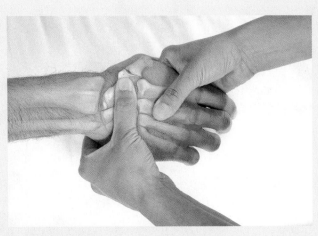

FIGURE 17.9e

The **pisiform** is a prominent bump on the anterior side of the wrist, below the base of the fifth metacarpal. It will feel like a small bony marble on the lateral side of the wrist. *Do you feel the tendon that attaches to the pisiform? (See Figure 17.9e ■)*

FIGURE 17.9f

Palpate the **distal row of carpals**—the trapezium, trapezoid, capitate, and hamate—on the posterior side of the wrist by lightly pressing the small bones proximal to the base of the five metacarpals, then flex and extend the wrist. *Do you feel the joints between the carpals and metacarpals open and close as you flex and extend the wrist? (See Figure 17.9f ■)*

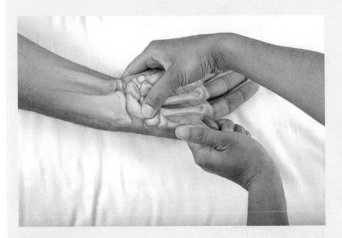

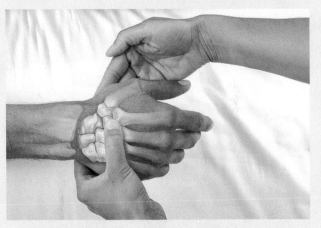

FIGURE 17.9g

Palpate the **trapezium** below the anterior side of the wrist at the base of the first metacarpal. Hold this spot, then cross your thumb toward the little finger. *Do you notice how crossing the thumb makes the trapezium easier to feel? (See Figure 17.9g ■)*

FIGURE 17.9h

Locate the small **trapezoid** below the base of the second metacarpal, on the distal surface of the wrist, then flex and extend the wrist. *Do you notice how the trapezoid is easier to feel with the wrist in flexion? (See Figure 17.9h ■)*

(continued)

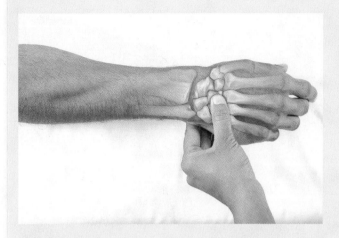

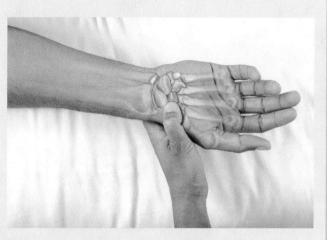

FIGURE 17.9i

To locate the **capitate,** flex the wrist, then slide from the lunate toward the base of the third metacarpal and you'll land on the capitate. Extend the wrist and notice how the capitate glides forward and seemingly disappears. *Are you on the posterior surface of the wrist? Do you feel the round head of the capitate when the wrist is flexed?* (See Figure 17.9i ▪)

FIGURE 17.9j

Palpate the **tubercles of the trapezium and scaphoid** at the base of the first metacarpal, on the anterior side of the wrist. The tubercles are too close together to palpate separately. *Do you notice the small bump the tubercles create in the center?* (See Figure 17.9j ▪)

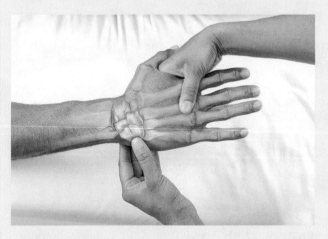

Palpate the **hamate** at the base of the fourth and fifth metacarpals, on the posterior side of the wrist. *Do you feel how wide the flat surface of the hamate is?* (See Figure 17.9k ▪)

FIGURE 17.9k

17.1.4 Metacarpals and Phalanges

The hand contains 19 miniature long bones—five metacarpals and 14 phalanges (Figure 17.10a ▪). Each of the five **metacarpals** has a relatively square *base,* a stout *shaft,* and a round *head.* The base of the metacarpals fit snugly against the distal carpals. Rather than being parallel to each other, the metacarpals fan out toward the fingers. The proximal, lateral surfaces of the metacarpals fit tightly against each other, which gives the palm of the hand greater stability. It is easier to palpate the metacarpals on the posterior surface of the hand, where they are closer to the skin, than on the palms.

Each of the four fingers contains three **phalanges** (singular: *phalanx*)—a *proximal, middle,* and *distal* phalanx—which become progressively smaller. As is typical of long bones, each phalanx possesses a base, a shaft, and a head. The small distal phalanges at the tips of the fingers taper into a flat, triangular shape. The concave surfaces on the

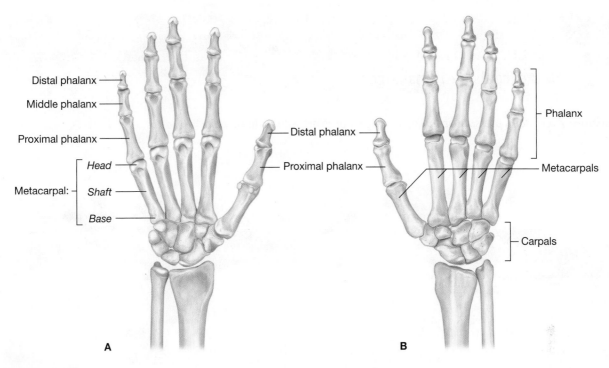

Distal phalanx
Middle phalanx
Proximal phalanx
Metacarpal:
  Head
  Shaft
  Base

Distal phalanx
Proximal phalanx

Phalanx
Metacarpals
Carpals

A   **B**

FIGURE 17.10

Bones of the hand: a) Posterior view b) Anterior view

proximal end of the proximal phalanges fit over the round convex heads of the adjacent metacarpals. A slight depression between the two condyles on the distal ends of the proximal phalanx and middle phalanx provides a groove for a flexor tendon running along the anterior surface of each finger (Figure 17.10b ■). The extensor tendons of the fingers lie flat against the posterior surface of the phalangeal shafts.

The thumb contains only a proximal phalanx and distal phalanx. The first metacarpal of the thumb has a saddle-shaped surface on its proximal end, which allows the thumb to move with a greater range of motion than the other four fingers. Tendons running along the anterior side of the thumb slide in a groove between two tiny sesamoid bones located at the base of the proximal phalanx.

BONE PALPATION
Metacarpals and Phalanges

Caution: Avoid deep pressure or pulling on fingers or joints with arthritic pain.

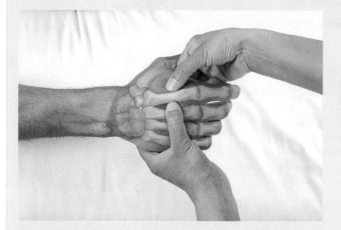

FIGURE 17.11a

Palpate the **metacarpals** on the posterior side of the hand by pressing along the shaft of the each bone, from the knuckles to the wrist. Then grasp each metacarpal through both the anterior and posterior sides of the hand. *Are you using a pincher grip to grasp each metacarpal? (See Figure 17.11a ■)*

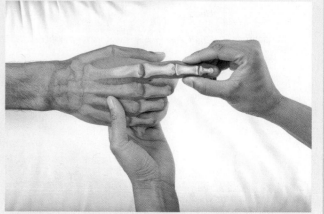

FIGURE 17.11b

Palpate each **phalange** by gently squeezing each finger along its sides, then squeezing it along the front and back. Compare the size of the phalanges of the thumb to the rest of the fingers. *Do you notice how each bone widens as you approach the joint? (See Figure 17.11b ■)*

17.2 JOINTS AND LIGAMENTS OF THE ARM AND HAND

The four joints of the elbow allow t≈he upper limb to bend and twist so that the hand can be brought toward the body. Like the knee, the elbow is also classified as a modified hinge joint because it flexes with a slight amount of axial rotation. The joints of the elbow should be easy to remember because each joint is named after its articulating bones. The four joints of the elbow and forearm are listed below, along with their joint classifications:

- Humeroulnar joint: hinge
- Humeroradial joint: hinge
- Proximal radioulnar joint: pivot
- Distal radioulnar joint: gliding

The many joints of the wrist and hand are also named according to their articulating bones, as well as their locations (Figure 17.12 ■). They are listed on the next page, along with abbreviations and joint classifications:

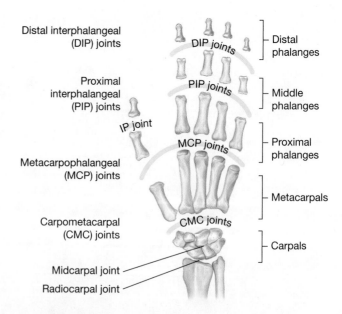

FIGURE 17.12

Joints of the wrist and hand

- Radiocarpal: ellipsoid
- Midcarpal: gliding
- Intercarpal (IC): gliding
- Carpometacarpal (CMC): gliding
- Metacarpophalangeal (MCP): ellipsoid
- Proximal interphalangeal (PIP): hinge
- Distal interphalangeal (DIP): hinge

17.2.1   Joints and Ligaments of the Elbow

A large and loose joint capsule encapsulates three joints at the elbow—the humeroulnar joint, humeroradial joint, and the proximal radioulnar joint. Although the fourth joint of the elbow—the distal radioulnar—is located near the wrist, it is classified as an elbow joint because it is mechanically linked to and moves with the proximal radioulnar joint. These two joints will be covered together in the next section. In movement of the elbow, the humeroulnar and humeroradial joints are mechanically linked and move together.

The **humeroulnar joint** is an articulation of the olecranon of the ulna with the trochlea of the humerus (Figure 17.13a-b ■). The jaw-like olecranon fits snugly around the trochlea and when the elbow flexes, the olecranon fossa turns around the trochlea like a wrench around a spool. Because the trochlea is wider on one side, the ulna joins the humerus at a slight angle, called the **carrying angle** of the elbow. The carrying angle, which is measured between the long axis of the humerus and the long axis of the forearm, averages 15 degrees (Figure 17.14 ■). When the arms hang vertically from the shoulders, the carrying angle causes the hands to rest slightly in front of the lateral line of the pelvis. The carrying angle also causes the elbow to flex in a plane slightly medial to the sagittal plane.

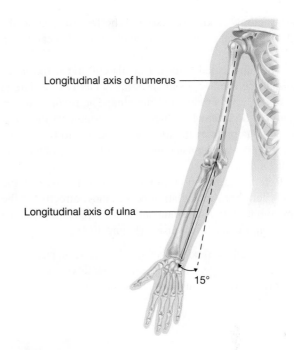

Longitudinal axis of humerus

Longitudinal axis of ulna

15°

FIGURE 17.14

Carrying angle of the elbow

As mentioned earlier, there is more than one joint in the elbow. The humerus articulates with both the ulna and radius in two of the three joints that reside within the same capsule. Directly lateral to the humeroulnar joint is the **humeroradial joint,** which is formed by the articulation of the radial head with the capitulum. The broad and loose joint capsule of the elbow encapsulates both the humeroulnar and humeroradial joints, which sit side by side.

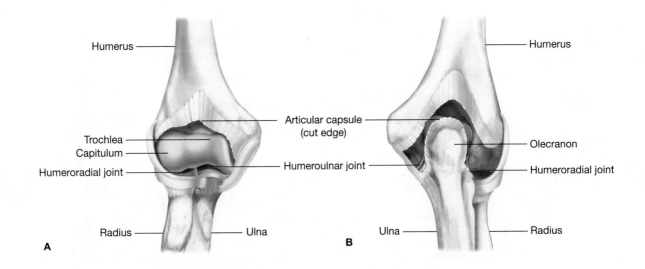

Humerus

Trochlea

Capitulum

Humeroradial joint

Articular capsule (cut edge)

Humeroulnar joint

Radius

Ulna

A

Humerus

Olecranon

Humeroradial joint

Ulna

Radius

B

FIGURE 17.13

Humeroulnar joint: a) Anterior view b) Posterior view

During elbow flexion, the slightly hollow surface on the end of the radial head glides around the rounded capitulum of the humerus.

The fan-shaped **lateral** (radial) **collateral ligament** connects the lateral epicondyle of the humerus to the lateral aspect of the olecranon and the ulna. The **medial** (ulnar) **collateral ligament** has three distinct segments that connect various parts of the medial epicondyle to the medial aspect of the olecranon and the coronoid process of the ulna (Figure 17.15 ■).

References to elbow motion refer to the part of the joint where bony articulation occurs most directly, at the humeroulnar joint. This uniaxial joint moves in one degree of motion: flexion or extension (Figure 17.16a-b ■).

- Active elbow flexion averages 145 degrees; passive flexion averages 160 degrees. Elbow flexion stops in a soft end-feel because tissue restricts further motion.

- Elbow extension averages 5 degrees and stops in a hard end-feel when the olecranon bumps up against the coronoid process. The elbow reaches a closed-pack position in extension.

17.2.2 Joints and Ligaments of the Forearm

Movement at one end the forearm always occurs with movement at the other end. Additionally, every movement of the elbow requires movement in both the proximal and distal radioulnar joints. The radius and ulna are connected along their length by a strong **interosseous membrane** (Figure 17.17 ■).

The **proximal radioulnar joint** is a pivot joint formed by the articulation of the radial head against the radial notch of the ulna. It is secured by an **annular ligament,** which wraps around the radial head and holds it in the radial notch of the ulna. A layer of cartilage under the annular ligament allows the radius to spin against the ulna with minimal

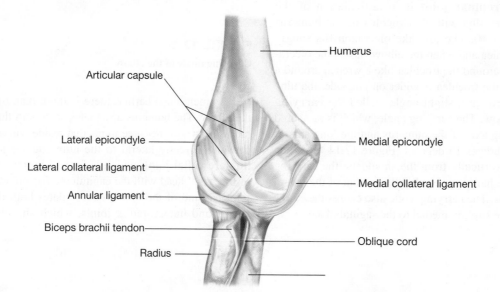

Humerus

Articular capsule

Lateral epicondyle

Lateral collateral ligament

Annular ligament

Biceps brachii tendon

Radius

Medial epicondyle

Medial collateral ligament

Oblique cord

Anterior

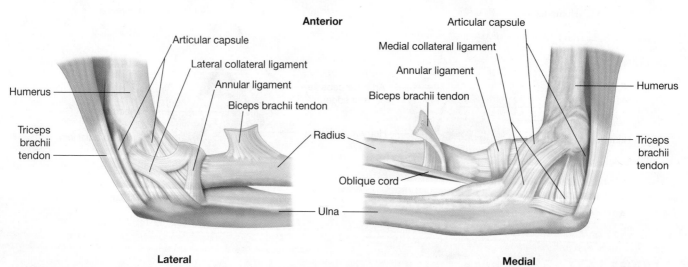

Humerus

Triceps brachii tendon

Articular capsule

Lateral collateral ligament

Annular ligament

Biceps brachii tendon

Radius

Oblique cord

Ulna

Lateral

Articular capsule

Medial collateral ligament

Annular ligament

Biceps brachii tendon

Humerus

Triceps brachii tendon

Medial

FIGURE 17.15

Ligaments of the elbow

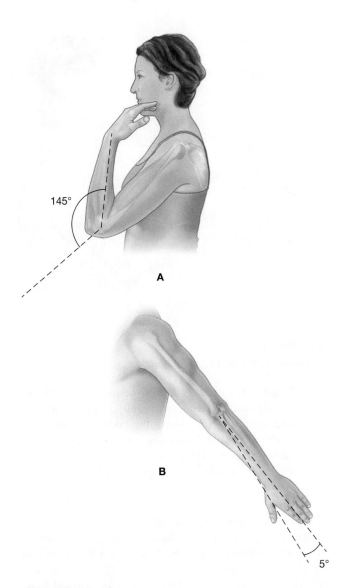

FIGURE 17.16

Range of elbow: a) Flexion b) Extension

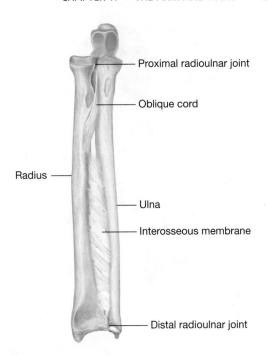

FIGURE 17.17

Radioulnar joints and interosseous membrane

friction during supination and pronation. Although the proximal radioulnar joint resides within the joint capsule of the elbow, it moves with the distal radioulnar joint during supination and pronation. The **distal radioulnar joint** is a fibrous joint formed by the articulation of the radius and ulna. A triangular-shaped fibrocartilage disk that lies against the distal surface of the ulna also cushions the distal end of this joint.

As the forearm supinates, it turns the palm to face up (Figure 17.18a ■). As the forearm pronates, it turns the palm to face down (Figure 17.18b ■). When the forearm reaches the end range of supination, the radius and ulna become parallel. As the forearm pronates, the radius twists around the ulna at the wrist. It is possible to supinate and pronate the forearm at the elbow with the hand fixed, causing the radius and ulna to twist around each other at the elbow and the shoulder to laterally rotate (Figure 17.19a-b ■). This range of movement can lock the elbow into a strained position and should be avoided when pushing or pulling, or even when resting the body weight on the hands. The forearm

can supinate an average of 90 degrees and pronate an average of 85 degrees (Figure 17.20 ■). The elbow circumducts within a range that allows the hand to move along the circumference of a cone (Figure 17.21 ■).

In a **neutral position of the forearm** in a standing posture, the thumb points forward when the elbow is extended and points up when the elbow is flexed. When a person walks, if the forearm is in a neutral position, the arms can swing freely in the sagittal plane. Postural holding patterns in the shoulders affect the position of the hands. When the thumbs point laterally, this indicates that the shoulders are

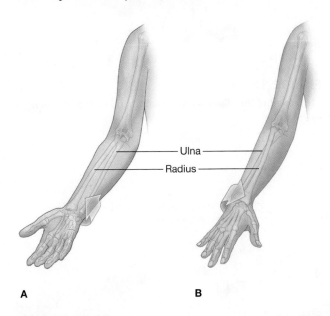

FIGURE 17.18

a) **Supination** b) **Pronation**

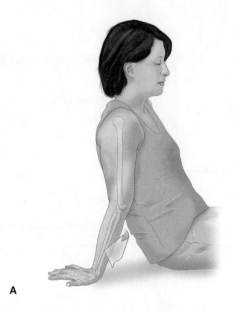

A

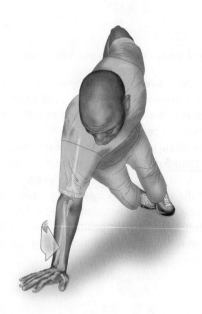

B

FIGURE 17.19

Movement of the elbow when the hand is fixed: a) Supination
b) Pronation

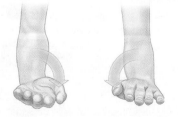

FIGURE 17.20

**The combined range of motion in supination and pronation
averages 175 degrees.**

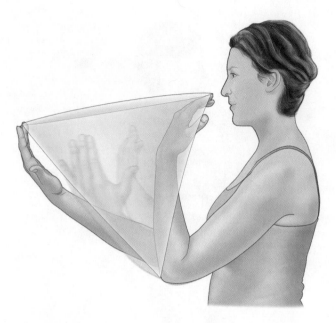

FIGURE 17.21

Arc of the elbow during circumduction

laterally rotated, which tends to hyperextend the elbows
and cause the arms to swing unnaturally in a sideways arc.
When the thumbs point toward the body, the shoulders
are medially rotated and the elbows might be chronically
flexed. Both patterns reflect muscular tension in the shoulders and reduce the efficiency of the overall gait pattern.

17.2.3   Joints and Ligaments of the Wrist

The wrist is actually made up of two joints. The ellipsoid
radiocarpal joint, which is the true wrist joint, is formed
by the articulation between the distal end of the radius and
the proximal carpal bones (Figure 17.22 ■). A secondary wrist articulation called the gliding **midcarpal joint**
is located between the proximal and distal row of carpal
bones. Although there are many bones in the midcarpal
joint, all of them are encapsulated by a continuous joint
capsule. Smaller gliding joints between the lateral surfaces
of the carpal bones, called the **intercarpal joints,** move
with a minimal degree of gliding motion and contribute to
the lateral stability of the wrist.

The radiocarpal joint is a biaxial joint that moves with
two degrees of motion (see Table 17.1 ■). It moves in a
range of flexion and extension and ulnar or radial deviation
(Figure 17.23 ■):

- Wrist flexion averages 80 degrees
- Wrist extension averages 70 degrees
- Ulnar deviation (abduction) average 45 degrees
- Radial deviation (adduction) averages 20 degrees

A combination of these four movements allows the
wrist to circumduct, moving the hand in a twirling motion
that inscribes an arc. We use this action to stir a bowl of
batter, twirl a sparkler, or use a rope like a lasso.

Ligaments on all four sides of the wrist attach the radius
and ulna to the carpals and restrict wrist motion in each

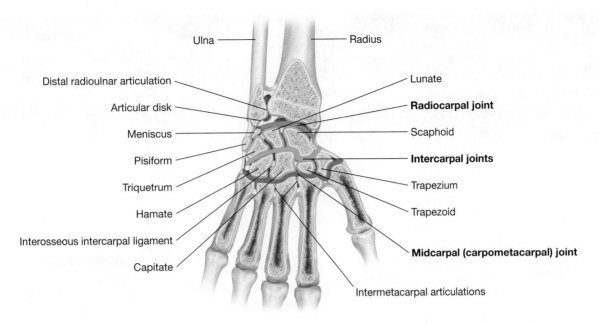

FIGURE 17.22
Joints of the wrist

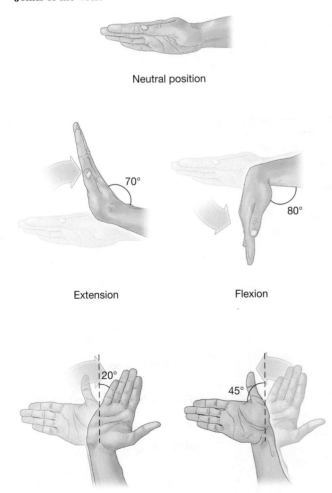

FIGURE 17.23
Wrist range of motion

direction (Figure 17.24a ■). A **radial collateral ligament** binds the styloid process of the radius to the scaphoid and trapezium and restricts excessive ulnar devation. An **ulnar collateral ligament** binds the styloid process of the ulna to the pisiform and triquetrum and restricts excessive radial deviation. Two thick and broad ligaments, the **palmar radiocarpal ligament** and **palmar ulnocarpal ligament,** connect the distal end of the radius and ulna to the carpals and restrict excessive wrist extension (Figure 17.24b ■). A thick, diagonal **posterior radiocarpal ligament** connects the radius to the scaphoid, lunate, and triquetrum and restricts excessive wrist flexion.

A broad, flat **transverse carpal ligament** (flexor retinaculum ligament) runs across the base of the palm, connecting the hamate and pisiform on the radial side to the scaphoid and trapezium on the ulnar side. This ligament forms the **carpal tunnel** located on the anterior side of the wrist and crosses the median nerve and the following 10 tendons (Figure 17.25 ■):

● Four tendons from the flexor digitorum profundus
● Four tendons from the flexor digitorum superficialis
● The flexor carpi radialis tendon
● The flexor pollicis longus tendon

A widespread condition that narrows the tunnel, called **carpal tunnel syndrome,** plagues people working in occupations that require repetitive hand movements, such as assembly line workers and those who use a computer keyboard and/or mouse for much of the work day. This common syndrome compresses the median nerve and the tendons running through the tunnel, causing inflammation and pain in the hand and wrist, numbness and tingling in the fingers, and weakness in the hand that manifests as the loss of grip strength.

TABLE 17.1	Range of Motion in the Wrist	
Wrist Motion	Range of Motion	End-Feel
Flexion	80 degrees	Firm
Hyperextension	70 degrees	Firm
Ulnar deviation (abduction)	45 degrees	Firm
Radial deviation (adduction)	20 degrees	Firm

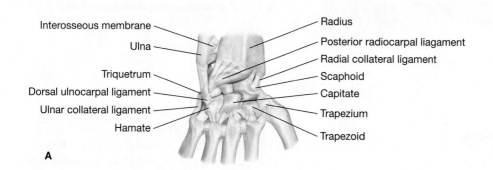

A

FIGURE 17.24

Ligaments of the wrist:
a) Posterior view b) Anterior view

B

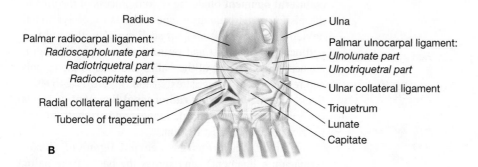

FIGURE 17.25

Carpal tunnel: cross section

BRIDGE TO PRACTICE
Preventing Carpal Tunnel Compression

You can prevent compression of the carpal tunnel by stretching the transverse carpal ligament. To do so, apply deep cross-fiber stripping between the base of the thumb and the base of the little finger. Passive stretching of the wrist and muscles whose tendons run through the tunnel is also important to prevent carpal tunnel compression. Avoid working on tissues over the carpal tunnel if it is inflamed.

EXPLORING TECHNIQUE
Passive Range of Motion for the Wrist

For each of the PROM steps below, begin with your partner supine or sitting. With your partner's forearm and hand in the neutral position, hold the forearm above the wrist in one hand and the palm in the other hand. Before you begin, read through these guidelines:

- Have your partner agree to report any pain or discomfort he or she feels during the motion. During the exercise, watch for signs of pain or discomfort and stop if you notice any pain reactions.
- Stabilize the wrist by holding the forearm above the wrist with one hand, and the palm of the hand with your other hand. The forearm can be either pronated or supinated. Keep the forearm and palm in the same plane as you move; avoid twisting the wrist.

- Hold the wrist in a neutral position, then apply traction. Maintain the traction as you move the wrist to avoid pinching structures in the wrist.
- Slowly move the hand along a linear pathway.
- When you feel you have reached the end range of motion, ask your partner if she or he feels a stretch, which will indicate you have reached the end range.
- Perform all the PROM tests on both wrists to make a bilateral comparison.

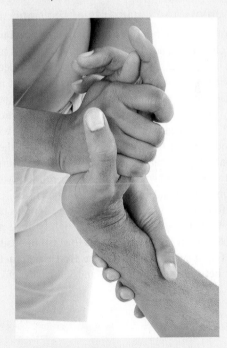

FIGURE 17.26b

b) PROM for wrist extension

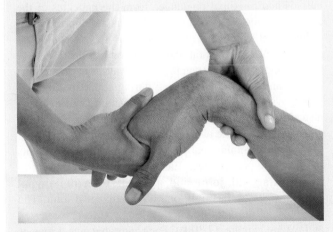

FIGURE 17.26a

a) PROM for wrist flexion

1. **Wrist flexion:** Begin by applying light traction, then passively flex the wrist until your partner reports a stretch (Figure 17.26a ■). *To what degree can the wrist be passively flexed?*

2. **Wrist extension:** Begin by applying light traction, then passively extend the wrist until your partner reports a stretch (Figure 17.26b ■). *To what degree can the wrist be passively extended?*

(continued)

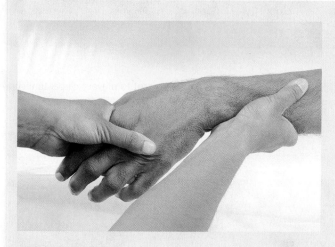

FIGURE 17.26c

c) PROM for ulnar deviation

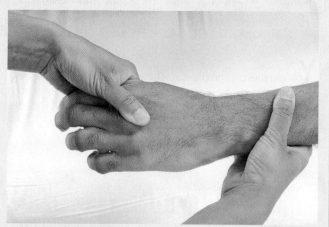

FIGURE 17.26d

d) PROM for radial deviation

3. **Ulnar deviation** (abduction): Begin by applying light traction, then passively side-bend the wrist toward the ulnar side until your partner reports a stretch (Figure 17.26c ■). *To what degree can the wrist be passively abducted?*

4. **Radial deviation** (adduction): Begin by applying light traction, then passively side-bend the wrist toward the radial side until your partner reports a stretch (Figure 17.26d ■). *To what degree can the wrist be passively adducted? Do you notice how much farther you can abduct the wrist than adduct it?*

17.2.4   Joints and Ligaments of the Hand

A series of small gliding joints called the **carpometacarpal joints** occupy the space between the distal carpals and the proximal metacarpals. The CMC joints are also collectively called the *midcarpal joint*. Although their range of motion is minimal, they contribute to a greater range of motion in the wrist. In this group of joints, the trapezium articulates with the first metacarpal; the trapezoid articulates with the second metacarpal; the capitate articulates with the third metacarpal; and the hamate articulates with the fourth and fifth metacarpals. The CMC joints are relatively stable gliding joints that contribute to wrist and hand stability.

The fourth carpometacarpal joint between the hamate and the fourth and fifth metacarpals is slightly more mobile than the other carpometacarpal joints to allow opposition of the little finger with the thumb. The **first carpometacarpal joint** between the trapezium and the first metacarpal

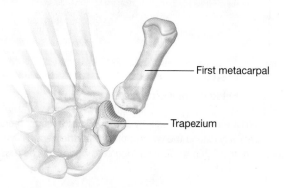

FIGURE 17.27

Saddle joint at base of thumb

is the highly mobile saddle joint at the base of the thumb (Figure 17.27 ■). This unique joint allows the thumb to fold across the palm toward the little finger in movements called **opposition** and **reposition.** The thumb flexes and extends in the same plane as the palm and abducts and adducts in a plane perpendicular to the palm (Figure 17.28 ■).

The **metacarpophalangeal joints** between the metacarpals and proximal phalanges form the knuckles of the hand. Each metacarpophalangeal joint is an ellipsoid (condyloid) joint with two degrees of motion: flexion and extension as well as abduction and adduction (Figure 17.29 ■). During abduction, the fingers move away from the midline of the hand (the middle finger); during adduction, the fingers move toward the midline of the hand. Each finger can also move in a combination of flexion, extension, abduction, and adduction, in the twirling motion of circumduction.

The **interphalangeal joints** are formed by articulations between the phalanges. Each finger has a **proximal interphalangeal joint** and a **distal interphalangeal joint**; the thumb has only one interphalangeal joint. The interphalangeal joints are uniaxial hinge joints that can flex and extend (Figure 17.30 ■). Each interphalangeal joint is covered by a small joint capsule that is stabilized on each side by tiny collateral ligaments that restrict accessory motions such as twisting and side-bending.

17.2.5   Hand Arches and Grips

The arches of the hand ensure the ability to grip and grasp things, allowing the hand to shape around variable objects. In a resting state, the hand curls into a natural, open curve with three arches. A **distal carpal arch** runs across the anterior

Labels on Figure 17.27: First metacarpal; Trapezium

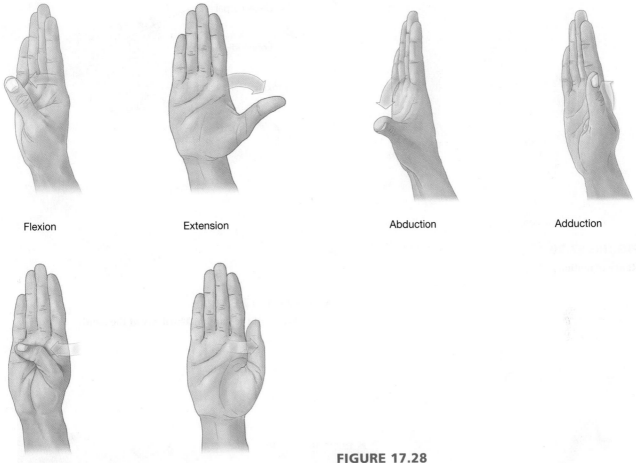

Flexion

Extension

Abduction

Adduction

Opposition

Reposition

FIGURE 17.28
Range of motion of the thumb

surface of the knuckles, between the heads of the metacarpals; a **proximal carpal arch** runs from the base of the thumb across the base of the metacarpals; a series of four **longitudinal arches** run from the base of each metacarpal along the inside of the corresponding finger (Figure 17.31a ■). The keystone of the central longitudinal arch is the third finger, third metacarpal, and capitate bone, which align along the midline of the fingers, hand, and wrist (Figure 17.31b ■).

The refined muscular control of the hands allows a person the dexterity to grasp or manipulate objects of different sizes and shapes in a variety of grips (Figure 17.32 a-e ■). There are two basic types of grips: a power grip and a precision grip. A person can grasp a tool or handle with a **power grip** that requires force, such as pounding a nail with a hammer or pulling a cart by its handle. There are several types of power grips. We use a **cylindrical grip** to hold onto a

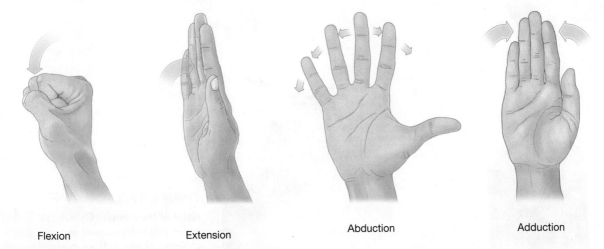

Flexion

Extension

Abduction

Adduction

FIGURE 17.29
Range of motion of MCP joints

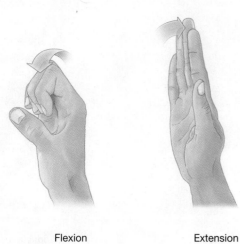

Flexion   Extension

FIGURE 17.30

Range of motion of IP joints

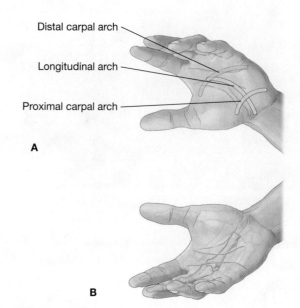

Distal carpal arch

Longitudinal arch

Proximal carpal arch

A

B

FIGURE 17.31

a) **Arches of the hand** b) **Third ray of the hand**

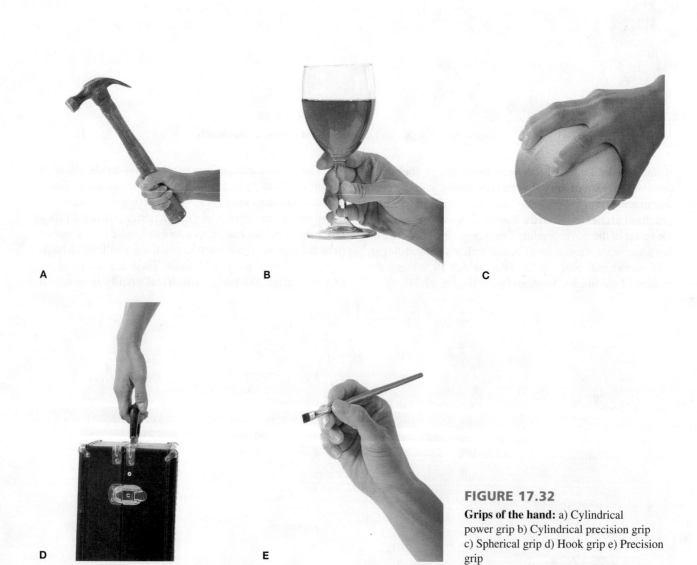

A

B

C

D

E

FIGURE 17.32

Grips of the hand: a) Cylindrical power grip b) Cylindrical precision grip c) Spherical grip d) Hook grip e) Precision grip

BRIDGE TO PRACTICE
Accessory Movements in the Fingers

The interphalangeal joints are susceptible to stress from accessory movements. For this reason, avoid twisting, side-bending, or pulling your client's fingers, especially on arthritic joints. Lateral or rotational movements of the fingers, or excessive traction, could injure damaged tissues and flare up symptoms of arthritis. Such unnatural movements could even injure healthy fingers. Petrissage and pressure point therapy on the muscles in the palm of the hand is effective for working with hand problems. Arthritic joints also respond well to joint approximation.

chinning bar, a **spherical grip** to hold a round object such as a ball, and a **hook grip** to hold the handle of a bag or suitcase. It is possible to sustain a hook grip for a long time without tiring because of the strength of the finger flexors.

A person uses a **precision grip** during activities that require fine motor control, such as drawing a picture or threading a needle. There are many types of precision grips. Consider the different ways you use your hand to hold a pen, a plate, or a penny.

17.3 MUSCLES OF THE ARM AND HAND

The muscles of the arm and hand are intricate and closely match the arrangement of muscles in the leg and foot. We look at this complex group of muscles according to their actions in the following five categories:

Elbow flexors and extensors:

- Flexors: *Biceps brachii, brachialis,* and *brachioradialis*
- Extensors: *Triceps brachii* and *anconeus*

Supinators and pronators:

- Supinators: *Biceps brachii* and *supinator*
- Pronators: *Pronator teres* and *pronator quadratus*

Wrist and finger flexors and extensors:

- Flexors: *Flexor carpi ulnaris, flexor carpi radialis, flexor digitorum superficialis, flexor digitorum profundus,* and *palmaris longus*
- Extensor: *Extensor carpi radialis longus, extensor carpi radialis brevis, extensor carpi ulnaris, extensor digitorum,* and *extensor indicis*

Muscles of the thumb:

- Extrinsic (long) muscles of the thumb: *Flexor pollicis longus, extensor pollicis longus, extensor pollicis brevis,* and *abductor pollicis longus*
- Intrinsic (short) muscles of the thumb: *Opponens pollicis, abductor pollicis brevis, adductor pollicis,* and *flexor pollicis brevis*

SELF-CARE
Grip Strength and Joint Alignment for Massage

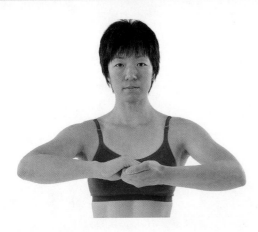

1. **Strengthening your finger flexors:** The flexed position of the fingers can be a powerful tool in massage. Strengthen your hook grip by practicing isometric finger pulls (Figure 17.33a ■). Hook your fingers together and pull for several seconds. As you do this exercise, make sure to keep your forearms aligned along the same axis and your palms in the same plane as your forearms. Avoid bending the wrists. You can also hang by your fingertips on a chinning bar or door frame.

FIGURE 17.33a

(continued)

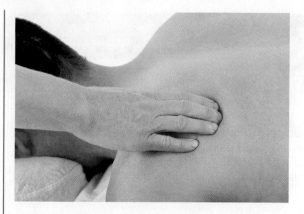

FIGURE 17.33b

2. **Pushing with the middle finger:** Cultivate a line of force through the middle arch of your hands by applying slow pressure with the middle finger (Figure 17.33b ■). As you do this exercise, be sure to keep your wrist extended and your middle finger lined up with the middle of your forearm.

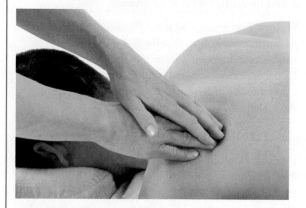

FIGURE 17.33c

3. **Hand-over-hand force:** Explore a hand-over-hand technique to apply finger pressure with maximum force (Figure 17.33c ■). Lean your body weight into your fingertips to increase your pressure.

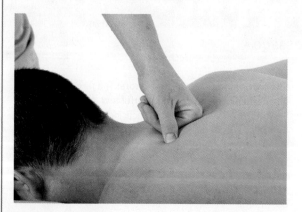

FIGURE 17.33d

4. **Stacking your joints:** Practice stacking the joints of your thumb in a straight line with your radius, then applying slow pressure through the thumb (Figure 17.33d ■). Stabilize your hand when using your thumb by resting your hand on a relaxed fist.

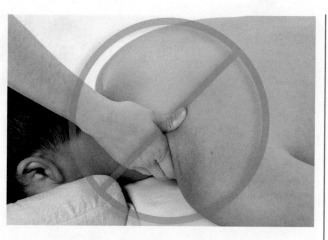

FIGURE 17.33e

5. **Protecting your thumb:** Avoid hyperextending your thumb, which could damage the joints (Figure 17.33e ■). If your thumbs hyperextend and you cannot get them straight when you apply direct pressure, use another hand position.

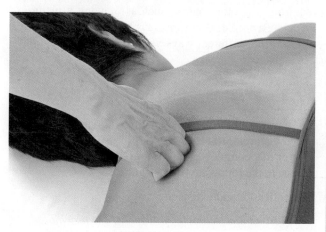

FIGURE 17.33f

6. **Using your knuckles:** Explore working with your knuckles (Figure 17.33f ■). The same alignment principles apply: Keep your wrist straight and your middle knuckle aligned with the center of your forearm.

Muscles of the hand:

- Between the metacarpals: *Palmar interossei, dorsal interossei,* and *lumbricals*
- Acting on the little finger: *Extensor digiti minimi, abductor digiti minimi, opponens digiti minimi,* and *flexor digiti minimi brevis*

Muscle-use patterns in the arms and hands usually reflect the types of activities and repetitive grips that a person uses during work-related activities. Looking at a person's repetitive hand movements during daily activities can shed light on the stress patterns that a client can develop in the arm muscles. For example, a potter pulls a pot up from a lump of clay by positioning the forearm in pronation and holding the hand in a straight-fingered pincher grip. This gives the forearm flexors and the lumbrical muscles of the hand an isometric workout, which can lead to stiffness and tightness in the hands and forearms. To counter this stress, a practitioner can stretch the transverse arches of the palm to widen the hand and the carpal tunnel, then stretch the pronator and flexor muscles of the forearm. Balance can then be restored to hand and forearm muscles by helping the potter client engage underused muscles—in this case, the finger extensors and supinators—with resisted movement exercises.

As you study the muscles of the arm and hand, consider how the hands work in various tasks. Assess the alignment of the joints for different tasks, determining which muscles might overwork and what range of movement would counterbalance the joint and muscle stress that the task requires.

As you palpate the fingers, keep in mind that no muscles attach directly on the fingers themselves. Although tendons and connective tissue membranes run along each finger, and small ligaments and joint capsules cover the joints in each finger, all muscles acting on the fingers are located in the palms of the hands or the forearms. To be effective, hands-on techniques to treat muscles of the fingers should be performed directly on the muscle tissue in either the palms of the hands and the forearms. Deep tissue work on the fingers themselves, such as linear stripping, could damage their small and intricate tissues. The same holds true for the toes.

17.3.1 Flexors and Extensors of the Elbow

Five muscles cross the elbow: three flexors—the *biceps brachii, brachialis,* and *brachioradialis*—and two extensors—the *triceps brachii* and *anconeus*. Both the triceps brachii and the biceps brachii also cross the shoulder, although their actions at the elbow are stronger. The brachioradialis attaches to the radial side of the wrist and acts on both the elbow and wrist.

A number of somatic writers have referred to the modern, sedentary culture as a flexion culture, meaning most daily activities take the body into flexion or encourage flexion. From bucket seats in our cars to soft couches that curl the spine, flexor muscles often become more developed than the extensors. This is particularly true around the elbow. Most people tend to use the flexors of the elbow more than the extensors. As a result, it is likely that you will encounter a number of massage clients with weak triceps and tight elbow flexors.

17.3.1.1 BICEPS BRACHII, BRACHIALIS, AND BRACHIORADIALIS

Each of the three flexors of the elbow—the biceps brachii, brachialis, and brachioradialis—works in a different capacity, depending on whether the forearm is supinated or pronated and whether or not flexion occurs against resistance (Figure 17.34 ■). The biceps contracts during supinated elbow flexion but not during pronation unless flexion occurs against resistance. When the forearm is pronated, the brachialis works as the prime elbow flexor. During quick movements or when the elbow is under heavy load, the brachioradialis works as a strong elbow flexor; otherwise, it is relatively silent during flexion. The biceps brachii and brachialis are innervated by the *musculocutaneous nerve;* the brachioradialis is innervated by the *radial nerve.*

The **biceps brachii** is a two-headed fusiform muscle with unique origins and insertions. The tendon of the short head runs directly from its origin on the coracoid process to its insertion on the proximal, anterior forearm below the crease of the elbow. In contrast, the tendon of the long head runs from its origin on the supraglenoid tubercle of the glenoid fossa into the joint capsule of the shoulder, then turns a corner and runs down the bicipital groove toward the same

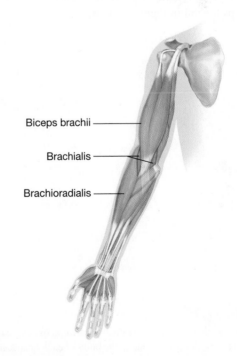

FIGURE 17.34
Biceps brachii, brachialis, and brachioradialis

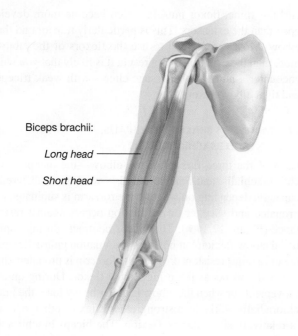

Biceps brachii:

Long head

Short head

FIGURE 17.35
Biceps brachii

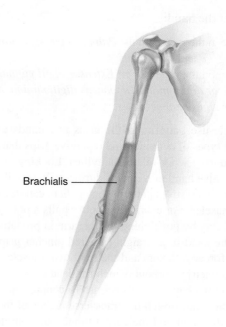

Brachialis

FIGURE 17.37
Brachialis

insertion (Figure 17.35 ■). The two heads converge into a cord-like tendon that bifurcates below the elbow, inserting into the posterior aspect of the tuberosity of the radius and on the fascia of the forearm flexors. Minimal contraction occurs in the long head of the biceps during shoulder flexion without resistance, but both heads contract forcefully during shoulder flexion against resistance. (See TrPs for the biceps brachii in Figure 17.36 ■).

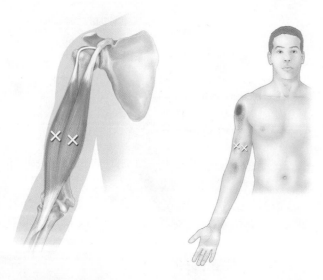

FIGURE 17.36

When overworked and dysfunctional, the **biceps brachii** can develop two trigger points, one in the belly of each head that can refer an aching pain over the anterior shoulder and into the crease of the elbow. Trigger points in the biceps brachii can restrict the range of motion in both the shoulder and the elbow.

The **brachialis** arises from an extensive origin along the lower half of the anterior humerus, then tapers into a flat tendon that wraps around the medial side of the upper forearm, inserting on the coronoid process and tuberosity of the ulna (Figure 17.37 ■). This somewhat flat yet powerful muscle lies under the biceps brachii and works as a forceful elbow flexor and an antagonist to the triceps brachii. (See TrPs for the brachialis in Figure 17.38 ■).

The **brachioradialis** arises from the upper two-thirds of the supracondylar ridge above the lateral epicondyle via a long, thin tendon attached to the base of the styloid process of the radius (Figure 17.39 ■). As mentioned earlier, the brachioradialis flexes the elbow during quick or loaded movements. It also stabilizes the forearm in a midposition between supination and pronation, with the thumb up, during ballistic elbow movement such as pounding nails. (See TrP for the brachioradialis in Figure 17.40 ■).

17.3.1.2 TRICEPS BRACHII AND ANCONEUS

The **triceps brachii** is a large bipennate muscle with a long head that arises from the infraglenoid tubercle of the scapula, a medial head that arises from the distal half of the posterior humeral shaft, and a lateral head that arises from the upper half of the posterior humeral shaft. All three heads of the triceps converge into a strong tendon that inserts on the posterior surface of the olecranon. The medial head lies deep to the other two heads and functions as a primary elbow extensor. The lateral head assists elbow extension, and all three heads contract during

FIGURE 17.38

When dysfunctional, the **brachialis** develop several trigger points scattered throughout its belly, which can refer pain over the anterior deltoid as well as pain, soreness, and numbness into the base of the thumb. Brachialis contractures can also entrap the brachial nerve.

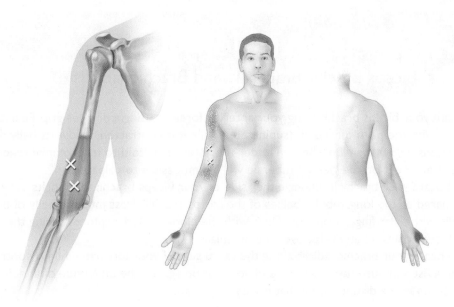

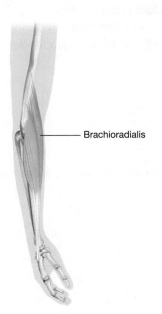

FIGURE 17.39

Brachioradialis

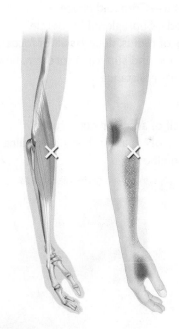

FIGURE 17.40

When dysfunctional, the **brachioradialis** can develop a trigger point in its belly directly below the crease of the elbow that can refer pain over the olecranon process and into the web of the thumb.

MUSCLE PALPATION
Biceps Brachii, Brachialis, and Brachioradialis

Palpate your biceps brachii along your anterior forearm using a pincher grip. Feel it contract by flexing the elbow with the palm turned up (supinated). While it is contracted, follow its belly down to its tendon and two insertions below the elbow and up under the anterior deltoid to its proximal tendon on the coracoid process. The attachment on the glenoid tubercle will be impossible to palpate.

Locate your brachialis under either side of your biceps brachii tendon. Its belly will feel large and meaty compared to the long, tubular bellies of the biceps brachii. Press into the belly of both the biceps and the brachialis with a flat-finger palpation. Then, with the elbow flexed, explore turning the palm up and down to feel the biceps contract and relax over the brachialis.

Locate your brachioradialis along the radial side of your forearm while it contracts. To get it to contract, make a fist and push the thumb side of your fist up against the underside of a table or desk. When it contracts, it pops up into a distinct bulge that is easy to palpate.

Biceps Brachii

O–Short head—Coracoid process
   Long head—Supraglenoid tubercle
I–Tuberosity of radius, deep fascia of forearm
A–Flexes elbow and supinates forearm, flexes GH
   joint against resistance

Brachialis

O–Lower half of anterior humerus
I–Coronoid process and tuberosity of ulna
A–Flexes the elbow

Brachioradialis

O–Upper two-thirds of lateral supracondylar ridge
I–Base of styloid process of radius
A–Flexes elbow under load and during rapid motion,
   stabilizes elbow during rapid motion

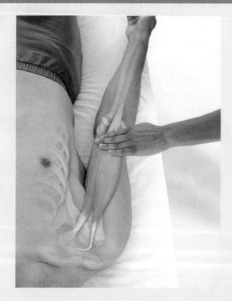

FIGURE 17.41a

Palpating the biceps brachii

With your partner in a supine position, palpate the **biceps brachii** using a pincher palpation to follow the muscle bellies down the anterior side of the upper arm (Figure 17.41a ■). Follow the tubular bellies down to its tendons directly below the elbow. *Do you feel the difference between the cord-like distal tendon and the meaty, tubular belly of the muscle?*

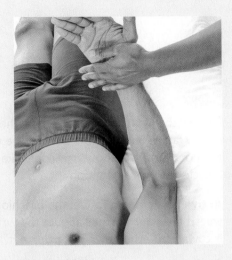

FIGURE 17.41b

Resisted movement of the biceps brachii

Active movement: Palpate the biceps while your partner holds the elbow in flexion, then alternately supinates and pronates the forearm. *Do you feel the biceps tendon at the elbow relax as your partner pronates?*

Resisted movement: Have your partner resist as you slowly press your partner's forearm in a down-ward direction (Figure 17.41b ■). By pressing above the wrist, you avoid engaging the wrist flexors.

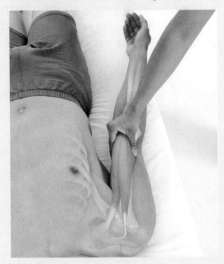

FIGURE 17.41c

Palpating the brachialis

Palpate the **brachialis** under both sides of the biceps brachii tendon (Figure 17.41c ■). You can also locate the meaty muscle between the triceps brachii and biceps brachii above the lateral epicondyle. *Are you palpating above the crease of the elbow? Do you feel how close the broad muscle belly of the brachialis is to the elbow?*

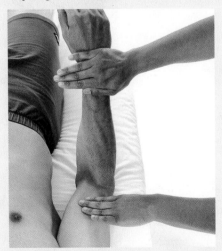

FIGURE 17.41d

Resisted movement of the brachialis

Active movement: Have your partner flex the elbow, then palpate the brachialis as your partner supinates and pronates the forearm. *When your part-ner pronates, can you feel the brachialis more clearly as the overlying biceps brachii relaxes?*

Resisted movement: Have your partner resist while you push the wrist down (Figure 17.41d ■).

(continued)

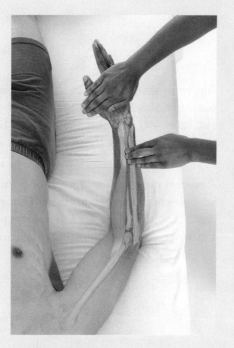

FIGURE 17.41e

Palpating the brachioradioalis contraction

Palpate the **brachioradialis** along the outer shaft of the radius between the base of the thumb and the crease of the elbow. It will feel like a thin, tubular muscle with a long tendon.

Active movement: To feel the brachioradialis contract, have your partner abduct the wrist by bending it toward the thumb as you palpate it.

Resisted movement: Hold your partner's hand as though you were shaking hands, then have your partner resist as you push your partner's hand down (Figure 17.41e ■). *Do you feel the brachioradialis pop up along the radial side of the forearm?*

resisted extension (Figure 17.42 ■). The long head of the triceps is a biarticular muscle that crosses two joints and assists shoulder extension and adduction. Although it is a powerful elbow extensor when pushing against resistance, the triceps brachii is frequently assisted by gravity in elbow extension, so it tends to be weak when not regularly used against resistance. (See TrPs for the triceps brachii in Figure 17.43 ■).

The **anconeus** is a small triangular muscle that arises from the posterior surface of the lateral epicondyle and inserts on the posterior side of the proximal ulna, below the olecranon. The primary role of the anconeus is as a stabilizer of the elbow, but it also assists the triceps brachii during slow elbow extension. During elbow extension, it should contract prior to the triceps brachii to stabilize the elbow joint. (See TrP for the anconeus in Figure 17.44 ■).

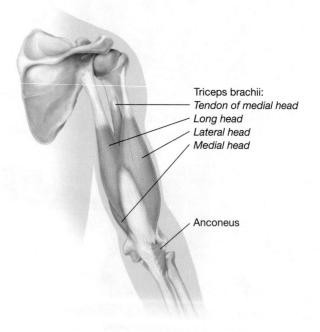

Triceps brachii:
Tendon of medial head
Long head
Lateral head
Medial head

Anconeus

FIGURE 17.42
Triceps brachii

FIGURE 17.43

When the **triceps brachii** develops active trigger points and becomes shortened, a person will be unable to abduct the shoulder and extend the arm overhead to touch the ear. When dysfunctional, the triceps brachii can develop six trigger points, each with a specific referral pattern:

a) Two trigger points along the belly of the long head can refer pain into the posterior shoulder and radial side of the posterior elbow.

b) A trigger point in the lateral side of the medial head slightly above the elbow can refer pain into the ulnar side of the posterior elbow. This trigger point is common when a person has "tennis elbow" (lateral epicondylitis), which is discussed in the section on the extensor carpi radialis brevis.

c) A trigger point deep in the medial side of the medial head slightly can refer pain into the ulnar side of the posterior elbow and the fourth and fifth fingers.

d) A trigger point in the tendon can refer pain over the olecranon process.

e) A trigger point deep in the middle of the belly of the lateral head can refer pain locally. Taut bands in the lateral head can entrap the radial nerve.

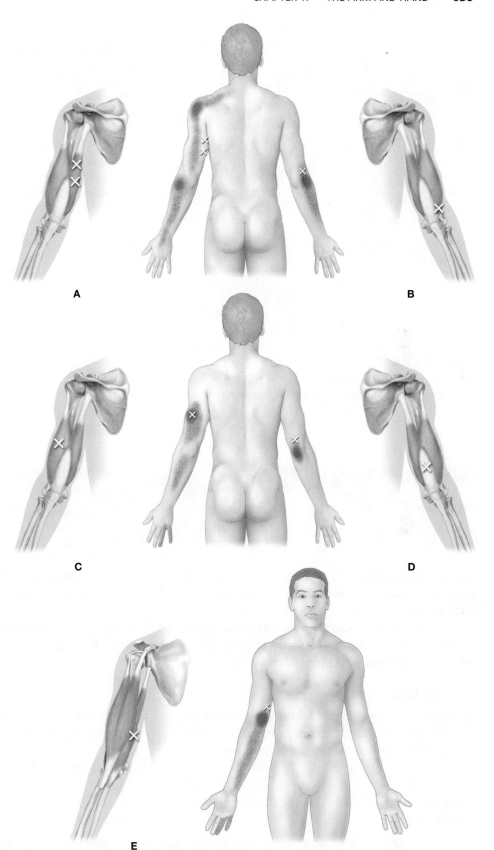

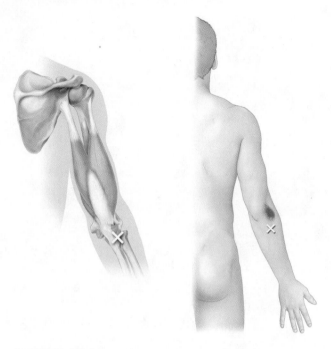

FIGURE 17.44

When dysfunctional, the **anconeus** can develop a trigger point in its belly that refers pain locally on the ulnar side of the posterior elbow.

17.3.2 Supinators and Pronators

Two muscles work as forearm supinators—the *biceps brachii* and the *supinator*—and two muscles work as forearm pronators—the *pronator teres* and *pronator quadratus*. The supinators and pronators turn the palm up and down to increase the range of dexterity in the hands. A typist uses the pronators to keep the palms facing the keyboard. In contrast, a waitress uses the supinator to carry a tray in the palm of the hand. To remember which is which, imagine the waitress "soup"-inating the forearm to carry a bowl of soup. The supinator muscle is innervated by the *radial nerve*. The pronators are innervated by the *median nerve*.

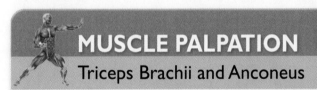

MUSCLE PALPATION
Triceps Brachii and Anconeus

Squeeze the large bulk of tissue in the triceps brachii along the back side of your upper arm. To feel it contract, press the ulnar side of your hand or fist down on a table while you explore the length and size of the triceps contraction.

Locate the superficial anconeus by pressing on the lateral side of the olecranon between the ulna and the lateral epicondyle. Slowly press your hand or fist into the table to feel the anconeus contract; as it contracts, you should feel the small bulge of its fibers.

Triceps Brachii

O—Long head—Infraglenoid tubercle of the scapula
    Medial head—Distal half of posterior humerus
    Lateral head—Proximal half of posterior
                humerus
I—Olecranon
A—All heads extend elbow, long head assists GH joint extension and adduction

Anconeus

O—Posterior surface of lateral epicondyle
I—Posterior surface of proximal ulna below olecranon
A—Stabilizes elbow, assists slow elbow extension

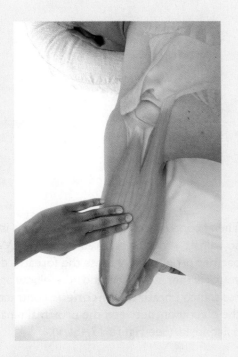

FIGURE 17.45a
Palpating the triceps brachii

With your partner in a prone position, locate the **triceps brachii** along the posterior shaft of the humerus (Figure 17.45a ■). Explore this large muscle from the elbow to the shoulder by grasping it along its length. Gently squeeze it and lift it away from the humerus. *Do you notice how the triceps brachii forms the muscular bulk along the back of the humerus? As you squeeze the triceps, do you feel where it attaches to the shaft of the humerus?*

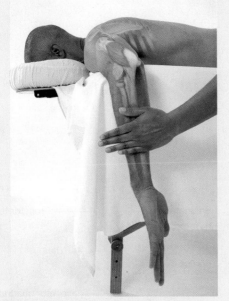

FIGURE 17.45b
Resisted movement of the triceps brachii

Active movement: Have your partner extend the elbow as you palpate the medial head of the triceps closest to the elbow. Then have your partner bend the elbow and raise the entire arm while you palpate. Its tendon bulge right below the posterior shoulder joint, between the teres major and teres minor tendons.

Resisted movement: Have your partner extend the elbow as you apply resistance on the forearm (Figure 17.45b ■).

(continued)

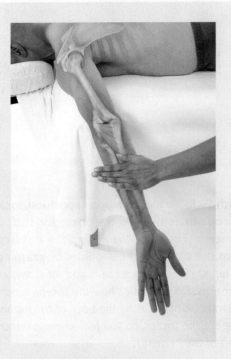

FIGURE 17.45c

Resisted movement of the anconeus

The anconeus is difficult to find when it is relaxed, so palpate it during resisted movement. With your partner prone, gently press the forearm down while your partner slowly extends the elbow against light resistance Locate the **anconeus** contraction below the olecranon, between the proximal ulna and lateral epicondyle. (See Figure 17.45c ■).

The **supinator** is a large muscle with a long origin that runs from the lateral epicondyle and the annular and radial collateral ligaments to the supinator crest along the lateral, proximal ulna (Figure 17.46 ■). In a relaxed state, the supinator spirals around the proximal end of the radius and inserts on the anterior, lateral side of the proximal third of the radius. Upon contraction, it rotates the head of the radius against the ulna to supinate the forearm. It works as the primary supinator of the forearm during elbow flexion and is assisted in supination by the biceps brachii during elbow flexion. (See TrP for the supinator in Figure 17.47 ■.)

The **pronator teres** has two origins: one directly above the common flexor tendon that hooks over the top of the medial epicondyle and a second on the medial border of the coronoid process of the ulna (Figure 17.48 ■). Its long fibers descend obliquely across the anterior, ulnar side of the proximal forearm and insert in the middle of the lateral side of the radius. This flat, strapping muscle pronates the forearm and assists elbow flexion against resistance. (See TrP for the pronator teres in Figure 17.49 ■.)

The **pronator quadratus** is a rectangular muscle crossing the anterior side of the forearm above the wrist. It runs from its origin along the anterior surface of the distal ulna to its insertion on the anterior surface of the distal radius. The pronator quadratus is strategically located to work as the primary pronator of the forearm. No trigger point has been identified for this deep, flat muscle and it is difficult to palpate because of its deep location.

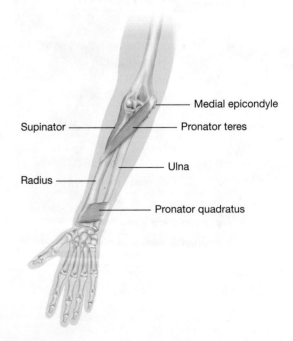

FIGURE 17.46

Supinator and pronators: in supination

FIGURE 17.47

When dysfunctional, the **supinator** can develop a trigger point near the radius that refers pain over the lateral crease of the elbow and into the web of the thumb. It becomes stressed and overloaded from quick movements that supinate the forearm, such as snapping a Frisbee or flipping a board. Chronic tension in the supinator can entrap the radial nerve, which runs through the belly of this muscle. Pain from supinator entrapment mimics pain from "tennis elbow" (lateral epicondylitis), which is discussed in the section on the extensor carpi radialis brevis.

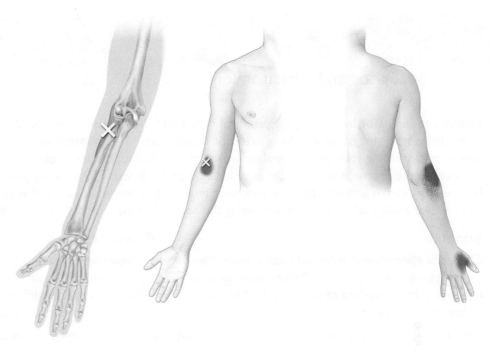

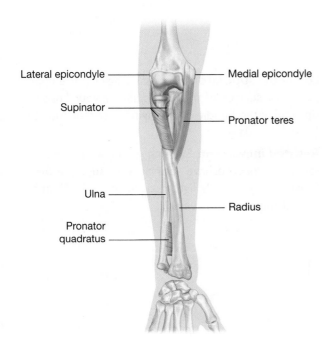

FIGURE 17.48

Supinator and pronators: in pronation

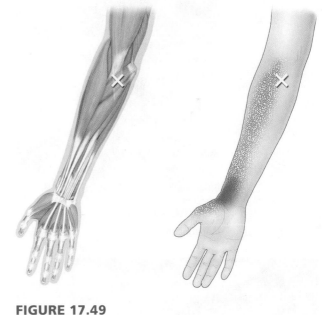

FIGURE 17.49

When dysfunctional, the **pronator teres** can develop a trigger point in the middle of its belly, which can refer pain down the radial side of the forearm into the wrist and thumb.

MUSCLE PALPATION
Supinator and Pronator Teres

Palpate the supinator by locating the proximal radius and the lateral epicondyle, then sink your fingertips under the dorsal side of the overlying extensor muscles into the supinator belly. Confirm your location on the supinator by turning your palm up and down. You should feel it alternately contract and relax.

Palpate the pronator teres on the anterior side of the forearm by pressing your fingertips into the tissues between the radius and ulna, then running your fingertips up and down along this space. The pronator teres will feel like a bulge of oblique fibers crossing the top half of the interosseous membrane.

Supinator

O–Lateral epicondyle, annular and radial collateral ligaments, supinator crest along lateral, proximal ulna
I–Anterior, lateral surface of proximal third of radius
A–Supinates forearm

Pronator Teres

O–Superior to medial epicondyle, on medial border of coronoid process
I–Middle of lateral surface of radius
A–Pronates forearm, assists elbow flexion

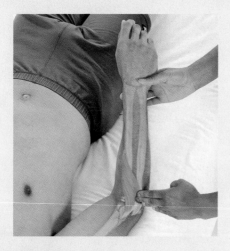

FIGURE 17.50a
Palpating the supinator

Locate the **supinator** by pressing against the upper, posterior surface of the radius, sliding your fingertips under the bundle of overlying extensor muscles (Figure 17.50a ■).

Resisted movement: Starting with your partner's forearm pronated, have your partner supinate the forearm as you apply light resistance to the thumb side of the back of the hand.

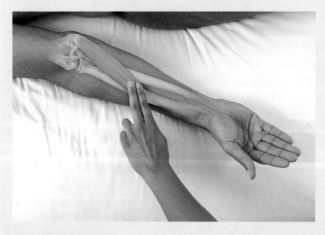

With your partner in a supine position, locate the **pronator teres** by sliding your fingertips up and down the anterior forearm, between the radius and ulna (Figure 17.50b ■). *Do you feel oblique fibers across the interosseous space several inches below the elbow?*

Active movement: Have your partner slowly turn the palm down to feel the pronator teres contract.

FIGURE 17.50b
Palpating the pronator teres

17.3.3 Flexors and Extensors of the Wrist and Hand

The muscles of the forearm are intricate and there is a relative symmetry between the superficial flexors and extensors of the wrist. The wrist flexors and wrist extensors share similar names and have a relatively square spatial arrangement around the wrist. The flexor carpi ulnaris and flexor carpi radialis run along the anterior side of the forearm and are mirrored by the extensor carpi ulnaris, extensor carpi radialis brevis, and extensor carpi radialis on the posterior side of the forearm (Figure 17.51 ■).

The fingers only bend in one direction, toward the palm, so it follows that the finger flexors would be stronger than the finger extensors. This logic is evident in the structure of the finger flexors compared to the finger extensors. A double layer of finger flexors—the flexor digitorum superficialis and the flexor digitorum profundus—are much larger and stronger muscles than their antagonist, the extensor digitorum. In addition, the group of flexors is twice the thickness of the group of extensors. Palpating individual muscles in the flexor group can be difficult because of their proximity, but it is possible to differentiate them by their actions.

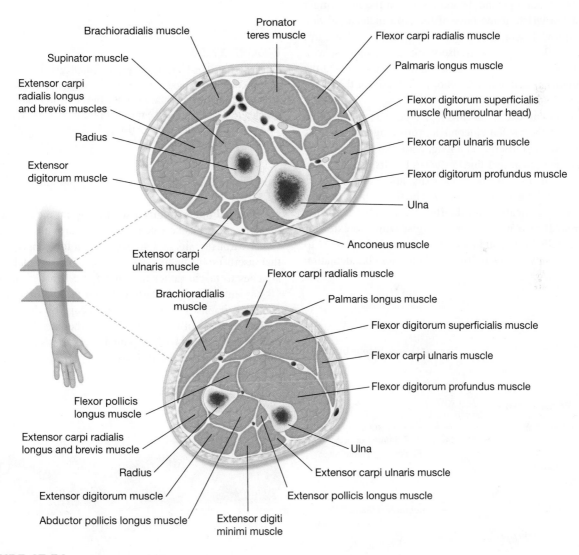

FIGURE 17.51

Cross section of the forearm: Note the relative symmetry of flexors and extensors of the forearm.

17.3.3.1 FLEXOR CARPI ULNARIS, FLEXOR CARPI RADIALIS, PALMARIS LONGUS, FLEXOR DIGITORUM PROFUNDUS, AND FLEXOR DIGITORUM SUPERFICIALIS

There are five flexors of the wrist and fingers located on the anterior side of the forearm. Four of them—the flexor carpi radialis, flexor digitorum superficialis and flexor digitorum profundus, and the palmaris longus—are innervated by the *median nerve.* The fifth flexor—the flexor carpi ulnaris—is innervated by the *ulnar nerve,* which also innervates part of the flexor digitorum profundus. All the flexor muscles share a common flexor tendon on the medial epicondyle of the humerus. As a group, they form the plump bundle of muscles that runs down the inside of the forearm (Figure 17.52 ■).

The **flexor carpi ulnaris** is a tubular muscle that arises from the medial epicondyle and inserts on the little finger side of the wrist, at the base of the fifth metacarpal and the pisiform. It works as a synergist with the flexor carpi radialis to flex the wrist. It also works as a synergist with the extensor carpi ulnaris to side-bend the wrist toward the body in ulnar deviation (adduction). (See TrP for the flexor carpi ulnaris in Figure 17.53 ■.)

The **flexor carpi radialis** is a bipennate muscle that arises from the medial epicondyle, runs diagonally across the forearm, and inserts via a long, cord-like tendon on the base of the second and third metacarpals. Its distal tendon runs along the medial side of the radial artery and serves as a guide for taking a person's pulse. The flexor carpi radialis works synergistically with the flexor carpi ulnaris to flex the wrist. It also works as a synergist with the extensor carpi radialis brevis and extensor carpi radialis longus to side-bend the wrist away from the body in radial deviation

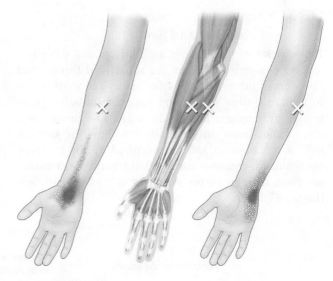

FIGURE 17.53

When dysfunctional, the **flexor carpi radialis** can develop a trigger point in the middle of the muscle that can refer pain to the radial side and center of the wrist; the **flexor carpi ulnaris** can develop a trigger point in the middle of the muscle that can refer pain to the medial side of the wrist.

(adduction). (See TrP for the flexor carpi radialis in Figure 17.53.)

The **palmaris longus** also arises from the medial epicondyle, then runs between the flexor carpi ulnaris and the flexor carpi radialis and spreads into a fan-shaped tendon that inserts on the palmar aponeurosis. This unusual muscle attaches to fascia rather than bone and is absent in about 10 percent of the population. When the palmaris longus contracts, it tenses the palmar fascia, cupping the palm and folding the base of the thumb toward the lateral side of the palm (Figure 17.54 ■). The palmaris also assists wrist flexion, although it is a weak flexor. (See TrP for the palmaris in Figure 17.55 ■.)

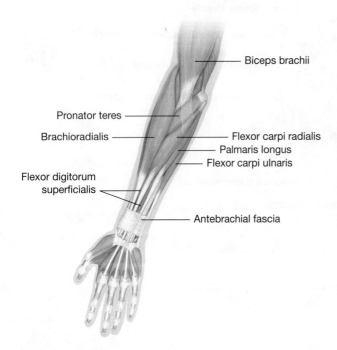

FIGURE 17.52
Flexors of the wrist and hand

Biceps brachii
Pronator teres
Brachioradialis
Flexor carpi radialis
Palmaris longus
Flexor carpi ulnaris
Flexor digitorum superficialis
Antebrachial fascia

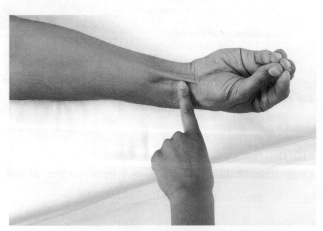

FIGURE 17.54
Palmaris contraction

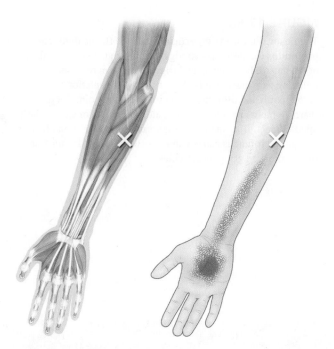

FIGURE 17.55

When dysfunctional, the **palmaris** can develop a trigger point in the middle of the muscle that can cause a distinct, prickling sensation in the center of the palm.

The **flexor digitorum superficialis** is a broad, bipennate muscle that lies under the flexor carpi ulnaris and flexor carpi radialis. It has an extensive origin that includes the medial epicondyle, the medial aspect of the coronoid process of the ulna, and the anterior shaft of the radius (Figure 17.56 ■). Its distal tendon divides into four tendons that each split into two tendons to insert on the sides of the middle phalanges of the four fingers. The flexor digitorum superficialis flexes the proximal interphalangeal joints. (See TrP for the flexor digitorum superficialis in Figure 17.58.)

A deeper **flexor digitorum profundus** is also a broad, bipennate muscle with an extensive origin. It arises along the middle, anterior surface of the proximal three-fourths of the ulna and the interosseous membrane (Figure 17.57 ■). Its distal tendon divides into four tendons that pass through the split tendon of the flexor digitorum superficialis to insert on the base of the distal phalanges of the four fingers. The flexor digitorum profundus flexes the DIPs. (See TrP for the flexor digitorum profundus in Figure 17.58 ■.)

A common and painful injury called **medial epicondylitis** is nicknamed "golfer's elbow" because it frequently occurs from repetitive strain to the flexor muscles during the forward swing. This condition results from the cumulative trauma that occurs when forceful, repeated contractions of the flexor muscles create microscopic tears in the common flexor tendon, which becomes inflamed and weakened. Over time the tendon, which is attached to the medial epicondyle, grows inflexible and scarred from chronic inflammation, exacerbating the condition. A person with medial epicondylitis develops weakness and pain in

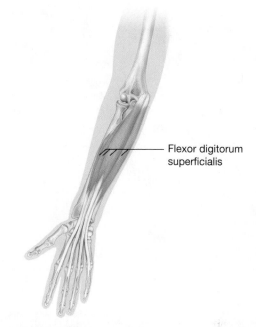

FIGURE 17.56
Flexor digitorum superficialis

the wrist during flexion and will lose grip strength. Treatment involves rest, ice, and cross-fiber stretching of the tendon, but only after the inflammation has subsided. If caught early enough, treatment can heal medial epicondylitis. The difficulty in treating golfer's elbow usually lies in getting a person to refrain from golfing and reinjuring it while the tissues heal.

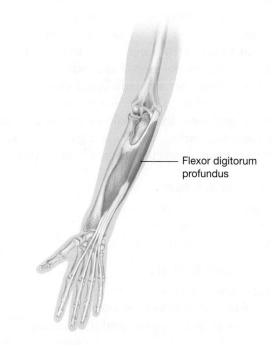

FIGURE 17.57
Flexor digitorum profundus

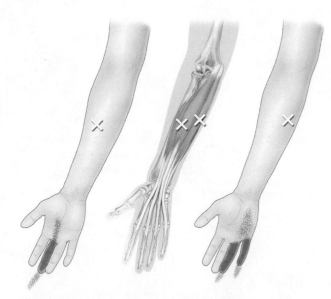

FIGURE 17.58

The **flexor digitorum superficialis** and the **flexor digitorum profundus** can develop two trigger points in the upper third of the muscle bellies: a lateral trigger point can refer sharp, lightning pain that extends along and past the anterior surface of the fourth and fifth fingers; a medial trigger point can refer sharp, lightning pain that extends along the anterior side of the middle finger. Both the flexor digitorum superficialis and flexor digitorum profundus can become overworked and dysfunctional from prolonged gripping activities.

MUSCLE PALPATION

Flexor Carpi Ulnaris, Flexor Carpi Radialis, Palmaris Longus, and Flexor Digitorum Superficialis and Profundus

To self-palpate the forearm flexors, turn your palm up, then strum across their common tendon directly below the medial epicondyle. Explore this plump, meaty group of muscles by squeezing and kneading with a broad pincher palpation, moving along the muscle bellies from the elbow toward the wrist.

It is difficult to distinguish individual muscles in this group with palpation, although you can locate their tendons at the wrist and follow them up into the forearm. You can also differentiate individual muscles in the group by their actions. Make a fist and flex the wrist to make the flexor tendons pop out below the wrist. The most prominent tendon in the center of the wrist is the flexor carpi radialis (see Figure 17.52). The flexor carpi radialis tendon runs medial to the palmaris longus tendon in the center of the wrist; the flexor digitorum profundus runs directly lateral to the palmaris longus tendon. The flexor carpi ulnaris is the most lateral tendon on the anterior forearm. Trace each tendon up into the belly of that muscle.

To feel the flexor carpi radialis and ulnaris contract, lay your hand across the anterior side of your other forearm, right below your elbow, and flex your wrist while keeping your fingers extended. To feel the flexor digitorum profundus and superficialis contract, extend your wrist, then curl your fingers while keeping your wrist extended. Because the flexor digitorum muscles are deep to the flexor carpi and ulnaris muscles, you should feel their contraction deeper in the forearm.

Flexor Carpi Ulnaris

O–Medial epicondyle of humerus
I–Base of fifth metacarpal and pisiform
A–Flexes wrist, adducts wrist (ulnar deviation)

Flexor Carpi Radialis

O–Medial epicondyle of humerus
I–Base of second and third metacarpals
A–Flexes wrist, abducts wrist (radial deviation)

Palmaris Longus

O–Medial epicondyle of humerus
I–Palmar aponeurosis
A–Assists wrist flexion, tenses palmar fascia

Flexor Digitorum Superficialis

O–Medial epicondyle, medial aspect of coronoid process, anterior shaft of radius
I–Sides of middle phalanges of four fingers
A–Flexes proximal interphalangeal joints of four fingers, assists wrist flexion

Flexor Digitorum Profundus

O–Anterior proximal surface of three-fourths of ulna, interosseous membrane

I–Base of distal phalanges of four fingers
A–Flexes distal interphalangeal joints of four fingers, assists wrist flexion

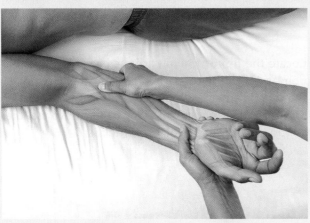

FIGURE 17.59a

Palpating the flexor muscles

With your partner in a supine position, locate the **flexor muscles** of the wrist and hand as a group by squeezing and kneading this plumb muscular mass below the medial epicondyle on the anterior side of the forearm (Figure 17.59a ■). Explore the flexors from the elbow down to their tendons at the wrist.

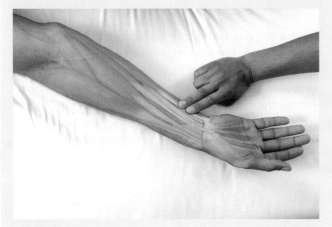

FIGURE 17.59b

Palpating the flexor carpi ulnaris

Locate the **flexor carpi ulnaris** by finding its tendon at the base of the fifth metacarpal and pisiform (Figure 17.59b ■). Follow the tendon toward the medial epicondyle, across the muscle belly. Strum across the forearm along its length to feel the contraction of the flexor carpi ulnaris.

Active movement: Have your partner flex and extend the wrist with a slight ulnar deviation.

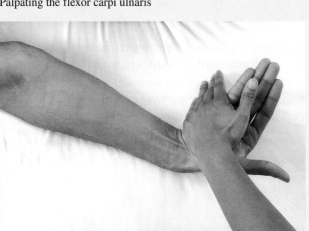

FIGURE 17.59c

Resisted movement of the flexor carpi ulnaris

Resisted movement: Have your partner flex the wrist with a slight ulnar deviation against resistance while you apply light pressure to the lateral side of the hand (Figure 17.59c ■).

(continued)

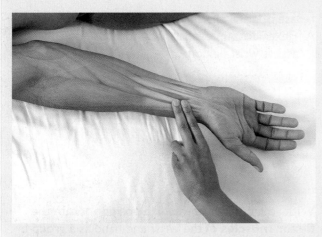

FIGURE 17.59d

Palpating the flexor carpi radialis

Locate the **flexor carpi radialis** by finding its tendon lateral to the palmaris tendon, at the base of the second and third metacarpals (Figure 17.59d ■). Strum across the forearm along its length to feel the contraction of the flexor carpi radialis.

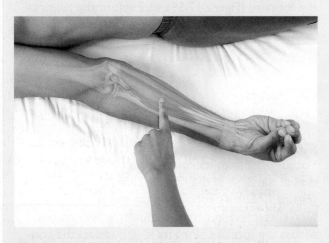

FIGURE 17.59e

Palpating the palmaris longus contraction

Locate the **palmaris** as it contracts by having your partner press the fingertips on one hand together. As the palmaris contracts, its tendon will pop out in the center of the wrist, but only if your partner has one. Follow the tendon toward the medial epicondyle, strumming across the forearm to feel the belly of the palmaris longus as it contracts (Figure 17.59e ■).

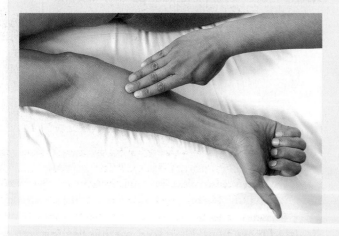

FIGURE 17.59f

Palpating the flexor digitorum contraction

To locate the **flexor digitorum superficialis** and **flexor digitorum profundus,** press your fingers across the middle of the forearm with a flat palpation. Then have your partner curl and relax the fingers several times (Figure 17.59f ■).

Resisted movement: Have your partner flex the fingers, then resist as you pull them into extension.

17.3.3.2 EXTENSOR CARPI RADIALIS LONGUS, EXTENSOR CARPI RADIALIS BREVIS, EXTENSOR CARPI ULNARIS, EXTENSOR DIGITORUM, AND EXTENSOR INDICIS

The extensors of the wrist and fingers lie along the posterior surface of the forearm (Figure 17.60 ■). Like their counterparts on the other side of the forearm, all the extensors share a common tendon. The common extensor tendon is located on the lateral epicondyle of the humerus. In this section we cover five extensor muscles—the extensor carpi radialis longus, extensor carpi radialis brevis, extensor carpi ulnaris, extensor digitorum, and extensor indicis—which are all innervated by the *radial nerve.* The extensor pollicis longus and extensor pollicis brevis will be covered under muscles of the thumb. The extensor digiti minimi will be covered under the muscles of the little finger.

The **extensor carpi radialis longus** arises from the supracondylar ridge of the humerus and tapers into a long tendon that inserts on the base of the second metacarpal. (See TrP for the extensor carpi radialis longus in Figure 17.61 ■.) This long muscle runs parallel to the brachioradialis and over its shorter namesake, the **extensor carpi radialis brevis,** which also arises from the common extensor tendon on the lateral epicondyle but inserts on the base of the third metacarpal. Both extensor carpi radialis muscles extend the wrist and work synergistically with the flexor carpi radialis to abduct the wrist. (See TrP for the extensor carpi radialis brevis in Figure 17.62 ■.)

The **extensor carpi ulnaris** also arises from the common extensor tendon on the lateral epicondyle and tapers into a cord-like tendon that inserts on the base of the fifth metacarpal. It extends the wrist and works synergistically

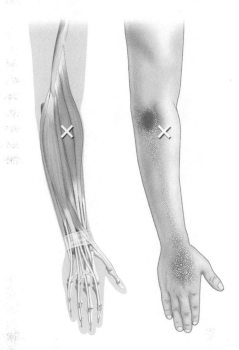

FIGURE 17.61

The **extensor carpi radialis longus,** when dysfunctional, can develop a trigger point directly below the elbow that can refer pain and tenderness to the lateral epicondyle and the radial side of the back of the wrist.

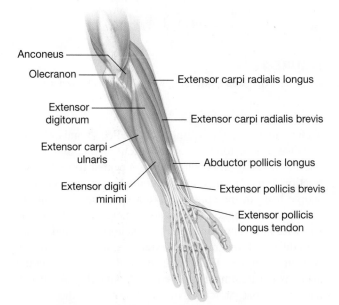

FIGURE 17.60

Extensor muscles of the wrist and hand

Labels for Figure 17.60:
- Anconeus
- Olecranon
- Extensor digitorum
- Extensor carpi ulnaris
- Extensor digiti minimi
- Extensor carpi radialis longus
- Extensor carpi radialis brevis
- Abductor pollicis longus
- Extensor pollicis brevis
- Extensor pollicis longus tendon

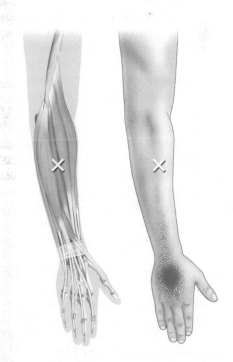

FIGURE 17.62

Of the two extensors, it is more likely for the **extensor carpi radialis brevis** to become dysfunctional and develop a trigger point in its muscle belly that can refer deep, prickly pain down the radius that concentrates over the dorsum of the hand.

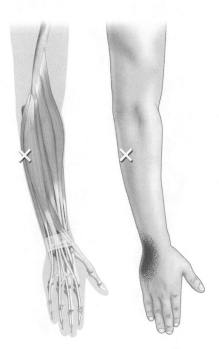

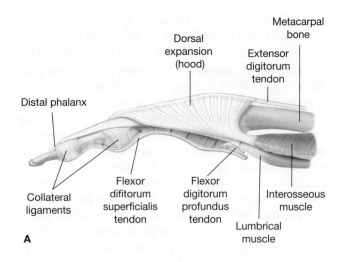

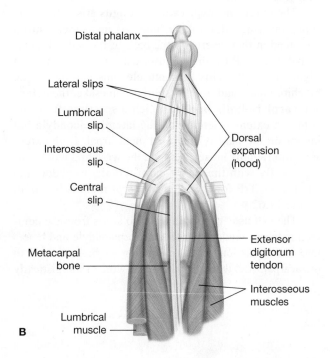

FIGURE 17.63

Although the **extensor carpi ulnaris** rarely has a trigger point, when it becomes dysfunctional, it can develop a trigger point over the middle of the muscle that can refer a circle of pain over the ulnar side of the back of the hand.

FIGURE 17.64

Extensor expansion tendons: a) Lateral view b) Posterior view

with the flexor carpi ulnaris to adduct the wrist. (See TrP for the extensor carpi ulnaris in Figure 17.63 ■.)

From its origin at the common extensor tendon on the lateral epicondyle, the **extensor digitorum** tapers into a large, flat tendon that splits into four prominent **extensor expansion tendons** that insert on the posterior surfaces of all three phalanges of the four fingers. The extensor expansion tendons are so named because they flare into a flat hood at the base of the proximal phalanges, proximal to where the interosseous tendons attach along each side and the lumbrical tendons attach along the medial sides (Figure 17.64a-b ■). Additionally, two tendinous slips arising from the underside of each expansion tendon secure it to the posterior surfaces of the proximal and middle phalanges. As its name implies, the extensor digitorum extends the finger; it also assists wrist extension. (See TrPs for the extensor digitorum in Figure 17.65 ■.)

The **extensor indicis** has an origin along the distal, posterior surface of the ulna and the interosseous membrane. Its insertion on the base of the proximal phalanx of the index (first) finger makes this small muscle a finger pointer; its sole function is to extend the index finger. (See TrP for the extensor indicis in Figure 17.66 ■.)

A frequent injury to the common extensor tendon, **lateral epicondylitis,** occurs with repetitive strains from activities requiring ballistic and repeated elbow extension,

such as tennis or fly-fishing. Also called "tennis elbow" because ardent tennis players often suffer this injury, lateral epicondylitis occurs when repeated forceful contraction of the extensor carpi radialis brevis causes microscopic tears in the common extensor tendon, leading to inflammation, tendon scars, and chronic soreness. A person with lateral epicondylitis experiences pain and weakness during elbow and wrist extension, and the condition worsens with use. The treatment for this condition is the same as the treatment for medial epicondylitis: rest, ice, and cross-fiber stretching of the tendon once the inflammation has subsided.

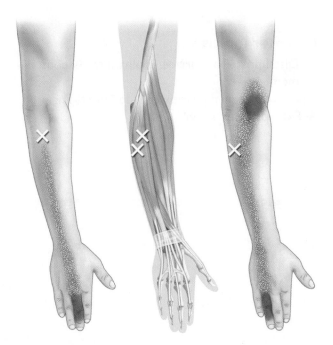

FIGURE 17.65

When dysfunctional, the **extensor digitorum** can develop two trigger points in the proximal end of the muscle: a proximal trigger point that refers pain to the top of the middle finger and a distal trigger point that refers pain to the crease in the elbow and the top of the fourth finger.

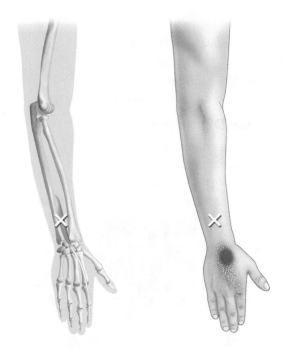

FIGURE 17.66

The **extensor indicis** can develop a trigger point in its belly and referred pain over the wrist from prolonged overuse, such as using the index finger to work a computer touchpad.

MUSCLE PALPATION

Extensor Carpi Radialis Longus, Extensor Carpi Radialis Brevis, Extensor Carpi Ulnaris, Extensor Digitorum, and Extensor Indicis

To self-palpate the forearm extensors, turn your palm down and grasp the plump, meaty group of muscles on the top of the forearm, directly below the elbow. Squeeze the extensors with a broad pincher palpation and explore lifting the muscle group from the elbow to the wrist.

To differentiate individual extensor muscles by actively moving them, lay your fingers across the back of your forearm. To locate the extensor carpi radialis muscles, hyperextend your wrist and palpate their tendons along the distal end of the radius. Follow the tendons up into the muscle bellies.

Keep your wrist hyperextended, then locate the extensor carpi ulnaris tendon along the distal end of the ulna and follow it into the muscle belly.

Straighten your wrist and hyperextend your fingers to feel the extensor digitorum contract. Follow its tendons, which will pop out along the back of your hand, from the wrist to the elbow.

Wiggle your index finger to feel the extensor indicis contract.

Extensor Carpi Radialis Longus

O–Lateral supracondylar ridge of humerus
I–Base of second metacarpal
A–Extends wrist, assists wrist abduction and elbow flexion

Extensor Carpi Radialis Brevis

O–Lateral epicondyle of humerus
I–Base of third metacarpal
A–Extends wrist, assists wrist abduction

(continued)

Extensor Carpi Ulnaris

O–Lateral epicondyle of humerus
I–Base of fifth metacarpal
A–Extends wrist, assists wrist adduction

Extensor Digitorum

O–Lateral epicondyle of humerus
I–Base of distal phalanges of four fingers
A–Extends fingers, assists wrist extension

Extensor Indicis

O–Distal posterior surface of ulna, interosseous membrane
I–Base of proximal phalanx of index (first) finger
A–Extends index finger

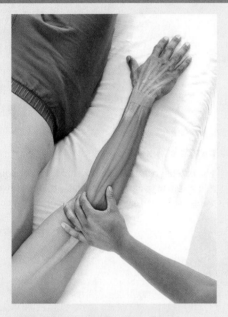

FIGURE 17.67a

Palpating the extensor muscle

With your partner in a supine position, palpate the **extensor muscles** of the wrist and hand as a group by squeezing and kneading this plump muscular mass with pincher palpation (Figure 17.67a ■). Explore this muscular mass directly below the crease of the elbow and work your way down toward the wrist.

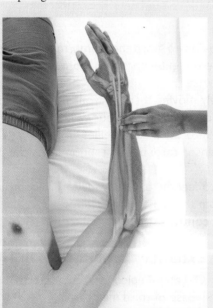

FIGURE 17.67b

Palpating the extensor carpi radialis and longus contraction

Locate the **extensor carpi radialis longus** and **extensor carpi radialis brevis** by having your partner hyperextend the wrist, then palpate along the radial side of the forearm from the wrist to the elbow (Figure 17.67b ■).

Resisted movement: Have your partner hold the wrist in extension and slight radial deviation while you apply light resistance to flex the wrist.

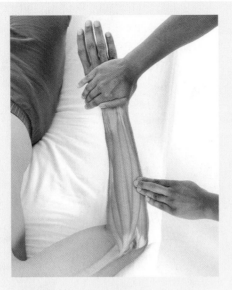

FIGURE 17.67c

Palpating the extensor carpi ulnaris contraction

Locate the **extensor carpi radialis ulnaris** by having your partner hyperextend the wrist, then palpate along the ulnar side of the forearm from the wrist to the elbow (Figure 17.67c ■). *As you move closer to the wrist, are you palpating over the ulna?*

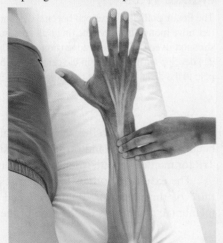

FIGURE 17.67d

Palpating the extensor digitorum contraction

To locate the **extensor digitorum,** press your fingers across the middle of the forearm, then have your partner wiggle the fingers while keeping the wrist extended, which will keep other wrist extensors quiet (Figure 17.67d ■). *Are you pressing through the overlying extensor carpi muscles to feel the contraction of the extensor digitorum?*

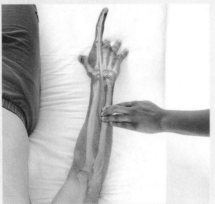

FIGURE 17.67e

Palpating the extensor indicis contraction

To locate the **extensor indicis,** press your fingers across the middle of the forearm, then have your partner move the index finger while keeping the wrist extended (Figure 17.67e ■). The tendon of the extensor indicis runs along the medial side of the extensor digitorum tendon along the first metacarpal. *Do you feel the muscle belly of the extensor indicis in the lateral third of the interosseous space?*

17.3.4 Muscles of the Thumb

Of all five fingers, the thumb possesses the broadest range of movement, which is made possible by the eight pollicis (meaning thumb) muscles devoted to this important digit. Each thumb has four long, extrinsic muscles that have origins in the forearm and insertions in the hand, and four short, intrinsic muscles that have both origins and insertions in the hand. The intrinsic muscles of the thumb create a bulge of muscle tissue at the base of the thumb called the **thenar eminence.** As mentioned earlier, the thumb flexes and extends in the same plane as the palm and abducts and adducts in a plane perpendicular to the palm. Keep this in mind while studying the movements of each of the thumb muscles.

17.3.4.1 EXTRINSIC MUSCLES OF THE THUMB

The extrinsic muscles of the thumb include the flexor pollicis longus, extensor pollicis longus and brevis, and the abductor pollicis longus. The extensor pollicis longus and brevis, as well as the abductor pollicis longus, have origins and insertions on the posterior surface of the forearm and hand and are collectively innervated by the *radial nerve* (Figure 17.68a ■). The flexor pollicis longus attachments are on the anterior side of the forearm, and it is innervated by the *median nerve* (Figure 17.68b ■). Because of their origins along the interosseous membranes, tenderness in the interosseous space between the radius and ulna could stem from muscle tension in the extrinsic muscles of the thumb.

The **flexor pollicis longus** is a bipennate thumb muscle that arises along the middle half of the interosseous membrane and attaches on the base of the distal phalanx of the thumb. It lies deep in the flexor digitorum superficialis.

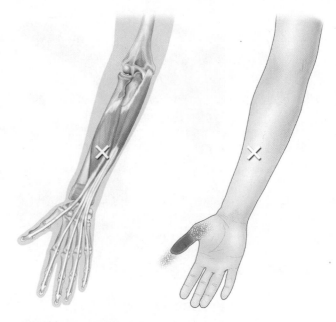

FIGURE 17.69

The **flexor pollicis longus** can become dysfunctional from repetitive motion that tires the finger flexors, such as prolonged and strenuous weed pulling or hedge trimming. When dysfunctional, it can develop a trigger point in the center of its belly that can refer pain to the distal phalanx of the thumb.

Its main function is to flex the distal phalanx of the thumb, bending it as one would do when pressing a button. (See TrP for the flexor pollicis longus in Figure 17.69 ■.)

The **extensor pollicis longus** arises from the middle third of the posterior ulnar shaft and the interosseous membrane and inserts on the base of the distal phalanx of

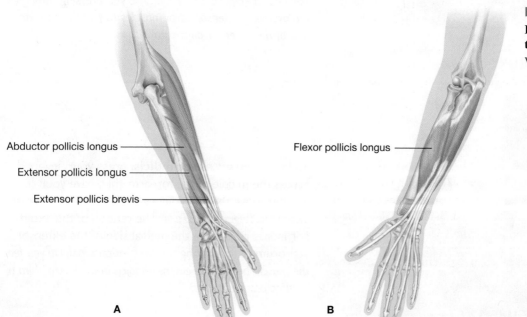

Abductor pollicis longus ——————

Extensor pollicis longus ——————

Extensor pollicis brevis ——————

Flexor pollicis longus ——————

A   **B**

FIGURE 17.68

Extrinsic muscles of the thumb: a) Posterior view b) Anterior view

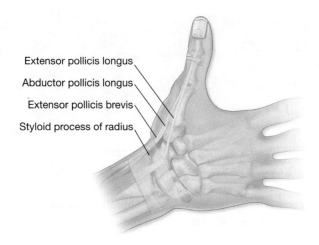

FIGURE 17.70
Anatomical snuffbox

Extensor pollicis longus
Abductor pollicis longus
Extensor pollicis brevis
Styloid process of radius

the thumb. It is innervated by the *radial nerve*. It extends the IP joint and assists extension of the wrist and the MCP joint of the thumb. It is the muscle that forms the lateral border of the "anatomical snuffbox" (Figure 17.70 ▪). The extensor pollicis brevis forms the medial border of the snuffbox. (See TrP for the extensor pollicis longus in Figure 17.71 ▪.)

The **extensor pollicis brevis** arises from the lateral half of the posterior radius and interosseous membrane and inserts on the base of the proximal phalanx of the thumb. It extends the thumb and abducts the hand. TrPs have not been identified for this muscle.

The **abductor pollicis longus** arises from the proximal half of the middle of the posterior surface of the radius and ulna and the interosseous membrane, then inserts on the base of the first metacarpal. Its primary actions are to abduct and extend the thumb; it also assists with wrist extension. (See TrPs for the abductor pollicis longus in Figure 17.72 ▪.)

17.3.4.2 INTRINSIC MUSCLES OF THE THUMB

The intrinsic muscles of the thumb include the adductor pollicis, flexor pollicis brevis, abductor pollicis brevis, and opponens pollicis. As a group, they form the meaty muscular bulge at the base of the thumb called the thenar eminence. The superficial heads of the flexor pollicis brevis, abductor pollicis brevis, and opponens pollicis are innervated by the *median nerve*. The adductor pollicis and deep head of the flexor pollicis brevis are innervated by the *ulnar nerve.*

The **adductor pollicis** forms the fleshy triangle in the web of tissue between the thumb and third metacarpal. It arises from the shaft of the second and third metacarpal and

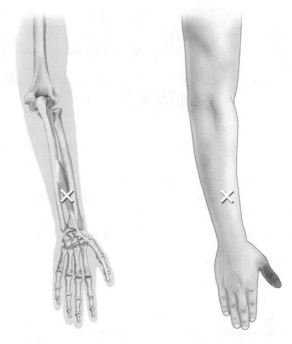

FIGURE 17.71

When the **extensor pollicis longus** becomes dysfunctional, a trigger point can develop in the center of its belly that can refer pain to the thumb.

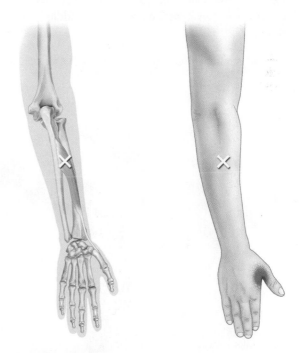

FIGURE 17.72

When dysfunctional, the **abductor pollicis longus** a trigger point can develop in center of its belly that can refer pain to the web of the thumb.

MUSCLE PALPATION

Flexor Pollicis Longus, Extensor Pollicis Longus, Extensor Pollicis Brevis, and Abductor Pollicis Longus

To self-palpate the group of extrinsic muscles of the thumb, run your fingertips along the posterior inner side of the radius from the wrist to the middle of the forearm. This muscle group creates a distinct bulge along the lateral half of the radius.

Hold your fingertips over the anterior side of the distal radius. Begin by flexing your thumb to locate the flexor pollicis longus. Next, extend the thumb to locate the extensor pollicis longus and extensor pollicis brevis. Finally, abduct the thumb to locate the abductor pollicis longus.

Flexor Pollicis Longus

O–Middle anterior shaft of radius, interosseous membrane
I–Base of distal phalanx of thumb
A–Flexes interphalangeal joint of thumb

Extensor Pollicis Longus

O–Middle third of posterior ulnar shaft, interosseous membrane
I–Base of distal phalanx of thumb
A–Extends interphalangeal joint of thumb, assists wrist extension, assists extension of saddle joint of thumb

Extensor Pollicis Brevis

O–Middle of lateral part of radius, interosseous membrane
I–Base of proximal phalanx of thumb
A–Extends thumb and abducts hand

Abductor Pollicis Longus

O–Middle of posterior surface of radius and ulna, interosseous membrane
I–Base of first metacarpal
A–Abducts and extends thumb, assists wrist extension

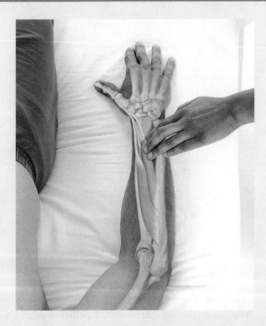

FIGURE 17.73a

Palpating the extrinsic muscles of the thumb

With your partner in a supine position, palpate the **extrinsic muscles of the thumb** as a group by running your fingertips along the medial edge of the distal half of the radius (Figure 17.73a ■).

Active movement: Have your partner move the thumb in all directions as you palpate both sides of the distal forearm.

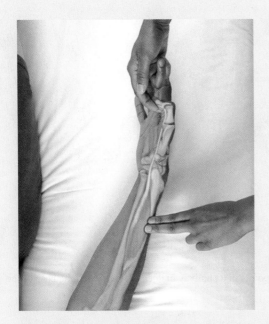

FIGURE 17.73b

Palpating the flexor pollicis longus contraction

Locate the **flexor pollicis longus** by placing your fingertips along the anterior side of the medial edge of the radius. Have your partner flex the distal phalanx of the thumb against your resistance to feel it contract (Figure 17.73b ■). *Are you palpating the distal end of the radius?*

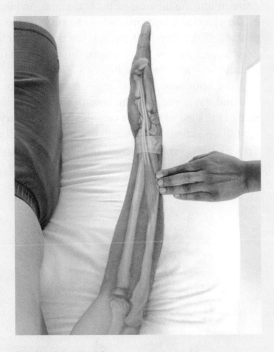

FIGURE 17.73c

Palpating the extensor pollicis longus and brevis contraction

Locate the **extensor pollicis longus** and **extensor pollicis brevis** by placing your fingertips along the posterior side of the medial edge of the radius, then have your partner extend the thumb (Figure 17.73c ■). Locate the **abductor pollicis longus** by placing your fingertips along the posterior side of the medial edge of the radius. *Is your partner moving his or her thumb like a hitchhiker?*

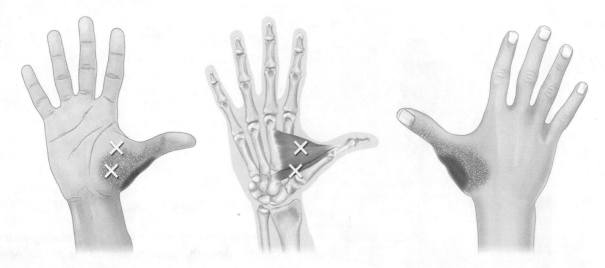

FIGURE 17.74

When dysfunctional, the **adductor pollicis** can develop two trigger points in its belly, which can refer pain to the base of the thumb.

the capitate, and it inserts on the medial side of the base of the thumb's proximal phalanx. Its main function is to adduct the thumb, drawing the thumb toward the palm in a powerful grasp. It also assists hand adduction. (See TrPs for the adductor pollicis in Figure 17.74 ▪.)

The **flexor pollicis brevis** has two small heads that arise from adjacent origins on the flexor retinaculum crossing the carpal tunnel and the trapezium and insert on the base of the proximal phalanx of the thumb. This muscle flexes the proximal phalanx and first carpometacarpal joint of the thumb. (See TrPs for the flexor pollicis brevis in Figure 17.75 ▪.)

The **abductor pollicis brevis** arises from the flexor retinaculum, the tubercle of the trapezium, and the tubercle of the scaphoid, and inserts on the base of the proximal phalanx of the thumb. It abducts the thumb as a hitchhiker muscle and assists thumb opposition. (See TrP for the abductor pollicis brevis in Figure 17.76 ▪.)

The **opponens pollicis** arises from the flexor retinaculum and the trapezium and inserts along the anterior surface of the shaft of the first metacarpal. Its primary action is opposition, drawing the thumb toward the little finger. (See TrPs for the opponens pollicis in Figure 17.77 ▪.)

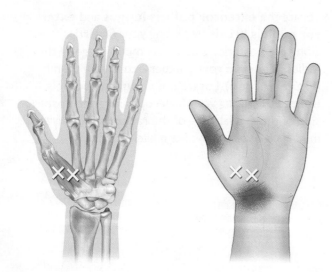

FIGURE 17.75

The **flexor pollicis brevis** can develop trigger points in two places, one in the muscle belly of each head, which can refer pain over its origin near the wrist and over the middle phalanx of the thumb.

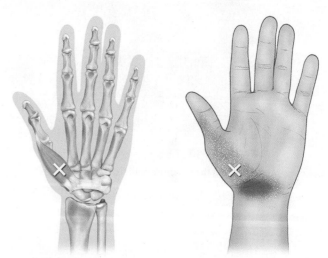

FIGURE 17.76

When dysfunctional, the **abductor pollicis brevis** can develop a trigger point in its belly, which can refer pain over its origin in the wrist and compress the carpal tunnel.

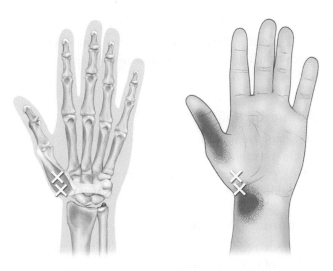

17.3.5 Muscles of the Hand

Muscles of the hand fall under several categories. We just looked at the intrinsic muscles of the thumb. In this section, we examine the muscles situated between the metacarpals and the intrinsic muscles of the little finger. Two muscle groups—the interossei and lumbricals—fill the webbing between the metacarpals. Three small muscles attach to the base of the little finger—the abductor digiti minimi, opponens digiti minimi, and flexor digiti minimi brevis. As a group, the digiti minimi muscles form the fleshy bulge of muscle tissue on the lateral side of the palm called the **hypothenar eminence,** which is less prominent than the thenar eminence at the base of the thumb.

FIGURE 17.77

When dysfunctional, the **opponens pollicis** can develop two trigger points in its belly that can refer pain from the wrist to the thumb and compress the carpal tunnel.

BRIDGE TO PRACTICE
Intrinsic Muscles of the Thumb

The intrinsic muscles of the thumb can become extremely tight and sore on anyone who works extensively with their hands holding or gripping tools, such as a dentist or a carpenter. On such clients, you may want to treat this area with pressure point therapy, myofascial stripping across the palm, and deep petrissage on the thenar eminence.

Because tendons of three intrinsic thumb muscles cross the carpal tunnel, if your client suffers from carpal tunnel syndrome, make sure to check these muscles for TrPs and treat them appropriately. Even if your client does not have carpal tunnel syndrome, if these muscles have chronic contractures, you could check and treat them for TrPs and stretch them with linear stripping as a preventative measure.

MUSCLE PALPATION
Adductor Pollicis, Flexor Pollicis Brevis, Abductor Pollicis Brevis, and Opponens Pollicis

Self-palpate the adductor pollicis with a pincher palpation in the webbing between the thumb and the palm of the hand. Gently squeeze this tissue, then adduct your thumb to feel it contract.

Locate the flexor pollicis brevis along the anterior surface of the first metacarpal at the base of the thumb. To feel it contract, press this area lightly while flexing the thumb, moving it in the same plane as your hand.

Move your fingers slightly lateral to the flexor pollicis brevis to locate the abductor pollicis brevis, which runs along the anterolateral surface of the first metacarpal. To feel it contract, press this area lightly while abducting your thumb.

(continued)

Press your fingertips over the base of the first metacarpal to locate the opponens pollicis, then feel it contract by crossing your thumb toward your little finger in opposition. The flexor pollicis brevis will also contract above it.

Adductor Pollicis

O–Shaft of second and third metacarpal, capitate
I–Medial base of proximal phalanx of thumb
A–Adducts thumb, assists hand adduction

Flexor Pollicis Brevis

O–Flexor retinaculum and trapezium
I–Base of proximal phalanx of thumb
A–Flexes the proximal phalanx and first carpometacarpal joint of thumb

Abductor Pollicis Brevis

O–Flexor retinaculum, tubercle of trapezium, tubercle of scaphoid
I–Base of proximal phalanx of thumb
A–Abducts thumb, assists thumb opposition

Opponens Pollicis

O–Flexor retinaculum and tubercle of trapezium
I–Shaft of first metacarpal
A–Thumb opposition

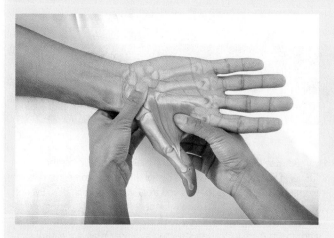

Locate the **adductor pollicis** by gently squeezing the webbing between the thumb and the palm of the hand close to the third metacarpal bone (Figure 17.78a ■). To feel it contract, have your partner move the thumb toward the index finger. *Do you notice how meaty and plump the fibers of the adductor pollicis are?*

FIGURE 17.78a
Palpating the adductor pollicis

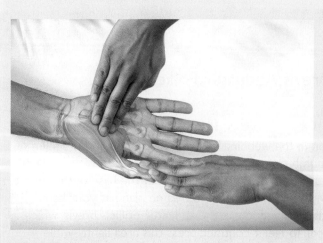

Locate the **flexor pollicis brevis** by pressing into the meaty tissue over the first metacarpal. To feel it contract, have your partner flex the thumb toward the index finger against your resistance (Figure 17.78b ■). *Are you pressing through the superficial layer of muscle to the second layer?*

FIGURE 17.78b
Palpating the flexor pollicis brevis contraction

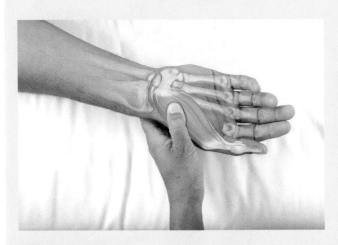

FIGURE 17.78c
Palpating the abductor pollicis brevis

Locate the **abductor pollicis brevis** by pressing your fingertips along the anterolateral surface of the first metacarpal (Figure 17.78c ■). To differentiate the abductor pollicis brevis from the flexor pollicis brevis, have your partner alternate between flexing and abducting the thumb. One assists the other in both actions, but you can feel which muscle fires first in each action. *Are you on the superficial layer of muscle?*

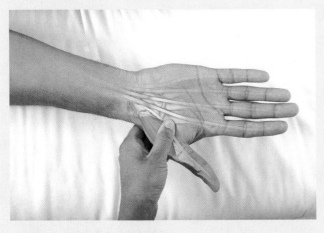

FIGURE 17.78d
Palpate the opponens pollicis

Locate the **opponens pollicis** at the base of the first metacarpal (Figure 17.78d ■). To feel it contract, have your partner fold the thumb toward the little finger. *Although adjacent muscles will contract, do you feel the opponens pollicis contract first?*

17.3.5.1 INTEROSSEI AND LUMBRICALS

The posterior interossei, palmar interossei, and lumbricals fill the webbing between adjacent metacarpals (Figure 17.79 ■). Both the interossei and the lumbricals are innervated by the *ulnar nerve.*

The **dorsal interossei** are small, bipennate muscles with muscular origins along the posterior sides of the shafts of all five metacarpals and tendinous insertions on the base of the second, third, and fourth proximal phalanges. Their distal tendons also blend into the hood of the extensor expansion tendon of the extensor digitorum, equipping these tendons to actively contribute to the extensor mechanism of the fingers and thumb. They also work as primary abductors of the fingers. (See TrPs for the dorsal interossei in Figure 17.80 ■.)

The smaller **palmar interossei** arise from muscular origins along the palmar sides of the proximal half of the metacarpal shafts and have similar tendinous insertions on the base of all of proximal phalanges except the middle (third) finger. As a group, the palmar interossei adduct the fingers and assist flexion of the metacarpophalangeal joints.

The **lumbricals** are unusual muscles because they attach to tendons rather than bone. They arise from the flexor digitorum profundus tendons in the palm and insert on the lateral sides of the extensor expansion tendons at the base of the proximal phalanges. This arrangement allows the lumbricals to generate an unusual action—they simultaneously flex the metacarpophalangeal joints while extending the interphalangeal joints (Figure 17.81 ■). Because of their deep location, the palmar interossei and lumbricals are difficult to directly palpate although you can approximate their locations in the palm of the hand.

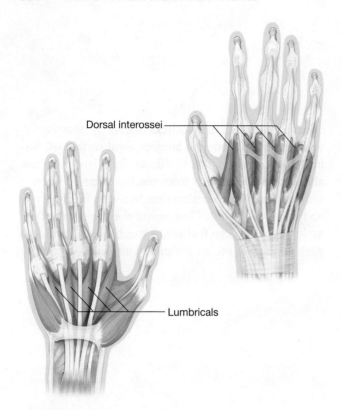

Dorsal interossei

Lumbricals

FIGURE 17.79
Interossei and lumbricals

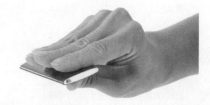

FIGURE 17.81
Lumbrical action

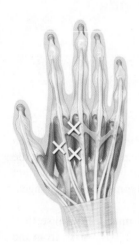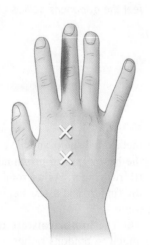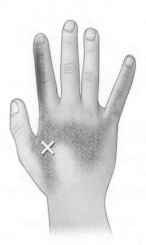

FIGURE 17.80
When overworked from prolonged gripping activities, the **dorsal interossei** can develop trigger points on the medial side of the second and third metacarpals that can radiate pain along the medial side of the same fingers. Prolonged gripping can also produce aching pain that mimics arthritic pain in the joints and makes simple hand movements such as writing or buttoning difficult.

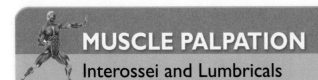

MUSCLE PALPATION
Interossei and Lumbricals

It is difficult to differentiate the lumbricals from adjacent tissues during palpation, although you can feel them contract. Press your fingertips into the palm of your other hand, then flex your knuckles while keeping your fingers straight (see Figure 17.81).

It is also difficult to directly palpate the interossei. Grasp the palm of your hand with a pincher grip, pressing into the space between two metacarpals, then abduct and adduct your fingers several times to feel them contract.

Dorsal Interossei
O–Posterior shafts of metacarpals
I–Base of second, third, and fourth proximal phalanges
A–Abduct the second, third, and fourth fingers

Palmar Interossei
O–Base of metacarpals, proximal anterior shaft of second, fourth, and fifth metacarpals
I–Base of first metacarpal, proximal anterior shaft of second, fourth, and fifth metacarpals
A–Adduct the fingers, assist flexion of the metacarpophalangeal joints

Lumbricals
O–Flexor digitorum profundus tendons in palm
I–Lateral sides of extensor expansion tendons at base of proximal phalanges
A–Flexes metacarpophalangeal joints while extending proximal and distal interphalangeal joints

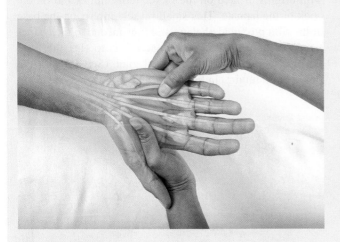

FIGURE 17.82

Pincher palpation of interossei and lumbricals

Locate the **interossei** and **lumbricals** with pincher palpation by gently squeezing both sides of the webbing between metacarpals (Figure 17.82a ▪). Have your partner subtly abduct and adduct the fingers to feel the interossei contract. *Do you notice how much easier it is to feel the interossei on the palm of the hand than on the posterior side of the hand?*

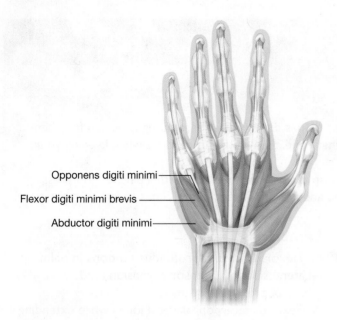

Opponens digiti minimi
Flexor digiti minimi brevis
Abductor digiti minimi

FIGURE 17.83

Anterior muscles acting on the little finger

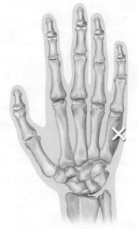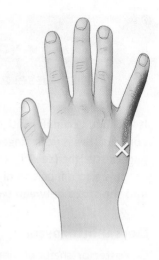

FIGURE 17.84

When overworked from prolonged gripping activities, the **abductor digiti minimi** can develop a trigger point in its belly that refers pain along the lateral side of the little finger.

17.3.5.2 MUSCLES OF THE LITTLE FINGER

There are four digiti minimi muscles that act on the little (fifth) finger. The extensor digiti minimi runs along the posterior side of the forearm and is innervated by the *radial nerve*. The other three muscles—the abductor digiti minimi, opponens digiti minimi, and flexor digiti minimi brevis—form the hypothenar eminence on the palm of the hand and are innervated by the *ulnar nerve* (Figure 17.83 ■). They can be easily palpated on the lateral side of the palm. When exploring the actions of the digiti minimi muscles, keep in mind that finger adduction and abduction involve respective movement of the fingers toward or away from the midline of the hand, which is the middle finger.

The **extensor digiti minimi** is a long, thin muscle that arises from the common extensor tendon on the lateral epicondyle and inserts via a long tendon to the posterior surface of the distal phalanx of the fifth finger. As its name implies, this muscle extends the fifth finger. Its distal tendon can be seen running lateral to the extensor digitorum tendon along the posterior side of the fifth knuckle.

The **abductor digiti minimi** arises from the pisiform and the tendon of the flexor carpi ulnaris and inserts on the medial side of the base of the fifth proximal phalanx. Its only function is to abduct the little finger. (See TrP for the adductor digiti minimi in Figure 17.84 ■.)

The **opponens digiti minimi** is a small, oblique muscle that shares an origin with the flexor digiti minimi brevis on the flexor retinaculum and the hook of the hamate. Its meaty fibers wrap around the lateral side of the fifth metacarpal and insert on the medial side of the shaft of this bone. When it contracts, the opponens digiti minimi rotates

the fifth metacarpal and draws the little finger toward the thumb in an oppositional motion. It also assists flexion of the fifth carpometacarpal joint. No TrP activity has been identified for this small muscle.

The **flexor digiti minimi brevis** has two small heads with origins located on the flexor retinaculum and on the hook of the hamate. This small muscle inserts on the base of the fifth proximal phalanx and runs medial to the abductor digiti minimi. Its primary action is to flex the little finger at the metacarpophalangeal joint. (See TrPs for the flexor digiti minimi in Figure 17.85 ■.)

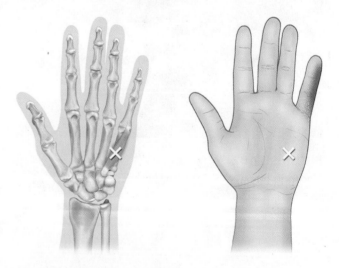

FIGURE 17.85

When the **flexor digiti minimi brevis** becomes stressed from overuse, it can develop a trigger point in the center of the muscle that can refer pain along the little finger.

Abductor Digiti Minimi, Opponens Digiti Minimi, and Flexor Digiti Minimi Brevis

Locate the abductor digiti minimi along the outside of your fifth metacarpal. Press into this meaty little muscle, then abduct your little finger to feel it contract.

To feel the opponens digiti minimi contract, press into the muscle along the inside of the base of the fifth metacarpal, then cross your little finger toward your thumb.

The flexor digiti minimi brevis lies over the opponens digiti minimi. To feel it contract, again press along the inside of the base of the fifth metacarpal, this time while flexing the MCP of the fifth finger.

Abductor Digiti Minimi

O–Pisiform and tendon of flexor carpi ulnaris
I–Medial side of base of fifth proximal phalanx
A–Abducts little finger, assists flexion of proximal phalanx of little finger

Opponens Digiti Minimi

O–Flexor retinaculum and hook of hamate
I–Medial side of shaft of fifth metacarpal
A–Draws little finger to thumb in opposition, assists flexion of fifth carpometacarpal joint

Flexor Digiti Minimi Brevis

O–Flexor retinaculum and hook of hamate
I–Base of fifth proximal phalanx
A–Flexes fifth metacarpophalangeal joint

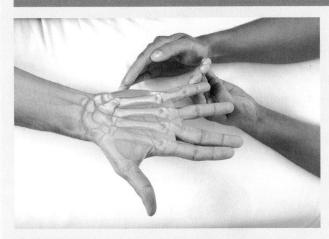

FIGURE 17.86a
Palpating the abductor digiti minimi contraction

Locate the **abductor digiti minimi** on the anterior surface of your partner's hand, along the outside of the fifth metacarpal. To feel it contract, have your partner abduct the little finger against your resistance (Figure 17.86a ■). *Are you pressing on the lateral side of the hand?*

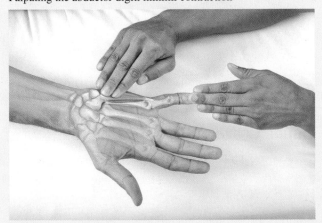

FIGURE 17.86b
Palpating the opponens and flexor digiti minimi contraction

Locate the **opponens digiti minimi** and the **flexor digiti minimi brevis** by pressing into the small muscular pad at the base of the fifth metacarpal, on the palm of the hand. To feel them contract, have your partner flex and cross the little finger toward the thumb against your resistance (Figure 17.86b ■). *Are you pressing on the hypothenar eminence?*

SELF-CARE
Stretching the Wrists and Thumbs

Caution: If you suffer from carpal tunnel syndrome or have inflammation around the wrist or thumbs, do not do these stretches because they could exacerbate your condition.

1. **Stretching the flexor muscles of your wrist:** Extend your forearm, then pull your wrist into extension (Figure 17.87a ■). Relax the muscles of the wrist that is being stretched. Hold for several seconds. Repeat on the other side.

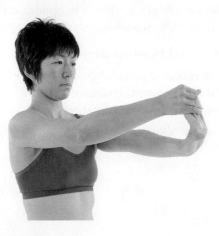

FIGURE 17.87a

2. **Stretching the extensor muscles of your wrist:** Extend your forearm, then lightly pull your wrist into flexion (Figure 17.87b ■). Relax the muscles of the wrist that is being stretched. Hold for several seconds. Repeat on the other side.

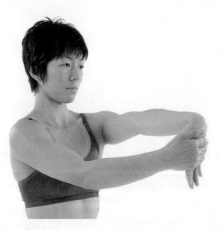

FIGURE 17.87b

3. **Stretching your thumb muscles:** Stretch the strong adductor pollicis muscle of your thumb by gently pulling it away from the midline of the hand and holding for several seconds (Figure 17.87c ■). Repeat with the other hand.

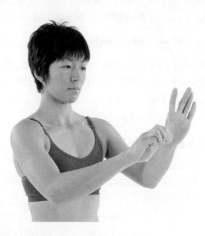

FIGURE 17.87c

4. Stretch the strong flexor pollicis muscle of your thumb by gently pulling it behind the hand and holding for several seconds (Figure 17.87d ■). Repeat with the other hand.

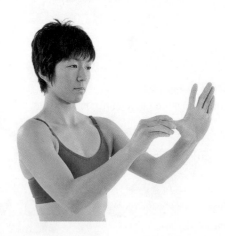

FIGURE 17.87d

CONCLUSION

The arms and hands provide a vital bridge between our bodies and the world, allowing us to carry out a vast range of communications, tasks, and manipulations. They are our key conduits of expression. We reach out with our hands, hug with our arms, and often communicate with hand and arm gestures. The arms and hands are also the primary working tools of a manual therapist, just as they are for the many other people who work with their hands. Musicians, artists, typists, toolmakers, and massage therapists experience firsthand (no pun intended) the incredibly articulate nature of the arms and hands.

Every action of the arms and hands is initiated in the brain and is carried out through the movement of the upper body. It would be difficult to move your hands without the arms and shoulders and even the spine, especially when practicing manual therapy. Keep this in mind whenever you reach, push, or pull. Let the action initiate in your trunk and shoulders, or allow it to sequence from your hands through your entire body. Drummers do this naturally, moving their whole bodies as they make music, which reduces the stress on the hands and wrists. As a massage therapist you can strive to do the same. No matter how small the stroke, moving your whole body behind your hands will allow the mechanical stresses of movement to be absorbed through and dissipated by all the joints and muscles of your body. Doing so will both enhance and protect the strength and intricate workings of your hands and arms over time.

SUMMARY POINTS TO REMEMBER

1. The arm is made up of three bones—the humerus, radius, and ulna.
2. There are eight carpal bones, five metacarpals, and 14 phalanges in the wrists and hands.
3. The elbow has four mechanically linked joints that move together in different combinations during flexion, extension, supination, and pronation. They are the humeroulnar joint, humeroradial joint, proximal radioulnar joint, and distal radioulnar joint.
4. The wrist, or radiocarpal joint, is a biaxial ellipsoid joint that can flex, extend, adduct (ulnar deviation), or abduct (radial deviation).
5. The midcarpal, intercarpal (IT), and carpometacarpal (CMC) joints are all gliding joints that provide minimal motion and maximal stability in the wrist.
6. The metacarpophalangeal (MCP) joints are ellipsoid joints that can flex, extend, abduct, and adduct the fingers at the knuckles.
7. A transverse carpal ligament covers the carpal tunnel at the base of the palm, which contains 10 tendons and the median nerve. The carpal tunnel is highly susceptible to inflammation and compression from repetitive movement and overuse.
8. Each finger has a proximal and distal interphalangeal (IP) joint, which are small hinge joints that can flex and extend.
9. The thumb has only one interphalangeal joint. This saddle joint at the base of the thumb between the first metacarpal and trapezium allows us to move the thumb in opposition and reposition.
10. Each hand has both distal and proximal carpal arches that run laterally across the palm, and four longitudinal arches that run from the metacarpals along each corresponding finger.
11. The arches of the hand give us the ability to grasp the hand around many different sizes and shapes of objects.
12. The three muscles that work as elbow flexors—the biceps brachii, brachialis, and brachioradialis—are opposed by the two elbow extensors—the triceps brachii and anconeus.
13. The forearm supinators—the biceps brachii and the supinator—are opposed by the forearm pronators—the pronator teres and pronator quadratus.
14. The five flexors of the wrist and fingers—the flexor carpi radialis, flexor carpi ulnaris, flexor digitorum superficialis, flexor digitorum profundus, and palmaris longus—are located on the anterior side of the forearm.
15. The five extensors of the wrist and fingers—the extensor carpi radialis longus, extensor carpi radialis brevis, extensor carpi ulnaris, extensor digitorum, and extensor indicis—are located on the posterior side of the forearm.
16. The wrist and finger flexors arise from a common flexor tendon on the medial epicondyle. The wrist and finger extensors arise from a common extensor tendon on the lateral epicondyle.
17. Eight pollicis muscles act on the thumb—four extrinsic, or long, muscles of the thumb (with origins in the forearm), and four intrinsic, or short, muscles of the thumb (with origins in the hand). The four intrinsic muscles of the thumb form the thenar eminence.
18. The interossei between the metacarpals allow abduction and adduction of the fingers; the lumbrical muscles flex the metacarpophalangeal joints while extending the interphalangeal joints.
19. Four small indicis muscles act on the little finger and form the hypothenar eminence.

REVIEW QUESTIONS

1. The eight carpal bones are the scaphoid, lunate,
   a. triquetrum, piriformis, trapezium, trapezoid, capitate, and hamate.
   b. triquetrum, pisiform, trapezium, trapezoid, capitate, and hamate.
   c. triquetrum, pisiform, talus, trapezoid, capitate, and hamate.
   d. triquetrum, pisiform, trapezium, trapezoid, capitate, and hallucis.

2. What is most frequently dislocated carpal bone and what type of accident usually dislocates it?

3. True or false (circle one). The hand is made up of 15 long bones: five metacarpals, five proximal phalanges, five middle phalanges, and five distal phalanges.

4. Identify two ways that the thumb differs from the other four fingers.

5. The three joints located inside the joint capsule of the elbow are the
   a. humeroulnar, humeroradial, and the proximal radioulnar joints.
   b. humeroulnar, humeroradial, and distal radioulnar joints.
   c. humeroulnar, humeroradial, and distal radiocarpal joints.
   d. humeroulnar, humeroradial, and the proximal radiocarpal joints.

6. The bony landmarks where the common extensor and common flexor tendons of the forearm muscles attach are the
   a. medial epicondyle and trochlea.
   b. radial tuberosity and lateral epicondyle.
   c. medial epicondyle and lateral epicondyle.
   d. olecranon and lateral epicondyle.

7. Which joint of the elbow is a pivot joint and what movements does it allow?

8. The ellipsoid joint of the wrist is called the _____ joint.

9. The 10 tendons of what four muscles pass through the carpal tunnel?
   a. flexor digitorum profundus, flexor digitorum superficialis, flexor carpi radialis, and flexor pollicis brevis
   b. flexor digitorum profundus, flexor digitorum superficialis, flexor carpi radialis, and palmaris longus
   c. flexor digitorum profundus, flexor digitorum superficialis, flexor carpi ulnaris, and flexor pollicis longus
   d. flexor digitorum profundus, flexor digitorum superficialis, flexor carpi radialis, and flexor pollicis longus

10. What is carpal tunnel syndrome and what five symptoms can it cause?

11. True or false (circle one). In the neutral position of the hand, the fingers rest in slight flexion.

12. The range of motion that the thumb has but the first toe does not have, and the joint that allows this range of motion is
    a. opposition and retraction, a range of motion made possible by the saddle joint at the base of the thumb.
    b. opposition and circumduction, a range of motion made possible by the saddle joint at the base of the thumb.
    c. opposition and reposition, a range of motion made possible by the saddle joint at the base of the thumb.
    d. opposition and reposition, a range of motion made possible by the ellipsoid joint at the base of the thumb.

13. The three flexors of the elbows are the
    a. biceps brachii, the brachialis, and the coracobrachialis.
    b. biceps brachii, the brachialis, and the brachioradialis.
    c. triceps brachii, the brachialis, and the brachioradialis.
    d. biceps brachii, the supinator, and the brachioradialis.

14. True or false (circle one). The biceps brachii is a strong elbow flexor when the hand is in a supinated position.

15. The primary action of the flexor digitorum profundus and flexor digitorum superficialis is flexion of the
    a. phalangeal joints.
    b. carpometacarpal joints.
    c. midcarpal joint.
    d. radiocarpal joint.

16. The primary antagonists to the flexor carpi radialis and flexor carpi ulnaris muscles are the
    a. extensor carpi radialis and extensor digitorum muscles.
    b. extensor carpi radialis longus and extensor carpi radialis brevis.
    c. extensor carpi ulnaris and extensor digitorum.
    d. extensor carpi radialis brevis and longus and the extensor carpi ulnaris.

17. The supinator can be palpated against the upper posterior surface of the
    a. radius under the overlying extensor muscles.
    b. ulna under the overlying extensor muscles.
    c. radius under the overlying flexor muscles.
    d. ulna under the overlying extensor muscles.

18. Tennis elbow is a common overuse injury also called _____ _____ *(two words)* that tears and inflames the _____ _____ *(two words)* tendon.

19. Identify which of the following statements is *not* true.
    a. Eight muscles are devoted solely to the movement of the thumb.
    b. The intrinsic muscles of the thumb form the hypothenar eminence.
    c. All of the thumb muscles have the word *pollicis* in their name.
    d. The thumb has four intrinsic and four extrinsic muscles.

20. Which are stronger, the finger flexors or extensors, and why?

Note

1. United States Department of Labor, Bureau of Labor Statistics. (2004). Events Causing Occupational Injuries. Retrieved June 12, 2011, from http://www.bls.gov/opub/ted/2004/mar/wk4/art05.htm.

18 Body Mechanics and Self-Care

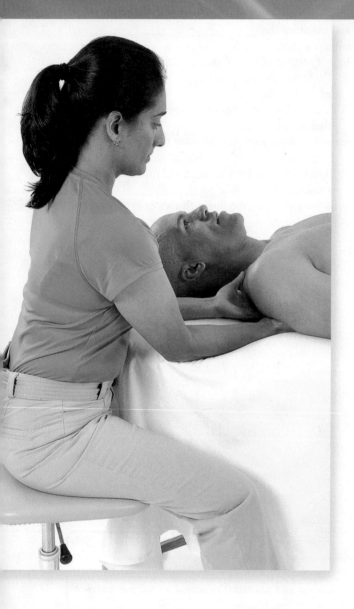

CHAPTER OUTLINE

Chapter Objectives

Key Terms

18.1 Skeletal Alignment

18.2 Relaxation, Breathing, and Fluidity

18.3 Moving Around the Massage Table

18.4 Force Applications and Hand Use

18.5 Ergonomics and Equipment

Conclusion

A basic understanding of the body can help people move more efficiently and avoid injury during work or play. Effective massage practitioners not only understand the body and how it moves, but embody that understanding in their own posture and movement.

Optimal posture, body awareness, and an ability to focus on how you move when doing bodywork are essential elements in the practice of massage. They allow you to model postural alignment and structural balance for clients. By maintaining a neutral spine and using your powerful trunk and hip muscles, you can safely lift, push, and pull. Physically centering the body in neutral spine can also help you leave

personal stresses at the door, free your energy to focus on the client and treatment, and set the form and tone you'll need for optimal body mechanics during each session.

Throughout this book we've emphasized experiential study by suggesting that you try exercises and movements on yourself as well as with a partner. This allows you to better understand kinesiology concepts by *feeling* them, using your body as the learning laboratory and your body awareness as the primary learning tool. With experiential understanding, you'll be able to put kinesiology to practical use for your clients and also for your own healthy body mechanics, helping you to create and maintain an effective massage practice.

CHAPTER OBJECTIVES

1. Explain the benefits of beginning a massage in a neutral, upright stance.

2. Describe effective lower limb alignment for body mechanics in massage.

3. Explain how core muscle engagement will improve body mechanics.

4. Describe the effect of hyperextended or flexed postures on body mechanics.

5. Discuss how keeping the sternum lifted supports the shoulder girdle.

6. Identify two guidelines for elbow and arm positioning while giving massage.

7. Describe how to actively relax muscles of the head and neck.

8. Describe how postural sway can be used to maintain a natural, fluid stance.

9. Explain how and why diaphragmatic breathing can support the shoulders and arms.

10. Discuss how and why to use complete movement sequences while giving massage.

11. Discuss how and why to face the direction of a stroke while giving massage.

12. Describe how and why to use a rocker base when making weight shifts.

13. Explain how to synchronize upper and lower body movements while giving massage.

14. Describe how to optimally align joints in the hands and forearms when applying force.

15. Describe two guidelines for maximizing leverage when applying force.

16. Discuss how and why to use optimal lines of force when pushing and pulling.

17. Discuss why varying hand positions when giving massage prevents injuries.

18. Describe optimal table height, chair and stool use, and client padding in massage.

KEY TERMS

Optimal posture

Neutral, upright stance

Base of support

Core stability

Shoulder symmetry

Scapula neutral

Weighted elbows

Active relaxation

Breath support

Complete sequences

Recentering in neutral

Facing direction of stroke

Rocker base

Upper–lower body synchronization

Moving through lunges

Using full-body motion

Stacking joints in arms

Leaning into pressure

Pushing from feet

Lines of force

Varying strokes

Optimal table height

Using stools

Padding clients

Sometimes practitioners concentrate so much on their clients that they forget the importance of taking care of themselves, or they don't think of themselves having the same needs as clients. Throughout this book there has been an emphasis on the importance of posture and movement in the health of the client. These aspects of kinesiology are also vital for the success and longevity of manual therapists. Our focus has been on developing clinical skills, but we have also encouraged you, the practitioner, to apply concepts of kinesiology to your own body mechanics and self-care. This is important because you are using your body to carry out the physical work required in this profession. As the title *Therapeutic Kinesiology* implies, learning about healthy patterns of muscle and joint function begins at home in your own self-study and body experience.

This last chapter is a reminder to use your knowledge of kinesiology to take care of your own body—in short, to practice what you preach. The more you understand and feel how your own body moves, the better equipped you will be to model and cultivate healthy patterns to your clients. Self-study helps you comprehend muscle and joint function on a deeper level; from your own personal experience. Each time you apply kinesiological concepts to your own body-use patterning, it reinforces the message you give to your clients about the importance of cultivating healthy posture and movement to improve general health and to prevent pain and injury.

In this chapter, we bring together concepts presented throughout the text about muscle and joint function. We apply these concepts to neuromuscular patterning in your own posture and movement. This chapter also serves as a general review for many of the self-care exercises and body mechanics tips that have been presented throughout the book, which are referenced here. As you go through this chapter, you may want to refer to earlier chapters to review concepts that were introduced previously.

Many of these body mechanics concepts overlap. You'll notice that one concept builds on another group in a progression aligned with the sequence of topics in the text. For example, good posture builds a foundation for efficient gait patterns, and the principles of gait apply to body mechanics in any activity. Keep in mind that although this material is specific to the practice of manual therapy, it can also be applied in client education and to activities of daily living.

18.1   SKELETAL ALIGNMENT

Effective body mechanics begin with optimal posture. Posture is an outward reflection of muscle-use patterns reflecting how the muscles align with the bones. There are many ways to approach postural education. Because the skeleton serves as a bony scaffold to which the postural muscles attach, in this approach we begin with a review of vertical alignment with an emphasis on the weight-bearing bones.

The pattern of bony alignment at the initiation of an action is usually carried throughout the entire movement sequence. People who sit with their shoulders hiked or rounded are likely to stand and walk with rounded shoulders. In that same dynamic, if a practitioner begins a massage with poor skeletal alignment held by a muscular holding pattern, that practitioner is likely to maintain the poor alignment and holding pattern throughout the entire massage. Since there is a tendency to carry faulty postures into daily activities, it is important to start a massage in the posture or stance that you want to maintain throughout the session. Hence, the first guideline for effective body mechanics relates to posture.

Keep in mind that as you work to change faulty postural patterns, a new posture will feel unnatural at first. The muscles become adapted to holding the body a certain way, so shifting to a more upright posture requires the muscles to work differently, which often feels like more muscular effort. For this reason, people who slouch find straightening the spine laborious and uncomfortable. The discomfort arises from lengthening myofascias that have adapted to shortened positions. Also, the neuromuscular circuitry of those who habitually slouch favors slouching, and until new pathways are established, habitual patterns dominate.

For the posture to change and improve, the tissues and nerve pathways must go through a period of adaptation. During this period, certain muscles need to stretch (which massage and bodywork can assist) and postural muscles need to contract. In addition, a person needs to be committed to self-awareness and change. Depending on the severity of the faulty posture and the habituation of the neuromuscular circuitry, as well as the diligence of the individual making the postural adjustments, the process can take considerable time, but it is well worth the time and effort.

18.1.1   Begin Massage with Optimal Posture in a Neutral, Upright Stance

Optimal posture is a position of the body in which the center of gravity (COG) of each weight-bearing mass—the head, thorax, and pelvis—align as close to the line of gravity (LOG) as possible. In ideal posture, the weight-bearing joints rest in a neutral, extended position. In contrast, the weight-bearing joints in a faulty posture are held in habitual flexion, hyperextension, or rotation. Optimal posture, with the bones aligned along the vertical axis, requires minimal muscular effort for sitting or standing. Any slight deviance from vertical requires muscular holding to keep the body from continuing to tip off center.

To practice effective body mechanics, a practitioner needs to minimize effort while maximizing force. This is done by beginning massage in an easy upright stance and working in this stance as often as possible (Figure 18.1 ■).

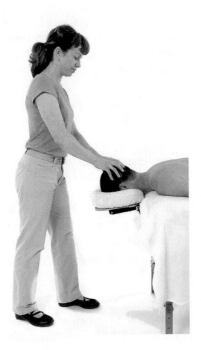

FIGURE 18.1

Start massage in a standing posture.

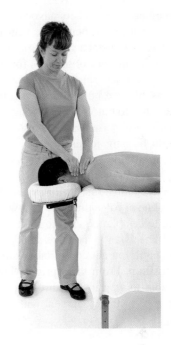

FIGURE 18.2

Stand over your base of support with the knees straight but not locked.

The direction that moves your body into a neutral upright posture will depend on which direction your postural patterns pull the body off its central axis. For example, a posteriorly tipped pelvis needs to shift anteriorly and vice versa. Here are some general cues for moving your body into a neutral posture:

- Rock your pelvis forward or back to move it to a level position.
- Elongate your neck (without raising your chin) so that your head rises up like a helium balloon.
- Lift your sternum to extend your thorax, but avoid overarching your lower back.
- Balance the weight on your feet between your heels, big toes, and little toes.

18.1.2 Center the Body over the Base of Support

In optimal posture, the body centers over the base of support; the feet form that base when you are standing (see the "Centering Your Body Over Your Feet" exercise in the chapter on posture) and the ischial tuberosities do so when you are sitting. As you stand, visualize the ankles, knees, and hips as three dots that line up along a vertical axis (Figure 18.2 ■). If your stance is too wide, the diagonal alignment of the legs can compress the sacrum. Also, the lower body will become fixated and it will be difficult to keep your joints aligned as you bend the legs to make weight shifts, which are needed to help you avoid torsion stresses in the ankles and knees.

Keeping your knees facing forward will help you move your lower limbs in the direction of your massage strokes, utilizing optimal gait mechanics as you move around your treatment table. When you walk, your hips, knees, and ankle usually face the direction you are walking. Likewise, face your legs in the same direction of your massage stroke to avoid rotations that can torque your joints and require excess muscular effort. The knees need to remain in the same plane as your feet to avoid twisting your joints, which could injure them (see the "Exercises for Lower Limb Alignment" exercise in the gait chapter). To keep the knees facing forward, imagine a headlight on each knee that illuminates the direction in which you are working.

18.1.3 Straighten the Knees but Avoid Locking or Bending Them

In a neutral, upright stance, keep your knees straight and avoid locking or bending them unless you have a health condition that requires a different posture. People with 5th lumbar disk problems, for example, often get pain relief from standing with one foot on a small stool.

If you are used to locking your knees, you can change this faulty habit by learning to unlock them without bending them. In such cases, locking the knees probably feels normal, so you will need to develop the awareness to feel the subtle difference between straight and locked knees. To develop this skill, notice how your knees feel in your usual lock-kneed posture, then practice the feeling of holding your knees straight until you can sense the difference (see the "Correcting Genu Recurvatum (Hyperextended Knees)" exercise in the knee chapter).

Some massage teachers advocate practicing massage from a low and wide bent-knee stance called the horse stance. This low stance is used in some martial arts to strengthen the muscles of the legs for defense maneuvers, but is not practical for use as a massage stance for a number of reasons. The horse stance requires a lot of excess muscular effort to hold. (See how long you can hold a bent-knee stance before your legs start shaking.) Also, holding the weight-bearing joints in flexion requires muscular contraction around the knees that compresses the knee joints, which will eventually damage the vulnerable structures of these joints. In addition, a bent-knee stance breaks the direct line of force through the lower limbs, which you will need to be able to push from the feet. If you are used to a bent-knee stance, practice standing with your knees extended until you get comfortable standing and working in this position. From this upright "human stance," you will be able to step in any direction easily as you give massage in a manner congruent with the biomechanics of bipedal gait.[1]

18.1.4 Engage Core Muscles to Lengthen and Stabilize the Spine and Torso

Once you've found your optimal postural stance, lightly contract your core muscles, which will provide postural support and spinal stability as you work. Exactly which core muscles you contract will depend on which ones are already engaged.[2] To feel which muscles you need to engage, scan your trunk from the base of your spine to your head. Here are some general guidelines for engaging the postural stabilizers:

- Use only one-third the maximum effort to contract your postural muscles.
- Lightly contract the transverse abdominis in your lower abdominal region, directly above the pubic bone (see the "Lower Back Protection with the Transversus Abdominis" exercise in the posture chapter).
- If you tend to have an excessive lordotic curve in your lumbar spine, engage the lumbar multifidus by drawing your lumbar vertebrae straight back (see the "Correcting a Lumbar Sway with Lumbar Multifidus Training" exercise in the spine chapter).
- Engage your lower trapezius to anchor your scapulae down your back and widen your chest (see the "Finding Scapula Neutral" exercise in the shoulder chapter). Make sure not to pinch your scapulae together.
- Engage your cervical stabilizers by lengthening your neck (see the "Neuromuscular Patterning to Engage the Neck Stabilizers" exercise in the head and neck chapter).

- Engage diaphragmatic breathing by inhaling into the lateral expansion of your lower ribs (see the "Coordinating Diaphragmatic Breathing with IAP" exercise in the thorax and respiration chapter).

18.1.5 Avoid Tendencies to Hyperextend the Spine

In an effort to stand up straight, many people overwork, pulling the shoulders back into scapular retraction and hyperextending the spine into an arched, rigid military posture. This overcorrection often throws the upper body behind the lower body and tilts the pelvis anteriorly. It overworks the extensor muscles along the back, often creating muscular tightness and pain along the spine.

A quick adjustment into the military posture also engages fast-twitch fibers in the extensor muscles, which tire quickly and ache from working in sustained contractions. To compensate for muscle fatigue and achiness, people who habitually hyperextend the spine eventually sit down and slouch for relief from pain, oscillating between a rigid posture and an unsupported one.

If your back tires even though you think you are sitting or standing straight, you are probably overworking the wrong muscles and may be hyperextending your spine (Figure 18.3 ■). To check this tendency and get visual

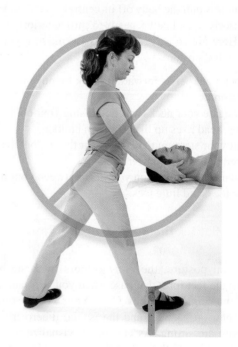

FIGURE 18.3

Avoid hyperextending the pelvis.

feedback about your pattern, look at a side view of your posture in a mirror. If your thorax is behind your pelvis, you will be able to observe it in the mirror. You can also feel your lower back to see if it is arched and your erector spinae muscles are overworking, in which case you will feel two mounds of muscles bulging along either side of your spine. Or have someone give you an axial compression test by applying a quick, light press down on your shoulders (see the "Axial Compression Tests to Assess Lines of Force" exploring technique exercise in the joint chapter) to get physical feedback. During the compression test, if your body is well-aligned, you will feel the compression transfer through joints in the core of your body, from your shoulders to your feet. If your thorax is behind your pelvis, your back will bend and arch.

If you tend to arch your back, put your hands on your lower back for feedback, then tilt your pelvis anteriorly and posteriorly several times. Reposition it in a place where the pelvis is level, your lower back lengthens, and your erector spinae muscles relax.

18.1.6 Keep the Sternum Lifted and the Shoulders Symmetrical

Keeping the sternum lifted is a great way to keep the thoracic spine extended. It will help you avoid slouching in the upper spine, which will prevent the kyphotic, rounded-shoulder posture that is easy to develop when working while leaning over a table. Lifting the sternum also prevents compression on the heart and lungs, allowing you to breathe more openly and fully. It widens the chest and provides more room for the organs, especially the heart, which lies directly under the sternum, anterior to the midthoracic vertebrae.

Keeping your sternum lifted also helps keep your shoulders symmetrical. Strive to maintain a sternal lift and shoulder girdle symmetry even when applying force with one hand. The reason this is important is to avoid twisting the upper spine, which can lead to neck and upper back pain. The best way to ensure the symmetry of the shoulders is by using your hands symmetrically, although this isn't always possible. When applying force with just one hand, keep your shoulders square, which will keep your scapulae and spine stable. Also keep your neck long and your head lifted.

If you tend to hold your spine in chronic flexion, lift your sternum and your heart using erector spinae muscles along the thoracic spine. As you do this, avoid hyperextending and arching your lower back. If you can, reposition the thorax without moving the pelvis.

18.1.7 Engage and Maintain the Scapula-Neutral Position

It is important to maintain the scapula-neutral position because it affects the alignment of your thoracic spine and neck. Maintaining scapula neutral will also help you avoid excessive scapular motion, which is important because scapular hypermobility and instability increases mechanical stress on the thoracic and cervical regions of the spine. It also weakens the lines of force from the spine and the arms.

Here are some guidelines for maintaining scapula neutral:

- Keep your clavicles horizontal and your sternum lifted.
- Keep your shoulders wide front and back.
- Position your scapulae so that they lie flat against your rib cage, but avoid hiking, rounding, or pinching your scapulae together.
- As you move your arms, focus on the motion occurring at the glenohumeral joints rather than the scapulothoracic joints.
- Breathe into the expansion of the ribs across your chest and under your armpits.
- Contract your lower abdominals lightly to maintain length in your lumbar spine, which, in turn, will support lift in your thorax.

Scapula neutral can be difficult to feel without direct feedback. If you can, when applying pressure with one hand or elbow, reach your other hand behind you to feel whether or not your scapula is lying flat against your ribs, then reposition your scapula as needed. Or have a partner give you feedback while you move your arms (see the "Assessing the Neutral Position of the Shoulder Girdle" exercise in the shoulder chapter) or while you give massage.

SELF-CARE
Stretching Chest Muscles and the Thoracic Spine

Here are several simple exercises you can use to stretch and relax your pectoralis muscles and restore symmetry to how you move your arms. These exercises are great for releasing muscular tension and balancing your shoulders between massage sessions.

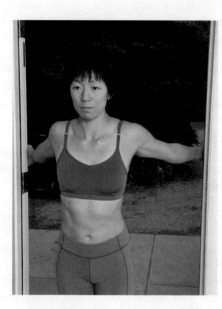

FIGURE 18.4a

1. **Doorway chest and arm stretch:** Stand in a doorway and hook your fingertips on both sides about chest level or lower (Figure 18.4a ■). Contract your lower abdominal muscles to keep your spine straight, then slowly lean forward to stretch your chest muscles. Make sure to keep your shoulders level and avoid hiking them. You can move your arms higher or lower to get a stretch in different areas. You could feel the stretch in your arms or chest, depending on where you need it most.

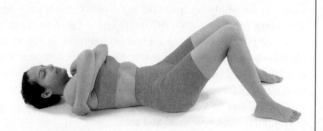

FIGURE 18.4b

2. **Constructive rest position with arm folds:** Lie on your back in a neutral spine position (also called the constructive rest position because it is a great position to relax in. Fold both arms across your chest (Figure 18.4b ■). Breathe into the ribs between your shoulder blades to relax that area. As you exhale, allow weight to sink into the back of your heart and thoracic spine. If you tend to have a rounded back and exaggerated thoracic kyphosis, place a small pillow under your mithoracic spine, then relax in this position. The pillow will help extend the thoracic spine.

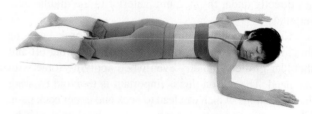

FIGURE 18.4c

3. **Upper homologous connection:** Lie prone with your head turned to one side. Put your arms out to your sides and bend your elbows at a right angle (Figure 18.4c ■). Flatten your palms and all 10 fingers on the floor. Relax your chest muscles in this position, allowing your chest to widen and flatten. Widen your elbows as your chest relaxes. If you are tight across the chest, limit your time in this position to 10 minutes or less because it slowly stretches the pectoralis myofascias, which could feel sore afterward.

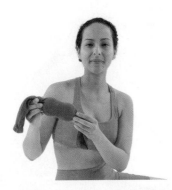

FIGURE 18.4d

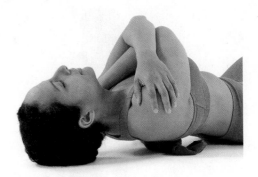

FIGURE 18.4e

4. **Midthoracic release with tennis balls:** Put two tennis balls in a sock, then tie a knot in the end of the sock to hold the balls together (Figure 18.4d ■). Place the tennis balls in a sock on the floor behind you, then lie with the middle of your thoracic spine on top of them (Figure 18.4e ■). Your spinous processes should be positioned in the space between the balls.

Breathe into that vertebral segment for a while, relaxing the weight of your spine into the balls. Reposition the tennis balls along your spine in any place you want to relax. *Caution: If you do place the tennis balls under the base of you occiput, be careful not to fall asleep in this position because it can put a lot of pressure on the occipital nerve.*

18.1.8   Allow the Elbows to Be Weighted and Keep the Arms Forward of the Body

Allowing the underside of your elbows and forearms to be heavy and weighted will keep your shoulders from hiking, which will help you maintain the neutral position of the scapulae (Figure 18.5a ■). Avoid lifting your elbows, which could overwork abductor muscles on the tops of your shoulders (Figure 18.5b ■).

Make sure to keep your elbows in front of your body or beside your body to avoid unnatural twisting of the shoulders or spine (Figure 18.5c ■). When the elbows migrate behind the body, a practitioner tends to retract the scapulae and pinch them together. If your elbows do get behind you, either turn your body to face your hands or step back a few steps to bring your arms in front of you (Figure 18.5d ■).

18.2   RELAXATION, BREATHING, AND FLUIDITY

Giving massage does require muscular effort, although it is important to differentiate relaxed effort from overworking. Keeping the body relaxed, breathing fully, and moving fluidly while giving massage can be tricky if you tend to overwork and focus so hard on achieving your goals that your muscular efforts create unnecessary muscular tension.

One challenge many people face when learning how to move in a relaxed manner is how to relax without becoming completely passive and collapsing the body. Another challenge involves how to move the body fluidly and with just the right level of muscular effort, not too much or too little. Here are a few guidelines to finding the right balance for active relaxation and fluid body movements.

18.2.1   Actively Relax the Muscles in the Head and Neck

One easy way to relax the muscles in the head and neck is to relax specific muscles in these areas, such as muscles of the throat, the tongue, and the frontalis muscle on the forehead. The throat is lined with constrictor muscles, so chronic tension in the throat can actually make a person feel like he or she is being choked. The tongue is a core muscle of the mouth and throat. Holding it plastered against the roof of the mouth has been associated with a high production of the beta brain waves, which occurs during concentrated thinking such as deliberating on a jury and scattered, agitated states associated with mind chatter. Relaxing the tongue, a tip that public speakers use to relax themselves before stepping up to the lectern, has been found to slow down beta brain waves and relax the whole body. Relaxing the frontalis muscle across the forehead has been associated with the production of alpha brain waves, which induce a calm yet awake state of mind.

Here are several directives for relaxing that you can apply while practicing massage and bodywork or during any activity:

- Allow your tongue to relax, falling away from the roof of your mouth so that your upper palate can float.
- Allow your jaw to be loose and slack.
- Maintain a small space between your back molars.
- Allow your forehead to be smooth and unwrinkled.
- Allow your eyes to be calm and to sink back.

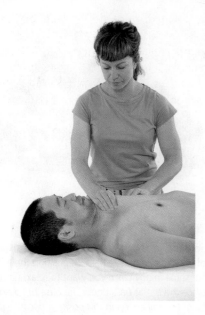

FIGURE 18.5a
Allow your elbows to be weighted.

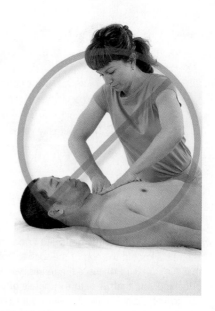

FIGURE 18.5b
Avoid working with your elbows lifted.

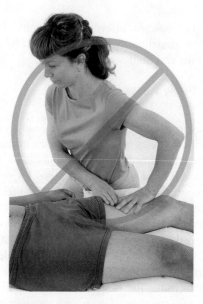

FIGURE 18.5c
Avoid working with your elbows behind you.

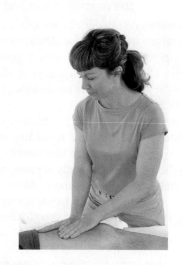

FIGURE 18.5d
Keep your arms in front of your body as you work.

18.2.2 Practice Postural Sway to Cultivate a Natural, Fluid Stance

The more aligned your body is during postural sway, the more efficient any subsequent movement will be as you give massage. From the dynamic movement of postural sway, you can simply initiate each stroke by swaying your body weight into your hands.

When you are getting ready to work and sensing your alignment, take a moment to feel the subtle postural sway. This will help you connect with an inner feeling of fluidity throughout your body (see the "Postural Sway for Fluid Body Mechanics" exercise in the posture chapter). If you start to feel stiff or tight while you are working, step back and take a moment to feel a subtle postural sway to reconnect with the innate fluidity of the human body.

You can practice postural sway anywhere and anytime that you find yourself standing still—in the checkout line at the store, while cooking in your kitchen, and especially when standing and working with clients in your treatment room.

18.2.3 Establish Breath Support for Shoulders and Arms with Diaphragmatic Breathing

The lateral expansion of the lower ribs is a benchmark for diaphragmatic breathing. When the diaphragm truly initiates the breath cycle, the inhalation sequences into an expansion of the trunk in all directions. As the breath expands the rib cage and lungs, breathing supports the shoulders from underneath (see "Breath Support for the Shoulder Girdle and Thoracic Spine" in the thorax and respiration chapter). Diaphragmatic breathing also creates an expansive, rhythmic flow of movement that you can tune into when you feel stiff. It can also energize you as you work by bringing in more oxygen.

Here are five cues to cultivate diaphragmatic breathing and breath support:

- Lightly contract your lower abdominals to counter the downward pressure of the diaphragm and prevent excessive abdominal distension on the inhalation.
- Allow each inhalation to fill and widen your lower ribs.
- Let each breath expand your rib cage and fill your chest.
- As the breath fills your chest, let your shoulders rest down on your rib cage like a coat sits on a hanger.
- During the exhalation, allow your spine to elongate as the respiratory muscles relax and the ribs sink down, like an umbrella closing around its center.

18.2.4 Move Slowly and with Awareness

Every now and then, a client needs a stimulating massage to increase tone, but this rarely occurs unless your job is to prepare an athlete for a sporting event right before it begins. Most massage and bodywork clients want to relax during a session. To help your clients relax and to help yourself work more effectively, slow down. Slowing down will give you time to feel how you are using your body as you work so that you can make adjustments as needed. Moving slowly with awareness will give you time to feel and listen to your client's body and how he or she responds, which could improve the efficiency of your work. Slow movement will also deepen your connection with your client.

Working slowly as you give massage also encourages you to use your muscles in clear contract–relax cycles so that you relax your arms and hands at the end of each stroke. It also encourages relaxation in both you and your client, which will ultimately enhance any myofascial and neuromuscular release techniques that you use. It is easy to feel that you need to rush because you have so much work to do, but your work will be more efficient if you move slowly and mindfully, making every move count.

18.2.5 Make Every Stroke a Complete Movement Sequence

On a fluid level, each massage stroke can be compared to squeezing a sponge underwater: You need to relax your hands at the end of the squeeze to allow fluid to flow back into the sponge. Taking a split-second pause at the end of a stroke and relaxing your hands not only allows the fluids to flow back into the client's tissues where you have been working, it allows the blood to flow back into your hands, too.

As you work, think of each stroke as a wave with a clear beginning, middle, and end. Feel the stroke rise and fall, then allow a moment of suspension or rest at the end of each stroke. The moment of rest at the end of the stroke will give your body time to recenter.

If you have trouble with fluidity, you may want to take up the practice of some kind of fluid dance form. If this is not possible, dance at home to your favorite music. Or even learn Tai Chi, a great martial art form to cultivate a sense of slow yet fluid body movement sequences. There are many Tai Chi videos available for home practice.

18.2.6 Occasionally Pause in a Neutral, Upright Posture to Recenter the Body and Mind

If you find yourself overworking and becoming tight while giving a massage, pause for a moment to recenter yourself and your body in an easy, upright posture. By keeping your attention or hands on your client, you can quietly pause without breaking the flow of massage. A good time to pause and recenter comes during the transition between working on one area and moving to another area.

Each time you take a centering moment, realign your spine in an upright position using the guidelines from the first section of this chapter. Make the subtle adjustments that you need to release tension and restore core muscular tone, such as relaxing your hands and shoulders, grounding your feet on the floor, and taking a deep diaphragmatic breath. Check the position of your joints to see if they are in a neutral alignment and adjust them accordingly. Also check your postural muscles to make sure they are still lightly contracted, especially in the lower abdominal region and along the spine. With practice, all these steps will become so quick and intuitive that what may seem like a long checklist here will only take a moment when you do it in your practice.

18.3 MOVING AROUND THE MASSAGE TABLE

The same principles that apply to gait mechanics apply to body mechanics in massage, especially when moving around the treatment table. For example, a person stands up to walk and initiates each step with a slight forward lean. Likewise, a manual therapist can begin a session in an upright standing posture and from this centered position, simply lean forward into the hands to begin the treatment.

Another example of gait mechanics in massage involves a body mechanics concept referred to as the "rocker principle." Each step a person takes while walking rocks the body from the back foot to the front foot. A massage therapist can use this same dynamic by spreading the feet in the direction of the massage stroke, then rocking forward on the front foot to deliver the stroke. We will revisit the rocker principle in this section as well as other gait concepts that you can use to improve the efficiency of how you move around the massage table as you work with clients.

18.3.1 Face the Direction of the Massage Stroke

In the same way that you face the direction in which you are walking, always keep your body facing the direction of your hands in a massage stroke (Figure 18.6a ■). Facing the direction of your stroke will help you keep your body facing the area that you are working on so that you avoid twisting your spine (Figure 18.6b ■). Facing your strokes also help you keep your body behind your hands, which is important for keeping the shoulders and hips square and level to avoid hiking your shoulders or hips.

When you need to change the direction of the stroke, simply turn your body behind your hands. To become more comfortable turning, practice long strokes down the arm or leg. When you reach the hand or foot, reverse your stroke by turning your whole body. When you reach the shoulder or hip, reverse your stroke again by turning your whole body. Massage up and down each limb several times until you can change directions without interrupting the flow of the massage.

18.3.2 Use a Rocker Base to Shift Body Weight when Stepping

Again, utilize gait mechanics by staggering your feet in the direction of your stroke, placing one foot in front of the other as you do when you are walking. This creates a rocker base between your feet that you can step back and forth across as you work.

To practice feeling your rocker base, stand with your feet under your body, then step forward on one foot (Figure 18.7 ■). With both knees straight but not locked and your feet in a stationary position, practice rocking back and forth between the back and front foot. As you rock forward,

notice how your pelvis lifts up and over the front foot, shifting your body weight from your back heel to your front toes. As the weight shifts up and over the toes of the back leg, this places you in an ideal position to push off from the back toes, which you can use when you need to increase your pressure. Switch legs and place your other foot in front so that you become familiar with using a rocker base on both sides.

As you explore rocking from one foot to another over a rocker base, imagine each stroke as a wave moving your pelvis up and over as you rock forward, then reversing and returning on itself as you rock backward. Here are some general guidelines for using a rocker base:

- Stagger your feet in the same direction as your massage stroke.
- Allow the length of your rocker to match the length of your stroke.
- Rock your trunk over your feet in sync with your massage stroke.
- Avoid holding your body in a stationary rocker position.
- Rock into a lunge when you need to sink down.
- Keep your knees under your hips and your feet under your knees.
- Keep your knees facing forward to avoid laterally rotating the hips because doing so can lead to rotator muscle spasms and sciatic nerve pain in the hip.[3]

18.3.3 Stay over the Base of Support to Remain Lifted over the Client

Stand over your front leg as you work, right next to the massage table. As you step over your front foot, the COG in your pelvis rises 1–2 inches, which places your trunk at its highest point (Figure 18.8a ■). This will help you keep your

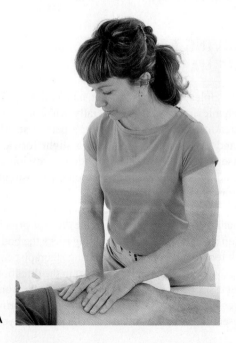

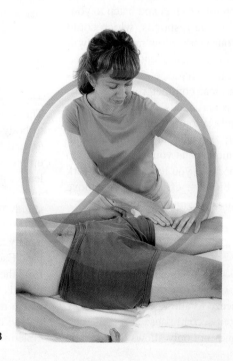

FIGURE 18.6

a) Face the direction of your stroke. b) Avoid facing away from your stroke.

A   B

FIGURE 18.7

Stand over a rocker base to make weight shifts.

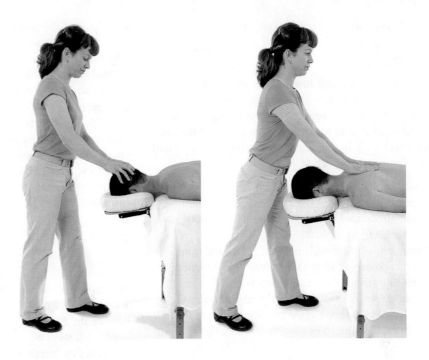

upper body up and over your client so that you can apply pressure down and in, just as a person gets up and over a kitchen sink to scour a pot, up and over a cutting board to chop vegetables, or up and over a ironing board to press clothes.

Let the movement of your body follow the movement of your hands as one dancer in a couple follows the lead of the other. For strokes on top of the client, use overcurves that get up and over your hands.

As you work, make sure to keep your trunk over the foot that is closest to the table. Be careful not to drop your body behind your standing leg, which will occur if your front leg ends up under the table (Figure 18.8b ■). Unless you are doing a long stroke in which you need to lunge, avoid wide stances because they can lower your center of gravity to a point that is too low to stay up and over your work (Figure 18.8c ■). Wide, low stances also require a lot of muscular work to hold, which reduces your economy of effort.

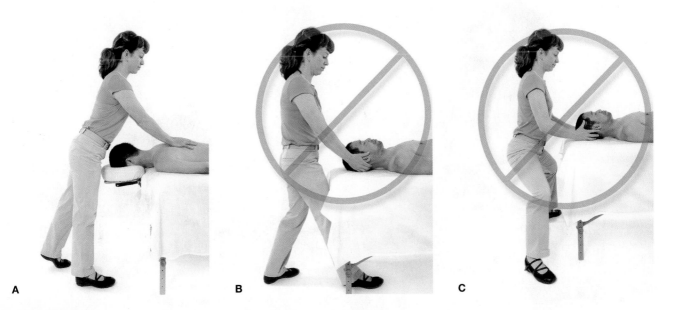

A   B   C

FIGURE 18.8

a) When standing, keep your weight over your front leg. b) Avoid placing your foot under the table. c) Avoid holding wide, low positions.

18.3.4   Match and Synchronize Upper Body Movement with Lower Body Movement

To promote an upper and lower body connection, move your lower body in sync with your upper body and arms in one smooth, full-body motion. Let your body movement mirror and support your hand movement in shape, size, and rhythm. This will help you maintain continuity of tone and movement through your whole body.

- If your stroke is short, take a small step.
- If your stroke is long, take a big step and lunge.
- If your stroke rocks back and forth, let your body also rock back and forth.
- If your stroke is curved, turn your pelvis and trunk in a curvilinear pathway that matches the direction, shape, and size of the massage stroke.
- If your stroke is shaped like a figure eight, move your hips like a figure eight and allow weight to transfer across the soles of your feet in a figure eight.

18.3.5   Take a Step when You Come to the End of a Reach

Sometimes, practitioners feel rushed and do not take the time to reposition the body to be able to reach within a reasonable distance. When people reach beyond their limit, a number of compensations occur that affect posture and stability. The thoracic spine usually flexes and the shoulder girdle lifts off the thorax to extend the arms beyond the base of support (Figure 18.9a-b ■). As the center of weight overextends, some part of the body will need to pull back to counterbalance the weight and keep the person from falling forward. The time you take to shift your body weight correctly as needed will be miniscule compared to the time it will take to deal with the problems that a faulty pattern will eventually create.

Once you arrive at the end of a stroke and have extended your arms as far forward as they can go, take a step to shift your base of support in order to reach farther. This way, your body follows the stroke and the arms pull the trunk forward. Always avoid overextending your spine by overreaching.

18.3.6   Move into a Lunge Rather than Assuming a Fixed-Lunge Stance

Whenever you need to lunge, move into the lunge rather than assuming a fixed-lunge position. As you are doing a long stroke, lean and step into a lunge. As you lunge, balance the COG in your pelvis over your front foot so that your trunk stays over your BOS.

Always lunge in the direction of your stroke to avoid twisting. When you lunge, place the foot in front that opens your lunge on the table side; otherwise, you'll have to twist your spine to reach across your leg (Figure 18.10a-b ■). As mentioned before, always stagger your feet in the lunge the same length of your stroke, keep the knee over the foot when you lunge to avoid twisting the joints, and keep your lumbar spine long and your lower abdominals contracted to avoid overarching and hyperextending your lower back.

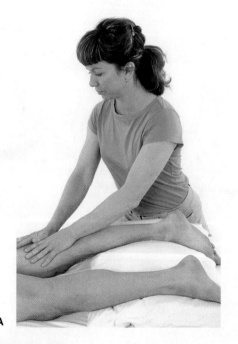
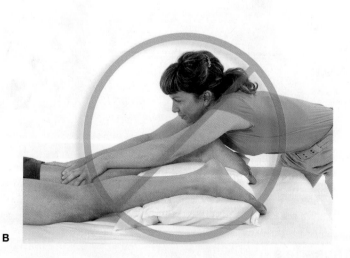

A   B

FIGURE 18.9

a) Shift your weight at the end of your reach. b) Avoid overreaching.

FIGURE 18.10

a) Lunge with your legs open to the table. b) Avoid lunging with your legs close to table.

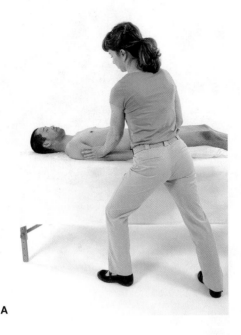
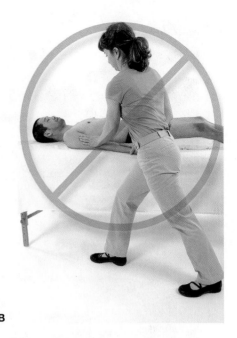

A

B

18.4 FORCE APPLICATIONS AND HAND USE

All forces that generate motion create some kind of mechanical stress in the body. In the chapter on biomechanics, the various effects of mechanical stresses were discussed. To review a few, pushing creates compression in the tissues, pulling creates tension and stretch in the tissues, and twisting or rotation creates torque in the tissues.

Every massage stroke involves some kind of force application. The key to using effective force application in massage is to generate the maximum force with the minimum stress on your body. In this section, we look at concepts to remember in order to maximize force while minimizing stress on your body as you work.

18.4.1 Make Every Stroke a Full-Body Movement

Apply each stroke with a full-body movement no matter how small or slow the stroke is. This will help you generate muscular effort with your whole body rather than just your arms, which will keep your arms from overworking. Move your hands in sync with the rest of the body, steering your hands with your body. During small, short strokes, your body movements can also be fairly small, perhaps comprising only a subtle sway or lean into your hands. During a long stroke, your entire body can move, ideally with a step and a lunge.

To feel how whole-body motion affects your quality of touch, try this hands-on experiment with a friend or colleague:

1. Massage a partner using your whole body, leaning into your hands to apply pressure and moving your body

in sync with your hands to shift your body weight in and out of each stroke. Ask your friend to notice how using body weight and whole-body movement feels.
2. Next, hold your body very still and continue to massage using only arm movement. Then ask your massage friend how it feels.

When doing this experiment in classes, students usually comment that the whole-body movement feels better, specifically because it feels deeper and more connected. In contrast, keeping the body still and only moving the arms creates a stiff and superficial quality of touch.

18.4.2 When Applying Pressure, Align the Fingers, Wrist, and Forearm

As much as possible, keep your middle finger aligned with the center of your forearm. This will help you keep your forearms and hands square by keeping your little finger aligned with the ulna and your index finger aligned with the radius. There will be times when you will need to deviate from center and adduct your wrist, such as when you use your thumbs (Figure 18.11a ■).

If you can align the joints of each finger with the corresponding metacarpal bone, you will be able to channel compressive forces through the center of your fingers into the wrist and up your forearm. Make sure to stack your joints when applying pressure with your fingers, especially your thumb. Avoid bending the thumb or fingers when applying pressure because compression through a bent joint can damage the joint structure (Figure 18.11b-c ■).

Practice force applications through your hands by leaning on your fingertips as though you were going to do a fingertips push-up. Make sure to keep your wrist extended and your fingers just slightly bent (Figure 18.12a ■).

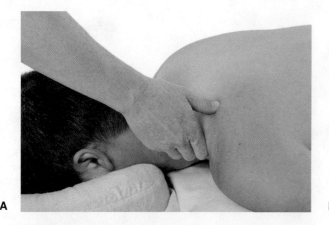

A

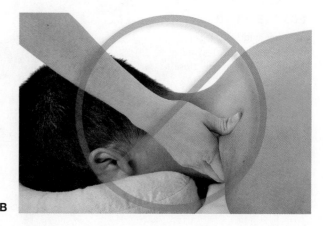

B

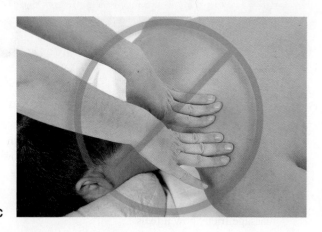

C

FIGURE 18.11

a) Keep your thumb straight when applying pressure. b) Avoid hyperextending the thumb. c) Avoid hyperextending of the fingers, especially during force applications.

This will engage the finger flexors, which increases grip strength. Practice applying fingertip pressure through slightly bent fingers by pressing the fingertips into the table, sensing the line of force into the center of the wrist. If you have a finger that hyperextends, explore different ways to straighten the joints as you press, such as using hand-over-hand pressure (Figure 18.12b ■). If your thumb hyperextends, figure out ways to use your thumb that will keep it straight (Figure 18.13a ■). You can also minimize the amount of compression on each thumb and double your force by using a thumb-over-thumb or thumb-beside-thumb pressure (Figure 18.13b ■).

18.4.3 To Apply Pressure, Lean the Whole Body into the Hands and Push from the Feet

To maximize leverage, use your body weight to apply pressure by leaning into your hands.[1] When you lean from your ankles, your whole body becomes the lever arm, and the longer your lever arm, the stronger your pressure.

Once you have leaned into your hands, you can increase pressure by pushing from your back foot. To engage the intrinsic muscles in your calf, slightly lift your heel and push with your toes as though you were stepping forward. Make sure to push with your whole body, from your core and feet, so that the compressive and tensional forces of pushing and pulling are absorbed through a series of linked joints from your hands to the feet, moving through your spine. This also allows the mechanical stresses created by movement to be distributed among and dissipated by as many body parts as possible.

When leaning, keep your spine aligned in neutral, in a plank position. If you are leaning into your hands, your client becomes a partial base of support, almost as if you were doing a table push-up (Figure 18.14 ■). Unless you are working with a brittle client, do not be afraid to lean on your client. It is impossible to do self-supported pushing, in other words, pushing without leaning. Lean at a 10- to 20-degree incline so that you can easily control pressing yourself back up to vertical.

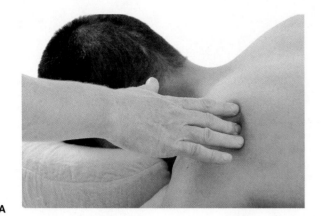

A

B

FIGURE 18.12

a) Using fingertip pressure b) Using hand-over-hand pressure

18.4.4 Use Optimal Lines of Force when Pushing and Pulling

A line of force is the pathway along which a force travels. Push or pull generates force. When pushing or pulling, keep as many joints extended as possible so that the forces transfer through the center of the joints. As mentioned earlier to push, lean with your spine extended and your arms straight. Push with a straight elbow so that the compressive forces of the push travel up the center of the arm into the shoulder girdle and down into the spine. Avoid locking the elbows (Figure 18.15a ■). To keep from locking your elbows, keep the olecranon processes facing sideways as you work (Figure 18.15b ■). If you lock your elbows while pushing, the line of force will get stuck in the elbow, which can damage the joint structure. The same dynamic is true for the locked knees.

If you need to bend as you push or pull, bend at your hips and knees rather than your spine or elbows. This way, compressive and tensional forces will translate through your arms and shoulders and into your spine.

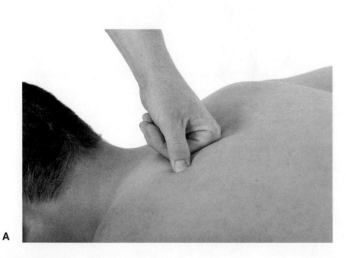

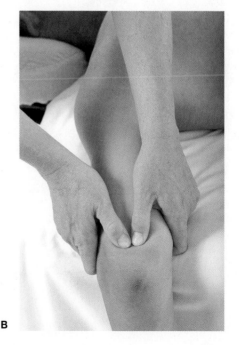

A

B

FIGURE 18.13

a) Using a fist to support thumb pressure b) Using thumb-beside-thumb pressure

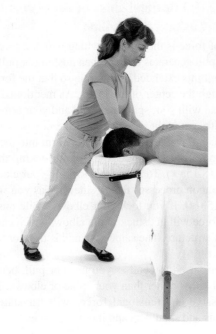

FIGURE 18.14

To increase pressure using body weight, lean on your client.

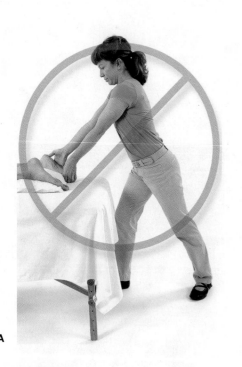

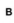

A

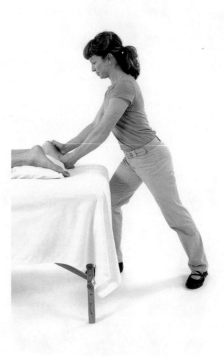

B

FIGURE 18.15

a) Avoid locking your elbows. b) To avoid locking your elbows, keep your elbows facing sideways.

EXPLORING TECHNIQUE
Push-Hands Exercise

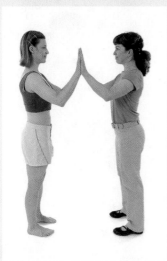 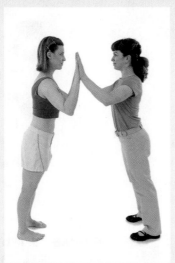 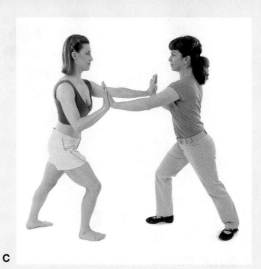

A   B   C

FIGURE 18.16

a) To begin push-hands exercise, touch hands. b) Then lean into each other with your full body weight. c) Explore push hands while walking and pushing back and forth.

To explore using optimal lines of force while pushing and pulling, here are two exercises to practice with a partner:

1. Practice this exercise with a partner to pattern pushing with your whole body in an optimally aligned position (Figure 18.16a ■).
2. Begin with both people standing in a neutral posture and touching palms with your arms slightly below shoulder height. Then slowly lean the weight of your bodies into each other's palms (Figure 18.16b ■).

3. Lunge as you lean with your spine in neutral, stepping into a rocker stance. Keep your scapulae connected to your back. Push from your back foot. Avoid tucking or flexing the hips and arching the back. Channel lines of compression through the skeletal system by connecting your hands to your feet through your core. Explore walking back and forth while pushing against your hands and pushing with your feet against the floor (Figure 18.16c ■).

EXPLORING TECHNIQUE
Pull-Back Exercise

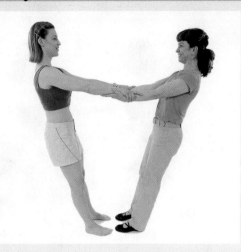

FIGURE 18.17a

To begin the pull-back exercise, grasp wrists, then lean back and balance.

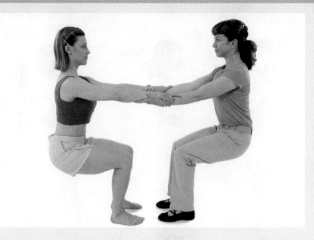

FIGURE 18.17b

Keep the spine straight while sitting down.

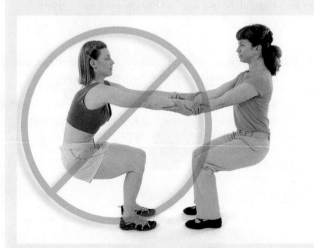

FIGURE 18.17c

Avoid hiking your shoulders as you pull back.

1. Practice this exercise with a partner to pattern pulling with your whole body with optimal alignment. Grasp each other's wrists. Slowly lean back at the same time to find a neutral balance point (Figure 18.17a ■).
2. Avoid arching the back or hiking the shoulders. Keep the shoulders connected to your back by contracting your latissimus dorsi, which will anchor your shoulders to your sacrum. Once you've found the neutral balance point where you are leaning back and supporting each other, slowly sit down together (Figure 18.17b ■).

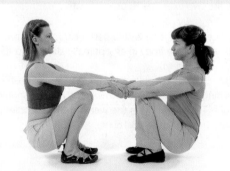

FIGURE 18.17d

Push down with your feet to come back up.

3. Keep your spine straight and vertical, taking your hips toward the ground with your spine moving along as the pathway of an elevator shaft, straight up and down. Make sure not to hike your shoulders or lock your elbows, which will break your line of pull (Figure 18.17c ■).
4. Once you've reached bottom, lean back with your arms straight, then push your feet down simultaneously to come back up (Figure 18.17d ■).

18.4.5 Vary Massage Strokes to Avoid Overusing Any One Hand Position

The quickest path to hand and wrist injuries is overusing one kind of hand position. There are many ways to use your hands. Each different hand position is like using a different tool. You'll want to have many tools in your toolbox, including thumbs, knuckles, fingertips, fists, palms, forearms, and elbows. If you tend to use one tool over and over again, it's important to start practicing using other options.

The finger flexors have incredible strength in a hook grip. You can adapt the hook grip as a hands-on tool we call the "claw," which involves pressing the fingertips into the tissue with the wrist extended and the fingers in slight flexion (Figure 18.18a ■). You can use the claw to plow the tissues when doing myofascial release, or to knead the tissues with circular motion or linear stripping. To strengthen your finger flexors, practice isometric finger pulls (Figure 18.18b ■).

18.4.6 Balance the Body by Alternating Opposing Strokes

In the chapter on biomechanics, we discussed balancing the body with reverse actions. For example, you can develop a stretch and strengthening routine that works the opposite muscles you use on the job, taking the shoulders into extension rather than flexion (see the "Balancing Your Body with Reverse Actions" exercise in the biomechanics chapter). You can also balance the way you use your arms as you work by alternating opposing strokes.

Any stroke that pushes compresses your joints. Any stroke that pulls decompresses your joints. Therefore, to balance your joints with opposing forces, alternate using pushing and pulling strokes.

Balance one-handed strokes by doing the same stroke with your other hand on the other side of the client's body. Dancers use this technique in classes, repeating each routine in the opposite direction, first moving across the floor from right to left, then from left to right. When you switch sides, make sure to do the same techniques on the other side using your other hand in the same manner. Strive to have your left-handed strokes mirror your right-handed strokes. This will help keep your muscle-use patterns symmetrical and prevent one-handed dominance. It will also ensure you do work evenly on both sides of your client's body.

After doing a lot of strokes with the thumbs that take the wrist into radial deviation, balance your body with strokes that use the lateral edge of your hand with ulnar deviation (Figure 18.19a-b ■).

Intermittently give your hands a break by using your forearms or elbows to apply pressure. You can lean on your forearms to apply deep, broad strokes down the back, hips, or legs. The forearms are also great tools for smaller practitioners to work with on larger clients. In addition, there are many effective shiatsu and Thai Massage techniques in which the practitioners apply pressure with the feet. Giving massage with the feet is a great way to use your body weight to generate pressure, while at the same time cultivating balance and agility in the lower body (Figure 18.20 ■).

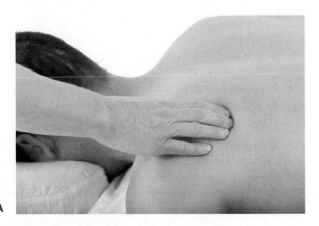

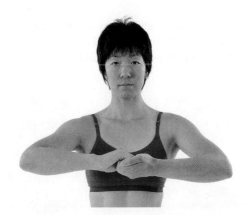

A   **B**

FIGURE 18.18

a) Using the "claw" b) Isometric finger-pull exercise

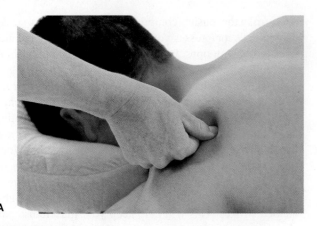

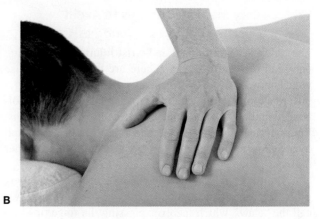

A

B

FIGURE 18.19

a) Thumb pressure with radial deviation b) Alternating stroke using ulnar deviation

18.5 ERGONOMICS AND EQUIPMENT

Taking the time to get the right massage equipment and set it up appropriately will greatly enhance your workplace ergonomics and make it much easier to use good body mechanics. There are several considerations to make when getting your equipment in place. In this section, we look at the key elements of table height; types of stools and chairs to use; how to use table pads, bolsters, and pillows; and where to place mirrors.

If you are just starting your practice, talk to seasoned therapists about equipment preferences before purchasing your equipment. They can give you invaluable information about what works for them that can save you time and money.

18.5.1 Table Height

A number of helpful guidelines are available for determining table height, but ultimately, you need to set your table at a height that is comfortable for you. You may

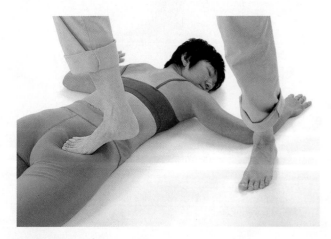

FIGURE 18.20

Working with the feet

need to experiment to find your own comfort level, which often changes over time as you practice different techniques. Position the top of your table at a height that allows you to easily reach the client from a comfortable standing position. The table usually needs to be lower for deep tissue work so that you can lean into your client more easily and use your body weight. The table usually needs to be higher for light massage techniques that require light pressure, such as lymph drainage or visceral manipulation.

Some teachers advocate positioning the top of the massage table to the height of the fingertips, knuckles, or wrists in a standing position, but it is important to take into account individual body proportions. If your arms, legs, or trunk tend to be long or short, such guidelines may not work for you. Here are two general guidelines:

- If you find yourself habitually bending your spine as you work, your table is probably too low (Figure 18.21a ■).
- If you find yourself habitually hiking your shoulders as you work, your table is probably too high (Figure 18.21b ■).

A hydraulic table will allow you to easily change your table height during a session, controlling it with a foot pedal control. However, these usually cost a lot more than a folding table and are difficult to move, so a hydraulic table will limit the use of your massage space to table massage only. If you want to practice floor techniques such as Thai massage or use the room to stretch in between clients, you'll probably want an adjustable table that is easy to fold up and put away.

Another element to consider when setting table height is that clients' bodies vary in depth. For larger clients, the table needs to be lower. Fortunately, a set table height usually works fine for the average client, so you should be able to work comfortably with a set table height. Once you get

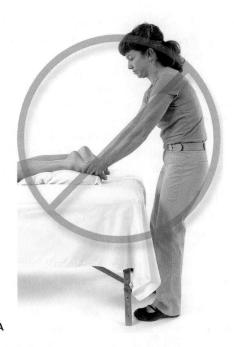

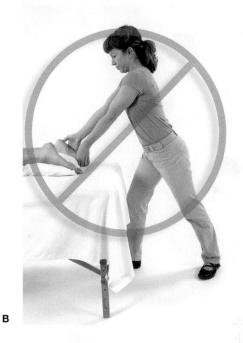

A   B

FIGURE 18.21

a) Avoid bending your spine from working with the table too low. b) Avoid hiking your shoulders from working with the table too high.

to know your clients and know when a larger client is coming, you can prepare by lowering your table for that session.

The body mechanics for performing basic Swedish petrissage strokes are similar to the body mechanics a baker uses while vigorously turning and kneading bread dough on a kitchen counter. The table height needs to position the top of the client's back at about the same height as the top of the bread dough would be on the countertop. To figure out this height, here's a simple exercise you can explore:

1. Stand in an upright posture.
2. Imagine a client on a massage table in front of you and give this imaginary client an air massage (like playing air guitar).
3. Note the height of the palms of your hands. Set your table at a height that lands about 5–6 inches—the average depth of a client's torso—below your palms.

18.5.2 Foot Stools and Folding Stools

A small foot stool can come in handy for several uses. Keep one under the center of your table to pull out for infirm clients to step on as they get on and off the table (Figure 18.22 ■). If you are a tall practitioner, your table height will probably be set pretty high, so a foot stool will come in handy for helping short clients get on a high table.

To get up and over your client so you can apply deeper pressure or acupressure along the spine, you can put one foot on a foot stool and your other knee on the table (Figure 18.23 ■). If you suffer from lower back pain,

propping one foot on a small stool can relieve pressure and pain on the lower back. Keep a plastic stool under your table that you can easily slide out with your toes to discreetly prop your foot on during a session.

If you practice seated techniques, folding stools are great to keep on hand. They also come in handy for house

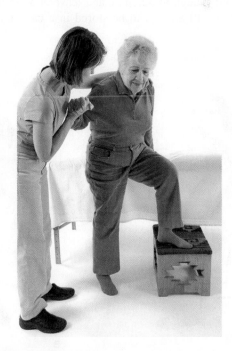

FIGURE 18.22

Use a step stool to help an infirm client get on and off the table.

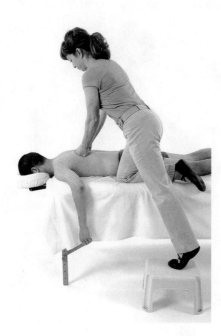

FIGURE 18.23

Using a step stool to work on the spine

calls, especially when you are unfamiliar with the room setup or know there will not be an appropriate chair in the room. Folding stools can also be helpful for working in hospitals or nursing homes because they give you flexibility in where you can sit around a hospital bed or cumbersome chair.[5] Lightweight stools are easy to carry, affordable enough to purchase and leave at a regular job site, and small enough to be stored in a car trunk or a closet.

18.5.3 Chairs and Seated Techniques

If you practice techniques done from a sitting position, it is helpful to have your table high enough that you can put your legs under it and rest your feet flat on the floor while you work. It should also be low enough that you can comfortably rest your elbows while still sitting upright (Figure 18.24a–c ■).

An adjustable stool or chair is ideal for working from a seated position, such as office chairs on wheels. Most massage stools do not have back supports but office chairs do, so consider whether or not you will need back support when working from a seated position. When picking out a chair, make sure the seat of your chair is level so that you can sit upright on it and keep your pelvis horizontal. Chair seats that tip down in the back tend, like bucket seats in a car, to place the pelvis in a posterior tilt, which puts excessive weight and pressure on the lumbar spine and can lead to back pain.

Rolling stools work best on carpeted floors where they are more stable; they will slide on wood, vinyl, or tile floors. (*Note:* Carpeted floors are usually preferable in a massage room because they are quiet, they help with shock absorption to cushion your joints as you work, and they protect clients from slipping when moving around the room in socks.)

When working in a sitting position, your ischial tuberosities (sit bones) are your base of support. Make sure to sit right on top of your sit bones and keep your pelvis level. If you need to lean forward, rock over your sit bones, leaning from your hips rather than arching the lower back or bending the spine (Figure 18.25a–c ■). To apply deeper pressure from a seated position, apply the same dynamics as you would use from a standing position. Stagger your feet in the direction of your stroke, lean your whole body into your

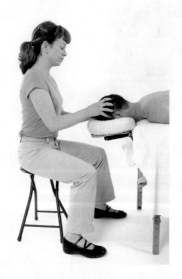

A

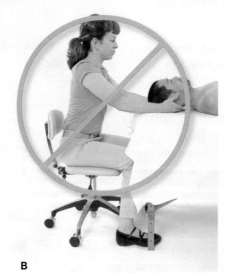

B

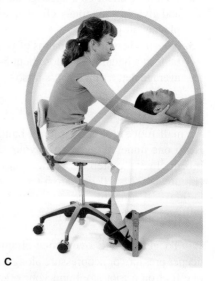

C

FIGURE 18.24

a) Appropriate chair height b) Chair is too low c) Chair is too high

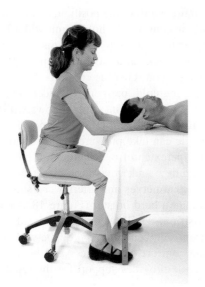
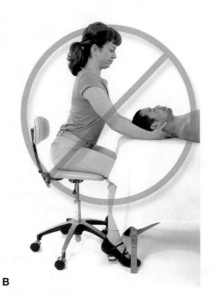
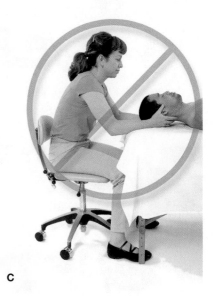

A   B   C

FIGURE 18.25

a) When leaning from a seated position, maintain a neutral spine. b) Avoid sitting with your spine hyperextended. c) Avoid sitting with your spine flexed.

pressure, and push from your back foot. When working on the top of the shoulder, you can generate greater pressure by using your forearm, which you can place perpendicular to the muscles (Figure 18.26 ■).

18.5.4 Table Pads, Bolsters, and Face Cradles

Some massage therapists like to put a foam pad on the table, which enhances the client's comfort as well as the therapist's. If you practice techniques in which you are

reaching under the client, the pad will allow you to slip your hand under the body more easily. A 3-inch-thick pad is recommended. Here are some other advantages of using foam pads:

- A foam pad provides a shock-absorbing cushion under your client, which will give you farther to sink during deep tissue applications (Figure 18.27 ■).
- Foam absorbs and radiates body heat, keeping your client warmer in cold weather.
- A foam pad can provide a quick way for adjusting your table height. If you run short on time to lower your table height, simply remove it before your next client arrives.
- If you like to alternate between table work and floor work, and have limited storage space, you can fold up your table and use your pad to work with clients on the floor.

The more comfortable a client is, the easier it will be for you to work on the client. Clients will shift around in

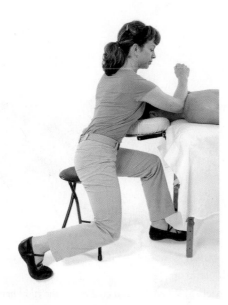

FIGURE 18.26

When using forearm pressure on the top of the shoulder, push with your back foot to increase your leverage.

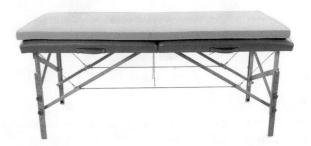

FIGURE 18.27

Consider using a foam pad on your table.

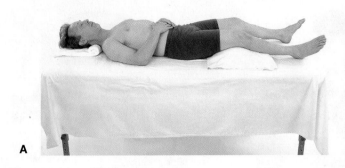

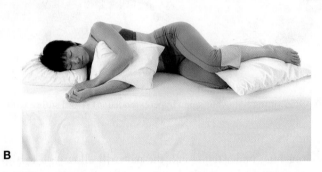

FIGURE 18.28

a) Using a soft pillow rather than a hard bolster under the knees will reduce pressure on the back of the knees. b) Use three pillows to comfortably pad and support a client in a side-lying position.

an effort to find a more comfortable position, or they will silently suffer while unconsciously holding muscular tension against a bolster that cuts into their shins or a face cradle that holds their necks at an awkward angle. With this in mind, make sure your client is comfortable. Ankle bolsters can be hard and cold, particularly under skinny, swollen, or injured knees and shins. Soft pillows will be more comfortable in all positions. In a prone position, a pillow under the ankle can take pressure off of the lower back if it tends to hyperextend from tightness or pain. In a supine position, a pillow under the knees places far less pressure on the popliteal nerves and arteries crossing the back of the knees than a hard bolster (Figure 18.28a ■). In a side-lying position, a pillow under the head will prevent the neck from side-bending, a pillow between the knees increases the comfort of the knees and hips, and a pillow over the chest provides support for the top arm (Figure 18.28b ■).

Face cradles can be torture on a client with an arthritic neck or suffering from chronic headaches. Many face cradles position the head too high, hyperextending the neck (Figure 18.29a ■). In this case, using a foam pad on your table will raise your client enough to effectively lower the cradle and position the head more comfortably (Figure 18.29b ■).

If your client has a hyperextended neck, causing the neck to arch and hyperextend when he or she is in a supine position, place a small towel or pillow under the head to lift it and lengthen the neck. If your client does not want to use a face cradle in a prone position but has trouble turning the

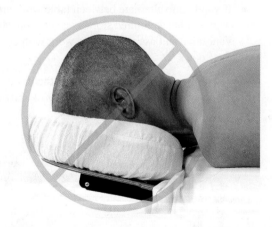

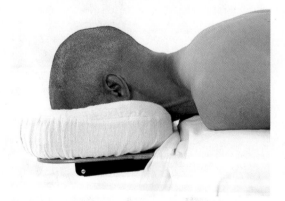

FIGURE 18.29

a) Avoid placing the face cradle too high because it hyperextends and strains the neck. b) When the face cradle is at the right height, the back of the neck will lengthen.

neck to one side, place a small towel or pillow on the side of the head and under the shoulder to reduce the degree of neck rotation (Figure 18.30 ■).

18.5.5   Mirrors for Feedback

A full-length mirror not only expands the size of a massage room, but when strategically placed in a workstation, it can provide you with invaluable feedback about your working posture. Everybody, including massage therapists and bodyworkers, has some kind of consistent postural challenge. Habitual postural problems tend to change slowly and need regular adjustments to feel normal. No matter how many times you readjust a chronically flexed thorax or swayed lower back, the pattern usually creeps in again when you are too busy to pay attention to your posture.

Though mirrors provide objective feedback and can be helpful for *occasionally* checking in on habitual patterns, be sure to note the emphasis on "occasionally" so that you do not become obsessive. You might check your mirror when you find yourself working in a stationary position, such as sitting to work on your client's head or doing deep tissue applications. Glance over to see if your spine is extended in a joint-neutral alignment, if your head is lifted and your neck elongated, and if your scapulae are lying flat against your rib cage in a neutral position. Then

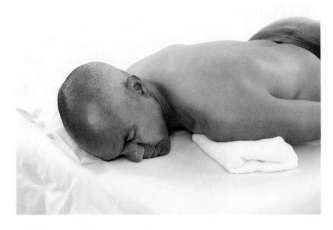

FIGURE 18.30

To reduce stress on your client's neck when the head is turned, put a towel under the shoulder and the side of the head.

make an adjustment and check again. If you use a mirror for feedback, you will probably begin to notice that you need to make the same postural corrections each time. Over time, these corrections will build muscle memory and will become easier to feel by just sensing where your body is in space rather than needing the visual feedback you get from a mirror.

SELF-CARE
Checklist for Body Mechanics in Massage

Here's a simple checklist you can use at the beginning of massage sessions to put the concepts listed in this section into practice:

1. Begin massage by standing in a neutral stance.
2. Align and ground your legs under your body.
3. Engage your core muscles.
4. Breathe into the width of your lower ribs to more effectively engage your diaphragm.
5. Sway a little to relax and feel fluid, intrinsic motion.
6. Stand next to the table and place your hands on your client and make a connection.
7. Slightly lean into your hands and begin the massage.
8. Find an easy rhythm that works for both you and your client.
9. Let your body follow your hands and face the direction of your stroke.
10. Move your whole body to move your hands.
11. Step forward into each stroke.
12. Stagger your feet in the direction of your stroke, which creates a rocker base.

CONCLUSION

Cultivating effective body mechanics is an inside job: Only you can help yourself. It is self-care in action, which requires persistent self-awareness of how you stand and use your body as you work. Applying kinesiology principles to your posture and movement will bring this work to life in your own experience and make your physical journey through daily activities easier and more enjoyable. Think of self-care as tuning up your vehicle of travel through life. Being an attentive driver will keep your muscles primed and your joints lubed so that you can keep your body on the road. It will minimize wear and tear on your body and give you a smoother ride through both work and play. After all, you only get one body and you need to make it last a lifetime. Therapeutic kinesiology applied to self-care and body mechanics can help you to be successful in this endeavor!

Notes

1. Foster, M. (200, April/May5). A Case for the Human Stance. *Massage and Bodywork Magazine,* pp. 72–81.
2. For more information about training postural muscles, see Chapter 9 in *Somatic Patterning: How to Improve Posture and Ease Pain,* by Mary Ann Foster (Longmont, CO: EMS Press, 2004).
3. Janet Travell warns against chronic hip rotation as a leading cause of sciatic nerve pain in massage therapists in her section on hip rotators in *Myofascial Pain and Dysfunction: The Trigger Point Manual: Vol. 2. The Lower Extremities* (Baltimore: Lippincott, Williams & Wilkins, 1999).
4. Turcahninov, R. and S. Ryason (2009). "*Science of Therapeutic and Stress Reducing Massage: Body Mechanics.*" Online Journal of Massage Science, accessed 8-1-2012 at <http://www.scienceofmassage .com/dnn/som/journal/0911/toc.aspx>.
5. Mary Rose discusses body mechanics specific to working in hospitals or nursing homes in her text *Comfort Touch: Massage for the Elderly and the Ill* (Baltimore: Lippincott, Williams, & Wilkins, 2010).

PEARSON myhealthprofessionskit™

Use this address to access the Companion Website created for this textbook. Simply select "Massage Therapy" from the choice of disciplines. Find this book and log in using your username and password to access interactive activities, videos, and much more.

Glossary

Abduction A movement of a limb, finger, or toe away from the midline of the body. See also *Adduction*.

Acceleration Describes the increasing velocity of a movement; also, a subphase of the swing phase of gait that occurs right after pushoff as the free leg swings in a downward arc. See also *Deceleration*, *Early swing*, *Velocity*.

Accessory movement See *Joint play*.

Actin A contractile protein inside the muscle fiber that makes up the thin filaments. See also *Myosin*.

Action potential A depolarization of the sarcolemma (cell membrane), which triggers the conduction of an electrical impulse through the muscle fiber.

Active insufficiency The point at which a biarticular or multiarticular muscle that is actively contracting has maximally shortened and cannot contract any farther; it can no longer produce tension and pull. See also *Passive insufficiency*.

Active motion Any movement that individuals perform of their own volition with no outside help. See also *Passive motion*.

Active pin and stretch A neuromuscular technique in which the practitioner maintains sustained pressure on a target muscle or tendon, then has the client actively move away from the point of pressure to stretch the muscle. See also *Pin and stretch*.

Active range of motion (AROM) The distance and direction (range), measured in degrees, that individuals can actively move their own joints using their own muscular power. See also *Passive range of motion*, *Range of motion*, *Resisted range of motion*.

Active restraints Contractile tissues that stabilize a joint, such as muscles and tendons. See also *Passive restraints*.

Active technique Describes any hands-on method requiring a client's active participation. See also *Passive technique*.

Active tension The tension generated by the contractile fibers in a muscle. See also *Passive tension*.

Activities of daily living (ADL) The natural movements that people use during the course of daily activities.

Acupressure points Specific points along a meridian, including motor points in muscles, which are treated using needles or direct pressure to improve the flow of energy along the meridian and also to relax muscular tension and relieve muscular pain.

Adaptive pattern See *Substitution pattern*.

Adaptive shortening The chronic tightness and fibrous buildup that occurs in a muscle as a result of being held in a shortened position for an extended period of time; total immobilization can eventually lead to the reabsorption of sacromeres. See also *Contracture*, *Stretch weakening*.

Adduction A movement of a limb, finger, or toe toward the midline of the body. See also *Abduction*.

Adhesive capsulitis A painful shoulder disorder in which inflammation adheres the joint capsule to adjacent ligaments and tendons and restricts movement; also called *frozen shoulder*.

Aerobic respiration The metabolic process in a muscle cell that requires oxygen to convert glucose into adenosine triphosphate (ATP). See also *Anaerobic respiration*.

Afferent neurons See *Sensory neurons*.

Agonist A term to describe a muscle that contracts to initiate an action; also called *prime mover*. See also *Antagonist*, *Fixator*, *Neutralizer*, *Synergist*.

Ambulation Walking.

Amphiarthrosis A semimoveable joint; a *fibrocartilage joint*. See also *Diarthrosis*, *Synarthrosis*.

Anaerobic respiration The metabolic process in a muscle cell that, in the absence of oxygen, converts glucose into adenosine triphosphate (ATP). See also *Aerobic respiration*.

Anatomical position A universal reference point from which we describe the position and movement of all body parts. In this position, the body is extended, with the palms facing forward and the legs slightly externally rotated. See also *Standing position*.

Anatomical stirrup A tendinous loop under the medial arch of the forefoot formed by the common insertions of the tibialis anterior and peroneus longus tendons; the muscles of the anatomical stirrup work as a steering mechanism to adapt the sole of the foot to uneven surfaces.

Angle of inclination The angle between the neck and the shaft of the femur, which averages 135 degrees.

Angle of pull See *Line of pull.*

Angle of torsion The angle between the neck of the femur and the axis that runs through the femoral condyles, which averages 15 degrees.

Angular motion See *Rotary motion.*

Antagonist A term used to describe a muscle working in opposition to an agonist. See also *Agonist, Fixator, Neutralizer, Synergist.*

Antalgic gait A gait dysfunction characterized by a shortened stance phase, which develops as a self-protective measure to avoid a painful range of motion. See also *Gait cycle.*

Anterior A positional term describing structures located closer to the front of the body than other structures or movement toward the front of the body. See also *Posterior.*

Anterior pelvic tilt (APT) A postural pattern that occurs when the top of the pelvis tips in a forward direction. See also *Posterior pelvic tilt.*

Anterior–posterior (AP) axis An imaginary straight line that runs between the front and back of the body, perpendicular to the frontal (coronal) plane. See also *Medial–lateral axis, Vertical axis.*

Anterolateral A diagonal view of the body from an anterior and lateral angle.

Aponeurosis A broad, flat, and dense sheet of fascia that provides attachment sites and support for intersecting layers of muscles, for example, the thoracolumbar fascia.

Appendicular skeleton The appendages and girdles in the human skeleton; made up of the 126 bones in the limbs (upper and lower) and girdles (shoulder and pelvis) and attaches to the axial skeleton. See also *Axial skeleton.*

Arthrokinematics Refers to the different types of movement that occur inside a joint; how the articulating surfaces of a joint move across each other. See also *Osteokinematics.*

Articulation A bony joint. See also *Joint.*

Assessment An estimation or determination of the significance or importance of something. In relation to a massage practice, an assessment is made to determine whether or not massage is indicated and what type of massage best suits the client's condition, needs, and preferences.

Association neurons See Interneurons.

Ataxic gait A gait dysfunction caused by neurological damage to the cerebellum with resulting ataxia and muscular flaccidity or spasticity; characterized by poor coordination, unsteadiness, and a wide step to compensate for poor balance. See also *Gait cycle.*

Autonomic nervous system (ANS) A division of the peripheral nervous system that regulates all *involuntary* or *automatic* organ functions; divided into the *parasympathetic nervous system* and *sympathetic nervous system.* See also *Peripheral nervous system, Somatic nervous system.*

Axial compression Compression along the body's vertical axis; vertical loading of the spine and lower limbs.

Axial plane See *Horizontal plane.*

Axial skeleton The central part of the skeleton that bears weight, made up of the 80 bones of the cranium, the vertebral column, thorax, sternum, sacrum, and coccyx. See also *Appendicular skeleton.*

Axis A line passing perpendicular to a plane. Also, the fulcrum of a lever; the point around which the lever pivots. See also *Lever.*

Backward rotation A posterior turn of the pelvis in the horizontal (transverse) plane. See also *Forward rotation.*

Ball-and-socket joint A triaxial synovial joint in which the ball-like spherical head of one bone sits in the cup-like socket of another bone.

Base of support (BOS) The part of a mass or body that is supporting weight. See also *Center of gravity, Line of gravity.*

Bend A mechanical stress that combines tensile and compressive stresses, leading to the bending of a structure or joint. See also *Compression, Shear, Tension, Torque.*

Biarticular muscle A muscle that crosses two joints. See also *Multiarticular muscle.*

Biaxial joint A type of synovial joint that can move in two planes, allowing it to flex, extend, adduct, abduct, and circumduct. See also *Nonaxial joint, Triaxial joint, Uniaxial joint.*

Bilateral axis An imaginary straight line that runs between the right and left sides of the body, perpendicular to the sagittal plane; also called the *medial–lateral axis.* See also *Anterior–posterior axis, Vertical axis.*

Biomechanics The applications of mechanical principles to living organisms, particularly to human movement.

Bone markings See *Bony landmarks.*

Bone strength The measure of a bone's resistance to fracture.

Bony landmarks Distinguishing features, such as tubercles, ridges, foramens, and grooves, found on skeletal system bones, with each kind of landmark reflecting its basic function; also called *bone markings*.

Broad-hand gliding   An open hand palpation technique using the entire palmar surface to feel the contours and tone of large muscle groups covering general areas, such as the spine. Gliding is a precursor to effleurage strokes. See also *Cross-fiber strumming, Fingertip palpation, Flat-finger palpation, Pincher palpation, Static contact.*

Bulging disk   A condition in which the annulus fibers of an intervertebral disk tear and the fluid in the center of the disk seeps laterally, causing swelling. See also *Herniated disk.*

Bursa (plural: *bursae*)   Small fibrous sac filled with synovial fluid, usually found under tendons to reduce friction.

Bursitis   Inflammation of a bursa.

Cadence   The speed of a gait pattern, measured by number of steps per minute.

Calcaneal valgus   When the distal end of the heel (calcaneus) turns away from midline. See also *Calcaneal varus.*

Calcaneal varus   When the distal end of the heel (calcaneus) turns toward the midline. See also *Calcaneal valgus.*

Cancellous bone   See *Spongy bone.*

Cardinal planes   The three primary planes that intersect the center of an object or body. See also *Frontal plane, Horizontal plane, Sagittal plane.*

Carpal tunnel syndrome   An entrapment of the median nerve in the wrist due to compression in the carpal tunnel, which can cause numbness, tingling, inflammation, pain in the hand and wrist, and loss of grip strength.

Carrying angle   An angle at the elbow between the long axis of the humerus and the long axis of the forearm, which averages about 15 degrees.

Cartilaginous joint   See *Fibrocartilage joint.*

Caudal   A positional term pertaining to structures located at or near the tail or posterior, inferior end of the torso.

Center of gravity (COG)   The point within a mass or body in which all the parts are exactly balanced; also called *center of weight.* See also *Base of support, Line of gravity.*

Center of weight   See *Center of gravity, Gravity.*

Central nervous system (CNS)   Made up of the brain and spinal cord. See also *Nervous system, Peripheral nervous system.*

Cephalad   A positional term pertaining to structures located at or near the head.

Chi   A term from traditional Chinese medicine translated generally as "life force" or "energy"; believed to flow through pathways or channels in the body called *meridians*; also called *ch'i, qi.*

Ch'i   See *Chi.*

Chondromalacia   The premature deterioration and softening of the patellar cartilage. See also *Patellofemoral joint pain syndrome.*

Chronic obstructive pulmonary disease   A pathology of the lungs from asthma, bronchitis, or emphysema that narrows the respiratory passageways, reduces the elasticity of lung tissues, and restricts breathing.

Circular friction   A hands-on technique in which a practitioner applies deep circular pressure over a targeted area of myofascial tissue. See also *Cross-fiber friction, Linear friction.*

Circumduction   A combined movement that inscribes a cone-like shape; combines the movements of flexion and extension, medial and lateral rotation, and abduction and adduction.

Classroom palpation   A tactile exploration used in educational settings for studying the human body; usually practiced with a focus on finding and assessing specific anatomical structures. See also *Therapeutic palpation.*

Closed kinetic chain   A movement in which the end of the kinetic chain is fixed. See also *Kinetic chain, Open kinetic chain.*

Close-packed position   A joint position in which the articulating surfaces of a joint reach maximum compression and the joint becomes maximally stable. See also *Loose-packed position.*

Collagen   The most abundant connective tissue fiber in the body. See also *Elastin fibers, Reticular fibers.*

Compact bone   A thin, protective layer of bone tissue with osteocytes arranged in tight, concentric rings called lamellae, which covers the outer layer of every bone; also called *cortical bone.* See also *Spongy bone.*

Compartment syndrome   A serious pathology caused by stiff and unyielding fascia around a pocket of muscles, which increases pressure, obstructs circulation, and can result in amputation or death if untreated.

Compensatory pattern   See *Substitution pattern.*

Compression   A mechanical stress that occurs when two forces press into the center of a structure from opposite directions. See also *Bend, Shear, Tension, Torque.*

Computer neck   See *Forward head posture.*

Concave–convex rule   Primary principle of joint arthrokinematics stating that, in joints that contain concave and convex joint surfaces, when the bone with the concave surface moves, the joint surface moves in the same direction as that bone; when the bone with the convex joint surface moves, the joint surface always moves in the opposite direction from that bone.

Concentric contraction   A muscular contraction in which the length of the muscle decreases; occurs when a contractile force exceeds the resistance to that force. See also *Eccentric contraction*.

Concurrent forces   Two or more forces that act on a body or object at the same point of application from different directions, creating a third resultant force, such as the air coming out of a bellows. See also *Concurrent movement*, *Linear forces*.

Concurrent movement   A movement during a contraction of a biarticular muscle when the muscle flexes one joint while being lengthened by the movement of the other joint, causing the muscle to slide toward the extended joint; also called *Parallel shift*. See also *Countercurrent movement*.

Condyloid joint   See *Ellipsoid joint*.

Congruent joint   A joint in which the space between opposing articulating surfaces is even and consistent. See also *Incongruent joint*.

Connective tissue   The most abundant of the four major tissues in the body (the other three are blood, bone, and cartilage). Connective tissue is made up of cells, fibers, and fluid; it provides a binding and supportive matrix for all bodily structures.

Contractility   A property of muscle tissue that allows muscles to generate contractile forces when adequately stimulated by motor nerves.

Contracture   A state of continual muscular contraction in which the crossbridges on the sliding filaments of the muscle fibers fail to unlink; also called a *spasm*.

Contralateral   One of the movement pathways along which patterns of early motor development occur; a term describing an action or structure as on or having to do with the opposite side of the body from another action or structure. See also *Homolateral*, *Homologous*, *Radial*, *Spinal*.

Coordination   In relation to human movement, the efficient and orderly recruitment of muscles during an action.

Coronal plane   See *Frontal plane*.

Cortical bone   See *Compact bone*.

Countercurrent movement   A movement during a concentric contraction of a biarticular muscle when the muscle acts on both joints to which it is attached by shortening into its center. See also *Concurrent movement*.

Counternutation   A nodding motion of the sacrum that rocks the top of the sacrum in a posterior direction. See also *Nutation*.

Coupled motion   Every spinal movement combines two actions; for example, flexion combined with rotation or extension combined with lateral flexion.

Cranial   Pertaining to the cranium.

Cranial nerves   Peripheral nerves that branch out of the brain stem and innervate the muscles and perceptual organs of the head and neck.

Cranial protraction   A movement of thrusting the chin forward, which flexes the lower cervical vertebrae while hyperextending the upper cervical vertebrae. See also *Cranial retraction*.

Cranial retraction   A movement of pulling the chin straight back, which flexes the upper cervical vertebrae while hyperextending the lower cervical vertebrae. See also *Cranial protraction*.

Creep   The progressive stretching that occurs when a viscoelastic tissue or other material is placed under sustained pressure, leading to a slow-motion plastic change.

Crossed-extensor reflex   A protective withdrawal reflex in which one leg flexes to pull away from a noxious stimulus while the other leg simultaneously extends to support the entire weight of the body; underlies contralateral movement.

Cross-fiber friction   A hands-on technique in which deep, transverse strokes are applied across a small area of tissue with a repetitive motion; also called *transverse friction*. See also *Circular friction*, *Linear friction*.

Cross-fiber strumming   A palpation technique in which a practitioner strums across muscles or bones in a perpendicular direction. See also *Broad-hand gliding*, *Fingertip palpation*, *Flat-finger palpation*, *Pincher palpation*, *Static contact*.

Curvilinear motion   Movement along a curved pathway. See also *Linear motion*, *Rotary motion*.

Deceleration   Describes the decreasing velocity of a movement; also, a subphase of the swing phase of gait that occurs as the free leg swings in an upward arc. See also *Acceleration*, *Late swing*, *Velocity*.

Deep   A positional term describing structures located farther away from the surface than other structures. See also *Superficial*.

Degrees of motion   The number of planes in which a joint can move. For example, an ellipsoid joint can move in two planes, therefore it has two degrees of motion. See also *Plane*.

Depression   A movement that is a return from elevation; can refer to lowering the scapula from an elevated position or opening the mouth. See also *Elevation*.

Developmental movement patterns   Early motor patterns crucial to normal brain development and neuromuscular organization; also called *neurological patterns*. See also *Neurological actions*, *Neurological pathways*.

Diagonal axis   A line between the opposite corners of a cube.

Diagonal plane   A plane that runs perpendicular to the diagonal axis.

Diarthrosis   A freely movable, synovial joint. See also *Amphiarthrosis, Synarthrosis*.

Diastasis recti   A split between the right and left sides of the rectus abdominis muscle that creates an abdominal separation; sometimes occurs with pregnancy.

Dimensional balance   Describes symmetry and proportion among the height, width, and depth of the body.

Dimensional cross   A structure made up of two axes positioned at right angles to each other.

Direct technique   Any therapeutic movement that takes the client in a direction that stretches the tissues and pulls them out of their shortened position. See also *Indirect technique*.

Distal   A positional term describing structures located farther away from the trunk than other structures. See also *Proximal*.

Dorsal   A positional term describing the top of the foot or structures located on the posterior surface (back) of the body. See also *Plantar, Ventral*.

Dorsiflexion   A movement of the ankle toward the dorsal (top) surface of the foot, closing the angle of the ankle. See also *Plantarflexion*.

Double-limb support   The period in a gait cycle in which both feet make simultaneous contact with the ground. See also *Stance phase*.

Downslip   A sacroiliac joint dysfunction that results in a slight downward motion of the iliac crest on one side of the pelvis. See also *Upslip*.

Downward rotation   A movement of the scapula that occurs when lowering the arm, which combines depression, retraction, and rotation. See also *Upward rotation*.

Drawer sign   An excessive anterior or posterior gliding motion of the proximal tibia that occurs when either of the cruciate ligaments have been damaged.

Drop-foot gait   A compensatory gait pattern caused by dysfunctional dorsiflexors, usually the tibialis anterior, causing the foot to drop on the ground on each step; a person with a drop-foot gait raises the knee higher than normal on the swing leg so that the foot clears the ground; also called *steppage gait*. See also *Gait cycle*.

Dynamics   A term used to describe mechanical principles that apply to a body in motion.

Early swing   The subphase of the swing phase of gait that occurs right after pushoff as the free leg swings in a downward arc; also called *acceleration*. See also *Swing phase*.

Eccentric contraction   A muscular contraction in which the length of the muscle increases; occurs when a contractile force is less than the resistance to that force. See also *Concentric contraction*.

Eccentric loading   A term to describe a muscle working eccentrically to support weight; can lead to stretch weakening and stretch injuries.

Efferent neurons   See *Motor neurons*.

Effort   The force applied to move a lever.

Effort arm   The distance between the point of force application and the axis of a lever.

Elasticity   The property of tissue to recoil or rebound after being deformed by a mechanical force; in muscle tissue, it causes a muscle to recoil and return to its normal resting length after being extended. See also *Elastic limit, Plasticity*.

Elastic limit   The stretching point at which an elastic tissue is unable to return to its original shape.

Elastin fibers   Connective tissue fibers that are elastic and are found in vast quantities in tissues that need to stretch, such as the skin and the urinary bladder. See also *Collagen, Reticular fibers*.

Elevation   Can refer to raising the scapulae or closing the jaw. See also *Depression*.

Ellipsoid joint   A biaxial synovial joint that has an ovoid surface, or condyle, which articulates with the elliptical cavity of the joint's other surface, allowing the joint to move in two planes; also called *condyloid joint*.

Endangerment sites   Locations in the body that have sensitive or delicate tissues, such as nerves or blood vessels, which could be damaged during massage and bodywork and should be approached with caution.

End-feel   The quality of restriction that a joint reaches when it cannot move any farther. Three normal end-feels are bony, capsular, and soft; all other end-feels indicate joint pathology.

Boggy end-feel   The quality of joint restriction characterized by a mushy, spongy feeling, usually from excess fluid or swelling in and around the joint.

Bony end-feel   The quality of joint restriction that occurs when bone meets bone, such as in elbow extension.

Capsular end-feel   The quality of joint restriction that occurs when connective tissues around a joint prevent further motion; also called *firm end-feel*.

Empty end-feel   The quality of joint restriction that occurs when joint movement causes pain that triggers muscular guarding, which prevents motion beyond a limited range; also called *spasm end-feel*.

Fibrotic end-feel   The quality of joint restriction characterized by a rapid buildup of tension, usually because of fibrotic thickening around the joint, perhaps due to scarring from injuries or surgeries.

Firm end-feel   See *Capsular end-feel*.

Hard end-feel   The quality of joint restriction characterized by an abrupt stop that occurs short of the normal end range, caused by an abnormal growth or bony restriction in the joint.

Lax end-feel   The quality of joint restriction that lacks an increase in tension and continues to stretch, causing the range of motion to exceed a normal range.

Soft end-feel   The quality of joint restriction that occurs when soft tissues prevent further motion, as in elbow or hip flexion.

Spasm end-feel   See *Empty end-feel.*

Equilibrium   Describes a condition in which all forces acting on a body are balanced.

Eversion   Turning the sole of the foot away from midline. See also *Inversion.*

Excitability   See *Responsiveness.*

Excursion   The distance a muscle can lengthen and shorten.

Exhalation fixation   A muscular holding pattern in which the rib cage is held in a deflated, sunken posture. See also *Inhalation fixation.*

Extensibility   A property of muscle tissue that gives it the capacity to be stretched or lengthened when acted upon by an outside force. See also *Elasticity, Plasticity.*

Extension   A movement that bends and opens the angle of a joint; a return from flexion. See also *Flexion.*

Extensor support moment   The point in the midstance phase of gait when the body begins to lean forward over the ankle, causing the knee and hip to simultaneously extend to prevent the lower limb from buckling under loading forces. See also *Stance phase.*

Extensor thrust reflex   A reflex that automatically and quickly extends the limbs. See also *Flexor withdrawal reflex.*

External rotation   See *Lateral rotation.*

Extrafusal fibers   The type of muscle fibers that function in a motor capacity to produce muscular contractions. See also *Intrafusal fibers.*

Fascia   A strong, pervasive tissue membrane made up of dense irregular connective tissue that wraps, supports, and binds all tissues.

Fast type IIA fibers   Medium-sized muscle fibers that metabolize energy through both oxidation and glycolysis, are moderately fatigue rapidly, and produce strong and fast contractions; also called *FOG fibers (fast oxidation glycolysis).* See also *Fast type IIB fibers, Slow type I fibers.*

Fast type IIB fibers   Large muscle fibers that metabolize energy through glycolysis, fatigue rapidly, and produce strong and fast contractions; also called *FG fibers (fast glycolysis).* See also *Fast type IIA fibers, Slow type I fibers.*

Feedback   A response or output from a process or structure that provides information about that process or structure. In massage and bodywork, a verbal or physical response from the client to the practitioner or vice versa.

FG fibers   See *Fast type IIB fibers.*

Fibrocartilage   A thick, dense cartilage found in the vertebral disks and menisci that is made up of thick interwoven layers of collagen fibers arranged in concentric rings.

Fibrocartilage joint   An amphiarthrotic joint in which dense connective tissue fibers and cartilage connect the bones, allowing minimal motion; also called *cartilaginous joint.* See also *Amphiarthrosis.*

Fibrous joint   A nonmovable, synarthrotic joint in which dense connective tissue fibers firmly bind and connect the bones. See also *Gomphosis, Synarthrosis, Syndesmosis.*

Fingertip palpation   A precise and targeted palpation technique using the tips of the fingers to apply direct pressure straight into a muscle belly or tendon. Fingertip palpation is a precursor to massage modalities based on pressure point techniques, such as shiatsu or trigger point therapy. See also *Broad-hand gliding, Cross-fiber strumming, Flat-finger palpation, Pincher palpation, Static contact.*

First-class lever   A lever that has the axis of motion located between the effort and the resistance. See also *Second-class lever, Third-class lever.*

Fixator   A term used to describe a muscle that contracts to prevent accessory joint motion. See also *Agonist, Antagonist, Neutralizer, Stabilizer, Synergist.*

Flat-back posture   See *Posture.*

Flat-finger palpation   A palpation technique using the palmar surface of the fingers to locate tissues that are easy to slip off of, such as thin, tubular muscle bellies or tissues covered with slippery fascia. See also *Broad-hand gliding, Cross-fiber strumming, Fingertip palpation, Pincher palpation, Static contact.*

Flexion   A movement that bends and closes the angle of a joint. See also *Extension.*

Flexor withdrawal reflex   A reflex that automatically pulls the limbs into quick flexion. See also *Extensor thrust reflex.*

Float moment   The period of time in a running gait in which both feet lose contact with the ground.

FOG fibers   See *Fast type IIA fibers.*

Foot angle   The degree of toe-out during gait.

Foot flat   The subphase of the stance phase of gait that occurs when the foot first comes into full contact with the ground. See also *Stance phase.*

Force   Any element that generates, affects, or alters movement.

Force couple   Two parallel forces that act simultaneously in opposite directions on the same joint.

Forced closure   Stabilization of the sacroiliac joint (SIJ) created by lower abdominal muscle forces. See also *Form closure.*

Force vector   In terms of contractile forces, the direction and magnitude of a muscular pull.

Force–velocity relationship   The inverse relationship between the amount of force a muscle can generate and the speed of the contraction.

Form closure   Stabilization of the sacroiliac joint (SIJ) created by the close-packed position of the joint. See also *Forced closure*.

Forward head posture   A habitual pattern of protracting the cranium by poking the chin forward, which creates faulty postural alignment and places the midcervical spine under excessive shearing stress; also called *computer neck*.

Forward rotation   An anterior turn of the pelvis in the horizontal (transverse) plane. See also *Backward rotation*.

Fracture   A break in a bone.

Friction   A force that occurs between two surfaces moving against each other, which decelerates the motion.

Frontal plane   Any vertical plane that divides the body or its parts into front (anterior) and back (posterior) sections; also called *coronal plane*. The primary movements of limbs relative to the frontal plane are abduction and adduction. See also *Horizontal plane, Sagittal plane*.

Frozen shoulder   See *Adhesive capsulitis*.

Fusiform muscles   Muscles with long, parallel fibers that are spindle-shaped, wide in the belly, and tapered on the ends into cord-like tendons. See also *Pennate muscles*.

Gait cycle   The movement of the lower limb through one stance phase and one swing phase; two steps or one stride. See also *Stride*.

Genu recurvatum   Hyperextension of the knee beyond a normal range of 5 to 10 degrees. See also *Genu valgus, Genu varum*.

Genu recurvatum gait   A gait dysfunction marked by a locking of the stance knee into hyperextension.

Genu valgus   An abnormally bent angle between the tibia and the femur at the knee; a knock-kneed alignment. See also *Genu recurvatum, Genu varus*.

Genu varus   An abnormally straight or inverted angle between the tibia and the femur at the knee; a bow-legged alignment. See also *Genu recurvatum, Genu valgus*.

Glide   The action of one articulating surface sliding across another.

Gliding joint   See *Plane joint*.

Global   Describes whole-body patterns or movement. See also *Local*.

Gluteus maximus lurch   A gait dysfunction caused by weakness or damage to the gluteus maximus muscle that results in a loss of control over hip extension, causing the stance hip to jackknife into flexion on heel strike, then lurch forward into hyperextension on midstance.

Gluteus medius lurch   See *Trendelenburg gait*.

Golgi tendon organs (GTOs)   Proprioceptors embedded in muscle tendons, along the musculotendinous junction, that register increased tension on a tendon when stretched and relay this information to the CNS, which triggers an inhibitory response that causes the muscle to relax.

Gomphosis   The fibrous, synarthrotic, peg-and-socket joints between the teeth and mandible. See also *Syndesmosis*.

Gravity   The attraction or pull of a mass toward the earth; a constant external force that gives mass weight. See also *Center of gravity, Line of gravity*.

Ground reaction force (GRF)   The force from the ground that pushes back against the downward force of a body against it.

Hallux valgus   A pattern of chronic adduction in the first toe that often develops into a painful bunion.

Heeloff   The subphase of the stance phase of gait that occurs when the heel lifts off the ground. See also *Stance phase*.

Heel strike   The subphase of the stance phase of gait that occurs when the heel first contacts the ground. See also *Stance phase*.

Herniated disk   A condition in which the annulus fibers of an intervertebral disk become so torn that the disk ruptures. See also *Bulging disk*.

Hinge joint   A type of uniaxial synovial joint in which the bony cylinder of one bone fits into the rounded trough of another bone, similar to the hinge on a door.

Homolateral   One of the movement pathways along which patterns of early motor development occur; a term describing an action or structure as on or having to do with another action or structure on the same side of the body; also called *ipsilateral*. See also *Contralateral, Homologous, Radial, Spinal*.

Homologous   One of the movement pathways along which patterns of early motor development occur; a term describing an action or structure as on or having to do with the same action or structure on both sides of the body. See also *Contralateral, Homolateral, Radial, Spinal*.

Horizontal abduction   A return of the arm from a position of horizontal adduction; also called *horizontal extension*. See also *Horizontal adduction*.

Horizontal adduction   A horizontal movement of the arm crossing the front of the body from an abducted position; also called *horizontal flexion*. See also *Horizontal abduction*.

Horizontal extension   See *Horizontal abduction*.

Horizontal flexion   See *Horizontal adduction*.

Horizontal plane   Any horizontal plane that divides the body or its parts into upper (superior) and lower (inferior) sections; also called *transverse plane*. The primary movement of the body relative to the horizontal plane is rotation. See also *Frontal plane*, *Sagittal plane*.

Hyaline cartilage   A thin, glassy, blue-white articular cartilage covering the articulating surfaces of bones in freely movable joints.

Hyperextension   Movement of a joint that extends the joint behind the frontal plane.

Hypermobility   An excessive range of joint motion. See also *Hypomobility*.

Hyperventilation   A condition that occurs when rapid breathing causes the amount of oxygen coming in to exceed the amount of carbon dioxide going out, causing a range of symptoms such as dizziness, lightheadedness, tingling, or fainting.

Hypomobility   A restricted range of joint motion. See also *Hypermobility*.

Hyperpronation   See *Pes planus*.

Hypersupination   See *Pes cavus*.

Ideokinesis   The process of using ideation or imagery to help change body movement or postural alignment.

Iliotibial band syndrome   An inflammatory condition of the knee that occurs when a tight iliotibial band becomes fibrotic and thickened, causing it to rub the lateral femoral epicondyle; a common cause of knee pain.

Incongruent joint   A joint in which the space between the opposing articulating surfaces is uneven. See also *Congruent joint*.

Indirect technique   Any therapeutic technique that, prior to lengthening the tissues, takes the client in a direction that approximates already compressed, shortened, or contracted tissues. See also *Direct technique*.

Inferior   A positional term describing structures that are below or lower than other structures. See also *Superior*.

Inhalation fixation   A muscular holding pattern in which the rib cage is held in an inflated, barrel-chest posture. See also *Exhalation fixation*.

Inner range   A range of joint motion in which the angle of the joint is maximally closed. See also *Midrange*, *Outer range*.

Insertion   One of the two places (along with the *origin*) where a muscle attaches to bone. The insertion is the distal attachment site and the site on the bone that moves during the joint motion. See also *Origin*.

Instantaneous axis of rotation (IAR)   The changing point of contact between the articular surfaces of a joint during joint motion.

Internal rotation   See *Medial rotation*.

Interneurons   Neurons that transfer signals between neurons in the brain and spinal cord; also called *association neurons*. See also *Motor neurons*, *Sensory neurons*.

Intra-abdominal pressure (IAP)   Pressure in the abdominal cavity from the contraction of surrounding muscles that helps support the trunk and prevent it from buckling under compression.

Intrafusal fibers   A type of muscle fibers that function in a sensory capacity to register stretch in a muscle; found inside muscle spindles. See also *Extrafusal fibers*.

Inversion   Turning the sole of the foot toward midline. See also *Eversion*.

Ipsilateral   See *Homolateral*.

Irregular dense connective tissue   A type of connective tissue made up of collagen fibers oriented in cross-hatched, multilayered sheets that form fascias and joint capsules. See also *Regular dense connective tissue*.

Irritability   See *Responsiveness*.

Isometric contraction   A muscular contraction in which the length of the muscle remains the same; occurs when the contractile force equals the resistance to that force. See also *Isotonic contraction*.

Isotonic contraction   A muscular contraction during which the length of the muscle changes; can be either an eccentric or concentric contraction. See also *Isometric contraction*.

Joint   A structure in which a bone articulates with another bone. See also *Articulation*.

Joint approximation   A therapeutic technique in which a practitioner presses the two articulating surfaces of a joint closer together.

Joint articulation   A therapeutic technique in which a practitioner performs passive joint motion using slow, specific movement, focusing on the quality of joint motion with the goal of improving joint arthrokinematics.

Joint capsule   A collar of dense, irregular connective tissue covering a synovial joint.

Joint instability   A condition of joint laxity in which a person is unable to control joint motion outside of a normal range. See also *Joint stability*, *Stability dysfunction*.

Joint mobility   The range of motion a joint can move without restrictions from surrounding structures.

Joint mobilization   A therapeutic technique in which a practitioner uses passive joint motion to restore normal joint position, stretch a stiff or hypomobile joint, relieve joint pain limiting active movement, or help a client recover from an injury or trauma.

Joint neutral   An extended position of a joint in which it is not flexed, rotated, or hyperextended.

Joint play   The range a joint can move or be moved that is beyond the normal range of motion; also called *accessory movement*.

Joint stability   The ability of joint structures to resist displacement. See also *Joint instability*.

Jump sign   A protective reflexive movement that a person has when pressure on a specific point in the body produces discomfort and pain; can be an indicator of a trigger point.

Kinematics   The study of the time and space elements associated with a moving body, such as speed and distance.

Kinesiology   The study of human movement with an emphasis on joint and muscle function.

Kinetic chain   A combination of successively linked joints connected by a series of muscles that make up a movement pathway. See also *Closed kinetic chain, Open kinetic chain*.

Kinetics   The study of the forces that act on the body to produce motion.

Kyphosis   A normal, posterior curve in the spine. See also *Lordosis*.

Kyphosis, excessive   An exaggerated posterior spinal curvature, usually in the thoracic spine. See also *Lordosis, excessive*.

Kyphotic curve   The posterior curve of the spine found in the thoracic and sacral areas. See also *Lordotic curve, Posture*.

Kyphotic-lordotic posture   See *Posture*.

Labral tear   A rupture of the labrum around the glenoid fossa of the shoulder or the acetabulum of the hip.

Labyrinth   A maze-like structure in the bones of the inner ear containing specialized proprioceptors that register positional changes in the head and neck, which result in shifts in ongoing adjustments to muscular tone related to balance and equilibrium responses; made up of the vestibule, three intersecting semicircular canals, and a snail-shaped cochlea.

Lateral   A positional term describing structures located farther away from the midline of the body. See also *Medial*.

Lateral flexion   A side-bending movement of the spine either to the right or left.

Lateral rotation   A movement of an appendicular joint as it turns away from midline of the body in an outward direction; also called *external rotation*. See also *Medial rotation*.

Late swing   The subphase of the swing phase of gait that occurs as the free leg swings in an upward arc; also called *deceleration*. See also *Swing phase*.

Law of acceleration   Newton's second law of motion, which states that the distance an object travels when set in motion is proportional to the force causing the movement.

Law of action and reaction   Newton's third law of motion, which states that for every action there is an opposite and equal reaction.

Law of inertia   Newton's first law of motion, which states that a body at rest or in linear motion tends to stay at rest or in motion unless acted upon by an external force.

Length–tension relationship   The ratio between the length of a muscle and the amount of contractile force it can generate at that length.

Lever   A simple machine that magnifies force. Every lever has three parts: an axis (fulcrum), effort (force), and resistance (load or weight). In the human body, the bones work as levers, the muscles produce force, and the joints serve as fulcrums in the production of movement. See also *First-class lever, Second-class lever, Third-class lever*.

Ligament   A short band of dense, regular connective tissue that connects bone to bone.

Linear forces   Forces applied along the same axis, either toward or away from each other. See also *Concurrent forces, Parallel forces*.

Linear friction   A hands-on technique in which a practitioner applies deep linear pressure along the fibers of a muscle; also called *stripping*. See also *Circular friction, Cross-fiber friction*.

Linear motion   Movement along a straight line through space; also called *translational motion* or *translatory motion*. See also *Curvilinear motion, Rotary motion*.

Line of force   A pathway along which a force passes from one joint to the next along a kinetic chain.

Line of gravity (LOG)   The direction of gravity's force or pull along the vertical axis; a plumb line. See also *Center of gravity, Gravity*.

Line of pull   The direction a muscular force exerts on a joint; also called *angle of pull*.

Listening touch   See *Static contact*.

Load   A mechanical force.

Local   Refers to structures or movement patterns in a specific area of the body. See also *Global*.

Long axis of a bone   See *Mechanical axis of a bone*.

Longitudinal axis   See *Vertical axis*.

Loose-packed position   Resting position of a joint in which its supporting ligaments become slack and its articulating surfaces have minimal contact; also called *open-packed position*. See also *Close-packed position*.

Lordosis   A normal, anterior curve in the spine. See also *Kyphosis*.

Lordosis, excessive   An exaggerated anterior spinal curvature, usually in the lumbar and cervical spine. See also *Kyphosis, excessive*.

Lordotic curve The anterior curve of the spine found in the cervical and lumbar areas. See also *Kyphotic curve*, *Posture*.

Lumbar pelvic rhythm The ratio of motion between the hips and lumbar spine during hip and trunk movements. See also *Scapulohumeral rhythm*.

Mass Anything that has weight and takes up space.

Mechanical advantage (M Ad) A measure of the efficiency of a lever, which is determined by dividing the length of the effort arm by the length of the resistance arm.

Mechanical axis of a bone An imaginary line that runs between the centers of the articulating joints on either end of a bone; the mechanical axis may or may not run through the shaft of a bone, depending on the overall shape of the bone; also called *long axis of a bone*.

Mechanical axis of the lower limb A vertical line that falls through the center of the hip, knee, and ankle.

Mechanical stresses Forces acting on the body. The five mechanical stresses are compression, tension, shear, torque, and bend.

Mechanics The branch of physics that deals with force and mass in relation to moving bodies.

Medial A positional term describing structures located closer to the midline of the body. See also *Lateral*.

Medial–lateral axis See *Bilateral axis*. See also *Anterior–posterior axis*, *Vertical axis*.

Medial rotation A movement of an appendicular joint as it turns toward the midline of the body in an inward direction; also called *internal rotation*. See also *Lateral rotation*.

Median plane The sagittal plane running through the body's midline from front to back that divides the body exactly into right and left halves; also called *midsagittal plane*. See also *Sagittal plane*.

Meridians Channels or pathways in the body, according to traditional Chinese medicine, through which *chi*, meaning "life force" or "energy," flows.

Midrange A range of joint motion at which the angle of the joint is halfway between its inner and outer range.

Midsagittal plane See *Median plane*.

Midstance The subphase of the stance phase of gait that occurs as the body weight shifts up and over the stance leg. See also *Extensor support moment*, *Stance phase*.

Midswing The subphase of the swing phase of gait that occurs when the free leg swings under the body. See also *Swing phase*.

Mindful touch Palpatory or therapeutic touch practiced with a conscious deliberation and sensitivity.

Mobility The movement of a body through space.

Mobilizer A general term to describe any muscle that generates joint motion. See also *Stabilizer*.

Moment arm The perpendicular distance between a muscle's line of pull and the axis of motion at the center of the joint.

Momentum A force acting as an impetus to a moving object, increasing its velocity.

Motility Intrinsic movement of the body generated by physiological rhythms and reflex mechanics.

Motor neurons Neurons that carry motor impulses from the brain and spinal cord (central nervous system) to the muscles; also called *efferent neurons*. See also *Interneurons*, *Sensory neurons*.

Motor point Point where the motor nerve enters the muscle and where a visible contraction can be elicited with minimal stimulation; generally located in the belly of the muscle.

Motor response A skeletal muscle response; a movement. See also *Sensorimotor loop*, *Sensory intake*.

Motor unit A motor neuron and all the muscle fibers it innervates.

Multiarticular muscle A muscle that crosses three or more joints. See *Biarticular muscle*.

Multiaxial joint See *Triaxial joint*.

Multiple motor unit summation See *Recruitment*.

Muscle energy techniques (METs) Manual therapy techniques that use active contraction to elicit a relaxation response in a muscle before stretching it. See also *Postisometric relaxation*, *Reciprocal inhibition*.

Muscle fascicle A bundle of muscle fibers wrapped in a connective tissue sheath called perimysium.

Muscle fatigue The state of a muscle when it stops contracting because it can no longer produce the energy needed to continue contracting.

Muscle fiber A muscle cell.

Muscle spindle Proprioceptive organ within the belly of skeletal muscles that is made up of 2–10 intrafusal fibers plus several types of sensory nerves encased in a spindle-shaped connective tissue capsule and embedded between extrafusal fibers; muscle spindles register and respond to changes in muscle length and the speed of these changes.

Muscle tone Describes the continuous involuntary, or passive, contraction of a resting muscle caused by unconscious nerve impulses.

Muscular balance The relative equality of length and strength in opposing muscles.

Muscular system The anatomical system made up of all the skeletal muscles and all their associated connective tissues, such as fascias and tendons.

Musculoskeletal Referring to the coordinated function of the muscular system and the skeletal system. See also *Neuromuscular*.

Myofascial meridians A term coined by anatomist and Rolfer Tom Meyers to describe the continuity of muscles and joints along specific kinetic chains and movement pathways addressed by a somatic manual therapy called *structural integration*.

Myofascial mobilization (MFM) See *Myofascial release*.

Myofascial release (MFR) A manual therapy technique in which a practitioner applies sustained force to myofascial tissues to mobilize and stretch restricted areas.

Myofascial system The muscular system with all its associated fascias.

Myosin A contractile protein inside a muscle fiber that makes up the thick filaments. See also *Actin*.

Myotatic reflex See *Stretch reflex*.

Nerve A group of fibers (made up of neurons) bundled together into cords that transmit impulses outside of the central nervous system.

Nerve plexus (plural: *plexi*) A group of intersecting nerve roots that strategically branch out toward the structures they innervate. See also *Peripheral nerve*.

Nervous system (NS) A network of neurons that transmits signals throughout the body and coordinates actions; in humans, the nervous system consists of a central nervous system and a peripheral nervous system. See also *Central nervous system, Peripheral nervous system*.

Neural tension The tension that occurs in a peripheral nerve when it loses extensibility along one area and tension increases in another area to equalize tension along the nerve.

Neurological actions The motor patterns of *yield*, *push*, *reach*, and *pull* that organize the neuromuscular system during early motor development. See also *Developmental movement patterns, Neurological pathways*.

Neurological pathways The movement pathways along which patterns of early motor development occur; these are the *radial, spinal, homologous, homolateral,* and *contralateral* pathways. See also *Developmental movement patterns, Neurological actions*.

Neurological patterns See *Developmental movement patterns*.

Neuromuscular Referring to the coordinated functions of the nervous system and the muscular system. See also *Musculoskeletal*.

Neuromuscular patterning Movement performed with the intention of reorganizing and improving muscle and joint function.

Neuromuscular system The combination of all of the tissues and mechanisms in the muscular system and the nervous system that work together to produce movement.

Neuron A nerve cell.

Neutral equilibrium Describes a body whose center of gravity remains level when the body shifts, such as a rolling ball.

Neutral position of the ankle A vertical position of the ankle in which the talus aligns over the calcaneus, between a position of inversion and eversion.

Neutralizer A term to describe a muscle that contracts to prevent a secondary movement of an agonist during an action. See also *Agonist, Antagonist, Fixator, Stabilizer, Synergist*.

Nociceptor A sensory nerve receptor that registers changes in temperature and pressure that reach a certain threshold as painful stimuli.

Nonaxial joint A type of synovial joint that cannot bend around an axis. See also *Biaxial joint, Triaxial joint, Uniaxial joint*.

Nutation A nodding motion of the sacrum that rocks the top of the sacrum in an anterior direction. See also *Counternutation*.

Objective findings The results of an assessment based on factual indicators that can be confirmed by two or more people. See also *Subjective findings*.

Open kinetic chain A movement in which the end of the kinetic chain is free. See also *Closed kinetic chain, Kinetic chain*.

Open-packed position See *Loose-packed position*.

Opposition A movement of the thumb folding across the palm toward the little finger. See also *Reposition*.

Optimal posture See *Posture*.

Origin One of the two places (along with the *insertion*) that a muscle attaches to bone. The origin is the proximal attachment site and the site on the bone that remains fixed when that muscle generates joint motion. See also *Insertion*.

Osteokinematics The study of the different types of joint movements, including flexion, extension, adduction, abduction, and rotation; the actions that can be observed as the muscles pull the two bones of a joint through space. See also *Arthrokinematics*.

Osteoporosis A degenerative condition is which bone absorption exceeds bone formation, decreasing bone density and strength and causing the bones to become brittle and susceptible to fracture.

Outer range The range of joint motion in which the angle of the joint is maximally opened. See also *Inner range, Midrange*.

Ovoid Describes a synovial joint in which a convex (ovoid, or egg-shaped) articulating surface fits into a concave articulating surface. See also *Sellar*.

Pacinian corpuscles Proprioceptive organs located in the skin, joints, and other parts of the body that detect rapid changes in pressure and vibration; those embedded in joint capsules convey information to the CNS on joint position. See also *Nocioceptors, Ruffini endings*.

Palmar A positional term describing the surface on the palm of the hand.

Palpation An examination of the body through touch.

Palpation techniques See *Broad-hand gliding, Cross-fiber strumming, Fingertip palpation, Flat-finger palpation, Pincher palpation, Static contact*.

Paradoxical breathing A reverse breathing pattern found in people with severe respiratory distress, which moves the chest in on the inhalation and constricts the rib cage, then moves the chest out on the exhalation and expands the rib cage. See also *Upper chest breathing*.

Parallel elastic components The noncontractile connective tissues around a muscle that provides passive resistance when a muscle is stretched. See also *Series elastic components*.

Parallel forces Separate forces of equal magnitude applied in the same plane either in the same direction or in opposite directions. See also *Concurrent forces, Linear forces*.

Parallel shift See *Concurrent movement*.

Parasympathetic nervous system (PSNS) A division of the autonomic nervous system that regulates slow, quiet organ functions such as digestion, elimination, and recuperation. See also *Autonomic nervous system, Sympathetic nervous system*.

Paravertebral Located along the anterior side of the vertebrae. See also *Prevertebral*.

Paresis Partial muscle dysfunction or paralysis. See also *Plegia*.

Passive insufficiency The point at which a biarticular or multiarticular muscle being passively lengthened at both ends is maximally lengthened and cannot stretch any farther. See also *Active insufficiency*.

Passive motion The movement of one person's joints by another person. See also *Active motion*.

Passive range of motion (PROM) The distance and direction (range), measured in degrees, that a person's joints can be passively moved by another person. See also *Active range of motion, Range of motion, Resisted range of motion*.

Passive restraints Noncontractile tissues that stabilize a joint, such as ligaments and the joint capsule. See also *Active restraints*.

Passive technique Any hands-on method that does not require a client's participation. See also *Active technique*.

Passive tension The elastic tension generated by the stretch of noncontractile connective tissues (also called parallel and series elastic components) in muscles. See also *Active tension*.

Patellofemoral joint pain syndrome Knee pain caused by poor patellar tracking; can lead to arthritis, inflammation, and recurring dislocation of the patella. See also *Chondramalacia*.

Patterning touch Intentional touch used to guide a client's active movement in order to change neuromuscular pathways and improve body patterns.

Pelvic girdle The bony structure made up of the pelvic bones, the sacrum, and the thighs.

Pelvic ring The circular bony structure made up of the sacrum and coxal bones.

Pennate muscles Muscles with fibers that run at oblique angles to their central tendons, like the fibers in a feather. A *unipennate* muscle looks like a feather with fibers only on one side of the tendon; a *bipennate* muscle closely resembles a feather with symmetrical fibers on each side of the central tendon; and a *multipennate* muscle looks like a fan of overlapping feathers. See also *Fusiform muscles*.

Perception How the brain interprets proprioceptive information about where the body is positioned in space or how it is moving; the brain uses perceptions to coordinate an ongoing stream of motor responses. See also *Proprioception*.

Periosteum Fascia covering bones that provides attachment sites for muscles and tendons.

Peripheral nerve A nerve outside the brain and spinal cord, located elsewhere in the body. See also *Nerve plexus*.

Peripheral nervous system (PNS) The part of the nervous system outside of the CNS that consists of the peripheral nerves; the PNS is further subdivided into the *autonomic nervous system* and the *somatic* (or *skeletal*) *nervous system*. See also *Central nervous system, Nervous system*.

Pes cavus Excessively high arches in the foot; also called *hypersupination*. See also *Pes planus*.

Pes planus A flattening of the medial arch of the foot; also called *hyperpronation*. See also *Pes cavus*.

Phasic stretch reflex See *Stretch reflex*.

Physiological movement The active range in which a person can move a joint motion, which is relative to the shape, size, and structure of each joint.

Piezoelectric effect A phenomenon that occurs when a material or tissue undergoes a mechanical stress that alters its electrical charge, causing electrical currents to spread through it.

Pin and stretch   A combined friction and myofascial release technique in which a practitioner pins one end of a restricted tissue layer or muscle to stabilize it, then uses linear friction to stretch the tissue away from the pinned end. See also *Active pin and stretch.*

Pincher palpation   A palpation technique in which the tissue being palpated, often a muscle belly, is grasped between the thumb and fingertips. See also *Broad-hand gliding, Cross-fiber strumming, Fingertip palpation, Flat-finger palpation, Static contact.*

Piriformis syndrome   A neuromuscular disorder that occurs when the piriformis muscle spasms and compresses the sciatic nerve, resulting in a range of symptoms that include pain, tingling, and numbness in the posterior hip, thigh, and down the back of the leg.

Pivot   A point, axle, or shaft around which something turns; the action of turning around a point.

Pivot joint   A type of synovial joint in which the rounded end of one bone projects into a ring-like shape of another bone, allowing the joint to turn.

Plane   An imaginary flat, two-dimensional surface in space. The three cardinal planes are sagittal, frontal (coronal), and horizontal (transverse).

Plane joint   A type of uniaxial synovial joint with fairly flat articulating surfaces that slide across each other; also called *gliding joint.*

Plantar   A positional term describing the surface on the bottom of the foot. See also *Dorsal.*

Plantar fasciitis   An inflammatory condition of the plantar fascia that causes a painful tightness and restricts motion in the longitudinal arches.

Plantarflexion   A movement of the ankle toward the plantar (bottom) surface of the foot, opening the angle of the ankle. See also *Dorsiflexion.*

Plasticity   The irreversible deformation of a tissue by a mechanical force that exceeds its elastic limit. See also *Elasticity, Extensibility.*

Plegia   Total muscle paralysis. See also *Paresis.*

Posterior   A positional term describing structures located closer to the back of the body than other structures. See also *Anterior.*

Posterior pelvic tilt (PPT)   A postural pattern that occurs when the top of the pelvis tips in a backward direction. See also *Anterior pelvic tilt.*

Posteromedial   A view of the body from an anterior and lateral angle.

Post-isometric relaxation (PIR)   A natural law that describes how a muscle undergoes a relaxation response after having been contracted; also a term for a muscle energy technique in which a muscle is contracted, then relaxed to elicit a post-isometric relaxation response, which enhances the subsequent stretch of that muscle. See also *Muscle energy techniques, Reciprocal inhibition.*

Postural stabilizers   The muscles with a primary function of providing postural support and joint stabilization through isometric contractions that occur in a stationary posture, independent of joint motion. See also *Mobilizer, Stabilizer.*

Postural sway   A postural reflex that occurs in a standing position and causes a subtle swaying motion of the entire body at the ankles.

Posture   The relative, observable, and measurable alignment of the many parts of the body's physical structure; can also refer to an observable attitude. As a verb it means to take a stance.

Flat-back posture   A posture marked by a posterior pelvic tilt, which tucks the pelvis and flattens the lumbar spine.

Kyphotic-lordotic posture   A posture marked by an anterior pelvic tilt and exaggerated spinal curvatures, with an exaggerated lordosis in the lower back and neck and an exaggerated kyphosis in the upper back.

Optimal posture   The upright position of the body in which the center of gravity of each weight-bearing body part aligns as close to the line of gravity as possible.

Round-back posture   A posture marked by an exaggerated kyphosis or "humpback" in the thoracic spine, usually due to chronic flexion in the entire trunk; a congenital type of round-back posture called *Scheuermann's disease* is caused by malformed thoracic vertebrae.

Sway-back posture   A posture marked by an anterior pelvic tilt, a lumbar lordosis, and a thoracic kyphosis.

Prevertebral   Located along the posterior side of the vertebrae. See also *Paravertebral.*

Prime mover   See *Agonist.*

Pronation   A movement of the forearm returning the palm of the hand from supination (facing upward) to a downward-facing position. A movement of the ankle and foot that lifts the lateral arch and combines eversion, dorsiflexion, and abduction. See also *Supination.*

Prone position   The position of a body lying on the abdomen, face down. See also *Supine position.*

Proprioception   The body's use of sensory receptors to create an awareness of posture, movement, balance, and the location of the body in space. See also *Perception.*

Proprioceptors   Sensory receptors in the muscles, tendons, and joints that receive information from the musculoskeletal system about changes in movement and position.

Proximal A positional term describing structures located closer to the trunk than other structures. See also *Distal*.

Proximal joints The joint in each limb nearest to the trunk in relation to other joints of the limb; the proximal joint in the upper limb is the glenohumeral joint (shoulder) and in the lower limb is the coxofemoral joint (hip).

Psoatic gait A antalgic gait caused by dysfunction of the psoas major muscle, its tendon, or its underlying bursa that is marked by chronic hip flexion and lateral rotation of the stance leg.

Pushoff The subphase of the stance phase of gait that occurs when the toes push off the ground; also called *toe-off*. See also *Stance phase*.

Q-angle The line of pull of the quadriceps on the knee.

Qi See *Chi*.

Radial One of the movement pathways along which patterns of early motor development occur; a term describing an action that initiates in the center of the body and sequences symmetrically out to the periphery. See also *Contralateral, Homolateral, Homologous, Spinal*.

Range of motion (ROM) The distance and direction (range), measured in degrees, that a joint can move between its flexed and extended positions. See also *Active range of motion, Passive range of motion, Resisted range of motion*.

Receptor neurons See *Sensory neurons*.

Reciprocal inhibition (RI) A natural law that describes how a muscle relaxes when the muscle opposing it contracts due to the reciprocal innervations of agonist and antagonist muscles in a reflex arc; also the term for a muscle energy technique that uses a contraction of an agonist to enhance the relaxation and subsequent stretch of an antagonist. See also *Muscle energy techniques, Post-isometric relaxation*.

Recruitment The process of increasing the number of motor units firing in a muscle; also called *multiple motor unit summation*. See also *Wave summation*.

Recruitment timing The order in which muscles fire during an action.

Reflex arc The most basic neuromuscular pathway that produces a rapid, automatic movement such as a flexor withdrawal reflex.

Regular dense connective tissue Connective tissue made up of collagen fibers oriented in parallel bundles; regular dense connective tissue makes up tendons and ligaments. See also *Irregular dense connective tissue*.

Remodeling A regenerative process in bone that involves the reabsorption of old tissue by specialized cells called *osteoclasts* and the production of new tissue by specialized cells called *osteoblasts*.

Reposition A movement of the thumb from opposition, a folded position across the palm, back to its original position. See also *Opposition*.

Resistance The weight or load that a lever moves; the force applied by a practitioner that a client can move against to stimulate muscular contractions.

Resistance arm The distance between the resistance, or weight, that a lever is moving and the axis or fulcrum of motion in the lever.

Resisted range of motion (RROM) In manual therapy, a range of joint motion performed against resistance. See also *Active range of motion, Passive range of motion, Range of motion*.

Respiration The intake of oxygen from external air into the body and the elimination of carbon dioxide from the body to external air.

Responsiveness A property of muscle tissue that gives it the ability to respond to stimuli from both inside and outside the body; also called *Excitability, Irritability*.

Reticular fibers Thin, delicate connective tissue fibers that provide a loose, supportive framework in organs such as the liver and the spleen. See also *Collagen fibers, Elastin fibers*.

Retinaculum A flat strip of fascia wrapping the ankles and wrists to hold the tendons close to the bone.

Reverse muscle action When the moving and fixed ends of the bones a muscle is attached to invert roles, causing the origin of a muscle to move toward the insertion as opposed to the insertion of the muscle moving toward the origin.

Rhomboidal muscle A flat, four-sided muscle with a quadrate or parallelogram shape. Its parallel fibers culminate in a flat tendon that attaches along a bony ridge or line.

Roll The movement when one articulating joint surface rolls across another.

Rotary motion A circular movement of a bone or body part around a fixed point; also called *angular motion* because it bends the moving joint into an angle. See also *Curvilinear motion, Linear motion*.

Rotation A joint movement in the horizontal plane around the vertical axis of the body.

Round-back posture See *Posture*.

Ruffini endings Proprioceptive organs embedded in the deep layers of the skin around joints that detect slow changes in the position or angle of the joint. See also *Nocioceptors, Pacinian corpuscles*.

Saddle joint A type of synovial joint in which each articulating surface has both a concave and a convex shape like a saddle, as in the joint between the first metacarpal and trapezium at the base of the thumb.

Sagittal plane Any vertical plane that divides the body or its parts into right and left sections; the primary movements of limbs relative to the sagittal plane are flexion and extension. See also *Frontal plane*, *Horizontal plane*, *Median plane*.

Sarcomere The contractile segments of a muscle fiber, compartmentalized by Z lines.

Scapula neutral A balanced resting position of the scapula in which it lays flat against the thorax and its medial border runs parallel to the thoracic spine.

Scapular winging A condition in which the medial border of the scapula is raised indicating a weakness of the serratus anterior muscle.

Scapulohumeral rhythm The ratio of movement between the glenohumeral and scapulothoracic joints during arm movements. See also *Lumbar pelvic rhythm*.

Scoliosis A lateral spinal curve that can occur anywhere in the spine.

Screw home mechanism See *Terminal rotation*.

Second-class lever A lever that has the resistance located between the effort and axis of motion. See also *First-class lever*, *Third-class lever*.

Sellar Describes a synovial joint in which each articulating surface has convex and concave shapes, creating either a saddle shape or two mounds and a valley. See also *Ovoid*.

Sensorimotor loop A constant cycle from sensory input to processing in the brain and/or spinal cord to motor output that produces movement responses.

Sensory intake The reception of stimuli from the sensory nerves. See also *Motor response*, *Sensorimotor loop*.

Sensory neurons Neurons that carry impulses from sensory receptors and proprioceptors to the brain and spinal cord; also called *afferent neurons* or *receptor neurons*. See also *Interneurons*, *Motor neurons*.

Sensory receptors Specialized cells and end organs in the body that relay sensory information along afferent nerves to the brain and spinal cord for processing.

Sequential movement Movement that sequences from one part of the body to another.

Series elastic components The non-contractile tissues within muscle tissue that contribute passive tension under stretch and elasticity during contraction, primarily tendons and connective tissues linking actin and myosin fibers. See also *Parallel elastic components*.

Shear A mechanical stress that occurs when two parallel forces press into a structure from opposite directions. See also *Bend*, *Compression*, *Tension*, *Torque*.

Shin splints An irritation of the tibial periosteum from overuse or repetitive jarring impact on foot strike, which causes excessive shear and pull in the interosseous membrane between the tibia and fibula.

Shoulder dislocation An injury to the glenohumeral joint in which the head of the humerus is pulled out of the socket. See also *Shoulder separation*.

Shoulder girdle An appendicular bony structure made up of the humerus, scapula, and clavicle bones that moves with the arms.

Shoulder separation An injury to the acromioclavicular joint that either strains, partially tears, or completely ruptures the joint ligaments and joint capsule. See also *Shoulder dislocation*.

Simultaneous movement A movement in which the whole body moves at the same time.

Skeletal muscle A type of muscle tissue that acts on the bones and joints and that can be voluntarily contracted, as opposed to cardiac or smooth muscle; also called *striated muscle*. See also *Smooth muscle*.

Skeletal nervous system See *Somatic nervous system*.

Skeletal system A body system made up of the bones, joints, cartilage, and ligaments providing support and a system of bony levers for movement.

Slow type I fibers Small muscle cells that metabolize energy through oxidation, are highly fatigue resistant, and produce slow, weak contractions; also called *slow fibers*. See also *Fast type IIA fibers*, *Fast type IIB fibers*.

Smooth muscle A type of muscle tissue found in organs that is controlled by the autonomic nervous system and contracts involuntarily. See also *Skeletal muscle*.

Soft end-feel See *End-feel*.

Somatic Comes from a Greek term meaning "of the body." In the context of body therapies, used to describe patterns of posture and movement that reflect underlying thoughts, emotions, and psychological processes.

Somatic dysfunction A condition of localized muscular imbalance that evolves into a generalized reflex dysfunction in the neuromuscular system. Begins with a local muscle or joint problem, often a mechanical problem associated with faulty posture and limited motion, which wears the system down to the point that neurological synapses and pathways start to change and become dysfunctional.

Somatic nervous system (SNS) A division of the peripheral nervous system that controls the skeletal muscles and *voluntary* movement; also called *skeletal nervous system*. See also *Autonomic nervous system*, *Peripheral nervous system*.

Spasm A state of continual contraction in which the crossbridges on the sliding filaments fail to unlink; also called a *contracture*.

Spasm end-feel   See *End-feel*.

Spin   A movement in which one articulating surface, usually a convex surface, rotates around another.

Spinal   One of the movement pathways along which patterns of early motor development occur; a term describing an action that sequences along the spine: of or pertaining to the spine. See also *Contralateral, Homolateral, Homologous, Radial*.

Spinal nerves   Peripheral nerves that branch out of the spinal cord at each vertebral segment to innervate the organs and skeletal muscles.

Spongy bone   The layer of bone under compact bone in which the osteocytes are loosely arranged along lines of tension called *trabeculae*; also called *cancellous bone* or *trabecular bone*. See also *Compact bone*.

Sprain   An injury to noncontractile tissues around a joint, such as ligaments and joint capsules. See also *Strain*.

Stability dysfunction   Loss of control of joint motion outside of a normal range of motion to such an extent that it causes tissue trauma. See also *Joint instability*.

Stabilizer   A general term to describe any muscle that prevents excessive joint play. See also *Mobilizer, Postural stabilizers*.

Stable equilibrium   When all forces and torques acting on the body are balanced, adding up to zero, so that shifting the body out of stability requires moving the COG. See also *Unstable equilibrium*.

Stance phase   The phase of gait in which the foot makes contact with the ground. The five subphases of the stance phase are heel strike, foot flat, midstance, heeloff, and pushoff (toe-off). See also *Swing phase*.

Standing position   Similar to the anatomical position, except with the palms facing toward the trunk rather than forward. See also *Anatomical position*.

Static contact   A general palpation skill that involves holding one or both hands on or around an area of the body using full-hand contact in an encompassing manner to assess the overall tone and density of the tissues; sometimes described as a listening touch. See also *Broad-hand gliding, Cross-fiber strumming, Fingertip palpation, Flat-finger palpation, Pincher palpation*.

Statics   Mechanical principles that apply to a body at rest.

Step   The distance in a gait cycle that begins when one foot makes contact with the ground and ends when the other foot makes contact with the ground. See also *Step width, Stride*.

Steppage gait   See *Drop-foot gait*.

Step width   The distance in a gait cycle between the sagittal pathways of each foot, measured at the heels. See also *Step, Stride*.

Stiffness   The measure of how much load it takes to elongate tissue within an elastic range.

Strain   An injury to contractile tissues around a joint, such as muscles or tendons. See also *Sprain*.

Strap muscle   A muscle with long, flat, parallel fibers that run the length of it; culminates in a wide, flat tendon. Can also be segmented, as in the rectus abdominis muscle.

Stretch injury   A muscle strain that occurs when the muscle is in an elongated position and overstretches.

Stretch reflex   A reflex mediated by the muscle spindle in response to lengthening of a skeletal muscle; also called *myotatic reflex*. There are two kinds of stretch reflexes: tonic and phasic. A gradual elongation in muscle length elicits a tonic stretch reflex, which results in a slow muscular contraction. A quick stretch of a muscle results in a phasic stretch reflex, which triggers protective contractions that prevent the muscle from overstretching and tearing.

Stretch weakening   Chronic weakness that occurs in a muscle as a result of remaining in a lengthened position.

Striated muscle   See *Skeletal muscle*.

Stride   The distance in a gait cycle made by two steps. See also *Step, Step width*.

Stripping   See *Linear friction*.

Structural integrity   A body state in which the joints are optimally aligned and the pulls of the muscles are balanced in each dimension.

Subjective findings   The results of an assessment based on a practitioner's feelings or interpretation rather than factual information. See also *Objective findings*.

Substitution pattern   When a muscle or muscles becomes chronically contracted to provide postural support for postural stabilizers that fail to fire; also called a *compensatory pattern* or *adaptive pattern*.

Superficial   A positional term describing structures located closer to the surface of the body than other structures. See also *Deep*.

Superior   A positional term describing structures that are above or higher than other structures. See also *Inferior*.

Supination   A movement of the forearm turning the palm of the hand from a downward-facing position to face up. A movement of the ankle and foot that lifts the medial arch and combines inversion, plantarflexion, and adduction. See also *Pronation*.

Supine position   The position of a body lying on the spine, face up. See also *Prone position*.

Sway-back posture   See *Posture*.

Swing phase   The phase of gait in which the foot loses contact with the ground and the lower limb swings. The three subphases of the swing phase are early swing (acceleration), midswing, and late swing (deceleration). See also *Stance phase*.

Sympathetic nervous system (SNS)　A division of the autonomic nervous system that pulls energy out of the viscera and sends it to muscles, speeding heart rate and respiration to put the body into action mode. See also *Autonomic nervous system, Parasympathetic nervous system*.

Synapse　A junction in the nervous system that allows electrical or chemical impulses to pass between neurons in the brain and spinal cord or between an axon and a receptor organ.

Synarthrosis　An immovable, fibrous joint; for example, the cranial sutures, gomphosis joints, and syndesmosis joints. See also *Amphiarthrosis, Diarthrosis*.

Syndesmosis　A type of synarthrotic joint in which the bones are bound together by a strong, fibrous membrane; for example, the tibiofibular and radioulnar joints. See also *Gomphosis, Synarthrosis*.

Synergist　A term to describe a muscle that assists the agonist during an action. See also *Agonist, Antagonist, Fixator*.

Synovial fluid　A viscous fluid that fills the space within freely movable joints and lubricates these joints.

Synovial joint　A freely moveable, diarthrotic joint with space between the articulating bones that is filled with synovial fluid. See also *Diarthrosis*.

Synovial sheath　An elongated tube of bursa that wraps and protects a tendon from friction. See also *Tenosynovitis*.

Temporomandibular dysfunction (TMD)　A disorder of the temporomandibular joint involving damage to musculoskeletal structures in and around the joint.

Tender point　A localized palpable nodule or band-like hardening in the muscle that, when placed under direct pressure, creates a localized pain response. See also *Trigger point*.

Tendonitis　Inflammation of a tendon. See also *Tenosynovitis*.

Tendon reflex　A protective reflex response mediated by the Golgi tendon organs that relaxes a muscle when its tendon reaches a certain degree of stretch.

Tenosynovitis　Inflammation of the synovial sheath wrapping a tendon. See also *Tendonitis*.

Tensegrity system　A system of tensional supports. In the human body, the myofascial network provides support as a three-dimensional tensegrity system.

Tension　A mechanical stress that occurs when two forces pull on a structure from opposite directions. See also *Bend, Compression, Shear, Torque*.

Terminal rotation　The movement that occurs during the last 30 degrees of knee extension, which involves lateral rotation of the proximal tibia against medial rotation of the distal femur and stabilizes the joint in a close-packed position; also called *screw home mechanism*.

Therapeutic palpation　A tactile exploration used in manual therapy for assessing the condition of anatomical structures and the movement functions of a client's body. See also *Classroom palpation*.

Third-class lever　A lever that has the effort or force located between the resistance and axis of motion. See also *First-class lever, Second-class lever*.

Thixotropic　The property of a gelatinous substance to respond to heat and cold by changing states from a solid to a gel and back again.

Thoracic outlet syndrome　A chronic pain condition caused by vascular and brachial nerve compression around the upper ribs in the upper thoracic area.

Tibial torsion　A medial twist of the distal end of the tibia relative to the proximal end of the tibia along the long axis of the bone.

Tissue layering　A palpation exercise in which each tissue layer is systematically palpated in a progression from the superficial layers to the deep layers.

Titin　An elastic filament inside a muscle fiber. See also *Actin, Myosin*.

Toe-off　See *Pushoff*.

Tonic stretch reflex　See *Stretch reflex*.

Torque　A mechanical stress that occurs when two or more forces perpendicular to the axis of the structure turn in opposite directions, resulting in rotation. See also *Bend, Compression, Shear, Tension*.

Torticollis　A scoliosis in the cervical spine resulting from damage to the sternocleidomastoid muscle. See also *Scoliosis*.

Trabecular bone　See *Spongy bone*.

Tracking　A clinical skill in which a practitioner pays attention to and follows many things going on at once, closely monitoring all of the details of a particular aspect that is being assessed in a client.

Tracts　Bundles of nerve fibers located in the brain and spinal cord.

Translation　A term to describe linear, gliding joint motion, usually used in reference to anterior or posterior displacement of the knee or the intervertebral joints.

Translational motion　See *Linear motion*.

Translatory motion　See *Linear motion*.

Transverse friction　See *Cross-fiber friction*.

Transverse plane　See *Horizontal plane*.

Trendelenburg gait A gait dysfunction caused by weakness or damage to the gluteus medius muscle that is marked by a lateral lurch of the pelvis over the stance leg; also called *gluteus medius lurch*.

Triangular muscle A muscle with fibers arranged in a fan-like shape that converge into a point. Its convergent fibers often twist into a spiral shape.

Triaxial joint A type of synovial joint that can move in three or more planes; also called *multiaxial joint*. See also *Biaxial joint, Nonaxial joint, Uniaxial joint*.

Trigger point (TrP) A localized palpable nodule or band-like hardening in the muscle that, when placed under direct pressure, refers pain to other areas of the body; can lead to movement dysfunctions. See also *Tender point*.

Trigger point therapy A hands-on treatment to alleviate muscular pain in which localized pressure is applied to a trigger point until symptoms subside.

Trochanteric bursitis Inflammation of the bursa located over the greater trochanter.

Uniaxial joint A type of synovial joint that can move in one plane, allowing it to flex and extend. See also *Biaxial joint, Nonaxial joint, Triaxial joint*.

Unstable equilibrium When a body can be shifted by minimal force, causing its center of gravity to shift. See also *Stable equilibrium*.

Upper chest breathing A respiratory pattern often caused by anxiety or emotional distress in which a person overcontracts abdominal muscles and lifts and expands the upper thorax during inhalation. See also *Paradoxical breathing*.

Upslip A sacroiliac joint dysfunction that results in a slight upward motion of the iliac crest on one side of the pelvis. See also *Downslip*.

Upward rotation A movement of the scapula that occurs when raising the arm, which combines elevation, rotation, and protraction. See also *Downward rotation*.

Vector In terms of kinesiology, a movement quantity defined by the magnitude and the direction of a force.

Velocity The speed of a body's movement in a specific direction. See also *Acceleration, Deceleration*.

Ventral A positional term describing structures located on the anterior surface (front) of the body. See also *Dorsal*.

Vertical axis An imaginary straight line that runs up and down along the body's relative line of gravitational pull, perpendicular to the horizontal plane; also called the *longitudinal axis*. See also *Anterior–posterior axis, Bilateral axis*.

Viscoelasticity A tissue property that combines the characteristics of viscosity and elasticity, giving the tissue fluid resistance to shear and flow (viscosity) and the spring-like ability to return to its original form (elasticity).

Viscosity The measure of a fluid's ability to resist stress or pressure, with thicker fluids being more viscous than thinner fluids.

Wave summation An increase in the strength of a muscle's contraction caused by an increase in the frequency of muscle stimulation. See also *Recruitment*.

Work The amount of force it takes to move an object a certain distance. In relation to the human body, work is usually defined as the amount of force the skeletal muscles produce to carry out an action.

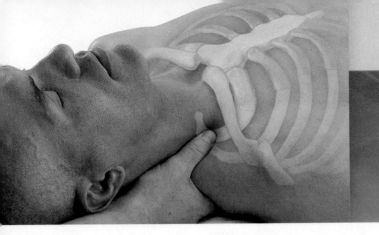

Answer Key

CHAPTER 1

Review Answers

1. Kinesiology is the study of human movement. Biomechanics is the study of mechanical concepts in human motion.
2. False
3. A
4. *Acceptable answers include:* Muscle contraction, friction, gravity, wind, water, and weight
5. B
6. D
7. True
8. True
9. A sequential movement travels from one muscle group and joint to the next in a consecutive chain; in a simultaneous movement, the whole body moves at once.
10. Superior, inferior, anterior, superficial
11. B
12. A
13. True
14. D
15. B
16. C
17. False
18. C

CHAPTER 2

Review Answers

1. D
2. B
3. The most abundant fiber in the skeletal system is collagen. It has the tensile strength of steel and also has a crimped fiber arrangement that gives it elasticity.
4. A
5. Compact (cortical) bone covers the outside of bone in a thin layer, whereas spongy (cancellous) bone is found inside the bone.

6. Trabeculae are the thin bony plates found in spongy bone that organize in geometric curves along lines of force and serves as pathways to transmit forces within a bone.
7. The five types of bones with examples of each one are long bones—femur, short bones—carpals, flat bones—ribs, irregular bones—vertebrae, and sesamoid bones—patella.
8. D
9. A
10. Three examples of bone markings are (1) condyle—a round, knuckle-like knob found on the end of a long bone in a joint, (2) crest—a narrow, sharp ridge, and (3) process—a prominent bony knob.
11. Hyaline cartilage covers the articular surfaces of the bones making up a synovial joint; fibrocartilage makes up the disks in the spine.
12. C
13. Fibrous joints—b, Fibrocartilage—c, Synovial—a
14. True
15. C
16. D
17. False
18. B

CHAPTER 3

Review Answers

1. Linear motion—c, rotary motion—a, curvilinear motion—b
2. Flexion, extension, and hyperextension occur in the sagittal plane. Abduction, adduction, and lateral flexion occur in the frontal plane. Lateral and medial rotation and spinal rotation occur in the horizontal or transverse plane.
3. D
4. A
5. False
6. C
7. Gliding is a nonaxial motion in which one bone slides across another.
8. False

9. So that they can visualize which direction to move the joint surfaces during passive joint motion in order to move a client within a safe range.
10. A
11. C
12. C
13. D
14. False
15. B
16. A practitioner would ask a client to demonstrate an active movement in order to see which range movement causes pain or to demonstrate a range of restricted motion.
17. Bony—b, firm—c, soft—a
18. B

CHAPTER 4

Review Answers

1. B
2. The flexor digitorum longus functions as a joint *flexor,* it is attached to the *digits* (fingers or toes), and it is *long.*
3. Strap muscles are long and flat.
   Fusiform muscles are long and tubular, shaped like a spindle.
   Rhomboidal muscles have a quadrate shape with four sides, similar to a parallelogram.
   Triangular muscles are fan-shaped with convergent fibers that often twist into a spiral.
   Pennate muscles have oblique fibers connected to a central tendon, like a feather.
4. False
5. D
6. C
7. A
8. B
9. True
10. C
11. B
12. The myofascial system is the skeletal muscles and all their associated fascias.
13. Adaptive shortening is the chronic tightness that occurs in a muscle as a result of remaining in a shortened position for extended periods. Stretch weakening is the chronic weakness that occurs in a muscle as a result of remaining in a lengthened position for extended periods. Faulty postures pull the body off of a neutral joint alignment, causing muscles on one side of the joints to chronically shorten while overstretching and stretch weakening opposing muscles.
14. D
15. Eccentric—c, concentric—b, isometric—d, isotonic—a
16. Agonist—c, antagonist—e, synergist—a, neutralizer—b, stabilizer—d
17. C
18. B

CHAPTER 5

Review Answers

1. A
2. Sensory (afferent) neurons—c, interneuron—b, motor (efferent) neurons—a
3. A peripheral nerve is covered with a fascial membrane called epineurium and is made up of bundles of nerve fibers called fascicles. Each fascicle is wrapped in fascia called perineurium and contains a group of single nerve fibers wrapped in fascia called endoneurium.
4. True
5. B
6. C
7. False
8. D
9. The components of a reflex arc include sensory receptors that pick up sensory information from sensory nerves and relay it to an integration center, which consists of singular or multiple synapses. The integration center then sends a signal to a motor nerve, which relays it to a muscle fiber, triggering a reflexive contraction.
10. True
11. Stretch injuries occur when a muscle is working under eccentric loading and the load on the muscle overcomes the force of the contraction, stretching the muscle while it is contracting. A common stretch injury that occurs when punters kick a football is that the agonist (quadriceps) contracts before the antagonist (hamstrings) can relax, straining the hamstrings by stretching it while it is contracting.
12. A
13. Pacinian corpuscles—c, Ruffini endings—d, nociceptors—a, semicircular canals—b
14. B
15. C
16. (1) Make sure the client is fully supported and comfortable. (2) Tell the client to inform you immediately of any pain or discomfort, then stop immediately. (3) Move the client slowly or apply pressure slowly using minimal effort. (4) Do not move any areas in which movement is contraindicated.
17. A
18. A trigger point is a tender point in a muscle that produces referred pain when compressed. Trigger points are treated with direct compression that is held until the client reports that the pain has subsided.

CHAPTER 6

Review Answers

1. Speed, direction
2. Acceleration is an increase in velocity. Deceleration is a decrease in velocity.
3. True

4. The line of pull is the direction that a muscular force places on a joint. As a muscle contracts, its line of pull changes as the joint bends and the angle of pull changes.
5. A
6. D
7. B
8. C
9. B
10. A
11. True
12. A
13. C
14. A lever is a simple machine that magnifies force and converts force to torque. Every lever has an axis, or fulcrum, around which it pivots; an effort or force that moves the lever; and a resistance or load that the lever moves against.
15. A third-class lever favors speed and distance over power and is commonly found in the human body.
16. False
17. D
18. C

CHAPTER 7

Review Answers

1. False
2. D
3. D
4. The spine resembles a curved column, the pelvis a braced arch, the shoulder girdle a hanging yoke, and the head a top load.
5. True
6. *Acceptable answers include:* Vertical axis, line of gravity, plumb line
7. C
8. B
9. *Acceptable answers include:* Substitution pattern, compensatory pattern
10. A stability dysfunction is a condition in which a person is unable to control joint motion beyond a normal range to the point that it causes tissue damage and injury.
11. A
12. Lordosis—c, kyphosis—a, scoliosis—b
13. A scoliosis in the neck is called a torticollis.
14. C
15. B
16. False
17. A
18. Two therapeutic applications for postural education are to improve body mechanics and to improve assessment skills.

CHAPTER 8

Review Answers

1. True
2. C
3. Double-limb support is the phase in a walking gait when both feet are on the ground at the same time.
4. A
5. During early swing the lower limb swings in a downward arc, during midswing the lower limb is directly under the hip, and during late swing the hip swings in an upward arc and the knee extends in preparation for heel strike.
6. A
7. True
8. D
9. Horizontal—a, sagittal—c, frontal—b
10. Shorter
11. C
12. False
13. Gluteus maximus dysfunction results in a gait pattern called the gluteus maximus lurch, which causes the stance hip to jackknife into flexion on heel strike, then lurch into hyperextension on midstance, creating an extreme backward-then-forward rocking motion of the trunk on the hips.
14. B
15. A
16. D
17. B
18. (1) A general assessment of the overall gait pattern, (2) a specific assessment of gait components, (3) an assessment of specific range of movement in each joint, (4) an assessment of which muscles are adaptively shortened and stretch weakened in a specific gait pattern.

CHAPTER 9

Review Answers

1. Touch
2. A massage and bodywork practitioner practices palpation to distinguish between normal and abnormal tissues and motion, protect the client by identifying areas that should not be worked, assess joints and muscles in order to improve skeletal alignment and muscular balance, and assess tissues in order to develop a treatment plan.
3. A
4. During palpation, a practitioner tracks the qualities of the tissues, including tone, density, and temperature; bilateral symmetry between muscles and bones on the right and left sides of the body; organic movements; physiological rhythms; reflex responses; and client responses such as relaxation or guarding, which can indicate areas of pain and injury.

5. True

6. B

7. In the classroom, students palpate to help learn to locate specific anatomical structures. In a practice, palpation is used with an open-ended orientation. A practitioner palpates to connect with clients, to feel what is going on in their bodies, and to make general assessments about structure and function.

8. Guidelines to improve the success of palpation include:
   a) Notice when you are second-guessing yourself or jumping to conclusions.
   b) Trust what you feel.
   c) Palpate slowly enough to take the time to feel but fast enough to not habituate to touching an area and numbing out.
   d) Keep your hands relaxed and sink into the tissues.
   e) Adapt your hand positions to the shape of the tissues.
   f) Look at anatomical pictures and skeletal models in order to more accurately visualize what you are palpating.

9. D

10. True

11. C

12. True

13. B

14. D

15. Muscles have a variety of different qualities and textures. All muscles are fibrous and somewhat plump from the fluids within them. They tend to have a meaty texture. They can range from being dense and substantial to being flat and ropey. If the muscles are fibrous and tense, they will be hard and numb. If they are injured or have active tender points in them, they can be sore and irritable. When they are responsive, muscles often relax when touched and pressed.

16. C

17. A

18. D

CHAPTER 10

Review Answers

1. C

2. A

3. B

4. The upper seven ribs are called true ribs because they attach anteriorly to the sternum via costal cartilage; ribs 8, 9, and 10 are called the false ribs because they have indirect attachments to costal cartilage; ribs 11 and 12 are called floating ribs because they lack any distal attachments and "float" in soft tissue.

5. Fibrocartilage

6. D

7. A practitioner would want to avoid applying strong pressure over the center of the costal arch because it could injure or break the small bony tip of the xiphoid process.

8. A

9. During respiration, each rib turns on its own axis; the lower and middle ribs turn in a bucket-handle motion; the upper ribs lift in a pump-handle motion; the inferior part of the sternum lifts in a sagittal motion.

10. C

11. D

12. True

13. C

14. B

15. False

16. B

17. *Acceptable answers include:* Deep or forced breathing, rigorous activity

18. Paradoxical breathing is a holding pattern in which the respiratory muscles work in a reverse action during breathing, constricting the chest wall on inhalation and expanding it on exhalation. This pattern occurs in people with severe respiratory distress, chronically obstructed airways, spinal cord injuries that cause paralysis of muscles below the diaphragm, and multiple rib fractures.

19. Upper chest breathing is a holding pattern caused by anxiety; paradoxical breathing is a dysfunction caused by severe respiratory distress from illness, injury, or paralysis.

20. When the diaphragm pushes down it distends the organs. Abdominal muscle tone provides resistance to the diaphragm, so that it can only move down so far, at which point the diaphragm levers off this resistance to expand the rib cage.

CHAPTER 11

Review Answers

1. The rearfoot is made up of the talus and calcaneus, the midfoot is made up of the navicular, cuboid, and three cuneiforms, and the forefoot is made up of the five metatarsals and the 14 phalanges.

2. The primary function of the tibia is to transfer weight from the knee to the foot.

3. C

4. D

5. B

6. C

7. The three bones of the talocrural joint are the distal tibial, the distal fibula, and the talus. The talocrural is a synovial hinge joint.

8. Subtalar, supination, pronation

9. C

10. False

11. The extrinsic muscles of the foot have origins in the leg and insertions in the foot; the intrinsic muscles of the foot have both origins and insertions in the foot.

12. A

13. D

14. B
15. Peroneus longus, peroneus brevis, lateral
16. C
17. True
18. Four layers
19. D
20. A

CHAPTER 12

Review Answers

1. False
2. The knee has two fibrocartilage disks (menisci) and 14 bursae.
3. D
4. A
5. The patellofemoral joint consists of the articulation between the posterior patella and the distal femur. The tibiofemoral joint consists of the articulation between the tibial plateau and the femoral condyles.
6. True
7. B
8. The function of the patella is to work as an anatomical pulley that deflects the pull of the quadriceps tendon away from the joint, which protects the joint from excessive friction and increases the mechanical advantage of the quadriceps.
9. B
10. C
11. 140, 5 to 10, 30, 40
12. Genu recurvatum is hyperextension of the knee past five to 10 degrees, which places abnormal stresses on the soft tissues of the knee by disturbing skeletal alignment.
13. A
14. True
15. C
16. D
17. The hamstrings are the primary knee flexors. The biceps femoris laterally rotates the knee in a flexed position; the semitendinosus and semimembranosus medially rotate the knee in a flexed position.
18. D
19. The popliteus unlocks the knee from the extended position.
20. C

CHAPTER 13

Review Answers

1. The four bones making up the pelvis are the two coxal bones, sacrum, and coccyx.
2. C
3. A
4. Coxofemoral

5. A
6. B
7. The iliofemoral ligament connects the coxal bone to the neck of the femur, the pubofemoral ligament connects the pubis to the neck of the femur, and the ischiofemoral ligament connects the posterior side of the acetabulum to the greater trochanter.
8. The six movements of the pelvis on the femur are the posterior tilt, anterior tilt, right lateral tilt, left lateral tilt, forward rotation, and backward rotation.
9. False
10. D
11. C
12. B
13. Nutation, counternutation
14. C
15. The distal tendon of the TFL is the iliotibial band (ITB). Because the ITB crosses the lateral side of the knee and inserts on the proximal tibia, when tight, it can compress the lateral side of the knee.
16. A
17. True
18. The piriformis attaches to the axial skeleton on the anterior side of the sacrum.
19. D
20. False

CHAPTER 14

Review Answers

1. The cervical spine is located in the neck and has seven vertebrae; the thoracic spine is located along the posterior rib cage and has 12 vertebrae; the lumbar spine is located in the lower back and has five vertebrae.
2. Spinal cord, movement, attachment sites, support
3. False
4. A
5. B
6. Fibrocartilage, vertebral bodies, intervertebral disks
7. A
8. The interbody (intervertebral) joints function as shock absorbers in the spine.
9. C
10. False
11. The cervical spine is the most freely moveable, the thoracic spine favors rotation, and the lumbar spine favors flexion.
12. D
13. C
14. B
15. Two superficial neck extensors are the splenius capitis and splenius cervicis.
16. D
17. Of the four abdominal muscles, the internal obliques and transversus abdominis attach to the thoracolumbar fascia.

18. Of the four abdominal muscles, the rectus abdominis is a primary trunk flexor.
19. B
20. B

CHAPTER 15

Review Answers

1. The eight bones of the cranium are the two parietal and the two temporal bones, as well as the frontal, occipital, sphenoid, and ethmoid bones.
2. B
3. True
4. Thyroid
5. Elastic, hyaline
6. The throat is made up of a series of cartilaginous rings that include the thyroid cartilage, the cricoid cartilage, and the trachea.
7. The hyoid bone is a U-shaped bone at the base of the mouth that is unique because it is suspended by a number of ligaments and tendons and is called a "floating bone." Its main function is to provide attachment sites for the suprahyoid and infrahyoid muscles that are active during chewing, talking, and swallowing.
8. A
9. D
10. C
11. The TMJ can move right or left in lateral excursion or deviation, anteriorly in protrusion, posteriorly in retrusion, up to close in elevation, and down to open in depression.
12. A
13. The atlantoaxial joint is a pivot joint with two parts. The medial part is located between the dens process and two small synovial cavities and the lateral part is made up of two facet joints with nearly horizontal articulating joint surfaces.
14. B
15. C
16. D
17. B
18. A
19. False
20. The suboccipitals connect the atlas and axis to the cranium and are continually active making small adjustments of the head on the neck.

CHAPTER 16

Review Answers

1. The three main bones making up the shoulder girdle are the humerus, clavicle, and scapula.
2. D

3. B
4. Glenohumeral, sternoclavicular, scapulothoracic
5. The glenohumeral ligament covers the joint capsule of the shoulder.
6. True
7. A
8. Adhesive capsulitis—d , shoulder dislocation—b, shoulder separation—a, clavicular fracture—c
9. False
10. B
11. Latissimus dorsi
12. D
13. Rhomboid
14. B
15. D
16. Supraspinatus
17. A
18. C
19. True
20. B

CHAPTER 17

Review Answers

1. B
2. The lunate is the most frequently dislocated carpal bone and it is most frequently dislocated during a fall on an outstretched hand (FOOSH).
3. False
4. The thumb has only has two phalanges while each of the four fingers has three phalanges and the thumb has a saddle joint at its base rather than an ellipsoid joint.
5. A
6. C
7. The proximal radioulnar joint, which allows supination and pronation of the forearm.
8. Radiocarpal
9. D
10. Carpal tunnel syndrome is the compression of the carpal tunnel, which can cause numbness, tingling, inflammation, pain in the hand and wrist, and loss of grip strength.
11. True
12. C
13. B
14. True
15. A
16. D
17. A
18. Lateral epicondylitis, common extensor
19. B
20. The finger flexors are stronger than the finger extensors because there are more of them.

Index

Note: Page numbers with *f* indicate figures; those with *t* indicate tables.

A

Abdominal muscles, 471–78, 472f
Abdominal separation, 473
Abduction, 52, 52f, 54, 54f
Abductor digiti minimi, 318–20, 318f, 666f, 666, 666f
Abductor hallucis, 317–20, 318f
Abductor pollicis brevis, 660, 660f, 663
Abductor pollicis longus, 656f, 657, 657f, 659, 660f
Acceleration, 130, 135, 185
Accessory movement, 62
Accessory muscles of respiration, 247–55, 249t. *See also* Scalenes
in forced exhalation, 249–50, 250f
in forced inhalation, 247, 249, 249f
serratus posterior inferior, 255, 255f, 257–58, 257f
serratus posterior superior, 255, 255f, 256f, 257–58
Acetabular labrum, 384–85, 385f
Acetabulum, 378f, 384, 385f
Achilles tendon, 73f, 272, 288, 300, 300f, 302
Acquired scoliosis, 169

Acromioclavicular (AC) joint, 565–68, 565f
Acromion process, 57, 57f, 554, 554f, 555
Actin filaments, 76–77, 77f
Actin molecules, 77
Action and reaction, law of, 135, 135f, 136
Action potential, 78
Active insufficiency, 91, 91f
Active motion, 63–64
Active motion skills, 116, 117f, 117t, 118
Active movement assessment, 210, 210f
Active pin and stretch technique, 123, 124f
Active range of motion (AROM), 61–62, 62f
Active relaxation, 679
Active restraints, 61
Active sitting, 152
Active technique, 16–17, 17f
Active trigger points, 119
Activities of daily living (ADL), 55
Adaptive pattern. *See* Substitution pattern
Adaptive shortening, 83, 83f
Adduction, 52, 52f, 54, 54f
Adductor brevis, 405–6, 406f, 408–11
Adductor hallucis, 323–26, 323f, 324f

Adductor longus, 73f, 405, 406f, 408–11
Adductor magnus, 73f, 406, 407f, 408–11
Adductor pollicis, 657, 660, 662
Adductor stretch, 431
Adductor tubercle, 333–34, 334f, 336
Adenosine triphosphate (ATP), 80
Adhesive capsulitis, 571–72, 571f
Aerobic respiration, 80
Agonist, 89–90, 89t
Alar cartilage, 498, 498f
Alar fascia, 82f
Alar ligaments, 509, 510f
Aligned knee bends, 190
Aligned lunges, 190–91
Aligning legs, 190
Alignment. *See* Gravity
All-or-none law, 78
Alpha motor neurons, 106
Alveoli, 240
Ambulation, 184. *See also* Gait
Amphiarthrosis joints, 34, 35f, 35t
Anaerobic glycolysis, 80
Anatomical position, 9–10, 10f
Anatomical snuffbox
extensor pollicis longus, 656–57, 657f
scaphoid, 614, 615f
Anatomical stirrup, 296, 296f
Anconeus, 640–42, 640f

Angle of inclination, 386–87, 386–87f
Angle of torsion, 387, 387f
Angular motion, 51, 51f
Ankle
neutral position of, 288, 288f
Ankle and foot joints, 279, 279t, 281–94
interphalangeal joints, 292, 292f, 294
intertarsal joints, 290
movement in three planes, 285, 285f
range of motion in ankle, 285, 285f, 285t, 286–87
subtalar joint, 284–85, 284f
talocrural joint, 282–84, 283–84f
tarsometatarsal joints, 290, 290f
tibiofibular joints, 282, 283f
transverse tarsal joint, 288–89, 288f
Ankle and foot ligaments
osteoligamentous plate, 279, 281f
plantar fascia and supporting ligaments, 281–82, 281f, 282f
Ankle and foot muscles, 294–327
extrinsic, 294–313
intrinsic, 294, 313–27
Ankle bones
posterior view, 270f

Ankle bones (*continued*)
regions of, 272*f*
surface anatomy of, 269*f*
talus, 272, 273*f*, 277*f*
Annular ligament, 622, 623, 623*f*
Annulus fibers, 448, 448*f*
Antagonist, 89*t*, 90
Antalgic gait, 196, 198
Anterior, 10, 11*f*
Anterior compartment, 295–300, 295*f*, 296, 296*f*, 297*f*
Anterior compartment syndrome, 297
Anterior cruciate ligament (ACL), 341, 341*f*
Anterior inferior iliac spine (AIIS), 377, 378*f*, 385*f*
Anterior inferior ischial spine (AIIS), 357
Anterior invertors, 267
Anterior longitudinal ligament, 456, 456*f*
Anterior pelvic tilt (APT), 166
Anterior-posterior axis (AP axis), 12, 12*f*
Anterior scalene muscle, 82*f*
Anterior superior iliac spine (ASIS), 377, 378*f*, 381
Anterior talofibular ligament, 283, 283*f*
Anterior tibiofibular ligaments, 282, 283*f*
Anterior triangle, 537, 537*f*
Anterolateral, 13, 15*f*
Anteromedial, 13
Anteversion, 387, 387*f*
Antigravity reflex, 108
Aorta, foramen for, 242, 242*f*
Aponeurosis, 81, 81*f*
Apophyseal joints. *See* Facet joints
Appendicular skeleton, 24, 24*f*
Approximation, 106, 107
Arches, 277, 279

inchworm articulation of, 321
plantar view, 277*f*
in stiff, flat feet, restoring, 280
Arcing exercise for spinal movement, 451–52
Arcuate ligament, 342
Areas of the body, 9, 10*f*
Arm, 9, 10*f. See also* Forearm
breath support for, with diaphragmatic breathing, 681
defined, 610
gait assessment, 203
stacking joints in, 685, 686*f*
surface anatomy of, 610*f*
Arm and hand bones, 610–20, 611*f*, 619*f*
carpals, 614–18, 615*f*
humerus, 610, 611*f*
metacarpals, 618, 619*f*
palpation of, 612–14
phalanges, 618–19, 619*f*
radius, 610, 611*f*
ulna, 610, 611*f*, 612
Arm and hand joints and ligaments, 620–31
elbow, 621–22, 621*f*, 622*f*
forearm, 622–24, 623*f*
hand, 620–21, 620*f*, 626, 628
hand arches and grips, 628, 630*f*, 631
supination and pronation, 623, 623*f*
wrist, 620–21, 620*f*, 624–26, 625*f*
Arm and hand muscles, 631–68
elbow flexors and extensors, 631, 633–40, 633*f*
hand muscles, 633, 661, 663–68
supinators and pronators, 631, 640, 642–44, 642*f*
thumb muscles, 631, 656–60, 656*f*

wrist and hand flexors and extensors, 631, 645–55, 645*f*
Artery in periosteum, 33*f*
Arthrokinematics, 56–61
close-packed and loose-packed positions, 60–61
concave–convex rule, 59, 59*f*
defined, 56
joint congruency and incongruency, 59–60
roll, glide, and spin, 57–59, 57*f*
Articular cartilage, 31, 32*f*, 35, 36*f*
Articular chain, 5
Articular pillar, 443, 443*f*, 446
Articular process, 442–43
Articulation, 34, 50, 66
Assessment
defined, 210
tools, palpation as, 210–11
Ataxic gait, 200–201
Atlantoaxial joint, 506, 509, 510*f*
Atlanto-occipital (AO) joint, 509, 510*f*
Atlanto-occipital (AO) joint rock, 542
Atlas, 443, 444*f*, 488
Auricle of the outer ear, 498, 499
Autonomic nervous system (ANS), 98, 99*f*
Avulsion fractures, 81
Axial compression, 42–43, 157, 163*f*
Axial movements, 50, 50*f*, 51–53
frontal plane, 52, 53*f*
horizontal plane, 52, 53, 53–54*f*
sagittal plane, 50, 50*f*, 51, 52*f*
Axial rotation of knee, 351, 355
Axial skeleton, 24, 24*f*
Axillary nerve, 580, 599

Axis, 12–13, 12*f*, 14*f*, 143, 443, 444*f*, 488
Axons, 98, 99, 100*f*

B

Back line, 114
Backward rotation, 53
Balance
exercise, 156, 157*f*
improving, 177
issues, working with clients with, 193
labyrinth mechanisms for maintaining, 110
Ball-and-socket joint, 38, 38*f*
Barefoot running, 182
Base of support (BOS)
center body over, 675, 675*f*
equilibrium and, 147, 147*f*
to remain lifted over client, 682, 683, 683*f*
in upright posture, 154
Belly breathing, 259
Bend, 40*f*, 41
Biarticular muscles, 90
Biaxial joints, 39, 39*t*
Biceps, 145*f*
Biceps brachii, 64, 73*f*, 74*f*, 633–38, 633*f*, 634*f*
Biceps femoris, 73*f*, 361, 363–65, 363*f*
Biceps femoris bursa, 340
Bicipital groove, 551, 551*f*, 553
Bilateral axis (medial-lateral axis), 12, 12*f*
Biomechanics, 4, 128–50
force, 135, 136–42
friction, 130–31
gravity, 130
inertia, 134
laws of motion, 134–35, 136
levers, 142, 143–48
lines of muscular pull, 131–32, 131–32*f*
reverse muscle action, 132–33, 133*f*, 134
terms and concepts, 130–34
velocity, 130
Bipedal gait, 184

Bipennate muscle, 74, 74f, 75f
Blood, 25, 25t
Blood vessels
  muscle, 82f
  tissue layering, 222, 224f
Body, orienting space within, 9–11
  anatomical position, 9–10, 10f
  areas of the body, 9, 10f
  directional terms, 10–11, 11f
Body in space, orienting, 11–14
  axis, 12–13, 12f
  diagonal planes, 13, 14f
  dimensional balance, 14, 15f
  planes, 12–13, 12f
Body mechanics in massage, checklist for, 697
Body-mind. See Somatics
Body of the sternum, 231, 232f
Bodywork, gait education in, 202, 203–4
Boggy end-feel, 65
Bolsters, 695–97, 696f
Bone, 25, 25t, 28–31. See also individual bones
  bony landmarks, 31, 31f
  compact, 28–29, 28f
  elasticity, 26, 27, 30–31
  fractures, 30–31
  muscle and, 82f
  remodeling, 30, 30f
  spongy, 29, 29f
  strength, 30–31
  tissue layering, 222, 223f
  types, 29–30
Bony end-feel, 64
Bow-legged alignment, 169, 169f, 189
Brachialis, 73f, 633f, 634–38, 634f, 635f
Brachial plexus, 102, 102f, 103f
Brachioradialis, 633f, 634–38, 635f

Brachioradialis, soft-end feel and, 64
Breathing, 681
Breathing exercises, 228
Breath support, 681
Broad-hand gliding, 215, 216f
Buccinator, 527f, 528, 528f, 530
Buccopharyngeal, 82f
Bulging disk, 448, 449f
Bursa, 36f
Bursae, 33–34, 34f, 338, 339, 339f
Bursitis, 34

C
Cadence, 188
Calcaneal tuberosity, 272, 275
Calcaneal valgus, 289, 290f
Calcaneal varus, 289
Calcaneocuboid joint, 288
Calcaneonavicular ligament, 281
Calcaneus, 272, 273f, 274f, 275, 277f
Cancellous (spongy) bone, 29, 29f, 36f
Capitate, 615, 615f, 618
Capitis, 462
Capitulum, 610, 611f
Capsular end-feel, 64, 64f
Cardiac muscle, 72
Cardinal planes, 12–13, 12f
Carotid sheath, 82f
Carpal arch, 628, 630f
Carpals, 30, 614–18, 615f
  distal row, 614, 617
  proximal row, 614, 616
Carpal tunnel, 625, 626f
Carpal tunnel syndrome, 625, 627
Carpometacarpal (CMC) joints, 626, 628, 629f
Carrying angle, 621, 621f
Cartilage, 25, 25t, 31–32, 32f
Caudal, 11, 11f
Cell bodies, 98, 99, 100f
Centering, 681

Center of gravity (COG), 39–40, 40f, 130, 147f, 154
Central nervous system (CNS), 98, 99f
Central tendon, 243, 243f
Cephalad, 11, 11f
Cerebral palsy (CP), 201
Cervical flexors, 459
Cervical hyperextension, 541–42, 541f
Cervical nerve, 585
Cervical nerves, 466, 537
Cervical spine, 440, 445
  lateral flexion, range of, 449, 450f
  motion in, 452–53, 511t
Cervical vertebra (C7), 82f
Cervicis, 462
Chairs and seated techniques, 694–95, 694–95f
Chest, center of gravity in, 39
Chest muscles, stretching, 678–79
Ch'i (qi), 112, 113f
Chinese energy meridians, 112, 113f
Chondrocytes, 25
Chondromalacia, 346
Chondrosternal junction, 235, 235f
Chronic lumbar flexion, 395
Chronic obstructive pulmonary diseases (COPDs), 259, 260
Chronic thoracic flexion, 161, 161f
Circular friction, 86, 86f
Circumduction, 54, 54f
  elbow, 54, 54f, 623, 624f
  in gait, 200, 200f
  glenohumeral joint, 559, 561f
  wrist, 624
Classroom palpation, 212–13
Clavicle, 30, 550f, 553
  fractures, 552

lateral rotation during shoulder elevation, 565, 565f
Claw, 691, 691f
Client-centered postural assessments, 174
Clinical applications for joint movement, 63–67
  active motion, 63, 64
  joint articulation, 66–67
  joint mobilization, 66
  passive motion, 64–65
  resisted range of motion, 66, 66f
Closed kinetic chain, 56, 56f
Close-packed position, 60–61
Coccygeal nerves, 380
Coccygeus, 422, 426f
Coccyx, 24f, 30, 375, 375f, 380, 380f, 384
Cochlea, 110, 110f
Collagen, 25, 26, 26f
Collateral ligaments of knee, 340–41, 340f
Colles' fracture, 31
Combined loading, 40f, 41
Comminuted fracture, 31
Compact (cortical) bone, 28–29, 28f, 33f
Compacted fracture, 31
Compartments of extrinsic muscles, 294–313, 295f
  anterior, 295–97, 295f
  deep posterior, 305–6, 306f
  lateral, 310–11, 310f
  posterior, 300–302, 300f
Compartment syndrome, 295
  anterior, 297
  lateral, 310
Compensatory pattern. See Substitution pattern
Complete fracture, 31
Complete sequences, 681
Compound (open) fracture, 31
Compression, 40–41, 40f
Concave–convex rule, 59, 59f

Concentric contraction, 87, 87*f*, 88*t*, 89*f*

Concentric contractions, 194, 195–96, 195*f*, 196*f*

Concurrent force, 137–38, 138*f*

Concurrent movement, 90, 90*f*

Condyle, 31

Condyloid (ellipsoid) joint, 38, 38*f*

Congenital scoliosis, 168–69

Congruent joint, 59–60

Connective tissue, 25–34
    cells in, 25, 25*t*
    composition and features of, 25, 25*t*
    dense, 25
    fibers in, 25–26, 25*t*
    fluids in, 25, 25*t*
    loose, 25

Connective tissue of peripheral nerves, 102

Connective tissue proper, 25, 25*t*

Connective tissue properties, 26–28
    elasticity, 26, 27
    piezoelectric effect, 27, 28
    plasticity, 27
    thixotropy, 26
    viscosity, 26, 27

Conoid ligament, 565

Contracted muscle, 75*f*

Contractile fibers, types of, 80–81, 80*t*

Contractility, 76

Contract–relax–antagonist–contract (CRAC), 122

Contract–relax–stretch, 122

Contracture, 80. *See also* Muscle contraction

Contralateral limb motion in gait, 192

Contralateral movement, 7, 8*f*

Coordination, 90

Coracoacromial (suprahumeral) arch, 565–66, 566*f*

Coracoacromial ligament, 565–66

Coracobrachialis, 599, 599*f*
    palpation of, 600–602
    trigger points, 600*f*

Coracoclavicular ligament, 565, 566*f*

Coracohumeral ligament, 559

Coracoid process, 554, 554*f*, 555

Core muscles, 164, 164*f*, 165

Core stability, 676

Corn-starch exploration, 27

Coronal suture, 501, 501*f*, 503

Coronoid fossa, 610, 611*f*

Coronoid process, 495, 495*f*, 498, 611*f*, 612

Corrugator, 525*f*

Cortical (compact) bone, 28–29, 28*f*, 33*f*

Costal arch, 31, 231, 232*f*, 233, 241, 242–45

Costal cartilage, 231, 232*f*, 235, 235*f*

Costalchondral junction, 235, 235*f*

Costal facets, 443, 443*f*

Costal joints, 235–238
    anterior, 235–36
    intercostal spaces between, 235, 235*f*
    posterior, 236

Costoclavicular ligament, 566, 567*f*

Costotransverse joints, 236, 236*f*, 237–38

Costotransverse ligaments, 236, 236*f*

Costovertebral joints, 236, 236*f*, 237–38

Countercurrent movement, 90, 90*f*

Counternutation, 396, 396*f*

Countersupport, exercises for, 136

Coupled motion, 447, 447*f*

Coxal (innominate) bones, 375, 375*f*

Coxa valga, 387, 387*f*

Coxa vara, 387, 387*f*

Coxofemoral joint, 384–94
    close-packed position of, 386, 386*f*
    femoral angulations, 386–87, 386*f*

Coxofemoral joint motion, 387–92
    of hip at pelvis, 387–89, 388*f*
    lumbar pelvic rhythm, 393–94, 393*f*
    of pelvis at hip, 389, 390*f*

Cranial, 11, 11*f*

Cranial bones, 488–94, 489*f*, 492*f*

Cranial mobilization, 503

Cranial nerves, 100, 101*f*

Cranial protraction, 452, 453*f*

Cranial retraction, 452, 453*f*

Cranialsacral therapy (CST), 501, 503

Cranial sutures, 501–3, 501*f*

Cranial vault, 488, 490, 491*f*

Creep, 84–85, 84*f*

Crest, 31, 31*f*

Crest of sacrum

Cricoid cartilage, 498, 499, 499*f*, 500

Crimping arrangement of collagen fibers, 26, 27, 27*f*

Crossed extensor reflex, 111

Cross-extensor reflex, 192

Cross-fiber friction, 28, 65, 85, 86*f*

Cross-fiber strumming, 215, 216*f*

Cross links, 26, 26*f*

Crouched gait, 201

Cruciate ligaments of knee, 340*f*, 341, 341*f*

Crus, 242

Cuboid, 273–74, 273*f*, 276, 277*f*

Cuboidnavicular joint, 290

Cuneiforms, 273, 273*f*, 274*f*, 277*f*, 290, 290*f*

Cuneocuboid joint, 290

Cuneonavicular joint, 290

Curvature of the spine, 166–67, 167*f*

Curvilinear motion, 51, 51*f*, 54

Cylindrical grip, 628, 630*f*

Cytoskeleton, 81

D

Deceleration, 130, 185

Deep, 11

Deep cervical muscles, 82*f*

Deep fascia, 32–33, 81, 81*f*, 218, 220, 220*f*

Deep infrapatellar bursa, 339, 339*f*, 340

Deep paravertebral muscle layer, 459

Deep peroneal nerve, 295, 310, 313, 313*f*

Deep plantarflexors, 266

Deep posterior compartment, 305–10, 306–7*f*

Deep-sea diving, 208

Deep six lateral hip rotators, 420–25, 420*f*

Deep tissue massage, 28

Deep tissue work, gauging pressure during, 78

Deep transverse metatarsal ligament, 282

Degree of motion, 38–39, 39*t*

Deltoid, 73*f*, 74*f*, 599, 599*f*, 600–602

Deltoid ligament, 283, 283*f*

Deltoid tuberosity, 551, 551*f*, 553

Demifacets. *See* Costotransverse joints

Dendrites, 98, 99, 100*f*

Dense connective tissue, 25, 25*t*, 32–34, 32*f*
    bursae, 33–34, 34*f*
    fascia, 32–33, 32*f*
    friction and deep pressure on, effects of, 28
    irregular, 32
    joint capsules, 33
    ligaments, 33
    periosteum, 33, 33*f*
    regular, 32
    synovial sheaths, 34, 34*f*
    tendons, 33

Dens process, 443, 444*f*

Depression, 53, 504, 505*f*, 506*f*

Depressor muscles
  anguli oris, 525*f*
  labii inferior, 525*f*
  septi, 526*f*
  tracing, 530

Diagonal line, 114, 114*f*

Diagonal line of pull, 132*f*

Diagonal plane, 13, 14*f*

Diaphragm, 240–46, 241*f*
  attachments sites, 241–42
  defined, 240–41
  intra-abdominal pressure, 245–46, 245*f*
  locating, tracking, and stretching, 242–43
  movement of, 243, 243*f*
  openings in, 242, 242*f*
  stitch in the side, 242, 243

Diaphragmatic breathing, 681

Diarthrosis joints. *See* Synovial joints

Diastasis recti in rectus abdominis, 473

Digastric, 530, 531*f*

Dimensional balance, 14, 15*f*

Dimensional cross, 14

Directional terms, 10–11, 11*f*

Direction of force, 136

Direct technique, 116

Displaced fracture, 31

Displacement of the knee, 340

Distal attachment, 75

Distal carpal arch, 628, 630*f*

Distal interphalangeal joint (DIP), 294, 628

Distal radioulnar joint, 623, 623*f*

Distal tibiofibular joint, 282

Dorsal, 11, 11*f*

Dorsal interossei, 326–27, 327*f*, 663, 664*f*

Dorsal layer, 294, 313–17

Dorsal root ganglion, 103*f*

Dorsal scapular nerve, 585

Dorsiflexion, 51, 52*f*

with fibular motion, 284, 284*f*
  PROM for, 284–85, 284*f*, 285*f*

Dorsiflexors, 266

Double condyloid joint, 347

Double-limb support, 185

Downslip of pelvis, 396, 396*f*

Down's syndrome, 201

Downward rotation, 55, 55*f*

Drawer sign, 341, 341*f*

Drop-foot gait, 199–200, 199*f*

Dural tube, 503

Dynamic postural reflexes, 155–56
  head righting, 156, 157*f*
  optical righting, 156, 156*f*
  postural sway, 155–56, 155*f*

Dynamics, 4

E

Ear. *See* Auricle of the outer ear

Early swing, 189, 189*f*, 194*t*, 195

Ear stones, 110

Eccentric contractions, 87, 87*f*, 88*t*, 89*f*, 194, 195, 195*f*, 196*f*

Eccentric loading, 161

Eckman, Paul, 523

Effort (E), 143

Effort arm (EA), 143, 143*f*, 145*f*

Elastic cartilage, 31, 32*f*

Elasticity, 76

Elastic limit, 27

Elastin fibers, 26

Elbow
  circumduction, 54, 54*f*, 623, 624*f*
  flexors and extensors, 631, 633–40, 633*f*
  joints and ligaments, 621–22, 621*f*, 622*f*
  palpation of, 612–14
  skeletal alignment, 679, 680*f*
  supination and pronation, 623, 624*f*

Elbow flexors and extensors, 631, 633–40, 633*f*
  anconeus, 640
  biceps brachii, 633–34, 633*f*, 634*f*
  brachialis, 633*f*, 634, 634*f*
  brachioradialis, 633*f*, 634, 635*f*
  triceps brachii, 634, 638, 638*f*

Electromyography (EMG), 164, 194

Elevation, 53, 504, 505*f*

Ellipsoid (condyloid) joint, 38, 38*f*

Empty end-feel, 65

Endangerment sites, 222, 224*f*

End-feel, 64, 64*f*, 65

Endolymph fluid, 110

Endomysium, 81, 82*f*

Endoneurium, 102, 103*f*

Energy sources for muscle contraction, 80

Envaginations of synovial lining, bursa that are, 338

Epicondyle, 31

Epimysium, 81, 82*f*

Epineurium, 102, 103*f*

Equilibrium, 147–48, 148*f*

Equilibrium responses (ER), 5

Erector spinae (ES), 460, 462–66, 462*f*

Ergonomics and equipment, 692–97
  bolsters, 695–97, 696*f*
  chairs and seated techniques, 694–95, 694–95*f*
  face cradles, 695–97, 696*f*
  mirrors for feedback, 697
  stools, foot and folding, 693–94, 693–94*f*
  table height, 692–93, 693*f*
  table pads, 695–97, 695*f*

Erythrocytes, 25

Esophagus, 82*f*, 242, 242*f*

Ethmoid bone, 488, 489*f*, 491*f*

Eversion, 52, 53*f*, 287

Evertors, 266

Excessive kyphosis, 160, 160*f*, 166, 167*f*

Excessive lordosis, 166, 167*f*

Excitability, 76

Excitatory nerve impulses, 109

Excursion, 74, 75*f*

Exhalation fixation, 255, 260*f*

Exploring foot position, 177

Extensibility, 76

Extension, 51, 52*f*

Extension of knee, 351, 351*f*

Extensor carpi radialis brevis, 651, 651*f*, 654

Extensor carpi radialis longus, 651, 651*f*, 654

Extensor carpi ulnaris, 651–52, 651*f*, 652*f*, 655

Extensor chain, 6, 6*f*

Extensor digiti minimi, 666, 666*f*

Extensor digitorum, 651*f*, 652, 653*f*, 655

Extensor digitorum brevis, 313, 313*f*, 315–17, 315*f*

Extensor digitorum longus, 74*f*, 296, 297*f*, 298–300

Extensor expansion tendons, 652, 652*f*

Extensor hallucis brevis, 313, 313*f*, 315–17, 315*f*

Extensor hallucis longus, 296–300, 297*f*

Extensor indicis, 651*f*, 652, 653*f*, 655

Extensor pollicis brevis, 656*f*, 657
  palpation of, 659

Extensor pollicis longus, 656–57, 656*f*, 657*f*, 659

Extensor retinaculum, 81*f*

Extensor support moment, 189
Extensor thrust reflex, 111
External acoustic meatus, 490, 492*f*, 493
External obliques, 73*f*, 232*f*, 246, 249–50, 249*t*, 250*f*, 473
External occipital protu- berance, 488, 489*f*, 490, 493
External (lateral) rotation, 52, 53*f*
Exteroceptors, 105
Extrafusal fibers, 106, 106*f*
Extrinsic abdominal mus- cles, 459
Extrinsic muscles of ankle and foot, 294–313
    compartments, 294–313, 295*f*
    tendons, 294, 294*f*
Extrinsic thumb muscles, 656–59, 656*f*
    abductor pollicis longus, 656*f*, 657
    extensor pollicis brevis, 656*f*, 657
    extensor pollicis longus, 656–57, 656*f*
    flexor pollicis longus, 656, 656*f*

F

Face cradles, 695–97, 696*f*
Facet, 31, 31*f*
Facet joints, 449–56, 450*f*, 506
Facial adhesions, 83
Facial bones, 489*f*, 495–98, 495*f*
Facial muscles, 517, 523–30, 523*f*, 524–28*f*
    actions of, 524–27*f*
Facial nerve, 513, 531
Facing direction of stroke, 682, 682*f*
Fall and recovery, 192–93, 193*f*
False ribs, 231, 231*f*
Fascia, 32–33, 32*f*
    continuity of, 81–86
    deep, 81, 81*f*, 82*f*

of infrahyoid muscles, 82*f*
    myofascial system, 81–86
    in neck, 82*f*
Fascial restrictions around bone, releasing, 33
Fascicles, 25, 26, 26*f*, 76, 82*f*
Fast glycolytic (FG) fibers, 80–81, 80*t*
Fast oxidative-glycolytic (FOG) fibers, 80–81, 80*t*
Feedback, 213–14
    mirrors for, 697
    neurological symptoms, 102
    passive joint movement, 103
    postural patterns, 173
Feet, 24*f*
    arches in, restoring, 280
    gait assessment, 203
    postural problems in, 169, 169*f*
    pushing from, 686, 688*f*
Femoral condyles, 333, 334*f*, 336
Femoral epicondyle, 333, 336
Femoral inclination, 386–87, 386–87*f*
Femoral nerve, 357, 399, 416
Femoral triangle, 405, 405*f*
Femur, 24*f*, 333, 334*f*
Fibers. *See* Muscle fibers
Fibrils, 25, 26*f*
Fibrocartilage, 32, 32*f*
Fibrocartilage joints, 34, 35*f*, 35*t*
Fibrotic end-feel, 65
Fibrous joints, 34, 35*f*, 35*t*
Fibula, 24*f*, 270, 270*f*, 271–72
Fibular collateral ligament, 36*f*, 340
Fibularis brevis. *See* Pero- neus brevis
Fibularis longus. *See* Peroneus longus

Fibularis tertius. *See* Pero- neus tertius
Fingers
    accessory movements in, 631
    little finger muscles, 666–67, 666*f*
Fingertip palpation, 215, 216*f*
Firm end-feel, 64, 64*f*
First carpometacarpal joint, 626, 628, 628*f*
First cervical nerve, 534
First lumbar nerve, 473
Fixators, 90
Flat-back posture, 167, 168*f*
Flat bones, 29*f*, 30
Flat-finger palpation, 215, 216*f*
Flatfoot, 288–89, 288*f*
Flexion, 51, 52*f*
Flexor carpi radialis, 646, 646*f*, 650
Flexor carpi ulnaris, 646, 646*f*, 649
Flexor chain, 6, 6*f*
Flexor digiti minimi bre- vis, 323*f*, 324–26, 325–26, 665*f*, 666, 666*f*, 667
Flexor digitorum brevis, 318, 318*f*
    palpation of, 319–20
Flexor digitorum longus, 306–10, 307*f*
Flexor digitorum profun- dus, 647, 647*f*, 648*f*, 650
Flexor digitorum superfi- cialis, 647, 647*f*, 648*f*, 650
Flexor hallucis brevis, 323, 323*f*, 324*f*, 325–26
Flexor hallucis longus, 306–10, 307*f*
Flexor pollicis brevis, 660, 660*f*, 662
Flexor pollicis longus, 656, 656*f*, 659
Flexor withdrawal reflex, 111
Floating ribs, 231, 231*f*, 233*f*

Float moment, 188
Fluidity, 681
FOOSH injury, 566, 566*f*
Foot
    angle, 188, 188*f*
    deep fascia of, 81*f*
    flexors, 89*f*
    joints (*See* Ankle and foot joints)
    ligaments (*See* Ankle and foot ligaments)
Foot bones, 270–77, 270*f*
    arches, 277, 279
    dorsal view, 273*f*
    fibula, 270–72, 270*f*
    lateral view, 274*f*
    medial view, 273*f*
    metatarsals, 273*f*, 274, 274*f*, 277*f*
    phalanges, 273*f*, 274, 274*f*, 277*f*
    plantar view, 277*f*
    posterior view, 270*f*
    regions of, 272*f*, 727
    surface anatomy of, 269*f*
    tarsals, 272–74, 273*f*, 274*f*
    tibia, 270–72, 270*f*
Foot flat, 188, 189*f*, 195
Foramen, 31, 31*f*
Foramen magnum, 488, 489*f*
Force, 5, 135, 136–42
    concurrent, 137–38, 138*f*
    force couple, 140–41, 141*f*
    force–velocity relation- ship, 141, 142
    linear, 137
    parallel, 137, 138*f*
    in pressure applica- tions, efficient use of, 139–40
    stress–strain curve, 141, 141*f*, 142
    torque, 138, 140–41, 141*f*
    vector, characteristics of, 136–37, 137*f*
Force applications and hand use, 685–92

alternate opposing strokes to balance body, 691, 692f
applying pressure, 685–86, 686–88f
full-body movement, 685
pushing and pulling, lines of force in, 687, 688f
vary massage strokes, 691, 691–92f
Force couple, 140–41, 141f
Forced closure, 395–96, 395f
Force vector, 136–37, 137f
Force–velocity relationship, 141, 142
Forearm, 9, 10f
cross section, 645f
deep fascia, 81f
defined, 610
joints and ligaments, 622–24, 623f
neutral position, 623, 624
palpation, 612–14
skeletal alignment, 679, 680f
supination and pronation, 623, 623f
Forefoot, 272f, 727
Form closure, 395
Forward head posture, 452, 453
Forward rotation, 53, 54f
Fossa, 31
Fracture, 30–31
clavicle, 552
rib, 236
scaphoid, 615f
Free bursae, 338
Friction, 130–31
Frontal bone, 488, 489f, 491f, 492
Frontalis, 73f, 513–16, 513f, 524f, 528
Frontal plane, 12, 12f, 13f, 52, 53f, 191, 192f
Front line, 114
Frozen shoulder, 571–72, 571f
Fusiform muscle, 72, 74f, 75f

G

Gait, 182–207
atypical gait patterns, 196–201
cadence, 188
cycle, 187
defined, 184
fall and recovery, 192–93, 193f
lower limb joint motion, 188–91, 189f
muscle activity in, 194–96
muscle patterns, 194t
pelvic movement in each plane, 191–92, 191–92f
stance and swing phases, 184–86, 185f, 187
step and stride length and width, 187–88, 187–88f
trunk rotation and contralateral limb motion, 192
Gait assessment, 201–4
education in bodywork, 202, 203–4
general, 201–2
specific, 201–2, 203
therapeutic applications for, 202
Gait patterns, atypical, 196–201
antalgic gait, 196, 198
holding patterns affecting gait, 196
muscle dysfunctions in gait, 198–200, 199f
neurological effects in gait, 200–201, 201f
range of motion limitations, 200, 200f
Gait phases
stance phase, 184–86, 185f, 187, 195, 195f
swing phase, 184–86, 185f, 187, 195–96, 196f
trunk and shoulders, 196
Galea aponeurosis, 81f
Galea aponeurotica, 513

Gamma motor neurons, 106
Ganglia, 98
Gastrocnemius, 73f, 89f, 300, 300f, 301f, 303–5, 362
Gastrocnemius bursa, 340
Gemellus inferior, 422, 424–25
Gemellus superior, 422, 424–25
Genioglossus, 530, 531f
Geniohyoid, 530, 531f
Genu recurvatum, 348, 349f, 350
Genu recurvatum gait, 198, 199f
Genu valgum, 169, 169f, 347, 348f
Genu varum, 169, 169f, 189, 347, 348f
Glenohumeral (GH) joint, 558–60, 558f
ligaments and bursae, 558, 558f, 559
motion, 559–60, 561f
Glenoid fossa, 554, 554f
Glenoid labrum, 558, 558f
Gliding motion, 57–59, 57f
Gliding (plane) joint, 38, 38f
Global movement, 9
Gluteal fold, 411, 411f
Gluteal muscles, 411–16, 411f
Gluteal nerve, 399
Gluteus maximus, 73f, 89f, 411, 411f, 412f, 414–16
weakness or inhibition, 413
Gluteus maximus lurch, 199, 199f
Gluteus medius, 73f, 411, 411f, 412f, 414–16
Gluteus medius lurch, 198–99, 199f
Gluteus medius stretch, 431
Gluteus minimus, 411, 411f, 413f, 414–16
Glycolysis, 80
Golfer's elbow, 647

Golgi tendon organs (GTO), 108–9
Gomphosis peg-in-socket joints, 34
Gracilis, 73f, 342, 345, 345f, 406, 407f, 408–11
Gracilis bursa, 340
Gravity, 5, 39–44, 130
center of, 39–40, 40f, 130, 147f, 154
line of, 39–40, 40f, 130, 147f, 154
lines of force, 41, 42–44, 42f
mechanical stresses, 40–41, 40f
optimal pressure and, 39–40, 40f
Greater horns of the hyoid, 498, 498f
Greater trochanter, 375, 377f, 381, 382
Greater tubercle, 551, 551f, 552
Greater wings of the sphenoid, 490, 491f, 494
Greenstick fracture, 31
Grip strength, 628, 630f, 631–32
Groove, 31
Grounding
exercises for, 136
horizontal, of body in recumbent position, 171f
Ground reaction force (GRF), 135, 135f
Ground substance, 25, 25t
Gutsmuths, Johann Friedrich, 2
Gymnastics, 2

H

Hair cells, 110
Hallux, 274
Hallux valgus, 317–18
Hamate, 615, 615f, 618
Hamstring, 89f, 140, 141f, 344, 361–62, 362f
balance, 428, 428f, 432
stretching, 91f, 430, 432

Hand, 24f
    arches and grips, 628,
        630f, 631–32
    bones (See Arm and
        hand bones)
    extensors, 631, 645–55,
        645f
    flexors (See Wrist and
        hand flexors)
    joints and ligaments,
        620–21, 620f, 626,
        628
    surface anatomy of,
        610f
Hand muscles, 633, 661,
    663–68
    interossei, 663, 664f
    little finger muscles,
        666–67, 666f
    lumbricals, 663, 664f
    palpation of, 667
Hard end-feel, 64f, 65
Harpist, hand dexterity
    and, 606
Head, 24f
    gait assessment, 203
    righting, 156, 157f, 484
    surface anatomy of,
        489f
    as top load, 159–60,
        160f
Head and neck bones,
    488–99
    cranial bones, 488–94,
        489f, 492f
    cricoid cartilage, 498,
        499
    facial bones, 489f,
        495–98, 495f
    hyoid, 498, 498f, 499f
    nose, 498, 498f
    outer ear, 498
    thyroid cartilage, 498,
        499f
    thyroid gland, 499, 499f
    trachea, 499, 499f
Head and neck joints, 499,
    500–509
    atlantoaxial joint, 506,
        509, 510f
    atlanto-occipital joint,
        509, 510f
    cranial sutures, 501–3,
        501f

temporomandibular
    joint, 503–6, 504f
Head and neck muscles,
    509, 513
    facial, 510, 517, 523–30,
        523f, 524–28f
    frontalis, 513, 513f
    infrahyoid muscles,
        531–32, 531–32f
    lateral pterygoid, 517,
        517f
    masseter, 517, 517f
    medial pterygoid, 517,
        517f
    occipitalis, 513, 513f
    prevertebral neck mus-
        cles, 537–38, 538f,
        541
    scalp, 510
    sternocleidomastoid,
        537–41, 537f
    suboccipitals, 532,
        534–35f, 534–36
    suprahyoid muscles,
        530, 531f
    temporalis, 513f, 514
    temporomandibular
        joint, 510
Head of humerus, 551,
    551f
Head of long bone, 31, 31f
Head of the femur, 376
Head of the fibula, 270,
    271
Heeloff, 189, 189f, 194t,
    195
Heel spurs, 198, 198f
Heel strike, 188, 189f,
    194t, 195
Hemi-pelvis, 173
Herniated disk, 448, 449f
Hiccups, 243
Hinge joint, 38, 38f
Hip
    abduction, 52, 52f, 391
    abductors, 399–404,
        400f
    adduction, 52, 52f, 392
    adductors, 404–11, 405f
    dislocations, 385
    extension of, 91f
    flexion, PROM for, 391
    hyperextension, PROM
        for, 392

lateral rotation, 52, 53f,
    392
medial rotation, 52, 53f,
    392
pain, anterior, 399
seniors with restricted
    hip motion, 398
Hip and pelvic muscles,
    399–432
    deep six lateral hip rota-
        tors, 420–22, 420f
    gluteal muscles,
        411–16, 411f
    hamstring balance, 428,
        428f, 432
    hip abductors, 399–404,
        400f
    hip adductors, 404–11,
        405f
    iliopsoas, 416–20, 417f
    pelvic floor, 426, 428
    perineal muscles, 422,
        426–28, 426f
    rectus femoris, 428,
        428f
    stretching, 431–32
Hip bones
    bony landmarks of,
        375–76, 376f
    palpation of, 381–84
Hip joints and ligaments,
    384–99, 385f
    coxofemoral joint,
        384–94
    hip problems, 396,
        397–99
    hip treatments, evaluat-
        ing, 389
    range of motion in hips,
        389t, 391–92
Homolateral movement,
    7, 8f
Homologous movement,
    7, 8f
Hook grip, 628, 630f, 631
Horizontal abduction, 53,
    54f, 559, 561f
Horizontal adduction, 53,
    54f, 559, 561f
Horizontal extension, 53,
    54f
Horizontal flexion, 53, 54f
Horizontal plane, 12, 12f,
    13f

Horizontal plane move-
    ment, 52, 53, 53–54f,
    191–92, 192f
Horizontal rotation of pel-
    vis, 191–92, 192f
Humeral head, 57, 57f
Humeroradial joint,
    621–22, 622f
Humeroulnar joint, 621,
    621f
Humerus, 24f, 29f, 550–51,
    550f, 610, 611f
Hyaline cartilage, 31, 32f,
    35, 36f
Hydrophilic, 25
Hyoid, 498, 498f, 499f,
    500
Hyperextended knee. See
    Genu recurvatum
Hyperextension, 51, 52f
Hypermobility, 62–63
Hyperpronation, 169, 169f,
    285, 286f, 288–89,
    288f
Hypersupination, 169,
    169f, 285, 286f, 288f,
    289
Hyperventilation, 260
Hypoglossal nerve, 531
Hypomobility, 62–63
Hypothenar eminence,
    661
Hypotonia, 200

I

Ideokinesis, 157
Iliac crest, 376, 378f, 381
Iliac fossa, 377, 378f, 382
Iliacus, 416, 417f,
    418–20
Iliococcygeus, 422, 426,
    426f
Iliocostalis, 464–66, 464f
    cervicis, 462f, 464
    lumborum, 462f, 464
    thoracis, 462f, 464
Iliofemoral ligament, 385,
    385f
Iliolumbar ligament, 457
Iliopsoas, 73f, 404,
    416–20, 417f
Iliotibial band (ITB), 73f,
    342, 342f, 344, 399,
    400f, 401, 402

Iliotibial band syndrome, 346
Ilium, 376, 377f
Inchworm articulation of arches, 321
Indirect technique, 116
Inertia, law of, 134
Inferior, 10–11, 11f
Inferior acromioclavicular ligament, 565, 566f
Inferior angle of scapula, 554, 554f, 557
Inferior attachment, 75
Inferior nuchal line, 489f, 490
Inferior pubic ramus, 377, 378f, 380
Infraglenoid tubercle, 554, 554f, 610
Infrahyoid muscles, 531–33, 531f
Infrapatellar bursa, 339, 339f, 340
Infraspinatus, 73f, 580, 581f
Infraspinous fossa, 554, 554f, 556
Inguinal ligament, 386
Inhalation fixation, 255, 259f
Inhibitory nerve impulses, 109
Initial swing, 185
Inner range joint position, 88, 89f
Insertion, 75
Inside line, 114–15, 114f
Instability, 62–63
Instantaneous axis of rotation (IAR), 59
Interbody joints, 448, 448f, 506
Intercarpal joints, 624, 625f
Intercondylar groove, 333
Intercostal nerves, 247, 247f
Intercostals, 246–48, 247f
  external, 246–47, 247f
  internal, 246–47, 247f, 249, 249f, 249t, 250f
  subcostales, 246, 247
Intercuneiform joint, 290

Intermediate cuneiform, 273, 273f
Internal obliques, 247, 249–50, 249t, 250f, 473
Internal (medial) rotation, 52, 53f
Interneurons, 99
Interoceptors, 105
Interossei, 663–65, 664f
Interosseous membrane, 282, 622, 623f
Interphalangeal (IP) joints, 292–94, 292f, 628, 630f
Interspinous ligaments, 457
Intertarsal joints, 290, 291
Intertransverse ligaments, 457, 457f
Intervertebral disks, 32, 448, 448f
Intervertebral joints, 448, 448f
Intra-abdominal pressure (IAP), 245, 245f
Intrafusal fibers, 106, 106f
Intraneural vessels, 103f
Intrinsic muscles, 294, 313–27, 313f
  dorsal, 313–17
  plantar, 317–27
  strengthening, 321
Intrinsic thumb muscles, 657, 660
  abductor pollicis brevis, 660
  adductor pollicis, 657, 660
  flexor pollicis brevis, 660
  opponens pollicis, 660
  palpation of, 661–63
Inversion, 52, 53f, 287
Irregular bones, 29f, 30
Irregular dense connective tissue, 32, 32f
Irritability, 76
Ischial ramus, 377
Ischial spine, 377, 378f
Ischial tuberosity, 377, 378f, 382
Ischiofemoral ligament, 385f, 386
Ischium, 376, 377, 377f

Isometric contractions, 87, 87f, 88, 88t, 89f, 194, 195, 195f, 196f
Isometric finger-pull exercise, 691, 691f
Isotonic contraction, 87, 87f

J
Joint, 34, 50. See also individual joints
  actions, naming, 55
  ankle and foot (See Ankle and foot joints)
  approximation, 37
  articulation, 50, 66–67
  capsule, 33, 35, 64
  cavity, 35
  instability, 163
  mobility, 61
  mobilization, 66
  neutral, 40
  play, 62
  proprioceptors, 109
  stability, 61
  thorax (See Sternocostal joints)
Joint classifications, 34–39, 35t
  fibrocartilage joints, 34, 35f
  fibrous joints, 34, 35f
  synovial joints, 35–36, 36f, 38–39
Joint movement, 48–69
  arthrokinematics, 56–61
  clinical applications for (See Clinical applications for joint movement)
  osteokinematics, 50–56
  passive, 59
  range of motion, 61–63
Jones, Lawrence, 116
Jugular notch, 231, 232f, 234
Jump sign, 120

K
Kegel exercise, 426
Kinematics, 5
Kinesiology, 4
Kinetic chains, 5–7
  assessing, 113–15

closed and opened, 56, 56f
  reflexive movement, 112–15, 113f
Kinetics, 5
Knee, 330–68
  bones, 333–37, 333f
  bursae, 338, 339f
  flexion of, 91f
  gait assessment, 203
  ligaments and tendons, 340–45, 340f, 342f
  meniscus, 338, 338f
  muscles of, 355–66
  palpation of, 336–37
  patellofemoral joint, 345–47, 345f
  position in skeletal alignment, 675–76
  postural problems, 169, 169f
  surface anatomy of, 335f
  tibiofemoral joint, 347–55
Kneecap. See Patella
Knee-jerk test, 106, 107
Knee ligaments, 340–45, 340f, 342f
  collateral, 340–41, 340f
  cruciate, 340f, 341
  palpation of, 343–44
Knee muscles, 355–66
  gastrocnemius, 362
  hamstrings, 361–62, 362f
  popliteus, 365, 365f
  quadriceps, 357–61, 358f
  sartorius, 362, 365
Knock-kneed alignment, 169, 169f
Kyphosis, 440. See also Excessive kyphosis
Kyphotic curve, 158, 159f, 453, 454, 454f
Kyphotic-lordotic posture, 167–68, 167f

L
Labral tear, 399
Labyrinth, 110, 110f
Lamboid suture, 501, 501f, 503

Lamellae, 28–29
Lamina, 442
Lamina groove, 442, 446
Larynx, 31
Latent trigger points, 119
Lateral, 10, 11*f*
Lateral border, 554, 554*f*, 557
Lateral collateral ligament (LCL), 283, 283*f*, 340, 340*f*, 343
Lateral (radial) collateral ligament, 622, 622*f*
Lateral compartment, 310–13, 310*f*, 311*f*
Lateral compartment syndrome, 310
Lateral cuneiform, 273, 273*f*
Lateral epicondyle, 610, 611*f*, 612
Lateral epicondylitis, 652
Lateral excursion, 504, 505*f*
Lateral flexion, 52, 53*f*
Lateral hip rotation, PROM for, 392
Lateral hip rotators, 420–422, 420*f* stretching, 423
Lateral line, 114, 114*f*
Lateral longitudinal arch, 277, 279
Lateral malleolar groove, 270, 270*f*, 272
Lateral malleolus, 269*f*, 270, 270*f*, 272
Lateral meniscus, 36*f*
Lateral patellar retinacula, 345, 345*f*
Lateral pelvic shift and pelvic tilt, 191, 192*f*
Lateral plantar nerve, 317, 320, 324, 326
Lateral pterygoid, 517, 517*f*, 519*f*, 520–22
Lateral (external) rotation, 52, 53*f*
Lateral rotator function in gait, 422*f*
Lateral temporomandibular ligament, 504, 504*f*
Late swing, 189, 189*f*, 196
Latissimus dorsi, 73*f*, 459, 574, 574*f*, 576*f*, 577–79

Law of acceleration, 135
Law of action and reaction, 135, 135*f*, 136
Law of inertia, 134
Laws of motion, 134–35, 136
  law of acceleration, 135
  law of action and reaction, 135, 135*f*, 136
  law of inertia, 134
Lax end-feel, 65
Leaning into pressure, 686, 688*f*
Left rotation, 52, 53*f*
Leg, 9, 10*f*
  aligning, 190
  deep fascia of, 81*f*
Lesser trochanter, 375
Lesser tubercle, 551, 551*f*, 552
Leukocytes, 25
Levator angulioris, 526*f*
Levator ani, 422, 426, 426*f*
Levatores costarum, 249*t*
Levator labii, 526*f*, 529
Levator scapula, 586, 587*f*, 588–92
Levator scapulae muscle, 82*f*
Levers, 143–48
  defined, 142
  equilibrium, stability, and mobility, 147–48, 148*f*
  in human body, 143–44, 144*f*
  mechanical advantage of, 144–45, 145–46*f*
  parts of, 142, 143
  pushing and pulling, 146
Lifting, proper, 148
Ligaments, 33, 222, 223*f*. *See also individual ligaments*
Ligamentum flavum, 457, 457*f*
Line, 31
Linea aspera, 376
Linear force, 137
Linear fractures, 30
Linear friction, 85, 86*f*
Linear motion, 51, 51*f*, 53–54

Line of gravity (LOG), 39–40, 40*f*, 130, 147*f*, 154
Lines of force, 41, 42–44, 42*f*, 687, 688*f*
  axial compression tests to assess, 42–43
  gravity, 41, 42–44, 42*f*
  in pushing and pulling, 687, 688*f*
  tests to assess, 42–43
Lines of pull, 74, 75*f*, 131–32, 131–32*f*, 133*f*
  in bipennate muscle, 75*f*
  fusiform muscle, 75*f*
Lister's tubercle, 610
Little finger muscles, 666–67, 666*f*
  abductor digiti minimi, 666, 666*f*
  extensor digiti minimi, 666, 666*f*
  flexor digiti minimi brevis, 666, 666*f*
  opponens digiti minimi, 666, 666*f*
Local movement, 9
Long bones, 29–30, 29*f*
Longissimus, 462, 462*f*, 463*f*, 465–66
  capitis, 462, 462*f*
  cervicis, 462, 462*f*
  lumborum, 462, 462*f*
  thoracis, 462, 462*f*
Longitudinal arches, 628, 630*f*
Longitudinal axis, 12, 12*f*
Long plantar ligament, 282
Long thoracic nerve, 585
Longus capitis, 537, 538*f*
Longus colli, 82*f*, 166*t*, 537, 538*f*
Loose connective tissue, 25, 25*t*
Loose-packed position, 60–61
Lordosis, 440
Lordotic curve, 158, 159*f*. *See also* Excessive lordosis
Lotion used to reduce friction, 131

Lower extremity (LE), 9, 10*f*
Lower limb, 9, 10*f*
  joint motion, 188–91, 189*f*
  mechanical axis of, 347, 347*f*
  misalignments, 169, 169*f*
  muscles in gait pattern capacities, 194
  sagittal tracking of, 197
Lower limb alignment exercises for, 190–91 gait assessment, 203
Lumbar multifidus, 164*f*, 166*t*, 175
Lumbar nerve plexus, 416
Lumbar nerves, 473
Lumbar pelvic rhythm, 393–94, 393*f*
Lumbar spine, 440, 446
  chronic flexion, 454, 455*f*
  motion in, 454, 455
  neutral spine, 455–56
Lumbar sway back, 469–70
Lumborum, 462
Lumbricals, 320, 320*f*, 322–23, 663, 664–65, 664*f*
Lunate, 614, 615*f*, 616
Lunging with legs, 684, 685*f*

M

Magnitude of force, 136, 137
Mandible, 495, 495*f*
Mandibular angle, 495, 495*f*, 497
Mandibular body, 495, 495*f*, 497
Mandibular condyle, 495, 495*f*, 507
Mandibular fossa, 490, 492*f*, 507
Mandibular ramus, 495, 495*f*, 497
Manubriosternal joint, 235, 235*f*

Manubrium, 231, 232*f*, 233–35, 235*f*, 241*f*, 551, 551*f*, 553
Marfan's syndrome, 201
Mass, 5
Massage
  checklist for body mechanics in, 697
  cadence in, 188
  lines of muscular pull in, 132
Massage stroke
  alternate opposing strokes to balance body, 691, 692*f*
  applying pressure, 685–86, 686–88*f*
  direction, 41
  facing direction of, 682, 682*f*
  full-body movement, 685
  pace of, 681
  varying, 691, 691–92*f*
Massage table, ergonomics and. *See* Ergonomics and equipment
Massage table, moving around, 681–85
  direction of stroke, 682, 682*f*
  lunging with legs, 684, 685*f*
  rocker base, 682, 683*f*
  shifting weight at end of reach, 684, 684*f*
  standing position, proper, 682–83, 683*f*
  upper-lower body synchronization, 684
Masseter, 73*f*, 517, 517*f*, 518*f*
Masseter stretch, 508
Mastoid process, 75, 75*f*, 490, 492*f*, 494
Maxilla, 495, 495*f*, 496
Mechanical advantage, 40
Mechanical advantage (M Ad), 144–45, 145–46*f*
Mechanical axis, 131, 131*f*, 347, 347*f*
Mechanical stresses, 40–41, 40f
Mechanics, 4

Medial, 10, 11*f*
Medial border, 554, 554*f*, 557
Medial collateral ligament (MCL), 283, 283*f*, 340*f*, 341, 343
Medial (ulnar) collateral ligament, 622, 622*f*
Medial cuneiform, 273, 273*f*, 276
Medial epicondyle, 610, 611*f*
Medial epicondylitis, 647
Medial hip rotation, PROM for, 392
Medial-lateral axis (bilateral axis), 12, 12*f*
Medial longitudinal arch, 277, 279*f*, 280
Medial malleolar groove, 270, 270*f*, 271
Medial malleolus, 269*f*, 270, 270*f*, 271
Medial meniscus, 36*f*
Medial plantar nerve, 317, 320, 323
Medial pterygoid, 517, 517*f*, 520–22, 520*f*
Medial (internal) rotation, 52, 53*f*
Medial tubercle of the talus, 272, 275
Median sacral crest, 378*f*, 380, 380*f*, 383
Media patellar retinacula, 345, 345*f*
Meninges, 503
Menisci, 32
Meniscus, 338–39, 338*f*
  distribution of weight, 338, 338*f*
  movement of, 355, 355*f*
  tracking and guiding motion of, 356
Mentalis, 525*f*
Meridians, 112–13
Metacarpals, 618, 619*f*, 620
Metacarpophalangeal (MTP) joints, 628
Metatarsals, 273*f*, 274, 274*f*, 277*f*, 278
Metatarsophalangeal (MTP) joints, 292–94, 292*f*

Microexpression Training Tool, 523
Microfibers, 76
Microfilaments, 76–78
Midcarpal joint, 624, 625*f*
Middle and posterior scalene muscles, 82*f*
Middle paravertebral muscle layer, 459
Midfoot, 272*f*, 727
Midrange joint position, 88, 89*f*
Midstance, 189, 189*f*, 194*t*, 195
Midswing, 189, 189*f*, 194*t*, 196
Military posture, 165, 165*f*
Mindful touch, 212
Mirrors for feedback, 697
Mitchell, Fred, Sr., 121
Mobility, 4, 147–48, 148*f*
Mobilizers, 90
Modified hinge joint, 347
Moment arm
  defined, 140, 140*f*
  of quadriceps, 345, 345*f*
Momentum, 135
Motility, 4
Motion. *See also* Movement; Range of motion (ROM)
  curvilinear, 51, 51*f*, 54
  glide, 57–59, 57*f*
  linear, 51, 51*f*, 53–54
  roll, 57–59, 57*f*
  rotary, 51–53, 51*f*
  spin, 57–59, 57*f*
Motion assessments and techniques, 116–19, 117*f*, 117*t*
  active motion skills, 116
  passive motion skills, 118
  resisted motion skills, 118, 119
Motor cortex, 104
Motor end plate, 100
Motor neurons, 79*f*
Motor (efferent) neurons, 99
Motor points, 100
Motor response, 210–11
Motor units, 78–80, 79*f*

frequency of stimulation, 79
muscle contracture and fatigue, 80
recruitment of, 79
Movement. *See also* Biomechanics; Joint movement; Motion; Reflexive movement
accessory, 62
applications in neuromuscular techniques, 115–24
construction worker's, 128
observation, 115
physiological, 62
restrictions, 66
Movement patterns, 4–9
  biomechanics, 4
  developmental, 7–8
  kinetic chains, 5–7
  kinetics and kinematics, 5
  mechanical forces of movement in manual therapy, 5
  mechanics, 4
  posture, 4–5
  whole-body, 9
Moving through lunges, 684, 685*f*
Multiaxial (triaxial) joints, 39, 39*t*
Multifidi, 466–67, 467*f*
  palpation of, 468–69
  training, lumbar sway back corrected with, 469–70
Multifidus, 89*f*
Multipennate muscle, 74, 74*f*
Multiple motor unit summation, 79
Muscle. *See also individual muscles*
adaptive shortening of, 83, 83*f*
approximation, 106, 107
attachments, 75–76, 75*f*
cardiac, 72
changing roles of (*See* Muscle functions)
continuity of, 81–86

Muscle (*continued*)
names, 72
parallel elastic components of, 86
postural stabilizers, 162–65, 166*t*
series elastic component of, 86–87, 87*f*
shapes, 72, 74, 74*f*
skeletal, 72–76
smooth, 72
stretch-weakened, 83, 83*f*
tissue, 72, 76
tissue layering, 220, 221–22
tone, 79
twitch, 78
Muscle activity in gait, 194–96
gait muscle patterns, 194*t*
stance phase, 195, 195*f*
swing phase, 195–96, 196*f*
trunk and shoulders, 196
Muscle contraction
contractile fibers, types of, 80–81, 80*t*
energy sources for, 80
motor units, 78–80
muscle fatigue, 80
muscle fibers, 76–78
muscle tissue, 76
sliding filament theory of, 78, 79*f*
structures and mechanisms in, 76–81
types of, 87–88
Muscle energy techniques (METs), 121, 122–24
general applications for, 122, 123
pin and stretch technique, 123, 124*f*
post-isometric relaxation, 121, 122–23
reciprocal inhibition, 111, 121, 122–23
Muscle fatigue, 80
Muscle fibers, 76–78, 79*f*. *See also* Motor units

arrangement of, utilizing, 73
contractile, types of, 80–81, 80*t*
defined, 76
microfilaments in, 76–78
sliding filament theory of muscle contraction, 78, 79*f*
wrapped by endomysium, 82*f*
Muscle functions, 88–91, 89*t*
agonist, 89–90
antagonist, 90
biarticular muscles, 90
coordination, 90
neutralizers, 90
passive and active insufficiency, 91, 91*f*
recruitment timing, 90
stabilizers, 90
synergists, 90
Muscles in action
ankle and foot, 266–67
arm and hand, 608–9
head and neck, 486–87
hip and pelvis, 372–74
knee, 332
respiratory, 230
shoulder girdle, 548–49
spine, 438–39
Muscle spindles, 106–8, 106*f*
Golgi tendon organs and, comparing, 108–9, 109*t*
reflex arc, 106, 107, 108*f*
stretch injuries, 108
stretch reflex, 107–8
Muscle tension, 86–88
active, 86–87, 87*f*
contraction and, 87–88, 87*f*, 88*t*
contraction types and, 87–88
joint position and, 88, 89*f*
length-tension relationship, 88, 89*f*
passive, 86
Muscular balance, 7

Muscular chain, 6
Muscular pull, lines of, 131–32, 131–32*f*
Muscular system, 70–94
anterior/posterior view of, 73*f*
changing roles of muscles, 88–91
continuity of muscle and fascia, 81–86
contractile structures and mechanisms in muscles, 76–81
defined, 72
muscle tension and contractile forces, 86–88
skeletal muscle, 72–76
Musculocutaneous nerve, 599
Musculoskeletal, 9
Musculotendinous junction, 108
Myelin sheaths, 104
Myers, Tom, 112, 113
Mylohyoid, 530, 531*f*
Myofascial mobilization (MFM). *See* Myofascial release (MFR)
Myofascial release (MFR), 84–86
creep, 84–85, 84*f*
piezoelectric effect, 85–86
stress and strain in, 142
viscoelasticity, 84–85
Myofascial system, 81–86, 83*f*
adaptive shortening of, 83, 83*f*
manual therapy for, 84–86
stretch-weakened, 83, 83*f*
three-dimensional integrity of, assessing, 115
Myofilaments, 76
Myosin filaments, 76–77, 77*f*
Myotatic reflex, 107

N

Nasal bones, 495–96, 495*f*, 498, 498*f*
Nasal cartilage, 498, 498*f*

Muscular chain, 6
Nasalis, 526*f*, 529
Navicular, 273, 273*f*, 274*f*
Navicular tuberosity, 273, 273*f*, 275
Neck
fascia, 82*f*
of femur, 375
flexion, 511, 512
gait assessment, 203
hyperextension, 511
passive range of motion, 511–12
proprioceptors, 110
rotation, 512
stabilizers, neuromuscular patterning to engage, 541–42
stretching, 512
surface anatomy of, 489*f*
Negative work, 87
Nerve, 100
Nerve plexus, 102
Nervous system (NS), 98–105, 101*f*
divisions of, 99*f*
neuromuscular patterns, 104
neurons, 98–100
peripheral nerves, 102–4
Neural tension, 102–4, 103*f*
Neurological actions, 7
Neurological chain, 6
Neurological pathways, 7
Neurological symptoms, feedback from, 102
Neuromuscular, 9
Neuromuscular junctions, 79*f*, 99, 100*f*
Neuromuscular patterning, 16–17, 104–5
to engage neck stabilizers, 541–42
patterning touch, 16
scapulohumeral rhythm, 572–73
sensorimotor loop and, 104–5
temporomandibular joint, 508–9
therapeutic kinesiology, 16–17

Neuromuscular (NM) system, 96–127
defined, 98
movement applications in neuromuscular techniques, 115–24
nervous system, 98–105
reflexes and basic movement pathways, 111–15
sensory receptors, 105–11
Neuromuscular (NM) techniques
motion assessments, 116–19
movement applications in, 115–24
muscle energy techniques, 121, 122–24
relaxation and, 101
trigger point therapy, 119–21, 120f
Neurons, 98–100, 100f
Neutral, upright stance, 674–75, 675f
Neutral equilibrium, 147, 147f
Neutralizers, 89t, 90
Newton, Sir Isaac, 134
Nociception, 109
Nociceptors, 109
Nonaxial joints, 39, 39t
Nonaxial movements, 50, 50f, 53–54, 54f
Nondisplaced fracture, 31
Normal resting muscle, 75f
Nuchal ligament, 456, 456f
Nucleus pulposus, 448, 448f
Nutation, 396, 396f

O

Objective findings, 211
Oblique capitis inferior, 534, 534f
Oblique capitis superior, 534, 534f
Oblique fractures, 31
Oblique popliteal ligament, 342, 342f, 343
Obliques, 473–78, 474f

contraction, 473, 473f
external, 473
internal, 473
Obturator externus, 421, 421f, 424–25
Obturator foramen, 377
Obturator internus, 421, 421f, 424–25
Obturator nerve, 420
Occipital bone, 488, 489f, 491f
palpation of, 493
trigger points, 513f
Occipital condyles, 490, 490f
Occipitalis, 513, 513f, 515–16
Occipitofrontalis, 513
Olecranon, 611f, 612, 613
Olecranon fossa, 610, 611f
Olecranon of ulna, hard-end feel and, 64f
Omohyoid, 82f, 531, 531f
Open (compound) fracture, 31
Open kinetic chain, 56, 56f
Open-packed position, 60–61
Opponens digiti minimi, 666–67, 666f
Opponens pollicis, 660, 661f, 663
Opposition, 628, 629f
Optical righting reflex, 156, 156f
Optimal posture, 674–75, 675f
Optimal table height, 692–93, 693f
Orbicularis oculi, 524f, 528–29, 528f
Orbicularis oris, 524f, 529
Origin, 75
Osteoblasts, 30, 30f
Osteoclasts, 30, 30f
Osteocytes, 25, 28
Osteokinematics, 50–56
axial movements, 50, 50f, 51–53
combined and miscellaneous movements, 54–55
kinetic chains, closed and opened, 56, 56f

linear, rotary, and curvilinear motion, 51, 51f
nonaxial movements, 50, 50f, 53–54
Osteoligamentous plate, 279, 281f
Osteons, 28, 28f
Osteoporosis, 31
Otoliths, 110
Outer ear, 498
Outer range joint position, 88, 89f
Ovoid joint, 36, 36f, 56
Oxidation, 80

P

Pacinian corpuscles, 109
Padding clients, 695–97, 695f
Pain
cycle, dynamics of, 163–64, 164f
patterns, stability dysfunction and, 162–63, 163f
posture and, 115, 115f
Palatine bones, 495–96, 495f
Palmar, 11, 11f
Palmaris longus, 646, 646f, 647f, 650
Palmar radiocarpal ligament, 625, 626f
Palmar ulnocarpal ligament, 625, 626f
Palmer interossei, 663
Palpation, 208–26. See also Tissue layering
active movement assessment, 210, 210f
art of, 211–13, 212f
as assessment tool, 210–11
broad-hand gliding, 215, 216f
classroom palpation vs. therapeutic palpation, 212–13
cross-fiber strumming, 215, 216f
defined, 210
fingertip, 215, 216f
flat-finger, 215, 216f

goals in therapeutic kinesiology, 211
as mindful, body-centered touch, 212
pincher, 215, 216f
round-robin, 214
science of, 210–11
tips, 213–15, 216–17f
tracking skills, 211
working with rather than on clients, 213
Palpation sites
abductor digiti minimi, 319–20
abductor hallucis, 319–20
abductor pollicis brevis, 663
abductor pollicis longus, 659
acromioclavicular joint, 567–68
acromion process, 555
adductor brevis, 408–11
adductor hallucis, 325–26
adductor longus, 408–11
adductor magnus, 408–11
adductor pollicis, 662
anconeus, 640–42
anterior compartment, 298–300
arm and hand bones, 612–14
auricle of the outer ear, 499
biceps brachii, 635–38
biceps femoris, 363–65
bones, thorax, 233–34
brachialis, 635–38
brachioradialis, 635–38
bursae, 339
capitate, 618
carpals, 616–18
coracobrachialis, 600–602
coracoid process, 555
coronal suture, 503
coronoid process, 498
costal joints, 237–38
cranial bones, 492–94
cranial sutures, 502–3
cricoid cartilage, 500

Palpation sites (*continued*)

deep posterior compartment, 307–10

deep six lateral hip rotators, 424–25

deltoid, 600–602

diaphragm, 244–45

elbow, 612–14

erector spinae, 465–66

extensor carpi radiali sbrevis, 654

extensor carpi radialis longus, 654

extensor carpi ulnaris, 655

extensor digitorum, 655

extensor digitorum brevis, 316–17

extensor digitorum longus, 298–300

extensor hallucis brevis, 316–17

extensor hallucis longus, 298–300

extensor indicis, 655

extensor pollicis brevis, 659

extensor pollicis longus, 659

external acoustic meatus, 493

external occipital protuberance, 493

extrinsic thumb muscles, 658–59

facial bones, 496–98

fibula, 271–72

flexor carpi radialis, 650

flexor carpi ulnaris, 649

flexor digiti minimi brevis, 325–26, 667

flexor digitorum brevis, 319–20

flexor digitorum longus, 307–10

flexor digitorum profundus, 650

flexor digitorum superficialis, 650

flexor hallucis brevis, 325–26

flexor hallucis longus, 307–10

flexor pollicis brevis, 662

flexor pollicis longus, 659

forearm, 612–14

frontal bone, 492

frontalis, 515–16

gastrocnemius, 303–5

gemellus inferior, 424–25

gemellus superior, 424–25

gluteus maximus, 414–16

gluteus medius, 414–16

gluteus minimus, 414–16

gracilis, 408–11

greater wings of the sphenoid, 494

hamate, 618

hand muscles, 667

hip bones, 381–84

hyoid, 500

iliacus, 418–20

iliocostalis, 465–66

inferior angle of scapula, 557

infrahyoid muscles, 532–33

infraspinous fossa, 556

intercostals, 248

interossei, 664–65

interphalangeal joints, 293

intertarsal joints, 291

intrinsic thumb muscles, 661–63

knee, 336–37

lamboid suture, 503

lateral border, 557

lateral compartment, 312–13

lateral epicondyle, 612

lateral pterygoid, 520–22

latissimus dorsi, 577–79

levator scapula, 588–90

ligaments of knee, 343–44

little finger muscles, 667

longissimus, 465–66

lumbricals, 322–23, 664–65

lunate, 616

mandibular angle, 497

mandibular body, 497

mandibular condyle, 507

mandibular fossa, 507

mandibular ramus, 497

mastoid process, 494

maxilla, 496

medial border, 557

medial pterygoid, 520–22

meniscus, 339

metacarpals, 620

metatarsals, 278

metatarsophalangeal joints, 293

multifidi, 468–69

nasal bones, 496

obliques, 475–78

obturator externus, 424–25

obturator internus, 424–25

occipital bone, 493

occipitalis, 515–16

olecranon, 613

opponens digiti minimi, 667

opponens pollicis, 663

palatine bones, 496

palmaris longus, 650

parietal bones, 492

pectineus, 408–11

pectoralis major, 595–97

pectoralis minor, 595–97

pelvic bones, 381–84

peroneus brevis, 312–13

peroneus longus, 312–13

phalanges, 278, 620

piriformis, 424–25

pisiform, 617

popliteus, 366

posterior compartment, 303–5

pronator teres, 644

psoas major, 418–20

quadratus femoris, 424–25

quadratus lumborum, 479–81

quadratus plantae, 322–23

radius, 613

rectus abdominis, 475–78

rectus femoris, 360–61

rhomboids, 588–90

rib, 233–34

rib cage, 233–34

rotator cuff, 583–85

sacral ligaments, 397–98

sagittal suture, 503

sartorius, 403–4

scalenes, 253–54

scaphoid, 616, 618

scapula, 555–57

semimembranosus, 363–65

semitendinosus, 363–65

serratus anterior, 588–90

serratus posterior inferior, 257–58

serratus posterior superior, 257–58

soleus, 303–5

spinalis, 465–66

spine of the scapula, 556

splenius capitis, 461–62

splenius cervicis, 461–62

squamous suture, 503

sternoclavicular joint, 567–68

sternocleidomastoid, 539–40

sternocostal joints, 237–38

styloid process of radius, 613

styloid process of ulna, 613

subclavius, 595–97

suboccipitals, 535–36

subscapular fossa, 556

subscapularis, 583–85

subtalar joint, 289

superior angle of scapula, 557

supinator, 644

supracondylar ridges, 612

suprahyoid muscles, 532–33
supraorbital margin, 493
supraspinatus, 583–85
supraspinous fossa, 556
tarsals, 275–76, 291
tarsometatarsal joints, 291
temporal bones, 493
temporal fossa, 493
temporalis, 515–16
temporomandibular joint, 507–8
tensor fascia latae, 403–4
teres major, 577–79
teres minor, 583–85
thyroid cartilage, 500
tibia, 271–72
tibialis anterior, 298–300
tibialis posterior, 307–10
trachea, 500
transverse tarsal joint, 289
transversospinalis, 468–69
transversus abdominis, 475–78
trapezium, 618
trapezius, 577–79
triceps brachii, 640–42
triquetrum, 616
ulna, 613
vasti muscle group, 360–61
vertebra, 444–47
wrist and hand extensors, 653–55
wrist and hand flexors, 649–50
zygomatic arch, 497
zygomatic bones, 497
zygomatic process, 494
Palpatory assessment, 115
Paradoxical breathing, 255
Parallel elastic components of muscle, 86
Parallel force, 137, 138f
Parallel shift, 90, 90f
Parasympathetic division, 98, 99f
Paravertebral muscles, 459

Paresis, 198
Parietal bones, 488, 489f, 491f, 492
Parkinsonian gait, 201
Partial fracture, 31
Passive insufficiency, 91, 91f
Passive joint movement, feedback during, 103
Passive motion, 63, 64–65
Passive motion skills, 117f, 117t, 118
Passive range of motion (PROM), 61–62, 62f
  ankle, 285, 285f, 285t, 286–87
  contraindications to practicing, 65
  hips, 370, 389t, 391–92
  knee, 352
  neck, 511–12
  shoulder girdle, 560, 562–63
  stretching, 65
  wrist, 627–28
Passive restraints, 61
Passive technique, 16
Patella, 30, 334, 337
Patellar ligament, 81f, 342, 345, 345f
Patellar motion and tracking, 345–46, 345f, 346f
  patellar contact during knee motion, 345, 346f
  patellar pathway, 345, 346f
  poor, conditions resulting from, 345–46
Patellar retinacula, 345, 345f
Patellofemoral joint, 340, 340f, 345–47, 345f
  knee alignment and Q angle, 347, 347f
  patellar motion and tracking, 345–46, 345f
Patellofemoral pain syndrome, 345
Patterning touch, 16
Pectineus, 73f, 404, 405, 405f, 406f, 408–11

Pectoralis major, 73f, 74f, 593, 593f, 595–98
Pectoralis minor, 247, 249, 249f, 249t, 593, 593f, 594f, 595–98
Pedicle, 442
Pelvic bones
  bony landmarks of, 376–78, 376f, 378f, 380
  palpation of, 381–84
  pelvic asymmetries, assessing, 378
  seated pelvic rock, 379–80
Pelvic floor, 426, 428
Pelvic girdle, 9, 10f, 384
Pelvic joints and ligaments, 394–96
  sacral ligaments, 394, 395, 395f, 397–98
  sacroiliac joint motion, 396, 396f
  sacroiliac joint stabilization, 395–96, 395f
Pelvic movement in gait, 191–92, 191–92f
  frontal plane movement, 191, 192f
  horizontal plane movement, 191–92, 192f
  sagittal plane movement, 191, 191f
Pelvic muscles. See Hip and pelvic muscles
Pelvic ring, 384
Pelvic rock, seated, 379–80
Pelvic tilt, 166
Pelvis, 24f
  as braced arch, 158–59, 159f
  center of gravity in, 39
  forward rotation of, 53, 54f
  gait assessment, 203
  hyperextending, avoiding, 676–77, 676f
  lines of thrust through, 384, 384f
Pennate muscles, 72, 74f
Perception, 105–6
Perichondrium, 235
Perimysium, 81, 82f

Perineal muscles, 422, 426–28, 426f
Perineum, 164f, 166t, 422. See also Perineal muscles
Perineurium, 102, 103f
Periosteum, 33, 33f, 222, 223f, 235
Peripheral nerves, 100, 101f, 102–4
  connective tissue of, 102
  cross section, 102, 103f
  neural tension, 102–4, 103f
  tissue layering, 222, 224f
Peripheral nervous system (PNS), 98, 99f
Peroneal trochlea, 274, 274f
Peroneus brevis, 311f, 312–13
Peroneus longus, 310–13, 311f
Peroneus tertius, 311, 311f
Pes anserine, 342, 345, 345f
Pes cavus, 169, 169f, 288f, 289
Pes planus, 169, 169f, 288–89, 288f
Phalanges, 273f, 274, 274f, 277f, 278, 618–19, 619f, 620
Phasic reflex, 107, 108
Phrenic nerve, 241
Physiological barrier, 62
Physiological movement, 62
Piezoelectric effect, 27, 28
Piezoelectric effect in myofascial release, 85–86
Pin and stretch, 86, 86f
Pin and stretch technique, 123, 124f
Pincher palpation, 215, 216f
Piriformis, 420, 421, 421f, 424–25, 426f
Piriformis syndrome, 421
Pisiform, 614–15, 615f, 617

Pivot joint, 38, 38f
Plane (gliding) joint, 38, 38f
Planes, 12–13, 12f
  cardinal, 12–13, 12f
  diagonal, 13, 14f
  mechanical movement in, 13f
  spinal movement in, 13f
Plantar, 11, 11f
Plantar aponeurosis, 282, 282f
Plantar fascia, 33, 281–82, 281f, 282f
Plantar fasciitis, 198, 282, 300
Plantarflexion, 51, 52f
  with fibular motion, 284, 284f
  PROM for, 284–85, 284f, 285f
Plantarflexors, 266
Plantar interossei, 326, 327f
Plantaris, 300, 300f, 302, 302f
Plantar layers, 294, 313, 313f, 317–27
  deepest layer of, 326–27, 327f
  second, 320–23, 320f
  superficial, 317–20, 317f
  third, 323–26, 323f
Plantar ligaments, 281–82, 281f, 282f
Plantar plate, 282, 282f
Plasticity, 27, 85
Platsyma, 531–32
Platysma, 82f
Plegia, 198
Plica, 109
Point of application
  of force, 136, 137
  of gravity, 130
Poland's anomaly, 173
Popliteal bursa, 340
Popliteal fossa, 334, 334f
Popliteal nerve, 365
Popliteus, 338, 365–66, 365f
Positive work, 87
Posterior, 10, 11f
Posterior compartment, 300–305, 300f, 301f

Posterior cruciate ligament (PCL), 341, 341f
Posterior inferior iliac spine (PIIS), 377, 378f
Posterior invertors, 267
Posterior longitudinal ligament, 457
Posterior pelvic tilt (PPT), 166
Posterior radiocarpal ligament, 625, 626f
Posterior superior iliac spine (PSIS), 377, 378f, 383
Posterior tibiofibular ligaments, 282, 283f
Posterior triangle, 537, 537f
Posterolateral, 13
Posteromedial, 13
Post-isometric relaxation (PIR) technique, 121, 122–23
Postural assessments, 169–74
  checklist for, 172
  client-centered, 174
  feedback about postural patterns, providing, 173
  observing postural patterns, 173
  skeletal alignment, 170–74
  topical landmarks, 170f
  views used to assess, 170–71, 171f
Postural education
  body mechanics, 174, 175
  exercises, 177
  imagery used in, 158
  integrating into bodywork sessions, 175, 176
  postural awareness and, 176
  postural corrections, challenges with, 176, 177
  therapeutic applications for, 174–77
Postural muscle contraction, 163–64, 163f

Postural observation, 115
Postural stabilizer muscles, 162–65
  core control, 164, 164f, 165
  functions of, 166t
  primary, 164, 164f, 166t
  stability dysfunctions and pain patterns, 162–63, 163f
  substitution patterns, 163–64, 163–64f
  training, 175
Postural sway, 108, 155–56, 155f, 680
Posture, 152–80
  chronic pain and, 115, 115f
  chronic thoracic flexion, 161, 161f
  components of, 154–61
  dynamic postural reflexes, 155–56
  movement systems in, role of, 160–61
  muscle patterns in, 162–65
  neutral, upright stance, 674–75, 675f
  optimal, 154, 154f, 160, 171f
  postural stabilizers, engaging, 676
  skeletal architecture in, 157, 158–60
  standing position at massage table, proper, 682–83, 683f
Posture, faulty, 165–69
  changing, steps in, 174
  client communication around, 174
  collapsed posture, 165, 167f
  excessive kyphosis, 160, 160f, 166, 167f
  excessive lordosis, 166, 167f
  flat-back posture, 167, 168f
  kyphotic-lordotic posture, 167–68, 167f
  lower limb misalignments, 169, 169f

military posture, 165, 165f
  round-back (kyphotic) posture, 168, 168f
  scoliosis, 166, 168–69, 168f
  sources of, determining, 173, 174
  sway-back posture, 167, 167f
  zig-zag pattern of, 171f
Pott's fracture, 31
Power, 135
Power grip, 628, 630f
Precision grip, 630f, 631
Pressure applications, force in, 139–40
Pretracheal, 82f
Prevertebral fascia, 82f
Prevertebral muscles, 459
Prevertebral neck muscles, 537–38, 538f, 541
Prime mover, 89–90
Prime mover contraction, 163–64, 163f, 164f
Procerus, 524f, 528
Process, 31
Pronation, 54f, 55
Pronation twist, 290, 290f
Pronator, 642, 642f, 643f
  in pronation, 643f
  in supination, 642f
Pronator quadratus, 642
Pronator teres, 642, 643f, 644
Prone position, 55
Proprioception, 105–6
Proprioceptors, 110
Protraction (abduction), 54, 54f
Protrusion, 504, 505f
Proximal, 10, 11f
Proximal attachment, 75
Proximal carpal arch, 629, 630f
Proximal interphalangeal joint (PIP), 294, 628
Proximal joints, 10
Proximal radioulnar joint, 622, 623f
Proximal tibiofibular joint, 282
Pseudo-winging, 586, 587f

Psoas major, 89*f*, 164*f*, 166*t*, 242, 242*f*, 416–20, 417*f*
Psoas minor, 417, 417*f*
Psoatic gait, 200, 200*f*
Pterygoids, 519*f*. See also Lateral pterygoid; Medial pterygoid
Pubic arch, 384, 385*f*
Pubic crest, 377, 378*f*, 382
Pubic symphysis, 394, 394*f*
Pubic tubercles, 378*f*, 380, 382
Pubis, 376, 377, 377*f*, 380
Pubococcygeus, 422, 426, 426*f*
Pubofemoral ligament, 385, 385*f*
Pull-back exercise, 146, 690
Pulling, 7
    exercise, 146
    lines of force in, 687, 688*f*
Push-hands exercise, 146, 689
Pushing, 7
    from feet, 686, 688*f*
    lines of force in, 687, 688*f*
Pushoff, 189, 189*f*, 194*t*, 195

Q
Q angle, 347, 347*f*
Quadratus femoris, 422, 424–25
Quadratus lumborum (QL), 242, 242*f*, 249, 249*t*, 471, 472*f*, 478–81, 478*f*, 479*f*
Quadratus plantae, 320, 320*f*, 321*f*, 322–23
Quadriceps, 89*f*, 357–61, 358*f*
    length assessment and stretch, 429
    lines of pull in, 345, 346
    moment arm of, 345, 345*f*

R
Radial bursa, 34*f*
Radial collateral ligament, 625, 626*f*

Radial movement, 7, 8*f*
Radial notch, 611*f*, 612
Radiate ligament, 236, 236*f*
Radiocarpal joint, 624, 625*f*
Radioulnar joint
Radius, 24*f*, 610, 611*f*, 613
    shaft of, 614
    styloid process of, 612, 613
    supination and pronation, 623, 623*f*
Ramus, 495, 495*f*. See also Mandibular ramus
Range of motion (ROM), 61–63
    active and passive, 61–62, 62*f*
    ankle, 285, 285*f*, 285*t*, 286–87
    carpometacarpal joints, 628, 629*f*
    cervical spine, 452–53, 511*t*
    gait patterns, atypical, 200, 200*f*
    hips, 389*t*, 391–92, 398
    hypomobility and hypermobility, 62–63
    joint stability and mobility, 61
    knee, 348, 348*t*, 349*f*
    measuring, 61, 61*f*
    restricted, 66, 66*f*
    scapulothoracic joint, 564*f*
    shoulder girdle, 559*t*
    spine, 450*t*
    thumb, 628, 629*f*
    tibiofemoral joint, 348–50, 348*t*, 349*f*
    wrist, 624, 626*t*
Ray, 290
Reach, shifting weight at end of, 684, 684*f*
Reaching, 7
Rearfoot, 272*f*, 727
Recentering in neutral, 681
Reciprocal inhibition (RI), 111, 121, 122–23
Reciprocal innervation, 111

Recruitment, 79
Recruitment timing, 90
Rectus abdominis, 73*f*, 140, 141*f*, 232*f*, 242, 244, 249–50, 249*t*, 250*f*, 472*f*, 473, 475–78
Rectus capitis anterior, 538, 538*f*
Rectus capitis lateralis, 538, 538*f*
Rectus capitis posterior major, 534, 534*f*
Rectus capitis posterior minor, 534, 534*f*
Rectus femoris, 73*f*, 74*f*, 132, 133*f*, 357, 358*f*, 360–61, 428, 428*f*
Rectus femoris stretch, 432
Rectus femoris tendon, 81*f*
Reflex arc, 106, 107, 108*f*
Reflexive movement
    kinetic chains, 112–15, 113*f*
    knee-jerk test, 106, 107
    in massage clients, 112
    meridians, 112–13
    pathways, 111–15
    reciprocal inhibition and, 111, 112*f*
    reflex arc, 106, 107, 108*f*
    stretch reflex, 107–8
    tendon, 109
    tonic labyrinthine reflex, 110
Regular dense connective tissue, 32, 32*f*
Relaxation, 679–80
    active, 679
    of head and neck muscles, 679–80
    postural sway, 680
    techniques, 101, 110–11, 116–24
Remodeling, 30
Repetitive strain injuries, 330
Reposition, 628, 629*f*
Resistance (R), 143
Resistance arm (RA), 143, 143*f*, 145*f*
Resisted motion skills, 117*f*, 117*t*, 118, 119

Resisted range of motion (RROM), 66, 66*f*
Respiration, 228–63. See also Thorax
    defined, 230
    muscles of, 230–31, 230*f*, 238–55
Respiratory motion and restrictive patterns, 255–60
    belly breathing, 259
    breathing to release tension, 258
    COPDs, 259, 260
    exhalation fixation, 255, 260*f*
    hyperventilation, 260
    inhalation fixation, 255, 259*f*
    paradoxical breathing, 255
    upper chest breathing, 255, 259
    weak abdominals, 259, 260*f*
Respiratory muscles, 230–31, 230*f*, 238–55
    accessory, 247–55, 249*t*
    diaphragm, 240–46
    intercostals, 246–47
    pleural sac, 238, 240, 241*f*
Responsiveness, 76
Reticular fibers, 26
Retinacula, 294, 294*f*
Retinaculum, 81
Retraction (adduction), 54, 54*f*
Retroversion, 387, 387*f*
Retrusion, 504, 505*f*
Reverse muscle action, 132–33, 133*f*, 134
Rhomboidal muscle, 72, 74*f*
Rhomboid major, 73*f*, 74*f*
Rhomboids, 585, 585*f*, 586*f*, 588–90
    agonist/antagonist relationships of, 586, 586*f*
    rhomboid major, 585, 585*f*
    rhomboid minor, 585, 585*f*

Rib, 29f, 30, 231–35, 231f, 232f
  dislocation, 236
  fracture, 236
  intercostal spaces between, 235, 235f
  motion, 238, 238f, 239
  palpation of, 233–34
  periosteum covering, 235
  separation, 236
  top rib ring, position of, 232f
Rib cage, 231–35, 231f, 232f
  flexibility of, 235, 235f
  function of, 230
  injuries to, 236
Ridge, 31
Right rotation, 52
Risorius, 527f, 530
Rocker base, 185–87, 682, 683f
Rolf, Ida, 112
Rolfing, 14
Rolf lines, 112, 113
Roll, 57–59, 57f
Rotary motion, 51–53, 51f
Rotated transverse processes, 453, 454f
Rotator cuff, 580–85, 580f
Rotatores, 466
Round-back (kyphotic) posture, 168, 168f
Round-robin palpation, 214
Ruffini endings, 109

S
Saccule, 110
Sacral canal, 380
Sacral foramen, 378f, 380, 380f, 383
Sacral hiatus, 380, 380f
Sacral ligaments, 394, 395, 395f, 397–98
Sacral motion, 396, 396f, 397–98
Sacral nerves, 420
Sacrococcygeal joint, 394
Sacrococcygeal ligament, 395, 395f

Sacroiliac joint (SIJ), 394, 394f
  flexibility in, 398
  sacroiliac joint motion, 396, 396f
  sacroiliac joint stabilization, 395–96, 395f
Sacroiliac ligament, 394, 395f, 397
Sacrospinous ligament, 394, 395, 395f
Sacrotuberous ligament, 394, 395f, 397
Sacrum, 24f, 30, 375, 375f, 378f, 380, 380f, 383
Saddle joint, 38, 38f
Sagittal plane, 12, 12f, 13f
Sagittal plane movements, 50, 50f, 51, 52f, 191, 191f
Sagittal suture, 501, 501f, 503
Sagittal tracking exercises, 330
Sarcolemma, 76, 77f
Sarcomere, 76, 76f
Sartorius, 73f, 74f, 342, 345, 345f, 362, 365, 402–4, 402f
Scalenes, 247, 249, 249t, 250–54, 252f
  action of, 251, 251f
  anterior view of, 250f
  fourth, 251f
  location of, 232f
Scaphoid, 614, 615f, 616, 618
Scaption, 569, 570
Scapula, 24f, 29f, 554–57, 554f
  coupled pulls of muscles turning, 585, 586f
  retraction and protraction of, 54, 54f
  upward rotation of, 55, 55f
Scapulae, 53
Scapula neutral, 568–73, 568f, 569f
  adhesive capsulitis, 571–72, 571f
  benchmarks of, 569, 569f
  finding, 602–3

scaption and shoulder abduction, 569, 570, 570f
scapulohumeral rhythm, 571, 571f, 572–73
Scapula neutral position, 677
Scapular plane, 568, 568f
Scapular winging, 586, 587f
Scapulohumeral rhythm, 393, 571, 571f
Scapulothoracic joint, 560, 562, 563–65
  collapsed posture, 563, 565, 565f
  movements at, summary of, 563
  range of motion, 564f
Scheuermann's disease, 168, 173
Schwann cell, 100f, 103f
Sciatic nerve, tibial portion of the, 361
Sciatic notch, 377
Scissors gait, 201, 201f
Scoliosis, 166, 168–69, 168f
Screw home mechanism, 355
Seated pelvic rock, 379–80
Seated techniques, 694–95, 694–95f
Self-palpation, 213, 213f
Sellar joint shape, 36, 36f
Semicircular canals, 110, 110f
Semimembranosus, 73f, 338, 362, 363–65, 363f
Semispinalis, 467, 467f, 468f
Semitendinosus, 73f, 342, 345, 345f, 361, 363–65, 363f
Semitendinosus bursa, 340
Seniors with restricted hip motion, 398
Sensorimotor loop, 104–5, 105f
Sensory intake, 210–11
Sensory (afferent) neurons, 99
Sensory receptors, 105–11

Golgi tendon organs, 108–9, 109f, 109t
joint proprioceptors, 109
labyrinth and neck proprioceptors, 110
muscle spindles, 106–8
proprioception and perception, 105–6
Sequential movement, 9
Series elastic component of muscle, 86–87, 87f
Serratus anterior, 73f, 166t, 232f, 247, 249, 249f, 249t, 586–90, 586f, 587f
Serratus posterior inferior, 249t, 255, 255f, 257–58, 257f
  in forced exhalation, 249, 250f
  in forced inhalation, 249, 249f
Serratus posterior superior, 249t, 255, 255f, 256f, 257–58
Sesamoid bones, 29f, 272, 273f, 274, 277f
Shaft of the femur, 333, 334f
Shaft of the fibula, 270, 271
Shaft of the tibia, 270, 271
Shear, 40f, 41
Shin splints, 297
Short bones, 29f, 30
Short extensors of toes, 313, 313f, 315f
Short plantar ligament, 282
Shoulder
  abduction, 57, 57f, 569, 570, 570f
  breath support for, with diaphragmatic breathing, 681
  dislocation, 560, 562f
  horizontal flexion and extension of, 53, 54f
  impingement, 57, 57f
  separation, 566, 566f
  symmetry in skeletal alignment, 677
Shoulder girdle, 9, 10f, 546–605

bony landmarks of, 552–53
breath support for, 240
neutral position of, 568–73, 568*f*, 569*f* (*See also* Scapula neutral)
passive range of motion, 560, 562–63
range of motion, 559*t*
slang terms for, 555
surface anatomy of, 551*f*
as yoke, 159, 159*f*
Shoulder girdle bones, 550–57, 551*f*
clavicle, 550*f*, 551
humerus, 550–51, 550*f*
scapula, 554–57, 554*f*
Shoulder girdle joints and ligaments, 558–73
acromioclavicular joint, 565–66, 565*f*
glenohumeral joint, 558–60, 558*f*
scapulothoracic joint, 560, 562, 563–65
sternoclavicular joint, 566–68, 567*f*
Shoulder girdle muscles, 573–603
coracobrachialis, 599, 599*f*
deltoid, 599, 599*f*
gait and, 196
latissimus dorsi, 574, 574*f*
levator scapula, 586, 587*f*
pectoralis major, 593, 593*f*
pectoralis minor, 593, 593*f*
rhomboids, 585, 585*f*
rotator cuff, 580–85, 580*f*
serratus anterior, 586, 586*f*
subclavius, 593, 593*f*
tension pulls of, 573, 573*f*
teres major, 576, 576*f*, 580
trapezius, 574, 574*f*

Simultaneous movement, 9
Skeletal alignment, 674–79
center body over base of support, 675, 675*f*
chest muscles, stretching, 678–79
elbows and forearms, 679
hyperextending the pelvis, avoiding, 676–77, 676*f*
knee position, 675–76
optimal posture, 674–75, 675*f*
postural stabilizers, engaging, 676
scapula neutral position, 677
sternum and shoulder symmetry, 677
thoracic spine, stretching, 678–79
Skeletal alignment, assessing, 170–74
faulty postures, determining sources of, 173, 174
muscular function and, 170–73
Skeletal architecture in standing position, 157, 158–60
head as top load, 159–60, 160*f*
pelvis as braced arch, 158–59, 159*f*
shoulder girdle as yoke, 159, 159*f*
spine as curved column, 157, 158, 159*f*
Skeletal muscle, 72–76
attachments, 75–76, 75*f*
defined, 72
names, 72
shapes, 72, 74, 74*f*
Skeletal nervous system, 98
Skeletal system, 22–46, 24*f*
alignment and gravity, 39–44
components of, 24
connective tissue, 25–34

defined, 24
functions of, 24
joint classifications, 34–39, 35*t*
Skin, 82*f*, 217, 219
Skull, center of gravity in, 39
Sliding filament theory of muscle contraction, 78, 79*f*
Slow oxidative (SO) fibers, 80, 80*t*
Slow type I fibers, 80, 80*t*
Slump test, 103–4, 104*f*
Smooth muscle, 72
Soft end-feel, 64, 64*f*
Soleus, 166*t*, 300, 300*f*, 301*f*, 303–5
Soleus, 73*f*
Somatic nervous system (SNS), 98, 99*f*
Somatics, 17–18
Spasm end-feel, 65
Sphenoid, 490, 491*f*
Spherical grip, 630*f*, 631
Spinal accessory nerve, 537
Spinal bones, 440–43
Spinal curves, 442*f*, 445
Spinal extensors, stretching and strengthening, 470–71
Spinal flexion, 447, 447*f*
Spinal hyperextension, 447, 447*f*
Spinalis, 462, 462*f*, 463*f*, 465–66
Spinalis cervicis, 462, 462*f*
Spinalis thoracis, 462, 462*f*
Spinal joints, 448–56
facet, 449–56, 450*f*
interbody, 448, 448*f*
Spinal ligaments, 456–57*f*, 456–58
Spinal movement, 7, 8*f*
Spinal muscles, 459–81
abdominal muscles, 471–78, 472*f*
on anterior side of spine, 459
contraction of, 459
erector spinae, 460, 462–64, 462*f*

layers covering spine, 459
quadratus lumborum, 478, 478*f*
splenius capitis, 459–60, 460*f*
splenius cervicis, 460, 460*f*
transversospinalis, 466–67, 467*f*
Spinal nerves, 100, 101*f*, 462, 466
Spine, 31, 31*f*, 436–83, 441–42*f*. See also Posture
arcing exercise for spinal movement, 451–52
balancing, 452
bones, 440–43
curvature of, 166–67, 167*f*
as curved column, 157, 158, 159*f*
curves, 442*f*, 445
joints, 448–56
lateral flexion of, 52, 53*f*
left rotation of, 52, 53*f*
ligaments, 456–58
muscles, 459–81
range of motion, 450*t*
of the scapula, 554, 554*f*, 556
surface anatomy of, 441*f*
vertebra, 443*f*
Spin motion, 57–59, 57*f*
Spinous process (SP), 440, 442, 443*f*
Spiral fractures, 31
Splenius capitis, 459–60*f*, 459–62
Splenius cervicis, 459*f*, 460–62, 460*f*
Spondylolisthesis, 167
Spongy (cancellous) bone, 29, 29*f*, 36*f*
Sprain, 63
Spring ligament, 272, 281
Squamous suture, 501, 501*f*, 503
Stability, 147–48, 148*f*
Stability dysfunction, 162–63, 163*f*

Stabilizer muscles. *See* Postural stabilizer muscles

Stabilizers, 89*t*, 90

Stable equilibrium, 147, 147*f*

Stacking joints in arms, 685, 686*f*

Stance phase, 195, 195*f*

Standing position, 10, 11*f*

Static contact, 215, 218

Statics, 4

Stellar joint, 56

Step, defined, 187

Step length, 187–88, 187–88*f*

Steppage gait, 199–200, 199*f*

Step width, 187–88, 187–88*f*

Sternoclavicular (SC) joint, 566–68, 567*f*

Sternoclavicular ligament, 566, 567*f*

Sternocleidomastoid (SCM), 13, 14*f*, 82*f*, 169, 537–41, 537*f*, 538*f*

anterior and posterior triangles, 537, 537*f*

contractions, 537, 537*f*

Sternocostal joints, 235–38, 235*f*

anterior, 235–36

intercostal spaces between, 235, 235*f*

junctions of, 235

manubriosternal, 235, 235*f*

palpation of, 237–38

posterior, 236

Sternohyoid, 531

Sternohyoid muscle, 82*f*

Sternothyroid muscle, 82*f*

Sternum, 24*f*, 75, 75*f*, 231, 232*f*, 233–34, 235, 235*f*, 241*f*, 677

Stilt walking, 22

Stitch in the side, 242, 243

Stools, foot and folding, 693–94, 693–94*f*

Strain, 63, 141–42, 141*f*

Strain–counterstrain, 116

Strap muscle, 72, 74*f*

Stress, 141–42, 141*f*

Stress fracture, 31

Stress–strain curve, 141, 141*f*, 142

Stretched muscle, 75*f*

Stretching

chest muscles, 678–79

diaphragm, 242–43

gastrocnemius, 303

hip and pelvic muscles, 431–32

iliotibial band, 401

lateral hip rotators, 423

levator scapula, 588

neck, 512

passive range of motion, steps in, 65

pectoralis major, 597–98

pectoralis minor, 597–98

posterior compartment, 303

posterior spinal ligaments, 457–58

soleus, 303

spinal extensors, 470–71

steps in PROM, 65

sternocleidomastoid, 540

targeted tissues only, 63

temporomandibular joint, 508–9

thoracic spine, 678–79

thumb muscles, 668

wrist, 668

Stretch injuries, 108

Stretch reflex, 107–8

Stretch weakness, 83, 83*f*

Striated muscle, 76, 76*f*

Stride, 187–88, 187–88*f*

Stripping, 85, 86*f*

Stroke. *See* Massage stroke

Structural integrity, 14

Stylohyoid, 530, 531*f*

Styloid process, 490, 492*f*, 612–13

Subacromial bursa, 34*f*, 57*f*, 559, 560*f*

Subclavius, 593, 593*f*, 594*f*, 595–97

Subcutaneous prepatellar bursa, 339*f*, 340

Subcutaneous tissue, 82*f*

Subdeltoid bursa, 34*f*, 559, 560*f*

Subdeltoid space, 559

Subjective findings, 211

Suboccipital nerve, 534

Suboccipitals, 166*t*, 532, 534–35*f*, 534–36

Subpopliteal bursa, 340

Subscapular fossa, 554, 554*f*, 556

Subscapularis, 580

palpation of, 583–85

trigger points, 582*f*

Subscapular nerve, 580

Substitution pattern, 163–64, 163–64*f*

Subtalar joint, 284–85, 284*f*, 289

Superficial, 11

Superficial (investing) cervical fascia of posterior (lateral) triangle, 82*f*

Superficial fascia, 82*f*, 217, 218, 219

Superficial muscle layer, 459

Superficial peroneal nerve, 310

Superior, 10–11, 11*f*

Superior acromioclavicular ligament, 565, 566*f*

Superior angle of scapula, 554, 554*f*, 557

Superior attachment, 75

Superior border, 554, 554*f*

Superior gluteal nerve, 411

Superior nuchal line, 489*f*, 490

Superior pubic ramus, 377, 378*f*

Supination, 54, 54*f*, 55

Supination twist, 290, 290*f*

Supinator, 642, 642*f*, 643*f*, 644

in pronation, 643*f*

in supination, 642*f*

Supine position, 55

Supracondylar ridges, 610, 611*f*, 612

Supraglenoid tubercle, 554, 554*f*, 610

Suprahyoid muscles, 530, 531*f*, 532–33

Supraorbital margin, 488, 489*f*, 493

Suprapatellar bursa, 340

Supraspinatus, 57*f*, 580, 581*f*, 583–85

Supraspinous fossa, 554, 554*f*, 556

Supraspinous ligaments, 456

Sustentaculum tali, 272, 273*f*, 275

Sway-back posture, 167, 167*f*

Sweigard, Lulu, 158

Sweigard's nine lines of movement, 158, 158*f*

Swing phase, 195–96, 196*f*

Sympathetic division, 98, 99*f*

Synapse, 99–100

Synarthrosis joints, 34, 35*f*, 35*t*

Syndesmosis joints, 34, 35*f*

Synergist, 89*t*

Synergists, 90

Synovial flexor tendon sheaths, 34*f*

Synovial fluid, 32, 36, 36*f*

Synovial joints, 35–36, 35*t*, 36*f*, 38–39

degrees of motion, 38–39, 39*t*

shapes of joint surfaces, 36, 36*f*, 38

structures and fluids, 35–36

types of, 38, 38*f*

Synovial membrane, 36, 36*f*

Synovial sheaths, 34, 34*f*

Synovium, 33

T

Table height, optimal, 692–93, 693*f*

Table pads, 695–97, 695*f*

Talocalcaneal ligaments, 285

Talocrural joint, 282–84, 283–84*f*

Talonavicular joint, 288
Talus, 272, 273f, 277f
Tarsals, 29f, 30, 272–76, 273f, 274f, 279, 279f, 291
Tarsal tunnel, 305–6
Tarsometatarsal joints, 290–91, 290f
Temporal bones, 490, 491f, 492f, 493
Temporal fossa, 490, 492f, 493
Temporalis, 73f, 513f, 514–16, 514f
Temporalis stretch, 508
Temporomandibular dysfunction (TMD), 506
Temporomandibular joint (TMJ), 53, 503–9, 504f
   disk position, 506f
   motion, 504–6, 505–6f
   tracking, 509
Temporomandibular ligament, 504, 504f
Tender points, 120
Tendon, 33, 82f
   of extrinsic muscles of foot, 294, 294f
   of knee, 340–45, 340f
   reflex, 109
   tissue layering, 222, 222f, 223f
Tendonitis, 34
Tennis elbow, 652
Tenosynovitis, 34
Tensegrity system, 81–83, 83f
Tension, 40f, 41
   breathing to release, 258
Tensor fascia latae (TFL), 73f, 399, 400, 400f, 403–4
Teres major, 73f, 576–79, 576f, 580
Teres minor, 580, 580f, 582f, 583–85
Terminal rotation, 355
Terminal swing, 185
Terrible triad injury, 341, 342f
Thenar eminence, 656
Therapeutic kinesiology, 2–20

active techniques, 16–17, 17f
body, orienting space within, 9–11
body in space, orienting, 11–14
defined, 15
movement patterns, 4–9
multi-systems approach, 15, 15f
passive techniques, 16
pattern recognition, 16
somatic nature of physical patterns, 17–18
Therapeutic palpation, 212–13
Thigh, 9, 10f, 357f
Thixotropy, 26
Thoracic nerves, 471, 473
Thoracic outlet syndrome (TOS), 251
Thoracic spine, 440, 445
   acupressure along, 453, 454f
   breath support for, 240
   flexion and rigidity, 236
   lateral flexion of, 453
   motion in, 453, 454f
   stretching, 678–79
Thoracis, 459, 462
Thoracolumbar fascia, 457
Thorax, 24f, 228–38
   bones of, 231–35
   deep fascia of, 81f
   defined, 231
   joints and ligaments of (See Sternocostal joints)
   rigidity, working with, 236
Thorax bones, 231–35
   palpation of, 233–34
   rib, 231, 231f, 238f
   rib cage, 230, 231, 231–32f, 235f
   surface anatomy of, 232f
Thumb muscles, 631, 656–60, 656f
   extrinsic, 656–57, 656f
   intrinsic, 657, 660
   range of motion, 628, 629f
   stretching, 668

Thyrohyoid, 531
Thyroid cartilage, 498, 499f, 500
Thyroid gland, 82f, 499, 499f
Tibia, 24f, 270f, 271–72, 334, 334f
Tibial collateral ligament, 36f, 341
Tibial condyles, 334, 334f, 337
Tibialis anterior, 73f, 89f, 296, 296f, 298–300
Tibialis posterior, 166t, 305, 306f, 307–10
Tibial nerve, 300, 305
Tibial plateau, 334, 334f, 336
Tibial portion of the sciatic nerve, 361
Tibial torsion, 270
Tibial tubercle, 334, 334f, 336
Tibial tuberosity, 334, 335f, 337
Tibiofemoral joint, 340, 340f, 347–55
   axial rotation of, 351, 353–54, 355
   flexion and extension of, 351, 351f
   movement of meniscus, 355, 355f
   range of motion, 348–50, 348t
Tibiofibular joints, 282, 283f
Tightness weakness, 83
Tissue. See also Connective tissue
   corn-starch exploration, 27
   cross-fiber friction and deep tissue massage, 28
   defined, 25
   stiff, unyielding, 26
   stiffness of, measuring, 28
Tissue layering, 215, 217–24
   blood vessels, 222, 224f
   bone, 222, 223f

deep fascia, 218, 220, 220f
defined, 217
endangerment sites, 222, 224f
ligaments, 222, 223f
muscle, 220, 221–22
periosteum, 222, 223f
peripheral nerves, 222, 224f
skin, 217, 219
static contact, 215, 218
superficial fascia, 217, 218, 219
tendons, 222, 222f, 223f
Titin, 77–78
Toe extensors, 267
Toe flexors, 267
Tonic labyrinthine reflex, 110
Tonic points, 112
Tonic reflex, 107, 108
Torque, 40f, 41, 138, 140–41, 141f
Torso, 9, 10f
Torticollis, 169, 169f
Trabeculae, 29, 29f
Trachea, 82f, 499–500, 499f
Tracing
   buccinator, 530
   depressor muscles, 530
   facial muscles, 528–30
   frontalis, 528
   levatorlabii, 529
   nasalis, 529
   orbicularis oculi, 529
   orbicularis oris, 529
   procerus, 528
   risorius, 530
   zygomatic muscles, 529
Tracking, 211
   diaphragm, 242–43
   meniscus, 356
   patellar motion, 345–46, 345f
   sagittal exercises, 330
   skills, 211
   temporomandibular joint, 509
Tracts, 100
Trampoline, jumping on, 48

Translation of the joint, 340

Translatory motion, 51, 51f

Transverse arch, 279, 279f, 280, 291

Transverse carpal ligament, 625, 626f

Transverse foramen, 443, 444f

Transverse fractures, 30–31

Transverse friction, 85, 86f

Transverse ligament, 509, 510f

Transverse process (TP), 442, 447

Transverse section of spinal cord, 79f

Transverse tarsal joint, 288–89, 288f

Transversospinalis, 466–69, 467f

Transversus abdominis, 163f, 164f, 165, 166t, 175, 241f, 242, 245, 246, 249–50, 249t, 259, 474–78, 475f

Transversus thoracis, 241f, 249, 249t, 250f

Trapezium, 615, 615f, 618

Trapezius, 73f, 82f, 459, 574–79, 574f, 575f
    imbalance in forward head posture, 574, 574f
    lower and middle, 164f, 166t, 175

Trapezoid, 615, 615f

Trapezoid ligament, 565

Travell, Janet, 421f

Trendelenburg gait, 198–99, 199f

Triangular (convergent) muscle, 72, 74f

Triaxial (multiaxial) joints, 39, 39t

Triceps, 73f

Triceps brachii, 634, 638, 638f, 639f

Triceps surae, 300, 422

Trigeminal nerve, 513, 517

Trigger points (TrPs), 80, 119–21, 120f
    abductor digiti minimi, 666f
    abductor pollicis brevis, 660f
    abductor pollicis longus, 657f, 660f
    active, 119
    anconeus, 640f
    anterior compartment, 296, 296f, 297f
    biceps brachii, 634f
    brachialis, 635f
    brachioradialis, 635f
    buccinator, 528, 528f
    coracobrachialis, 600f
    deep posterior compartment, 306, 306–7f
    deltoid, 599f
    dorsal interossei, 664f
    extensor carpi radialis brevis, 651f
    extensor carpi radialis longus, 651f
    extensor carpi ulnaris, 652f
    extensor digitorum, 653f
    extensor indicis, 653f
    extensor pollicis longus, 657f
    facial muscles, 528, 528f
    flexor carpi radialis, 646f
    flexor carpi ulnaris, 646f
    flexor digiti minimi brevis, 666f
    flexor digitorum profundus, 648f
    flexor digitorum superficialis, 648f
    flexor pollicis brevis, 660f
    flexor pollicis longus, 656f
    gluteus maximus, 412f
    gluteus medius, 412f
    gluteus minimus, 413f
    hip adductors, 404
    iliocostalis, 464f
    iliopsoas, 404
    infraspinatus, 581f
    in intercostal muscles, 247, 247f
    interossei, 664f
    latent, 119
    lateral compartment, 310, 311f
    lateral pterygoid, 519f
    latissimus dorsi, 576f
    levatorani, 426f
    levator scapula, 587f, 591, 592
    longissimus, 463f
    masseter, 518f
    medial pterygoid, 520f
    multifidi, 467f
    obliques, 474f
    occipital bone, 513f
    opponens pollicis, 661f
    orbicularis oculi, 528, 528f
    palmaris longus, 647f
    pectoralis major, 593f
    pectoralis minor, 594f
    piriformis, 421f
    platsyma, 532
    posterior compartment, 300, 301f
    pronator, 643f
    pronator teres, 643f
    quadratus lumborum, 479f
    rectus abdominis, 472f
    rhomboids, 586f
    sartorius, 402f
    scalenes, 251, 252f
    semispinalis, 468f
    serratus anterior, 587f
    serratus posterior inferior, 255, 257f
    serratus posterior superior, 255, 256f
    spinalis, 463f
    splenius cervicis, 459f, 460, 460f
    sternocleidomastoid, 538f
    subclavius, 594f
    suboccipitals, 534f
    subscapularis, 582f
    supinator, 643f
    supraspinatus, 581f
    temporalis, 514f
    teres major, 576f
    teres minor, 582f
    trapezius, 574, 575f
    triceps brachii, 639f
    zygomatic muscles, 528, 528f

Trigger point (TrP) therapy, 120–21

Triquetrum, 614, 615f
    palpation of, 616

Trochanter, 31, 31f

Trochanteric bursitis, 398, 400

Trochlea, 610, 611f

Trochlear notch, 611f, 612

Troponin complex, 77

True ribs, 231, 231f

True winging, 586, 587f

Trunk, 9, 10f
    gait assessment, 203
    muscles during gait, 196
    rotation in gait, 192

T-tubules, 76, 77f

Tubercle, 31, 231f, 251, 253

Tuberosities, 31, 31f
    calcaneal, 272, 275
    of cuboid bone, 274f
    of fifth metatarsal, 273f, 274, 274f, 276, 277f
    of first metatarsal, 273f
    ischial, 377, 378f
    navicular, 273, 273f, 275

Type IIA fibers, 80–81, 80t

Type IIB fibers, 80–81, 80t

U

Ulna, 24f, 610–13, 611f
    shaft of, 612, 613
    styloid process of, 611f, 612, 613
    supination and pronation, 623, 623f

Ulnar bursa, 34f

Ulnar collateral ligament, 625, 626f

Uniaxial joints, 39, 39t

Unipennate muscle, 74, 74f, 75f

Unloaded, 40, 40f

Unstable equilibrium, 147, 147f

Upper chest breathing, 255, 259

Upper extremity (UE), 9, 10*f*
Upper limb, 9, 10*f*
Upper–lower body synchronization, 684
Upper trapezius, 247, 249, 249*t*
Upslip of pelvis, 396, 396*f*
Upward rotation, 55, 55*f*
Urogenital diaphragm, 426
Using full-body motion, 684
Utricle, 110

V
Varying strokes, 691, 691–92*f*
Vasti muscle group, 357–61
  vastus intermedius, 357, 358*f*
  vastus lateralis, 357, 359*f*, 361
  vastus medialis, 357, 359*f*, 361
  vastus medialis oblique (VMO), 357
Vasti stretch, 431
Vastus lateralis, 73*f*
Vastus medialis, 73*f*
Vastus medialis oblique, 166*t*
Vaulting gait, 200, 200*f*

Vector, 135, 136
Vector force, 136–37, 137*f*
Velocity, 130
Vena cava, foramen for, 242, 242*f*
Ventral, 11, 11*f*
Vertebra, 29*f*, 30, 443*f*, 444–47
Vertebral body, 442
Vertebral border, 554, 554*f*
Vertebral column, 24*f*
Vertebral foramen, 442
Vertical (longitudinal) axis, 12, 12*f*
Vertical oscillation of pelvis in sagittal plane, 191, 192*f*
Vestibule, 110, 110*f*
Visceral fascia, 33, 82*f*
Visceroceptors, 105
Viscoelasticity, 84–85
Viscosity, 26, 27
Vitruvian Man, 14, 14*f*

W
Waddling gait, 199
Wave summation, 79
Weak abdominals, 259, 260*f*
Weighted elbows, 679, 680*f*
Weight-training, 70
Wolff's law, 30

Work, defined, 144
Wrist
  circumduction, 624
  joints and ligaments, 620–21, 620*f*, 624–26, 625*f*, 626*f*
  passive range of motion, 627–28
  range of motion, 624, 626*t*
  stretching, 668
Wrist and hand extensors, 651–55
  extensor carpi radialis brevis, 651, 651*f*
  extensor carpi radialis longus, 651, 651*f*
  extensor carpi ulnaris, 651–52, 651*f*
  extensor digitorum, 651*f*, 652
  extensor expansion tendons, 652, 652*f*
  extensor indicis, 651*f*, 652
Wrist and hand flexors, 631, 645–55, 645*f*
  flexor carpi radialis, 646
  flexor carpi ulnaris, 646
  flexor digitorum profundus, 647, 647*f*
  flexor digitorum superficialis, 647, 647*f*

medial epicondylitis, 647
palmaris longus, 646
Wry-neck, 169, 169*f*

X
Xiphoid process, 231, 232*f*, 233, 235*f*, 242, 242*f*, 244

Y
Yellow marrow, 33*f*
Yielding, 7
Y ligament, 385, 385*f*
Yoga, 96, 436

Z
Zig-zag posture, 167, 167*f*
Z-line, 76, 76*f*
Zona orbicularis, 385
Zygomatic arch, 495, 495*f*, 497
Zygomatic bones, 495, 495*f*, 497
Zygomatic muscles, 527–29, 527*f*, 528*f*
Zygomatic process, 490, 492*f*, 494